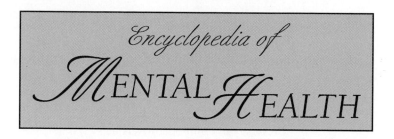

Encyclopedia of

MENTAL HEALTH

Volume 1   A–Di

Encyclopedia of MENTAL HEALTH

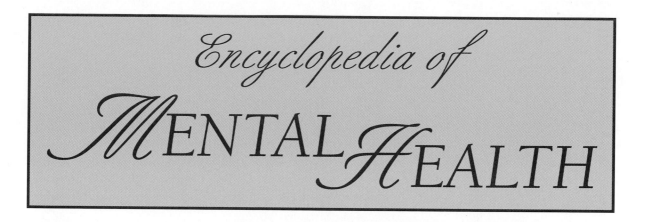

Volume 1   A–Di

Editor-in-Chief

HOWARD S. FRIEDMAN

Department of Psychology
University of California, Riverside

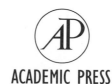

ACADEMIC PRESS

SAN DIEGO   LONDON   BOSTON   NEW YORK   SYDNEY   TOKYO   TORONTO

This book is printed on acid-free paper. ∞

Academic Press
a division of Harcourt Brace & Company
525 B Street, Suite 1900, San Diego, California 92101-4495, USA
http://www.apnet.com

Academic Press Limited
24-28 Oval Road, London NW1 7DX, UK
http://www.hbuk.co.uk/ap/

Library of Congress Card Catalog Number: 98-84208

International Standard Book Number: 0-12-226675-7 (set)
International Standard Book Number: 0-12-226676-5 (volume 1)
International Standard Book Number: 0-12-226677-3 (volume 2)
International Standard Book Number: 0-12-226678-1 (volume 3)

PRINTED IN THE UNITED STATES OF AMERICA
99 00 01 02 03 MM 9 8 7 6 5 4 3 2

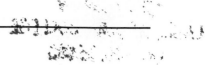

Contents

VOLUME II

About the Editor-in-Chief

HOWARD S. FRIEDMAN is Professor of Psychology at the University of California, Riverside. He also holds adjunct appointment as Clinical Professor at the University of California San Diego Medical School. Dr. Friedman attended Yale University, graduating magna cum laude with honors in psychology. He was awarded a National Science Foundation graduate fellowship at Harvard University, where he received his Ph.D. in 1976.

Professor Friedman is a thrice-elected Fellow of the American Psychological Association and a Fellow of the Society of Behavioral Medicine. He has received research grants from the National Institute of Mental Health, the American Cancer Society, and the American Heart Association, and he directs a project on health and longevity funded by the National Institute on Aging. Friedman is author of many influential scientific articles in leading journals and was named a "most-cited psychologist" by the publishers of the Social Science Citation Index. His books include the textbooks *Health Psychology* and *Personality;* three edited scholarly volumes, *Personality and Disease* (Wiley, reprinted in Japanese), *Interpersonal Issues in Health Care* (Academic), and *Hostility, Coping, and Health* (APA); and the authored comprehensive trade analysis titled *The Self-Healing Personality* (Henry Holt, reprinted in French and German). Dr. Friedman's research centers around the relations of mental and physical health, with a special focus on expressive style. His wide-ranging interests and integrative orientation served him well in editing this Encyclopedia. Friedman has taught undergraduates, graduate students, medical students, and postdocs. In 1995, Professor Friedman received the Distinguished Teaching Award from the University of California, Riverside.

About the Executive Advisory Board

NANCY E. ADLER is Professor of Psychology, Departments of Psychiatry and Pediatrics at the University of California, San Francisco, where she is also Vice-Chair of the Department of Psychiatry and Director of the Center for Social, Behavioral, and Policy Sciences. She has served as director of the graduate program in health psychology at UCSF and of an NIMH-sponsored postdoctoral training program, "Psychology and Medicine: An Integrative Research Approach." At UCSF, she is also Chair of the Committee on Curriculum and Educational Policy for the School of Medicine and a member of the Executive Committee for the Center of Excellence on Women's Health and the Center for Integrative Medicine, the Committee on Indirect Cost Recovery, Chancellor's Task Force on Health Care Reform, Academic Planning and Budget (Vice-Chair), and Strategic Planning Board.

Dr. Adler is a Fellow of the American Psychological Society and the American Psychological Association. She has served as President of Division 34 (Population and Environmental Psychology) of APA and received the Superior Service Award from that division. She is a member of the Society for Experimental Social Psychology, the Academy of Behavioral Medicine Research, and the Society for Behavioral Medicine. She recently served on a blue-ribbon panel to review the Intramural Research Program at the National Institute of Mental Health and has served on advisory committees for the National Institute of Child Health and Human Development. She has served on the editorial boards of *Journal of Population and Environment, Health Psychology, Journal of Applied Social Psychology,* and *Journal of Health Psychology* and as associate editor of *Health Psychology and Women's Health: Research in Gender, Behavior, and Policy.* She has been awarded the UCSF Chancellor's Award for Advancement of Women and has been elected to membership in the Institute of Medicine of the Natural Academy of Sciences.

Dr. Adler has focused on the utility of decision models for understanding health-risking behaviors. Her research has examined adolescent decision-making regarding contraception, conscious and preconscious motivation for pregnancy, and perception of risk of sexually transmitted diseases. She has also conducted research on the psychological responses of women following therapeutic abortion.

ROSS D. PARKE is a Distinguished Professor of Psychology and Director of the Center for Family Studies at the University of California, Riverside. Prior to his UCR position, he taught at the Universities of Wisconsin and Illinois and held a research position at the Fels Research Institute. He is past president of Division 7 of Developmental Psychology and is the 1995 recipient of the G. Stanley Hall Award for outstanding contributions to developmental psychology from this APA division. In 1997 he was elected a fellow of the American Association for the Advancement of Science. He has been editor of *Developmental Psychology* and associate editor of *Child Development* and is currently editor of the *Journal of Family Psychology.* Professor Parke is author of *Fatherhood* and co-author of *Child Psychology: A Contemporary Viewpoint* (now in its 5th edition). He has edited or co-edited many other volumes, including *The Family, Review of Child Developmental Research,* Vol. 7, and most recently was co-editor of *Exploring Family Relationships with Other Social Contexts.* His research has focused on early social relationships in infancy and childhood, and he is known for his early work on the effects of punishment, aggression, and child abuse, as well as for his pioneering work on the father's role in infancy and early childhood. His current work fo-

cuses on the links between family and peer systems as well as on the impact of economic stress in families of various ethnic backgrounds.

CHRISTOPHER PETERSON is Professor of Psychology and Director of Clinical Training at the University of Michigan, Ann Arbor. Author of several research monographs and textbooks on clinical and introductory psychology, his research interests include cognitive influences on achievement, depression, and physical well-being. In 1993, two of his articles on explanatory style were identified by *Current Contents* as "citation classics." He has additionally served on the editorial boards of *Psychological Bulletin, Journal of Abnormal Psychology,* and *Journal of Personality and Social Psychology.* He is also a member of the American Psychological Association Media Referral Service.

ROBERT ROSENTHAL is the Edgar Pierce Professor of Psychology and Chair of the Department of Psychology at Harvard University, and former director of the clinical psychology program at the University of North Dakota. A fellow of the American Association for the Advancement of Science and the American Psychological Society, Dr. Rosenthal is the author of over 350 articles and over 25 books. His areas of interest include self-fulfilling prophecy, the effect of teachers' expectations on students' performance, nonverbal communication, and methodology and data analysis of behavioral research. Dr. Rosenthal has been the recipient of several awards and citations, including the 1960 Sociopsychological Prize of the American Association for the Advancement of Science, the First Prize Cattell Fund Award of the APA, a Distinguished Career Contribution Award from the Massachusetts Psychological Association, the Donald Campbell Award of the Society for Personality and Social Psychology, the 1993 AAAS Prize for Behavioral Science Research, and a 1996 Distinguished Scientist Award of the Society of Experimental Social Psychology.

RALF SCHWARZER is Professor of Psychology and Chair of the Department of Organizational and Health Psychology at the Freie Universität Berlin. Dr. Schwarzer is a fellow of the American Psychological Association (APA), as well as a member of the International Association for Applied Psychology (IAAP), International Council of Psychologists (ICP), European

Health Psychology Society (EHPS), European Association of Personality Psychology (EAPP), and German Psychological Association (DGfP). He is an executive board member of the International Society of Health Psychology Research (ISHPR), a former president of the international Stress and Anxiety Research Society (STAR), former vice-president of the Health Psychology Division of the German Psychological Association and currently (1996–1998) is the president of the European Health Psychology Society (EHPS).

Dr. Schwarzer's research interests lie primarily in the areas of educational and health psychology, including instructional processes, self-efficacy, anxiety, stress, coping, health behaviors, and social support. Within these areas, he is on the editorial boards of seven major journals, and was founding editor of *Anxiety, Stress, and Coping: An International Journal.*

ROXANE COHEN SILVER is an Associate Professor in the Department of Psychology and Social Behavior in the School of Social Ecology at the University of California, Irvine. She has also served as the coordinator of the Health Psychology Ph.D. Program at UC Irvine since its inception. A member of the American Psychological Association, American Psychological Society, Society of Experimental Social Psychology, and Society for Personality and Social Psychology, Dr. Silver studies how individuals cope with stressful life experiences, such as loss of a spouse or child, divorce, childhood sexual abuse, physical disability, and natural disaster. Her work also examines the long-term effects of traumatic life experiences and considers how beliefs and expectations of the social network impact on the coping process.

DAVID SPIEGEL is Professor of Psychiatry and Behavioral Sciences at Stanford University School of Medicine and Director of the Psychosocial Treatment Laboratory. Author of over 200 journal articles and book chapters, he was the first to scientifically demonstrate that group support results in significantly enhanced survival time for cancer patients. He also studies immediate reactions to life-threatening events, dissociative symptoms, and posttraumatic stress disorder.

A fellow of the American College of Psychiatrists and the American Psychiatric Association, Dr. Spiegel is also a member of the editorial boards of *The Journal of Psychosocial Oncology, Psycho-Oncology,* and *Health Psychology,* a consulting editor to the *American Journal of Clinical Hypnosis,* an associate editor for *The Journal of Psychotherapy: Practice and Research,* and an advisory editor to *The International Journal of Clinical and Experimental Hypnosis.*

Dr. Spiegel was awarded the 1995 Edward A. Strecker Award from the Institute of the Pennsylvania Hospital and Jefferson Medical College for significant contributions to American psychiatry. He was 1996–1997 Burroughs Wellcome Visiting Professor of the Royal Society of Medicine in Great Britain. He is the recipient of the Schneck Award for significant contributions to medical hypnosis from the Society for Clinical and Experimental Hypnosis, the Treya Killam Wilber Award from the Cancer Support Community, and the One From the Heart Award from Med-Peninsula Hospice. He was given the Kaiser Award and the Academic Faculty Member Residency Program Award for Excellence in Teaching at Stanford University School of Medicine.

Preface

A number of scientific and intellectual trends have converged to change vastly our understanding of mental health. Our conceptions of mental health and mental dysfunction have broadened to take into account new knowledge about the genetic, biological, developmental, social, societal, and cultural nature of human beings. This is the first encyclopedia to bring together these emerging trends, to paint a sometimes-startling picture of mental health.

What are these trends? First, our understanding has moved well beyond the artificial nature–nurture dichotomy. We know more about the biological underpinnings of mental states and behavior, but we also better understand how these biological tendencies unfold in family, social, and cultural environments. Second, we have moved beyond the old "mental" versus "physical" ("mind vs body") dichotomies. To a greater extent than previously imagined, there is a strong reciprocal relation between our general health and activity and our cognitions, moods, and mental well-being. Third, the experts increasingly recognize the complementary importance of prevention and treatment. A simple model of treating mental "disease" is often ultimately futile without associated prevention efforts, but yet prevention cannot sensibly ignore the need for efficacious treatments. Fourth, we now emphasize primary mental health promotion—the structural, environmental, family, and cultural contexts of mental health. In healthy environments, the incidence

and consequence of mental disturbance decline. Fifth, the best scholars now recognize meaningful variations across ages, genders, cultures, families, and societies. That is, to understand fully and improve significantly a person's mental health, we need to know about that person's biological and personal make-up, and also about his or her age, family, work, and position in society.

CONTENTS

The *Encyclopedia of Mental Health* thus encompasses all levels of analysis, from the molecular and biological, through the social and family, to the cultural. We have therefore included coverage of key topics not traditionally found in such a reference work. We of course include topics like depression, schizophrenia, mood disorders, mental retardation, dementia, panic attacks, somatization, conduct disorder, dissociative disorders, obsessive–compulsive disorder, epilepsy, Alzheimer's disease, phobias, biofeedback, and therapy—cognitive therapy, behaviorist therapy, psychoanalytic therapy, constructivist therapy, and more. But we also examine the close links to behavioral medicine, health psychology, and other aspects of physical health. Interestingly, we add extensive coverage of the validity (or invalidity) of psychiatric diagnosis (and *DSM-IV*), including standards for psychotherapy, models of normality, and psychiatric epidemiology.

Stress is increasingly recognized as a complex interaction of the person, the environment, the social support structure, and the culture. Many of our articles thus deal with the mental health aspects of such topics as stress and coping, posttraumatic stress, cardiovascular reactivity, commuting, infertility, rape, cancer, burnout, support groups, death and dying, grief, bereavement, religious influences, social support, and social networks. Relatedly, neurology sits at the intersection of physical and mental health, and so there is good coverage of such topics as autism and pervasive developmental disorder, headache, pain, attention deficit disorder, aphasia and alexia, brain plasticity, body rhythms and body clocks, brain imaging, and the evolutionary basis of mental health.

Aside from the striking breakthroughs at the genetic and molecular levels, perhaps the greatest current interest is in the family and developmental context for mental health and mental impairment. We include a truly exceptional and extensive discussion of the various relevant issues, including expert articles on psychosocial development, childhood stress, child sexual abuse, cognitive development, childhood wellness, parenting, marital health, divorce, couples therapy, fathers, child custody, day care and child care providers, extended families, family therapy, cooperation and competition, attachment, television viewing, and various aspects of mental health promotion across the life span. Such articles should certainly be of value to parents, educators, attorneys, pediatricians, social workers, and anyone else involved with the mental health of children and families. There is also significant attention to mental health in middle age and among the aged.

We have considerable concentration on normal and abnormal motivations, habits, and emotions— anger, intrinsic motivation, emotional regulation, hardiness, gambling, smoking, alcohol problems, substance abuse, impulse control, criminal behavior, adherence, conflict resolution, subjective well-being, and self-esteem.

In modern industrial nations, tremendous amounts of money and effort are expended on issues revolving around body image, exercise, and diet, and so we include extensive discussion of physical activity, sports, exercise, anorexia and bulimia, body image, dieting, obesity, the physiological control of eating, and nutri-

tion and mental health. Sophisticated presentations of the relations between hormonal changes and sociocultural influences appear in articles on gender differences, stress in pregnancy, premenstrual syndrome, and menopause.

Increased understanding of the theoretical, structural, cultural, and societal bases of and influences upon mental health is seen in significant chapters on mental hospitals and deinstitutionalization, legal issues of institutionalization, homelessness, socioeconomic status, unemployment, urbanization, healthy environments, societal influences (social causation), racism and mental health, ethnicity, homosexuality, managed care, mental health services research, and the ethics of research in the mental health field. Such factors are of high importance in achieving a full understanding of mental health, but are often overlooked.

Finally, we have not neglected those fascinating topics that usually would not be considered psychiatric pathology but seem integral to understanding mental health nonetheless—such issues as shyness, deception, creativity, play, loneliness, self-fulfilling prophecies, mental control, positive illusions, procrastination, optimism, nonverbal communication, human–computer interaction, charisma, humor, and wisdom. As an illustration, take a look at the article on hypnosis. A true appreciation of mental health necessitates familiarity with these strikingly modern understandings.

In sum, what is especially distinctive about this encyclopedia is its movement beyond pathology to a heavy emphasis on the various intersecting forces that constitute mental health. We explicitly emphasize the "health" part of "mental health." Wherever possible, implications for the promotion of health are articulated. Indeed, we believe that this comprehensive, modern view of mental health is available nowhere else!

DISTINGUISHED SCHOLARS

With the assistance of the outstanding editorial board, we have secured contributions by the most distinguished scholars and practitioners. Many are founders of their fields, and they are justly famous. But many contributors represent the brilliant new generation of mental health scholars. Importantly, I have encouraged the contributors to write about what is most important. We thus have a reference work rooted in the present and looking toward the future, rather than bogged down in obsolete notions and topics.

AUDIENCE

This encyclopedia is aimed at a wide range of reference users, including college students; students in the health professions; popular writers and reporters; allied professionals such as lawyers, social workers, and corporate researchers; and the many educated men and women who seek to read up in a concise fashion on specific topics of interest in their own public or corporate library. Emphasis has been placed on clarity and accessibility.

I thank Nikki Levy, our acquisitions editor at Academic Press, and Barb Makinster, her very able assistant, who helped make all this possible. Naturally, I also thank the many, many highly distinguished scientists and clinicians who devoted the time to make this endeavor worthwhile.

I am extremely proud and pleased to bring this remarkable encyclopedia to fruition. I am confident that it will prove a valuable resource to all of us—scholars, practitioners, students, and laypersons—in the mental health and behavioral science communities.

Howard S. Friedman

How to Use the Encyclopedia

The *Encyclopedia of Mental Health* is intended for use by students, research professionals, and practicing clinicians. Articles have been chosen to reflect major disciplines in the study of mental health, common topics of research by professionals in this domain, and areas of public interest and concern. Each article serves as a comprehensive overview of a given area, providing both breadth of coverage for students, and depth of coverage for research and clinical professionals. We have designed the encyclopedia with the following features for maximum accessibility for all readers.

Articles in the encyclopedia are arranged alphabetically by subject. Complete tables of contents appear in all volumes. The index is located in Volume 3. Because the reader's topic of interest may be listed under a broader article title, we encourage use of the Index for access to a subject area, rather than use of the Table of Contents alone. For instance, the topic area of recovered/repressed memories is covered under the article title "Standards for Psychotherapy." Because a topic of study in mental health is often applicable to more than one article, the Index provides a complete listing of where a subject is covered and in what context. As an example, the topic of aging and mental health is covered in a number of articles including "Aging and Mental Health," "Assessment of Mental Health in Older Adults," and "Emotion and Aging."

Each article contains an outline, a glossary, cross-references, and a bibliography. The outline allows a quick scan of the major areas discussed within each article. The glossary contains terms that may be unfamiliar to the reader, with each term defined *in the context of its use in that article*. Thus, a term may appear in the glossary for another article defined in a slightly different manner or with a subtle nuance specific to that article. For clarity, we have allowed these differences in definition to remain so that the terms are defined relative to the context of the particular article.

The articles have been cross-referenced to other related articles in the encyclopedia. Cross-references are found at the first or predominant mention of a subject area covered elsewhere in the encyclopedia. Cross-references will always appear at the end of a paragraph. Where multiple cross-references apply to a single paragraph, the cross-references are listed in alphabetical order. We encourage readers to use the cross-references to locate other encyclopedia articles that will provide more detailed information about a subject.

The Bibliography lists recent secondary sources to aid the reader in locating more detailed or technical information. Review articles and research articles that are considered of primary importance to the understanding of a given subject area are also listed. Bibliographies are not intended to provide a full reference listing of all material covered in the context of a given article, but are provided as guides to further reading.

A

Adolescence

Grayson N. Holmbeck

Loyola University Chicago

Adolescence A transitional developmental period between childhood and adulthood which is characterized by a host of biological, psychological, and social role changes. Although the period is typically viewed as spanning the age range of 10–20, the actual onset and endpoint of adolescence vary depending on individual differences and the manner in which one assesses the onset and endpoint.

Adolescent Psychopathology Includes problem behaviors that develop during adolescence due to difficulties in managing the important developmental tasks of this period. They can include internalizing (e.g., depression, suicide, anxiety, eating disorders) or externalizing forms of psychopathology (e.g., conduct disorders, aggression).

Contexts of Adolescence Include contexts which shape the impact of the primary changes of adolescence. For example, how parents and peers respond to the physical and cognitive changes of adolescence will have an effect on how these primary changes are experienced. Contexts include family, peer, school, and work settings.

Primary Changes of Adolescence Include changes in the biological, cognitive, and social role domains. Although the timing and nature of these changes vary across culture, they are viewed as universal and as occurring temporally prior to the other changes that typically characterize the adolescent period (e.g., changes in identity development, autonomy, etc.).

Secondary Changes of Adolescence Include the following psychological issues of adolescence: identity, achievement, sexuality, intimacy, autonomy, and attachment. Most of these issues are of concern at all periods in a person's life, but they have special significance during the adolescent developmental period. The manner in which the individual manages each of these issues is impacted upon by the primary changes and contexts of adolescence.

ADOLESCENCE is a transitional period between childhood and adulthood which is characterized by a host of biological, psychological, and social role changes. Scholars who have written about adolescence from a psychoanalytic perspective have viewed this developmental period as a time of storm and stress when extreme levels of conflict with parents result in a reorientation toward peers. Despite disconfirming empirical evidence, it appears that public policy and the public's beliefs are still in line with this perspective. The main purpose of this article is to describe an empirically based framework for understanding adolescent development. This framework is based on the notion that there are primary changes that occur during adolescence (i.e., pubertal, cognitive, and social role changes), all of which impact on a set of secondary changes (i.e., changes in identity, achievement, sexuality, intimacy, autonomy, and attachment). The primary changes have an impact on the secondary changes *via* the contexts in which adolescents develop (i.e., family, peer, school, and work settings). An additional purpose of this article is to discuss the implications that developmental psychology has for clinical interventions with adolescents.

I. A FRAMEWORK FOR UNDERSTANDING ADOLESCENT DEVELOPMENT

Scholars who have written about adolescence from a psychoanalytic perspective have viewed this developmental period as a time of storm and stress when extreme levels of conflict with parents result in a reorientation toward peers. Given that such views have been based on clinicians' observations of adolescents with adjustment difficulties, it is not surprising that recent research involving large representative samples of adolescents has not supported these early storm and stress notions. Despite such disconfirming empirical evidence, it appears that public policy and the public's beliefs are still in line with the psychoanalytic perspective. Moreover, those who write for mass media publications will often invoke concepts such as rebelliousness, parent–adolescent conflict, early onset of sexual behaviors, and identity crises to make points about the negative nature of adolescence.

The main purpose of this article is to describe an empirically based framework for understanding adolescent development. This framework is based on the notion that there are primary changes that occur during adolescence, all of which impact on a set of secondary changes. The primary changes have an impact on the secondary changes *via* the contexts in which adolescents develop, namely, family, peer, school, and work settings. This framework is presented in Figure 1. In this framework, concepts such as sexuality and identity are not afforded primary status, but instead are viewed as "secondary changes." The biological, cognitive, and social role changes of adolescence are viewed as "primary changes." Although the timing and nature of these primary changes vary across culture, they are viewed as primary because they are universal and because they occur temporally prior to the secondary changes that characterize the adolescent period. The goal of this first section is to provide a brief overview of the research findings which relate to each of the concepts included in the framework. At the end of this section, several examples which make use of the framework are provided.

It is critical to note at the outset that there are a host of factors which will impact on the connections that occur between the different components of the framework for understanding adolescent development. For example, mesosystemic factors include bidirectional effects between contexts, such as between family relationships and child functioning in the school setting. Exosystemic factors include effects on adolescent de-

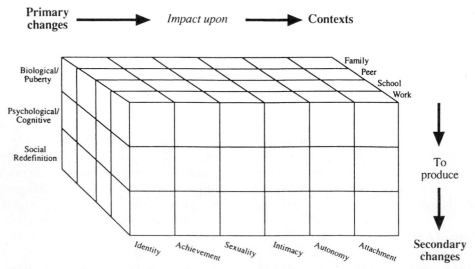

Figure 1 A framework for understanding adolescent development. [Adapted from J. P. Hill (1980). "Understanding Early Adolescence: A Framework." Center for Early Adolescence, Carrboro, NC.]

velopment which arise from environments where parents spend their time, such as the parents' work setting. Finally, the meaning of the primary changes, contexts, and secondary changes of adolescence will vary across different cultures (i.e., a macrosystemic factor), thus influencing the interconnections between the components of the framework.

A. Primary Changes of Adolescence

From infancy until late adolescence, children experience dramatic intraindividual changes across a number of domains, namely, biological, psychological, and social (see Fig. 1). It is important to note that changes within and across these domains are asynchronous and vary between individuals in terms of both rate and pattern.

1. Biological/Pubertal Changes

More than any other stage of life except the fetal/neonatal period, adolescence is a time of substantial physical growth and change. Changes in body proportions, voice, body hair, strength, and coordination are found in males and changes in body proportions, body hair, and mencheal status are found in girls. Crucial to the understanding of this process is the knowledge that the peak of pubertal development occurs 2 years earlier in the modal female than in the modal male and that there are substantial variations between individuals in the time of onset, the duration, and the termination of the pubertal cycle. Thus, not only is there intraindividual variation in terms of the onset of the different pubertal changes but there is interindividual variation in the many parameters of these changes as well. Both pubertal status (an individual's placement in the sequence of predictable pubertal changes) and pubertal timing (timing of changes relative to one's age peers) should be taken into account.

Unlike the newborn, adolescents are aware of these changes and this awareness may be pleasing or horrifying; lack of information about puberty/sexuality can contribute to emotional upset. On the other hand, pubertal changes are not traumatic for the majority of adolescents. Most of the psychological effects of pubertal changes are probably not direct, but rather are mediated by the responses of the adolescent or the responses of significant others to such changes. Sig-

nificant others may assume, for example, that physical changes indicate development in psychological areas. At present, however, there are no known direct links between physical and psychological development.

2. Psychological/Cognitive Changes

Jean Piaget has provided us with a comprehensive theory of cognitive development that has general applicability to infants, children, and adolescents. Piaget has enumerated a series of four stages of cognitive development, each of which is assumed to be: (1) qualitatively different than the stage before or after, (2) a structured whole in a state of equilibrium, (3) universal across cultures, and (4) part of an invariant set of stages. It is worth noting that there is some controversy regarding the usefulness and accuracy of Piagetian theory and there exist alternative theories of adolescent thinking. One of these theories, which highlights the role of social interactions in cognitive development, is discussed below. [See COGNITIVE DEVELOPMENT.]

According to Piaget, the sensorimotor period (birth to 2 years of age) involves a series of substages whereby the infant develops from "a bundle of reflexes" to one who can physically manipulate his/her world with a set of organized and progressively more advanced set of behaviors. Preoperational children (2 to 7 years of age) can use mental images to represent events but are limited (in comparison to their older peers) in that they tend to be highly "egocentric." These children do not view others as having perspectives different from theirs and their speech is not tailored to the listener. The thinking of children in the concrete operational period (ages 7 to 11) is more dynamic and involves what Piaget refers to as cognitive operations. Thought is more in tune with the environment and is increasingly logical and flexible.

Though less overtly observable, the cognitive changes of adolescence are probably as dramatic as the physical changes. Piaget is credited with the identification of adolescence as the period of formal operational thinking. Adolescents who have achieved such thinking abilities are able to think more complexly, abstractly, and hypothetically. They are more able to think in terms of possibilities and they are increasingly able to think about the future. Some adolescents can think about their own thinking (meta-cognition). Interestingly, however, this latter skill is not without potential difficulties. Some have suggested that the adolescent may become obsessed with this new ability. Even if not obsessed, adolescents are not fully developed in a social cognitive sense and may misperceive others as equally interested in their own thoughts and actions but as unable to understand their emotional experiences (i.e., adolescent egocentrism).

According to Piaget, development does not occur in a vacuum, but rather is fostered or hindered via interactions with the social world. This viewpoint has led several researchers to explore the interface between cognitive development and social relations (i.e., social cognitive development). The development of role-taking and empathy skills, the role of affect in understanding people versus things, attributional processes in social situations, and prosocial behavior are a few of the research areas that have interested developmental and social psychologists working in this area.

Although too numerous to discuss in detail, many other theories of psychological development have also been suggested. Kohlberg describes six stages of moral reasoning with two stages comprising each of the following three levels: preconventional, conventional, and principled (or postconventional). People at lower stages tend to be rule- and obedience-bound whereas people at higher stages recognize the arbitrary nature of rules and laws and that such laws can be changed if they are unjust. These postconventional individuals base their decisions on a universal set of ethical principles as well as on their own conscience. Kohlberg's notions are social cognitive in nature in that experiences with the social world shape development. Loevinger's theory of ego development is also a stage theory which involves increasing levels of maturity. Stages differ along dimensions of impulse control, maturity of interpersonal relations, and cognitive style. Research with Loevinger's Sentence Completion Test has revealed, for example, that adolescents at higher levels of ego development evidence less psychopathology. [See MORAL DEVELOPMENT; PERSONALITY DEVELOPMENT.]

3. Changes in Social Role

A variety of changes in the social status of children occurs during adolescence. Although such social redefinition is universal, the specific changes vary greatly across different cultures. In some nonindustrial societies, public rituals (i.e., rites of passage) take place soon after the onset of pubertal change. Norms for appropriate social behaviors are altered at this time and the adolescent is now viewed as an adult. In Western industrialized societies, the transition is less clear, but analogous changes in social status do take place. Changes can occur across four domains: interpersonal (e.g., changes in familial power status), political (e.g., late adolescents are eligible to vote), economic (e.g., adolescents are allowed to work), and legal (e.g., late adolescents can be tried in adult court systems). In addition, adolescents are able to obtain a driver's permit and can get married. Homeleaving in late adolescence also serves to redefine one's social role.

Given that the primary changes of adolescence have now been discussed, the next section concerns the contexts of adolescence.

B. Normative Contextual and Environmental Changes

Contextual changes during childhood and adolescence can occur in the following domains: family, peers, school, and work (see Fig. 1). Changes in each domain will be reviewed, in turn.

1. Changes in Family Relationships

Not only does the family play a principal role in the socialization of an adolescent, but there are developmental changes in this role as well. Recent research suggests that *both* parents and siblings appear to play significant and unique roles in this process. The role of fathers in adolescent development is beginning to receive attention as are the effects of divorce and maternal employment on adolescent adjustment. [See FAMILY SYSTEMS.]

Although those from the family therapy tradition have shown an interest in dimensions of parenting and family functioning, an extensive developmentally oriented literature exists that concerns parenting behaviors and their corresponding adolescent adjustment outcomes. Based on factor-analytic studies of parental warmth and control, a two-dimensional classification scheme of parenting has been developed which includes the following parenting patterns: authoritarian–autocratic, indulgent–permissive, authoritative–reciprocal, and indifferent–uninvolved.

Authoritative parents are similar to authoritarian

parents in their emphasis upon explicit standards and guidelines, the difference being that the former are likely to be more affectionate and to permit more say in the construction and application of rules. Permissive parents are those that do not clearly state or explain their rules and are more likely to submit to their children's demands. Regarding socialization outcomes, authoritarian and authoritative parenting have been found to have a negative and a positive impact, respectively, on children's (and especially boys') social competence, initiative, spontaneity, moral development, motivation for intellectual performance, self-esteem, and locus of control. Permissive parents tend to have children who are more aggressive and impulsive. [*See* PARENTING.]

Adolescence is a time of transformation in family relations. Changes in adolescent attachment and autonomy as well as changes in the life circumstances of the parents themselves have an impact on the adolescent and the family system. Families with young adolescents are more likely to engage in conflict over mundane issues (rather than basic values) than are families with older or younger children; parents and adolescents tend to have roughly one conflict every 3 days. On the other hand, *most* adolescents negotiate this period without severing ties with parents or developing serious disorders. Despite the lack of serious relationship trauma during adolescence, there does appear to be a period of increased emotional distance in parent–adolescent relationships during early adolescence, particularly during the peak of pubertal change. A therapist who works with an adolescent should be aware that transformations in attachments to parents are to be expected during adolescence and that some normative familial problems may arise because of difficulties in negotiating this transition.

2. Changes in Peer Relationships

Most now agree that an adolescent's peer relationships are necessities rather than luxuries and that these relationships have a positive impact on cognitive, social–cognitive, linguistic, sex role, and moral development. Indeed, there is considerable support for the hypothesis that children and adolescents with poor peer relations are at risk for later personal and social difficulties (e.g., dropping out of school and criminality). One might argue that quality relationships with parents can take the place of peer relationships or at least buffer any negative effects of problematic relationships with other adolescents. On the other hand, research findings suggest that it is often through interactions with age-mates that an individual is able to learn skills such as cooperation and empathy. In short, peer relationships appear to provide a *unique* contribution to adolescent adjustment.

Peer relationships during childhood and adolescence appear to evolve through a series of developmental stages. Stage theories of interpersonal understanding and social perspective-taking have been proposed. Some have argued that an individual's personality is best understood by an examination of his/her interpersonal interactions. Harry Stack Sullivan, for example, describes his notion of "chumship" and maintains that this (typically) same-sex friendship is a critical developmental accomplishment. It is with this relationship that the young adolescent presumably learns about intimacy, and this friendship serves as a basis for later close relationships.

Although we have stressed, as have others, that families and peers provide unique contributions to development and adjustment, it is also true that the family can provide a secure base for a child's exploration into the world of peers. Healthy family relations are a necessary basis for the development of healthy peer relations, especially in light of the following findings: (a) children and adolescents usually adhere to their parents' values even during increases in peer involvement, (b) parent and peer values are typically quite similar, especially with regard to important issues, and (c) differences between parent and peer values are more likely when adolescents have distant relationships with their parents *and* when they associate with peers who endorse and exhibit antisocial behaviors. Thus, we must be careful not to treat the world of peers and the world of the family as separate. Each affects the other, with both contributing uniquely to adolescent development and adjustment.

3. Effects of the School Context

Another context of adolescent development is the school environment. Scholars have argued not only that we should be interested in the school's effect on cognition and achievement, but that we should also look at the school as an important environment for the development of one's personality, values, and social relationships.

With increasing age, children are exposed to more complex school environments. Movement between schools (such as between elementary and junior high school) can be viewed as a stressor, with multiple school transitions producing more deleterious effects. Past research suggests that children (and particularly girls) who switch from an elementary school into a junior high school (as opposed to staying in a K–8 school) will show significant self-esteem decrements and that recovery in self-esteem is not likely for a sizeable number of these girls. Boys and girls who make such a transition also evidence decrements in grade point average and extracurricular activities. Presumably, these adjustment difficulties are due, at least in part, to movement from a protected environment (elementary school) to an impersonal environment (junior and senior high school).

The school environment also impacts on adolescent development. The physical setting of the school, limitations in resources, philosophies of education, teacher expectations, curriculum characteristics, and interactions between teacher and student have been found to be related to a host of adolescent outcomes, and these findings are maintained even after social background is held constant. For example, high school students appear to profit from nonauthoritarian teaching approaches. We know that smaller schools and less authoritarian school environments promote commitment on the part of the student (i.e., fewer students drop out) and that the high rate of drop outs in some school districts indicates that the environment has not been well matched to student needs.

4. Effects of Working

The last context that will be considered is the work environment. Although more than 80% of all high school students in this country work before they graduate, little research has been done on how work impacts on adolescent development or the adolescents' relationships with significant others.

The research that has been done suggests that the work environment has important positive *and* negative effects on adolescent development. Although adolescents who work tend to develop an increased sense of self-reliance, they also tend to (a) develop cynical attitudes about work, (b) spend less time with their families and peers, (c) be less involved in school, (d) be more likely to abuse drugs or commit delinquent acts,

and (e) have less time for self-exploration and identity development. The primary problem seems to be the monotonous *and* stressful nature of adolescent jobs.

C. Secondary Changes of Adolescence

As discussed earlier, there are a number of psychosocial issues that are impacted upon by the primary changes of adolescence as well as the nature of the adolescent's contextual environment. The secondary changes that will be discussed in this section are as follows: identity, achievement, sexuality, intimacy, autonomy, and attachment (see Fig. 1).

1. Identity

A major psychological task of adolescence is the development of an identity. Adolescents develop an identity through periods of role exploration and role commitment. One's identity is multidimensional and includes self-perceptions and commitments across a number of domains, including occupational, religious, sexual, and political commitments. Development occurs at different rates across each domain. Although the notion that all adolescents experience identity crises appears to be a myth, identity development is recognized as an important adolescent issue.

Research in the area of identity development has isolated at least four identity statuses which are defined with respect to two dimensions: commitment and exploration. These identity statuses are as follows: identity moratorium (exploration with no commitment), identity foreclosure (commitment with no exploration), identity diffusion (no commitment and no systematic exploration), and identity achievement (commitment after extensive exploration). A given adolescent's status can change over time, reflecting increased maturation and development or, alternatively, regression to some less adaptive identity status.

When an adolescent systematically explores various roles prior to making a serious commitment to any one role, the adolescent is in a state of identity moratorium. This can often involve a painful and deliberate decision to take time off from current stressors to create breathing space for exploration. This person is not drifting aimlessly—instead, the adolescent searches systematically as a preparation for commitment. The adolescent who is identity foreclosed has not made an autonomous choice. A commitment to a role has taken place, but the adolescent has made the commitment with little or no exploration. Such individuals typically adopt an identity that has been prescribed by important people in their life (i.e., parents, friends). It could be said that such people miss out on their full range of potential. The adolescent who is identity diffused has an incomplete sense of self, with no commitments to an identity. Such a person lacks beliefs and principles and tends to "live for the moment." Roles are tried on quickly but are abandoned just as quickly. Finally, the identity achieved individual has made a firm commitment after a period of exploration.

Regarding gender and cultural differences, it appears that the process of identity formation differs for males and females. Identity development in males appears to involve struggles with autonomy and themes of separation whereas identity development in females is more likely to be intertwined with the development and maintenance of intimate relationships. Researchers have also explored the possibility that identity development may proceed in different ways for different socioeconomic and ethnic groups. Adolescents low in socioeconomic status, for example, are usually unable to explore options (given their financial constraints), thus making them less likely to experience a period of identity moratorium.

2. Achievement

Decisions made during one's adolescence can have serious consequences for one's future education and career. Some adolescents decide to drop out of school whereas others complete their education and graduate from high school. Some decide to continue on to college or graduate school. For those who remain in school, it is during high school that most adolescents are, for the first time, given the opportunity to decide which classes they want to take. Such decisions present the adolescent with new opportunities but also limit the range of possible employment and educational options available to the adolescent. After graduation from high school, adolescents typically decide whether they want to pursue more education or whether they wish to seek full-time employment—a decision which is certainly affected by one's socioeconomic status. Finally, adolescence is a time of preparation for adult work roles, a time when vocational training begins. Given the complexity of achievement decisions, adolescents benefit from the cognitive

changes that characterize this developmental period. Those who have developed these abilities are at an advantage when they begin to make education- and career-related decisions.

It has been suggested that adolescents will exert more or less effort in school depending on their level of achievement motivation (which is considered to be a relatively stable personality trait) and their fear of failure (which produces anxiety in achievement-related situations). These two drives come into conflict (i.e., an approach–avoidance conflict) with the former making it more likely that the adolescent will engage in achievement-related behaviors and the latter making it less likely that the adolescent will engage in such behaviors. Others have stressed the importance of one's attributions concerning successes and failures in predicting whether an adolescent will exhibit achievement-related behaviors. Past research suggests that some adolescents attribute their successes and failures to internal factors (e.g., one's innate intelligence), whereas other adolescents tend to attribute their successes and failures to external factors (e.g., the difficulty or fairness of a test).

In terms of gender differences, boys are more likely than girls to enroll in higher level math and science classes—despite similar ability levels in these areas. Scholars studying such differences have argued that parents are differentially supportive of boys and girls in these academic areas, with most parents being more supportive of boys' efforts. Moreover, it appears that girls are socialized to expect that they will not do well in mathematics classes. In general, girls are more likely than are boys to make internal attributions in failure situations.

3. Sexuality

Most children have mixed reactions to becoming a sexually mature adolescent. Parents also have conflicting reactions to such increasing maturity. Despite the importance of this topic, we know very little about normal adolescent sexuality, primarily due to the difficulty in conducting studies on this topic.

There are a host of factors which are associated with the onset and maintenance of sexual behaviors. Pubertal changes of adolescence have both direct and indirect effects on sexual behaviors. Direct activational effects of hormones exert an influence on sexual interest and behaviors (particularly for boys). Regarding indirect effects, visible secondary sex characteristics are social stimuli that signal the physical maturity of the adolescent to potential dating partners. Ethnic and religious differences in the onset of sexuality also exist. Finally, personality characteristics (e.g., the development of a sexual identity) and social factors (e.g., parent and peer influences) also serve as antecedents to adolescent sexual behaviors. [*See* SEXUAL BEHAVIOR.]

Unfortunately, sex education programs in this country have not been entirely successful at impacting on adolescent contraceptive knowledge or behaviors. Many of these programs are too brief to have any lasting impact on students. Partnerships between schools and family planning clinics, increased access to contraceptive services at appropriate ages, a reduction in the media's mixed messages regarding teenage sexuality, and a more secure legislative position regarding consent for contraception would all be helpful in reducing the fertility rate, delaying the onset of sexual activity, and preventing high-risk sexual behaviors. Sensitivity to cultural issues and the targeting of particularly at-risk groups would also be important additions to available programs. The increasing rates of sexually transmitted diseases among adolescents and the fact that many young adults with AIDS (acquired immune deficiency syndrome) probably became infected as adolescents would suggest that adolescent sexuality is deserving of considerable national attention (from researchers, school administrators, public policy advocates, and public health officials).

4. Intimacy

It is not until adolescence that one's friendships have the potential to become intimate. An intimate relationship is characterized by trust, mutual self-disclosure, a sense of loyalty, and helpfulness. Intimate sharing with friends increases during adolescence as does adolescents' intimate knowledge of their friends. All relationships become more emotionally charged during the adolescent period and adolescents are more likely to engage in friendships with opposite-sex peers than are children. Girls' same-sex relationships are described as more intimate than are boys' same-sex relationships. Having intimate friendships is adaptive; adolescents with such friendships are more likely to have high self-esteem. Some scholars have proposed that friendships change during the adolescent period because of accompanying social–cognitive changes.

The capacity to exhibit empathy and take multiple perspectives in social encounters makes it more likely that friendships will become similarly more mature and complex. [*See* LOVE AND INTIMACY.]

5. Autonomy

Autonomy is a multidimensional construct in the sense that there is *not* just one type of adolescent autonomy (i.e., there are at least three types: emotional autonomy, behavioral autonomy, and value autonomy). Emotional autonomy is the capacity to relinquish childlike dependencies on parents. Adolescents increasingly come to de-idealize their parents, see them as people rather than simply as parenting figures, and be less dependent on them for immediate emotional support. Despite such increases in emotional distance between parent and child during the adolescent period, research with healthy adolescents suggests that autonomy from mothers and fathers does not develop at the expense of their relationships with their parents.

When adolescents are behaviorally autonomous, they have the capacity to make their own decisions, to be less influenced by others, and to be more self-governing and self-reliant. Being autonomous in this way does not mean that adolescents never rely on the help of others. Instead, they are able to recognize those situations where they have the ability to make their own decisions versus those situations where they will probably need to consult with a peer or parent for advice. Susceptibility to peer pressure increases to a peak in early adolescence, due in part to an increase in peer pressure prior to early adolescence and an accompanying decrease in susceptibility to parental pressure.

Finally, the development of value autonomy also occurs during the adolescent period. Adolescents' views of moral, religious, and political issues become more complex and abstract. Adolescents are also increasingly likely to have values of their own rather than simply internalizing their parents' or peers' values. As noted earlier, however, value sharing is common between parents and adolescents, with adolescents tending to select as friends peers that have the same values as their parents.

6. Attachment

The last secondary change that will be considered is attachment. As suggested earlier, past research suggests that one task of adolescence is to gain increasing levels of behavioral autonomy without sacrificing the attachment that one has to his/her primary caregivers (an attachment that developed between infant and parent many years earlier). Interestingly, parental disapproval is anticipated to be more upsetting than peer disapproval by most adolescents. Discontinuities in the parent–child relationship during the transition to adolescence tend to occur against a backdrop of relational continuity (with respect to level of connectedness, warmth, and cohesiveness between parents and adolescents). Over the course of adolescence, the attachment relationship between parent and adolescent tends to be transformed from one of unilateral authority to one of mutuality and cooperation. [*See* ATTACHMENT.]

D. Use of the Framework for Understanding Adolescent Development

Having reviewed the different components of the Framework for Understanding Adolescent Development, a few examples of how this framework can be used to understand the behavior of adolescents are provided. Recall, that the primary changes of adolescents impact on the contexts of adolescence which, in turn, influence the secondary changes of adolescence.

Example 1   Suppose that a young preadolescent girl begins to physically mature much earlier than her age-mates. Such early maturity will impact on her peer relationships. For example, early maturing girls are more likely to date and initiate sexual behaviors at an earlier age than are girls who mature on time. Such impacts on male peers will influence her own self-perceptions in the areas of identity and sexuality.

Example 2   Suppose that a young adolescent boy has recently begun to develop cognitively and is now able to take multiple perspectives in social interactions, think hypothetically, and conceive of numerous possibilities for his own behaviors. Such increased cognitive skills will impact on his familial relationships insofar as he is now able to imagine how his relationships with his parents could be different. He begins to challenge the reasoning of his parents and requests more decision-making power in his family. The accompanying changes in his relationships with his parents will also impact on his level of behavioral autonomy, the nature of his attachments to his parents, and his identity.

Example 3   A 16-year-old girl has just obtained a driver's license and has decided that she will look for her first job to earn some spending money. Because she is now 16 years old, she has recently gained a number of privileges that she did not have before (i.e., her social role has changed). She takes a job in a fast food restaurant several miles from home and, because she now has a driver's license, she can get to work on her own. Her experiences at her job produce increases in feelings of autonomy and achievement as she begins to develop an occupational identity.

As can be seen by these examples, this framework is very useful in describing and understanding the behaviors of individual adolescents as well as promoting a more general understanding of adolescent development. Now that several examples of the framework have been provided, the discussion now turns to the next section of this article, which concerns the implications of developmental psychology for clinical interventions with adolescents.

II. IMPLICATIONS OF ADOLESCENT DEVELOPMENT FOR CLINICAL INTERVENTIONS WITH ADOLESCENTS

After providing a rationale for examining the interface between developmental psychology and treatment, two types of knowledge that appear to have implications for the treatment of adolescents and for treatment-based research are examined: (a) knowledge of developmental norms, level, and transitions, and (b) knowledge of developmental psychopathology.

A. Rationale

Clinical child psychologists often mistakenly endorse what has been termed the *developmental uniformity myth*—the assumption that children and adolescents of different ages and developmental level are more alike than they are different and that all can be handled similarly in the treatment setting. Many scholars writing in this area have maintained that most existing treatments for adolescents are not sensitive to the developmental level of the client. Given that many are concerned with the lack of interface between developmental psychology and treatment, it is surprising that so few developmentally gauged treatments have been designed. Although developmental psychology and psychopathology have been brought together in the new field of *developmental psychopathology*, there is room for greater consideration of treatment issues.

B. Using Knowledge of Developmental Norms, Level, and Transitions

In the first portion of this article, a variety of normative intraindividual and contextual changes that occur during adolescence were discussed. Given the primacy of change during the second decade of life, it appears that researchers and therapists who are knowledgeable about normal and maladaptive development are at a great advantage when attempting to design a treatment, determine the conditions under which a treatment is efficacious, and/or apply a given treatment. In short, the quality of adolescent treatment is likely to "move up a notch or two" when knowledge of developmental psychology is taken into account.

Although the existing clinical literature has not been attentive to normal development, this does not mean that efforts which do take developmental factors into account do not exist. In this section, research efforts and discussions of clinical practice that have attempted to take developmental norms, level, and transitions into account in the design, assessment, or implementation of treatment approaches are discussed.

I. Developmental Norms and Treatment

Knowledge of developmental norms serves as a basis for making sound diagnostic judgments, assessing the need for treatment, and selecting the appropriate treatment. In terms of diagnosis, both overdiagnosis and underdiagnosis can result from a lack of knowledge of developmental norms. A clinician who lacks the knowledge that a behavior is typical of the adolescent age period (e.g., interest in sexuality) is much more likely to overdiagnosis and to inappropriately refer such an adolescent for treatment. With regards to underdiagnosis, it is a common belief (as discussed earlier) that adolescents have stormy and stressful relations with their parents and that "detachment" from parents is the norm. On the other hand, research has not supported this notion—it appears that approximately 20% (rather than 100%) of adolescents have such relationships with their parents. It is interesting to speculate about the clinical implications of such erroneous "storm and stress" beliefs. Some have warned

that adolescents who are experiencing severe identity crises or extreme levels of conflict with their parents are not experiencing normative adolescent "growing pains." A clinician who overlooks this possibility will underdiagnose the psychopathology owing to storm and stress beliefs.

Some changes during adolescence are normal and these have implications for the selection of treatments. Given the adolescent's normal developmental trend toward greater autonomous functioning, certain treatments are more appropriate for this age group. Self-control strategies are probably more useful with older adolescents than are behavioral programs where parents are employed as behavior change agents. Also, different cognitive problem-solving strategies are relevant at different ages.

2. Cognitive Developmental Level and Treatment

The importance of cognitive development as a moderator of treatment effectiveness has been stressed by many but has rarely received empirical attention. Given that most efforts thus far have been in the form of theoretical discourse, rather than empirical study, it appears that this is a new research area that shows great promise for the future. Some have argued that treatment effectiveness will be moderated by the developmental level of the adolescent. For example, children at different cognitive developmental levels will have different understandings of traumas such as sexual abuse and divorce.

Although the developmental differences in adolescents' understandings of major life events have been discussed in this literature, we need more information concerning the actual type of intervention strategy to employ. What is needed are developmentally gauged, step-by-step strategies that could be employed after assessing a child's cognitive developmental level. It would be helpful if clinicians could develop alternate forms of their treatments that could be appropriately applied to those of varying developmental level.

In the area of adolescent pregnancy, for example, few intervention programs have considered the cognitive developmental level of the adolescent. Given the availability of contraception and sex education classes, many are puzzled by the "irrationality" of adolescent contraception nonuse. The reasoning behind the link between adolescent cognitive development and contraceptive use involves the notion that adolescents who are less cognitively mature may not appreciate the seriousness of contraceptive nonuse, anticipate the difficulties that will be encountered in the future if pregnancy results, or properly evaluate the probability of pregnancy. The less cognitively mature mate may also not "take the role" of his partner and, as a consequence, may not take seriously the risk of pregnancy or the consequences for the female if she should become pregnant. It is important to note that, as yet, there is little empirical evidence for connections between level of adolescent cognitive development and sexual decision-making.

3. Developmental Transitions and Treatment: The Importance of Prevention Efforts

Past research suggests that an adolescent who must confront multiple life changes and transitions simultaneously (e.g., school change, pubertal change, early dating, geographical mobility, and major family disruption) is at risk for adjustment difficulties. For example, an adolescent who has just moved to a new school may be unable to seek emotional support at home if his/her parents are also going through a divorce (two life changes which are frequently linked).

What implications do these findings have for treatment? This line of research suggests that prevention efforts are needed for adolescents who are about to experience multiple transitions. The focus of such prevention should be on the development of appropriate adolescent coping strategies. Here the focus would be on coping *with future events* rather than focusing on coping with *current* stressors. Indeed, how often are sixth graders prepared (in any way) for their upcoming move to junior high school? More to the point, could we not easily target children who are about to experience multiple life changes? Finally, are different coping strategies going to be helpful with children and adolescents at different developmental levels? Prevention could be applied in conjunction with changes in developmental level as well. The obvious application of this notion is to sex education. If they are cognitively ready, should we not educate preadolescents about sexuality and contraception *before* they are reproductively mature?

In sum, although there has been much more discussion of the interrelatedness of developmental level and child psychotherapy than actual research, it appears plausible that our treatment strategies could be im-

proved by incorporating findings from developmental research into our clinical work.

C. Using Knowledge of Developmental Psychopathology

Developmental psychopathology is a field concerned with the continuity and discontinuity of certain psychological maladies (i.e., the developmental transformations in the types and nature of psychopathology—all of which have important implications for treatment). The nature and frequency of most disorders appear to vary across age level. For example, the findings of current research suggest that the nature of attention-deficit hyperactivity disorder (ADHD) varies with age, with the various components of the disorder (i.e., impulsivity, inattention, and hyperactivity) being exhibited in varying degrees at different ages. That is, inattention and impulsivity appear to continue into adolescence and adulthood, whereas gross motor disturbance is most likely to peak in early to middle childhood. Regarding depression, adolescent girls tend to exhibit symptoms of withdrawal, whereas younger depressed girls are less likely to exhibit this symptom. Age differences have also been noted for other disorders falling within both the externalizing and internalizing categories (e.g., conduct disorders and anxiety, respectively). [*See* ATTENTION DEFICIT HYPERACTIVITY DISORDER (ADHD).]

Just as there is discontinuity across age in the manifestation of certain disorders, there is considerable continuity as well. Most depressed adults, adolescents, and children evidence distortions in their perceptions of their own abilities and they tend to make attributions for negative events that are both internal and global. Thus, at least for depression, it may be that there is cognitive continuity. [*See* DEPRESSION.]

Roughly half of all adolescent disorders are continuations of those seen in childhood. Those that are new during adolescence (e.g., anorexia) tend to be quite different than those that began during childhood. There are increases in the rates of the following disturbances during adolescence, relative to rates during childhood: depression, bipolar affective disorders, attempted suicide, completed suicide, and schizophrenia. There are increases in the frequency of antisocial activities but not in the number of individuals involved. Animal phobias become less common during adolescence and agoraphobia and social phobias become more common. The incidence of enuresis and encopresis is also less during adolescence. It is critical to note, however, that most adolescents do *not* develop mental disorders and that the actual percentage of adolescents who do show symptoms (most estimates are between 10 and 20%) is only slightly higher (perhaps less than 5% higher) than the rates for children or adults. Antisocial behavior tends toward continuity insofar as antisocial adults have almost always been antisocial children. Depressed adults tend not to have been depressed children—with the onset of depression being less common in childhood. Finally, schizophrenia disorders are often not preceded by psychotic disorders during childhood. [*See* AGORAPHOBIA; ANTISOCIAL PERSONALITY DISORDER; SCHIZOPHRENIA; SUICIDE.]

In short, there is not a simple continuous relationship between childhood and adolescent disorders. Clinicians would want to have this knowledge of developmental psychopathology to enable them to develop hypotheses about the course of a given child's disturbance. Is it likely that the disturbance will change or abate or stay the same over time? Is the disturbance typical of the problems that are usually seen for a child of that age? Without answers to these questions, the therapist may be prone to apply inappropriate treatments or to be overly concerned about the presence of certain symptoms.

III. CONCLUDING COMMENTS

In this article, a framework for understanding adolescent development was discussed and examples of interconnections between the different parts of the framework were provided. Implications of developmental psychology for the treatment of adolescents were also discussed. The importance of knowledge in the following areas, for both researcher and therapist alike, was stressed: knowledge of developmental norms, level, and transitions, and knowledge of developmental psychopathology. Unfortunately, it appears that there is still an appreciable lack of interface between developmental psychology and clinical treatment—and this applies to those who do research as well as to those who do clinical work with adolescents. Therefore, we must teach clinicians (and parents and teachers) to "think developmentally" so that the integration of these two areas may proceed.

This article has been reprinted from the *Encyclopedia of Human Behavior, Volume 1.*

BIBLIOGRAPHY

Feldman, S. S., & Elliott, G. R. (Eds.) (1990). "At the Threshold: The Developing Adolescent." Harvard University Press, Cambridge, MA.

Hende, W. R. (Ed.) (1991). "The Health of Adolescents." Jossey-Bass, San Francisco, CA.

Hill, J. P. (1980). "Understanding Early Adolescence: A Framework." Center for Early Adolescence, Carrboro, NC.

Lerner, R. M., Petersen, A. C., & Brooks-Gunn, J. (Eds.) (1991). "Encyclopedia of Adolescence." Garland, New York.

Steinberg, L. (1989). "Adolescence," 2nd ed. McGraw-Hill, New York.

Van Hasselt, V. B., & Hersen, M. (Eds.) (1987). "Handbook of Adolescent Psychology." Pergamon, New York.

Aggression

Raymond W. Novaco

University of California, Irvine

Aggression Behavior intended to cause psychological or physical harm to someone or to a surrogate target. The behavior may be verbal or physical, direct or indirect.

Aggressive Cues External or internal stimuli that elicit aggressive behavior by virtue of their learned association to it.

Anger A negatively toned emotion, subjectively experienced as an aroused state of antagonism toward someone or something perceived to be the source of an aversive event.

Cathartic Effect The lowering of the probability of aggression as a function of the direct expression of aggression toward an anger-instigator. The lowering of arousal associated with such catharsis is more or less immediate and can be reversed by re-instigation.

Escalation of Provocation Incremental increases in the probability of aggression, occurring as reciprocally heightened antagonism in an interpersonal exchange.

Excitation Transfer The carryover of undissipated arousal, originating from some prior source, to a new situation having a new source of arousal, which then heightens the probability of aggression toward that new and more proximate source.

Frustration Either a situational blocking or impeding of behavior toward a goal or the subjective feeling of being thwarted in attempting to reach a goal.

Hostility An attitudinal disposition of antagonism toward another person or social system. It represents a predisposition to respond with aggression under conditions of perceived threat.

Inhibition A restraining influence on the occurrence of aggression. The restraint may be associated with either external or internal factors.

Symbolic Learning of Aggression The acquisition of aggressive behavior through observation and symbolic communication, as opposed to learning through the reinforcement of emitted behavior.

Violence Seriously injurious aggressive behavior, typically having some larger societal significance.

AGGRESSION is behavior that is intended to produce harm or damage to someone or to something functioning as a substitute for that personal target. Intention and harm-doing are key attributes in defining aggressive behavior, which may be physical, verbal, or symbolic in form. The intended harm or damage may be physical or psychological in nature. This article addresses aggression as a human behavioral phenomenon; thus it foregoes consideration of animal research and of biological factors. It identifies what are recognized as key psychological determinants of human aggression, including situational factors, developmental antecedents, and motivational processes; and it reviews how aggression is learned, maintained, and regulated. As mental health is the general subject of this volume, considerable attention is given to aggression in a clinical and societal context. Aggressive behavior in conjunction with clinical disorder and among clinical populations is described, as well as approaches to treatment.

I. AGGRESSION AS A SOCIETAL ISSUE

Aggressive behavior is easily at the forefront of our attention, as violence has become a prominently recognized social problem. Taking certain glances at our contemporary world, the view is unflattering and suggestive of a Hobbesian view of the state of nature—as a war of all against all. While Rousseau and other social philosophers have, in contrast, argued that compassion and "moral sense" are instinctual, human nature is surely flawed, and aggression features prominently in that less than perfect make-up. The human capacity for violence is indeed a central shortcoming, but closer scrutiny of human societies reveals significant achievements in science, literature, art, and medicine. Aggression should be understood contextually, and part of that context is temporal perspective.

Because of electronic technology, violence is very salient. However, our contemporary world is perhaps no more violent now than it has been since preclassical times. To be sure, the Assyrians, Romans, Turks, European monarchies, Mongolians, and Zulus, to take a few dynastic examples, perpetrated ample brutality here and there. But in the present era of rapid communication, consciousness about violence threatens our sense of personal and community well-being, particularly with heightened intergroup conflict as a backdrop.

Contemporary societies are confronted with the apparent intractability of violence, which remains so because of its functional value. Without denying the contribution of biological factors to the occurrence of aggression, human aggression is an inevitably learned behavior, because of its instrumentality. From Machiavelli, to Hobbes, to Freud, to animal ethologists, and to the overwhelming majority of social scientists, aggression has been conceived to be acquired and maintained because it works. It functions in self-defense and in maintaining order in world affairs. While the functionality of aggression obviates its eradication, it is yet always in need of regulation, because of its capacity to erode the social fabric or to produce catastrophe.

Because of the survival functions served by aggres-

sion and by anger, its most important activator, aggression is an inevitable element of human behavior. Indeed, while concerns about violence are commonplace, the occurrence of violence remains a relatively low base rate phenomenon, compared to so many other aspects of human behavior. When contrasted with the likelihood of occasions of kindness, curiosity, inquisitiveness, problem-solving, navigation, rule-following, and so on, exposure to violence is fortunately quite low in probability. The problem with such a comparison, however, is that violence is a very consequential phenomenon—its end product has lasting significance.

Because of the instrumental value of aggression (it can be used to get what is wanted), there will always be some proportion of humans who act violently. While, on the one hand, violence is a low base-rate phenomenon, on the other hand, it does not take many people to be violent to have a serious social problem. Therefore, society is structured so that forces external to the person inhibit aggressive behavior, and socialization is shaped to internalize prohibitions against aggression. The regulation of aggression, thus, centrally involves inhibitory control.

The erosion of external and internal inhibitory controls raises the probability of aggression. That is, the occurrence of aggressive behavior is not only a function of factors that activate ("push" and "pull") aggression; it is also a product of factors that disinhibit ("release") aggression by lowering inhibitory control. To understand the likelihood of aggressive behavior, both activation and inhibition must be taken into account. Activational factors are things such as anger, incentives, and situational cues for aggression. Types of inhibitory factors are expectations of punishment, values counter to aggression, and consideration of the consequences of one's behavior. Both societal restraints and internalized personal restraints are needed to minimize and regulate aggression. The situational attenuation or progressive erosion of these restraining factors, such as by substance abuse or by desensitization to the awfulness of violence, weakens inhibitory control, and thereby disinhibits aggression. [*See* CONTROL.]

II. THE FUNCTIONALITY OF AGGRESSION

The central maintaining influence on the occurrence of aggressive behavior is its functional value for survival.

Although animal behavior is not a key subject in this article, it can be said that among the most basic observations of the functions of aggression are those that have been observed in ethological investigations, i.e. the study of animal behavior in nonlaboratory, naturalistic conditions. Most generally, ethologists distinguish two types of aggressive behavior: that between members of the same species (intraspecific aggression) and that between members of different species (interspecific aggression). The latter form is also known as predation. The concept of "fighting" is restricted to intraspecific aggression.

Both forms of aggression, fighting and predation, can be seen to have species-preserving functions. Predation obviously has functional value for the predator's nutritional needs. However, predatory aggression also has functional value for prey populations. Predation maintains ecological balance by maintaining optimal population size, preventing the depletion of food supplies, overcrowding, and excess bacteria in the habitat of the prey species. It also removes weak members of a species who are unable to escape, thus acting as a selective agency for the breeding of healthy offspring. Even parasites have species-preserving functions for the host—their presence increases resistance in the host species. External parasites also promote the development of social bonds by influencing mutual grooming behavior by conspecifics. The presence of predators generally encourages social aggregation, as it is more difficult to concentrate on a single member of the flock, herd, or school. Social organization is also encouraged for purposes of defense, best reflected in the social structure of primates.

Intraspecific aggression or fighting among members of the same species also has multiple species-preserving functions. Aggression works to establish a rank-order of group members, creating a social hierarchy that promotes peace within a community. A dominance hierarchy constitutes a social structure that lowers the probability of fights initiated by lower-ranking members against higher-ranking ones, and dominant animals also intervene to stop fights between peripheral animals and juveniles. The social structure does provide for better defense against outside attack, and it also plays a critical role in sexual selection. Fights between rivals contribute to selective breeding, ensuring that the most capable animals will be more likely to procreate. In addition, by virtue of its spacing-out effects, fighting also prevents the exhaustion of natural resources through territoriality.

Among animals, most intraspecific conflicts are typically settled by a complex system of signals, often stereotyped in form and ceremonial in appearance. Thus, "fighting" can be highly ritualized, not involving injury or even contact. Importantly, while it is not uniformly the case, lethality is restrained by strong inhibitory mechanisms associated with appeasement or submission signals. Animals with particularly effective weapons (e.g. wolves, rattlesnakes, and rams) have been observed to have strong inhibitions against killing a conspecific. The inhibition seems to be an active process and can have a distinctly sudden onset; however, there is no absolute reliance on the inhibition. Animals are killed by their conspecifics.

For humans, aggression clearly has survival functions for personal defense in the face of threats to well-being. It also has instrumental value in acquiring resources, particularly when the likelihood of punishment is low; and in a social system having values receptive to aggression, aggressive behavior facilitates the acquiring and maintaining of status. Within the larger society, there can be subcultures having a distinct set of values, norms, and symbols; violent subcultures, such as gangs, endorse or promote violent behavior as a normative response for dealing with problem situations. Enculturation in such social environments leads not only to the acceptance of violence, but to the learned expectation that the use of aggression is the way to solve conflict and that status derives from the capacity to use aggression.

More generally, however, conflict (i.e., antagonistic exchange between persons or systems competing for resources) itself has functional attributes. The presence of conflict within a system structures that system (e.g. political parties or the branches of government). Conflicts between systems increase system cohesion, as system members become unified against an external threat (e.g., "evil empires" or "Great Satans"). Conflicts also enable a system to adapt to its environment, in that the resolution of conflict can rearrange the system in an adaptive manner (e.g., battles over civil rights can produce a stronger constitution and a more accommodating society). At the societal level, the occurrence of violence serves as a danger signal to the system. It can be a catalyst for important societal change by forcing attention to the state of critical variables, such as employment, political representation, or moral degradation. Violence can raise the salience of the need for unification, as well as be a means of achieving the destruction and reconstruction of a system.

This array of personal instrumental purposes and of societal functions served by aggressive behavior render as inevitable its acquisition and activation. Indeed, the very persistence of aggressive behavior is indicative of its functionality. Therefore, thoughts about the eradication of aggression are misguided. Civilization seeks to regulate aggression, not to eliminate it. Despite political posturing to the contrary, aggression is part of the natural order.

III. DETERMINANTS OF AGGRESSION

The determinants of aggressive behavior have been a major subject of analysis, and much emphasis has been placed on observable events. However, the defining characteristic of aggression, as given at the outset of this article, is that it is behavior *intended* to cause harm or damage. "Intent," which is not directly observable but must be inferred, is now generally recognized as a defining property of aggression; but this was not always so. Some conceptions of aggression, guided by a strict behavioristic philosophy, had sought to define it independently of things not directly observable, such as "intent." Hence, some rather awkward definitions of aggression emerged in the 1960s and 70s, such as "a response that delivers noxious stimuli."

To accommodate such mechanistic language, stipulations had to be given that made reference to violations of social rules so as to disqualify "noxious stimuli delivery" done in official social roles (e.g., a dentist drilling a tooth or a parent enforcing discipline). In an overzealous effort to emulate physics, sectors of scientific psychology sought to eliminate "cognitive fictions" as useless hypotheticals—the fact that physicists do not directly see "black holes" or subatomic particles, like a neutrino or an antineutrino, is never the sort of thing such polemics considered. To make a long story short, the cumbersome efforts to define aggression without reference to intent have not been fruitful. The intention to cause harm or damage is generally accepted as a defining characteristic of aggression.

On matters of definition, it is helpful to bear in mind that definitions are not keys to the essence of things; they are rules for using words in a language. They have validity to the extent that they are useful and coherent. Aggression quite usefully and coherently is defined in terms of intention to cause or seeking to inflict harm or damage. Whether or not the behavior actually does cause harm or damage does not matter. If a projectile is intended to hit someone but passes the person without notice, this is of no consequence with regard to the classification of the throwing or shooting as aggressive behavior—despite it being of great consequence to the target. Conversely, behavior that produces harmful injury but was not intended to do so, is not aggression. It might be negligence, discourtesy, or simply an accident, but it is not aggression. Aggressive behavior is deliberate in inflicting injury or damage unwanted by its target.

One of the most important things to realize about aggression is its multifactorial production—that is, there are many determinants or causes of aggression. Moreover, these determinants exist in a wide range of environmental fields, from the macrosocial (e.g., sociopolitical conflicts, regional economic strains, or societal values) to the physiological (activation in brain structures, such as the hypothalmus and the amygdala, or imbalances in neurotransmitters, such as serotonin). Particular conceptions or theories of aggression will give emphasis to particular types of causal variables and causal mechanisms, and this variation is often a matter of differing *levels of analysis.*

Empirical investigations proceed at different levels of observation, in accord with seeking to study microlevel to macrolevel phenomena. The investigative approaches to aggression that are utilized by various academic disciplines, from the biochemical to the anthropological, are adopted in correspondence with the phenomena being studied. Obviously, one does not use a microscope to study economic strain or do biochemical assays to study sociocultural transmission of values about the use of aggression in conflict resolution. Academic disciplines construct terms, propositions, and methods suited to the observational elements and the dynamic properties that are sought to be described and explained.

When seeking to identify determinants of aggression, one must be clear on levels of analysis and avoid reductionism—that is, the idea that observations and theories existing at a more micro level are more "basic" or "fundamental" and, thereby, more "causal." Instead, there must be coordination of theoretical concepts and methods, on the one hand, with the phenomena to be observed and explained, on the other. The fact that there may be microlevel correlates of macrolevel phenomena does not provide sufficient conditions for "reducing" the macro to the micro, as the former cannot be fully translated and represented by the latter. For example, one can by no means fully understand the dynamics of job loss and its effects on aggression by the study of serotonin in the brain; conversely, macrolevel theory about social strain will not be very useful in telling us why Rocky is more aggressive than Bob or why Rocky is angry from 2:00 to 2:30 P.M., but not for the rest of the afternoon.

The effort to identify psychological determinants of aggression has produced a number of important factors, many of which are quite hypothetical in nature. They are "hypothetical" in the sense that the identified factor and the way that it affects aggression are not directly observed but are instead inferred from observations of human behavior. Statements about determinants or causes are embedded in particular theories, so it is always important to recognize the theoretical context. While the hypothetical quality of identified causes of aggression is perhaps most obvious for "aggressive instinct," this is also the case for the other determinants given below.

A. Instinct

Early psychodynamic theorizing, especially that of Freud, placed emphasis on instinctual forces as determinants of aggression. Freud postulated that human aggression was a product of the death instinct. He arrived at this idea, which was a major theoretical change for him, following World War I, which produced massive carnage on battlefields. For example, in 1916, the British and German armies fought the battle of the Somme (which occurred in the region of that river in France), and the French and German armies fought the battle of Verdun (in the region of that town in northeast France). Collectively, more than a million soldiers died in those two battles. In the wake of the catastrophes of this war, Freud asserted that aggression was the product of the innate savageness of human beings. He theorized that the death instinct can be directed outward as a way of diverting its self-destructive aims—thereby accounting for aggressive behavior. He also claimed that any restrictions on outwardly expressed aggression increase self-destruction—which is the basis for the psychodynamic view of depression as anger turned inward and for pop psychology ideas of ventilating anger. Freud also postulated that aggressive instinct could be neutralized by life instinct forces (erotic or constructive tendencies) or be displaced in safe venues, such as work, sport, games, or humor. Some animal ethologists, such as Konrad

Lorenz, and post-Freudian psychoanalysts, such as Karl Menniger, also promoted the view that human aggression was caused by instinctual forces. However, there is considerable consensus among contemporary aggression scholars, including those who study its biological components, that aggression is primarily a learned or acquired behavior, rather than being innately or instinctually determined.

B. Frustration

The scientific study of the determinants of aggression received its impetus from a behavioristic model that was strongly influenced by an important aspect of Freudian theory, which was that aggression or hostility is aroused when libidinal impulses are blocked or frustrated. Inspired by this idea, a group of social scientists at Yale in 1939 generated the landmark monograph, *Frustration and Aggression,* which asserted that the occurrence of frustration always leads to aggression and that aggression was always a consequence of frustration. Also embedded in their conception was the idea that aggression was "instigated" by a state of internal drive. While this motivational state was seen to be learned or acquired, rather than instinctual, aggression was nonetheless viewed as being impelled by a force from within. Not long afterwards, the argument was modified to stipulate that aggression is only one of the responses to frustration and that response probabilities were ordered by the persistence of frustration. The longer the frustration persists, the more probable the aggression becomes.

While there has been considerable debate regarding the aggression inducing properties of frustration, there is consensus that frustration increases the probability of aggression when it is a violation of an expectancy for goal attainment, especially if the frustration is perceived to be arbitrary. For example, job loss due to redundancy can generate aggressive inclinations because it can be assumed to be aversive, to entail ongoing experiences of negative affect, and to be especially so when the job loss is unexpected and viewed as lacking fairness.

C. Aversive Experiences

Frustration, unfortunately, is an inherently ambiguous concept, referring both to external circumstances and to an internal state. More parsimoniously, it has been argued that the key attribute of frustrating situations is that they are aversive. Exposure to aversive events, especially those that persist, that threaten survival, or that thwart efforts to attain important goals, will activate aggressive behavior through its instrumental functions and through its association with anger. Various theoretical models have been proposed to account for the mediational processes. However, the common denominator is that aversive events (unpleasant occurrences that would otherwise be avoided) motivate aggressive behavior through evolutionary links to the survival value of vigorous motor activity. Conditions of perceived endangerment, recognized as threats to well-being, evoke excitatory reactions and strong motor responses. By virtue of conditioned association with survival-threatening events, less urgent annoyances also elicit aggression, commonly when mediated by anger that "justifies" the aggression.

D. Anger

As a normal emotion that has considerable adaptive value for coping with life's adversities, anger can facilitate perseverance in the face of frustration or injustice. Because anger arousal can mobilize psychological resources and can energize behaviors that take corrective action, the capacity for anger is needed as a survival mechanism. Anger provides for personal resilience. It is a guardian of self-esteem, it potentiates the ability to redress grievances, and it can boost determination to overcome obstacles to personal happiness and aspirations. Nevertheless, because anger can activate aggression, anger control is indispensable to aggression control. Also, because anger can interfere with information processing and thus adversely affect prudent thought, anger often needs to be regulated for efficient functioning. [See ANGER.]

The relationships of anger to aggressive behavior is that anger is a significant activator of aggression and has a mutually influenced relationship with it, but anger is neither necessary nor sufficient for aggression to occur. Just because someone is angry does not mean that this person will act aggressively, and when aggression does occur, it does not mean that the person was angry to begin with. The level of anger does influence the probability of aggression, and, because anger and aggression occur in a dynamic interactional context, the occurrence of aggression will, in turn, influence the level of anger.

One aspect of this dynamic reciprocity occurs in conjunction with what is called the "cathartic effect," which is the lowering of the short-term future probability of aggression as a function of the direct expression of aggression toward an anger-instigator. The idea of tension reduction via outward expression of "blocked" emotions is fundamental to psychodynamic therapies and has its roots in the writings of Aristotle, who thought that in watching tragedies, members of the audience would be purged of pity, fear, and anger by vicariously experiencing the tragic performance. In the history of research of aggression, catharsis has been a controversial topic since the famous 1939 *Frustration and Aggression* monograph, whose authors postulated that the occurrence of any act of aggression would reduce the instigation to aggression. Indeed, the likelihood of subsequent aggression does decrease following the expression of aggression, but this is an immediate consequence and occurs only when the person has been made angry and the aggression is directed at the anger instigator. Because anger arousal can be re-instigated, the cathartic effect is a short-term phenomenon. Moreover, as the direct expression of aggression reduces the aroused anger, aggression is then reinforced as a way of dealing with aversive events.

A distinction is often made between "hostile" versus "instrumental" aggression to differentiate aggressive behavior enacted for the purpose of doing harm/damage to the attacked person/target from aggression motivated by noninjurious goals, such as economic gain or status enhancement. This is a bogus distinction, as aggression is inherently instrumental (including being an expression of anger), so the idea of noninstrumental aggression makes little sense. Other relabelings of this distinction, such as "annoyance-motivated" versus "incentive-motivated" or "reactive" versus "proactive" have been offered. These bifurcated classifications of aggression that hinge on ambiguously differentiated goal distinctions can be bypassed by simply thinking of aggression as occurring with or without anger.

E. Situational Cues

In addition to being activated by the internal "pushing" force of anger arousal, aggression also occurs by being elicited or "pulled" by external stimuli having a conditioned association with aggression. Aggressive cues are situational stimuli that are infused with meaning by virtue of their association with aggression. Things can have aggressive meaning by virtue of their intrinsic properties, such as is the case with weapons or a violent movie scene, or for their symbolic significance, such as social group identifiers or fighting words. External stimuli may also function as aggressive cues by being associated with previously obtained rewards for aggression.

Stimuli that have been associated with unpleasant events, especially traumatic ones, can also pull for aggression. Particular sounds, especially loud and sudden ones, and particular words, scents, movements, and appearances that have been associated with aversive experiences can instigate aggression. In posttraumatic stress disorder (PTSD), otherwise neutral situational cues take on strong aggressive meaning through their association with survival threat, as occurs in the context of combat or criminal violence victimization. The triggering of aggression in response to the subsequently encountered cue may be understood as an attempt to remove the aversive stimulation. With regard to PTSD, the occurrence of aggression (a survival response) may represent context-inappropriate functioning. That is, the person behaves as though he or she is in a survival situation when this is not the case. [See POSTTRAUMATIC STRESS.]

F. Symbolic Activators

Just as animals territorialize space and use aggression in defense of that territory to ensure survival, humans respond to encroachments of personal space with aggressive behavior. For humans, however, weapons enable territorial warfare to occur with less trespassing; moreover, humans territorialize ideas as well as real estate. Human aggression is largely driven by cognitive or symbolic mediators. Thus, in addition to behaving aggressively in response to threats of personal space, humans respond aggressively to threats of personal worth.

Aggressive behavior is directed by attention. To get angry about something or to respond aggressively to a perceived threat, you must pay attention to it. These antagonistic responses are often the result of selective attention to cues having high provocation value. This cue salience may involve a negativity bias in prioritizing focus or in processing information about someone or something. A principal function of cognitive systems is to guide behavior, and attention itself is guided by integrated cognitive structures, known as schemas or scripts, which incorporate rules about environment–behavior relationships. What receives attention is a product of the cognitive network that assigns meaning to events and the complex stimuli that configure them. A person's "mental sets" or expectations will guide the attentional search for cues relevant to particular needs or goals. When a repertoire of aggression or anger schemas has been developed, events (e.g., being asked a question by someone) and their characteristics (e.g., the *way* the question was asked, *when* it was asked, or *who* asked it) are encoded or interpreted as having meaning in accord with the preexisting schema. Because of their survival function, the threat-sensing aspect of aggression schemas can preempt other information processing.

As people monitor their physical and social environment for threats to their resources or their self-esteem, as well as for opportunities to acquire more resources or esteem enhancement, they operate with expectations about how events and the behavior of others will unfold. As discussed above, thwarted expectations are frustrative and can induce aggression. Further, when antagonism, opposition, or annoyance is expected, this can lead to selective perception of situational cues in line with an aggressive script. Also, when aggression is expected to be instrumental in achieving desired outcomes, it will occur in anticipation of those rewards. When punishing consequences or retaliation are anticipated, aggression is restrained. Situational cues can prime or activate an aggressive script and set it in operation.

Whether or not aggression occurs is very much a matter of how circumstances are appraised. Since the writings of the Stoic philosophers of the classical period, behavior has been understood to be strongly determined by personal interpretations of events. The concept of appraisal is that of interpretation, judgment, or meaning embedded in the perception of something—not as a cognitive event occurring after that something has happened. The appraisal of provocation is *in* the seeing or hearing. Appraisal, though, is an ongoing process, so various reappraisals of experience will occur and will correspondingly affect whether or not the probability of aggression is lessened, maintained, or intensified. Rumination about provoking circumstances will of course extend or revivify anger reactions. As well, the occurrence of certain thoughts can prime semantically related ideas that are part of an aggression schema.

Perceived malevolence is one of the most common forms of aggression-inducing appraisal. When another person's behavior is interpreted as intending to be harmful to oneself, anger and aggression schemas are activated. In turn, receiving information about mitigating circumstances (e.g., learning that the person was fatigued and working overtime) can defuse the appraisal of personal attack and promote a benign reappraisal.

Perceiving malevolence or attributing aggressive intent in appraising someone else's behavior pulls for aggression by involving the important theme of justification, which includes the externalization of blame. When harm or injustice has been done, social norms of retaliation and retribution are engaged. Aggression is thereby "justified" either as a response to perceived grievous transgressions or as a preemptive strike. Justification is a core theme with regard to the activation of anger and aggression, being rooted in ancient religious texts, such as the Bible and the Koran, as well as classical mythologies about deities and historical accounts of the behavior of ancient rulers. Aggression is viewed as a means of applying legitimate punishment for transgression or as a way of correcting the unjust circumstances. An embellished justification functions well in exoneration of blame for destructive outcomes of aggression.

G. Inhibition

The occurrence of aggression is not only a function of activational or instigational forces, it is also affected by inhibition. Instigation and inhibition can be thought to operate in an algebraic manner, although no formula for this has been established. Nevertheless, aggression is inhibited by the anticipation of punishment. The punitive consequences may be legal sanctions, direct retaliation, social disapproval, or self-reproach. Of course, while external punishment for aggression is codified in the social contract, it is typically the internalization of societal controls that guides civility. Socially acquired personal moral codes and self-monitoring are more pervasive regulators of aggressive behavior than externally imposed punishments.

The anticipation of punishment for acting aggressively against a certain target can result in the aggressive action being displaced—that is, directed against a substituted target, for which punishment is less

likely. The displacement of aggression to a substitute target is otherwise called indirect aggression. The idea of "taking out one's frustrations on something else" refers to aggression being restrained against some primary instigator and then being displaced to another target. Some incidents of domestic violence can be viewed in such terms. For example, someone who feels thwarted or insulted by a supervisor at work or perhaps is frustrated by other types of personal setbacks at work may then direct aggression toward a partner at home where the harm-doing behavior can more easily escape social censure. Similarly, a highly distressed and very angry hospitalized patient may engage in self-mutilation rather than attack a member of the ward nursing staff. The inhibition of direct aggression also may affect the form of aggression, as well as the chosen target. Verbal abuse, ridicule, or sarcasm can substitute for physical attack.

H. Disinhibition

Because aggression is controlled by external and internal restraints against harm-doing, the weakening of such restraints thereby increases the likelihood of aggressive behavior. This is called disinhibition, and it thus pertains to a releasing effect. Indeed, the ingestion of substances that impair cognitive functioning, such as alcohol or other drug use, decreases the capacity of inhibitory control, particularly in the face of perceived provocation, but there are a number of other disinhibitory mechanisms.

One mechanism for disinhibition is exposure to unpunished aggressive behavior by others, especially if there is some novelty involved. A child in a playground watching one classmate bop another over the head with a plastic water bottle, without being detected or reprimanded by a supervisor, will be less inclined to refrain from having such fun himself. Cinematic models, as well as real-life models in violent subcultures, can demonstrate aggression in ways that connote its normality, especially with high rates of exposure to the fictional or real models. Forms of aggressive behavior, then, lose their prohibited status.

Heightened physiological arousal is another disinhibitory factor, as it serves to override cognitive control mechanisms, such as considering mitigational information or consideration of the consequences of one's actions. When physiological arousal is high, the person becomes tunnel-visioned, failing to recognize potentially important bits of secondary information ("peripheral cues"). An aroused person is also biased in processing information that is suggestive of threat and is inclined to act impulsively. Importantly, the state of arousal may be heightened by the carryover of undissipated arousal originating from some prior source. That is, there can be "excitation transfer" from an earlier arousing experience, such as a stressful event, to a new situation having its own arousal activator. This additive effect then heightens the probability of aggression toward that new and more proximate source.

Disinhibition also can be facilitated by diffusion of responsibility and lessened self-awareness (deindividuation), such as occurs in large crowds during a street disturbance or during a football/soccer match. Generally, people lose self-restraint when they are not mindful of who they are and of their place in a rule-governed society. The disengagement of internal restraints may be accompanied by dehumanization of the target or victim of the aggression.

A behavior setting may be contextually conductive to aggression by virtue of its disinhibiting characteristics. On a highway, especially at night, there is considerable anonymity and opportunity to escape. The expectation of punishment is thereby diminished. Moreover, in settings where fighting is somewhat common, such as in certain bars, its commonality gives shape to a social script. In settings such as highways and bars, the disinhibition of aggression can be further amplified by the presence of weapons, which serve as cues for aggression. While riots are typically triggered by some precipitating event that gives justification to destructive behavior, the physical/psychosocial context and historical scripting facilitate disinhibition.

IV. THE DEVELOPMENT OF AGGRESSIVE BEHAVIOR

For the most part, human aggression is an acquired behavior. However, individual differences in aggression appear during infancy and early childhood, as manifested in temperament and rough-and-tumble play. There is growing evidence of an inherited predisposition to aggression, determined from longitudinal studies of twins reared apart and of adopted children, whereby a person's aggressive behavior as an adult has been found to be more concordant with biological par-

ents than with adoptive parents. Evidence for an inherited predisposition for aggression can also be found in animal studies of selective breeding. Nonetheless, genetic predispositions are just that—something to which the child's early learning experiences will give shape. Whether the predisposition is potentiated, exacerbated, buffered or neutralized is a function of the socialization process.

The acquisition or learning of aggression occurs primarily in family relationships, among peers, and in media exposure. The process of acquisition most generally involves observational learning through exposure to aggressive behavior and to values supporting enacted aggression, including reinforcement and punishment contingencies. This is contextually driven, as a child raised in an environment replete with deprivation, frustration, victimization, and instability will have many opportunities to develop aggression and to not learn inhibitory control. The rewards for aggression tend to be in the present; in contrast, the rewards for aggression control tend to be in the future. When someone discounts or devalues the future, aggression is a more likely.

The family and home environment furnish the central opportunities for the development of aggression. Family interactions patterns, involving siblings as well as parents, provide models of aggressive behavior and direct opportunities to learn how aggression functions in meeting needs. In observing how parents respond to distress or conflict, children learn aggression as a prepotent response to aversive events. Parent or caretaker behavior, such as occurs in a disciplinary confrontation, may model coercion as a way of achieving compliance. Displays of coercive power in the form of physical punitiveness and verbal abuse, as opposed to reasoning and firm discipline motivated by love, will breed aggression. Moreover, when the parent or caretaker is rejecting of the child and fails to provide security, warmth, and affection, the child learns that mistreatment is normative. Having an aggressive sibling facilitates the development of aggression and its escalation. There is considerable evidence that children raised by parents who are physically punitive and emotionally rejecting are more likely to have aggressive behavior problems. Insecurity and impulsive aggression easily develop from harsh, erratic, and inept discipline during formative years. [See PARENTING.]

The home is by no means the only arena for the learning of aggression. While parents and extended family members are the primary socializing agents during childhood, interactions with peers become increasingly important. Specific aggressive behaviors are learned in playing with other children, as well as rules for enacting those behaviors of tormenting, chasing, pushing, and hitting, including norms of retaliation. Particularly in interacting with peers, as well as with siblings, children learn that aggressive counterattack is successful. While aggressive children may be rejected by many nonaggressive peers, they do form affiliations with other aggressive children. Thus, their aggressive behavior alienates them from aggression-neutralizing, prosocial influences, and they then also acquire further training in harm-doing behavior. Their camaraderie with others who share their antisocial inclinations exacerbate their conflicts with the gatekeepers of society. The escalating problem of youth violence in American society is very much about gang culture, which provides the reward and value structure for shaping and maintaining aggression, ostensibly in the service of security and status.

The observational learning process that applies to the acquisition of aggression from witnessing aggression enacted by parents, siblings, and peers also applies to the modeling that occurs in media exposure. It has been soundly established that exposure to violence on television is associated with subsequent aggressive behavior. The effects of exposure to televised violence have been demonstrated in controlled experiments conducted in laboratory and field settings, which have been concerned with relatively short-term influences, and in naturalistic studies that have been longitudinal. The naturalistic studies have shown that television violence viewing habits are related to concurrent aggression and to aggressive behavior many years later and that this effect, while modest in magnitude, is independent of other influences, such as social class and intelligence. [See TELEVISION VIEWING.]

The aggression-inducing influence of media exposure is both enduring and reciprocal. Viewing violent programming has long-term effects on behavior, and aggressive children become inclined to watch violent television. Thus, there is a cyclical process involved—that is, exposure to television violence stimulates aggression, and the development of aggressive behavior patterns leads to more violence viewing. For children, the aggressive behavior habits and the television viewing have detrimental effects on academic and social

skills, which in turn increase the tendency toward aggression. This is a deviation-amplification cycle.

The process of observational learning, whether through real or fictional models, can be understood in terms of the development of cognitive scripts for aggression—that is, mental programs for processing information that are conducive to aggressive behavior. People encode information about environment-behavior transactions in the form of scripts that become guides for behavior in situations resembling those of the encoding. Cognitive scripts develop through paying attention to, encoding, and retaining in memory the event-response-outcome sequences. The script then becomes a guide for behavior and social problem-solving. It can be rehearsed, reinforced, and elaborated over time as its enactment generates consequences. Aggressive scripts, which are activated in conjunction with situational cues, can be highly automatized in their operation. Learned scripts are resistant to change. As development proceeds from childhood to adulthood, subsets of learned scripts can be abstracted to more general scripts that function as personal rules for aggression as social behavior.

V. PERSONALITY AND AGGRESSION

There is considerable consistency in aggressive behavior over time. At about 8 years of age, children show characteristic patterns of aggression that remain relatively stable during childhood and adolescence and are predictive of adult aggression. In longitudinal studies, it has been found that aggression at ages 8 and 9 (experimenter-rated, peer-rated, and teacher-rated) is predictive of self-reported aggression and criminal violence in late adolescence and adulthood. While some aggressive antisocial children will "normalize" as they grow older, highly aggressive children, whether girls or boys, tend to become highly aggressive adults. The development of cognitive structures conducive to aggressive behavior, as learned and elaborated over the life course, may account for this stability.

Among the early manifestations of problematic aggressive behavior is bullying in school. Bullies have a positive view of violence and its use, they need to dominate others, and they have little empathy for their victims. Boys who bully tend to be physically stronger than their peers, are impulsive, and are *not* characterized by anxiety, insecurity, or low self-esteem. As bullying is part of a more generalized pattern of antisocial behavior (school bullies are also aggressive to teachers, parents, and siblings), they are at increased risk for later criminality. Similarly, proneness to aggression that persists through adolescence is accompanied by other forms of antisocial behavior, such as substance abuse, reckless driving, and theft.

Behavioral violation of social norms in disregard for the rights of others, as a recurrent pattern from adolescence, is a key feature of the "antisocial personality" clinical diagnostic classification. Indeed, aggression and lack of impulse control occur conspicuously in several personality disorders. When enduring dispositions or trait characteristics, because of their inflexible or maladaptive nature, cause significant impairment in social and occupational functioning or subjective distress, they are thought to constitute personality disorders. Such conditions represent long-term functioning and are not episodic. In addition to antisocial personality disorder, paranoid and borderline personality disorders involve considerable features of anger and aggressive behavior. However, aggression features most prominently in the antisocial personality. Repeated aggression is a core element, along with lying, impulsivity, recklessness, and remorselessness. Such behavior patterns, of course, produce nonfriendly responses from other people, which thus provide "justification" for continued antisocial behavior and lack of empathy for the feelings of other people or respect for their rights. [See ANTISOCIAL PERSONALITY DISORDER.]

Associated with the classification of antisocial personality disorder is the concept of psychopathy, which has emerged as an important predictor of violent behavior. While psychopaths indeed have the impulsive, antisocial, unstable and deviant life-style behavioral features of antisocial personality disorder, they are further distinguished by core enduring traits. Psychopaths are characterized by a slick, charming, and manipulative style, combined with callousness and shallow emotions, which enables them as social predators. They tend to be serious criminal offenders who are grandiose, egocentric, and lacking in anxiety, as well as guilt. They have low frustration tolerance and are impulsive, but they can be planful and premeditated in using aggression and are inclined to put themselves in situations where violence might be needed. Char-

acteristically, they fail to take responsibility for their actions; instead, they blame others and rationalize their behavior. Psychopathy is significantly related to violent recidivism. [See PSYCHOPATHOLOGY.]

Chronically aggressive persons may very well go looking for reasons to act aggressively, because they welcome the opportunity to inflict harm. Such persons lack inhibitory controls. Undercontrolled individuals tend to account for a high proportion of violent incidents; however, in addition to these chronically aggressive persons, there are also others who are typically quite overcontrolled in their personal style, yet enact serious aggression. The overcontrolled offender routinely buries resentment and then in one instance lashes out in response to aggressive cues. The aggressive act, which is often one of extreme proportion, is completely uncharacteristic of the person, who has typically exercised high levels of control and inhibition. While the aggression may seem impulsive, as in a sudden murder, it may be the product of recurrent anger excessively inhibited and fueled by rumination about grievances. For such overcontrolled individuals, preoccupation with violence in fantasy may be an important predictive factor.

In addition to antisocial personality, psychopathy, and the overcontrolled type, other personality characteristics have been found to be associated with aggression, albeit less problematic in severity. The tendency toward irritability (antagonistic reactions to minimal provocations), emotional susceptibility (distress in response to mild frustrations), and rumination (dwelling on misfortune or slights) are personality characteristics that are predisposing for aggression. Reactive aggression also has been found for persons who are known as "Type A," which is a shorthand term for the coronary-prone behavior pattern of time-urgency, hard-driving competitiveness, and generalized hostility. The Type A or coronary-prone personality has a tendency toward impatience and irritability, which is in contrast to Type B individuals who are more relaxed and easy-going. The Type A person is reactively aggressive in the sense that the aggression occurs in response to provocation. Indeed, it is the hostility and proneness to anger component that constitutes the central risk factor for coronary heart disease. When individuals who are high in generalized hostility are confronted with a stressful demand, they have strong cardiovascular responses in blood pressure, neurohormonal secretions, and cholesterol. The aggressiveness of Type As may be further magnified by other hormonal factors, such as testosterone. [*See* TYPE A–TYPE B PERSONALITIES.]

VI. AGGRESSION AND MENTAL DISORDER

Aggression occurs in conjunction with many psychiatrically classified disorders, some of which are discussed above in the context of personality, as well as the conduct disorders of childhood and adolescence. Those personality and conduct disorder conditions centrally concern problems of impulse control. Another impulse control dysfunction is that of intermittent explosive disorder, which involves discrete episodes of serious aggression enacted in a way that is out of proportion to any psychosocial stresses that may have been implicated and is not accounted for by any other mental disorder.

Highly stressful events that are of a traumatic nature, such as military combat, criminal assault or rape, severe accidents, and natural disasters, can produce posttraumatic stress disorder (PTSD). The key features of PTSD are intrusive reexperiencing of trauma, avoidance of reminders and emotional numbing, and heightened arousal manifested in hypervigilance, hyperstartle, and irritability. Aggression and anger occur as part of the arousal symptom cluster. Anger and aggression are indeed a central feature of PTSD, and, in conjunction with this disorder, can be understood as context-inappropriate activation of "survival mode" functioning.

Repeated exposure to traumatic events, such as those occurring in combat or child abuse victimization, can produce dissociative amnesia that sometimes involves enraged attacks or self-harm for which the person has no recall. In another type of dissociation, aggression sometimes appears in a dissociated identity (multiple personality). While the alternate personality is hostile, controlling, and destructive, the primary personality is passive, dependent, and depressed.

Depression itself often involves anger and aggression. In bipolar mood disorders, anger and aggression can occur as part of the psychomotor agitation and irritability in a manic episode, and aggression is certainly manifested in a self-directed form by the suicidal behavior of depressed persons. Self-mutilation and suicidal behavior are also common features of borderline personality. [*See* BORDERLINE PERSONALITY DISORDER; DEPRESSION; MOOD DISORDERS.]

General medical conditions sometimes produce disturbances in mental states, and aggression appears in some of these psychiatric disorders, such as delirium, dementia, and psychosis. For example, in dementia, paranoid ideation may lead to false accusations and to verbal and physical attacks. As well, severe head trauma can cause brain damage dementia with associated impulsive aggression and anger outbursts. Head trauma often occurs as a result of sensation-seeking, high-risk behavior by young males. Acute brain syndromes that produce aggression are also induced by chemical substances. The disinhibition of aggressive impulses is a common feature of intoxication due to alcohol, barbiturates, cocaine, and amphetamines. Delusion disorder linked to amphetamine use may involve suspiciousness and paranoia that can subsequently lead to violence against perceived enemies. Phencyclidine (PCP) intoxication entails high-amplitude responses coupled with an imperviousness to pain that make for unpredictability as well as belligerent, assaultive behavior. Withdrawal conditions in substance abuse syndromes have irritability as a common feature. Persons with substance abuse disorders present a significantly higher risk for violence in the community. Lastly, with regard to neurological dysfunction, aggression enhancement may be the result of brain damage produced by perinatal difficulties, particularly when combined with an unstable family environment. [*See* DEMENTIA; PRENATAL STRESS AND LIFE SPAN DEVELOPMENT; SUBSTANCE ABUSE.]

Aggression is indeed associated with schizophrenia and psychotic symptoms, particularly ideation about the threat of personal harm and beliefs about the override of personal control by external forces. Overt expressions of both verbal and physical aggression occur especially during acute phases of psychosis. While aggression can be observed in several types of schizophrenia, it is especially prominent in paranoid schizophrenia, as persecutory delusions and heightened threat perceptions are predisposing for violence. Strongly suspicious and inclined to perceive malevolence, the paranoid person is primed for aggression. During an acute episode of psychosis, delusions and hallucinations combine with excitement, panic, and interpersonal detachment. The person can feel an overwhelming urge to attack, thought to be directed by a force outside his or her control. The motivation to do violence may also be heightened by grandiose beliefs of heroic responsibility to avenge against evildoers. [*See* SCHIZOPHRENIA.]

The evidence for the relationship of schizophrenia and other major mental disorders to violence is substantial and is derived in part from studies of the behavior of mentally disordered persons before they are hospitalized, while they are hospitalized, and after their discharge from the hospital; in some instances of this latter type of study, psychiatric patients are compared with normal community residents. In addition to these studies concerning persons who are at some point institutionalized, mental disorder has been found to be a risk factor for violence in epidemiological studies of persons in the open community. Generalizing across a number of major studies of community populations and controlling for the association of violence with substance abuse and demographic factors, such age, sex, and socioeconomic status, persons who are mentally disordered are more likely to be violent than non-mentally disordered persons.

The assaultive behavior of psychiatric patients in institutional settings is also noteworthy. Violence in psychiatric hospitals has been established as a serious problem in North American and European institutions. Generalizing across many studies involving different types of institutions and observational intervals, violence by patients in mental hospital wards is quite prevalent, as it occurs on average among one-fourth of the patients. Assaultive behavior by psychiatric patients in both private and public facilities presents an enormous challenge for hospital staff who are charged with providing treatment to remedy such behavior while guarding against physical harm to themselves. Attacks on hospital personnel by psychiatric patients produce not only physical and emotional injury to the staff member, but also have very significant financial costs for the institution and detrimental effects on the treatment milieu.

VII. TREATMENT INTERVENTIONS

Precisely because of the instrumental value of aggression, it is a difficult problem for which to provide treatment. Aggression is a time-honored means of controlling things and people. Aggressive individuals do not want to surrender their means of survival and of getting what they want, hence they resist change. Moreover, anyone serving as a therapist or counselor for such clients must face the risk of becoming the target of verbal or physical aggression. People having recurrent problems with aggressive behavior thus tend to be treatment-resistant and to activate negative sentiment in treatment providers.

Therapeutic interventions for aggression seek to replace the destructive behavior routines with constructive social behavior. Most approaches incorporate an educational component that teaches problem-solving and encourages prosocial behavior. Intervention approaches are typically guided by a theoretical orientation to aggression and its detriments.

Psychodynamic approaches to the treatment of aggression follow principles of ego psychology and emphasize the development of internal control mechanisms to manage impulses. Attention is given to unresolved conflict or trauma in childhood experiences, which are then worked through in the context of the therapeutic relationship. Considerable value is placed on cathartic expression of distressed feelings, which may occur in play or fantasy, as well as direct disclosure. Aggressive energy is sought to be displaced or redirected to safe activities, such as sport, work, games, and humor. Aggression-neutralizing influences, such as love, kindness, and constructive social activities are encouraged. [*See* PSYCHOANALYSIS.]

Behavioral approaches seek to manage the contingencies that shape and maintain aggression, particularly those in the home and school environment. Much attention is given to functional analysis of the aggressive behavior and to parent/teacher training regarding child discipline, including detailed procedures for the administration of rewards and punishments according to negotiated behavioral contracts. The central aim is to decrease the motivation for aggression by reducing its payoffs. Behavior therapy methods may also involve training in relaxation, communication, respectful assertiveness, and other social skills. [*See* BEHAVIOR THERAPY.]

Cognitive-behavioral approaches focus on cognitive and affective (anger) mediators of aggression, while incorporating many elements of behavior therapy, such as training in self-monitoring, relaxation, and social skills. Cognitive-behavioral therapies centrally seek to modify cognitive styles of processing information about social situations and to enhance anger-regulatory coping skills. They strongly emphasize self-regulation, cognitive flexibility in appraising situations, and the learning of prosocial values and scripts. Making extensive use of therapist modeling and client rehearsal, provocation proneness is modified by restructuring cognitive schemas, by increasing the capacity to regulate arousal, and by facilitating the use of constructive coping behaviors. [*See* COGNITIVE THERAPY.]

Systematic research on the effectiveness of interventions for aggression have primarily been conducted in conjunction with the use of behavioral and cognitive-behavioral approaches. Effectiveness is enhanced by approaching the context of the aggression, whether it be a family, school, or treatment institution, as a system having a dynamic social and physical environment.

BIBLIOGRAPHY

Archer, J., & Browne, K. (1989). *Human aggression: Naturalistic approaches*. New York: Routledge.

Berkowitz, L. (1993). *Aggression: Its causes, consequences, and control*. New York: McGraw Hill.

Dollard, J., Doob, L. W., Miller, N. E., Mowrer, D. H., & Sears, R. R. (1939). *Frustration and aggression*. New Haven: Yale University Press.

Geen, R. G. (1990). *Human aggression*. Milton Keynes: Open University Press.

Howells, K., & Hollin, C. R. (1989). *Clinical approaches to violence*. New York: John Wiley & Sons.

Huesmann, L. R. (1994). *Aggressive behavior: Current perspectives*. New York: Plenum Press.

Monahan, J., & Steadman, H. J. (1994). *Violence and mental disorder: Developments in risk assessment*. Chicago: University of Chicago Press.

Potegal, M., & Knutson, J. F. (1994). *The dynamics of aggression: Biological and social processes in dyads and groups*. Hillsdale, NJ: Erlbaum.

Zillmann, D. (1979). *Hostility and aggression*. Hillsdale, NJ: Erlbaum.

Aging and Mental Health

Margret M. Baltes

Free University of Berlin

Ann L. Horgas

Wayne State University

Alzheimer's Disease One type of dementia that is irreversible, progressive, and life-threatening. It involves a progressive loss of cognitive ability, self-care skills, and personality, and ultimately leads to death.

Dementia An acquired mental health syndrome that affects multiple cognitive domains especially memory, judgment, and abstract thought. Dementia has many causes, some of which are reversible.

Cohort Effects The effects of socioenvironmental contexts that a group of people born at the same historical time experiences during their lifetime.

Epidemiology The study of the distribution of mental or physical disorders in specified populations and of the factors that influence that distribution. This may lead to specifications of risk patterns for the occurrence of disorders.

Life-Span Developmental Theory A psychological theory that describes a perspective toward human development from birth to death.

Plasticity Changes in biological or behavioral systems that are caused by environmental modifications.

Psychopathology The study of mental disorders, their causes, manifestations, and treatments.

Resilience A concept in developmental psychopathology that describes the ability of people to avoid negative outcomes despite existing risk factors or to regain normal development after setbacks.

Risk Factor Any condition or event that increases the likelihood of the development of a disorder or deviancy.

Selective Optimization with Compensation (SOC) This metamodel describes three processes that facilitate the adaptation to internal or external changes during development, particularly in old age.

MENTAL HEALTH OF THE ELDERLY is not worse than that of other age groups, despite the many losses or risk factors in old age. After a brief overview about the major mental diseases in old age, risk factors related to psychopathology are described. The major thrust is directed toward explaining why, with the exception of dementia, there is not more psychopathology in old age. We describe protective factors that help to increase the resilience of old people. The model of selective optimization with compensation (SOC) is proposed as an explanation of adaptive processes.

I. INTRODUCTION

Why bother about the mental health of the elderly? Why is it an individual and societal concern with high priority? Much has been written about the elder-boom in all industrialized countries. It is, indeed, a revolution when one considers the numbers. There were about 3 million people over the age of 65, representing 4% of the population, in the United States at the turn of the twentieth century. At the turn of the twenty-first century, there will be about 32 million older adults representing 13% of the population. This increase in the old population is most dramatic in the group over 85 years of age. This group represents 1.3% of the population today (a sixfold increase since the beginning of this century) and is estimated to increase to 3% by the year 2030.

Without any doubt, for the first time, society faces an increasing number and proportion of elderly people who live longer. Thus, any age-correlated illnesses or problems will, by definition, increase as well. Does this imply that longevity is bought at the cost of illness? There are two opposing perspectives on quantity versus quality of life, the pessimistic perspective, held by many demographers, and the more optimistic compression of morbidity perspective. In other words, the question is whether the added years are healthy, vital years or sick years burdened with disability and impairments. The model of compression of morbidity represents the optimistic view. The argument is that (a) the maximum life span is fixed, and (b) most diseases in old age are chronic diseases that are the product of lifestyle and bad health habits. Educating people toward healthier lifestyles will either delay the manifestation of chronic diseases or avoid their manifestation altogether. Morbidity could be compressed into the time just before death, thus extending health and vitality to newly won years.

In contrast, pessimists paint a catastrophic picture: the increase in years is but an increase in sick years. In this context, the concept of "active" life expectancy has been coined, suggesting that only some years of the extended life expectancy are active and vital years. The outcome of this debate is still unresolved, although each side can claim data supporting its position and only the future will show.

What is the state of mental health in the population of people over 65 years of age? At first glance, one would expect on the basis of increasing biological vulnerability and concomitant stress an increasing likelihood of psychopathology in old age. Current data unanimously show, however, that this is not the case; elderly adults suffer no more psychopathology than the younger age groups in our population. Therefore, the main question in need of answers is how the elderly manage and what protective factors they enlist to combat the many risk factors.

When dealing with mental health in the elderly, we have to examine some major issues related to aging.

Although there is an increasingly negative balance between gains and losses in old age, there is also great heterogeneity among older adults and much reserve capacity or plasticity in old age. Whereas the first issue underlines the plight of old age, the second one tells us that people do not age similarly and that within a person aging can take on many different faces. Moreover, the third issue tells us that even in old age there are resources that can serve as protective factors in the battle against losses. That is, the elderly are highly resilient and are able to grow despite, or perhaps because of, losses and plights.

It should also be emphasized that in old age, mental health is not only a medical question but a philosophical one as well that touches on the meaning of a good life. Mental health or wellness is not just the absence of psychopathology. To be well in old age will mean different things to different people, and freedom from disease might represent only a small part of it. A much larger portion of well-being is likely to be associated with continuing to have goals and striving to meet them. It is important, therefore, to treat psychopathology, or disease for that matter, in old age from a contextualistic, systemic perspective. In this vein, we discuss psychopathology in old age in the context of risk and protective factors and present a model that can be used to combat the risk factors and make the most use of the protective factors.

II. EPIDEMIOLOGY OF MENTAL DISORDERS IN OLD AGE

The notion that most elderly are lonely, anxious, depressed, isolated, forgetful, and unhappy is a very common public opinion. This stereotype is definitely wrong, as shown by most field studies concerned with the psychopathology, or lack thereof, in old age across different countries. Prevalence rates of mental disorders fluctuate between 20% and 40%; the fluctuation is related to measurement issues (see later). Across all adults over the age of 65 living in the United States, about 22% meet the criteria for some type of emotional or cognitive disorder. These prevalence rates are consistent with reports that 17 to 22% of those over age 18 have a developmental, emotional, or behavioral problem. Thus, the proportion of the population with a mental disorder appears to be relatively stable across the life span, although the occurrence of specific disorders varies by age. Indeed, if cognitive impairment is excluded, the prevalence of mental illness is actually lower in advanced age. In the Epidemiologic Catchment Area (ECA) Study, adults over the age of 65 had the lowest prevalence rate (12.3%) of any Diagnostic Interview Schedule (DIS) disorder. Recent data from the Berlin Aging Study (BASE), an intensive interdisciplinary study with a representative sample of 70 to 105-year-old adults stratified for age and gender, indicated a prevalence rate of 24% for psychopathology. [*See* EPIDEMIOLOGY: PSYCHIATRIC.]

A. Dementia

Dementia can be considered the most prevalent mental illness in old age. Defined as an acquired impairment affecting multiple cognitive domains, especially memory, judgment, and abstract thought, dementia interferes with one's physical, mental, and social functioning. The most frequent type of dementia is Alzheimer's disease. There is a strong age and gender relationship with dementia. In the ECA study, an overall rate of severe cognitive impairment of 4.9% among those over the age of 65 is reported. This figure, however, obscures the age-related increase in dementia across age groups within late life. The prevalence of *severe* cognitive impairment is 2.9% among 65- to 74-year-olds, 6.8% among 75- to 84-year-olds, and 15.8% among those 85 and over. When considering *mild* cognitive impairment, rates were higher: 13% among 65- to 74-year-olds, 19.5% among 75- to 84-year-olds, and 24% among those 85 and over. In data from BASE, the overall rate of dementia (mild and moderate) was 14%. Although also showing a highly significant age correlation, the prevalence rates for age groups are somewhat different from the ECA rates but are more consistent with a recent Canadian national study: 0% in the 70 to 74 age group, about 8% in the 75 to 79 age group, 11% in the 80 to 84 age group, about 25% in the 85 to 89 age group, 32% in the 90 to 94 age group, and more than 40% in the 95+ age group. The Commission of the European Community Concerted Action on the Epidemiology of Dementia (EURODEM) pooled prevalence rates across Europe and reported the following rates of dementia: 0.3% among those aged 65 to 74, 3.2% among those aged 75 to 84, and 10.8% in those 85 and older. Differences in prevalence rates are most likely due to differences in the samples (i.e., including only severe vs. se-

vere and moderate cases or mostly young–old vs. also old–old) and in the diagnostic procedures. In contrast to field studies, for instance, participants in BASE underwent an intensive psychiatric examination.

Gender differences in dementia have been frequently reported, but the direction of the effect is not always clear. Some reports show cognitive impairment among the 65- to 74-year-old adults to be more common among men (4.2%) than women (1.9%). However, if those over age 85 are considered, women have higher rates of dementia. This may be due to the fact that there are few men in samples of the very old. There is also, however, the possibility of a cohort effect rather than a gender effect. Because education is inversely related to the incidence of dementia, older women— having had, on average, less education than men in those cohorts—would be diagnosed more frequently with dementia. In BASE, with its stratified sample, this gender difference in dementia can be fully explained by educational status. Gender differences also vary according to the type of dementia. Alzheimer's disease, for instance, is equally prevalent for men and women, whereas vascular dementia is more common among men. The latter is associated with cardiovascular disease (e.g., heart disease and hypertension), diabetes, and smoking—risk factors that vary by gender and that also contribute to the life expectancy in men. [*See* ALZHEIMER'S DISEASE; DEMENTIA.]

B. Depression

One of the most equivocally discussed mental disorders among elderly adults is depression. It is important, first of all, to be clear about the use of terms, for instance, to distinguish between clinical depression (e.g., major depression) and depressive symptoms (sometimes referred to as subacute depression or dysphoria). In contrast to popular perceptions, clinical depression is less frequent in old age compared with younger ages, but depressed affect and depressive symptoms show an age-related increase after middle-age. Estimates of the prevalence of depression in those over age 65 vary widely. Epidemiological studies in the United States report that 2.5% of older adults meet the diagnostic criteria for either major depressive disorder or dysthymic disorder (e.g., depressed mood). In contrast, 27% of the elderly participants in these same studies had some subdiagnostic depressive symptoms. Similarly, within BASE, 5% of the participants were diagnosed with major depression, and 18% demonstrated depressive symptoms. [*See* Depression.]

In contrast to dementia, there is no increase in these prevalence rates with age in the elderly population. Empirical findings with regard to the existence of gender differences are equivocal. In general, women show higher rates of depression than men.

Several studies suggest that this gender difference narrows in advanced age such that men and women have equally high levels of depressive symptoms after the age of 80. In BASE, the gender effect remains significant even after controlling for social, marital, and residential status.

Age and gender effects are also noted in one potential outcome of depression—that of suicide. Older adults commit 17% of all suicides; depressive disorders were present in two thirds of these cases. Elderly white males, particularly those suffering from chronic pain and illness, show an increased risk of suicide from age 60 to 85. Recent reports in the United States indicate a rapid increase in suicide rates among nonwhite older men and elderly individuals of Asian heritage [*See* Suicide.]

C. Anxiety Disorders

Anxiety disorders, although exhibiting similar prevalence rates as depression, have received little attention. Anxiety disorders, encompassing phobias, panic attacks, and generalized anxiety disorders, affect 5.5% of persons over the age of 65. Between 10% and 20% of elderly adults are reported to experience clinically significant symptoms of anxiety. Anxiety disorders are more prevalent in younger age groups and tend to first appear early in life; that is, new onset of anxiety disorders in advanced age are relatively rare. Women are more likely than men to suffer from anxiety. Data from the ECA studies on specific anxiety disorders suggest that phobias may be the most common psychiatric syndrome in elderly women and the second most common in elderly men. [*See* Anxiety; Panic Attacks; Phobias.]

III. SUMMARY AND METHODOLOGICAL PROBLEMS

With the exception of cognitive impairment and dementia, old age is not associated with greater risk of psychopathology. Disorders such as depression and anxiety are the most common forms of mental conditions in this age group, but their prevalence is not significantly higher than at other ages in the life span. The prevalence of dementia increases markedly across the age decades beyond 65, and, at age 80, is the most frequent mental disorder of old age. In general, women have been reported to be at higher risk for mental disorders, although these findings are not always consistent. Furthermore, some gender differences can be explained by other variables, notably educational, marital, residential, and social status. [*See* Gender Differences in Mental Health.]

A note about nursing home residents might be of interest. Most of the data presented have not distinguished between community-dwelling and institutionalized elders. It should be noted that the rates of mental illness among nursing home residents are considerably higher, leading some authors to conclude that nursing homes have become major treatment sites for mentally impaired elders. Estimates of mental disorders in nursing homes suggest that between 59% and 94% of all residents have at least one diagnosable mental condition. Approximately 56% of all nursing home residents in one study were diagnosed with primary degenerative dementia. In addition, between 33% and 80% of nursing home residents have symptoms of depression. Studies that include institutionalized older people thus will show higher prevalence rates for dementia and depression.

Prevalence rates of mental disorders in late life are influenced by several other methodological and measurement factors. One of the fundamental issues in diagnosing mental disorders is the challenge of differential diagnosis. This includes differentiating between normal and pathological aging as well as between different disorders. Discriminating between normal age-related cognitive changes, for instance, from early signs of dementia is known to be highly problematic. In addition, the clinical manifestations of mental health problems in later life may differ from those of younger persons, so that presenting symptoms are less distinguishable. Furthermore, co-morbidity of physical and mental disorders is the norm rather than the exception in late life. These multiple conditions, especially when treated with multiple medications, may exacerbate or obscure other physical and mental conditions.

With regard to measuring mental disorders, it has been consistently reported that older adults perform differently from younger or middle-aged adults on many psychodiagnostic instruments. The use of age-sensitive measures and the development of age norms for standardized tests is a necessary step in distinguishing between pathology and age-associated changes. Another issue influencing the estimates of mental disorders in late life is that of statistical power. Because of the shorter life expectancy of men, the numbers of older and particularly of very old men in field studies are limited. Therefore, statistical comparisons between men and women often lack sufficient statistical power necessary to detect reliably gender and age differences in mental disorders.

Finally, age differences may be confounded with cohort differences. A general cohort effect is evident with regard to depression in that more recent cohorts show higher rates of depressive disorders, earlier ages of initial onset, and higher rates of relapse than those born earlier in this century. Sociocultural changes since World War II, including urbanization and changing family structures, have been cited as possible contributing factors. As shown earlier, cohort effects may also influence the prevalence of dementia, especially with regard to the confounding of age, gender, and education effects. Whether future cohorts of women with educational levels equal to men will show diminished rates of dementia remains a question for the future.

With all of these methodological problems, it is obvious that longitudinal and prospective research designs are required to untangle these issues. Most research on aging and psychopathology is, however, cross-sectional. Moreover, measurement of change requires that we not only know what we want to measure but that we also consider the notion of equivalence of measures over time and the possibility of changes in distributions and norms. Despite or perhaps because of these caveats, it is important to ask, What are the risk factors for mental disorders in old age?

IV. RISK FACTORS FOR MENTAL DISORDERS IN LATE LIFE

From a life-span developmental perspective, risk factors can be characterized into three broad categories of influence systems: age-graded, history-graded, and non-normative. These influences create a context within which individuals act and react, and are likely to have an important impact on mental disorders in late life. Non-normative risk factors are those that are idiosyncratic; that is, they do not occur univer-

sally. These may include things like financial losses or crises, winning the lottery, divorce, or death of spouse, family members, or friends. Age-graded influences are those that occur for most people at specific points in the life course, such as retirement, attending school, and so on. The third set, history-graded influences, represents events that are experienced by all cohorts at a specific historical period. Such events can be epidemics such as AIDS, nuclear threats such as Chernobyl or Three Mile Island, wars, or introduction of a national health insurance.

However, this categorization of events is not fixed and immutable. Going to college, for instance, represents a normative, age-graded life event for many young adults at around age 18. This same life event—entering college—may be considered a non-normative event for someone in middle or later adulthood. Furthermore, what is non-normative at one point in time in society—for example, divorce—might become an age-graded event at another point in time in society. Also, what is a non-normative influence at a younger age might be an age-graded influence in old age, especially when one considers some of the negative life events such as widowhood, physical illness, or financial changes. Moreover, non-normative and age-graded events are influenced by the specific time in history in which they occur. For example, given the shorter life expectancy at the turn of the century, widowhood may have been a normative life event for 40-year-old women, whereas today it is considered non-normative for this age group.

In old age, non-normative and age-graded influences become increasingly negative and pose a threat to adaptation, well-being, and life satisfaction. Because of the number and co-occurrence of many of these influences, resources and reserves are quickly overtaxed, which places older adults at increased risk for psychopathology. Some of the major risk factors are discussed in the following section.

A. Physical Illness, Functional Impairments, and Correlates

There is a clear age-associated increase in physical illness and disabilities in late life. Physical health is intricately tied to well-being among older adults. Illness, disability, and functional limitations are associated with lower life satisfaction and more psychological symptoms. Losses in functional health often decide one's residential status, whether to live independently or to be institutionalized, which, in turn, can influence mental health.

Age-related pathologies, such as cancer, cardiovascular disease, metabolic disorders, or chronic pain, have been associated with late-life depression and dementia. Lower physical health and social support were found to be the strongest predictors of new cases of depression in those over age 55. Cardiovascular diseases have been associated with panic disorders and dementia. In the Berlin Aging Study (BASE), the age correlation with psychopathology can be fully explained by physical morbidity: depression is shown to be significantly related to impairment in mobility and in activities of daily living; dementia is significantly related to cardiovascular multimorbidity and sensory impairments. In concert, the data speak against a pure age-mediated co-occurrence of psychopathology. Thus, for many elderly, physical morbidity and mental co-morbidity is the norm rather than the exception among older adults. This association can result from a number of different mechanisms: physical conditions can lead to mental disturbances, mental conditions can exacerbate physical symptoms; the co-occurrence of physical and mental disorders can lead to a decline in physical status; or psychosocial factors can result in the inability to manage physical conditions. Regardless of the source of the relationship, physical and mental health are inextricably entwined and one cannot be reliably assessed without attention to the other.

Not surprisingly, co-morbidity is also associated with high rates of multiple prescription medication use to treat both physical and mental conditions. Polypharmacy places elders at risk for potentially serious adverse drug reactions and drug–drug interactions. The behavioral manifestations of adverse drug effects among elderly adults include depression, confusion, sedation, and functional and cognitive impairments. Thus, medications themselves may have a serious negative impact on mental health in late life and compound the difficulties associated with differential diagnoses of physical and mental health conditions.

Finally, although objective, clinical evaluations of health are often believed to be the "gold standard," subjective appraisals of health are also important influences on elderly adults' wellness. Not only are perceived health ratings reliable proxies for objective health indicators, subjective health has been shown to be a significant predictor of mortality, cognitive functioning, and well-being. As such, subjective health may represent a separate, but related, risk factor for mental health status in late life.

B. Psychosocial Influences

Aside from physical and functional health problems, psychosocial factors can also function as risk factors. There is much research about the risk for psychopathology as a consequence of low education and income, institutionalization, widowhood, and social isolation. We have previously alluded to the inverse relationship between education and dementia. This is not to say that the highly educated are less likely to experience decline and dementia. The highly educated start their decline at a higher level of functioning, with more resources than less educated elders so that diseases such as Alzheimer's disease can be compensated for longer and its manifestation delayed. Social isolation and widowhood seem particularly related to depression. Overall, it should be mentioned that people from the lower social class stratum seem to experience more critical life events, which may explain the relationship between lower social class and psychopathology. [See SOCIOECONOMIC STATUS.]

C. Conclusion

The aging paradox—many losses, high vulnerability, and fewer resources, on the one hand, and no increase in psychopathology on the other hand—needs explanation. Given the number of potential losses in old age and the number of demands and tasks confronting a person who becomes more and more vulnerable, the reported prevalence rates do not reflect the expected increase in psychopathology in old age. What protective factors are at work? How are risk factors overcome or coped with?

V. PROTECTIVE FACTORS INCREASING RESILIENCE IN OLD AGE

What do the elderly possess that allows most of them to age at least "normally," if not always "successfully," well into their 80s? A great number of psychological mechanisms have been reported in the literature: social support and its protective effect in times of crises, self-efficacy and personal control and their protective impact in dealing with conflicts and losses, protective personality traits as well as the protective notion of possible selves, the merits of downward social comparison, and protective coping mechanisms. In the context of developmental psychopathology, the concept of "resilience" has been used extensively to refer to the fact that there are children growing up in the worst of circumstances who become "normal" adults; children who despite early childhood adversities do not succumb to any kind of psychopathology or delinquency. It was only recently that the concept of resilience was introduced into the gerontological literature (i.e., Staudinger and colleagues). The presence of resilience in old age would explain why elderly people are, on average, satisfied with their lives even more so than the young. [*See* COPING WITH STRESS; SOCIAL SUPPORT.]

From a life-span perspective, resilience is a type of reserve capacity, a resource that can maintain or restore functioning with the help of a number of protective factors and mechanisms. The goal, thereby, is threefold: (a) to enable the elderly to live independently and in an autonomous manner, (b) to live in a self-responsible and self-determined manner, and (c) to live a life that is satisfying. Two sets of factors that make realization of these criteria feasible are behavioral and social–emotional competence. The former includes, for instance, cognitive functioning and everyday functioning; the latter competence includes management of emotion and self, personal control, and social integration.

A. Behavioral Competence

I. Cognitive Functioning

Current understanding in the gerontological literature is that cognitive aging is highly multifaceted and multidimensional. There is a strong negative correlation—albeit tremendous interindividual variation—between age and dimensions of fluid intelligence, such as problem-solving ability, but not between age and dimensions of crystallized intelligence, such as vocabulary. Thus, crystallized intelligence, that is, experience and culture, can offset the loss in the mechanics and allow the elderly to continue to grow. The differential maintenance of various aspects of cognitive functioning may serve as an important resource against psychopathology in late life.

2. Everyday Functioning

The positive relationship between everyday functioning, everyday activities, and well-being has long been reported by gerontologists. Activity theory in its many variations is a prime example. There is, albeit equivocal, support for a relationship between level of activity and well-being among elders. Some authors have been able to specify this relationship by demonstrating that it is not the level of activities that is the crucial variable but rather whether activities are self-selected. In our own research, we have defined everyday functioning as the orchestration of skills and abilities to manage everyday demands effectively and efficiently. We have shown that there are basically two components of everyday competence. Basic competence comprises all activities that are necessary for survival. These are highly automatized and routinized activities, such as eating. Expanded competence encompasses all leisure, social, and complex instrumental activities (like banking). They are very much a function of individual preferences, motivations, skills, and experiences. By using regression analyses, we find that both level and variety of optional activities, as well as whether these activities are engaged in with others, have a positive effect on well-being and satisfaction in aging and on positive affect. In contrast, resting and sleeping and less time spent in presumably pleasurable leisure activities were associated with higher levels of depression, even after controlling for physical pain.

B. Social–Emotional Competence

I. Emotion and Self Management

It seems plausible that a person whose positive emotions dominate, or whose positive and negative emotions are balanced, can better deal with life's problems. Negative emotions such as anxiety, irritation, and others are thought to be indicators of stress. There is not much research on emotion and aging. There are findings in the American literature showing that elderly do not have fewer emotions, but become better in dealing with emotions. Findings from BASE demonstrate that elderly do experience more positive emotions than negative ones, but that there is, nevertheless, an increase in negative emotions across the ages 70 to 105. Several strands of research lend themselves as explanatory paradigms for the maintenance of positive emotions, for example, socioemotional selectivity theory, coping mechanisms such as accommodative coping and secondary control, and social integration, to name a few.

2. Social Integration

The literature on social network and its effects is voluminous. Similar to scholars' first assumptions that more control is better or help is always beneficial, social contact has also been regarded as having positive effects only. Instead, a highly differentiated picture has emerged because of the equivocalness of empirical findings. Differentiations are made between quantity and quality of contact, objective and subjective support, instrumental and emotional support, type of network members, received and perceived support, and so on. There is no doubt that elderly spend more time alone than any other age group, but this does not necessarily permit the inference that they, as a group, are lonely or isolated. Reducing one's social network might have a protective function, in that it assists emotion and self management. To explain this relationship, Laura Carstensen, a Stanford psychologist, has developed the socioemotional selectivity theory. It says that with age, the regulation of emotion and the protection of one's self assumes greater prominence among the social motives that govern social interaction. When the future becomes limited, people initiate or avoid social contact largely because of its potential for meaningful, emotionally rich experiences that demand careful selection of social partners. In this view, smaller social networks reflect a distilling of the social world such that the most rewarding relationships are maintained and less rewarding relationships are discarded. At the same time, emotionally close social contacts help preserve one's self. Self-concept maintenance requires the selection of social partners who provide a self-verification function not a self-doubt function. [See SOCIAL NETWORKS.]

3. Personal Control and Mastery

Control has been regarded as a basic need of humans, and research has shown that people are motivated to maintain control. The perception of being in control is beneficial, and depriving individuals of control can result in passivity, negative affect, and depression. Control seems to act as a mediator of the effects of stress on health. How this effect works has many explanations and no consensus among experts. Because vulnerability increases with age, the operating range to deal with stress shrinks and the type of stresses

change. Old age presents many uncontrollable losses, which makes primary control obsolete and requires new or other forms of control such as secondary control, proxy control, or accommodative coping. There is research to show that elderly favor an accommodative coping style over an assimilative one, thus permitting the elderly to acknowledge unavoidable and uncontrollable losses and events that need adjustment, not resistance.

Proxy control, that is, actively delegating control to others, is regarded as a mechanism to maintain self-efficacy in the face of unavoidable and irreversible losses. Delegating control to others at the cost of becoming dependent on others can nevertheless be a very powerful mechanism to maintain domains in danger of decline or loss. Baltes and her colleagues used a social learning framework to demonstrate that dependency can be an instrument for control. By exhibiting dependent behaviors, the elderly person exerts control over the social environment, gains social contact, and avoids isolation. [See CONTROL.]

The metamodel of *selective optimization with compensation* (SOC), which has been developed by Margret Baltes and Paul Baltes in the context of successful aging, seems well suited to provide an explanatory umbrella for these different strands of research.

VI. SELECTIVE OPTIMIZATION WITH COMPENSATION

The basic assumption of the SOC model is that the three processes—selection, optimization, and compensation—form a system of behavioral action or outcome-oriented functioning. First, *selection* involves goals or outcomes that give direction to behavior and its development. By selection, a given individual samples from a population of possibilities or opportunities. Selection refers to a restriction of one's involvement to fewer domains of functioning as a consequence of new demands and tasks or as a consequence of or in anticipation of losses in personal and environmental resources. Selection may mean avoidance of one domain altogether or it can mean a restriction in tasks and goals within one domain or in a number of domains. Thus, an elderly person experiencing the terminal illness of a spouse may completely give up the domain of sexuality, or may restrict some goals and involvements in the social network at large but make no changes in the domain of leisure activities and family. Although selection connotes a reduction in the number of high-efficacy domains, tasks, goals, and so on, it does not necessarily suggest continuation of previous goals and domains, albeit in smaller numbers. Selection can also include new or transformed domains and goals.

Selection implies that an individual's expectations are readjusted and reassessed. Selection can be proactive or reactive. Selection encompasses both environmental changes (e.g., relocation), active behavior changes (e.g., reducing the number of commitments), or passive adjustment (e.g., avoiding climbing stairs). Proactively, people can monitor their functioning, predict future changes and losses (e.g., death of the spouse), and make efforts to look and search for tasks and domains that will remain intact after losses. Selection is reactive when unpredictable or sudden changes force either the person to make a selection or others to make a selection for the person. If a stroke suddenly and severely impairs a person, a decision to remain at home might not be viable, but the person can engage in other selection processes such as which institution, how much and what kind of self-care, what type of rehabilitation and what activities to engage in, what television program to watch, and when to write a letter or make a telephone call.

Terms such as secondary control and accommodative coping are thought of as selection strategies for losses in competence or for uncontrollable events. In both instances, people reorganize goal structures and goal hierarchies so that they achieve a fit between personal competence and environmental demands. The mechanism of downward social comparison seems to be extremely useful in adjusting one's reference points. In the face of difficulties and irreversible losses, downward comparison allows people to adjust and maintain a positive evaluation of the self. The adaptive task of the person is to concentrate on and select those domains, tasks, goals, and expectations that are of high priority and involve a convergence of environmental demands, individual motivations, skills, and biological capacity.

Compensation, the second component factor facilitating mastery of loss in reserves, becomes operative when specific behavioral capacities or skills are lost or reduced below the level required for adequate functioning. Compensation is the response to a loss *in goal-relevant means.* The question here is: Do I have other means to reach the same goal, to accomplish the same outcome in a specific domain? Losses in specific behavioral capacities loom particularly large when situations and goals require a wide range of activity and a high level of performance (e.g., competitive sports, rush hour traffic, accumulation of daily hassles, and situations that require quick thinking and memorization). The need for compensation in old age stems mostly from person- or environment-associated changes in means–ends resources. Examples of these are changes in means–ends resources (plasticity) caused by aging or a move into a new ecology that may imply a change in person–environment fit.

Compensatory efforts can be automatic or planned. In a domain that includes a large number of activities and means, if a goal is well elaborated, the person will not experience much trouble in counterbalancing or compensating for a specific behavioral deficiency. If the deficiency is large in scope or if the domains and goals are defined by one or very few activities, compensatory efforts will be more difficult. Compensation is not necessarily dependent on existing behaviors or means. Compensation sometimes requires the acquisition of new skills or means not yet in the person's repertoire. An avid reader who becomes blind might learn braille in order to continue reading or might divert to listening to "books on tape."

Thus, compensation differs from selection in that the target, domain, task, or goal is maintained, but new means are enlisted to compensate for a behavioral deficiency in order to maintain or optimize prior functioning. The element of compensation involves aspects of both the mind and technology. Psychological compensatory efforts include, for example, the use of new mnemonic strategies or external memory aids when internal memory mechanics or strategies prove insufficient. The use of a hearing aid is an example of compensation by means of technology. The world of the disabled is full of technical means that compensate for impairments and make a more or less independent and successful life possible. Not only technical means, but also human means are often needed to achieve compensation. The assistance of a hand or arm when walking, a hired worker who does the cooking, or a companion who does the writing may provide the compensatory means that enables elderly people to pursue their lives as fully as possible.

Findings from self-efficacy theory suggest compensatory processes in the form of proxy control. In contrast to secondary control, described earlier as a selection strategy, proxy control allows the elderly person to maintain specific goals, but instead of reaching them through active behaviors performed by themselves, they obtain them through passive behaviors and delegate the active ones to others.

Third, *optimization* involves the probability, level, and scope of desirable outcomes or goal attainment (minimization of losses and maximization of gains). Therefore, the central themes of optimization are to generate and refine means (resources) associated with the generation and production of goal attainment (desired outcomes). Optimization and growth may relate to the development of existing goals and expectations (e.g., in the domain of generativity). They may also reflect new goals and expectations in line with developmental tasks of the third phase of life, such as acceptance of one's own mortality.

How much selection and compensation must be invested to secure maintenance and stimulate optimization is an empirical question. Recent literature in gerontology suggests that many elderly people, in principle, have the necessary resources and reserves to optimize functions but face restrictive or overprotective environments that inhibit optimization. There is no doubt that the process of optimization will be contingent to a large extent on stimulating and enhancing environmental conditions. Thus, society plays a central role in providing environments that facilitate optimization. In fact, the success of relatively simple interventions suggests that the elderly often live in a world of underdemand rather than overdemand. Optimization depends on available possibilities and opportunities, unless older people actively forge new terrain and frontiers.

Within gerontology, a host of evidence for optimization comes from intervention studies. These provide evidence for plasticity and growth possibilities when environmental conditions stimulate practice, training and exercise, attention, and task motivation in both the psychological domain, such as in the areas of cognition (e.g., memory performance or social behavior), as well as the biological domain in diverse areas (e.g., lung functions, cardiovascular system, etc.). These diverse studies have demonstrated that old people are able to profit from "optimizing" environments. Specifically, physical exercise has been shown to improve biological functioning and well-being; cognitive intervention can increase well-being and even help to ameliorate the impact of dementia on daily living; behavioral interventions can reverse chronic dependent behaviors and increase autonomy. Studies of control-enhancing interventions demonstrate substantial improvement in activity level, health, and life satisfaction after minor institutional modifications.

VII. OUTLOOK

We have shown that there is an aging paradox. Despite increasing losses and vulnerability, psychopathology does not increase in old age, with the exception of dementia. We have demonstrated that the elderly have at their disposal a range of processes and mechanisms—in short, resources—that help offset the detrimental effects of losses. This is true at least for the young old, from ages 65 to 85. After 85, and particularly in the 90s, there seems to be a general trend toward more negative moods, more negative affect, and lower life satisfaction. Thus, viewing aging from a systemic perspective, age poses more and more stress the older one gets. This has implications not only for the very old themselves, but also for their environment, their social partners, and their caregivers. The metamodel of selective optimization with compensation describes processes by which elderly adults as well as their partners can cope with these stresses and maintain a higher level of well-being and mental health that stereotypical views of aging would predict.

BIBLIOGRAPHY[1]

Baltes, M. M. (1996). *The many faces of dependency in old age.* New York: Cambridge University Press.

Baltes, P. B., & Baltes, M. M. (Eds.). (1990). *Successful aging: Perspectives from the behavioral sciences.* New York: Cambridge University Press.

Baltes, P. B. (1993). The aging mind: Potential and limits. *The Gerontologist, 33,* 580–594.

Carstensen, L. L. (1993). Motivation for social contact across the life span. A theory of socioemotional selectivity. In J. Jacobs (Ed.), *Nebraska Symposium on Motivation: Developmental perspectives on motivation* (Vol. 40, pp. 209–254). Lincoln, NE: University of Nebraska Press.

---

[1] We apologize for the fact that much research is cited in this entry without citing the respective scholars. The references presented here are but a minuscule fraction of the number of authors who should be cited.

Carstensen, L. L., Edelstein, B. A., & Dornbrand, L. (Eds.). (1996). *The practical handbook of clinical gerontology.* Newbury Park, CA: Sage.

Cicchetti, D., & Cohen, D. (Eds.). (1995). *Manual of developmental psychopathology.* New York: Wiley.

Copeland, J. R. M., & Abov-Saleh, M. T. (Eds.). (1994). *The psychiatry of old age.* London: Wiley.

Ebrahim, S., & Kalache, A. (Eds.). (1996). *Epidemiology in old age.* London: BMJ.

Futterman, A., Thompson, L., Gallagher-Thompson, D., & Ferris, R. (1995). Depression in later life: Epidemiology, assessment, etiology, and treatment. In E. E. Beckham & W. R. Leber (Eds.), *Handbook of depression* (2nd ed., pp. 494–525). New York: Guilford Press.

Gatz, M., Kasl-Godley, J. E., & Karel, M. J. (1996). Aging and mental disorders. In J. E. Birren & K. W. Schaie (Eds.), *Handbook of the psychology of aging* (4th ed., pp. 365–382). San Diego, CA: Academic Press.

Lutz, W. (Ed.). (1994). *The future population of the world. What can we assume today.* London: Earthscan.

Mayer, K. U., & Baltes, P. B. (Eds.). (1996). *Die Berliner Altersstudie* [The Berlin Aging Study]. Berlin: Akademie Verlag.

Smyer, M. A. (Ed.). (1993). *Mental health and aging: Progress and prospects.* New York: Springer.

Agoraphobia

Geoffrey L. Thorpe

University of Maine

Cognitive Therapy A system of psychotherapy focused upon identifying and restructuring dysfunctional thoughts and schemas linked to psychopathology.

Exposure *in Vivo* The structured treatment of anxiety disorders by systematic confrontation of feared external situations to reduce avoidance behavior and anxiety.

Exposure to Somatic Cues Extends the methods of exposure *in vivo* to those internal cues and bodily sensations associated with panic attacks.

Limited Symptom Attack An anxiety episode with a few subjective anxiety symptoms, insufficient in number to qualify as a panic attack.

Panic Attack A discrete period of intense fear, not explained by a continuing organic factor, that arises rapidly with at least 4 anxiety symptoms from a 13-item list specified in the *DSM-IV*.

Pharmacological Dissection The identification of qualitatively separate anxiety patterns by examining the differential effects of certain medications.

AGORAPHOBIA is an anxiety disorder characterized by marked fear of entering crowded, public places; of traveling away from home, especially by public transportation; of feeling trapped or confined; and of being separated from a place or person associated with safety. Sudden, brief episodes of extreme anxiety—panic attacks—are commonly associated with agoraphobia, and may lead to avoidance of situations in which they occur. Often there is a "fear of fear" pattern, in which the bodily sensations of mounting panic are themselves a source of anxiety. Generally more debilitating than specific or social phobias, agoraphobia causes some people to remain entirely housebound. As a syndrome of anxiety elements in physiological, behavioral, and subjective domains, agoraphobia represents a distinct disorder with a typical clinical presentation and course. It usually arises in early adult life, with a prevalence in the Western world of approximately 2.5%; there is a significant preponderance of females in surveys of agoraphobia in clinical and community settings. Since about 1970, clinical researchers have developed effective pharmacological and psychological treatments to reduce or eliminate agoraphobic avoidance behavior and panic attacks.

I. AGORAPHOBIA: PAST AND PRESENT

The term "agoraphobia" was introduced by the German psychiatrist C. F. O. Westphal (1822–1890) in a classic monograph of 1871, *Die Agoraphobie*. He chose the term to describe the abnormal fears of a series of three men who experienced anxiety episodes when walking alone in public places. Feared situations included city squares, concert halls, churches, open streets and fields, crowded rooms, and traveling by carriage, bus, or train; typical anxiety symptoms were trembling, heart palpitations, and "an immediate breakout of intense anxiety," or feeling "strange all at once, almost like a 'hangover.'" Westphal gave prominence to the patients' fear of walking alone in streets or across squares, and therefore used agoraphobia to denote "fear of spaces"; however, he acknowledged that the term was not exhaustive because it did not embrace all features of the disorder. Contemporary commentators have noted that the Greek "agora" refers to a marketplace or place of assembly, and find Westphal's choice of term felicitous in aptly describing the chief situational fears associated with agoraphobia today.

Despite the enthusiasm of some American psychiatrists, interest in agoraphobia waned in the years following the publication of *Die Agoraphobie*. The taxonomist Emil Kraepelin later described a patient similar to those of Westphal, but referred neither to him nor to agoraphobia. The field of psychiatry rapidly became dominated by the psychoanalytic paradigm at the turn of the century, and, while agoraphobia received some attention from psychoanalysts, it was viewed as but one of many psychogenic disorders, not meriting particular notice. Sigmund Freud was more interested in all-encompassing theories of psychosexual development and neurotic symptom formation than in the classification of specific syndromes.

The development of behavior therapy in the 1950s by Joseph Wolpe and others was closely connected with the study of phobias and other anxiety disorders; interest in agoraphobia revived with American and British research on systematic desensitization and related methods in the 1960s, and with the publication of Isaac Marks' *Fears and Phobias* in 1969. Systematic desensitization produced disappointing outcomes with agoraphobia, but treatment based on graduated or full-flooded real-life exposure to relevant situations was successful in reducing avoidance behavior and anticipatory anxiety. [*See* ANXIETY PHOBIAS.]

The work of Donald Klein on "pharmacological dissection" suggested that benzodiazepines are helpful in relieving anticipatory anxiety, whereas monoamine oxidase inhibitors and tricyclic compounds attenuate panic attacks. Such findings raise the question of different, co-existing anxiety patterns in agoraphobia.

This progress in psychological and pharmacological treatment of agoraphobia in the 1970s influenced the diagnostic classification itself in the United States, so that in 1980 agoraphobia appeared for the first time as a distinct category. Further developments in the 1980s gave prominence to the panic attack as the central feature of agoraphobia and, indeed, of panic disorder, a parallel syndrome not marked by phobic avoidance of situations. Psychological treatment of both syndromes focused on therapeutic exposure to panic sensations, and on encouraging patients to make more realistic and benign ascriptions as to the source of their anxiety; exposure to somatic cues and cognitive therapy have become the leading psychological interventions.

II. DESCRIPTIVE PSYCHOPATHOLOGY AND EPIDEMIOLOGY

A. Description of Agoraphobia

People with agoraphobia usually fear, and often avoid, situations in which it would be difficult or embarrassing to obtain help if overwhelmed by anxiety. Such situations include (a) traveling away from home, especially by bus, train, or car; (b) crowded, public places, such as government buildings, supermarkets, concert halls, shopping malls, and places of worship; and (c) confined places, such as elevators, the dentist's or beautician's chair, and—when driving—passing through tunnels, over bridges, or along a limited-access highway. Agoraphobia is commonly associated with highly distressing attacks of panic that appear to arise spontaneously and unpredictably, often—but not always—in the situations typically feared and avoided. When confronted by such typical agoraphobic situations as a large auditorium or a crowded shopping mall, a person with the disorder may experience rapid heartbeat, a compelling urge to escape from the situation, apprehensions about dying or losing control, and a sense of depersonalization or unreality. A "fear of fear" pattern often develops in which the appearance of any bodily sensation associated with anxiety engenders fear of an impending panic attack, thus arousing further anxiety. Some people with agoraphobia restrict their lives substantially, sometimes to the point of remaining housebound, in order to avoid the anxiety or panic aroused by entering public places.

For many patients, dysphoric mood, somatoform disorders, interpersonal conflict, or substance abuse accompany agoraphobia. Untreated, agoraphobia tends to follow a chronic, fluctuating course. It is common for people with agoraphobia to experience daily variations in anxiety severity; most describe having "good days" and "bad days." For some patients, there may be weeks or months of near-normal functioning followed by a resurgence of the original symptoms. For others, gradual improvement leading to complete recovery may occur without professional intervention, but this is not typical. In one study, patients interviewed 8 years following successful treatment reported general maintenance of improvement with some interim exacerbations. When agoraphobic problems had reappeared temporarily, the most common context was acute objective stress such as the loss of employment or a bereavement.

B. Diagnostic Classification

The psychiatric taxonomy accepted in the United States is the *Diagnostic and Statistical Manual of Mental Disorders* (DSM), published since 1952 by the American Psychiatric Association and revised in 1968, 1980, 1987, and 1994. Before 1980, agoraphobia was not listed as a distinct disorder in the DSM classification, but could be found among lists of the Greek names for specific phobias in textbooks on psychiatry and abnormal psychology. By the time the third edition of the DSM was published in 1980 it had become clear that agoraphobia was in no sense a specific phobia— its prevalence, its resistance to treatment, its distressing and disabling consequences, and the broad range of its symptoms all clearly set it apart from such focal fears as phobias of heights, snakes, blood, or the number 13.

Agoraphobia does include fear of situations (shopping malls, crowded buses, public meetings, etc.), but patients show varied patterns of specific fears, and there is no standard list of situations that must be feared for the diagnostic criteria to be met. Given that it is quite typical in agoraphobia for the patient to fear having a definite appointment, or even the ringing of the doorbell, it is difficult indeed to specify exactly what external situation constitutes the phobic stimulus. Some commentators note that what is chiefly feared in agoraphobia is the absence of safety signals, not the presence of disturbing objects. Most recently, "fear of the panic attack" (or, in patients who do not panic, fear of limited symptom attacks or circum-

scribed anxiety episodes) has been cited as a central feature of agoraphobia. The significance of the panic attack in many cases of agoraphobia further sets it apart from the specific phobias.

In the 1980s, with such considerations in mind, the compilers of the DSM considered listing agoraphobia as a distinct diagnostic category. Renewed interest in agoraphobia in turn sparked interest in the panic phenomenon, and it was soon recognized that the overlapping of agoraphobia and panic attacks allowed several possible patterns: Agoraphobia with or without panic attacks, and panic attacks with or without agoraphobia. Accordingly, in the *DSM-III* of 1980 agoraphobia appeared in two forms, with and without panic attacks, and panic disorder was allotted a distinct category. The most recent changes were seen in the *DSM-III-R* of 1987 and the *DSM-IV* of 1994, both of which gave precedence to panic in the syndrome that includes panic attacks and agoraphobia.

C. The *DSM-IV* Classification

Agoraphobia appears twice in the *DSM-IV*, as *panic disorder with agoraphobia* and as *agoraphobia without history of panic disorder;* both are found among the anxiety disorders. The *DSM-IV* lists separate criteria sets for "Panic Attack" and for "Agoraphobia." These are not diagnostic categories in themselves.

1. Panic Disorder with Agoraphobia

The essential elements of this diagnosis are the presence of Panic Attacks and Agoraphobia, as defined in the criteria sets. Panic attacks are recurrent, distinct episodes of extreme anxiety or distress, not explained by the presence of a continuing organic factor. Panic attacks include at least 4 of a 13-item list of typical anxiety symptoms, which by definition are initially unexpected and are not produced in response to stimuli associated with specific or social phobias. The list of typical symptoms in a panic attack includes shortness of breath, dizziness, heart palpitations or rapid heart rate, trembling or shaking, sweating, the sensation of choking, depersonalization or derealization, and fear of dying, losing control, or developing an acute mental illness. By definition, the anxiety symptoms in a panic attack arise suddenly and rapidly increase in intensity. An organic factor may have been influential in early panic attacks (for example, the patient may have experienced dizziness as a result of a viral infection of the vestibular system, or depersonalization following ingestion of an illicit drug) but, by definition, the attacks will have continued despite successful treatment or removal of the initiating organic factor. [See PANIC ATTACKS.]

To meet criteria for panic disorder with agoraphobia, the patient with this diagnosis also has agoraphobia, of course, which is chiefly defined by fear of situations in which it could be difficult to obtain help if a panic attack arose, leading to avoidance or marked distress. The diagnosis applies even if the person's fear and avoidance of situations are not attributed to fear of having a panic attack.

2. Agoraphobia without History of Panic Disorder

A person with this disorder has never had problems that meet criteria for panic disorder. Instead, he or she fears, and may avoid, situations in which it would be difficult or embarrassing to leave in the event of the sudden onset of anxiety, which may represent a "limited symptom attack" that would not include the range of symptoms associated with a panic attack. Agoraphobia entails difficulties with travel: either avoidance of travel altogether, or being able to travel only with the aid of a trusted companion, or despite significant discomfort.

Finally, it should be noted that patterns meeting criteria for panic disorder but not agoraphobia are classified as *panic disorder without agoraphobia;* patterns consistent with panic disorder but in which an organic factor initiates and maintains the problems are classified as *anxiety disorder due to a general medical condition.*

D. Epidemiology

Appropriate methodology requires assessing the prevalence and correlates of agoraphobia in the general community as well as in clinic samples (which tend to be unrepresentative). Because of recent changes in the taxonomy, allowance has to be made for the different terms and criteria in studies conducted in different decades. Accordingly, the most informative studies have separated the agoraphobic syndromes from panic disorder without history of agoraphobia and have used accurate community survey techniques. In the studies cited, about half of the respondents with agoraphobia

would be classified as having panic disorder with agoraphobia, and half as having agoraphobia without history of panic disorder. However, in clinical samples of agoraphobia, panic disorder with agoraphobia predominates, justifying extensive coverage of panic in discussions of treatment.

The largest and most authoritative epidemiological investigation to include assessment of anxiety disorders was the Epidemiological Catchment Area study, reported in the 1980s. The fully structured Diagnostic Interview Schedule was used in a survey of 18,572 appropriately sampled adults in five communities in the United States (New Haven, Baltimore, St. Louis, Durham, and Los Angeles). The life-time prevalence of agoraphobia was estimated as 4.8%. A smaller study with similar methodology conducted in the former West Germany showed a life-time prevalence of 5.7% for agoraphobia; a similar Canadian study gave 2.9%. A rate of 6.9% was found for a Hispanic population in Puerto Rico with a Spanish form of the interview schedule. Generally, the estimates of the 6-month prevalence of agoraphobia in these studies were one or two percentage points lower than the life-time estimates.

Overall, the findings on the prevalence of agoraphobia are consistent across countries and cultures in studies using the same instrument and careful sampling procedures. Across studies, the life-time prevalence of agoraphobia, with or without panic attacks, is about 5%; the 6-month prevalence is about 4%. However, by 1997 most experts, including the authors of the *DSM-IV,* had concluded that these estimates were inflated. A more realistic general prevalence estimate for agoraphobia is 2.5%. Yet, whichever prevalence rate is accepted, these rates are markedly higher in women than in men; for the five sites in the Epidemiological Catchment Area study the ratio of women to men with agoraphobia was 2.7:1.

Agoraphobia is associated with more severe impairment than other phobias and has a markedly higher comorbidity rate for depression. Substance abuse, hypochondriasis, somatization disorder, and personality disorders are often associated with agoraphobia. The usual course is chronic. The age of onset in agoraphobia varies but is usually in the 20s or 30s with a mean of about 28 years. There is no general agreement on an association between agoraphobia and specific childhood experiences. Maternal overprotection has been studied, but findings are mixed. [See PERSONALITY DISORDERS; SUBSTANCE ABUSE.]

The estimated morbidity risk of anxiety disorders in the first-degree relatives of patients with agoraphobia is 32%; there is also a greater risk of an alcohol disorder. Concordance rates for panic disorder with and without agoraphobia are significantly higher in monozygotic than in dizygotic twins; a Norwegian study showed 31% concordance in 32 monozygotic twins but 0% in 53 dizygotic twins. Such results have been taken to indicate some genetic predisposition for agoraphobia and panic disorder.

III. ETIOLOGICAL THEORIES

A. Biological Theories

The observations that anxiety syndromes seem to run in families and that pharmacological treatment can be helpful have understandably led to considerable interest in biological mechanisms underlying agoraphobia and related disorders. Attention has been paid to the heritability of agoraphobia, to possible biological variables increasing vulnerability to agoraphobia, and to potential specific mechanisms that may explain agoraphobia.

There is general agreement that a predisposition toward agoraphobia (and panic) may be inherited, but it is not possible to predict who will develop agoraphobia even among people with a number of close relatives with the disorder. (It is also widely accepted that mental disorders in general defy attempts to fit a classical model of single-gene heredity.) Agoraphobia probably conforms to a diathesis-stress model in which an inherited vulnerability is necessary, but not sufficient, for the eventual appearance of the syndrome. That would require the additional operation of certain environmental factors in interaction with the predisposing conditions.

Physiological variables distinguishing agoraphobia from normal functioning, and from less pervasive anxiety disorders like specific phobia, include resting heart rate and forearm blood flow (both higher in agoraphobia) and skin conductance (higher and more variable in agoraphobia). However, such findings have not produced clear conclusions with implications for etiology or treatment.

The most promising candidates for the inherited vulnerability factor (if there is but one) in people with agoraphobia can be described as personality traits such as neuroticism, emotionality, trait anxiety, or "nervousness." Studies of animals and humans have consistently indicated a genetic component in emotionality; it is well known that rats can be bred for emotional reactivity, for example, and in the human studies, there is even stronger evidence for the heritability of trait anxiety or neuroticism than there is for the heritability of anxiety disorders.

Neuroticism is thought to result from lability of the limbic system, of the autonomous nervous system, or of specific neurotransmitter processes. For example, one animal study showed that rats bred for emotionality had more brain benzodiazepine receptors than rats bred normally. Malcolm Lader has noted that many of the data on panic may be explained by positing an instability or hypersensitivity of central noradrenergic mechanisms centering on locus coeruleus function. Despite these observations, few definite conclusions may be drawn from the many physiological and endocrinological studies. The best-supported generalization is that patients with agoraphobia and related anxiety disorders have chronically overaroused central nervous systems and are slow to habituate to noxious stimuli.

Several physiological processes and physical disorders produce symptoms like those of panic, arousing interest in possible mechanisms for agoraphobia. These include hyperventilation, asthma, limbic seizures, abnormalities of thyroid function, hypoglycemia, and mitral valve prolapse. Of particular interest has been the phenomenon of provocation of panic by sodium lactate infusions; people with a history of panic disorder, but not those without prior experience of panic, tend to react to the infusion with panic. Furthermore, pharmacological treatment by means of imipramine can abolish the lactate provocation of panic. Although such observations may appear to confirm a biological basis for panic disorder (and, therefore, of at least one of the agoraphobic syndromes), the mechanism is a subtle one that interacts with environmental and cognitive factors. The lactate provocation of panic can also be blocked by psychological treatment; hence, it would be misleading to focus exclusively on biological processes in interpreting panic phenomena.

There is as yet no clear evidence of a particular biological variant that explains all of the features of agoraphobia. There is likely to be an inherited predisposition toward a labile limbic or autonomic nervous system, associated with chronic overarousal and slow habituation. This diathesis may in turn interact with certain behavioral and cognitive mechanisms to produce agoraphobic syndromes. David Barlow has pointed out that "The fact that language and meaning structures are the most common stimuli for anxiety in humans requires a complex neurobiological system."

B. Psychodynamic and Interpersonal Theories

Psychoanalytic theory proposes that mental experience and behavior are influenced profoundly by the dynamic interaction of largely unconscious intrapsychic forces. All disorders are viewed as having important unconscious determinants, but this is particularly poignant in such disorders as agoraphobia because of the pivotal importance of anxiety to psychoanalytic theory. Early childhood experiences, particularly interactions with parents and other significant people, are given prominence not only because they form the prototypes for adult social interactions, but also because they influence the development of the mental apparatus itself. Particularly relevant to agoraphobia are the person's inner representations of other people. It is vital to one's sense of safety and security to develop stable "object relations," or internal representations of others. If object relations are disturbed, due, for example, to a poor quality or consistency of early actual relationships, then the person may be vulnerable to insecurity and anxiety later in life. Studies have shown that in humans and animals early separation from parents can be linked to agoraphobia-like behavior.

Freud's initial theory of anxiety dealt with its somatic aspects. He described "anxiety neurosis" as an *actual* neurosis ("condition of the nerves"), not a psychoneurosis, because it results from undischarged neural excitation (caused by emotional trauma, for example). To Freud, such actual neuroses involve disturbed bodily processes, particularly difficulties in breathing. He later described psychoneuroses in which undischarged tension results from unacceptable ideas rather than from external stimulation.

Eventually Freud turned his attention away from physical explanations of anxiety and emphasized its role as an ego function that is aroused in response to danger, a sense of helplessness when confronted by internal or external threat. Relevant to agoraphobia, Freud's ideas are consistent with the views that the ego responds with anxiety to (1) real danger, (2) physiological processes involving the autonomic nervous system, and (3) the arousal of emotions like anger or frustration.

An important issue for clinicians taking a psychodynamic approach is to separate manifestations of anxiety that stem from biological disturbances from those that stem from intrapsychic problems, such as an underlying conflict or a disorder of object relations. Psychodynamicists argue that, because environmental stimuli influence neurophysiological reactivity, and because the *meaning* of those stimuli mediates their impact, there is an important role for psychodynamic hypotheses and therapy in application to agoraphobia.

An integrative theory put forward by Alan Goldstein and Dianne Chambless in 1978 uses behavioral and psychodynamic concepts to explain the various phenomena of agoraphobia, including typical personality factors and interpersonal styles. It is argued that the person with agoraphobia (a) fears panic attacks rather than particular places; (b) has difficulties with self-sufficiency, independence, and assertiveness; (c) is unable to trace the antecedents of emotional feelings when they arise; and (d) develops the initial symptoms of agoraphobia in a climate of interpersonal conflict. The interaction of these factors produces agoraphobia. The typical patient in this model is a woman who feels trapped in a troubled marriage. Although she wishes to leave, she lacks the necessary autonomy, independence, and self-sufficiency to make leaving a realistic option. Dealing directly with her feelings and asserting her opinions toward her husband are unfamiliar and difficult for her, so she attempts to tolerate this unsatisfactory situation. An argument with her husband early in the day elicits dysphoric mood but not a specific, identifiable emotion. Out in public later in the day, she still feels ill at ease, but is unsure of the origin of this feeling. Waiting in line somewhere (or using an elevator, traveling through an underpass, etc.), she feels trapped, and at some level this is reminiscent of being trapped in the unsatisfactory marriage. A panic attack suddenly arises. She later begins to avoid places similar to the site of the panic attack. Eventually becoming housebound, she is no longer able to contemplate leaving her husband, and this has the advantage of settling the matter so that she is no longer troubled by her mixed feelings about leaving.

This view of agoraphobia draws attention to the potential role of adjunctive treatments like assertiveness training, marital therapy, or therapeutic work on recognizing and identifying feeling states. The work of some behavior therapists attests to the value of assertiveness training in programs for agoraphobia, and marital therapy has brought benefit to at least some patients with agoraphobia, as judged by anecdotal reports. However, marital distress has not been shown to have general etiological significance in agoraphobia.

C. Behavioral and Cognitive Theories

1. Conditioning Theories

The most familiar behavioral theory of the etiology of agoraphobia calls attention to classical conditioning as a possible mechanism. According to this view, previously innocuous stimuli such as streets, shops, and crowds acquire fear-eliciting properties through systematic pairing with noxious events. Although these noxious events are usually not specified, there are various plausible possibilities, such as witnessing an accident while in town, or being taken ill while shopping. Suddenly becoming ill, for example, creates reflex responses of distress and discomfort. By their pairing with the stimuli that elicit distress, certain stimuli in the immediate environment could become conditioned stimuli that on later occasions call forth anxiety as a conditioned response.

An immediate objection to classical conditioning as an explanation of agoraphobia is that extinction of the acquired anxiety would be expected when the person encounters the newly feared situations without the original noxious stimuli. However, Mowrer's two-factor theory posits the operation of a second process, instrumental or operant learning, to explain the persistence of conditioned fear. Once fear is acquired by means of classical conditioning, avoiding the feared situations will be reinforced because avoiding these situations means removing anxiety. At the same time, avoidance of conditioned stimuli prevents the exposure to them that would be necessary to allow extinction to occur.

So many objections have been raised to two-factor theory in this context that it can no longer be supported as a general explanation of agoraphobia. In agoraphobia, levels of fear and avoidance behavior are not closely correlated, yet two-factor theory explains avoidance behavior as motivated by conditioned fear. Conditioning does not explain the common phenomenon of daily fluctuations in anxiety severity, or the fact that general stress is often associated with an exacerbation of agoraphobia. It is not clear from two-factor theory why agoraphobia so often represents a syndrome of fears of travel, crowds, confinement, and so forth, if indeed conditioning takes place haphazardly and involves whichever stimuli happen to be prepotent at the time. Conditioning theories do not obviously explain the comorbidity of agoraphobia with depression or hypochondriasis. Even the survivors of serious accidents or natural disasters do not necessarily develop an anxiety disorder, despite having been subjected to highly anxiety-provoking experiences. By contrast, most people with agoraphobia cannot recall having had an aversive experience with the situation or object they fear. Conditioned fear is very difficult to produce in humans in laboratory experiments, and there are many contradictory findings. Several attempts to replicate landmark studies of classical fear conditioning in humans were notorious failures.

There is the paradox that, although unadorned conditioning accounts of agoraphobia have been discredited, treatments that seem based on extinction procedures have been quite successful. Exposure *in vivo*, in which the patient learns to confront agoraphobic situations without leaving at the onset of anxiety, can be helpful in overcoming a pattern of avoidance of situations *and* can attenuate panic attacks. However, the success of such treatment does not confirm a two-factor theory account of the etiology of agoraphobia.

When the panic attack itself is considered to be the noxious event that allows classical conditioning of fear to external situations, the conditioning explanation becomes more credible. That leads to the proposition that it will be most helpful to explain the origin and maintenance of panic attacks. A panic attack may be viewed as the result of a vicious circle or upward spiral in which, at each point, stimuli associated with anxiety elicit conditioned anxiety responses, which in turn produce further anxiety-eliciting stimuli. This is an interoceptive conditioning view in which it is assumed that the conditioned stimuli are the bodily sensations that result from initial anxiety arousal, and that each conditioned response has a greater amplitude than its immediate predecessor. It follows from this view of panic attacks that it will be helpful therapeutically for the patient to confront anxiety sensations themselves rather than simply the external situations in which they commonly arise. If the patient fears the bodily sensations of anxiety (heart pounding, dizziness, shortness of breath, and so forth), then the exposure principle would predict that systematic confrontation of these sensations will ultimately diminish their power to evoke anxiety.

Problems with this view of panic attacks include the following. If any arousal of anxiety leads inexorably to a vicious circle that culminates in a panic attack, then people with panic disorder would never experience limited episodes of mild or moderate anxiety. However, it is usual for panic disorder patients to display moderate levels of generalized anxiety between their panic attacks. The theory also fails to explain who will be vulnerable to the escalation of mild anxiety into panic attacks. The cognitive therapy approach to which we turn next attempts to address this problem.

2. Cognitive Theories

Aaron Beck's cognitive therapy rests upon several theoretical assumptions that center upon the individual's appraisal of events. Such appraisals range from fleeting "automatic thoughts" in the form of accessible, though covert, verbalizations (e.g., "Oh, no. I knew I'd get anxious if I came to the mall, and I feel slightly dizzy already!") to deeper and more enduring "cognitive schemas," not necessarily verbalized, reflecting a more fundamental attitude (e.g., strange feelings could indicate a serious medical catastrophe).

Central to the application of cognitive therapy assumptions to panic attacks is the patient's appraisal of the bodily sensations or somatic cues connected with mounting anxiety. David Clark has argued that people with panic disorder have developed cognitive schemas concerning vulnerability to medical catastrophes, and he and others have demonstrated that people with panic disorder show cognitive biases in that direction. (The notion of fear of medical catastrophes as one variant of agoraphobia was introduced by Joseph Wolpe in 1970.) This model complements the conditioning of somatic cues model by indicating who is vulnerable to panic and why not all anxiety episodes culminate in panic. Variations in cognitive appraisals between and within individuals may account for the unpredictability of panic attacks. In Clark's model, the sequence begins when the client experiences sensations from a flushed face or pounding heart. It is immaterial to the model whether these sensations result from pathologi-

cal (developing a fever in response to an infection) or normal (having run up the stairs) processes. Next, the patient makes a "catastrophic misinterpretation" of the bodily sensations, viewing them as signals of a medical disaster such as a heart attack. The misinterpretation itself arouses increased anxiety, and the vicious circle continues when further alarming appraisals are made.

3. A Comprehensive Model

Perhaps the most comprehensive contemporary theory is that of David Barlow, who suggests that panic results from activation of an ancient alarm system, and is the basic emotion of fear, while anxiety is a more general cognitive-affective structure. Panic occurs in response to three types of alarm. *True alarms* are panic attacks elicited by genuine danger. *False alarms* are panic attacks in the absence of objective danger, and result from a genetically determined predisposition in interaction with an accumulation of general stress. (Anyone may experience a false alarm, not only people with anxiety disorders.) *Learned alarms* are panic attacks that are triggered by cues, which may be particular objects, as in specific phobia, or internal physiological changes, as in panic disorder. Anxious apprehension also plays a part in explaining the development of anxiety disorders; a cognitive schema containing propositions concerning anxiety elicits negative affect when triggered, and the sequence of events that follows includes directing attention to internal self-evaluations, increased arousal, narrowing of attention, and hypervigilance concerning sources of apprehension.

In summary, Barlow's model of agoraphobia is his model of panic disorder with the addition of the development of agoraphobic avoidance. Biological vulnerability interacts with objective stress to produce an initial uncued panic attack, or false alarm. The connection of the panic attack with interoceptive cues leads to the development of cued learned alarms. As a result, there is a psychological vulnerability characterized by anxious apprehension about future panic attacks. Next, panic attacks are triggered unpredictably by a combination of autonomic and cognitive symptoms of anxiety with additional somatic cues. Depending on the presence or absence of safety signals and various cultural and environmental factors, avoidance behavior may develop, giving rise to the panic disorder with agoraphobia syndrome.

IV. ASSESSMENT AND DIAGNOSIS

The assessment of agoraphobia in clinical practice proceeds through several stages. First, the diagnosis is established. Second, identification of the specifics of a patient's level of distress and disability allows development of an individualized treatment plan. Third, evaluating concomitant problems or issues, ranging from diagnosable disorders to matters of life circumstances, permits employment of adjunct treatments or influences the sequence in which treatments for agoraphobia are provided. Fourth, monitoring the patient's progress throughout the course of therapy is essential in determining response to treatment and alerting the clinician to needed procedural changes.

A. Diagnosis

People with agoraphobia may be self-referred, referred by friends or relatives, or referred by other professionals. It is not uncommon for a patient to seek treatment having made a self-diagnosis of agoraphobia after reading a magazine article or viewing a television presentation about agoraphobia. It is also quite common for a patient to be referred to a mental health professional by emergency room staff after one or more visits for urgent treatment during panic attacks. Because many people with agoraphobia are either entirely housebound or have a limited range of travel, clinicians working with this disorder become accustomed to making home visits, at least in the early stages of assessment and treatment.

Because there are several physical conditions that give rise to symptoms like those of agoraphobia, it is important that the patient receive a physical examination before mental health interventions begin. If anxiety persists despite successful treatment of a precipitating or complicating physical condition, then treatment of agoraphobia proceeds. It should be noted that having certain physical conditions is not incompatible with having agoraphobia, but accompanying physical disorders demand attention first.

Assessment is needed to identify other psychiatric disorders that may co-exist with agoraphobia, including mood, somatoform, substance use, and personality disorders. Also relevant for assessment are issues like marital conflict, social skills deficits, and difficulty with personal autonomy that may not require a formal di-

agnosis but may yet be important foci for intervention. By no means do all people who experience anxiety when in public places or who have had panic attacks have problems that meet diagnostic criteria for agoraphobia syndromes. Social and specific phobias may center upon some of the situations commonly avoided in agoraphobia, and panic attacks may occur in mood disorders, psychosis, and in people without psychiatric disorders. Treatments usually employed with agoraphobia may be misdirected in these other diagnostic contexts.

B. Assessing the Range and Extent of Agoraphobia

Simply applying the appropriate diagnostic label is insufficient to guide treatment. The clinician seeks to know the patient as a unique individual and accordingly conducts the usual psychosocial history and mental status examination. Beyond that, the nature and extent of the agoraphobic problems will need to be charted in sufficient detail to allow formulation of an appropriate individual treatment plan and continued evaluation of progress toward treatment goals.

The Anxiety Disorders Interview Schedule—IV (ADIS-IV) is the most widely used structured interview protocol in the assessment of agoraphobia and other anxiety disorders. Developed by Barlow and his colleagues, the ADIS-IV allows detailed and accurate characterization of the person's anxiety problems and permits authoritative diagnosis in *DSM-IV* terms. The instrument is primarily employed in research trials to ensure uniformity of diagnostic practices. Although the complete protocol is too lengthy for routine clinical use, subsets of the ADIS-IV may be used appropriately and conveniently in most clinical settings.

Self-report questionnaires like the Fear Questionnaire, the Anxiety Sensitivity Index, and the Mobility Inventory are all useful for treatment planning and charting progress in respect of the specific agoraphobic symptoms. Questionnaires on other related issues, such as assertiveness, depression, or marital harmony, are generally helpful in initial evaluations and may be germane to the issues of particular clients throughout the course of treatment.

It is highly desirable to have the patient self-monitor general anxiety, panic attacks, and agoraphobic avoidance daily. Individualized forms may be used so that details of the specifics of the patient's situation may be accommodated therein. For example, daily ratings may be made of a patient's degree of avoidance of, fear in, and self-confidence about each item in a customized graded hierarchy of feared situations. Daily ratings of the frequency and intensity of panic attacks allow the patient to record the circumstances surrounding each episode, situational, cognitive, and interpersonal.

The nature of agoraphobia allows the use of a hierarchically ordered behavioral test for most patients. This takes the form of an unaccompanied journey—walking, driving, or using public transportation—to take in as many situations relevant to the patient's fear and avoidance as is feasible. The clinician asks the patient to proceed as far as possible, and takes the distance actually traveled as a helpful datum in sampling current levels of agoraphobic avoidance.

Physiological monitoring has been a customary component of research trials designed to provide generalizable information on treatment effectiveness, but is far less common in routine clinical practice. The typical finding that measures of anxiety in the different domains—self-report, behavioral observation, and psychophysiological—do not covary as might be predicted should not daunt the clinician unduly. When all such measures are available, it is recommended that treatment proceed until clear reductions have been seen in each measurement modality.

V. TREATMENT

A. Pharmacological Treatment

Pharmacological treatment has several advantages for the patient and significant progress has been made in this area since 1970, improving the general outlook for agoraphobia. Many people with agoraphobia have their first clinical contacts with physicians, either in emergency rooms following an initial panic attack or in family practice settings, and medication is readily available and convenient to use. (Despite this, surveys show that the general public and people with agoraphobia tend to disfavor drug therapy.)

Agoraphobia subsumes anxiety and avoidance behavior, and is often associated with dysphoric mood if not clinical depression. The medications most commonly used, and extensively studied, in the treatment of agoraphobia are those that are generally prescribed for anxiety and depressive symptoms.

I. Tricyclic Compounds

Together with the monoamine oxidase inhibitors, the tricyclic compounds are chiefly used in treating depression, but the term "antidepressants" commonly applied to them may be misleading in this context because there is controversy about their role in agoraphobia treatment (do they attenuate dysphoric mood, facilitating other treatments, or do they act specifically to block panic attacks?).

Imipramine has been the most extensively studied, but the related tricyclics desipramine and clomipramine may be similar in effectiveness. Early studies appeared to show that imipramine reduced panic attacks, but patients continued to avoid agoraphobic situations.

Later studies demonstrated imipramine's superiority to placebo medication and indicated that it brought additional benefit when added to behavioral treatment. However, this additional benefit was not attributable to the blockade of panic. When imipramine is used in conjunction with the anti-therapeutic recommendation to avoid confronting feared situations, improvement in mood, but not in agoraphobia, is the result. Empirically, imipramine plus exposure therapy seems more effective than either treatment alone. It has been argued that inconsistencies in research findings with imipramine may result from marked differences in doseage across studies.

2. Monoamine Oxidase Inhibitors (MAOIs)

The MAOIs phenelzine and iproniazid have received most attention. Whereas some studies have shown little if any difference between phenelzine and placebo in application to agoraphobia, another has shown that phenelzine reduces general disability and avoidance behavior. In that study phenelzine was more effective than imipramine. For reasons that are unclear, phenelzine appears to potentiate self-initiated exposure.

3. Benzodiazepines and Triazolobenzodiazepines

The benzodiazepines are minor tranquilizers that have been extensively prescribed for various forms of anxiety and stress reactions, clinical and subclinical, for decades. Donald Klein's initial work on imipramine had suggested that it is specific for blocking panic, whereas the benzodiazepines are effective only with generalized or anticipatory anxiety. Later work suggests that high doses of benzodiazepines may be effective in treating panic attacks. The recent development of high-potency benzodiazepines like alprazolam and clonazepam has brought substantial benefit in the treatment of agoraphobia and panic. Alprazolam, a triazolobenzodiazepine, has been the subject of a multi-center world-wide double-blind study of people with panic disorder (with and without agoraphobia). Fifty percent of the alprazolam patients and 30% of placebo patients were panic-free 3 weeks after the start of the trial.

Strong withdrawal reactions after discontinuance of alprazolam pose a significant problem, as does the phenomenon of "rebound panic" in which a minority of patients may experience even worse panic attacks after withdrawal from medication than before treatment.

4. Summary

Imipramine, phenelzine, and alprazolam are helpful in the treatment of agoraphobia. The related medications desipramine, clomipramine, tranylcypromine (an MAOI), and clonazepam have received less attention but may be as helpful. Some medications not noted above, like the beta-blocker propranolol, have been shown ineffective for agoraphobia. By the late 1990s the selective serotonin reuptake inhibitors and other new medications have been widely prescribed for people with agoraphobia, and there is a ferment of pharmacological research activity. The mechanisms underlying successful pharmacological treatment are unclear.

B. Psychological Treatment

Psychodynamic approaches to agoraphobia have received far less attention than biological, behavioral, and cognitive approaches in recent decades, and there is no corpus of empirical research on psychodynamic formulations of etiology or on the results of psychodynamic treatment. However, its proponents suggest that psychodynamic approaches are particularly germane to some of the common clinical issues in agoraphobia, and applying psychodynamic reasoning could be especially fruitful in this context. It is argued that these approaches may be particularly helpful with treatment-resistant patients, in guiding the strategy of supportive psychotherapy, and in using the therapeutic relationship in a supportive context and as a potential therapeutic tool.

Behavior therapists treating agoraphobia in the late 1950s and early 1960s emphasized its commonalities with the phobias, and sought to reduce situational fear and avoidance behavior by means of techniques effective for specific phobia. In the 1970s the differences between agoraphobia and other phobias began to be recognized, and treatment by systematic desensitization was replaced by imaginal flooding and exposure *in vivo*. Attention was paid to panic attacks as well as to avoidance behavior. Since the 1980s the focus has been on direct psychological treatment of panic attacks.

I. Treatment of Agoraphobic Avoidance Behavior

Despite initial enthusiasm for Joseph Wolpe's technique of systematic desensitization as a therapeutic breakthrough for phobias, its application to agoraphobia in controlled clinical trials in the 1960s brought disappointing results. The technique was largely abandoned as treatment for agoraphobia when developments in the 1970s established flooding in fantasy and graded practice in real life as effective treatments. Researchers in Vermont led by Stuart Agras showed that graded practice—with or without praise for specific accomplishments—could quickly reduce agoraphobics' avoidance of unaccompanied journeys away from the clinic. This work converged with that of Isaac Marks in the United Kingdom to identify exposure *in vivo* as the central ingredient of psychological treatment for agoraphobic avoidance.

Procedural variations such as brief or prolonged exposure duration, massing or spacing of treatment sessions, and terminating exposure at the point of increasing or decreasing anxiety were examined assiduously by clinical researchers, but the consensus is that these technical details are less important than the general recommendation to confront, rather than avoid, feared situations. This exposure principle is as well-founded as any in the entire field of mental health work.

Improved functioning after exposure treatment for agoraphobia has been shown to persist for several years post-treatment. Not all patients accept or remain in exposure treatment; the attrition rate during therapy has been estimated at 12%. Of those who complete a course of treatment, approximately 70% have successful outcomes.

Exposure treatment may proceed intensively and rapidly. In some studies, an entire course of treatment was completed in 2 weeks of prolonged, daily sessions. While the data on adverse complications from rapid treatment are equivocal, particularly those concerning the possibility of social and marital disruptions, gradual treatment is recommended in order to facilitate patients' thorough consolidation of therapeutic gains at each step. Treatment of avoidance through exposure preferably includes weaning patients from "safety signals," items like written instructions from the therapist, bottles of minor tranquilizers (even empty ones), or canes or umbrellas that are carried more for their associations with a sense of security than for any more obviously practical benefit.

2. Treatment of Panic

The current diagnostic classification assigns central importance to panic attacks in most cases of agoraphobia seen in clinical settings. If panic is primary, and avoidance behavior a secondary complication thereof, then treatment could logically be directed at panic phenomena. This is not incompatible with treatment of avoidance by exposure, which can itself reduce panic attacks. But, as David Barlow has put it, "treating avoidance behavior will always be necessary. Nevertheless, the primary goal should be the treatment of panic."

The essential technique in the psychological treatment of panic is *exposure to somatic cues*, or reproduction of and confrontation by the bodily symptoms that the patient associates with panic attacks. The patient is asked to create sensations of panic deliberately in treatment sessions. Running in place, voluntary hyperventilation, and spinning around in a swivel chair are examples of procedures for creating such sensations. Clinicians match particular procedures to patient's most troublesome symptoms; someone who is most troubled by dizziness will practice spinning around, while someone disturbed by the sensations of a rapid heart-rate will run up and down the stairs.

In early trials, this approach has brought the most impressive results yet seen in the treatment of panic and agoraphobia, the success rates approaching 100% in some studies. Advances in methodology that have allowed the daily monitoring of panic attacks have permitted accurate tracking of panic attack frequency. "Percentage of patients panic free" has become a standard datum to report in contemporary treatment trials.

The success of exposure to somatic cues as treatment for panic has prompted a reinterpretation of some early studies that lacked a theoretical context at the time. Inhalation of carbon dioxide as treatment for generalized anxiety, the "running treatment" for agoraphobia, the utility of imaginal flooding to phobia-irrelevant themes in reducing phobic sensitivity, and the lactate provocation of panic as treatment for anxiety episodes—all found in the literature of the last few decades—may be readily understood today as consistent with the exposure principle in its most recent application to panic sensations.

The efficacy of exposure to somatic cues has been attributed to various theoretical processes. These include the exposure principle, possibly resting upon the extinction or habituation of conditioned anxiety responses to panic sensations, or upon the development of coping skills by the patient. The success of the method is consistent with the specific hypothesis that chronic hyperventilation underlies panic disorder. It is also consistent with the cognitive therapy view that the patient makes catastrophic misinterpretations of the bodily sensations of panic, ascribing to them morbid significance as harbingers of a medical emergency.

Parallel to exposure to somatic cues is *cognitive therapy* in the contemporary treatment approach to panic. Consistent with David Clark's model of an interaction of sensitivity to somatic cues and catastrophic misinterpretation thereof, patients are engaged in a cognitive treatment process of collaborative empiricism in which implicit schemas construing panic sensations as signals of dire illness are carefully assessed, gently challenged, and empirically tested. Cognitive therapy involves exploring, in a sympathetic and accepting way, the specific idiosyncratic cognitions that are assumed to underlie emotional distress. Wherever possible, real-life "experiments" are undertaken in attempting to challenge unrealistic assumptions. There is no standard, structured format that must be applied systematically to all patients; rather, the principles of cognitive therapy guide a creative treatment approach with each individual. The results of preliminary trials of cognitive therapy have been as encouraging as those of exposure to somatic cues, and the combination of these treatments has brought the best outcomes.

3. Comprehensive Treatment of Agoraphobia

In addition to the central psychological treatment approaches of exposure *in vivo*, exposure to somatic cues, and cognitive therapy, relaxation training and breathing retraining have been found helpful in the treatment of agoraphobia and are recommended as optional components of a treatment plan. There is a consensus that in the typical case of panic disorder with agoraphobia treatment should proceed employing all of these techniques in sequence, beginning with self-paced exposure *in vivo*. Some authorities argue that, because it is not associated with deleterious side-effects or complications from withdrawal, psychological treatment should be used first, and pharmacological treatment brought in as necessary subsequently.

VI. CONCLUSIONS AND PROSPECTS

Although it is fragmented by the current nomenclature into two distinct disorders, agoraphobia is a coherent syndrome with a range of symptomatology extending far beyond the limited compass of specific phobias. Recognized since 1871 as an unusually debilitating anxiety disorder, agoraphobia has only recently yielded to effective pharmacological, behavioral, and cognitive treatments.

The conclusion of a recent Consensus Development Conference on the Treatment of Panic Disorder, sponsored by the National Institutes of Health and the National Institute of Mental Health in the United States, are pertinent and may be summarized as follows. Although perhaps most patients receiving psychological treatment are also taking medication, little is known about the effectiveness of combined pharmacological and psychological treatment. Not enough is known about the mechanisms of action of contemporary treatments, patient factors predicting success or permitting matching to the most appropriate treatment, the long-term effectiveness of the new treatments for panic, and the value of treatment for associated mental health problems and issues.

Also in need of further attention by clinicians and researchers are the following. Whereas pharmacological treatment is readily available, it is difficult for many patients to gain access to psychological treatment, especially in rural areas. Innovations in service delivery are needed, and studies should address the viability of psychological treatment of agoraphobia from remote sites by means of the latest communications technology. Many communities are underserved by mental health professionals, and people who are housebound by agoraphobia have even greater difficulties than most people in gaining access to needed psychological services.

This article has been reprinted from the *Encyclopedia of Human Behavior, Volume 1*.

BIBLIOGRAPHY

Barlow, D. H. (1988). "Anxiety and Its Disorders." Guilford Press, New York.

Beck, A. T., Emery, G., & Greenberg, R. L. (1985). *Anxiety disorders and phobias: A cognitive perspective.* New York: Basic Books.

Chambless, D. L., and Goldstein, A. J. (Eds.) (1982). "Agoraphobia: Multiple Perspectives on Theory and Treatment." Wiley, New York.

Gournay, K. (Ed.) (1989). "Agoraphobia: Current Perspectives on Theory and Treatment." Routledge, London.

Hecker, J. E., and Thorpe, G. L. (1992). "Agoraphobia and Panic: A Guide to Psychological Treatment." Allyn and Bacon, Boston.

Hecker, J. E., Losee, M. C., Fritzler, B. K., & Fink, C. M. (1996). Self-directed versus therapist-directed cognitive-behavioral treatment for panic disorder. *Journal of Anxiety Disorders, 10,* 253–265.

Knapp, T. J. (Ed.) and Schumacher, M. T. (Trans.) (1988). "Westphal's 'Die Agoraphobie'." University Press of America, Lanham, MD.

Marks, I. M. (1987). "Fears, Phobias, and Rituals: Panic, Anxiety, and Their Disorders." Oxford University Press, New York.

Mathews, A. M., Gelder, M. G., and Johnston, D. W. (1981). "Agoraphobia: Nature and Treatment." Guilford, New York.

Thorpe, G. L., and Burns, L. E. (1983). "The Agoraphobic Syndrome: Behavioural Approaches to Evaluation and Treatment." Wiley, Chichester, UK.

Walker, J. R., Norton, G. R., and Ross, C. A. (Eds.) (1991). "Panic Disorder and Agoraphobia: A Comprehensive Guide for the Practitioner." Brooks/Cole, Pacific Grove, CA.

Alcohol Problems

Melanie E. Bennett and William R. Miller

The University of New Mexico

Alcohol Dependence Severe problem drinking that involves heavy use of alcohol despite the experience of serious alcohol-related consequences. The individual might drink more than intended, make unsuccessful attempts to stop drinking, spend substantial amounts of time drinking, and neglect other responsibilities due to drinking. Physiological symptoms of tolerance (need for more alcohol to feel intoxicated) and withdrawal (physiological reactions when alcohol is stopped or reduced) often develop.

Harmful Drinking The use of alcohol that causes the drinker to experience negative consequences. Such consequences can be physical, legal, social, occupational, or interpersonal in nature.

Public Health Model A model for describing how various factors interact to increase risk for alcohol problems. This model incorporates aspects of the agent, host, and environment in describing risk.

Social Learning Theory A theory that emphasizes the role of individuals and experiences in the social world as important determinants of behavior.

Targeted Prevention Strategies Prevention strategies aimed at particular groups who are at high risk for developing alcohol problems.

Universal Prevention Strategies Prevention strategies that target a large population such as all people in a particular city.

ALCOHOL PROBLEMS represent several ways in which alcohol has a negative impact on an individual's life. Some alcohol problems are severe and involve substantial consumption of alcohol, which results in multiple physical and psychosocial problems. Other alcohol problems are less severe—an individual experiences some negative consequences as a result of his or her drinking, but these difficulties have not impacted the individual's overall functioning.

I. WHAT IS ALCOHOL HEALTH?

In order to understand the problematic use of alcohol, it is helpful first to consider what constitutes a state of health with regard to its use. Alcohol has held a common, even honored, place in the daily life of many cultures for thousands of years. It has been an element central to religious observances in Judeo-Christian and other faiths, and has often been part of important social and cultural events as well. Wine has long been recommended to promote physical health, and indeed recent scientific evidence indicates a consistent association between moderate drinking and longevity, although the reasons for this link are still poorly understood.

At the same time, it is abundantly clear that heavier drinking is often associated with devastating consequences to the individual and to society. Alcohol is involved in about half of all traffic fatalities, and a substantial proportion of fatal falls, drownings, deaths by fire, homicides, and suicides. Excessive drinking is also closely linked to violence, crime, injuries, and a plethora of chronic diseases.

The relationship of alcohol to health can thus be understood as a continuum. At one end of the continuum are abstainers, those who do not drink alcohol at all, who constitute more than one-third of adults in the United States. Such people obviously have no negative consequences related to their own drinking. Next are moderate problem-free ("normal") drinkers. The average consumption for this large group is about three or four drinks per week. They fall largely within the limits for safe drinking recommended by the National Institute on Alcohol Abuse and Alcoholism: not more than two drinks per day for men, and not more than one drink per day for women, with some alcohol-free days each week. Because alcoholic beverages differ in content, it is important here to define what constitutes "one drink." A useful definition is that one standard drink contains one-half ounce of ethyl alcohol. Table I shows how this alcohol content changes for different alcoholic beverages.

When moderation is exceeded, or when one drinks at all in dangerous situations, one enters the realm of risky drinking, which includes both acute and chronic risk. Acute risk has to do with the immediate effects of intoxication. Even low levels of alcohol in the bloodstream, for example, can significantly impair driving ability. The only safe blood alcohol level behind the wheel is zero. A small amount of impairment from intoxication can also be lethal when combined with ac-

Table II Approximate Hours from First Drink to Zero Alcohol Concentration Levels for Men

Number of drinks	Weight in pounds							
	120	140	160	180	200	220	240	260
1	2	2	2	1.5	1	1	1	1
2	4	3.5	3	3	2.5	2	2	2
3	6	5	3.5	4	3.5	3.5	3	3
4	8	7	6	5.5	5	4.5	4	3.5
5	10	8.5	7.5	6.5	6	5.5	5	4.5

One drink = 10 oz. of beer or 4 oz. of wine or 1 oz. of liquor (100 proof).

tivities such as water sports, skiing, hunting, climbing, or using power tools, where minor misjudgments can have major consequences. There is no known safe level of drinking during pregnancy. Perhaps one of the most dangerous aspects of intoxication is that above very moderate doses, perception and judgment are among the first abilities to be impaired. This can and does result in errors of perception regarding one's ability or (lack of) impairment, and in decisions and judgments that themselves lead to risky consequences. Tables II and III show how long it takes to eliminate alcohol completely from one's body, illustrating how even small amounts of alcohol can remain in and possibly impair functioning.

Chronic risk, on the other hand, has to do with the long-term effects of drinking. Heavy drinking is closely linked to a wide range of health problems, at least doubling the risk for heart disease, cancers of

Table I Standard Drink Equivalents

One drink is equal to:

Ounces of alcohol	Alcoholic beverage	Percent alcohol content
10 ounces	beer	5%
4 ounces	table wine	12%
2.5 ounces	fortified wine	20%
1.25 ounces	80 proof liquor	40%
1 ounce	100 proof liquor	50%

Table III Approximate Hours from First Drink to Zero Alcohol Concentration Levels for Women

Number of drinks	Weight in pounds							
	120	140	160	180	200	220	240	260
1	3	2.5	2	2	2	1.5	1.5	1
2	6	5	4	3	3.5	3	3	2.5
3	9	7.5	6.5	5.5	5	4.5	4	4
4	12	9.5	8.5	7.5	6.5	6	5.5	5
5	15	12	10.5	9.5	8	7.5	7	6

One drink = 10 oz. of beer or 4 oz. of wine or 1 oz. of liquor (100 proof).

many types, and hypertension. Risks for liver disease and for cancers of the mouth and gastrointestinal system are greatly increased by drinking above moderate levels.

Harmful drinking is when negative consequences from drinking actually occur. In addition to adverse effects on physical health and appearance, common types include legal problems, social consequences, damage to relationships, financial problems, and emotional disturbance. Because alcohol is a depressant drug, depression is often caused or exacerbated by heavy drinking. In college students, drinking level has a strong and negative relationship to grade point average. Memory problems are common in heavy drinkers, and the occurrence of memory blackouts is associated with brain impairment from alcohol. A majority of crimes resulting in imprisonment are committed under the influence of alcohol, which is also associated with domestic violence.

Alcohol dependence occurs as a person develops a pattern of alcohol use that results in substantial impairment in functioning. The person's life becomes more and more entangled with drinking. Typically, alcohol dependent people are quite able to "hold their liquor," showing less apparent intoxication from drinking than might be expected in the average person. Such tolerance is misleading, however, because while it appears that the person is unaffected, in fact he or she has a sufficiently high blood alcohol level to cause serious acute and chronic risk. Drinking occupies more of the person's time, and becomes increasingly important so that it is unpleasant to be away from alcohol. Gradually, the body adjusts to the presence of alcohol, so that sobering up results in unpleasant experiences such as hangovers, insomnia, agitation, or nervousness, sweating, and trembling. In the extreme, alcohol can produce a withdrawal syndrome stronger and considerably more life-threatening than that associated with heroin addiction. Other features of alcohol dependence include drinking more or for a longer time than intended, failed attempts to reduce or stop drinking, and foregoing other important activities in favor of drinking.

II. NORMAL DEVELOPMENT AND EPIDEMIOLOGY OF ALCOHOL PROBLEMS

What is the normal course of human development with regard to alcohol? The answer to this question is quite specific to culture. In some cultures, the normal course is lifelong abstention from alcohol. In France, on the other hand, heavy drinking is common among adults, resulting in one of the world's highest levels of alcohol-related health problems. In Mexico, binge drinking is common among males, whereas women are usually abstainers.

Large general population surveys reveal that a majority of Americans drink alcohol. In 1992, researchers conducting the National Health Interview Survey interviewed more than 40,000 people about their alcohol consumption. At one end of the continuum, about one-third of men and one-half of women were classified as abstainers—individuals who drink less than once per year or not at all. Most individuals were classified as either light drinkers, consuming 1 to 13 drinks per month, or moderate drinkers, consuming 4 to 13 drinks per week. Fewer individuals were classified as heavier drinkers (14 or more drinks per week), although men were more likely to report heavier drinking than women (19% versus 7%, respectively).

Although most Americans drink without negative consequences, a significant minority of individuals are found at the harmful end of the use continuum. Recent surveys estimate that 15.3 million individuals meet criteria for alcohol abuse ("harmful drinking"), dependence, or both. Drinking at these levels becomes increasingly dominated by men, who drink more often, in greater quantities, and report more frequent episodes of intoxication than women. In fact, studies find that men are more than three times more likely to be diagnosed with alcohol abuse or dependence at any age than are women. Table IV presents alcohol consumption norms for adults in the United States for both men and women. These figures illustrate women's greater likelihood of drinking moderately or not at all compared with men.

In addition to gender, drinking patterns are affected by age. After little or no drinking during childhood, alcohol use increases sharply during adolescence and peaks in young adulthood. Young adults drink in greater quantities, show the highest rates of binge drinking and problems related to alcohol use, and show the highest rates of alcohol abuse and dependence of any age group. With adulthood, drinking tends to decrease, with most young adults "maturing out" of problem drinking in their later twenties. The percentage of abstainers increases with age, although it is thought that heavier drinkers may be more likely to

Table IV Alcohol Consumption Norms for U.S. Adults, in Percentages (Percentage of Adults Who Drink This Amount or More)

Drinks per week	Total	Men	Women
0	65	71	59
1	42	54	32
2	34	46	23
3	32	43	22
4	29	39	18
5	23	33	14
6	22	32	13
7	20	30	11
8	19	29	11
9	18	27	10
10	17	25	9
11	16	25	9
12	15	23	8
13	14	23	7
14	13	21	6
15	13	20	6
16	12	19	6
17	11	18	5
18	10	16	4
19	9	15	4
20	9	14	4
21	8	12	4
22	8	12	4
23–24	7	12	3
25	7	11	2
26–27	6	11	2
28	6	10	2
29	5	9	2
30–33	5	8	2
34–35	5	7	2
36	4	7	2
37–39	4	6	2
40	4	6	1
41–46	3	5	1
47–48	3	4	1
49–50	2	3	1
51–62	2	3	1
63–64	1	3	<0.5
65–84	1	2	<0.4
85–101	1	1	<0.1
102–159	<0.5	1	<0.1
160+	<0.2	<0.5	<0.1

Source: National Alcohol Survey, Alcohol Research Group, Berkeley. Courtesy of Dr. Robin Room.

One drink = 10 oz. of beer, 4 oz. of wine, or 1 oz. of liquor (100 proof).

show stability of heavy drinking over time. This decrease in the number of people who use and abuse alcohol continues into older adulthood. Adults over age 65 have the lowest rates of alcohol abuse, dependence, and alcohol-related negative consequences of any age group. Some longitudinal research suggests that drinking patterns remain fairly stable over time, with the decreased rates of use and problems in older adulthood being attributable to increased mortality of heavy drinkers.

Along with gender and age, a growing literature documents differences in alcohol use and problems across racial/ethnic groups. Although studies of general population samples indicate that consumption and problems are greatest during the young adult years, studies have found that minority groups do not always follow this pattern. For example, Blacks have been found to show low rates of heavy drinking in young adulthood, followed by increased rates of heavy drinking and problems in their adult years. Importantly, rates of abstinence are higher among Blacks of all ages, especially among Black females. Research has also found variations by age from general population samples in patterns of drinking among Hispanics. In a way that is similar to non-Hispanic Whites, heavy drinking and associated problems increase during the young adult years among Hispanics. Hispanic men, however, show a smaller decrease in heavy drinking and problems from young adulthood to adulthood than that found among general population samples. For Hispanic men, heavy drinking and negative consequences remain high into middle adulthood, and Hispanic men show higher rates of alcohol abuse and dependence than other racial/ethnic groups over this time as well. In addition, Hispanic women show higher rates of abstention at all ages than non-Hispanic White women. Importantly, research with Hispanic samples is complicated by the practice of studying individuals of Mexican, Cuban, and Puerto Rican descent together, ignoring the substantial cultural and geographic differences among these groups as well as their different rates of drinking and attitudes toward alcohol use.

American Indians tend to show higher rates of alcohol problems than the general population, with a death rate from alcohol dependence that is more than five times higher than the rate for other races. Patterns vary widely by tribal affiliation, however, with some tribes drinking more than the general population average and others drinking less. Alcohol use among

American Indians is highest and is associated with the greatest number of negative consequences through young and middle adulthood, with a decline in consumption in the forties. [*See* ETHNICITY AND MENTAL HEALTH.]

III. ETIOLOGY OF ALCOHOL PROBLEMS

Whatever the population, it is clear that a significant minority of individuals drink in an excessive or harmful way. What causes alcohol problems? Historically, this question too often has been answered by pointing to a single cause. In the nineteenth century, drunkenness was the mark of a sinful person who lacked morals or will power. More recently, alcohol problems have been attributed to genetics, an alcoholic personality, or a "dysfunctional" family. It is clear, however, that there are many causes of alcohol problems, which develop out of interacting biological, environmental, and cognitive factors that begin early in life and continue over the course of development. At various points in development, different factors have more or less of an influence on drinking behavior.

A. Biological Factors

Much research has shown that genetics play a role in the development of alcohol problems. This research studies individuals with varying degrees of genetic relatedness to individuals with alcohol problems, and observes the rates at which these different relatives develop alcohol problems themselves. For example, family pedigree studies look at biological relatives of alcohol dependent adults; twin studies examine the rates at which identical and fraternal twins both develop alcohol problems; adoption studies follow children of alcohol dependent individuals who have been adopted by individuals without alcohol problems. The results of contemporary genetic studies strongly support a role for genetics in the development of alcohol problems, particularly among sons of alcohol dependent parents, who are three to four times more likely to develop alcohol problems than sons of nonalcohol dependent parents.

Knowing that genetics plays a part in the development of alcohol problems, researchers have now turned their attention to identifying those processes or deficits that might be genetically transmitted and contribute to alcohol problems. Alcohol problems are often conceptualized as stemming from biologically based difficulties in temperament and self-regulation, defined by Diaz and Fruhauf in 1991 as the ability to "plan, guide, and monitor one's own behavior flexibly according to changing circumstances." Self-regulation becomes more sophisticated over the course of development. As children are required to function more independently, they learn skills to help them evaluate situations and change behavior such as self-monitoring of functioning, evaluating functioning in comparison to a standard, and designing and implementing behavior change if needed. Some children make this transition readily, while others fail to become competent self-regulators. Temperamentally difficult children—those showing poor behavioral control, hyperactivity, and impulsivity—are thought to have poor self-regulation. Such children can be difficult to parent. Their heightened activity interferes in the development of self-control skills, as well as in the formation of strong relationships with others such as parents who would help them develop these skills. As individuals develop and are required to behave more autonomously, individuals who are poor self-regulators may be less able to change their behaviors to meet new challenges. As a result, they rely on external sources of regulation such as alcohol and drugs, which in turn tend to impair self-regulation still further. A large body of research has shown that temperamentally difficult children show a greater likelihood of developing alcohol problems as adults. [*See* GENETIC CONTRIBUTORS TO MENTAL HEALTH.]

B. Environmental Factors

Although genetic and biological processes contribute to the development of alcohol problems, environmental factors are also strongly involved. Difficulties in temperament and self-regulation can be thought of as risk factors that interact with personal and environmental factors to lead to the development of alcohol problems. Social learning models of alcohol use and problems emphasize the importance of social reinforcers—reactions from others in the social world that either reward or punish particular behaviors. Positive reactions serve to reinforce drinking behavior, while negative reactions punish such behavior. Also important to such a model are personal, internal events that guide an individual's perception of the external world, such as attitudes and expectations about drinking.

What environmental factors might be important to drinking behavior? There are multiple levels of environmental influence—more immediate influences include family members and peers, while farther removed factors include aspects of society, culture, and religion. Family and peers strongly influence drinking behaviors by setting examples, altering availability of alcohol, and by encouraging or discouraging alcohol use. Much evidence suggests that adolescents and young adults tend to hold attitudes toward alcohol and show drinking behaviors that are like those of their parents and peers: young individuals who drink tend to have parents and peers who drink. Through these links with drinking others, young people observe the positive features of drinking, learn how to drink, and receive positive feedback for their drinking. Similarly, peer influence appears to have a particularly strong impact on drinking in adolescence and young adulthood. Heavy-drinking youth typically are involved with similarly heavy-drinking peers. Such drinking networks may serve to teach adolescents and young adults how to drink, model appropriate (or inappropriate) drinking behavior, and reward such behavior with attention, movement into a higher social status, and an identity as a drinker. [See ADOLESCENCE.]

Along these lines, Jessor describes a problem–behavior theory in which proneness both to problem drinking and to other problem behaviors in youth results from an interaction of personality, environmental, and behavioral systems. Personality proneness to problem behavior includes a low value on academic achievement, a high value on independence, and greater tolerance for deviance coupled with lower expectations of attaining goals and lower self-esteem. Environmental stressors include low parental support and control along with high peer engagement in and approval for deviance. Together these factors have been described as a style of unconventionality. This unconventionality makes for problematic behaviors and stressful interactions with others.

Importantly, environment includes more than just an individual's home and peer experiences. Characteristics of the person and the immediate environment occur within a larger social context. Cultural ideas about alcohol use, societal attitudes toward intoxication, and laws about the purchase and consumption of alcohol all interact with an individual's biological, environmental, and cognitive makeup. For example, during

Prohibition in the United States, when attitudes were distinctly anti-alcohol and purchasing liquor was illegal, people drank less and experienced fewer alcohol problems. Patterns of alcohol use and problems vary by religious group affiliation. Jews tend to report a high prevalence of drinking but very low rates of alcohol problems, while Catholics tend to report higher rates of both drinking and heavy drinking. An especially important societal influence in modern society is the media. Both visual and print media provide a variety of models of and reinforcers for alcohol consumption. Messages about the positive effects of alcohol (it's fun and everyone is doing it) are delivered via television, movies, radio, billboards, and magazines. Drinkers are shown as attractive, socially adept, and healthy. In contrast, messages regarding the potentially harmful effects of alcohol on physical and psychological functioning are rarely shown.

C. Cognitive Factors

Recently, the alcohol field has become interested in a third set of factors that influence and are influenced by an individual's biology and environment. Cognitive factors—beliefs about alcohol and its use, one's ability to cope with stress, and ideas about what sorts of things might help a person with their problems—become increasingly important in decisions to engage in risky or harmful drinking. The young adult who has difficulty with self-regulation, is engaging in multiple problem behaviors, and experiences poor interactions with others is then faced with the more adult task of coping, a skill that has been found to be lacking in adolescents and young adults who drink heavily. In explaining differences between normal- and problem-drinking adolescents, some researchers describe a stress-coping perspective in which adolescents who drink the most are using alcohol to cope with high levels of stress and few external rewards. Studies in this area have shown that teens who drink heavily report more life stressors along with poorer coping skills than teens who drink moderately.

In making a decision about how to cope with a stressor or a problem, beliefs about the effects of alcohol appear to be another important cognitive factor. Alcohol expectancies are beliefs that alcohol use will have positive outcomes, such as increased feelings of relaxation, assertion, or general well-being. Alcohol expectancies have been found to be related to differences in drinking behavior in adolescents and adults—individuals who drink more report more positive expectations or beliefs about alcohol and its effects. Moreover, individuals who develop alcohol problems report stronger alcohol expectancies than normal drinking adults. Positive experiences have been found to exist before a child's direct experience with alcohol, suggesting a role for expectancies in developmental models of alcohol problems. Importantly, alcohol expectancies may connect coping and stress: problem drinking develops from using alcohol to cope with stress by those individuals who lack other means of coping and who perceive alcohol as being able to help resolve bad feelings. Research has shown some support for this view, finding that poor coping is linked to problem drinking in individuals with strong, positive alcohol expectancies. Thus at highest risk for problem drinking is the individual who, when faced with stress, shows low coping self-efficacy (I can't cope) and has strong positive expectancies about the effects of alcohol (Alcohol will help me cope). [*See* COPING WITH STRESS.]

Rogers' protection–motivation theory emphasizes a person's perception of risk as crucial to the decision to engage in harmful behavior such as problem drinking. According to this view, health behaviors are guided by perceptions of threat and coping. First, a person must evaluate the likelihood of threat (Will drinking cause bad things to happen to me?) and the severity of the threat (If drinking causes bad things to happen to me, how bad will these things be?). Engaging in the maladaptive response, in this case harmful or risky drinking, is influenced by the interaction of rewards (feeling good, having fun, social approval) and consequences. Second, the individual makes a coping appraisal, a judgment about what alternatives are available and one's ability to engage in alternative behavior (Are there things to do besides drinking and can I do them effectively?). Rogers stresses the importance of self-efficacy, an individual's appraisal that he/she is capable of implementing and carrying out the behavior change. Problem-drinking individuals tend to evaluate the threat of problem drinking as low, the severity of potential consequences as low, the alternatives to drinking as unpleasant, and their ability to implement change as minimal. [*See* SELF-EFFICACY.]

Thus multiple influences over the course of development interact to produce threats to alcohol health. Alcohol problems can evolve out of inherited difficulties in temperament and self-regulation that lead an individual to engage in problem behaviors and poor interactions with others. With this foundation, a developing person is ill-equipped to cope with the stressors and problems that accompany the transition to adulthood. The balance of rewards that accompanies drinking and the perception of minimal threat contribute to an individual's maintaining problem alcohol use.

Recently, researchers have become interested not only in the question of who is going to show alcohol problems at one point in time, but also in who is going to continue to have alcohol problems at many points in time. Remember that although young adults experience the highest rates of alcohol use and related problems, these rates decrease substantially in adulthood. These trends suggest that most young adults "mature out" of problem drinking upon entering adulthood. Different reasons for this "maturing out" have been suggested, most prominently that the assumption of adult roles such as work and marriage, along with a decrease in problem drinking among peers, leads young adults to moderate their use into patterns of typical social drinking. Individuals with alcohol problems, however, tend to report that they began drinking and experiencing negative consequences at a young age, so that rather than maturing out, some individuals will continue problem-drinking patterns from youth into adulthood. Some researchers have suggested that these patterns represent different problem-drinking typologies. According to this view, individuals who continue problem drinking over time are likely to be at the greatest risk for developing severe problems in adulthood; thus it is important to identify which young adults will be the ones to continue problem drinking into adulthood. Recent research suggests some qualities that may characterize individuals who will continue problem drinking from youth to adulthood, including having a higher degree of behavioral undercontrol, engaging in other problem behaviors in addition to problem drinking, and using alcohol to relieve negative feelings.

IV. THE CHANGING NATURE OF ALCOHOL PROBLEMS OVER TIME

The above discussion highlights some of the many factors that influence the development and continuation of alcohol problems over time. It is important to remember that alcohol problems vary widely: some individuals develop risky, harmful, or dependent patterns, and some cycle in and out of these various use patterns. Rather than being stable, alcohol problems change and develop over time and show a range of outcomes. Vaillant has provided the clearest illustration of this variability in his research on the natural history of alcohol problems. He has followed a large sample of men for more than 50 years, 110 of whom had experienced alcohol abuse at some point in their lives. These men drifted in and out of alcohol problems: some were abstinent for long periods of time, others relapsed to heavy or risky drinking, and others returned to dependent patterns of drinking. In his most recent follow-up of these men, now in their 70s, Vaillant stressed that alcohol abuse can have different paths for different people, sometimes progressing to more severe drinking, sometimes remitting, and most often varying in severity over time. Vaillant's data illustrate that within an individual problem-drinking path there are many twists and turns, with periods of harmful and risky drinking interspersed with periods of moderate problem-free drinking or abstinence.

V. RISK AND PROTECTIVE FACTORS

What factors put individuals at increased risk for alcohol problems? A public health model offers a useful framework for describing different types of risk factors and illustrating how they interact to influence outcomes. As with other complex disease processes, this approach highlights three kinds of risk factors—agent, host, and environment—to be considered in understanding the development of alcohol problems. The *agent* in infectious diseases is a bacterium or virus, but in this case the agent is alcohol. Alcohol has its own destructive properties, much like a particular virus can cause specific symptoms and damage. Yet in most diseases, only some individuals who are exposed to the agent actually come down with the disease. Similarly, only some individuals who are exposed to alcohol develop problems, highlighting the importance of *host* factors—individual characteristics that increase or decrease risk of alcohol problems. There are many such factors that are involved, including biological and psychological influences. One of the most important is gender. Men are more often drinkers and show a greater likelihood of drinking at a risky or harmful

level at all ages. A family history of alcohol problems also is a significant risk factor. Evidence from family, twin, and adoption studies suggests that a genetic vulnerability contributes to alcohol problems in some individuals, especially in sons of alcoholic fathers. Yet even identical twins may differ in whether or not they develop alcohol problems, indicating the role of environmental factors in addition to agent and host factors. Age also constitutes a significant risk factor for problem drinking—young adults show the greatest use and greatest number of alcohol-related problems of any age group. In his study of the natural history of alcohol problems, Vaillant found that more than half of the individuals who would meet diagnostic criteria for alcohol abuse did so by age 31.

Other host characteristics include temperament, coping skills, expectancies, and other psychopathology. As described earlier, temperamentally difficult children show a greater likelihood of developing alcohol problems as adults. Relatedly, individuals with alcohol problems tend to show poorer coping skills and to use alcohol to cope with the pressures and stresses that face them. As discussed earlier, individuals with strong, positive expectancies for alcohol (expecting alcohol will help relieve bad feelings) are more likely to drink and to develop alcohol problems. Finally, research shows that experiencing a psychological problem such as depression or anxiety greatly increases risk for developing an alcohol problem.

A third relevant domain is the environment. As discussed earlier, environment can be defined in a number of ways. Immediate environmental risk factors for alcohol problems include heavy or other problem-drinking family members who not only contribute possible genetic influences but also serve as role models for alcohol use and create a stressful home environment that may contribute to alcohol use. For adolescents and young adults, peer influences are among the most important—being part of an alcohol-using peer group increases risk for alcohol problems in these populations. Aspects of the larger environment are also relevant. Heavy-drinking communities show greater rates of alcohol-related problems. Cultures that sanction liberal use of alcohol likewise show higher rates of risky and harmful drinking. Stress may also be an important environmental risk factor: research suggests that severe and prolonged stress appears to be an important factor in problem drinkers returning to drinking after a period of abstinence.

While there are characteristics that put people at increased risk for alcohol problems, there are also factors that protect individuals in the face of these risks. Protective factors are not merely the opposite or lack of risk factors. Rather, they are influences that moderate the links between risk factors and alcohol outcomes such that an individual may be exposed to risk but show resiliency and avoid problem alcohol use. Several protective factors have been identified in adolescents and young adults, including close and positive relationships with parents, adolescent conventionality, parental adjustment, and success in school. Religious affiliation and involvement appears to be a strong protective factor. Individuals who report strong religious beliefs or high levels of religious commitment consistently show lower levels of alcohol use and fewer alcohol-related problems. In contrast, individuals with alcohol problems are less likely to report firm religious beliefs or involvement. In addition, social support has been found to play an important protective role: individuals engaged in supportive relationships with others appear less likely to develop alcohol problems, and social resources are thought to offset other potentially harmful stressors and risks. It also makes a difference whether one's social group supports abstinence, moderation, or risky and heavy drinking. [See PROTECTIVE FACTORS IN DEVELOPMENT OF PSYCHOPATHOLOGY; SOCIAL SUPPORT.]

VI. CONTINUUM OF INTERVENTION FOR ALCOHOL PROBLEMS

From the previous discussion, it is clear that alcohol problems encompass a range of risk factors and difficulties that vary along a continuum of severity. All individuals are exposed to some risk factors; many individuals experience multiple risk factors that make them increasingly vulnerable. Some individuals are just beginning to develop problems with alcohol; others already have well-developed dependence. Such diversity necessitates a variety of intervention strategies. Any single type of prevention program is not likely to reach all who are at-risk, and one brand of treatment will not be effective for all problem drinkers.

At one end of the continuum are universal prevention strategies, designed to target a large population with the goal of reducing the incidence of alcohol problems; for example, by increasing awareness of

risks and promoting alternatives to alcohol use. A target population might be all individuals in a particular city, school district, or university campus. An example of a universal prevention strategy is instituting an excise tax on alcoholic beverages that makes alcohol more expensive, with the result that people purchase less. Print and electronic media campaigns are also designed to reach large groups of people with their alcohol-related messages. Universal prevention strategies target everyone in a population, regardless of their level of risk for developing problems.

Other interventions focus on individuals who are at high risk for developing problems. Termed *targeted* prevention strategies, such interventions are aimed at particular groups who have not yet developed a problem but are at increased risk due to their exposure to particular or multiple risk factors. Examples of such high-risk groups are children of parents with alcohol problems, adolescent boys with behavior problems, and college students with poor grades. The goal of targeted prevention is to stop a problem before it starts, or at least early in its development, by intervening with those at highest risk. For example, programs in college dormitories, fraternities, and sororities are aimed at providing information to individuals at high risk for drinking and related problems.

Prevention is aimed at individuals who have not yet developed problems. Once an individual is identified as having an alcohol problem, the focus of intervention shifts toward treatment. Individuals identified as already having an alcohol problem may be referred for some sort of intervention or treatment. However, only a small percentage of individuals with alcohol problems ever receive formal treatment. A critical bridge between developing problems and receiving treatment is the person's motivation for change. Strengthening the commitment to change constitutes an important first step, and may need to be addressed before treatment takes place. Effective methods are available for enhancing motivation for change. Among the important elements of such interventions are providing personal feedback about drinking, empathic listening, acknowledging a range of alternatives for working toward behavior change, and emphasizing personal responsibility and ability to make change happen. Such motivational interventions are designed to help an individual become more aware of the impact of his/her drinking and to instill a commitment to change.

This discussion has emphasized the diversity of alcohol problems along a continuum of severity. The implication of this diversity is that what is helpful or appropriate for a drinker just beginning to develop an alcohol problem will differ from the most effective treatments for more severe, dependent drinkers. Individuals who are just beginning to show signs of problem alcohol use might fit the description of "risky' or "harmful" drinkers who are drinking heavily or in potentially dangerous situations. Intervention with these individuals is aimed at recognizing a problem early and preventing it from reaching diagnostic levels. For example, businesses have employee assistance programs where personnel are trained to recognize the early signs of alcohol problems in their employees. Other early identification strategies include urine drug-screening programs, justice system referrals, screening during routine health care, and programs for impaired drivers. Individuals at the beginning stages of problem development are often helped by brief interventions—motivational strategies that help individuals see their increasing involvement with alcohol and the negative consequences they may experience as a result. These interventions are usually one or two sessions of alcohol-related counseling and advice to reduce drinking. Some brief interventions involve providing clients with reading and other educational materials that review drinking patterns and ways to reduce drinking. Studies have consistently found that such brief interventions help problem drinkers reduce their alcohol use.

What about individuals who are far enough along the continuum to have developed more severe alcohol problems? There now exist a range of promising and effective approaches for use with different types of drinkers. As individuals with alcohol problems frequently have difficulties in many areas of functioning, several interventions are often combined. For drinkers with more severe problems, detoxification may be necessary to overcome the acute effects of alcohol withdrawal. With proper supervision, an addicted drinker is through the worst withdrawal within a week, and modern medical care can prevent the more uncomfortable and dangerous symptoms of alcohol withdrawal. Detoxification, however, is not treatment. Simply detoxifying a dependent drinker is unlikely to have any long-term effect on drinking.

Various medications have been tested in treating alcohol problems. One of the most popular of these is disulfiram (Antabuse)—a medication that produces a negative physical reaction (nausea, vomiting) when alcohol is ingested. Naltrexone (ReVia) also appears to

be a promising agent in reducing relapse and craving. Medications, however, are only an aid in treatment, and are unlikely to be effective when given without other treatment.

Some view alcohol problems as a lack of coping skills. Skills-training approaches view alcohol use as a maladaptive coping strategy, and teach appropriate coping skills as an alternative to drinking. Social skills training is used to help individuals with alcohol problems to interact effectively with other people, to cope with positive and negative feelings, and to handle stressful situations in the environment. The community reinforcement approach similarly emphasizes the need for the drinker to be prepared to cope with stress, and to establish a rewarding, alcohol-free life-style. Efforts are made to get individuals connected to community resources, social supports, employment, and other activities that would contribute to a rewarding life-style without alcohol. From this perspective, the focus is not only on stopping alcohol use but also on helping people to acquire skills and make changes that will support an alcohol-free life-style.

Alcohol problems often affect family functioning. Behavioral marital therapy (BMT) regards the marital relationship as crucial in the maintenance and change of an individual's drinking behavior. BMT is designed to improve communication skills, teaching spouses how to reinforce changes in drinking behavior, and ways to cope with drinking-related situations and feelings. There are also effective approaches to help concerned family members and friends of individuals with alcohol problems, even if the drinker is unwilling to accept help. These concerned others often wish to help their loved one but lack the knowledge and skills to do so. Concerned family members can be helped to engage the problem drinker in treatment. Such treatments also attend to the needs of the family members themselves—to distance themselves from the drinker and to learn skills for coping with stress and other negative feelings.

Recovery from alcohol problems typically involves relapse. Effective treatment often includes attention to the people, places, and things that are likely to trigger alcohol use in the future. Marlatt's relapse-prevention (RP) incorporates cognitive-behavioral strategies aimed at anticipating slips and considering how to handle high-risk situations. Specifically, RP stresses anticipating and working to prevent relapses and realistically considering how to recover and learn from relapses if they occur. To this end, clients identify specific high-risk situations and outline a plan for making it through without drinking.

For individuals with less severe drinking problems, strategies to teach skills for moderate drinking are sometimes used. Moderation training programs are designed for risky or heavy drinkers who might not participate in treatment aimed at total abstinence, but who could benefit from reducing their alcohol use. For example, behavioral self-control training (BSCT) teaches clients skills for moderating their drinking. BSCT makes use of behavioral principles of self-control and teaches ways to self-monitor drinking, to set goals for decreasing consumption, and to implement alternative coping skills. BSCT and programs like it may be used with either abstinence or moderation goals.

The above interventions all involve the individual with alcohol problems seeking assistance from a trained professional. Although outcome studies strongly support the efficacy of these treatment strategies, the fact remains that most individuals with alcohol problems never receive professional help and yet "recover" without formal intervention. Many of these drinkers will seek help not from professionals but from others with similar problems. Particularly in North America, mutual-help groups serve as a major source of help and support for many individuals with alcohol problems. The largest and best-known of these groups is Alcoholics Anonymous (AA), serving over two million members in 150 countries around the world. AA emphasizes commitment to abstinence and renewed spirituality recognizing the strength of a "higher power" as necessary to the change process. Other self-help groups, such as Women for Sobriety, SMART Recovery, Rational Recovery, and Moderation Management, emphasize personal control and responsibility in overcoming alcohol problems.

VII. CONCLUSION

Alcohol problems encompass a range of difficulties. Some individuals with alcohol problems experience minor difficulties in a one area of functioning. Other individuals experience substantial impairment in mul-

tiple life areas due to their alcohol use. In this article, we have reviewed factors that put people at risk for alcohol problems, as well as theories that seek to explain how alcohol problems develop. There now exists a range of interventions for individuals at all levels of the alcohol problems spectrum. Future research will add to our knowledge of alcohol problems and yield important new information about how such problems develop and how they can be most effectively treated.

ACKNOWLEDGMENT

Preparation of this article was supported in part by National Institute on Alcohol Abuse and Alcoholism Grant K05-AA00133.

BIBLIOGRAPHY

Blane, H. T., & Leonard, K. E. (Eds.). (1987). *Psychological theories of drinking and alcoholism.* New York: Guilford Press.

Diaz, R. M., & Fruhauf, A. G. (1991). The origins and development of self-regulation: A developmental model on the risk for addictive behaviors. In N. Heather, W. R. Miller, & J. Greely (Eds.), *Self-control and the addictive behaviors.* Sydney: Maxwell Macmillan Publishing.

Hester, R. K., & Miller, W. R. (Eds.). (1995). *Handbook of alcoholism treatment approaches: Effective alternatives* (2nd ed.). Boston, MA: Allyn & Bacon.

Jessor, R. (1987). Problem-behavior theory, psychosocial development, and adolescent problem drinking. *British Journal of Addiction, 82,* 331–342.

Marlatt, G. A., & Gordon, J. R. (1985). *Relapse prevention.* New York: Guilford Press.

Miller, W. R., & Rollnick, S. (1991). *Motivational interviewing: Preparing people to change addictive behavior.* New York: Guilford Press.

Monti, P. M., Abrams, D. B., Kadden, R. M., & Cooney, N. L. (1989). *Treating alcohol dependence: A coping skills training guide.* New York: Guilford Press.

National Institute on Alcohol Abuse and Alcoholism. (1993). *Eighth special report to the U.S. Congress on alcohol and health.* Rockville, MD: U.S. Department of Health and Human Services.

Rogers, R. W. (1983). Cognitive and physiological processes in fear appeals and attitude change: A revised theory of protection motivation. In J. T. Cacioppo & R. E. Petty (Eds.), *Social Psychophysiology* (pp. 153–176). New York: Guilford Press.

Vaillant, G. E. (1983). *The natural history of alcoholism: Paths to recovery.* Cambridge, MA: Harvard University Press.

Alzheimer's Disease

Mark W. Bondi

California State University San Marcos,
San Diego Veterans Affairs Medical Center, and
...iversity of California, San Diego

Kelly L. Lange

San Diego State University, and
University of California, San Diego

Neurotransmitters Chemical substances in the brain that relay messages between neurons.

Semantic Memory A general fund of knowledge, consisting of overlearned facts and concepts, which are not dependent upon contextual cues for retrieval.

ALZHEIMER'S DISEASE (AD) appears to be the most common cause of dementia, accounting for more than 50% of all dementia cases. AD is a progressive degenerative brain disorder that is characterized by neocortical atrophy, neuron and synapse loss, and the presence of senile plaques and neurofibrillary tangles. The plaques and tangles were first identified and reported in 1907 by the German physician and neuropathologist Alois Alzheimer. In his initial case he autopsied a 51-year-old patient who had recently died (from what we now term dementia) and discovered the presence of several histopathologic alterations, two of which were the neuritic plaques and the neurofibrillary tangles. Today they remain the two classic hallmarks of the disease and constitute the basis for the neuropathologic diagnosis of Alzheimer's disease. The dementia of AD is characterized by severe amnesia with additional deficits in language, "executive" functions, attention, and visuospatial and constructional abilities. Patients may also experience changes in affect or personality and impairment of judgment. This article will provide an overview of the clinical, pathological, neuropsychological, and affective features associated with AD.

I. CLINICAL FEATURES

A. Definition of Dementia

Dementia refers to a syndrome of acquired intellectual impairment of sufficient severity to interfere with social or occupational functioning, caused by brain dysfunction. According to the American Psychiatric Association's *Diagnostic and Statistical Manual of Mental Disorders,* Fourth Edition, "Dementia of the Alzheimer's Type" involves memory impairment and cognitive deficits in at least one other domain, demonstrated by aphasia, apraxia, agnosia, or impaired executive functioning. These symptoms must not be due to other neurological disorders, medical conditions resulting in dementia, or substance abuse. The cognitive impairments must have a gradual onset and a progressive decline and be severe enough to significantly interfere with social or occupational functioning. Furthermore, the cognitive impairment must represent a significant decline from a previously higher level of functioning, and it must not occur exclusively during the course of delirium (see Table I). [*See* DEMENTIA.]

Prior to the *DSM,* however, in 1984, the Work Group on the Diagnosis of Alzheimer's Disease, established by the National Institute of Neurological and Communicative Disorders and Stroke and the Alzheimer's Disease and Related Disorders Association (NINCDS-ADRDA), developed criteria for the clinical diagnosis of *probable* and *possible* AD (see Table II). Since then the NINCDS-ADRDA clinical criteria have been tested against autopsy verified diagnoses and found to be quite effective.

B. Diagnosis and Course of Alzheimer's Disease

Because dementia is associated with more than 50 different causes of brain dysfunction (see Table III), and there are no known peripheral markets for Alzheimer's disease, a definitive diagnosis continues to require histopathological verification of the presence of characteristic neurodegenerative abnormalities at autopsy (i.e., neuritic plaques and neurofibrillary tangles). However, documentation of the presence of dementia and the exclusion of all other known poten-

Table I   DSM-IV Diagnostic Criteria for Dementia of the Alzheimer's Type

A. The development of multiple cognitive deficits manifested by both
  1. memory impairment (impaired ability to learn new information or to recall previously learned information);
  2. one (or more) of the following cognitive disturbances:
      a. aphasia (language disturbance);
      b. apraxia (impaired ability to carry out motor activities despite intact motor function);
      c. agnosia (failure to recognize or identify objects despite intact sensory function);
      d. disturbance in executive functioning (i.e., planning, organizing, sequencing, abstracting).
B. The cognitive deficits in Criteria A1 and A2 each cause significant impairment in social or occupational functioning and represent a significant decline from a previous level of functioning.
C. The course is characterized by gradual onset and continuing cognitive decline.
D. The cognitive deficits in Criteria A1 and A2 are not due to any of the following:
  1. other central nervous system conditions that cause progressive deficits in memory and cognition (e.g., cerebrovascular disease, Parkinson's disease, Huntington's disease, subdural hematoma, normal-pressure hydrocephalus, brain tumor);
  2. systemic conditions that are known to cause dementia (e.g., hypothyroidism, vitamin B_{12} or folic acid deficiency, niacin deficiency, hypercalcemia, neurosyphilis, HIV infection);
  3. substance-induced conditions.
E. The deficits do not occur exclusively during the course of a delirium.
F. The disturbance is not better accounted for by another Axis I disorder (e.g., Major Depressive Disorder, Schizophrenia)

Note. DSM-IV refers to the *Diagnostic and Statistical Manual for Mental Disorders,* 4th edition. From American Psychiatric Association, 1994.

tial causes allows probable or possible Alzheimer's disease to be clinically diagnosed during life with some certainty (i.e., current estimates are approximately 90% or better).

Patients with Alzheimer's disease often live for many years following their diagnosis, dying eventually from conditions like pneumonia, sepsis, or other fatal conditions to which people of advanced age are prone. The duration of the disease from the time of diagnosis to death can be as little as 2 years or as long as 20 years or more, although the average length ranges between 7 and 10 years.

Table II NINCDS-ADRDA Criteria for Definite, Probable and Possible Alzheimer's Disease

I. Definite Alzheimer's disease:
 Clinical criteria for Probable AD;
 Histopathologic evidence of AD (autopsy or biopsy).
II. Probable Alzheimer's disease:
 Dementia established by clinical exam and documented
  by mental status testing;
 Dementia confirmed by neuropsychological testing;
 Deficits in two or more areas of cognition;
 Progressive worsening of memory and other cognitive
  functions;
 No disturbance of consciousness;
 Absence of systemic or other brain diseases capable of
  producing a dementia.
III. Possible Alzheimer's disease:
 Atypical onset, presentation, or progression of a dementia
  syndrome with a known etiology;
 A systemic or other brain disease capable of producing
  dementia is present but not thought to be the cause of the
  dementia;
 A gradually progressive decline in a single intellectual func-
  tion in the absence of any other identifiable cause.
IV. Unlikely Alzheimer's disease:
 Sudden onset of symptoms;
 Focal neurological signs and symptoms;
 Seizures or gait disturbance early in the course of the illness.

From McKhann et al. (1984). Clinical diagnosis of Alzheimer's disease: Report of the NINCDS-ADRDA Work Group, Department of Health and Human Services Task Force on Alzheimer's Disease. *Neurology, 34,* 939–944.

C. Epidemiology

1. Prevalence and Incidence of Alzheimer's Disease

Estimates of the prevalence of dementia vary widely due to differences in definitions, sampling techniques, and the sensitivity of instruments used to identify cases. However, Cummings and Benson calculated the average of prevalence estimates across studies and suggested that approximately 6% of persons over the age of 65 have severe dementia, and an additional 10% to 15% have mild to moderate dementia. Also, the prevalence of the syndrome of dementia doubles approximately every 5 years after age 65. Not surprisingly, the prevalence of dementia is higher among hospital and nursing home residents than among those living within the community.

Table III Causes of Dementia

I. Cerebral neuronal degenerative disorders:
 Alzheimer's disease;
 Pick's disease;
 Parkinson's disease;
 Huntington's disease;
 Progressive supranuclear palsy;
 Dementia lacking distinctive histopathology.
II. Acquired cerebral disorders (some of which may be reversible):
 Vascular dementia: Multi-infarct dementia; Binswanger's
  disease;
 Multiple sclerosis;
 Intracranial neoplasms;
 Trauma (e.g., subdural hematoma; dementia pugilistica;
  diffuse axonal injury);
 Hydrocephalus;
 Transmissible spongiform encephalopathies (e.g.,
  Creutzfeldt-Jakob disease).
III. Other potentially reversible dementias:
 Metabolic disorders; Chronic drug intoxication; Alcoholism;
  Malnutrition (e.g., vitamin B_{12} deficiency);
 Infections: HIV (AIDS); Neurosyphilis; Tuberculous or bac-
  terial meningitis; Cryptococcosis; Acute viral encephalitis;
 Dementia syndrome of depression.

Note: A complete listing would include many more disorders; those listed above serve to illustrate that dementia results from many different etiologies

Adapted from Berg & Morris, in Terry, Katzman, & Bick (1994).

2. Risk Factors for Alzheimer's Disease

A number of reliable risk factors for Alzheimer's disease have been identified. First, age is the single most important risk factor for dementia. Population-based studies in many different countries have confirmed that the prevalence of the most common causes of dementia (i.e., Alzheimer's disease and vascular dementia) rises in an approximately exponential fashion between the ages of 65 and 85. Second, it has been suggested that women have a slightly greater risk for Alzheimer's disease than men, due in part to its higher prevalence in women. The greater risk for women, however, may be a factor of their longer life expectancy, since incidence rates for Alzheimer's disease have not shown differences between men and women. [*See* AGING AND MENTAL HEALTH; GENDER DIFFERENCES IN MENTAL HEALTH.]

Third, uneducated individuals over the age of 75 have about twice the risk for dementia as those who

Table IV Genetics of Alzheimer's Disease

Chromosome	Protein	Percentage of AD	Age of Onset
21	Amyloid Precursor Protein	<1	45–60
19	Apolipoprotein E	30–50	60+
14	Presenilin 1	1–2	32–56
1	Presenilin 2	<1	40–85

have completed at least a grade school education. Low lifetime occupational attainment, associated with little education, may also yield a greater risk for Alzheimer's disease. Education and occupational achievement may act as a surrogate for brain or cognitive reserve that helps to delay the onset of the usual clinical manifestations of the disease.

Fourth, the risk of developing dementia is increased approximately fourfold by a family history of Alzheimer's disease in a first-degree relative (i.e., mother, father, brother, or sister). Given some of the findings of specific point mutations on the amyloid precursor protein gene of chromosome 21 and linkage studies identifying gene loci on chromosomes 1, 14 and 19, there is now little question that this familial association is genetically based (see Table IV). Furthermore, the epsilon-4 allele of the apolipoprotein E gene (ApoE-ε4) located on chromosome 19 has recently been identified as another risk factor for dementia because of its over-representation in patients with Alzheimer's disease. [*See* GENETIC CONTRIBUTORS TO MENTAL HEALTH.]

Finally, the risk of developing Alzheimer's disease is doubled for individuals with a history of a single head injury that led to a loss of consciousness or hospitalization. This finding, however, may be confined to those Alzheimer's patients with previous head injuries who also carry at least one ApoE-ε4 allele. Recent research has demonstrated that individuals with a history of head injury who lack the presence of the ApoE-ε4 allele are not at increased risk for Alzheimer's disease.

If one assumes that these aforementioned risk factors are simply additive at the population level, then the attributable risk of developing Alzheimer's disease from these known factors appears to be between 40% and 50% (and probably more given the recent addition of ApoE-associated risk).

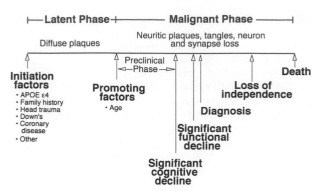

Figure 1 Chronic disease model of Alzheimer's disease. Adapted from Katzman and Kawas (1994), in Terry, Katzman, & Bick (Eds.), *Alzheimer disease,* with permission of Raven Press.

Thus, current views suggest that Alzheimer's disease is a chronic disease, much like cancer or heart disease, in which an individual is predisposed by genetic factors, traumatic events, or other unknown factors toward entering a malignant phase. Intracellular events will eventually lead to neuritic degeneration, the formation of neurofibrillary tangles, and neuron and synapse loss. Over a period of time, the neural degeneration gradually reaches a level that initiates the clinical symptoms of the dementia syndrome. This framework for understanding the development of AD suggests that cognitive deficits associated with the disease also appear gradually (see Fig. 1).

D. Neuroimaging in Alzheimer's Disease

A variety of neuroimaging techniques have been used to study and characterize Alzheimer's disease. Some of the most recent techniques include structural and volumetric analysis of the brain with magnetic resonance imaging (MRI), computation of regional cerebral metabolism with positron emission tomography (PET), regional cerebral blood flow with single photon emission computed tomography (SPECT), and determination of regional biochemical concentrations with magnetic resonance spectroscopy (MRS).

MRI studies of Alzheimer's disease patients reveal a decrease in brain volume, apparently due to gyral atrophy and ventricular dilatation. However, gyral atrophy and enlarged ventricles are also found in normally aging brains, lending minimal diagnostic value to structural images early in the course of the disease. Future research targeting hippocampal or entorhinal cortex, however, may yield more sensitivity to early stage Alzheimer's disease.

Functional imaging studies with PET and SPECT have found significant differences between Alzheimer's disease patients and healthy older adult control subjects. Temporoparietal and frontal cortical regions have shown significant glucose metabolic reductions, with relative sparing of visual and sensorimotor cortex. Furthermore, significant relationships have been found between neuropsychological impairment in AD and the degree of hypometabolism found by PET. In addition, Haxby (in Rapoport, Petit, Lays, and Christen) measured cerebral metabolism with PET in Alzheimer's patients and found differing patterns of decreased metabolism in the association cortex. The individual patterns of decreased metabolism correlated with neuropsychological test scores purported to reflect processing in particular brain regions. The decreased neocortical metabolism was found even in patients in the earliest stages of dementia of the Alzheimer type, in whom neuropsychological testing revealed no deficits other than amnesia. This finding suggests that PET imaging can be useful in the early detection of AD.

As a marker of cerebral blood flow in Alzheimer's disease, SPECT also demonstrates similar regional reductions to that of PET, although its spatial resolution is not as high. However, its significantly lower cost allows for its more widespread use. In addition, SPECT studies have attempted to trace neurotransmitter receptor changes in Alzheimer's disease patients (e.g., muscarinic receptors; dopaminergic D2 receptors), although results have been mixed to date.

Findings in MRS studies suggest that this technique may also be sensitive to the early detection of Alzheimer's disease. For example, an increase in the biochemical concentration of myo-inositol has been found in patients with mild to moderate Alzheimer's disease. Myo-inositol serves several functions in the brain, one of which may involve the deposition of neuritic plaques characteristic of Alzheimer's disease. Increases in myo-inositol concentration have not been found in patients with other dementing illnesses or in normally aging individuals.

Thus, preliminary findings from a number of recent studies suggest that MRI, PET, SPECT, and perhaps MRS can provide complementary information to the usual diagnostic procedures and may contribute to the early and more specific detection of the disease.

It should be emphasized, however, that although the usefulness of structural or functioning neuroimaging procedures appear promising, each of these costly techniques remains experimental and has not been shown to be as accurate as the clinician's judgment in the differential diagnosis of Alzheimer's disease. Future longitudinal studies are needed to determine the prospective accuracy of early diagnosis through structural and functional neuroimaging techniques, particularly studies that will be able to provide neuropathologic confirmation. [See BRAIN SCANNING/ NEUROIMAGING.]

II. NEUROPATHOLOGICAL FEATURES

Alzheimer's disease is primarily characterized by two particular histological findings in the brain: neuritic plaques and neurofibrillary tangles (see Fig. 1). Other associated features include neurotransmitter reductions, particularly acetylcholine and norepinephrine, as well as neuron and synapse loss.

A. Neuritic Plaques

Neuritic plaques are complex deposits of amyloid protein and glial cells. These extracellular deposits collect most heavily in portions of the entorhinal cortex and hippocampal formation, two brain areas critical for memory and learning of new information. Neuritic plaques are also found throughout the cortical mantle of the neocortex, with a predilection for association regions (see Fig. 2).

B. Neurofibrillary Tangles

Neurofibrillary tangles are networks of insoluble proteins which collect inside neurons and result in a breakdown in the structure of the neuron's cytoskeleton (see Fig. 3). The protein networks become so complex over time that normal cell metabolism and nutrient flow become impossible and the cell eventually dies. As with plaques, tangles accumulate most densely in the entorhinal and limbic regions of the brain, although tangles are also found in many structures that project to the cerebral cortex such as the nucleus basalis of Meynert, locus ceruleus, midline thalamic nuclei, as well as in some hypothalamic nu-

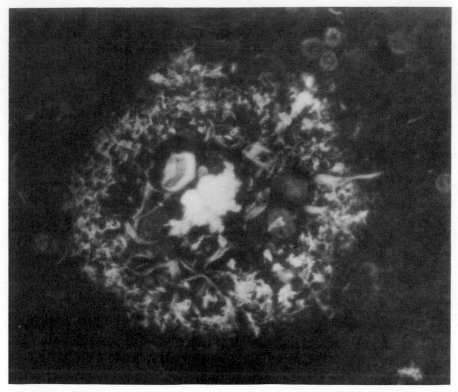

Figure 2 Microscopic stain of a neuritic plaque. Plaques consist of dystrophic neurites and glial elements with or without a dense central core of insoluble amyloid protein.

clei and the ventral tegmental area, and dorsal raphé nucleus.

C. Distribution of Neuropathological Changes

In addition to plaques and tangles, pathological changes in Alzheimer's disease include neocortical atrophy (see Fig. 4), neuron loss, and synapse loss (see Fig. 5). These changes occur primarily in the hippocampus, entorhinal cortex, and in the association cortices of the frontal, temporal, and parietal lobes. Although the temporal progression of the neuropathological changes of Alzheimer's disease are not fully known, recent studies suggest that the hippocampus and entorhinal cortex are involved in the earliest stage of the disease, and that frontal, temporal, and parietal association cortices become increasingly involved as the disease progresses.

D. Major Neurochemical Alterations

In addition to these cortical changes, subcortical neuron losses occur in the nucleus basalis of Meynert and in the locus ceruleus, resulting in a decrement in neocortical levels of cholinergic and noradrenergic markers, respectively.

E. Lewy Body Variant of Alzheimer's Disease

Another neuropathologic condition in demented patients is characterized by the typical cortical distribution of senile plaques and neurofibrillary tangles of Alzheimer's disease, the typical subcortical changes in the substantia nigra, locus ceruleus, and dorsal vagal nucleus of Parkinson's disease, and, in addition, Lewy bodies that are diffusely distributed throughout the

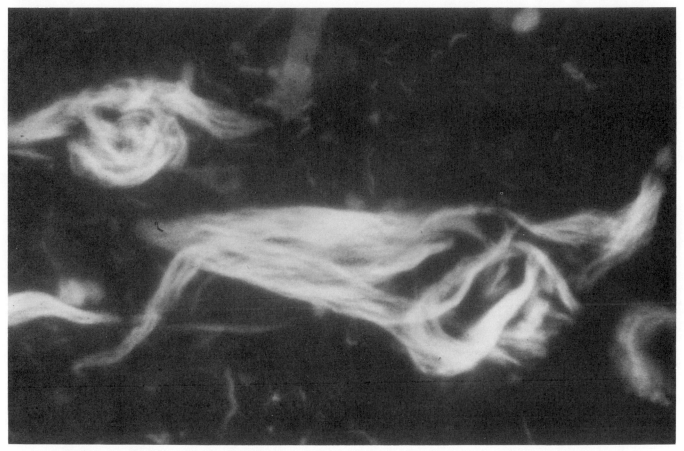

Figure 3 Microscopic stain of a neurofibrillary tangle. Tangles result from the accumulation of abnormal components of the neuronal cytoskeleton and create disruptions in the structure and function of the neuron.

neocortex. Although only recently identified, this neuropathologic condition is not rare and may occur in approximately 25% of all demented patients.

The clinical manifestation of this disorder, which is sometimes known as the Lewy body variant of Alzheimer's disease, is similar to that of Alzheimer's disease in many respects, and these patients are often diagnosed with probable or possible Alzheimer's disease during life. However, retrospective studies indicate that Lewy body variant of Alzheimer's disease may be clinically distinguishable from "pure" Alzheimer's disease. While both disorders are associated with a severe and progressive dementia, there may be an increased prevalence of mild extrapyramidal motor findings (e.g., bradykinesia, rigidity, masked facies)

and hallucinations in patients with Lewy body variant of Alzheimer's disease, as well as a more rapid course.

III. NEUROPSYCHOLOGICAL DEFICITS

A. Memory

Failure of recent memory is usually the most prominent feature during the early stages of Alzheimer's disease. Accordingly, much of the neuropsychological research concerning the early detection of Alzheimer's disease has focused on memory. Numerous studies have shown that measures of the ability to learn new information and retain it over time are quite sensitive

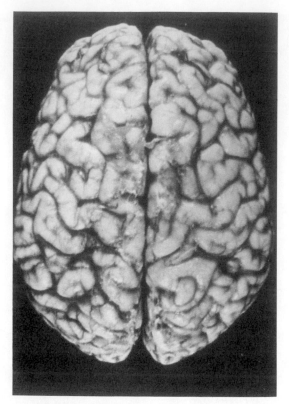
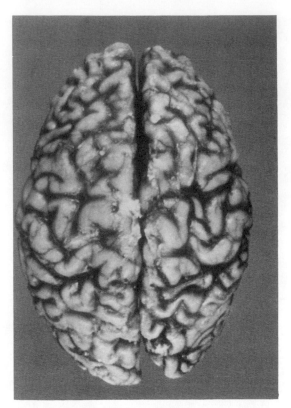

Figure 4   Gross examination of the brain of a nondemented older adult (shown on left) and that of an Alzheimer's disease patient (shown on right) demonstrates sulcal widening and gyral atrophy.

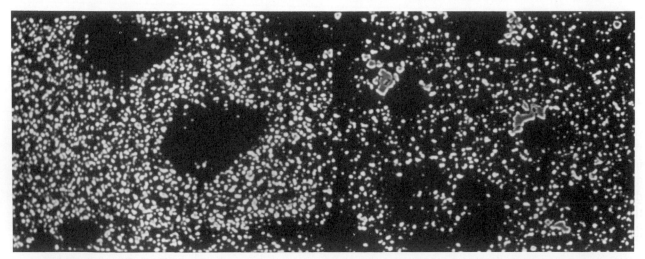

Figure 5   Synaptic loss in Alzheimer's disease. With the advent of immunostaining techniques to label and image synapses, an area of frontal cortex of a nondemented older adult (shown on left) displays abundant numbers of synapses, whereas the frontal cortex of an Alzheimer's disease patient (shown on right) has significant reductions in synaptic density. Reprinted from Terry, Masliah, & Hansen (1994), in Terry, Katzman, & Bick (Eds.), *Alzheimer disease,* with permission of Raven Press.

in differentiating between mildly demented patients with clinically diagnosed AD and normal older adults.

1. Explicit Memory

Explicit, or declarative, memory, which refers to the conscious recollection of previously acquired information, is the type of memory assessed by classic, clinical tests of recall and recognition. One common dichotomous classification of explicit memory, the distinction between episodic and semantic memory, is based on the type of information stored in memory. Episodic memory contains context-linked information in which retrieval depends upon spatial and temporal cues. For example, remembering whether one took one's last dose of a medication requires retrieval of an episodic memory (i.e., where and when one took the medicine). Semantic memory, in contrast, refers to information that is context-free and usually overlearned. Thus, recollection that $3 \times 2 = 6$, that Hawaii is in the Pacific, and that the colors of the American flag are red, white, and blue, can be achieved without recalling the episode (or spatiotemporal context) in which that information was acquired.

Although of general heuristic value in understanding anterograde amnesia (i.e., impaired learning and retention of new information after occurrence of cerebral insult), the episodic-semantic distinction's application to retrograde amnesia (i.e., impaired recollections of information acquired before cerebral insult) is more problematic. For this reason, loss of remote memory (or retrograde amnesia) in Alzheimer's disease is discussed briefly before episodic and semantic memory are discussed.

2. Remote Memory

Retrograde amnesia is temporally graded in early Alzheimer's disease. In other words, events from the distant past, such as the patient's childhood, are remembered more easily than events from more recent past, such as middle adulthood. As the disease progresses into later stages, the patients' retrograde amnesia loses its temporal gradient, and a deficit is seen in retrieval of all explicit memory, regardless of when the information was encoded.

3. Episodic Memory

Episodic memory involves the storage and recollection of temporally dated autobiographical events that depend upon temporal and/or spatial contextual cues

for their retrieval. Memory difficulties in the earliest stages of Alzheimer's disease become apparent when patients are confronted with everyday tasks requiring the use of episodic memory, such as tracking medication regimens, paying bills on schedule, and keeping abreast of recent events in the news. Because of its prevalence in the early stages of AD, episodic memory disturbance is considered to be a necessary (but not sufficient) feature for the clinical diagnosis (see Table I).

Memory impairments, even in patients in the early stages of the disease, are apparent on clinical and experimental memory tasks that require the learning and retention of either verbal or nonverbal information over a series of trials. This severe anterograde amnesia appears to primarily result from a failure in consolidation that is mediated by damage to the hippocampus and entorhinal cortex, and neurotransmitter changes in the cholinergic system. This inability of Alzheimer's patients to transform to-be-remembered information into a form suitable for long-term retention cannot be circumvented by effortful or elaborative processing at the time of acquisition. This contrasts with normal elderly, who have been shown to benefit from engaging in elaborative or semantic processing of information during the study phase of free recall tasks.

Further evidence of patients' deficiencies in storage (i.e., consolidation) is provided by their severe impairments on recognition as well as on recall tasks and by their very limited improvement in acquisition over repeated learning trials (see Fig. 6). The numerous observations that Alzheimer's patients tend to recall only the most recently presented stimuli (i.e., heightened recency effects) support the notion that these patients have great difficulty in transferring information from short- to long-term storage.

In addition to their difficulties in storing new information, patients also tend to evidence rapid forgetting of what little they do initially learn. The rapid forgetting is apparent for both verbal and nonverbal information and has been shown to be even more rapid in Alzheimer's disease than in amnesia. Recent findings suggest that this feature of memory loss is most important for the early and differential diagnosis of Alzheimer's disease and can be obtained through measures of delayed recall (e.g., number of words recalled after a few minutes delay) and savings scores (e.g., percent retained over a period of time).

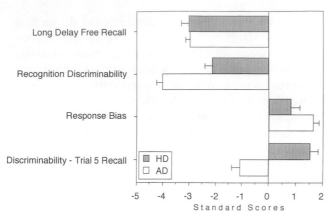

Figure 6 Standard scores of patients with Alzheimer's disease and Huntington's disease on the California Verbal Learning Test, a standardized memory test. Despite comparable poor delayed recall between Alzheimer's and Huntington's patients, the two groups differ in recognition memory, response bias, and a third measure assessing both retention over time and potential benefits of a recognition format over free recall—the difference between recognition memory performance and recall on trial 5 of the initial learning trials. Adapted from Delis et al. (1991). Profiles of demented and amnesic patients on the California Verbal Learning Test: Implications for the assessment of memory disorders. *Psychological Assessment, 3,* 19–26, with permission of the American Psychological Association.

Intrusion errors, or errors representing the intrusion of previously learned information into the attempted recall of new material, represent a consistent behavioral marker of dementia in Alzheimer's disease and are evident on tests of memory for verbal and figural information. However, some caution should be exercised when using such errors in a clinical setting. Intrusion errors in isolation do not represent an exclusive finding in AD since they also occur in patients with other forms of dementia (e.g., Huntington's disease) and in some patients with circumscribed amnesia (e.g., Korsakoff's syndrome). Furthermore, measures of error types have not proven to be the most sensitive cognitive indices for the detection of dementia. Thus, the occurrence of intrusion errors on episodic memory tests should be considered one indicator of a significant memory disturbance and should serve to initiate a thorough search for the processes underlying the patient's impairments.

4. Semantic Memory

While the episodic memory impairment in Alzheimer's disease has been studied in great detail, the semantic memory deficits associated with the disorder have only recently been extensively investigated. It has been known for some time through clinical characterizations of Alzheimer's disease that language deficits, such as word-finding difficulties in spontaneous speech and mild anomia, often occur during the course of the disease. Similarly, decrements in patients' general fund of knowledge concerning common facts of history, geography, arithmetic, and science have been observed and reported. Despite these observations, systematic study of patients' semantic knowledge was lacking. Fortunately, investigators have now begun to examine the language and knowledge deficits in Alzheimer's disease within the framework of current models of the representation of semantic knowledge that were developed in the field of experimental cognitive psychology.

It is often assumed that semantic knowledge is organized as a complex network of associated concepts, and that within the network, concepts that have many attributes in common are more strongly associated than those that share fewer attributes. These strongly related concepts are thought to form conceptual categories made up of exemplars that share many attributes. The attributes not only provide a means of grouping concepts into categories, but also provide a means of distinguishing among the various exemplars that constitute a given category. Thus, dog and lion are both categorized as animals because they share attributes such as being alive, being mobile, and being able to reproduce, but they can be distinguished from each other by such attributes as domesticity, size, and shape. A number of recent investigations suggest that this organization of semantic memory is disrupted in patients with AD, possibly due to damage to the association cortices that are thought to store the concepts and associations that constitute semantic knowledge (see Fig. 7).

There are a number of characteristics of the semantic memory impairment in Alzheimer's patients. First, patients exhibit a disproportionately severe fluency deficit when generating exemplars from a semantic category (e.g., animals) as compared to generating words from a phonemic category (e.g., words beginning with "F"). Their category fluency performance is characterized by an increased propensity to produce category labels relative to specific exemplars. Second, AD patients are impaired on object-naming tasks and produce a significantly greater proportion of semantically based errors than normal older adults and patients with Huntington's disease. In particular, Alzheimer's patients tend to refer to specific objects by their superordinate category names (e.g., "bird" for peli-

ENC

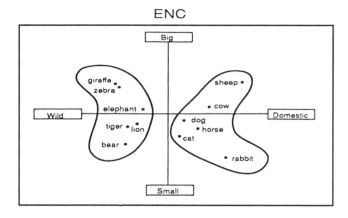

HD

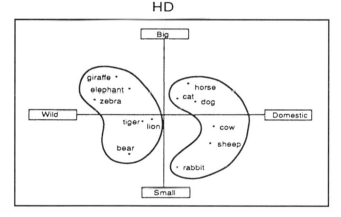

DAT

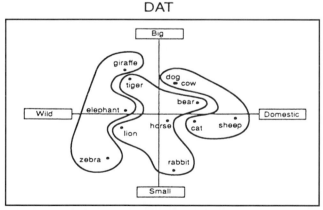

Figure 7 Cognitive maps of elderly normal controls (ENC), patients with Huntington's disease (HD), and patients with Alzheimer's disease (AD) obtained from multidimensional scaling analysis (MDS) and ADDTREE clustering analysis. The position of each animal is determined by MDS; animals in the same cluster, according to ADDTREE cluster analysis, are encircled together. ENC and HD maps have two clusters based on domesticity and size. The map for Alzheimer's patients contain three disorganized clusters. Reprinted from Chan et al. (1993). An assessment of the semantic network in patients with Alzheimer's disease. *Journal of Cognitive Neuroscience, 5,* 254–261, with permission of MIT Press.

can). Third, patients with Alzheimer's disease demonstrate a deficit in sorting items on the basis of subordinate, but not superordinate, attributes. Fourth, there is a correspondence in items missed by AD patients across tasks designed to access semantic knowledge through different modes of input and output. Lastly, there is a deterioration in the organization of semantic knowledge in patients that can be consistently demonstrated by alterations in cognitive maps that reflect the semantic relationships used in categorizing concepts.

Taken together, these findings suggest that there is a true loss of semantic knowledge in Alzheimer's disease, and that the nature of semantic memory deterioration in AD is consistent with a bottom-up breakdown in which specific attributes of a semantic category are lost before more general superordinate knowledge. This loss of semantic knowledge disrupts the normal organization of semantic memory in AD patients and results in aberrations in their network of semantic representations.

5. Implicit Memory

Tests of episodic and semantic memory generally require that prior episodes or events, or previously acquired knowledge, be explicitly and consciously recollected. However, recent research indicates that some forms of learning and memory occur implicitly, without conscious recollection. This implicit knowledge is expressed indirectly throughout the performance of the specific operations comprising a task. Classical conditioning, lexical and semantic priming, motor skill learning, and perceptual learning have all been considered forms of implicit memory. In all of these instances, individual's performances are facilitated "unconsciously" by the prior exposure of stimulus material.

As is the case for episodic and semantic memory, the distinction between explicit and implicit memory receives neurobiological and neuropsychological support from studies of patients with amnesia. Severely amnesic patients are impaired on tests of explicit memory, but perform normally on implicit memory tests. For example, amnesic patients can acquire and retain motor skills (e.g., playing a series of notes or tune on a piano) without any memory for the training experiences. Similarly, amnesic patients will often evidence decreased visual identification thresholds for previously presented words they cannot recall or recognize on explicit memory tests. It is presumed that the initial visual presentation of the words activated some unconscious trace that later facilitated the visual identification of the stimuli without affecting conscious attempts to recollect the materials.

Although the specific neurological substrates of explicit memory have been extensively described, little attention has been given to the brain structures responsible for various forms of implicit memory. While damage to the mesial region of the temporal lobes, the medial diencephalon, and the basal forebrain all result in severe impairments in explicit memory, little is known about the brain structures that mediate various forms of verbal and pictorial priming and skill learning. However, recent studies of the performances of Alzheimer's and Huntington's patients on lexical and pictorial priming as well as on skill-learning tasks have resulted in some new insights into this neuropsychological issue. The findings emanating from these studies have indicated that Alzheimer's and Huntington's patients matched for overall level of cognitive decline can be dissociated with implicit memory tasks that involve the priming of semantic knowledge and the initiation of central motor programs. This double dissociation suggests that portions of the association cortex and the basal ganglia mediate quite different forms of implicit memory. More specifically, the association cortices, which are damaged in Alzheimer's disease, appear to be vital for implicit tasks that seem to rely upon the integrity of semantic knowledge, whereas the basal ganglia, which are damaged in Huntington's disease, are most important for implicit tasks that involve the generation and modification of central motor programs to guide behavior.

B. Attention/Concentration

In addition to memory deficits, patients with Alzheimer's disease also experience deficits in attentional and concentration abilities. It has been hypothesized that impairment in working memory results in difficulty maintaining attention to complex or shifting sets. In fact, subtle impairments in the earliest stages of AD may be seen on complex attentional tasks depending upon divided and shifting attention. Some patients in the early disease stages do not have attentional problems, but such deficits typically emerge and increase in severity as the disease progresses.

C. Language

Deficits in some aspects of language increase in severity throughout the course of Alzheimer's disease. Certain language abilities tend to remain intact, however. Patients exhibit little impairment in articulation abilities, and they also have little of the severe grammatical deficits seen in other neurological disorders, such as Broca's aphasia. With relatively few phonetic and syntactic deficits, the fluency of patients' spontaneous speech and oral reading typically remain intact. In the later stages of the disease, some patients have difficulty producing complex syntax in spontaneous speech. Similarly, patients' auditory comprehension of complex sentences with abstract components may become impaired as dementia increases in severity.

Difficulty with word finding is seen early in Alzheimer's patients, although usually not as early as memory deficits. Patients experience a progressive anomia directly evident on tests of confrontation naming, such as the Boston Naming Test. Patients often circumlocute as they search for particular targets. They also make semantic errors, as described earlier, such as providing picture names that are actually the categories to which pictures belong (e.g., saying "bird" for the target "pelican") and providing names for pictures that are meaningfully associated to the target (e.g., saying "sweeping" for the target "broom").

Alzheimer's patients also exhibit semantic deficits on tests of category fluency. This is a disproportionately severe fluency impairment exhibited by patients when generating exemplars from a specific category compared to generating words that begin with a particular letter.

D. Spatial Cognition

Impairments in spatial cognition are evident in some patients with mild Alzheimer's disease, and in nearly all patients in the later stages of the disease. Degeneration of the parietal lobe is the likely cause of these deficits. Early in the disease, patients experience a more severe and progressive disorientation in space relative to time. This results in the wandering behavior and confusion about location seen frequently in patients. Spatial disorientation appears to be a result of combined impairment in both memory and visuospatial skills.

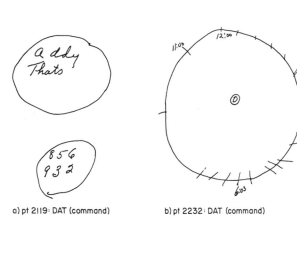

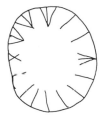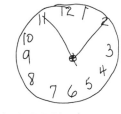

a) pt 2119: DAT (command) b) pt 2232: DAT (command)

c) pt 2179: DAT (command) d) pt 2179: DAT (copy)

Figure 8 Examples (a) and (b) depict conceptual errors in the clock drawings of patients with Alzheimer's disease (DAT). Examples (c) and (d) represent a single patient's attempts to draw the clock to command (c) and to copy (d). Reprinted from Rouleau et al. (1992). Quantitative and qualitative analyses of clock drawings in Alzheimer's and Huntington's disease. *Brain & Cognition, 18,* 70–87, with permission of Academic Press.

A progressive decline in drawing ability is also characteristic of patients with Alzheimer's disease. An early onset of impairment is often seen on complex tasks. For example, patients are significantly impaired compared to healthy older adults when asked to draw a clock or when copying complex geometric designs such as the Rey-Osterrieth Complex Figure. In their drawings, patients tend to make more omission, confabulatory, and perseverative errors, and when drawing a clock AD patients often make conceptual errors (see Fig. 8). Finally, qualitative differences in the types of errors made on tests of visuoperceptive ability may help differentiate normal aging from patients in the early stages of Alzheimer's disease.

E. Executive Function

Although patients are typically aware of their earliest symptoms, such as memory problems, there is an increasing loss of insight as Alzheimer's disease progresses. Gradually patients are unable to recognize their cognitive impairments and to judge the quality of their own behavior. In addition, preservations and intrusions are evident in patients' daily behavior early in the disease. Progressive decline in patients' executive function is also seen in their ability to think abstractly and to solve problems, with deficits occurring early in the course of the disease.

IV. AFFECTIVE AND PERSONALITY CHANGES

Personality changes represent one of the most common alterations in Alzheimer's disease, affecting upward of 75% of patients at some time during the course of the disease. Changes can vary widely in a number of ways such as disengagement or disinterest in one's surroundings, disinhibition or inappropriate social behavior, psychosis, delusions, or other disruptive behaviors. Affective changes can occur as well. Although major depression is uncommon, dysphoric affect can occur with some regularity in Alzheimer's disease (e.g., 50% report symptoms of sadness or demoralization), and anxiety is reported in approximately 50% of patients as well. Hallucinations, which occur in approximately 25% of Alzheimer's cases, are typically visual or auditory in nature, although gustatory, olfactory and haptic hallucinations have also been reported. Delusional preoccupation is not uncommon either. For example, "capgras syndrome," in which the individual believes that his or her family member has been replaced by an imposter, represents one of the most common types of delusional disturbances. Finally, agitation is also one of the most frequently cited symptoms in patients (up to 75%), which creates tremendous burden for caregivers. In sum, abnormal behaviors as a consequence of affective or personality changes in Alzheimer's patients are quite common and typically give rise to more caregiver-related burden than do the cognitive sequelae. [*See* PERSONALITY.]

V. DIFFERENTIATION OF ALZHEIMER'S DISEASE FROM OTHER ETIOLOGIES

A. Alzheimer's Disease Versus Normal Aging

Individuals in the early stages of Alzheimer's disease are by definition impaired in two or more cognitive functions, although the most effective neuropsychological measures for distinguishing between these subjects and healthy older individuals are those that assess the ability to learn new information and retain it over time. For example, in direct comparisons of the effectiveness of measures of learning, retention, confrontation naming, verbal fluency, and constructional ability for differentiating between very mildly demented patients with probable AD and normal elderly individuals, a number of studies have demonstrated the highest diagnostic accuracy (approximately 90%) with delayed free recall measures. Similar results have also been obtained with confirmation by subsequent postmortem histopathologic evidence of Alzheimer's disease in patients who were psychometrically classified as mildly impaired and in none of those classified as normal elderly.

Although measures of learning and retention are the most effective neuropsychological indices for differentiating between mildly demented and normal elderly individuals, measures of language, "executive" functions, and constructional abilities also have some diagnostic value. For example, performances of mildly demented patients with probable Alzheimer's disease and normal elderly control subjects on several types of verbal fluency tasks demonstrate that the semantic category fluency task has greater than 90% sensitivity and specificity for the diagnosis of dementia. Similarly high sensitivity and specificity rates for the differentiation of normal older adults from those patients with Ad has been shown on tests of executive function such as the Stroop Color-Word test, Trailmaking, and on a modified version of the Wisconsin Card Sorting Task.

In addition to detecting subtle cognitive impairment in the early stages of a dementing illness, neuropsychological testing is important for tracking the progression of cognitive decline throughout the course of the disease. Several studies have shown that brief, standardized mental status examinations can effectively document general cognitive decline. Nevertheless, despite the effectiveness of mental status examinations for assessing general cognitive decline, comprehensive neuropsychological testing is often required to track the progression of dementia, particularly when it is necessary to detect changes in specific cognitive domains, or to evaluate the efficacy of a potential treatment. A number of studies have shown that tests of memory and other neuropsychological functions are sensitive to the cognitive decline that occurs between the mild and moderate stages of dementia severity. However, these studies have also shown that neuropsychological measures other than memory are most effective in this regard. Because even mildly demented patients often have severe memory deficits that result in near floor performance on tests of free recall, measures of recognition memory, verbal fluency, confrontation naming, and praxis may be better studied for staging dementia severity or tracking its progression.

B. Alzheimer's Disease versus Depression

A continuing problem for health care professionals involves the diagnosis of older adults who present with signs of both cognitive impairment and depression. In these individuals, a determination must be made whether the patient is experiencing cognitive difficulty secondary to a mood disorder or whether the patient has developed a depressive syndrome secondary to a dementing illness such as Alzheimer's disease.

Kaszniak and Christenson (in Storandt and VandenBos) highlight that research findings concerning neuropsychological test performance of patients with depression and cognitive impairment remains small and difficult to interpret. The "dementia syndrome of depression" likely represents a heterogeneous mixture of different patient groups. Some of these patients may have a combination of a primary dementing illness and depression, and they will remain cognitively impaired following effective treatment of their depression. Others may have cognitive impairment secondary to their depression and will demonstrate improvement of both cognition and mood following effective treatment. However, even among this second group, some patients may manifest a clear progressive dementia over time despite initial improvements in mood. Thus, it is not surprising to find that depressed patients form clusters of different patterns of performance on various neuropsychological tests, such as the California Verbal Learning Test. In reviews of the research literature relevant to differentiation of dementia from

Table V Qualitative Features in Neuropsychological Test Data that are Helpful in Differentiating Alzheimer's Disease from Dementia Syndrome of Depression

Measure	Alzheimer's Disease	Dementia Syndrome of Depression
Recognition memory	Impaired	Relatively intact
False positive recognition memory errors	Greater	Fewer
"Don't know" errors (controversial)	Unusual	Usual
Performance on "automatic" encoding tasks	Impaired	Intact
Effort in attempting to perform tasks	Good	Poor
Performance on tasks of similar difficulty	Consistent	Variable
Semantic organization	Unhelpful	Helpful
Prompting	Less helpful	Helpful
Awareness of impairment	Impared	Intact

Note. From Kaszniak & Christenson, in Storandt & VandenBos, 1994.

depression (see Kaszniak and Christenson), attempts have been made to determine those quantitative and qualitative aspects of neuropsychological test performance that may be helpful in this diagnostic task. Those features most frequently identified by these authors are listed in Table V.

Kaszniak and Christenson caution that these neuropsychological test features should be viewed as guidelines for increasing or decreasing suspicion of a patient having Alzheimer's disease versus the dementia syndrome of depression, rather than as providing definitive diagnoses. Recent research suggests that differentiating patients with dementia syndrome of depression from those with vascular dementia due to subcortical infarctions, or other subcortical dementias, may be particularly difficult. Investigators have found that, among a group of depressed patients, the California Verbal Learning Test revealed a subgroup demonstrating the same pattern of deficits as those seen in patients with Huntington's disease, which is typically regarded as a prototypical subcortical dementing illness. [*See* DEPRESSION.]

C. Alzheimer's Disease versus Subcortical Dementia

A considerable amount of recent research has been directed toward identifying the pattern of cognitive changes that might distinguish between Alzheimer's disease and dementia associated with other neurodegenerative diseases. Much of this research has been carried out within the framework of a "cortical-subcortical" distinction, which holds that different patterns of primary neuropsychological deficits are associated with neurodegenerative diseases that predominately involve regions of the cerebral cortex (e.g., Alzheimer's disease, Pick's disease) or that have their primary locus in subcortical brain structures (e.g., Huntington's disease, Parkinson's disease, progressive supranuclear palsy). Studies that address this distinction usually compare and contrast neuropsychological test performance of patients with AD (a prototypical cortical dementia) and that of patients with Huntington's disease (a prototypical subcortical dementia) (see Table VI).

In addition to these differences in the general neuropsychological features of Alzheimer's disease and dementia associated with Huntington's disease, numerous studies utilizing concepts and experimental procedures of cognitive psychology suggest that there is a fundamental difference in the nature of the memory impairment that occurs in each disorder. Alz-

Table VI Neuropsychological Features Associated with Cortical and Subcortical Dementia

Cortical Dementia (e.g., Alzheimer's Disease)	Subcortical Dementia (e.g., Huntington's Disease)
• Failure in storage (amnesia)	• Retrieval deficit (forgetfulness)
• Severe retrograde amnesia	• Mild-to-moderate retrograde amnesia
• Rapid forgetting	• Relatively normal rate of forgetting
• Impaired recall and recognition memory	• Relatively normal recognition memory
• Numerous intrusion errors	• Few intrusion errors
• Deterioration of semantic knowledge	• Intact structure of semantic knowledge
• Intact skill learning	• Impaired skill learning

Note. Adapted from Butters, Salmon, & Butters, in Storandt & Vandenbos, 1994.

heimer's patients exhibit a severe deficit in episodic memory (i.e., temporally dated autobiographical episodes that depend upon contextual cues for their retrieval) that appears to result from ineffective consolidation (i.e., storage) of new information, whereas the memory disorder of Huntington's patients is thought to result from a general difficulty in initiating a systematic retrieval strategy when recalling information from either episodic or semantic memory (i.e., overlearned facts and concepts that are not dependent on contextual cues for retrieval).

Although Huntington's patients also exhibit difficulty in learning and recalling information on free recall tasks, evidence of a general retrieval deficit is provided by a marked improvement in their performance when memory is tested with a recognition format, and by their ability to retain information over a delay in near normal fashion, quite unlike that of AD patients (see Fig. 6).

Patients with cortical and subcortical dementia syndromes can also be differentiated by their performances on tests of remote memory. Several studies indicate that in early stages of DAT, remote memory loss is temporally graded with memories from the distant past (i.e., childhood and early adulthood) better remembered than memories from the more remote past (i.e., mid and late adulthood). In contrast, patients with Huntington's disease or Parkinson's disease suffer only a mild degree of retrograde amnesia that is equally severe across all decades of their lives. These results suggest that the remote memory deficit of patients with subcortical dementia is another reflection of a general retrieval deficit that equally affects recollection of information from any decade of their lives, whereas the temporally graded remote memory loss of Alzheimer's patients is indicative of a failure to adequately consolidate information through repeated processing, rehearsal, or re-exposure.

In addition to their distinct patterns of performance on tests of episodic and remote memory, patients with cortical and subcortical dementia syndromes differ markedly with regard to presence and severity of language deficits. AD patients, for example, are noted for mild anomia and word-finding difficulties in spontaneous speech, and evidence suggests that this deficit is indicative of a loss of semantic knowledge and a breakdown in the organization of semantic memory. In contrast, patients with Huntington's disease generally retain their language abilities. For example, these patients perform at near normal levels on tests of con-

frontation naming, and the errors they produce are often visuoperceptually based rather than semantically based. Although Huntington's patients perform poorly on tests of verbal fluency, they are equally impaired regardless of the semantic demands of the task, suggesting that their poor fluency performance is more likely to be related to their general deficiency in initiating an effective retrieval strategy than to a true language deficit.

Another major distinction that can be drawn between patients with cortical and subcortical dementia syndromes is the different patterns of spared and impaired abilities they exhibit on various implicit memory tasks. Implicit memory has been described as being mediated by a distinct memory "system" independent from the conscious, episodic memory system. Neuropsychological and neurobiological evidence for this distinction is provided by numerous studies that have demonstrated preserved implicit memory in patients with severe amnesia arising from damage to hippocampal formation or to diencephalic brain regions.

Studies comparing patients with cortical and subcortical dementia on various priming tasks have shown that Alzheimer's patients, but not Huntington's patients, are significantly impaired on lexical, semantic, and pictorial priming tests. In contrast to the priming results, Huntington's patients, but not Alzheimer's patients, are impaired on motor skill learning, prism adaptation, and weight biasing tasks that involve generation and refinement (i.e., learning) of motor programs to guide behavior.

VI. CLINICAL MANAGEMENT OF ALZHEIMER'S DISEASE

A. Management of Behavioral Disturbances

Alzheimer's patients experience a variety of behavioral disturbances, which place great demands on caregivers in finding ways to effectively manage them. Psychiatric symptoms, wandering, and aggressive behaviors, ranging in severity, are common in patients. Patients may also become frustrated with their own impairments, for example, when trying to communicate or remember things. More severe changes in behavior are evident in the later stages of the disease, when patients are no longer able to handle their daily functioning needs, like eating, bathing, and toileting.

Management of these behavioral symptoms is often attempted by teaching caregivers behavioral modification techniques. Simplifying the stimulation available in patients' environments, offering frequent reminders and reassurances, abiding by a consistent routine, and providing patients with enjoyable activities also help to keep the patient comfortable and content. To aid in coping with the stress of managing these symptoms, support groups for caregivers of Alzheimer's patients are available nationwide. Because the responsibilities of caregiving for patients with AD are so great, however, the services offered by nursing homes often provide care for patients whose families are unable to handle the tasks on their own.

B. Pharmacologic Treatment

Psychotropic medications may be used to manage behavioral disturbances in Alzheimer's patients. Antipsychotic drugs, such as Haldol, can minimize delusions, hallucinations, and agitation experienced by patients. Antidepressants, like Prozac, are used to improve patients' moods and energy level. Valium and other anti-anxiety medications are prescribed to manage agitation and anxiety. Unfortunately, many psychiatric medications can also further compromise cognitive functioning, especially those with strong anticholinergic properties.

Recent research has focused on testing medications that may slow the progression of Alzheimer's disease. Tetrahydroaminoacridine (THA), or Cognex, is a drug that purportedly suppresses the breakdown of acetylcholine in the hopes of slowing patients' cognitive decline. Unfortunately, Cognex, the first drug approved for the treatment of Alzheimer's disease, has not appeared to be clinically effective in the majority of patients for whom it is prescribed. Other current research is focusing on the role of neurotrophic factors, estrogen, calcium, and antioxidants in the progression of Alzheimer's disease. [*See* PSYCHOPHARMACOLOGY.]

VII. SUMMARY

Alzheimer's disease is the most common cause of dementia, currently affecting nearly 4 million people in the United States. Estimates project that its prevalence will rise to approximately 14 million by the year 2050. Whether one views AD from an individual, family, or public health perspective, its devastating consequences will continue to escalate and affect us either directly or indirectly in many ways. In short, Alzheimer's disease will increasingly become the dominant disorder in late life.

Cognitive changes associated with this dementia include progressive impairments in memory, attention, language, spatial cognition, and executive function, some of which occur in the earliest stages of the disease. Patients also experience changes in behavior, affect, and personality. The cognitive, behavioral, and affective changes result in an increasing dependency of Alzheimer's patients on others in their day-to-day functioning.

The disease is characterized by a number of neuropathological changes, including the presence of neurofibrillary tangles and neuritic plaques, loss of neurons and synapses, neocortical atrophy, and alterations in neurotransmitter levels. A definitive diagnosis can be made only at autopsy or with a brain biopsy, upon detection of sufficient numbers of neurofibrillary tangles and neuritic plaques. As no effective treatment or cure for Alzheimer's disease is currently available, strategies for the management of disease symptoms focus on behavioral modification and the use of psychiatric medications where appropriate.

Fortunately, sustained efforts on a number of research fronts (i.e., molecular biological, genetic, cognitive, and behavioral) have helped to improve our understanding of Alzheimer's disease and ultimately may lead to effective treatments for the prevention and cure of this complex and devastating disease.

ACKNOWLEDGMENTS

Preparation of this chapter was supported in part by funds from the National Institute on Aging (AG12674) and the Medical Research Service of the Department of Veterans Affairs.

BIBLIOGRAPHY

American Psychiatric Association (1994). *Diagnostic and statistical manual of mental disorders* (4th ed.). Washington, DC: Author.

Birren, J. E., Sloane, R. B., & Cohen, G. D. (Eds.). (1992). *Handbook of mental health and aging*. San Diego: Academic Press.

Craik, F. I. M., & Salthouse, T. A. (Eds.). (1992). *The handbook of aging and cognition*. Hillsdale, NJ: Lawrence Erlbaum Associates.

Cummings, J. L., and Benson, D. F. (1992). *Dementia: A clinical approach* (2nd ed.). Boston: Butterworth-Heinemann.

Grant, I., & Adams, K. M. (Eds.). (1996). *Neuropsychological as-*

sessment of neuropsychiatric disorders (2nd ed.). New York: Oxford University Press.

La Rue, A. (1992). *Aging and neuropsychological assessment.* New York: Plenum.

Parks, R. W., Zec, R. F., and Wilson, R. S. (Eds.). (1993). *Neuropsychology of Alzheimer's disease and other Dementias.* New York: Oxford University Press.

Rapoport, S. I., Petit, H., Leys, D., & Christen, Y. (Eds.). (1990).

Imaging, cerebral topography, and Alzheimer's disease. Berlin: Springer-Verlag.

Storandt, M., & VandenBos, G. R. (Eds.). (1994). *Neuropsychological assessment of dementia and depression in older adults: A clinician's guide.* Washington, DC: American Psychological Association.

Terry, R. D., Katzman, R., & Bick, K. L. (Eds.). (1994). *Alzheimer disease.* New York: Raven Press.

Amnesia

John F. Kihlstrom* and
Elizabeth L. Glisky

University of Arizona

Alcoholic Blackout Amnesia without loss of consciousness, in which the intoxicated person retains the ability to perform certain "automatized" behaviors without any subsequent memory for the episode.

Amnesia A special case of forgetting in which the memory loss is greater than would be expected under ordinary circumstances. Anterograde amnesia affects memory for events occurring after the instigating event; retrograde amnesia affects memory for events occurring before the instigating event.

Amnesic Syndrome A profound deficit in learning and memory usually associated with bilateral damage to the diencephalon or to the medial portions of the temporal lobe. It always involves an anterograde amnesia and may involve a retrograde amnesia as well.

Functional Amnesia A significant loss of memory attributable to an instigating event, usually stressful, that does not result in insult, injury, or disease affecting brain tissue. Its most common forms are psychogenic amnesia, psychogenic fugue, and multiple personality disorder.

Infantile and Childhood Amnesia An amnesia observed in adults, affecting memory for personal experiences occurring in the first 5–7 years of life. Infantile amnesia commonly covers the period before language and speech develop.

Posthypnotic Amnesia A retrograde amnesia induced by means of hypnotic suggestion; it may be canceled by a prearranged reversibility cue.

Transient Global Amnesia A benign and temporary amnesia characterized by sudden onset, apparently caused by momentary vascular insufficiencies affecting brain tissue.

Traumatic Retrograde Amnesia A retrograde amnesia resulting from a concussive blow to the head; most of the affected memories are eventually recovered, except for a "final RA" affecting the accident itself.

AMNESIA may be defined as a special case of forgetting, in which the loss of memory is greater than would be expected under ordinary circumstances. A head-injured patient is no longer able to learn things that he was once able to master easily; a patient with psychogenic fugue loses her identity as well as her fund of autobiographical memories. Amnesia includes frank pathologies encountered in neurological and psychiatric clinics, such as Korsakoff's syndrome, Alzheimer's disease, traumatic retrograde amnesia, and multiple personality disorder. But it also includes abnormalities of memory observed ubiquitously, such as infantile and childhood amnesia, the exaggerated forgetfulness associated with healthy aging, and the memory failures associated with sleep and general anesthesia. These naturally occurring pathologies of

*John F. Kihlstrom is presently at the University of California, Berkeley.

memory have their counterparts in amnestic states induced in otherwise normal, intact individuals by means of experimental techniques, such as electroconvulsive shock in laboratory rats and posthypnotic amnesia in college sophomores.

Experimental research on memory began with the publication of Ebbinghaus' *Uber das Gedachtniss* in 1885, but the clinical description of amnesia dates from even earlier. Korsakoff described the amnesic syndrome that bears his name in 1854. And in 1882 Ribot published *Les Maladies de la memoire,* with a detailed description of the consequences for memory of brain insult, injury, and disease, as well as a theory of memory and amnesia. On the basis of his observations, and Hughlings Jackson's principle that ontogeny recapitulates phylogeny, he concluded that brain disorder produces a progressive loss of memory that affects memories in the reverse order of their development. Thus, in traumatic retrograde amnesia, memories for events occurring immediately before the accident are most likely to be lost. This principle, now known as Ribot's Law, does not always hold, but it was an important first step in the journey from clinical description to scientific theory.

For reasons that are not completely clear, clinical and experimental study of amnesia languished for the first half of the 20th century, but was revived by Talland's 1965 monograph *Deranged Memory,* which reported an extensive psychometric and experimental study of patients with Korsakoff syndrome. Talland's work ushered in a new age of research in which clinicians and experimentalists joined forces under the banner of *cognitive neuropsychology*—a discipline that attempts to integrate evidence obtained from the intensive study of brain-damaged patients with theories of normal cognitive function. In this article, we provide a summary of this research, as it pertains to the major disorders of memory—pathological and normal, natural and artificial—and discuss the role of this research in the contemporary psychology of memory.

I. THE AMNESIC SYNDROME

The amnesic syndrome represents a profound deficit in learning and memory; it is by far the most commonly studied pathology of memory. Its characteristic feature is a gross anterograde amnesia (AA), meaning that the person cannot remember events that have occurred since the time of the brain damage. Short-term memory (as measured by digit span, for example) is unimpaired; but after even a few moments' distraction, these patients cannot remember what they have said or done, or what has been said or done to them, just recently. In the classic cases, the patient's cognitive deficits are specific to long-term memory: general intelligence, perception, reasoning, and language functions are spread. But this anterograde amnesia is associated with several different etiologies, and careful examination indicates that these disparate origins are associated with somewhat different patterns of memory and cognitive deficit.

One form of the amnesic syndrome, now known as *diencephalic amnesia,* was first described by Korsakoff in association with alcoholism. At the time, chronic alcoholics frequently suffered from a deficiency of vitamin B_1 (thiamine) which results in bilateral damage to structures of the diencephalon, including the upper portion of the brainstem, the mammillary bodies, the dorsomedial nucleus of the thalamus, and the mammillothalamic tract (unilateral lesions produce "material-specific" amnesias for verbal or nonverbal memories, depending on which hemisphere is damaged). Although this disease is now effectively prevented by the introduction of vitamin-enriched commercial foods, other etiologies, including vascular insufficiencies, tumors, and fronto-temporal brain damage can have similar effects. These patients typically show a retrograde amnesia (RA) as well as AA, meaning that they also have difficulties in remembering events from their premorbid life, especially those from the years immediately preceding their disease. Remote memory, such as for childhood events, is apparently preserved. Note that such a pattern conforms to Ribot's Law.

Another form of amnesic syndrome, known as *temporal lobe amnesia,* stems from bilateral lesions in the medial portion of the temporal lobe, and especially the hippocampus, entorhinal cortex, and surrounding structures (again, there are also material-specific amnesias resulting from unilateral damage to these structures). The most famous case is Patient H. M., who displayed a profound AA after surgical resection of his medial temporal lobes, including the hippocampus, in a desperate attempt to relieve intractable epileptic seizures. Other cases have been caused by brain tumors, ischemic episodes, head trauma, and herpes encephalitis. Temporal-lobe patients always show AA; when they show RA, it is not always as extensive as in diencephalic patients.

There is also a *frontal-lobe amnesia,* which is qualitatively different from the amnesic syndrome. Frontal-lobe patients are not globally amnesic, but they frequently show deficits on tasks requiring memory for temporal order, as well as memory for the source of newly acquired knowledge. They also lack *metamemory* capabilities—they have little appreciation of the contents stored in their own memories, or in the availability of appropriate memory strategies. Patients who have frontal damage in addition to diencephalic or medial-temporal lobe damage experience their greatest difficulties on memory tasks requiring strategic planning and organization.

Finally, *transient global amnesia* is a temporary (typically lasting several hours) condition characterized by sudden onset. It closely resembles the permanent diencephalic and medial-temporal lobe amnesias, in that it involves both AA and RA, but, as its name implies, it is brief. The condition, while frightening, is benign: after remission, there are no signs of permanent brain damage (and little risk of another episode in the future). Transient global amnesia appears to be caused by temporary vascular insufficiency affecting brain tissue; interestingly, many cases appear in association with physical exertion or mental stress.

In the absence of permanent brain damage, something akin to the amnesic syndrome may be observed in cases of *alcoholic blackout.* Blackout involves amnesia without loss of consciousness. The intoxicated individual may engage in conversation or perform other actions normally, but after regaining sobriety, he or she will have no memory for the episode. Blackouts are most commonly observed in chronic alcoholics, though they do occur to nonalcoholics who are severely intoxicated. In any case, blackout is most likely to occur when the person ingests large quantities of alcohol rapidly, especially when fatigued or hungry. Alcohol folklore suggests that the amnesia is an instance of state-dependent retrieval—that the memories return when the person resumes drinking. However, laboratory research clearly indicates that the memories covered by blackout are unrecoverable, and thus that the amnesia reflects an encoding deficit. Sedative drugs, such as the barbiturates and benzodiazepines, also produce irreversible AA. [*See* ALCOHOL PROBLEMS.]

The different patterns of task performance offer clues about the nature of the memory deficit in the amnesic syndrome. In principle, any instance of forgetting may be attributed to a failure at one or more of three stages of memory processing: encoding (the creation of a memory trace of a new experience), storage (the retention of trace information over time), and retrieval (the recovery of trace information for use in ongoing experience, thought, and action). Logically, a syndrome that affects memory for postmorbid but not premorbid events is most likely due to encoding failure. And, in fact, it has been suggested on the basis of laboratory experiments with lesioned rats and monkeys that the hippocampus and other structures in the medial-temporal lobe mediate that consolidation and storage of new memories. An alternative formulation assumes that representations of the various elements of an event are distributed widely in the cortex, and that the hippocampus creates a "cognitive map" to index and bind them together. In either case, the occurrence of AA means that the hippocampus is crucial for memory formation, even though the memories themselves are not stored there.

What about the RA? Some degree of RA is usually, but not always, observed in the amnesic syndrome. Logically, damage to a structure that consolidates and organizes new memories should have no effect on old memories. In some cases, RA may reflect the disruption of premorbid memories that were incompletely consolidated at the time of disease onset; this would produce a temporal gradient, but the extent of RA observed would seem to imply that proper consolidation requires weeks, months, or years instead of seconds, minutes, or hours. On the other hand, if the hippocampus serves a binding and indexing function, its destruction will create an RA by effectively preventing the retrieval of memories that remain available in storage; this would produce an amnesia for remote as well as recent memories and would not necessarily produce a temporal gradient. Finally, in some cases what appears as RA may in fact be AA, reflecting the slow onset of an insidious disease process and producing the appearance of a temporal gradient; this suggestion is particularly plausible in the case of diencephalic amnesia associated with chronic alcohol abuse, but cannot account for amnesias of sudden onset.

The nature of RA in the amnesic syndrome remains unresolved. In the final analysis, it is important to remember that in real life outside the laboratory, pure cases of amnesic syndrome are exceedingly rare. Patients may suffer primary damage to one area, but collateral damage to another, and the precise combination of lesions may determine the presence and extent of RA.

Even conclusions about encoding deficits must be qualified to some extent. At first glance, the AA observed in the amnesic syndrome appears to be a complete inability to acquire new information. However, closer examination indicates that certain aspects of learning and memory are spared even in the densest cases of amnesia. Thus, Patient H. M. has learned to solve the Tower of Hanoi puzzle, but he does not recognize the puzzle as familiar. Amnesic patients who study the word *ELATED* do not remember it just minutes later; but when presented the stem *ELA-* and asked to complete it with the first word that comes to mind, they are more likely to produce *ELATED* (as opposed to *ELASTIC* or *ELABORATE*) than would be expected by chance. The ability of amnesic patients to acquire cognitive and motor skills, and to show priming effects in word-stem completion, shows that they are able to acquire new information through experience, although, somewhat paradoxically, they are not aware that they possess this knowledge.

The limits of such learning are still being studied, but already they have motivated a distinction between two expressions of episodic memory, *explicit* and *implicit*. Explicit memory (EM) refers to the conscious recollection of a previous episode, as in recall or recognition. By contrast, implicit memory (IM) refers to any change in experience, thought, or action that is attributable to such an episode, such as skill learning or priming. The dissociation between EM and IM in amnesic patients indicates that some forms of learning and memory are preserved. According to one view, amnesics suffer from a specific inability to encode declarative knowledge about specific events, but retain an ability to acquire procedural (or other nondeclarative) knowledge. This would account for their ability to acquire new cognitive and motor skills. Preserved priming has been attributed to the automatic activation of declarative knowledge structures that were stored prior to the brain damage, or to the encoding of new episodic representations in a primitive perceptual memory system that lacks the kinds of information (e.g., about the meaning of an event, or its spatiotemporal context) that would support EM.

II. TRAUMATIC RETROGRADE AMNESIA

Another form of amnesia occurs as a consequence of head trauma. A very severe blow to the head can bruise gray matter and shear white matter, producing both cortical and subcortical damage that may result in AA and RA similar to that observed in the amnesic syndrome. Even in the absence of such damage, some blows to the head can result in a concussion or temporary cessation of electrical activity in the cortex and loss of consciousness. The recovery of consciousness begins with the return of simple reflexes, then the gradual return of purposeful movement, and then speech (this pattern would be predicted by Ribot's Law). After the victim appears fully oriented, he or she will display an AA for some time, as well as an RA for the accident itself and the events leading up to the accident. Typically, the AA is immediate, i.e., it will start at the time of the trauma. But if the loss of consciousness is delayed, the onset of the AA will be delayed as well. Such *lucid intervals* suggest that the AA is a result of vascular complications that may take some time to develop.

The RA is characterized by a temporal gradient, meaning that it is densest for events nearest the time of the accident—another example of Ribot's Law at work. However, the gradient is broken by *islands of memory* consisting of isolated events, not necessarily personally important, that are remembered relatively well. The extent of the RA is correlated with the extent of the AA. Although the memories covered by the AA are permanently lost, apparently reflecting an encoding deficit, the RA gradually remits. It was once thought that this recovery began with the earliest memories and proceeded forward, which again would be predicted by Ribot's Law. Although the most recent events are generally recovered last, more careful studies show that the shrinkage of amnesia is accomplished by filling in the gaps that surround the islands of memory, leaving a *final RA* covering the accident itself and the moments or minutes leading up to it, and perhaps a few *islands of amnesia*. The shrinkage of amnesia clearly indicates that traumatic RA is a disorder of retrieval, and that the islands of memory act as anchors to support the recovery process. However, the final RA may reflect either a loss of memory from storage or more likely a disruption of consolidation.

A nontraumatic form of retrograde amnesia is observed in psychiatric patients who are administered *electroconvulsive therapy* (ECT) for acute affective disorder. In ECT, electrical stimulation (e.g., 100 V, 500 mA for 500 msec), delivered from surface electrodes applied over the temporal lobe, induces a convulsive, tonic–clonic seizure not unlike those of grand mal epilepsy; after a short series of such treatments (e.g., 6–10 sessions over 2–3 weeks), patients often experience a rapid return to their normal mood state (ECT is not a cure, as episodes of depression or mania may recur).

Because they are anesthetized when the treatment is delivered, patients experience no pain or distress from the convulsions themselves; because they receive muscle relaxants, the convulsions do not result in bone trauma. However, the seizure does produce both AA and RA as adventitious consequences (i.e., unrelated to treatment success). The RA shows the same sort of temporal gradient observed following concussive blows to the head. Because there is less memory impairment (though no difference in treatment outcome) with unilateral than with bilateral electrode placement, ECT is usually delivered to the nondominant hemisphere. The RA gradually clears up (except for the moments before ECT is actually delivered), but memories affected by the AA cannot be recovered.

The amnesia induced by ECT shows a dissociation between EM and IM similar to that observed in the amnesic syndrome. In one experiment, patients who studied a list of words within 90 minutes following administration of ECT showed a deficit in recognition, but no deficit in priming on a word-stem completion test. In another study, patients who read word strings presented in mirror-reversed fashion before delivery of ECT later showed an advantage in reading those words, even though they failed to recognize these words as familiar.

What about the memories covered by the final RA? Although electroconvulsive shock may disrupt encoding processes, it does not appear to remove the memory traces from storage. The relevant evidence comes from studies of the effects on memory of *electroconvulsive shock* (ECS) administered to animals. A common research paradigm is called one-trial, step-down, passive avoidance learning. A rat is placed on a shelf above an electrified floor. If the animal steps down, it receives a footshock and jumps back up on the shelf. Under ordinary circumstances, the animal will not return to the floor; it learns in one trial to avoid the shock by doing nothing. But in the experiment, the animal received a dose of ECS similar to that delivered to patients in ECT. After the animal recovers, it steps down onto the floor after being placed on the shelf— as if it has forgotten all about the shock.

ECS-induced amnesia shows a temporal gradient similar to that observed in other forms of traumatic retrograde amnesia. If the ECS is delayed from the time of the original learning experience, there is less amnesia than if it is administered immediately afterward. But the extent of amnesia also depends on how memory is measured. The amnesic animal steps down immediately, as if the footshock never happened. At the same time, it shows a marked increase in heart rate. Moreover, if the animal receives *reminder treatments*, such as tail shock in another environment or immersion in circulating ice water, it will remain on the shelf and avoid the floor. The *desynchrony* between behavioral and psychophysiological indices of fear is analogous to the dissociation between EM and IM observed in human amnesic patients; and the effectiveness of reminder treatments shows that at least some aspects of the forgotten event have been preserved. Memories covered by the final RA may never be accessible to conscious recollection, but they may nonetheless be expressed as implicit memories.

III. FUNCTIONAL AMNESIAS

Clinically significant amnesias are not confined to cases of organic brain syndrome. Psychiatrists and clinical psychologists also encounter forms of *functional amnesia* in a group of mental illnesses known as the *dissociative disorders*. Functional amnesia may be defined as a loss of memory that is attributable to an instigating event (often, mental stress) that does not result in insult, injury, or disease to the brain. For example, victims of violent crimes such as rape, or other sorts of traumatic stress, often display an amnesia for the event itself. Although this might be an AA reflecting encoding deficits caused by high levels of arousal, there is often an RA covering the events leading up to the trauma as well—sometimes extending to a large portion of the person's life. Because there is no evidence of head injury, such memory failures are labeled as *psychogenic amnesia.* Compared to traumatic retrograde amnesia, psychogenic amnesia appears to be more extensive and longer lasting. Clinical lore holds that psychogenic amnesia can be reversed by hypnosis or barbiturate sedation, but evidence for the reliability of recollections produced by these techniques is largely lacking. [*See* DISSOCIATIVE DISORDERS.]

Another dissociative disorder, *psychogenic fugue,* entails a more extensive loss of autobiographical memory, covering the whole of the person's life, a loss and/or change in identity, and sometimes physical relocation (from which symptom the syndrome derives its name). Such cases often come to the attention of police and health providers when a person cannot identify himself; or when she comes to herself in a strange place and does not know how she got there. Interestingly, fugue patients lose self-knowledge and autobiographical memory, but they do not seem to lose their fund of semantic memory, or their repertoire of procedural knowledge.

Upon recovery the patient is left with an amnesia covering the events of the fugue state itself, and retains no knowledge of whatever identity he or she may have adopted in that state. Examination of such cases after they are resolved often reveals an instigating episode of psychological stress.

Multiple personality disorder (MPD), in which two or more personalities appear to inhabit a single body, alternating control over experience and action, also involves a disruption of memory and identity. One of these personalities is often "primary," in that it is the one that has been manifest the longest and known by most other people. Most important in the present context, the various personalities appear to be separated by an amnesic barrier that prevents one alter ego from gaining access to the memories of another. In many cases, the amnesia is asymmetrical, in that Personality A may be aware of Personality B, but not the reverse. The amnesia largely affects identity and autobiographical memory; as a rule, the various personalities share semantic memory and procedural knowledge in common. The most widely accepted theory of MPD holds that it develops in defense against abuse, trauma, or deprivation in early childhood. [*See* CHILD SEXUAL ABUSE; PERSONALITY DISORDERS.]

Reports of MPD were relatively common in the clinical literature before 1920, and then virtually disappeared. There has been a resurgence of MPD, bordering on epidemic, in recent years. However, it is not clear how many of these are iatrogenic in nature or simply misdiagnosed. Where the alternate personalities are initially elicited through hypnosis or other special techniques, or when an amnesic barrier is absent, the case is suspect. MPD is sometimes offered as an insanity defense, claiming that a second personality is actually responsible for crimes of which the first personality is accused. MPD raises interesting issues of criminal law: in principle, the actions of one personality may be outside another personality's ability to control; interpersonality amnesia may prevent the accused from assisting in the defense; and techniques intended to elicit testimony from a personality may violate constitutional safeguards against self-incrimination. However, MPD has rarely proved successful as a defense against criminal charges.

There are several experimental studies that confirm the existence of interpersonality amnesia in MPD. Thus, for example, one alter ego is often unable to recall or recognize a list of items studied by another. Interestingly, there is some evidence that IM may be spared in these cases. Thus, one alter ego may show savings in relearning, interference, transfer of training, or priming effects involving a list studied exclusively by another one. Although the available research is somewhat ambiguous, in general it seems that the amnesic barrier is permeable in the case of implicit memories.

Just as the amnesic syndrome finds its experimental analog in drug-induced amnesia, and traumatic retrograde amnesia in ECT and ECS, the functional amnesias seen clinically have their laboratory parallel in posthypnotic amnesia. Following appropriate suggestions and the termination of hypnosis, many subjects cannot remember the events that transpired while they were hypnotized. After the hypnotist administers a prearranged cue, the critical memories become accessible again; the fact of reversibility marks posthypnotic amnesia as a disruption of memory retrieval. The amnesia does not occur unless it has been suggested (explicitly or implicitly), and memory is not reinstated merely by the induction of hypnosis; thus, posthypnotic amnesia is not an instance of state-dependent memory. Response to the amnesia suggestion is highly correlated with individual differences in hypnotizability: while hypnotic "virtuosos" typically show a very dense amnesia, their insusceptible counterparts show little or no forgetting. [*See* HYPNOSIS AND THE PSYCHOLOGICAL UNCONSCIOUS.]

Like the organic amnesias, posthypnotic amnesia is selective. The subject may forget which words appeared on a study list, but retains the ability to use these words in speech and writing. Skills acquired in hypnosis transfer to the posthypnotic state, and suggestions for amnesia have no impact on practice effects. Subjects who learn new factual information while hypnotized may retain it despite suggestions for amnesia, but these same subjects may well forget the circumstances in which this knowledge was acquired—a phenomenon of *source amnesia* that has also been observed in the amnesic syndrome. Finally, there is good evidence that priming effects are preserved in posthypnotic amnesia. That is, subjects who cannot remember words from a study list are more likely to use those words as free associations or category instances than would be expected by chance. Thus, posthypnotic amnesia shows the familiar dissociation between EM and IM.

Because functional amnesia occurs in the absence of brain damage, and because posthypnotic amnesia occurs in response to suggestion, questions inevitably arise about malingering, simulation, and behavioral compliance. Unfortunately, it is difficult to distinguish between genuine and simulated amnesia in either clinical or experimental situations. Claims of amnesia are readily accepted when there is palpable evidence of brain damage. It should be understood, however, that evidence of a significant interpersonal or sociocultural component does not necessarily mean that functional amnesia is faked. Rather, it means that functional amnesia is complex. Hypnosis may be a state of altered consciousness, but it is also a social interaction; thus, it should not be surprising to discover that the subject's response to amnesia suggestions will be influenced by the precise wording of the suggestion, the discourse context in which it is embedded, the subject's interpretation of the hypnotist's words, and perceived social demands. The social context is probably important in the organic amnesias, but its role is magnified in their functional counterparts.

IV. AMNESIA THROUGH THE LIFESPAN

Some forms of amnesia occur naturally in the course of psychological development. For example, adults rarely remember much from their early childhoods; the earliest memory is typically dated between the third and fourth birthdays, and is limited to a relatively small number of isolated fragments until about 5 or 7 years of age. The appearance of childhood amnesia is not merely an artifact of the long retention interval between childhood encoding and adult retrieval; something special seems to happen to memories for childhood events. Infantile amnesia, covering the first year or two of life, may be attributed at least in part to the lack of language and to the immaturity of the neocortex and other critical brain structures. However, the exact mechanism for childhood amnesia, covering the years after the second birthday, remains uncertain.

The classic explanation for childhood amnesia was proposed by Freud. In his view, during the phallic stage of psychosexual development the child resolves the Oedipus complex by repressing infantile sexual and aggressive impulses, as well as any thoughts, images, and memories that might be related to them. Since (according to the theory) all the young child's mental life is concerned with these topics, all of early childhood is repressed—except a couple of banal *screen memories* that aid repression by giving the person something to remember. Recall that the major goal of psychoanalysis is to lift the repressive barrier so that patients can acknowledge and cope realistically with their primitive instinctual urges. Other theories emphasize the relationship between cognitive processes employed at encoding and retrieval. For example, Schachtel proposed that memories encoded by pre-oedipal, primary-process modes of thought cannot be retrieved by post-oedipal, secondary-process schemata. A similar account can be offered from Piaget's perspective, emphasizing the incompatibility between sensory-motor and preoperational encodings and the retrieval processes characteristic of concrete and formal operations. Note that all these theories predict that memories of childhood experience should be accessible to young children, who have not undergone the "five-to-seven shift." In contrast, some theorists have argued that young children simply do not possess the information-processing capacity—specifically, the ability to pay attention to two things at once, like an event and its episodic context—required to encode retrievable memories. In this case, the prediction is that children will know little more about their childhood histories than adults do. [*See* COGNITIVE DEVELOPMENT.]

It should be noted that infantile and childhood amnesias affect only memories for personal experiences. Children acquire a vast fund of information, and a considerable repertoire of cognitive and motor skills, which they carry into adulthood. Whether this selectivity reflects merely the effects of constant rehearsal, or reveals a dissociation between EM and IM similar to that observed in the clinical amnesias, is not clear.

At the other end of the life cycle, it appears that even the healthy aged have difficulty learning new information and remembering recent events. Aging has little effect on primary or short-term memory, as reflected in digit span or the recency component of the serial-position curve; but it has substantial effects on secondary or long-term memory, especially after moderately long retention intervals. Again, the deficit primarily affects episodic memory: the elderly do not lose their fund of semantic information (although they may be slower on such tasks as word-finding) and their repertoire of procedural knowledge remains intact, provided that they have been able to maintain these skills through practice.

At the same time, it should be noted that episodic-semantic comparisons almost inevitably confound type of memory with retention interval. Memories for recent experiences have, by definition, been encoded recently; most semantic knowledge was acquired while the individual was relatively young. Surprisingly, little is known about the ability of older individuals to learn new vocabulary or acquire new world knowledge. The aged do show an impairment in episodic memory for remote events, but it is not clear whether this reflects age differences in retrieval processes or simply the effects of the retention interval and opportunities for proactive and retroactive interference.

A relatively recent topic in research on aging memory compares EM and IM. Compared to the young, the aged show definite impairments on EM (especially free recall, less so on recognition); but they show less deficit, or none at all, on IM tasks such as stem-completion. Part of the reason for their problems with EM may lie in the difficulty that the elderly have in processing contextual information. Spatial context, temporal context, and source are necessary for distinguishing one event from another, and thus crucial to conscious recollection. Whether this difficulty is specific to contextual features of events, or merely a reflection of a more general limitation on cognitive resources, is unclear.

Memory problems are confounded in the dement-

ing illnesses often associated with aging, e.g., Alzheimer's disease (AD). The severe memory problems associated with AD are likely related to the increase of neuritic plaques and neurofibrillary tangles, particularly in medial temporal regions of the brain. These changes, as well as neuronal loss and depletion of neurotransmitters in other cortical and subcortical areas, contribute to the extensiveness of the disease process. Both AA and RA emerge early in the course of these diseases and progressively worsen. In contrast to the amnesic syndrome, however, the memory deficit in dementia affects primary as well as secondary memory and forms part of a larger cluster of deficits affecting a broad swath of cognitive and emotional life, including the loss of premorbid semantic and procedural knowledge as well as episodic memory. In the latter stages of their illness, demented patients may show *anosognosia* or a lack of awareness of their deficits. [*See* ALZHEIMER'S DISEASE; DEMENTIA.]

Does the abnormal forgetting observed in aging and dementia extend to implicit as well as explicit memory? Research on this question is still at a very early stage, but already it seems fairly clear that implicit memory is relatively spared in normal aging. Thus, elderly subjects will fail to recognize studied words, but show priming effects on word-fragment completion. With respect to AD and other forms of dementia, however, some controversy remains. There is some evidence of intact motor-skill learning in AD patients, but there is also evidence of impaired performance on priming tasks. The issue is complicated by the fact that AD is a progressive illness. Although impairments in explicit memory may be observed quite early in the course of the disease, deterioration of implicit memory may wait until later stages.

V. AMNESIAS OF EVERYDAY EXPERIENCE

Amnesia is a symptom of neurological or psychiatric disorder, but it is also something that occurs in the ordinary course of everyday living. The most familiar example is sleep. A great deal transpires while we are asleep, including events in the external environment and endogenous activity such as dreams, nightmares, and (in some cases) episodes of somnambulism (sleepwalking) and somniloquy (sleeptalking), but virtually none of this is remembered in the morning. In fact, our inability to remember what has been happening is often the phenomenological basis for inferring that we have been asleep. Similarly, attempts at sleep learning have been almost uniformly unsuccessful, leading investigators to conclude that we are able to learn during sleep only to the extent that we stay awake. [*See* Sleep.]

Most investigators explain sleep-induced amnesia in terms of an encoding deficit or consolidation failure. According to this view, the low levels of cortical arousal characteristic of sleep effectively impair complex information-processing functions. Thus, events in the environment are not noticed, relevant information in memory is not retrieved, and traces of new experiences are not encoded in retrievable form. Some evidence favoring this view comes from studies of memory for dreams. Sleepers who are awakened during REM sleep almost invariably report a dream, apparently by virtue of retrieval from primary memory; but dreams are rarely reported upon awakening in the morning, a task that requires access to trace information in secondary memory. However, subjects will remember a dream in the morning if they awaken directly out of REM sleep. And dreams reported during REM awakenings will be accessible in the morning, provided that the dreamer has remained awake long enough to rehearse the dream before returning to sleep. [*See* Dreaming.]

Most evidence of sleep-induced amnesia comes from studies of EM, leading to speculation that evidence of memory for sleep events, including successful sleep learning, might be obtained with measures of IM. Research on this topic has only just begun, but the available evidence is negative. When care is taken to ensure that there is no evidence of cortical arousal indicative of awakening, subjects show neither EM nor IM for events that occurred while they were sleeping. Even if positive evidence for sleep learning were obtained, it would almost certainly not be as efficient as learning in the normal waking state.

Amnesia is also an important component of general anesthesia induced in surgical patients. Clinically, the success of general anesthesia is indicated by the patient's lack of response to instructions, suppression of autonomic and skeletal responses to incisions and other surgical stimuli, and absence of retrospective awareness of pain and other events occurring during surgery. Thus, by definition, amnesia is a consequence of adequate general anesthesia. But, as with sleep, the amnesia is always assessed in terms of EM, leaving

open the possibility that even adequately anesthetized patients might show IM for surgical events. Some anecdotal evidence favoring this proposition is provided by occasional cases in which patients awaken from surgery with an inexplicable dislike of their surgeon— an attitudinal change which is plausibly traced to unkind remarks made about the patient by members of the surgical team.

In recent years, this question has been the object of considerable investigation, and in fact research employing paradigms derived from studies of the amnesic syndrome has sometimes, but not always, provided evidence of spared IM. Thus, patients who are presented a list of words during surgery sometimes show significant priming effects. Such effects are not always obtained, however; and even when they are obtained, they are relatively small. Certainly the scope of information processing during general anesthesia cannot compare to what is possible when the patient is awake and properly oriented; for example, IM after anesthesia may well be limited to the processing of the physical properties of stimuli, but not their meaning. What accounts for the different outcomes across the available research is not clear. Perhaps some anesthetic agents impair EM but spare IM, while others impair both. Such a result might yield interesting insights about the biological foundations of memory.

VI. THEORETICAL AND PRACTICAL IMPLICATIONS

Research on amnesia is intrinsically interesting, but it also has theoretical and pragmatic implications. At the theoretical level, amnesia engages our attention because it seems to carve nature at its joints. Amnesia is selective, and the difference between those aspects of memory that are impaired in amnesia and those that are spared promises to provide information about the processes underlying memory functioning and the organization of memory into different systems. Such conclusions are based on the *logic of dissociation*. In *single dissociations*, variable A affects performance on task Y but not task Z; in *double dissociations*, variable A affects Y but not Z, while variable B affects Z but not Y; in *reversed associations*, changes in A increase Y and decrease Z, while changes in B decrease Y and increase Z; in *stochastic independence*, performance on task Y is uncorrelated with performance on task Z. All other things being equal, differences such as these suggest that the tasks in question differ in qualitative terms. If they were only quantitatively different, they would be correlated with each other and influenced by the same variables.

Such dissociations are commonly observed in amnesia. For example, the fact that the amnesic syndrome affects the recency portion of the serial-position curve, but not the primacy component, has been cited as evidence that primary (short-term) and secondary (long-term) memory are qualitatively different memory systems, perhaps with different biological substrates (one affected by the brain lesion, the other not). Evidence from amnesia also has been used to support other structural distinctions: between declarative and procedural knowledge and, within the domain of declarative knowledge, between episodic and semantic memory. Thus, amnesic patients have difficulty learning new factual information, but retain an ability to acquire new cognitive and motor skills; and if they do retain new factual knowledge, they display an amnesia for the circumstances in which this information was acquired. Logic and experience tell us that when something breaks, it tends to do so along natural boundaries, which form lines of least resistance. When a disorder of memory separates past memory from new learning, procedural and declarative knowledge, or episodic and semantic memory, it tells us that these distinctions, conjured in the minds of theorists, actually mean something in the real world. The fact that these kinds of dissociations are observed in all sorts of amnesia—not just the amnesic syndrome, but in traumatic retrograde amnesia, psychogenic amnesia, and posthypnotic amnesia as well—strengthens the conclusion that the theoretical distinctions are psychologically and biologically valid.

Of particular interest in recent theory are the various dissociations between explicit and implicit expressions of episodic memory. To date, three broad classes of theories have been proposed to explain these dissociations; each has several exemplars. According to the *activation* view, the activation, by a current event, of pre-existing knowledge representations is sufficient for IM; but EM requires elaborative activity, in which individually activated structures are related to each other. According to the *processing* view, IM is an automatic consequence of environmental stimulation, while EM occurs by virtue of controlled processes that

are limited by attentional resources. According to the *memory systems* view, IM reflects the activity of a perceptual representation system, which holds information about the form and structure of the objects of perception, and EM reflects the activity of an episodic memory system that represents knowledge about the meaning of events and the context in which they occur.

Research on the amnesic syndrome, including studies of both human patients and animal models, indicates that the medial-temporal lobe, including the hippocampus, entorhinal cortex, and perirhinal and parahippocampal cortex, forms the biological substrate of explicit memory. But the diencephalic form of amnesic syndrome seems to indicate that the mammillary bodies and the dorsomedial nucleus of the thalamus are also critical for memory. As research continues, investigation of amnesia will make a unique and valuable contribution to understanding the relation between explicit and implicit memory, and the biological foundations of each.

At the same time, evidence of preserved memory functioning offers new insights concerning amelioration and rehabilitation in cases of amnesia. Loss of explicit memory has debilitating consequences for afflicted individuals in everyday life. They are often unable to keep track of events, remember appointments or schedules, engage in educational or vocational pursuits, or manage home activities. Attempts at rehabilitation have frequently focused on restoration of damaged explicit memory processes either through the use of repetitive drills or by teaching patients mnemonic strategies such as visual imagery or verbal elaboration. These retraining attempts have met with limited success. There is no evidence that exercising damaged neural or cognitive mechanisms leads to positive outcomes; and although patients have sometimes been able to acquire a few pieces of information by using mnemonic techniques, they do not use the strategies spontaneously in everyday life.

On the other hand, rehabilitation strategies that have focused on providing compensatory devices designed to bypass problems in daily life have been somewhat more promising. External aids such as notebooks, diaries, alarm watches, and environmental labels have enabled some amnesic patients to function somewhat more independently, although use of such devices often requires considerable amounts of training and practice. The microcomputer, potentially a powerful prosthetic for people with memory impairments, has yet to be extensively used for this purpose.

The finding that implicit and procedural memory often remain intact even in cases of severe amnesia has recently prompted researchers to begin to explore ways in which these preserved processes might be exploited beneficially for rehabilitation purposes. Cuing techniques, which take advantage of amnesic patients' ability to respond normally to word-stem or fragment cues, have been used successfully to teach individuals new factual information such as vocabulary as well as procedural tasks such as data-entry and word-processing. Continued research in this direction, paralleling more theoretically based research concerning preserved memory functions in amnesia, should enable further progress toward improving the ability of amnesic individuals to function effectively in their everyday lives.

ACKNOWLEDGMENTS

Preparation of this article, and the research that supports the point of view represented herein, was supported by Grants MH35856 from the National Institute of Mental Health and AG09195 from the National Institute of Aging, the McDonnell-Pew Program in Cognitive Neuroscience, and the Flinn Foundation. We thank Terrence Barnhardt, Jeffrey Bowers, Jennifer Dorfman, Martha Glisky, Michael Polster, Barbara Routhieaux, Victor Shames, Michael Valdiserri, and Susan Valdiserri for their comments.

This article has been reprinted from the *Encyclopedia of Human Behavior, Volume 1.*

BIBLIOGRAPHY

Eich, E. (1990). Learning during sleep. In "Sleep and Cognition" (R. R. Bootzin, J. F. Kihlstrom, and D. L. Schacter, Eds.). pp. 88–108. American Psychological Association, Washington, DC.

Glisky, E. L., and Schacter, D. L. (1989). Models and methods of memory rehabilitation. In "Handbook of Neuropsychology" (F. Boller and J. Grafman, Eds.), Vol. 3, Part 5, pp. 233–346. Elsevier, Amsterdam.

Kihlstrom, J. F., and Schacter, D. L. (1990). Anaesthesia, amnesia, and the cognitive unconscious. In "Memory and Awareness in Anaesthesia" (B. Bonke, W. Fitch, and K. Millar, Eds.), pp. 21–44. Swets & Zeitlinger, Amsterdam.

Schacter, D. L., and Kihlstrom, J. F. (1989). Functional amnesia. In "Handbook of Neuropsychology" (F. Boller and J. Grafman, Eds.), Vol. 3, pp. 209–231. Elsevier, Amsterdam.

Shimamura, A. P. (1989). Disorders of memory: The cognitive science perspective. In "Handbook of Neuropsychology" (F. Boller and J. Grafman, Eds.), Vol. 3, Part 5, pp. 35–74. Elsevier, Amsterdam.

Squire, L. R., Knowlton, B. J., and Musen, G. (1993). The structure and organization of memory. *Annu. Rev. Neurosci.* **44,** 453–495.

Tulving, E., and Schacter, D. L. (1990). Priming and human memory systems. *Science* **247,** 301–306.

Anger

Dolf Zillmann

The University of Alabama

Aggression   The infliction of pain, minor or severe injury, permanent mutilation, or total destruction on another person or organism.

Anger   The noxious experience of annoyance for which someone or something is held accountable and that inspires hostile and aggressive dispositions and actions toward the instigating agents or conditions.

Cautious Disengagement   A strategy of anger and aggression control based on the detection of symptoms of escalating arousal that creates the conditions under which violence is imminent.

Cognitive Deficit   The transitory mental incapacitation associated with intense emotional experiences. In acute anger, for instance, cognitive deficit manifests itself in the preoccupation with immediate retaliatory actions and the inability to consider the nonimmediate consequences of such actions.

Excitation Transfer   The summation of arousal from different sources that fosters overly intense and often inappropriate reactions to immediate stimulation, such as provocation and endangerment.

Excitatory Escalation   The incrementation of arousal in acute emotional states. In anger, for instance, excitation increases with repeated provocations during conflict, eventually producing the conditions for rage and impulsive aggression.

Hostility   The disposition to inflict harm on another person or organism and/or the actual infliction of harm to these agents. Harm is broadly conceived as anything that fosters annoyance and related forms of mental anguish.

Rage   A state of intense emotional experience associated with uncontrolled destructive behavior.

ANGER and its dispositional properties are detailed in this article, along with the essential expressive and motivational components of the anger experience. In a psychobiological analysis, the utility of anger in early human evolution is specified, and the loss of much of this utility in contemporary societies is traced. The cognitive and excitatory manifestations of anger, especially the interdependencies between these processes, are then elaborated in a psychophysiological and neuroendocrine examination. Strategies are presented for the control of the escalation of anger and the prevention of aggressive outbursts with their destructive behavioral consequences. Finally, the pathogenic effects of anger are addressed. Special attention is given to the consequences of dysfunctional anger for coronary artery and heart disease.

I. CONCEPTIONS OF ANGER

Anger is a universal experience. Its profound role in human affairs has been documented in the earliest recorded cultures, and there is every reason to believe that it pervaded interactions in preliterate societies and even in the earliest groupings of hominids. It has remained abundant and obtrusive in contemporary society, crossing all ethnic boundaries as well as personality distinctions. Although substantial individual and situational variation in the manifestations of anger is apparent, virtually nobody can claim not to have experienced the transitory state referred to as anger.

If the experience is universal, the conception of the experience is not. Different cultures have focused on different aspects of the experience, and they have differently judged, in moral terms, the expression of anger. Morally derived rules for the expression of anger aside, different conceptions of anger also abound in contemporary Western societies, and no single conception of anger could be considered generally accepted.

Imagine, for instance, a student who received a bad grade for an exam. A student who expected a good grade might be discontent with his professor, blame him for the grade, and feel angry toward him. However, a student who recognizes his inferior performance might blame himself and thus feel anger toward himself. It would seem legitimate for him to say that he is angry at himself. Some psychiatrists and psychologists have embraced this common-language concept of self-directed anger. Others have not. Anger, in these others' view, has to have an external inducing agent, and it has to be directed at that agent. Self-directed anger, they suggest, is more appropriately characterized as frustration, irritation, or annoyance with oneself.

The student in our illustration could, of course, also blame himself, but respond with disappointment and sadness to his failure. This possible reaction reveals that anger, more than other response alternatives, implies a tendency to do something about the situation that caused it. Disappointment and sadness imply an inducing condition, but do not seem to carry with them a disposition to act on this condition. If anything, the concepts convey inaction and withdrawal. Frustration, irritation, and annoyance are similarly linked to inducing conditions, but also indicate little by way of action toward these conditions. If action is indicated, it is self-directed. The proverbial frustrated person who pulls her hair in distress or despair comes to mind. Such self-directed attacks seem to justify the application of the anger concept. Unlike disappointment and sadness, frustration, irritation, and annoyance appear to have a dispositional component that

urges action—although this action tends to be inwardly directed or is without direction.

The fact that anger proper has a strong dispositional component that is squarely directed at the agent held accountable for instigating the experience is readily illustrated. Imagine a person unable to collect a soft drink from a vending machine that took his money. The person is apt to pound the machine with his bare fists. Imagine a housewife who, after cleaning all day long, finds that the puppy soiled the new couch. She is liable to kick the dog. Imagine a lady who has been stood up by a date. She is bound to decide on punitive action and is likely to execute it at a later time. Or imagine a husband in an argument with his wife as she discloses affairs with several men. His anger is likely to erupt in violent action against his wife and possibly against her lovers.

Anger, then, appears to have a dispositional component that (a) favors action over inaction and that (b) is directed at the agents deemed responsible for the anger experience. With the exception of self-directed anger, anger characteristically addresses external agents.

It is generally agreed that anger is a noxious experience that motivates actions that are designed to terminate this experience or, at least, diminish its intensity. Anger is thus viewed as an emotion with an experiential and a dispositional component. It is also agreed that anger, as an emotion, is associated with physiological arousal that determines its experiential and dispositional intensity. Coercion and destruction "in cold blood" are thought to be inconsistent with anger and emotional upheaval. A state of physiological arousal is a necessary, although clearly not a sufficient, condition of anger. [*See* EMOTIONS AND MENTAL HEALTH.]

Conceptualized in these terms, it should be clear that the experience of anger is difficult to separate from its dispositional component. Empirical efforts at separating experience and disposition have been of dubious value. Conceptually, a distinction can be drawn. It is also of dubious value, however. Recent theorizing makes the consciousness of anger dependent upon the stream of cognition, expressed linguistically in mature language users, at the time of the emotion. This makes it likely that idiosyncratic covert verbal dispositional reactions (such as "You bastard, I'll show you!" or simply "F. . . you!") are primarily responsible for persons' cognizance of their anger.

The covert verbal flow may, of course, involve self-directed hostility ("God, I'm stupid!") or it may be specific to experience ("Boy, does he make me mad!"). The point to be made is that dispositional recognition may often precede experiential recognition, which indicates the futility of separating the two naturally confounded components.

What is it that induces the emotion of anger? Broadly speaking, it is the threat to a person's physical, social, and mental welfare. Direct physical assault defines one extreme. The possibility of diminished self-esteem the other. In between are all endangerments of the body and all threats thereof. The loss of social standing and power, as well as the threat thereof, are similarly potent inducers of anger. So are actual or threatened attacks on a person's possessions or things held dear, such as houses and cars, friends and pets, tastes and convictions of any kind, as well as aesthetic preferences. Much of the latter is a matter of personal judgment and may seem petty when compared to physical assaults. It would be a grievous mistake, however, to conclude that threats of nonphysical harm would be less important in the evocation of anger than actual physical endangerments. Imagine someone who challenges another's musical taste or sense of humor. Especially when presented condescendingly, it undoubtedly can infuriate the offended party.

Perceptions of injustice done to self and intimate affiliates may be considered the primary inducers of anger in modern society. Violations of generally accepted rules of conduct, however trivial, are bound to evoke anger when they can be construed as deliberate. For instance, a man's reluctance to bend down to retrieve an earring dropped by his date is likely to foster anger and the termination of the date. Nothing seems as anger-provoking, however, as perceived injustice in the distribution of incentives. Imagine two employees who are both granted a substantial raise in salary. If one, for whatever reason, perceives that his competitor's raise should have been lower and his own higher, anger will be acute, and residual anger will linger for indefinite periods—all this despite having been benefited by a raise in salary. It is this human capacity for moral reasoning that can be considered pivotal in the evocation of much anger.

What is it that the emotion of anger motivates? Oddly, it is the capacity for moral reasoning that again creates major problems. Those who have this capacity are inclined to retaliate, attempting to recompense aversion suffered with a similar or higher amount of aversion inflicted upon their annoyer. The intent to punish those who have wronged and thus angered us is, of course, a manifestation of moral reasoning. This reasoning tends to make us unforgiving for anger suffered. In particular, the morally derived urge to "get even" inspires hostile action even when such action is unlikely to have utility beyond relieving the experience of anger.

Although the dispositional component of anger is mostly seen as the instigator of hostile and punitive action, anger need not be expressed in these terms. Anger may be suppressed and thus may be without aversive, destructive consequences for others. Anger may also be redirected and it may intensify efforts at correcting the conditions that induced it. Self-directed anger about a poor performance on an exam, for instance, could be rechanneled and inspire a commitment to put more effort into preparing for the next exam. Such redirection of an angry disposition tends to be applauded as a constructive use of anger. It should be recognized, however, that the hostile expression of anger can also be constructive—though in a different way. Depending on the specific social circumstances, verbal and physical retaliation may restore lost esteem, prestige, and power. At the very least it offers the shortest route to recovery from a noxious experience and the restoration of feelings of well-being. On the other hand, if the hostile expression of anger fails to restore losses and it prompts further conflict, if it even escalates the conflict, acting on anger becomes counterproductive. Not acting out anger, but suppressing it, may seem a constructive option under the indicated circumstances. However, as we shall see, inaction has its cost, and it may not be as constructive an option as it appears to be. [See SELF-ESTEEM.]

Consideration of these aspects of the experience of anger and its behavioral expression suggests the following set of working definitions.

Anger is an emotion characterized by the intertwined operation of an experiential and a dispositional response component. Physiological arousal is a necessary but not a sufficient condition for acute anger. The dispositional component of anger favors action over inaction without, however, compelling action. The behavioral expression of anger favors hostile action over nonhostile alternatives without, however, compelling hostile action. Whether the suppression or expression of anger is constructive or counterproductive is a function of social circumstances.

II. THE PSYCHOBIOLOGY OF ANGER

The fact that acute anger is invariably associated with a state of physiological arousal and agitation is thought to have its roots in the evolution of humankind. For early hominids who encountered physical danger, be it in the form of hostile others of their own kind or of predators and similar tooth-and-claw-equipped animals, it was undoubtedly advantageous to be quasi-instantaneously supplied with energy for effective coping—either to attack the threat and ward it off or to escape from it and thereby ward it off. The well-known fight-and-flight paradigm expresses the essentials of this process: The recognition of danger is viewed as triggering a rapid bodily energization that is to serve vigorous action for the relatively short period of fighting or fleeing. Meticulous analyses of fighting in various mammalian species show, in fact, that vigorous skirmishes rather quickly deplete the immediately generated energy supplies and exhaust the animals. [See EVOLUTION AND MENTAL HEALTH.]

Getting aroused, agitated, and energized when scared or angry in the confrontation with endangering conditions, thereby being prepared for superior coping through fight and flight, appears to have served humans well in earlier times. Being aroused when afraid or aggravated had utility. Some degree of this utility has been retained in vigorous displays of anger and in the performance of violent action. For instance, temper tantrums still signal the depth of an angry reaction, even the strength of the willingness to fight physically to resolve an issue. Such signaling can intimidate opponents and persuade them to yield and compromise. The seemingly raw expression of anger in a fit of bad temper thus can be seen as a coercive strategy that is effective on occasion. More importantly, going on a violent rampage and beating someone into submission, when this can be done with impunity or under conditions where attainable benefits outweigh repercussions, also constitutes effective strategy—but apparently only as long as the stipulated conditions prevail, which they hardly ever do. However, the utility of such archaic vigorous action

as a means of coping with threats and dangers, and of resolving social conflict, has been lost for the most part. The conditions of life in contemporary society have severely compromised the adaptive value of getting aroused in preparation for fight and flight. Responding with emotional agitation to threats to self-esteem, social status and power, or economic security not only tends to lack adaptive utility, but is often counterproductive. Rather than assisting coping, the supply of energy for action is likely to be maladaptive, creating rather than resolving problems. More often than not, responding with acute anger to provocation has less utility than more controlled, cautious, thought-out reactions. For example, the burst of energy in response to an erroneous bill from the Internal Revenue Service is bound to fuel irritation and anger, but probably functions as an impediment to successful, clarifying negotiations with representatives of the institution. Analogously, such provision of energy is a hindrance rather than a help for an angry employee who feels he has been wronged by his boss, a mother who is annoyed with her screaming baby, or a student who suffered humiliation before his peers by an undiplomatic professor. The fight–flight arousal reaction, finally, also does not help us resolve broad social problems, such as global pollution. The burst of energy is neither helpful in solving these problems through attack, nor by running away from them. [See COPING WITH STRESS.]

The psychobiological analysis of anger thus suggests that, although most aggravations of life in contemporary society cannot be averted or combated with physical force, the archaic agonistic reaction tendencies exert their influence nonetheless. As in earlier days, we do get excited when provoked; and we are being prepared to hit and run, even though this preparation offers no way out. We still get hot under the collar and erupt in angry expression when staying calm and collected in devising conflict-resolving strategies would better serve our welfare and self-interest.

It is this archaic response tendency, then, that the psychobiological analysis implicates with the problems and the mismanagement of much acute anger. As we shall see, the psychophysiological examination of this archaic condition reveals its secrets and thereby provides us with means for the construction of strategies to minimize and possibly remove its influence on the experience of anger, along with its consequences for overt aggression.

III. THE PSYCHOPHYSIOLOGY OF ANGER

In emotion theory, the experience of anger is thought to be controlled by three basic interdependent response components. First, there is a *dispositional* component that directs overt behavior. This component integrates reflexive, acquired, and planned motor reactions. At the elementary level are reactions such as raising the arms to cover the face in order to protect it against rapidly approaching objects. Yelling and screaming, slamming the fist on the table, and grabbing an annoyer by the throat are learned and usually well-practiced reactions. Other reactions may have been contemplated but not practiced, their enactment awaiting opportune circumstances. Second, an *excitatory* component exists that serves the energization of the dispositionally guided behavior. Third, an *experiential* component functions as a monitor of overt action. Higher brain processes are enlisted to plan the expression of affect and the performance of actions, to assess their appropriateness and effectiveness during execution, and to redirect or terminate the actions if necessary. This component is thus burdened with the correction of behavior that is initially controlled by more elementary or basal processes.

To illustrate: A patron of a fine restaurant, who had piping hot coffee spilled over his hand by a clumsy waitress, might scream in pain and cover his hand protectively—as if to prevent further assault on it. Such reactions are the result of spontaneous, unlearned dispositional guidance. He may then experience intense agitation and feel infuriated, this being the result of the excitatory factor. As a consequence of his intensely felt anger he might shout vulgarities at the waitress, especially so if such expression is frequently used and constitutes a habit. Behavior guidance reverts to acquired dispositions in this case. Finally, our angry diner, by surveying the facial reactions of his companions and other patrons to his hostility, might recognize the inappropriateness of his hostile action, redirect his behavior, and profusely apologize to his annoyer. This would be the result of the experiential or monitoring function that, in this case, served as a corrective.

In order to comprehend emotions, the emotion of anger in particular, it is imperative to understand the operation and interplay of the indicated response components. There are critical differences, first of all, in the volitional control of these components. The experiential component can be seen as manifesting such control. Activity in the neocortex mediates cognition that expresses itself in the assessment and evaluation of external and, to a lesser degree, internal circumstances. Monitoring and judgment provide behavioral guidance, guidance that is imposed on the dispositional component.

Motor behavior may be reflexive, learned, or follow scripts and prescriptions. Incipient reactions that are mediated by mechanisms of learning, for instance, can readily be halted and redirected by the monitoring function. As in our scalded-patron example, initial rage, once deemed inappropriate, can be stopped and corrected with apologies. Overt expression and action, then, are to a high degree under volitional control.

In contrast, evocation, regulation, and withdrawal of excitatory reactions largely elude volitional control. These processes are organized in ancient structures of the brain, the limbic system, and are comparatively rigid. Moreover, they are humorally mediated, which makes them sluggish and lethargic. Excitatory processes are essentially controlled by hormones released into systemic blood, where they are active until metabolized. The humoral mediation of excitation, then, is mechanical in the sense that, once a reaction is triggered, it runs its course. Monitoring cannot turn off this process, once in motion. It can, however, foster reinterpretations of the anger-inducing conditions and thereby slow and halt the so-called counterregulation of excitation.

Because the time course of excitatory reactions is crucial in disarming the destructive potency of acute anger, we shall briefly discuss the specific mediation of the essential excitatory processes associated with anger and related emotions.

A. Excitation in Anger

Emotions, anger in particular, that appear to favor the resolution of conflict and the termination of annoyance by immediate vigorous actions are associated with substantial excitatory activity that is mediated primarily by the adrenomedullary system, but also by the adrenocortical system.

Activity in the adrenomedullary system, through the release of catecholamines and their fast but short-lived hyperglycemic effect, provides energy for essentially one behavioral engagement. The energization is said to be phasic or episodic. It is energy for one fit of angry expression or one course of vigorous hostile action.

Activity in the adrenocortical system, mainly through the release of glucocorticoids and their hyperglycemic effect, also generates energy, but does so for extended periods of time. This energization is said to be tonic. Such tonic energization is part of the coping response to social and environmental stressors.

In the production of their sympathomimetic effect, the two systems operate in an integrated fashion. Heightened activity in the adrenocortical system usually defines the undercurrent for acute anger and other agitated emotions. It places the organism in a state of increased action readiness. It creates, among other things, superior conditions for anger and aggressive responsiveness, and it does so tonically. Agonistic reactions build on this foundation. Phasic excitation from heightened activity in the adrenomedullary system combines with tonic excitation, and this combination creates agonistic reactions of potentially great intensity.

The correspondence between the duration of tonic or phasic excitation, on the one hand, and the time course of the stimulation that induces the excitatory reactions under consideration, on the other, is usually very poor. This poorness of fit, which is mainly the result of the humoral nature of the mediating agents, proves to have significant consequences for anger and angry aggression.

Stressful stimulation fosters heightened adrenocortical activity only after a considerable latency period. More importantly, the activity may persist for hours and days after the termination of the stressful stimulation. Individuals suffering from stress induced by conditions external to specific conflicts thus carry adrenocortical activity along into these conflicts. It is this circumstance that increases their vulnerability to anger escalation and to impulsive aggression. [*See* STRESS.]

Anger-inducing stimulation fosters heightened activity in the adrenomedullary system also only after some latency. The latency is a matter of seconds, however, and has little practical significance. The period of time during which the excitatory reaction persists is again more important. The time beyond the cessation of annoyance and provocation is a matter of minutes. These minutes may seem unimportant, but turn out to be crucial in the escalation of anger and angry aggression.

Table I Neuroendocrine, Autonomic, and Behavioral Differentiation of Anger and Fear

Response Component	Acute Emotion	
	Anger	Fear
Limbic System Mediation	Amygdalar Central Nucleus	Amygdalar Basal Nucleus
Neuroendocrine Pattern		
Norepinephrine	markedly up	slightly up
Epinephrine	slightly up	markedly up
Renin	markedly up	uncertain
Testosterone	markedly up	uncertain
Cortisol	normal	slightly up
Autonomic Pattern		
Blood Pressure	markedly up	slightly up
Heart Rate	markedly up	slightly up
Behavioral Manifestation	fight, effort	flight, effort

Note. Adapted from Henry, J. P. (1986). Neuroendocrine patterns of emotional response. In R. Plutchick & H. Kellerman (Eds.), *Emotion: Theory, research, and experience. Vol. 3. Biological foundations of emotion* (pp. 37–60). Orlando, FL: Academic Press.

It should be mentioned that other hormones and hormonal systems, such as testosterone of the pituitary gonadal axis, are also involved in the potentiation of anger and angry aggression. Table 1 summarizes the excitatory mediation of anger in comparison with that of fear.

B. Excitatory Escalation in Anger

Escalating conflict can be conceptualized as a sequence of provocations, each triggering an excitatory reaction that materializes quickly and that dissipates slowly. If a second sympathetic reaction occurs before the first has dissipated, the second reaction combines with the tail end of the first. Moreover, if a third reaction occurs before the second and first reactions have dissipated, this third reaction combines with the tail ends of both earlier reactions. From this follows the principle that any excitatory reaction to provocation late in the escalation process rides the tails of all earlier excitatory reactions. It also follows that the combination of residual sympathetic excitation from earlier provocations with the excitation in response to a subsequent provocation will produce anger and angry aggression of an intensity that appears to be incommensurate with the subsequent provocation. Sympathetic excitation is at artificially high levels, and these overly high levels are bound to foster overly intense feelings of anger and a propensity for overly intense outbursts of violence.

C. Transfer of Excitation into Anger

The excitatory escalation of anger is greatly complicated by the fact that portions of excitation from sources other than provocation can enter into the bulk of excitation that fuels episodes of anger and outrage. Whereas the excitatory patterns of emotions can show marked differences (e.g., between fear and elation), emotions characterized by sympathetic dominance in the autonomic nervous system share all essential elements. Commonality of excitatory components has been proposed for the trichotomy of fight, flight, and sexual behavior. Expressed in terms of emotion, anger, fear, and sexual excitedness are seen as sharing the behavior-energizing mediation and hence their excitatory patterns. Because of this sharing, excitation induced by fear or sexual excitedness should readily combine with excitation uniquely associated with anger. Under the assumption that we do not carefully trace from where our excitation comes, the confounding of excitation goes unnoticed.

From such theorizing it follows that residual excitation from fear or sexual excitedness should be capable of intensifying experiences of acute anger as well as the intensity of violent outbursts. More important here, such intensification has been amply documented by pertinent research.

D. Cognition in Anger

The primary function of cognition is to guide behavior. A most immediate objective of such guidance is the avoidance of harm and the minimization of aversion. The attainment of gratifications is often an attached objective.

Regarding the evocation of anger, cognition initially serves to monitor for threats to the individual's welfare and well-being. Such threats, once recognized, are subjected to an appraisal that determines their severity. For instance, a seemingly offensive remark or a confrontational disagreement in a discussion are screened for hostile intent, or harsh performance criticism from the boss is evaluated in terms of both its justification and its social consequences. Such appraisal thus concerns the circumstances that evoked anger as well as the damage done by the incident.

If this appraisal shows the anger-provoking action to be deliberate, unwarranted, and unjust (which, given the self-serving nature of the assessment, it usually does), cognition further serves the preparation of counterreactions. This preparation entails the anticipation of affective and social consequences from (a) the open expression of anger, (b) the expression of hostile intent and threats, and (c) the perpetration of retaliatory action in verbal or physical form. Depending upon these preappraisals, great anticipated aversion and severe repercussions will demand the inhibition of angry expression and retaliatory measures. Anticipated relief and gratification as well as minimal or no repercussions, on the other hand, will yield fits of expressed anger and retaliatory action. The anticipation of consequences is, of course, subject to miscalculation. An employee, for instance, who thought that an obvious misjudgment on the part of his boss could be corrected by an angry rebuttal, may learn otherwise and come to suffer the wrath of additional misjudgment. [See EMOTION AND COGNITION.]

Finally, appraisals are not applied just once, but repeatedly. Anger is commonly instigated in dynamic, reciprocal social exchanges. There is an ongoing give and take by the involved parties. The circumstances thus need to be continually appraised, preappraised, and reappraised.

E. Cognition–Excitation Interdependencies in Anger

Acute anger is consistently evoked by aversive treatments that (a) are perceived to be deliberately and purposely inflicted and (b) are deemed unwarranted and unfair in the sense of violating prevailing conventions for social exchanges under given circumstances. Deliberate and unwarranted aversive treatments are apparently viewed as threats to personal welfare, and as endangerments of sorts they invariably trigger excitatory reactions. It is generally held that the magnitude of these reactions determines the intensity of felt anger. The stronger the activation of the adrenomedullary system, the stronger the agitation that fuels anger, and the higher the propensity for angry outbursts that can escalate to destructive violence.

It would appear that much of this excitatory activity

could be controlled, either by preventing its development or by facilitating its decay, if aversive treatments could be presented as unintentional and not in violation of rules of conduct. If information to that effect existed, the conveyance of this information should produce the indicated curtailment of excitation, associated anger, and the propensity for violent outbursts.

We shall present an experimental investigation to illustrate these interdependent processes. Students were severely provoked by a rude, abusive experimenter. Later on, they were given an opportunity to express their anger and to retaliate. In one condition, the students received no information about circumstances that could have made their tormentor's behavior appear less assaultive. His rudeness seemed deliberate, and the students had no alternative to appraising it as a personal attack. In the other conditions, information of mitigating circumstances was provided. The rude experimenter was said to be under a lot of stress from his preliminary doctoral examination. In one of these conditions, the students received the mitigating information prior to being mistreated. In the other, they received it after the mistreatment.

In the case of prior communication about mitigating circumstances, any seemingly hostile action on the part of the experimenter was preappraised. His actions could be attributed to stress and frustration deriving from conditions unrelated to the students' behavior. His rudeness did not have to be construed as a personal attack, and the students did not have to ready themselves for such an attack. Compared with the control condition in which mitigating information had not been communicated, the students should appraise the situation as less threatening. As a result, their excitatory reactions should be subdued, their experience of anger should be less intense, and they should be less inclined to take strong retaliatory actions.

In the case of the later communication of the same mitigating information, the students had suffered the full impact of the experimenter's rudeness. Excitatory reactions were comparatively strong, and the experience of anger was intense. The reception of the mitigating information eventually fostered a reappraisal of the circumstances. This reappraisal should remove the personal, deliberate, and arbitrary component from the mistreatment. Once such recognition materializes, excitation, now expendable, should start to dissipate, and the intensity of the experience of anger should diminish. However, as related research has shown that intensely felt anger may instigate retaliatory intentions and that these intentions may be executed "in cold blood" long after recovery from acute anger, reappraisals can not be expected to curtail retaliatory actions as effectively as preappraisals.

In the experiment, excitatory activity was monitored at critical times between provocation and retaliation. Sympathetic excitation was ascertained in peripheral manifestations (blood pressure, heart rate). The findings, summarized in Figure 1, show that students who had prior knowledge of mitigating circumstances were relatively unperturbed by the mistreatment they received. Sympathetic excitation never reached high levels, and it dissipated to particularly low levels. In contrast, the mistreatment prompted extreme excitatory reactions in students without such prior knowledge. The communication of mitigating information after the mistreatment apparently fostered a reappraisal that initiated and accelerated excitatory recovery. Excitation quickly fell below levels in the control condition in which students had not received mitigating information. But the reappraisal clearly failed to lower excitedness to levels compa-

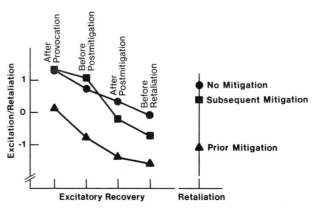

Figure I The effect of mitigating information on excitatory reactions to provocation and on retaliatory hostility. The provision of mitigating information prior to provocation (labeled Prior Mitigation) prevented strong excitatory reactions and intense feelings of anger, and it kept retaliation to a minimum. The subsequent provision of mitigating information (labeled Subsequent Mitigation or Postmitigation) accelerated the decay of excitation, but it failed to reduce retaliation effectively. Excitation and retaliation are expressed in z scores for ease of comparison. (From Zillmann, D. (1979). *Hostility and aggression.* Hillsdale, NJ: Erlbaum. Reprinted with permission.)

rable with those in students who had prior knowledge of the mitigating circumstances.

The severity of retaliatory actions proved to be proportional to levels of sympathetic excitation at the time these actions were taken. Students who received mitigating information prior to being mistreated showed considerable compassion for their tormentor. On the other hand, students who had received this information after having suffered the full blow of this treatment were almost as punitive with their tormentor as those who never learned of mitigating circumstances.

It should be pointed out that a commitment to retaliatory action that is made during the initial experience of anger is not always sustained postemotionally. In fact, individuals, once relaxed, might deem preposterous the intentions that they contemplated in the heat of passion. On the other hand, the intensity of originally felt anger may be partly revived in the reconfrontation with annoyers, and initial retaliatory intentions might be reactivated as well.

Granted remaining uncertainty about the long-term persistence of hostile, retaliatory intentions, the research at hand clarifies the influence of cognition on excitation associated with anger, and it provides a sound basis for the construction of strategies to control anger and the hostile behavior it motivates.

F. Cognitive Deficit in Acute Anger

The cognitive-deficit concept addresses the apparent inability of extremely excited and agitated persons to conceive and execute rational, effective courses of action. The deficit seems to manifest itself in all emotions associated with hypersympathetic activity. As a behavioral emergency develops and elevated sympathetic activity readies the body for fight or flight, but the environmental and social conditions are such that neither attack nor escape routes are immediately apparent, the actions taken are often patently counterproductive. People in acute fear, for instance, are known to panic and tend to do whatever others are seen doing. In earthquakes and fires, crowds often come to harm at congested exits without ever having tried others that were open and in full view. Phobic behavior is generally marked by nonproductive action selections. The same holds true for acute anger and rage. Just imagine an infuriated youngster who picks a fight with a bully of superior strength and fighting

skills, only to get his nose bloodied. Or imagine an enraged and re-enraged employee who, some time after being laid off, goes to shoot his former fellow workers and then takes his own life.

Although illustrations of strategically poor and ineffective cognitive guidance in states of rage are plentiful, the deficit concept is to be used with caution. Research suggests that this deficit is relative and selective rather than absolute. In anger, attention is focused on the immediate circumstances of threats, and the cognitive machinery is preoccupied with preparing instant reactions to them, motor reactions in particular. Such overattention comes at a cost: the relative neglect of less immediately relevant conditions, such as delayed consequences of actions taken. The cognitive deficit, then, concerns due consideration of the aftermath of anger and angry action, especially of repercussions in the form of social reproach and contingent aversive and punitive treatments.

The available research evidence suggests that during all acute emotional states attention and information processing concentrate on immediately present events—the so-called *here and now*. In anger, aversion is felt and more aversion is anticipated, prompting the planning and, conditions allowing, the execution of actions capable of terminating felt aversion and averting anticipated additional aversion. If anger in all its physical manifestations were not to materialize, individuals would be free to contemplate numerous behavioral options as well as immediate and future consequences. As acute anger develops, however, and individuals become preoccupied with the immediate situation, consideration of the implications of their actions and of future events is temporarily relegated to insignificance. It is common knowledge that persons seething with anger are concerned with immediacy to a point where they "don't give a damn" about what happens to them, as a result of actions taken in anger, tomorrow and thereafter. Their anticipatory skills concerning future coercive and punitive contingencies seem greatly diminished, indeed. Relative time (i.e., the immediacy versus future remoteness of aversive conditions) thus emerges as a relevant consideration in the anger impairment of cognition.

Another important consideration derives from stress research, specifically from the examination of anxieties. It has been proposed that worrying expresses exaggerated self-concern. Such self-concern also typifies acute anger. Analogous to anxiety, anger tends to foster a preoccupation with bad things that could happen to oneself. Little, if any, attention is given to suffering by others, especially by parties who issued threats and continue to pose dangers. This is another way of saying that, in acute anger, empathic sensitivities deteriorate and become defunct. As empathic sensitivities would stand in the way of inflicting anger-inspired harm upon annoyers, this proposal accords well with psychobiological conceptions. More importantly, however, the loss of empathy and its potential inversion to counterempathy in the face of despised and hated persons has been demonstrated in pertinent research.

The deterioration of empathic sensitivity seems of paramount importance in the consideration of anger escalation. In the initial stages of conflict, a particular provocation may have little impact because the person reacting to it is still capable of taking the opponent's perspective. At advanced stages, after this ability has faded, the same provocation may be deemed contemptuous behavior, if not an intolerable assault. In general, the later in a provocation sequence a specific provocation occurs, the greater its emotional impact is likely to be. This reasoning, it should be noticed, projects evaluative changes on the basis of altered conditions for information processing. More

specifically, it suggests that, because of changed judgmental conditions, provocations late in the escalation sequence will have a disproportionally strong effect on anger.

Finally, it has been proposed that the catecholamine and testosterone rush associated with acute anger fosters an illusion of power and invulnerability. Interoception of muscular tension may prompt exaggerated assessments of physical preparedness and strength, and such assessments may trivialize perceptions of risk and vulnerability. If so, the anticipation of success or failure with coping reactions should shift away from failure and move toward success. Anticipation of oppositional actions should be similarly trivialized. One's own physical, aggressive power, then, should be overestimated, whereas that of opponents should be underestimated. All these judgmental partialities should become manifest at exceedingly high levels of sympathetic activity. And all, it should be noticed, favor hostile and aggressive actions over noncoercive and nonaggressive alternatives. Table 2 summarizes the various processes involved in the discussed escalation from anger to acute anger and rage.

The physiological mechanics of the indicated cognitive changes during escalating anger have been the subject of much speculation. It has been suggested, for instance, that small amounts of the catechola-

Table II Stages in the Escalation of Anger

	Provocation		
Response	Stage 1	Stage 2	Stage 3
Cognitive	Exhaustive appraisal of circumstances and consequences; balanced judgment;	Selective appraisal of circumstances and consequences; increased self-concern; diminished empathy;	Severely limited appraisal of circumstances and consequences; excessive self-concern; lack of empathy; illusion of power and invulnerability;
	irritation.	annoyance, anger.	spite, hatred; reversion to established and habitual behavior.
Excitatory	Low, moderate; increment upon recognition of endangerment.	Moderate, high; residues from earlier stage;	High, excessive; residues from earlier stages;
		heightened readiness for action.	acute readiness for vigorous action.
Behavioral	Cautiously assertive, nonimpulsive, argumentative.	Strongly assertive, unyielding, hostile, aggressive.	Impulsive, explosive, irresponsible, reckless, violent.

Note. From Zillmann, D. (1994). Cognition-excitation interdependencies in the escalation of anger and angry aggression. In M. Potegal & J. F. Knutson (Eds.), *The dynamics of aggression: Biological and social processes in dyads and groups* (pp. 45–71). Hillsdale, NJ: Erlbaum.

mines that mediate sympathetic excitation in the peripheral structures, especially epinephrine and norepinephrine, cross the brain blood barrier and affect central processes that favor immediate action against threats and dangers. It has also been suggested that particularly active areas of the cortex (i.e., groups of neurons engaged by mental efforts) attract a disproportional flow of blood and energizing hormones, this at the expense of support to regions less called upon to perform. However, with regard to acute anger, the operation of such specific, cognition-mediating processes has not as yet been demonstrated.

We shall use an experiment again to summarize the workings of cognitive incapacitation in acute anger. In this investigation, male students were or were not strongly prearoused by invigorating strenuous physical exercise. The exercise consisted of riding a bicycle ergometer. This task had been shown to be affectively neutral, neither enjoyable nor irritating, tiresome, or unreasonable. The students were then provoked by a male experimenter's abusive behavior, and they were eventually provided with an opportunity to express their anger and to retaliate against their annoyer. Just prior to getting the opportunity to vent their anger and retaliate, a female confederate had occasion to enter the laboratory, calling the experimenter to the phone. He left with a snide remark, giving her a chance to comment on the fact that he was under a lot of stress from exams toward his doctorate.

At moderate levels of excitation, such mitigating information should be received, processed, applied to the circumstances, and ultimately curtail anger and retaliatory actions. Such anger-reducing effect of mitigating information has been observed in numerous investigations. At very high levels of excitation, however, the effect should not materialize because of cognitive incapacitation. The findings confirmed these expectations. In accord with the earlier observations, the conveyance of mitigating information strongly reduced anger and retaliation at moderate levels of excitation. At exceedingly high levels of excitation, in contrast, the conveyance of mitigating information proved to be without appreciable effect on anger and hostility. The implicit refusal to consider mitigating information when enraged is graphically presented in Figure 2.

Unanticipated data from this investigation suggest that mitigating information is similarly received but is processed differently at different levels of excitation.

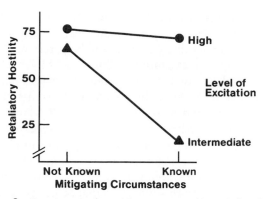

Figure 2 Impairment of cognitive response guidance in hostile behavior associated with high levels of sympathetic excitation. At intermediate levels of excitation, the conveyance of mitigating information diminished anger and retaliation. At high levels of excitation, such conveyance had no appreciable effect. (From Zillmann, D. (1979). *Hostility and aggression*. Hillsdale, NJ: Erlbaum. Reprinted with permission.)

The prearoused students apparently comprehended the information, but rejected it vehemently. Upon the confederate's revelation of stress from exams, these prearoused students uttered assessments like "That's just too bad!" Other utterances expressed the same sentiment, but in so doing used the strongest vulgarities the English language has to offer. Regardless of the intensity of the language used, however, the comments suggest that acutely angry, extremely excited and agitated persons become unforgiving and obsessed with retaliatory desire. They are determined to "get even" with their tormentors, and they appear to become oblivious to consequences such as social condemnation of their actions and likely reprisals by their opponents.

IV. THE CONTROL OF ANGER

Sociological accounts of destructive violence that is precipitated by anger and rage invariably point to the involvement of two critical conditions. (a) Acute anger and rage are rarely commensurate with the object of conflict and appear to be fueled by experiences outside the conflict proper. (b) Judgment-impairing drugs, mostly alcohol, heighten the propensity for rage and destructive violence. These truisms are readily explained by the psychophysiological analysis of anger. [*See* ALCOHOL PROBLEMS.]

Much anger may well derive from initially trivial

disagreements. To the extent that parties in conflict deem other's disagreement threatening, excitation will increase; further disagreement will be perceived more threatening, and excitation will increase to yet higher levels; and so forth. More likely, however, parties in conflict bring with them excitation from sources entirely unrelated to present conflicts. Research has shown, for instance, that following especially demanding, stressful days at work, professionals are prone to erupt in anger and even become violent in family interactions, seemingly upon minimal provocation. On days with a more manageable workload, these professionals were peaceful and unresponsive to the same provocations. Most important here, when given a chance to relax upon returning home from stressful work, they also managed provocations rather well. The physical manifestations of severe stress, then, along with the likely rumination in cognitions associated with the experience of stress, greatly facilitated and intensified angry and hostile reactions.

However, stress is by no means the only condition capable of facilitating anger and its consequences. As a rule rather than the exception, excitation that prevails at times of provocation confounds contributions from various sources. For instance, a mother, being agitated from an argument with her husband, is more likely to snap at her unruly toddler, possibly hitting the child, than when she is calm and collected. A father, excited from watching his favorite sports program, is more likely to bark and lash out at his son, who comes to tell him that he has ruined the family car, than when reading a similarly involving book. Anger is further potentiated by the use of drugs, such as alcohol. All drugs that foster impaired cognition enhance, of course, the cognitive deficit that is incurred at high levels of excitation. Less obvious is that, when sexual intimates have a row, their anger can be intensified by elements of sexual excitedness. Or that someone who is elated from winning a tennis match is prone to overreact to provocation, due to the so-called testosterone rush that is common to elation and anger.

All this is to say that, if explosive anger is to be controlled, strategies must aim at preventing (a) the build-up of excitation from singular or multiple sources and (b) the impairment of cognition that mediates the consideration of nonimmediate circumstances. Strategies embracing this dual objective have been developed for the management of anger. We shall outline their essential directives.

Social conflict that generates anger and angry aggression is dyadic in principle. Persons are angry at other persons, and anger may or may not be reciprocated. Irrespective of the uni- or bi-directionality of anger, consideration of control must address both one's own anger and that of others.

Effective self-instruction in anger management must establish and hone sensitivity to, and the comprehension of, the hostile intentions and aggressive propensities of all parties in conflict. Efforts at controlling anger, however, must be primarily self-directed, as the control over one's own behavior is potentially more effective because it does not entail the risk of faulty assumptions about another's responding. Additionally, in devising strategies for the control of anger it is necessary to recognize and distinguish domains of anger that demand specific treatments. In our presentation of control directives, we shall focus on three such domains: (a) preventing the escalation of anger, (b) averting violence, and (c) coping with post-confrontational anger.

A. Preventing the Escalation of Anger

Directive 1 If at all possible, preattribute annoying events and information about annoying events to motives and circumstances that make the induction of annoyance appear unintentional and devoid of malice, and reattribute annoying events and information about annoying events in the same manner.

Acutely angry persons invariably perceive their emotional behavior to have been deliberately provoked, with hostile purpose, by the target of their anger. As a result, they consider the expression of their anger justified and feel righteous about it. Targets of anger, on the other hand, tend to perceive the emotional behavior of those directing their anger at them as incoherent, arbitrary, and unjustified. The bridging of this perceptual and evaluative gap is imperative. Targets of others' anger are thus advised to search for mitigating circumstances of what may appear to be a deliberate personal attack. The detection of mitigating conditions—matters such as sheer awkwardness, erroneous suspicions, emotional upheaval and stress from alternative sources, even physical pain—prior to annoying revelations and happenings will help to prevent strong excitatory reactions and thus curtail anger. If this detection comes after the evocation of a strong excitatory reaction and acute anger, it will initiate the dissipation of excitation and thereby diminish anger and the propensity for violent reactions.

Directive 2 If a provocation is perpetrated under conditions that render it innocuous or less threatening than apparent, convey information about such mitigating conditions at the earliest possible time.

Those who annoy others without meaning to do so must be quick to indicate that their actions are not deliberate or purposeful. If distressing treatments are inflicted without malintent, prompt apologies and a show of remorse are likely to curtail angry reactions, even to control retaliatory inclinations. Prompt apologies, presumably because they convert an apparent assault into a mishap and thereby eliminate apprehensions, have been found to be more effective in holding down anger about a mistreatment than the later removal of the mistreatment's undesirable consequences. However, the research also indicates that apologies become ineffective as the severity of annoying treatments increases.

Third-party intervention (i.e., intervention by persons being neither instigators nor targets of anger) is less effective. Third parties may well succeed in convincing an angry person that the provocative behavior derives from conditions other than malevolence, such as ignorance or clumsiness. However, efforts at diminishing others' anger through the reappraisal of harm done (e.g., "It's not that bad." "You'll be alright!" "Aren't you overreacting?") are likely to fail, because angry persons tend to construe such efforts as a belittlement of their grievances. In fact, efforts of this kind may prove counterproductive in that what is judged to be belittlement is likely to function as an added annoyance that intensifies the experience of anger.

If social conflict cannot be averted and annoyance and acute anger directed at oneself and directed by oneself at others is unavoidable, control strategies focus on the perception of cues of the angry persons' excitatory state.

Directive 3 Monitor excitedness of self and others and, upon the detection of notable increments in excitedness of self or others, disengage cautiously.

This stratagem calls for a cooling time. Based on the supposition that emotion-laden confrontational debate is unlikely to yield constructive resolutions of social conflicts, there is little point in continuing to argue and in risking further escalation of excitedness and anger. Hence, upon noticing increased excitedness of self interoceptively (e.g., pounding of the heart, accelerated heartbeat, shortness of breath, or muscular tenseness) or exteroceptively (e.g., trembling hands or loudness of voice) or of others in external manifestations (e.g., loudness of voice or general agitatedness), acquiescing withdrawal offers itself as sound strategy.

Identifying one's own and others' stress-based agitation (i.e., tonic arousal rather than phasic, emotional excitedness) is equally important. Social withdrawal after extended stressful stimulation, because it allows excitatory recovery and cognitive adjustment, is an effective conflict-minimizing strategy. [*See* SOLITUDE.]

Cautious disengagement should not be confused with demonstrative withdrawal, nor with communicative passivity. Literally walking away from open conflict, especially without saying anything, is likely to be interpreted as defiance that further infuriates angry persons.

Difficult as it may be not to pursue one's own vital interests and to act within one's rights, emotional conflict is best resolved by signaling, to the extent possible (i.e., without becoming dishonest and deceptive), an understanding, even limited acceptance, of the others' point of view.

Directive 4 In escalating conflict, convey sympathy with the others' agony. Without breaching credibility, indicate that their point of view has merit and that their goals are legitimate and actions toward them justified.

It should be clear that cautious disengagement that entails acquiescing efforts does not mean yielding to unreasonable demands. Acquiescence is accomplished through communication, not by acting in compliance with the disputed demands. However, if communicative acquiescence is considered a form of yielding, such yielding is temporary only. It is in the interest of equitable conflict resolutions that a strategy of temporary acquiescence is recommended. On the premise that equitable resolutions cannot be achieved with acutely angry, highly agitated parties, the call for a disengagement period during which anger-associated excitation is allowed to dissipate amounts to postponement, not abandonment, of negotiations. The resolution of conflict is merely delayed until excitation returns to levels that are more conducive to rational argumentation and compassion with disagreeing others.

These recommendations apply equally to conflict with angry persons who are intoxicated by alcohol or drugs with similar cognition-impairing effects.

Directive 5 In escalating conflict, monitor intoxication in angry persons, and disengage cautiously whenever observation confirms mental debilitation.

The premise is again that equitable resolutions cannot be achieved with acutely angry, cognitively impaired parties, and that negotiations better be delayed.

B. Averting Violence

If a strategy of cautious disengagement is advisable in the control of anger and its escalation, it is imperative in the prevention of angry aggression. In dealing with intensely angry, enraged persons, the foremost consideration must be to defuse the danger of violence. This objective is best served by disengagement to the point of physical separation from or of the feuding parties. Targets of others' acute anger, in particular, should cautiously but quickly extract themselves from confrontations in which violent outbursts seem imminent. [See AGGRESSION.]

First, however, persons interacting with excessively aroused, enraged others should abandon mediational efforts, no matter how well intended.

Directive 6 Under conditions of imminent violence, abandon attempts to reattribute infuriating events and information about such events to ulterior causes. Refrain from reasoning and arguing with infuriated persons.

Persistence in disagreeing, no matter how valid objections and explanations may be, is not likely to calm down truly enraged persons. In fact, such persistence tends to heighten, rather than reduce, the propensity for violence because each disagreement adds annoyance and consequently increases excitation and the experiential intensity of anger. Cognitive impairment is likely to increase along with these changes.

Directive 7 Monitor the excitatory, emotional intensity of the behavior of infuriated persons and, upon detection of extreme agitation, extricate yourself and others from the confrontation with them. Equally important, extricate yourself and others from the confrontation with extremely infuriated persons whose mental debilitation from intoxication is apparent.

The crucial insight leading to these recommendations is again that constructive resolutions of conflict cannot be achieved with persons who seethe with anger, whose mental faculties are impaired by toxins, and who seem prone to erupt in violent action. Fortunately, the period of rage and acute propensity for violent action is comparatively short-lived. Enraged persons have to calm down eventually, if only for reasons of excitatory exhaustion and homeostasis. Until

such excitatory normalization manifests itself, the acquiescing, accommodating, even compassionate treatment of enraged persons that characterizes the process of careful extrication from the confrontation is the strategy that holds the greatest promise of preventing violence. Once normalization has come about, this technique may be abandoned, and negotiation for equitable conditions may resume.

For persons who seek to control their own angry aggression, but who failed to prevent the escalation of their anger, it is imperative to avoid confronting the target of their anger at this time and to delay a reconfrontation until excitation has normalized. In case acute anger materializes during confrontation, or confrontation is unavoidable, immediate withdrawal from that confrontation is indicated. The avoidance of mentally debilitating toxins, such as alcohol, is suggested as well.

The strategy of cautious disengagement might, of course, be called upon repeatedly. Especially in conflict among intimates, parties may be re-enraged whenever particular issues come up for consideration and discussion. If conditions for rational negotiation cannot be established at all, violence-preventing disengagement might have to become a final, permanent solution.

C. Coping with Postconfrontational Anger

After the successful extrication from acute but unresolved conflict, strategy focuses on the facilitation of excitatory recovery and the normalization of mental functioning. Numerous techniques have been offered to accomplish these ends.

Relaxation and meditation have been suggested as viable procedures, and some degree of success has been ascribed to them. In light of recent findings concerning mood management, the effectiveness of these techniques may be questioned, however. Acutely angry persons tend to be cognitively preoccupied with their experiential state, with its causal circumstances as well as with the preparation of retaliatory actions. Their rumination is motivationally driven, and intentional self-distraction (as in meditation) is bound to suffer the frequent intrusion of spontaneous, ruminative thought. Relaxation is similarly nondistracting and hence also unlikely to effectively break the rumination cycle. Experimental research on the persistence of anger has failed to indicate any benefit of the provision of time and the opportunity to relax. Most acutely angry men are apparently so eager to get even with those who mistreated them that they use any time provision to reflect on retaliatory strategies rather than on nonaggressive means of coping. Needless to say, such reflection perpetuates anger cognitively, and it maintains the high levels of excitation associated with acute anger. Some research indicates, in fact, that acutely angry men do not want to be distracted from their anger as long as there is a chance to retaliate. In contrast, most angry women seem to use time for reflection to contemplate nonaggressive means of coping, and they consequently manage to control their anger and aggressiveness. This gender difference raises the question of whether it is more adaptive, in the long run, to habitually sustain and express anger or to find nonaggressive response options that diminish and terminate anger. [See MEDITATION AND THE RELAXATION RESPONSE.]

Different postconfrontational ruminations have different health implications. Recent research on cardiovascular disease suggests very strongly that unproductive, dysfunctional rumination in anger and aggressive thoughts is pathogenic, whereas productive, functional rumination in anger and aggressive thoughts is not. This is to say that anger, its expression and associated action, do not pose a health risk if provocations are effectively rebuffed, punitively recompensated, and corrected in this sense. On the other hand, anger, its expression and all associated aggressive efforts, are pathogenic if ineffective. The extreme form of such ineffectiveness is, of course, when anger cannot even be expressed, and the angry person is forced to hold it back.

The other, related revelation from recent research on anger and cardiovascular disease concerns the degree to which persons believe to be in control of their social environment by their own action. Even if such control is illusory, believing to have it is adaptive. Analogously, even if the lack of control is illusory, believing not to be in control is pathogenic. The implications of this are obvious.

Directive 8 Unless provocation can be promptly recompensated or such recompensation is believed to be readily administered, avoid rumination in angry and aggressive thoughts.

The recommended avoidance of rumination is best, and perhaps most conveniently, accomplished by exposure to potent distractors. Work on mood management has shown that intervention in anger is more effective, the stronger the distracting stimulation, and the less affinity this stimulation has with anger, its inducement, and its consequences. Moreover, it has been shown that rather unexciting but engaging stimulation is capable of reducing anger effectively. Hedonically opposite stimulation holds the greatest promise, however, of neutralizing emotions. Anger is difficult to sustain during prolonged pleasant stimulation and experiences.

Directive 9 In order to terminate unproductive angry rumination, partake in pleasant, absorbing, and comparatively unexciting activities that have no affinity with anger and aggression.

Practically speaking, angry persons should seek out pleasant company and do something with them that is highly engaging and that does not pertain to their anger. They should resist the temptation to share their grievances with good friends and take comfort in their friends' siding with them. As a form of overt rumination, such sharing of grievances invites and ensures the perpetuation of anger, and it often complicates later efforts to resolve persisting conflicts. Angry persons also should seek beneficial diversion through entertainment. Particular types of music, drama, and comedy, for instance, are known to have considerable intervention power. Highly distracting entertainment choices are plentiful, as the only inadvisable choice concerns items laden with conflict, provocation, abuse, anger, and violence. [See HUMOR AND MENTAL HEALTH.]

V. ANGER AND PATHOLOGY

As indicated already, research on anger and cardiovascular disease has converged on two conditions that constitute appreciable health risks: (a) the habitual unproductive rumination in anger, and (b) the belief or the knowledge of not being able to control the circumstances causing recurrent anger.

It is apparently adaptive, and thus healthy, to be able to act effectively against anger-provoking agents and events—or at least, to be able to believe to be able to do so. Additionally, having this ability, or believing to have it, makes rumination in anger productive: plans can be laid for corrective, retaliatory, and punitive action, the planning being on the joyful rather than distressing side.

There is, on the other hand, the overwhelmed person, knowing or believing that nothing of consequence can be done about frequently suffered annoyances and grievances. All such a person can do is to mull over mistreatments and recognize the futility of counteractions. Anger is indefinitely perpetuated and held back. It is this condition of prolonged anger that has been implicated with increased risk of cardiovascular disease.

It has been observed with considerable consistency that the suppression of anger is related to high blood pressure, both systolic and diastolic, in men and women of diverse ethnic origin. It is thus conceivable that persons who frequently harbor contempt, without ever expressing their feelings of anger, develop excessive blood pressure, thereby placing themselves at risk of cardiovascular complications. In considering the etiology of such complications, it appears that at excessive blood pressures the inner walls of arteries, as the result of hemodynamic and chemical injury, suffer deposition of atheromatous plaque. The catecholamines, which are prominently involved in the emotion of anger, are considered particularly atherogenic because they mobilize free fatty acids and related lipids that, in case anger is not acted upon, are in excess of metabolic requirements. Deposition eventually produces the vascular problems associated with coronary artery and coronary heart disease, but also with cerebrovascular disease such as carotid atherosclerosis.

The risk of such complications has fostered a reassessment of the merits of assertiveness. Assertiveness that proves unproductive, yielding endless conflicts and concessions, is obviously inadvisable. It ensures frequent anger and its suppression. In terms of health, it is a risky proposition, indeed. The recommendation to practice yielding without emotional upheaval in situations of conflict may sound cynical but prove supportive of good health. It is apparently adaptive to know when to quit fighting, such as in pursuit of unattainable goals. Modifying one's assertiveness, then, by bringing it in line with expectations and demands that can be met and backed by effective assertive actions, would seem to be sound strategy.

Before advocating a yielding disposition as superbly adaptive, however, it should be mentioned that the evidence concerning the relationship between suppressed anger and cardiovascular disease has not gone without challenge. The correlational nature of the research demonstrations invites alternative explanations. One of these explanations simply suggests that hypertensives, who have been characterized as hotheaded, rash, daring, impatient, tense, emotional, and often angry, respond to provocations more readily, more frequently, and more intensely than do normotensives. Therefore, hypertensives have occasion to experience, remember, and ultimately report a greater number of anger experiences that did not find expression. It is thus conceivable that cardiovascular disease is associated with both frequently suppressed anger and frequently expressed and acted-on anger.

The latter linkage is supported by research showing that hostile Type A persons, who must vigilantly monitor their social environment because of their distrust of others, excrete larger amounts of the gonadal hormone testosterone than do Type B persons. Excessive testosterone levels are also pathogenic in facilitating atherosclerosis. A proneness for coronary disease has thus also been proclaimed for hostile, cynical persons, especially men.

It would seem prudent, then, to consider implicated with an increased risk of cardiovascular disease both the frequent suppression of anger and excessive assertiveness that manifests itself in the overly frequent experience of suppressed and expressed anger. Aiming for the fewest, shortest, and least intense experiences of anger thus emerges as sound strategy. In terms of health, it seems that anger simply does not pay.

BIBLIOGRAPHY

Averill, J. R. (1982). *Anger and aggression: An essay on emotion.* New York: Springer-Verlag.

Berkowitz, L. (1993). *Aggression: Its causes, consequences, and control.* Philadelphia: Temple University Press.

Johnson, E. H. (1990). *The deadly emotions: The role of anger, hostility and aggression in health and emotional well-being.* New York: Praeger.

Novaco, R. W. (1986). Anger as a clinical and social problem. In R. J. Blanchard & D. C. Blanchard (Eds.), *Advances in the study of aggression* (Vol. 2, pp. 1–67). Orlando, FL: Academic Press.

Siegman, A. W., & Smith, T. W. (Eds.). (1994). *Anger, hostility, and the heart.* Hillsdale, NJ: Erlbaum.

Tavris, C. (1989). *Anger: The misunderstood emotion* (Rev. ed.). New York: Touchstone.

Wegner, D. M., & Pennebaker, J. W. (Eds.). (1993). *Handbook of mental control.* Englewood Cliffs, NJ: Prentice Hall.

Zillmann, D. (1979). *Hostility and aggression.* Hillsdale, NJ: Erlbaum.

Anorexia Nervosa and Bulimia Nervosa

Melissa Pederson Mussell

University of St. Thomas
University of Minnesota

James E. Mitchell

University of North Dakota Medical School
Neuropsychiatric Research Institute

Anorexia Nervosa A type of eating disorder associated with failure to maintain a minimally healthy body weight.

Binge Eating Eating large amounts of food in a discrete period of time accompanied by a sense of loss of control of food intake.

Bulimia Nervosa A type of eating disorder involving recurrent episodes of binge eating and compensatory behaviors (e.g., purging, fasting, or excessive exercise).

Eating Disorder A category of psychiatric disorders involving disturbances in eating patterns and attitudes toward food and body image.

Purging A method of compensating for dietary intake, most commonly by self-induced vomiting, laxative abuse, or diuretic abuse.

ANOREXIA NERVOSA AND BULIMIA NERVOSA are two of the most commonly recognized eating disorders. The term "eating disorder" encompasses a variety of psychological/psychiatric disorders involving disturbed eating patterns and attitudes toward food and body image. Unhealthy weight control practices and intense body image distortion or disparagement are central features of eating disorders.

I. OVERVIEW OF EATING DISORDER TERMS

The word "nervosa" indicates that each of these conditions is a "nervous disorder." Psychological difficulties are likely to be involved in the development of these disorders, and also are likely to be exacerbated by the eating-disordered behavior. "Anorexia" means "lack of appetite." The hallmark feature of anorexia nervosa (AN) is failure to maintain a minimally normal body weight. The meaning of the term "bulimia" is "ox hunger," or "hungry as an ox." Bulimia nervosa (BN) is characterized by recurrent episodes of binge eating (i.e., eating large amounts of food accompanied by a sense of loss of control) and compensatory behaviors (e.g., purging, fasting, or excessive exercise). Overlap between the symptoms of these disorders occurs in some individuals. Furthermore, individuals may engage in disturbed eating behaviors and/or indicate intense body image disparagement, but not meet full criteria for AN or BN. Detailed information about diagnostic criteria are provided later in this chapter. It is important to note that eating-related behaviors may be best conceptualized as existing along a continuum ranging from "healthy" to "unhealthy" eating-related behaviors and body image.

II. CONTINUUM OF HEALTH RELATED TO EATING DISORDERS

The pursuit of and preoccupation with beauty represent a central feature of the female sex-role stereotype. Therefore, it is possible that attractiveness, and specifically body image, have a greater influence on self-concept for women than for men. Although standards of beauty have varied widely across time and cultures, the mass media have contributed to the development of a more uniform standard of beauty.

Unfortunately, the current images of women that are portrayed in the media often represent unrealistic weights and shapes for most women. In a classic study, Garner and colleagues demonstrated a consistent decrease in body weights and measurements of two (albeit arguable) standards of beauty (e.g., Miss America pageant winners, and Playboy centerfolds) over two decades (1950s to 1970s). Fashion models are now 23% thinner than average women, compared to 8% thinner than average woman three decades ago. Indeed, models who depict the in-vogue "waif" look are likely to have a body weight consistent with criteria for AN.

Given the preponderance of images of thinness as the ideal for beauty that are depicted in the media, it is not surprising that many females would perceive their bodies as inadequate. Because women naturally have more body fat than men, even those who are of normal body weight may judge themselves as overweight. In a recent national survey, over 40% of females reported having a negative body image. Although almost one-half of young girls reported wanting to lose weight in one survey, only 4% actually were found to be overweight. Women are far more likely to rate their ideal figure to be significantly thinner than actual size than are men.

Therefore, perceptions that one is overweight may be potentially more distressing for women and may lead to attempts to control body weight and shape through methods such as dieting. Female college students report dieting at much higher rates than their male counterparts. In a recent large-scale national survey data from the Centers for Disease Control and Prevention, containing a sample of over 60,000 adults, 38% of female and 24% of male adults reported to be trying to lose weight, and 44% of females versus 15% of males in high school sample of over 11,000 students reported to be trying to lose weight. [SEE DIETING.]

The high prevalence rates of negative body image attitudes and dietary behaviors found among females has been referred to as "normative discontent." Therefore, although not necessarily "healthy," it may in fact be "normal" for women in Western cultures to hold disparaging views toward their bodies and to engage in activites aimed at modifying their weight and shape. However, body image disparagement and dieting behaviors may pose as risk factors for the development of an eating disorder. Initial degree of body image dissatisfaction has been found to predict increased eating disturbance in longitudinal studies of adolescent girls and to predict eating disordered behavior in adults. Similarly, the interaction between body image and other risk factors (e.g., pressure for thinness) increased probability of reporting eating disturbance in female athletes. In a study of adult ballet students, body dissatisfaction and dietary restriction were found to predict eating-disordered symptoms.

Therefore, individuals who derive self-esteem primarily or exclusively based on the perception of body image may be at increased risk for development of an eating disorder. It has been argued that individuals who develop eating disorders unquestionably accept and internalize societal messages about thinness as the ideal for female attractiveness. Excessive dietary restraint, often used as a means to modify body weight and shape in an attempt to more closely correspond to a thin ideal of beauty, has been posited to increase the potential for development of binge eating. Secondary symptoms of semi-starvation resulting from prolonged dietary restriction or fasting, such as increases in preoccupation with food, urges to binge eat, and depressed mood, may lead to further exacerbation of body image disparagement and disturbed eating. Although body image concerns and dieting practices are commonplace for many women, when body image disparagement and eating disturbances become extreme and begin to interfere with functioning or to compromise health, an eating disorder may be diagnosed. [See BODY IMAGE; SELF-ESTEEM.]

III. DIAGNOSTIC CRITERIA

Although the symptoms of the various eating disorder syndromes overlap considerably and often are characterized as along a continuum, classification of specific eating disorders is based on criteria as outlined in the *Diagnostic and Statistical Manual of Mental Disorders (DSM-IV)*. [*See* DSM-IV.]

A. Anorexia Nervosa

The primary distinguishing feature of anorexia nervosa (AN) is the refusal to maintain a minimally normal body weight (i.e., at least 85% of expected body weight considering age and height). Despite their excessively low-weight status, individuals with AN exhibit intense fear of gaining weight. Such individuals experience their body weight or shape in a distorted manner (e.g., size distortion) and often indicate intense distress regarding body image. Body weight or shape unduly influences self-evaluation, often being the primary determinant of self-esteem. Absence of three or more consecutive menstrual cycles (i.e., amenorrhea) is also required to make a diagnosis of AN. Perhaps the feature that presents the greatest challenge in accurately assessing and effectively treating this disorder is the adamant denial of the seriousness of maintaining an excessively low body weight. Individuals with AN may also engage in recurrent binge eating and purging (i.e., self-induced vomiting, abuse of laxatives, or diuretics), which is classified as the binge eating/purging subtype of AN. Absence of recurrent binge eating and purging characterizes the restricting type of AN.

B. Bulimia Nervosa

Within the past two decades bulimia nervosa (BN) only has been recognized as a distinct clinical disorder. The primary feature of BN is recurrent binge eating (i.e., eating large amounts of food in a short time period accompanied by a sense of loss of control) followed by methods of inappropriate compensation. Compensatory methods include purging (i.e., self-induced vomiting, or abuse of laxatives, or diuretics), fasting, or excessive exercise. Symptom frequency for a diagnosis of BN entails binge eating and compensatory behavior(s) occurring on average at least twice a week for a 3-month period. Perception of body shape and weight unduly influencing self-evaluation also is required for the diagnosis of BN. A diagnosis of BN is not given to individuals who receive a diagnosis of AN, because

that diagnosis takes precedence. Subclassification of BN is based on type of recurrent compensatory methods, referred to as purging and nonpurging types.

C. Eating Disorders Not Otherwise Specified

A large number of individuals engage in disturbed eating behaviors, but do not meet strict diagnostic criteria for AN or BN, in which case a diagnosis of eating disorder not otherwise specified (ED-NOS) may be appropriate. Examples of symptom constellations that might meet the criteria for ED-NOS include bulimic behavior occuring less frequently than two times per week or purging in the absence of binge eating behavior. Another example of ED-NOS, binge eating disorder (BED), which is characterized by recurrent binge eating in the absence of compensatory behaviors, has been listed in the appendix of *DSM-IV* as a diagnosis warranting further research.

IV. EPIDEMIOLOGY

Although increasing prevalence combined with increased recognition of eating disorder problems for women has contributed to the perception that eating disorders have become an "epidemic," this is not supported by epidemiological research. However, the high prevalence of eating disorders is well documented, with women representing the majority of those afflicted. Although these disorders are most commonly seen in women, approximately 5% to 10% of individuals who develop AN or BN are men. Research on AN and BN indicate that these disorders are most often found among Caucasian adolescent and young adult females in industrialized countries espousing the idealogy of Western culture. The most recent figures indicate that from .10% to 1.0% of young females have AN. Prevalence rates are higher for BN, ranging from 1% to 3% of young women when using stringent diagnostic criteria. [*See* EPIDEMIOLOGY: PSYCHIATRIC.]

Increased rates of AN and BN have been associated with certain professions (e.g., fashion models, ballet dancers) that emphasize thinness. Elevated rates of eating disorders have also been found among individuals involved in competitive athletics, particularly those in which maintenance of a low body weight is competitively advantageous (e.g., gymnastics, running, wrestling). It is possible that participation in such activities poses as a risk factor in the development of an eating disorder. Alternatively, some individuals with established eating disorders (or body image disparagement) may be drawn to such activities, in order to use compulsive exercise as a socially condoned form of dietary compensation in efforts to maintain or achieve a low body weight.

V. PSYCHOLOGICAL AND SOCIAL IMPAIRMENT

Body image disturbance is a central feature of AN and BN. Body size overestimation among individuals with AN and BN has been empirically documented. Among individuals with AN and BN, marked fluctuations of body image disparagement frequently occur, which may precipitate and/or result from intensified eating disordered behavior.

Increased psychological distress often is found among individuals with an eating disorder. Relatively high rates of comorbid psychopathology (especially affective disorders) have been reported for samples of individuals with AN. In addition, problems with past or present substance abuse are not uncommon among eating disordered samples. Individuals with eating disorders also display a pattern of cognitive abnormalities, such as a dichotomous thinking style. Low self-esteem and difficulties in interpersonal relationships are often reported by individuals seeking treatment for eating disorders.

The extent to which these psychological and social difficulties may be involved in the development of eating disorders remains unclear and could be clarified by prospective, longitudinal studies. However, it is important to note that many of these symptoms are ameliorated with treatment that results in reduction or cessation of eating disordered behaviors.

VI. MEDICAL COMPLICATIONS

Several thorough reviews are available providing detailed accounts of adverse medical sequale of eating disorders. Although prevalence rates for AN are relatively low, the medical consequences can be grave. Mortality rates for AN at long-term follow-up range from 6% to 20% and up to one-fourth of anorectic individuals develop severe, chronic disabilities resulting from the disorder. The results of prolonged malnutrition found in AN include certain visably recognizable symptoms, including obvious weight loss, dry hair and skin, alopecia (i.e., hair loss), and excessive lanugo hair (e.g, fine, downy body hair). Cold intolerance, sleep disturbances, headaches, and fatigue are common among individuals with AN. Prolonged protein depletion resulting from chronic malnutrition results in additional symptoms, detectable through laboratory examinations. Abdominal pain and bloating, and constipation are often reported by individuals with AN, which may be due to delayed gastric emptying. Constipation also may result from laxative abuse and starvation. Among the most serious consequences of AN are osteoporosis, growth stunting, and cardiac complications. [*See* FOOD, NUTRITION, AND MENTAL HEALTH.]

Although mortality rates for BN are low, fatalities have been documented as a result of gastric rupture after binge eating, esophageal perforations (i.e., Boerhooves syndrome), and cardiomyopathy due to chronic ingestion of Ipecac. Fluid loss due to recurrent purging can result in dehydration and electrolyte imbalance, potentially leading to cardiovascular disturbances. Recurrent vomiting may result in esophageal erosion. Constipation and abdominal bloating and pain may result from binge eating.

VII. DETECTION AND ASSESSMENT

Several factors contribute to the secretive nature of eating disorders, including denial of the seriousness of symptoms, embarrassment regarding the symptoms, and/or fear of the consequences of relinquishing the disturbed behaviors (i.e., potential weight gain or increased anxiety). Consequently, eating disorders often go unnoticed and can be challenging to assess, although warning signs are often present. Secretive eating, refusal to eat in public, and frequent dieting may be indicative that an individual is struggling with some form of an eating disorder; these symptoms are usually found in individuals with either AN or BN. Behavioral indications of purging behavior include spending excessive amounts of time in bathrooms or frequently going to a bathroom immediately following eating. Excessive or compulsive physical activity may also indicate the use of exercising as a form of dietary compensation. The use of stringent diets or fasting for extended periods of time may signal the presence of an eating disorder. Substantial changes in body weight, including weight fluctuations, or continued weight gain or loss may also be indicative of an eating disorder.

Emaciation is usually the primary physical indication of AN. Measurements of body weight obviously aids in determining if an individual is below 85% of expected weight; however, individuals with AN may drink excessive amounts of fluid or wear concealed weights in an attempt to manipulate assessment of body weight. Overactivity (e.g., continuous body movement or pacing) is often observed among individuals with AN. As described above, some of the additional detectable signs of AN include dry skin and hair, lanugo, and alopecia. Ammenorhea may also indicate the possibility of AN, although the use of oral contraceptives may complicate the detection of this symptom.

Although frequent weight fluctuations may signal the presence of BN, many individuals with BN are of normal weight and appear relatively healthy. Although BN is usually less easily detected than AN, certain signs may aid in its detection. One indication of recurrent self-induced vomiting, sometimes referred to as a "Russell's sign," is the development of callouses or scarring on the back of the hand resulting from abrasion during self-induced vomiting. This symptom may not be present in those individuals who primarily use alternative forms of purging (i.e., laxative, diuretic, or enema abuse), who have nonpurging BN, or who after prolonged vomiting have come to do so reflexively. Self-induced vomiting may also contribute to hypertrophy of the salivary glands, creating a swollen appearance of the neck and face (i.e., "puffy cheeks"). Although this symptom may be fairly pronounced in some women, it is not detectable in the majority of individuals with BN. Additional signs include the presence of small skin hemorrhages (i.e., facial petechiae) or conjunctival hemorrhages that may result from forceful vomiting. Dental enamel erosion, most pronounced on the inside surface of the upper teeth, is another indication of purging that may produce protrusion of dental fillings or discoloration (i.e., darkening) of the teeth. This symptom, which is easily detected during dental examinations, may be overlooked during routine physical examinations unless specifically assessed. Edema may be present for those who abuse laxatives or diuretics. Individuals with BN often present with complaints of "bloating," constipation, or lethargy. Laboratory tests may be used to detect electrolyte imbalance, although such abnormalities are detected in only approximately 40% of individuals with BN.

VIII. TREATMENT

A. Psychotherapy

Psychotherapy is commonly used in the treatment of eating disorders. One form of psychotherapeutic intervention, cognitive behavioral therapy (CBT) has been the most extensively studied. Based on the work of Beck for the treatment of depression, CBT is a time-limited, present-focused, solution-oriented form of therapy. This approach is based on "collaborative empiricism" in which the client and therapist actively work together using an experimental approach to resolve a specified problem. As applied to eating disorders, the primary focus is on modifying disordered eating behaviors and distorted cognitions about food, weight, and shape. A combination of behavioral techniques, cognitive interventions, and emphasis on relapse prevention are integrated in this approach. The efficacy of CBT has been demonstrated in several studies of BN. Favorable reduction rates of binge eating (ranging from 77% to 93%) and purging (74% to 94%) have been reported for five of the most recent, large studies. Methods used in behavior therapy (BT) also are commonly integrated in CBT treatment for individuals with eating disorders. Studies comparing BT with CBT have generally demonstrated that the addition of cognitive interventions to behavioral methods are associated with similar or greater clinical gains. [See BEHAVIOR THERAPY; COGNITIVE THERAPY.]

The efficacy of an alternative type of psychotherapy, Interpersonal Psychotherapy (IPT), recently has been demonstrated in treating individuals with BN, as well as BED. IPT is time-limited, present-focused, and solution-oriented. IPT differs from CBT in that the emphasis of treatment is on modification of interpersonal interactions, rather than eating disordered behavior or cognitions.

Another therapeutic approach that has been investigated is supportive-expressive therapy, a short-term, nondirective, dynamically informed modality that conceptualizes core conflicts in terms of interpersonal issues. Although supportive-expressive therapy was found to be effective in reducing binge eating in this study, CBT was found to be associated with greater improvements in many aspects of eating disturbance and psychopathology, and a higher rate of remission in bulimic symptoms.

Alternative psychotherapeutic approaches to treating individuals with eating disorders recently have been well articulated, although no controlled outcome studies have yet to be conducted. The relative efficacy of psychodynamic therapy is unclear given the absence of empirical data. However, this approach may be beneficial for clients who have not derived benefit from less intensive interventions, such as CBT. Feminist therapists have convincingly argued for the importance of considering sociocultural and political issues in designing interventions for individuals with eating disorders. The potential efficacy of psychotherapeutic interventions incorporating feminist perspectives warrant future empirical investigation. [See PSYCHO-ANALYSIS.]

Although favorable results have been reported using psychotherapy, particularly CBT and IPT, several limitations of this body of research warrant discussion. Despite the substantial rates of symptom reduction and remission reported in these studies, it is important to note that approximately one-third to one-half of participants remained symptomatic at the end of treatment. Furthermore, strict inclusion criteria utilized in research studies such as these limit the generalizability of the findings, which may not be representative of the majority of individuals seeking treatment for BN. Data are not available regarding the relative efficacy of individual versus group administration of CBT or IPT. Additional research comparing the relative efficacy of alternative psychotherapeutic approaches is warranted. However, this body of literature provides support for the efficacy of using solution-focused psychotherapeutic interventions such as CBT and IPT in treating individuals with BN.

Despite the fact that AN has received attention from clinical researchers for several decades, little empirical data are available regarding efficacy of psychotherapy for this disorder. To a large extent, the paucity of AN treatment research is attributable to the logistical difficulties involved in implementing controlled studies with this population. Only four outpatient

psychotherapy studies of AN have been reported to date, with some suggestions of effectiveness. The potential benefits of using behavioral modification programs (which overlap to a certain extent with CBT interventions) during inpatient hospitalization has received support in several studies. Although limited empirical data are available regarding the relative efficacy of individual versus family therapy in treating individuals with eating disorders, some therapists have convincingly articulated the potential benefits of using family approaches in working with eating disordered individuals. Some empirical support exists for using family therapy for younger individuals with AN. Additional research is needed to investigate various psychotherapeutic interventions for treating individuals with AN, and relapse prevention strategies, given the substantial rate of relapse in those who initially respond to treatment. [See FAMILY THERAPY.]

B. Medication

Antidepressant medications have been found to effectively reduce binge eating and purging symptoms in several BN studies. Four controlled trials involving outpatient samples have demonstrated the superiority of serotonin-reuptake inhibitors (SRIs) in comparison to placebo in reducing bulimic symptoms, although one impatient trial failed to support added benefit for the drug. These medications generally have been found to be well-tolerated. Therefore, fluoxetine hydrochloride (Prozac) administered at daily doses of 60 mg (higher than the recommended dose of 20 mg used to treat individuals with major depressive disorder) is considered by some the first choice for pharmacotherapy for BN. The use of tricyclic antidepressants or monoamine oxidase inhibitors also is supported by research. Although the side effects of these classes of medications may be more problematic for many individuals than the SRIs, they may be beneficial treatment strategies for those individuals who do not respond to the use of SRIs. In addition, some clinicians prefer the second generation tricyclics, such as despiramine, as the initial intervention owing to the lower cost of the medication.

Despite the relative efficacy of antidepressant medications compared to placebo in reducing bulimic symptoms, it is important to note that rates of bulimic symptom remission at end of treatment range from 4% to 20% in most studies. These rates of symptom remission are lower than those reported in psychotherapy outcome studies. Augmenting psychotherapy with pharmacotherapy may seem indicated in some cases, although results from research on this are mixed. Three studies have reported no benefit to adding antidepressant treatment regimen to psychotherapy on outcome in eating variables, and the results are equivocal in one study. There is some suggestion that certain other symptoms, such as those of depression, may benefit from the combination of interventions.

Little empirical data are available from investigations of the benefits of pharmacotherapy in promoting weight restoration in individuals with AN. Approximately a dozen controlled trials have been conducted on variety of medications, yielding often ambiguous results. Benefits have been demonstrated for the use of amitriptyline in one study and for cyproheptadine in two studies. However, the majority of placebo-controlled studies, investigating the efficacy of these and other medications (e.g., antipsychotics, clonidine, cisapride, lithium, and tetrahydrocannabinol) have not demonstrated efficacy in promoting weight restoration. [*See* Psychopharmacology.]

C. Nutritional Counseling

Nutritional counseling is often regarded as a necessary therapeutic component for treatment of individuals with eating disorders. Healthy meal planning is the cornerstone of this approach, which involves providing objective nutritional information about the types and amounts of food necessary to achieve or maintain adequate nutrition and healthy weight. Behavioral strategies are also employed to increase the likelihood of successfully adhering to nutritional recommendations. Nutritional counseling is essential for the treatment of AN, which requires an increase in caloric intake to promote gradual weight restoration at a rate of 1 to 3 pounds per week. Nutritional counseling is also useful for treating BN to help stabilize the dietary chaos that often promotes binge eating.

D. Hospitalization

At times sufficient medical danger exists (e.g., dehydration, severe electrolyte imbalance, gastrointestinal bleeding, severe emaciation, suicidal ideation) to require inpatient hospitalization. Goals of hospitalization include interruption of weight loss (usually if less than 70 to 75% of ideal body weight), progress toward restoration of healthy body weight, cessation of binge eating or vomiting, treatment of medical complications, and treatment of comorbid conditions (e.g., depression or substance abuse). Hospitalization also may be indicated if clinical benefits are not obtained from adequate outpatient therapy. This may be required for severely underweight individuals who, evidence starvation-induced impaired cognitive functioning.

Day treatment, or partial hospitalization, may be recommended following inpatient discharge or as an alternative to hospitalization. This type of treatment allows patients to receive therapy during the day without requiring an overnight stay. This type of treatment is more economical than inpatient hospitalization and is less socially disruptive. Additional benefits of this type of treatment include allowing the patient to pursue work or education while obtaining intensive treatment, and providing a structured atmosphere during meal times.

IX. PREVENTION

Given the prevalence of these disorders and the seriousness of the psychological and medical sequelae, the prevention of eating disorders is an important area that requires increased attention. Such efforts often involve providing psychoeducational information in school-based settings aimed at reducing unhealthy dieting behavior and enhancing body acceptance, often involving critical analysis of messages conveyed through mass media. A number of eating disorder studies have been conducted to investigate the effectiveness of primary prevention programs. However, an unfortunately consistent finding across such studies is that although knowledge about eating disorders often increases, behavioral changes (i.e., reductions in unhealthy dietary practices) have not been detected among participants. Failure to observe the desired behavioral outcomes of primary prevention programs may be attributable, in part, to a variety of methodological challenges, including the validity of self-report assessments and the relatively low baseline frequency of eating disordered behaviors (e.g., self-induced vomiting) among the general adolescent population. However, it is also possible that, in order to have a significant impact, prevention efforts may need to be delivered to individuals at a younger age (i.e., elementary school). Increased understanding of the complex etiology of AN and BN may be required in order to develop more comprehensive and effective prevention strategies. In addition, relatively little attention has been devoted to investigating the effectiveness of secondary prevention of eating disorders. As such, effective strategies to assist in identifying individuals who are experiencing initial symptoms of an eating disorder and facilitating appropriate treatment remain an important area to be developed.

X. SUMMARY

Stringent diagnostic criteria show that the prevalence for any single eating disorder is rather low. However, combining prevalence rates across various types of disorders reveals that up to 5 to 10% of women may be afflicted with a diagnosable eating disorder (i.e., AN, BN, or ED-NOS). Serious medical, psychological, and social consequences are associated with these disorders.

The treatment of individuals with eating disorders often requires a multifaceted approach (e.g., psychotherapy, pharmacotherapy, nutritional counseling, medical management) involving members of several professional disciplines (e.g., dieticians, psychologists, psychiatrists, internists) and various settings (e.g., inpatient, outpatient, day treatment, residential).

Literature on the treatment of these disorders indicates that substantial progress has been made in the last few decades. However, a sizable subgroup of individuals with either AN or BN do not adequately respond to established therapies, or do respond but subsequently relapse. Much additional work is needed in predicting treatment response, matching individuals to treatments, and developing relapse prevention strategies. Furthermore, effective primary and secondary prevention strategies remain to be established.

BIBLIOGRAPHY

Brownell, K. D., & Fairburn, C. G. (Eds.). (1995). *Eating disorders and obesity.* New York: Guilford Press.

Fairburn, C. G. & Wilson, G. T. (Eds.). (1993). *Binge eating: Nature, assessment and treatment.* New York: Guilford Press.

Fallon, P., Katzman, M. A., & Wolley, S. C. (Eds.). (1994). *Feminist perspectives in eating disorders.* New York: Guilford Press.

Garner, D. M. & Garfinkel, P. E. (Eds.). (1997). *Handbook of treatment for eating disorders.* (2nd ed.). New York: Guilford Press.

Mitchell, J. E. (Ed.). (1990). *Bulimia nervosa.* Minneapolis, MN: University of Minnesota Press.

Smolak, L., Levine, M. P., & Striegel-Moore, R. (Eds.). (1996). *The developmental psychopathology of eating disorders: implications for research, prevention and treatment.* Mahwah, NJ: Lawrence Erlbaum.

Striegel-Moore, R.H., Silberstein, L.R., & Rodin, J. (1986). Toward an understanding of risk factors for bulimia. *American Psychologist, 41,* 246–263.

Thompson, J.K. (Ed.). (1996). *Body image, eating disorders, and obesity.* Washington, DC: American Psychiatric Association.

Antisocial Personality Disorder

Robert G. Meyer and Daniel Wolverton

University of Louisville

Sarah E. Deitsch

University of Kentucky

Burnout   The notion that the passage of time, repetition, or aging generates a behavior change.

Criminal Personality   A concept that overlaps with that of antisocial personality disorder. It is more inclusive as it refers to more criminal behavior patterns.

Primary–Secondary Psychopathy   A further delineation of the concept of psychopathy. Primary psychopaths show even lower levels of anxiety, avoidance learning, and remorse, and higher levels of violence and sensation-seeking.

Psychopath   A term that also overlaps but is more narrow in focus than the antisocial personality disorder. Psychopaths show even less remorse and ability to profit from experience, and more violence, glibness, callousness, and sensation-seeking.

Psychopathy Checklist—Revised (PCL-R)   The premier instrument for the assessment of psychopathy.

Recidivism   The return to a prior criminal-antisocial behavior pattern.

Sensation-Seeking   A need for increased stimulation of various sorts, as well as an increased need for thrills and danger.

ANTISOCIAL PERSONALITY is arguably the most important personality disorder, in terms of both impact on society and complexity of psychological and legal issues. The concept of the antisocial personality disorder is confused by the common usage of three overlapping terms: the criminal personality, the antisocial personality, and the psychopath (sociopath). The criminal personality is a sociological term, not a DSM category. As we will see, it includes a variety of different personalities who are involved in some way in criminal activity. Many different personality types function as criminals in our society; of these, the antisocial personality, or the related term "psychopath," is only one specific psychological syndrome. Antisocial personalities apparently account for no more than about 30% of the overall prison population.

I. CHARACTERISTICS OF THE CRIMINAL

Several overall patterns characterize the criminal. Four principal characteristics of the criminal lifestyle are (1) irresponsibility, (2) self-indulgence, (3) interpersonal intrusiveness, and (4) social rule breaking. The young or "apprentice" criminal is typically motivated by peer influence, combined with stimulation-seeking, which gradually give way to more antisocial components as the criminal career develops. More specifically, the majority of offenses are caused by individuals aged 21 and younger, and approximately 80% of adult chronic offenders were chronic offenders before age 18. Criminals tend to be male, at about a 5:1 ratio, up to as high as 50:1 in some specific categories of aggressive crime. With the rise in feminism, we are increasingly closer to gender parity in "white-collar crime," but the high ratio of males has persisted in aggressive crimes. As to the general causes of crime, both poor sociocultural conditions and heredity are major factors, while more specific factors are cold, rejecting, harsh, inadequate, and/or inconsistent parenting; a high level of stimulation-seeking; psychopathy; impulsivity; low intelligence, especially low verbal intelligence; mesomorphic body type; and a history of hyperactivity, handicap, and/or being abused as a child. [See CRIMINAL BEHAVIOR.]

Psychodiagnostician Edwin Megargee and several colleagues have developed an ongoing research program that has generated an excellent typology of the criminal personality. Using data primarily from the MMPI, they differentiated 10 criminal types in one prison population. On the basis of behavioral observations, social history data, and other psychological tests, they obtained validation for this classification and subsequently extended its use to other prison populations. Most importantly from the perspective of good research design, researchers working indepen-

dently of Megargee established the validity of the system in other prisons, and others have independently validated similar patterns. It is clear from this and other data that there is no single criminal type. Their empirically derived and applicable system is likely to remain the standard one for many years. Another helpful way of conceptualizing different criminal "paths" is provided in Table I.

II. ANTISOCIAL PERSONALITY DISORDER— PSYCHOPATH TERMINOLOGY

The term *antisocial personality* reflects an evolution through a number of terms, the most widely known of which has undoubtedly been "psychopath." In about 1800, Philippe Pinel coined the term *Manie sans délire* to reflect the fact that these individuals manifest extremely deviant behavior but show no evidence of delusions, hallucinations, or other cognitive disorders. While Pinel was certainly including several personality disorder categories other than the antisocial personality in his descriptions, James Prichard's label of "moral insanity," denoted in 1835, is a clear forerunner of the antisocial personality grouping. This general conceptualization grew in acceptance, and late in the 19th century the label *psychopathic inferiority,* introduced by Johann Koch, became the accepted term. Later variations included "psychopathic character," "psychopathic personality," and "psychopath."

Table I Tracks to Various Antisocial Patterns

The aggressive/versatile track leading to "cafeteria style" offending, including violent, property, and/or drug offenses/abuse	The nonaggressive antisocial track leading to more specialized offending including property and drug offenses/abuse
Characteristics	*Characteristics*
Higher rate of genetic, prenatal and/or birth disorders	Lower rate of genetic, prenatal and/or birth disorders
Onset of conduct problems in preschool years	Onset in late childhood or early to middle adolescence
Aggressive and concealing problem behaviors	Mostly nonaggressive conduct problems
More hyperactive/impulsive/attention problems	No appreciable hyperactive/impulsive/attention problems
Poor social skills	Capable of social skills
Poor peer relationships	Association with deviant peers
Academic problems	Sporadic or minimal academic problems
High rate of instigation of offenses	Low rate of instigation of offenses
Low remission rate	Higher remission rate, at least for delinquency
More males than females	Higher proportion of females than in aggressive/versatile path
Higher rate of drug abuse	Lower rate of drug abuse
Higher rate of stimulation-seeking	Lower rate of stimulation-seeking

Source: Adapted in part from R. Loeber (1990), *Clin. Psychol. Rev.* **10**, 1–42.

Expositions by a number of individuals, particularly by Hervey Cleckley, brought the term into common usage.

Despite the foundation for the condition, the first (1952) edition of the American Psychiatric Association's *Diagnostic and Statistical Manual of Mental Disorders (DSM-I)*, the generally accepted "bible" of mental disorder classifications, muddied the issue by substituting the term "sociopathic personality" to cover the patterns that had traditionally be subsumed under the psychopath label. "Sociopathic" was used to emphasize the environmental factors allegedly generating the disorder and to de-emphasize the moralistic connotations that had become encrusted on the old terminology. Nevertheless, both concepts remained in lay and professional usages. The confusion was further heightened with the 1968 revisions of the *Diagnostic and Statistical Manual (DSM-II)*, which included neither term; instead, the *DSM-II* substituted the label "antisocial personality disorder." Although this new term carries an inherent implication of specifically criminal behavior, many professionals believed that it was a clear improvement in that it emphasized observable behavioral criteria: that is, to patterns of observable, definable behavior that conflict chronically with agreed-upon societal norms.

The trend toward objective criteria for the application of the term continues in the latest revisions of the *Diagnostic and Statistical Manual,* and the term "antisocial personality" disorder is also retained. It would be helpful if a specific psychopathic disorder diagnosis was included in the *DSM*, especially if references to overt criminality were minimized. Incidentally, if the individual is younger than 18, the appropriate diagnosis is conduct disorder.

From early on, studies have found that the term "psychopathic personality" is meaningful and useful in diagnosis. Also, in an early, landmark study, Spitzer and his associates (1967) checked for the diagnostic reliability of all of the standard mental health diagnostic categories, and found the highest level of agreement ($r = .88$) in the respondents' ability to label persons in the category of antisocial personality.

As we see, there is considerable overlap between the terms "antisocial personality disorder" (the present official *DSM* term), the "psychopath," and the "sociopath." Throughout this article, we will use the overall term "antisocial personality," recognizing that the psychopath (or sociopath) is typically seen as a sub-

group of this category. [*See* DSM-IV; PERSONALITY DISORDERS.]

III. CHARACTERISTICS OF THE ANTISOCIAL PERSONALITY (AP)

The essential characteristic of the antisocial personality disorder (AP) is the chronic manifestation of antisocial behavior patterns in amoral and impulsive persons. They are usually unable to delay gratification or to deal effectively with authority, and they show narcissism in interpersonal relationships. The pattern is apparent by the age of 15 (usually earlier) and continues into adult life with consistency across a wide performance spectrum, including school, vocational, and interpersonal behaviors.

A consensus of the research on the specific characteristics of the antisocial personality (and this research typically focuses on that narrower range of individuals seen as psychopathic) presents the following, i.e., relative to normals, they are (a) less physiologically responsive (e.g., by EKG, GSR, and EMG measures) to fearful imagery; (b) less psychologically responsive to social disapproval; (c) less responsive psychologically to affect-laden words, i.e., they respond cognitively but not affectively; (d) perseverate in behaviors with negative consequences even when they are intellectually aware of these consequences; (e) show more evidence of "cortical immaturity" but not significantly greater indices of brain dysfunction; and (f) show higher levels of sensation- and thrill-seeking behaviors.

Although the *DSM-IV* discusses only the overall category of AP, there is good evidence that it can be further subdivided into categories of primary psychopath and secondary psychopath. Primary psychopaths are distinguished by the following characteristics: (1) they have very low levels of anxiety, avoidance learning, or remorse; (2) they are even more refractory to standard social control procedures; (3) they are higher in sensation- and thrill-seeking behaviors, particularly the "disinhibition" factor that refers to extroverted, hedonistic pleasure seeking.

Both the secondary and the primary psychopath are quite different from those individuals who are antisocial because they grew up in and adapted to a delinquent subculture. These delinquent individuals are normal in relation to the subculture they were reared in; they follow (often almost obsessively) the rules and mores of this group. They can be as conformist as the good middle class, middle management person. As we have already noted, not all criminals are psychopaths, and not all psychopaths are criminals.

Cleckley (1955), a particularly influential early theorist, asserted that psychopaths are often intellectually superior, and this concept has unduly influenced attitudes toward the AP. However, Cleckley was clearly in error here; such a characterization best fits the unique subsample that he usually encountered with in his clinical practice. It is not surprising that those rare psychopaths who (a) were willing to participate and stay in therapy and, especially, who (b) could pay a private therapist's fees would be brighter than the average psychopath. As a whole, all subgroups of antisocial personalities actually show lower than average scores on intelligence tests. This is logical considering their inability to adjust to school, and is especially so if genetic dysfunction and/or brain immaturity are involved.

Violent crimes of nonpsychopaths are often characterized by extreme emotional arousal and frequently occur in situations of domestic dispute. They are more often perpetrated against women who are known to the aggressor and can be loosely characterized as "crimes of passion." On the other hand, the violent crimes of psychopaths are less affectively laden, being perpetrated most commonly against men unknown to the aggressor. Violence of psychopaths is often callous and cold-blooded, frequently stemming from a dispassionate search for revenge or retribution and displays of machismo.

IV. HERITABILITY OF PSYCHOPATHY

Cesare Lombroso's very early theory that one can tell a criminal by certain physical features, such as a low forehead, has been discarded. However, though some still believe the genetic effect is not very strong, most modern researchers have shown that criminal behavior is affected by heredity, thus providing strong, though indirect, support for the belief that the AP also is affected by heredity.

V. DIFFICULTIES IN STUDYING THE PSYCHOPATH

There is a reasonable concern that some of the research data available on AP's are not based on ade-

quate sampling techniques. Two populations are a favorite target of researchers: (1) persons (often college students) who score high on the Psychopathic Deviate (Pd (4)) scale of the Minnesota Multiphasic Personality Inventory (MMPI) and (2) incarcerated criminals. There are problems with both groups. Individuals high on the Pd scale (as is true for a significant number of psychology graduate students and medical students) may be creative, productive individuals who are contributing positively to society even though they do not accept some of the standard social mores.

The use of an incarcerated criminal population is also a questionable practice. First, it assumes that the great majority of AP's are unsuccessful and, second, that they are lodged in prisons. There are data (some cited earlier) that refute both of these assumptions, and logic would argue otherwise. The most critical error lies in the assumption that the criminal population is largely composed of AP's. Anyone familiar with prisons is all too aware of the polyglot of individuals in residence.

VI. ASSESSMENT MEASURES WITH AP

Numerous tests, e.g., MMPI-2, provide a narrow or indirect evaluation of psychopathy. However, empirical evidence gathered over the course of the past 10 years indicates that Hare's Psychopathy Checklist (PCL) and its revised form (PCL-R) offer one of the most promising methods of assessing psychopathy directly and comprehensively, yet reliably. The PCL-R is a 20-item revision of the original 22-item scale (Hare, 1980) designed to measure not only behaviors, but also inferred personality traits central to the traditional clinical conceptualization of psychopathy. Assessment is based on a semistructured interview (about 90–120 minutes) and a review of file information. The interview serves not only as a source of information about the subject, but also allows the examiner an opportunity to observe the person's interpersonal style. [See PERSONALITY ASSESSMENT.]

Scoring is based on a three-point scale (0, 1, or 2). Scoring criteria are well delineated and allow satisfactory interrater reliability of .83 for a single rating and .92 for the average of two ratings. The total score can range from 0 to 40 with higher scores indicating a closer match to the psychopathic prototype. Although scores fall along a continuum, a cutting score of 30 is recommended as the best diagnostic indicator and this cutoff is currently being used in most studies of forensic populations. In such populations the mean score is usually between 20 and 25 with a standard deviation of approximately 7.

The psychometric properties of the PCL-R have been well documented and there is extensive evidence to support the measure's reliability and validity. Also, the base rate of psychopathy and the psychometric properties of the PCL for adolescents are similar to those obtained with adult male offenders.

In addition, it does not appear that shortening the test severely compromises the positive psychometric properties, especially in civil populations. The PCL:SV, a 12-item screening version of the PCL-R, has been tested on both criminal and civil populations and has shown good psychometric properties. It has slightly lower reliability than the full-length version, with which it correlates at about .80. Testing is based on a 30- to 45-minute interview and less extensive file information. Scores range from 0 to 24 with a score of 18 or higher being a good indicator of psychopathy. While this measure is easier to administer and flexible enough to be used in a variety of populations, the full-length version is still the best measure in forensic populations and should be used whenever this is feasible.

VII. PCL-R-GENERATED CONCEPTS

There is substantial evidence that psychopathy, as measured by the PCL-R, consists of two stable, main factors, and both factors show good interrater reliability and internal consistency. The more behaviorally oriented Factor 2 demonstrates slightly higher reliability than Factor 1 which is not surprising since there is less subjectivity involved in the scoring of Factor 2 items. However, greater internal consistency is shown by items loading on Factor 1 which is consistent with the idea of a core set of psychopathic personality traits. The factor components are as follows:

Factor 1:
(1) Glibness/superficial charm,
(2) egocentricity/grandiose sense of self-worth,
(3) pathological lying,
(4) conning/lack of sincerity,
(5) lack of remorse,
(6) shallow affect,
(7) callousness/lack of empathy,
(8) failure to accept responsibility.

Factor 2:
(1) Need for stimulation/proneness to boredom,
(2) parasitic lifestyle,
(3) poor behavioral controls,
(4) early behavior problems,
(5) lack of realistic long-term plans,
(6) impulsivity,
(7) irresponsibility,
(8) juvenile delinquency,
(9) revocation of conditional release.

Factor 1 is positively related to clinical ratings of psychopathy and with personality measures of narcissism, dominance, and Machiavellianism. It is negatively correlated with nurturance, agreeableness, empathy, anxiety, and *DSM* diagnoses of avoidant and dependent personality disorders. Factor 2 is related to disruptive prison behavior, drug and alcohol problems, and *DSM-IV* APD. It is negatively correlated with conscientiousness, socialization, SES, employment, education, and IQ.

There is evidence that the diagnosis of psychopathy via the PCL-R predicts recidivism even after such variables as criminal history, previous conditional release violations, and relevant demographic characteristics have been controlled. The behavioral and lifestyle variables of Factor 2 are important in the prediction of general recidivism, while the personality characteristics that compose the first factor are more important in predicting violent recidivism. This finding is consistent with the view that violent psychopaths are more persistent and instrumental in their use of violence than nonpsychopaths.

Yet, while the PCL-R demonstrates impressive incremental validity in predicting violence, especially considering the severe restriction of range under which it functions, the usefulness of the PCL-R should not be overgeneralized. One should not infer from extant supporting research that the PCL-R is able to consistently predict violent behavior in the general population. So far, it appears that the usefulness of the psychopathy construct in predicting violence presupposes some history of violent behavior.

VIII. THE PSYCHOPATH AND THE MAJOR THEORETICAL ORIENTATIONS

This section presents conceptualizations of the psychopath within the framework of the dominant theoretical orientations in psychology, e.g., psychodynamic, learning/behavioral, cognitive, existential, and finally biological, followed by a proposed etiological model.

A. Psychodynamic Concepts

Blending psychodynamic and ethological perspectives, psychodynamic theorists such as John Bowlby have argued for the selective advantage of strong emotional attachments on the part of young animals toward their primary caregivers. Studying children in orphanages who had been reunited with their parents after long separations, Bowlby extended these ethological theories to humans and elaborated on a number of pathological attachment styles, e.g., clinging–dependent, anxious–ambivalent, and avoidant.

Clearly the attachment style of the psychopath would be "avoidant," since an inability to form meaningful attachments with others is a cardinal symptom of psychopathy. Given the frequency of lax, inconsistent, and often violent parenting in the families of psychopaths, it is not surprising that a budding antisocial would learn that social independence, self-sufficiency, and even interpersonal manipulation are the best defenses in a hostile, unsupportive, unnurturing world. To remain unattached is the best prevention against frustrated attachment. [See ATTACHMENT.]

This viewpoint may account for the psychopath's peculiar blend of affective blandness interspersed with occasional fits of angry, gratuitous violence. The great majority of the time, the psychopath is the ultimate "well-defended" person—cold, unfathomable, and unflappable. The angry, frustrated inner child is usually buried so deeply that it is seldom available to the others, or to the psychopath himself.

His developmental needs for nurturance, trust, and acceptance gone sorely unmet in childhood, the psychopath rises above his blocked needs by developing a "moving against" interpersonal style. Feeling profoundly inferior at one psychological level, the psychopath "rises above" others by dragging them down—manipulating, exploiting, humiliating, and perhaps even physically tormenting them to this end. Generally lacking education and socially accepted skills, the psychopath may even come to take special pride in his talent for antisocial and criminal pursuits.

B. Learning/Behavioral Concepts

The issue of conditionability is noted earlier in this chapter. To amplify, the learning viewpoint also em-

phasizes early experience with primary caregivers, but frames these interactions more in terms of reinforcement and punishment. The basic notions here are that the parents of psychopaths are inconsistent and punitive in their parenting behavior. The apparently random quality of the caregivers' behavior teaches the young psychopath that others' treatment of him is not contingent upon his behavior. Moreover, because he is so frequently punished, and most often on a noncontingent basis, he eventually becomes enured to punishing consequences in general. Child-rearing patterns such as these may contribute to the fact that adult psychopaths do not learn from the punishing consequences of life mistakes, as well as the finding that, in learning experiments, psychopaths ignore negative consequences and focus only on potential rewards.

C. Cognitive Concepts

At first glance, the cognitive model seems to have little to add to the discussion of the origins of psychopathy. Especially as articulated in the early writings of Aaron Beck and Albert Ellis, this model has focused less on etiology and more on here-and-now intervention. However, the following existential model certainly provides a cognitive perspective. Also, consider the underlying cognitive schemas that Beck finds to be facilitative of psychopathic behavior, as discussed in the upcoming treatment section.

D. Existential Concepts

It is interesting to view the psychopath from this perspective because of its heavy emphasis on such notions as guilt, anxiety, and freedom. From a point of view influenced by Friedrich Nietzsche's writings, the psychopath is the most free person in the world (this may sound odd given the frequency with which psychopaths are incarcerated). Because he has suppressed it, or is not capable of experiencing it, he is not encumbered by the guilt and anxiety which would interfere with free, self-determined action in the world—he is not a "lamb." He has transcended the conflict and discontent befalling most who struggle to have their needs met in the context of a prohibiting society. He is willing to live with "dirty hands."

Existentialists often focus not only on freedom, but also on death, isolation, and meaninglessness. We might even admire the psychopath in terms of his ability to confront, accept, and embrace death in the form of reckless and dangerous behavior; we might admire his ability to embrace his ultimate isolation and "go it alone"; and we might even grudgingly come to respect his having grasped the purposelessness of existence and then choicefully imposed his own meaning on it, however cruel and perverse its manifestations might be.

But upon closer examination, we see that the psychopath does not really comfortably fit within the existentialist model. He has not really grappled and struggled with the conflicts inherent in choicefulness, e.g., the anxiety which follows from passing up opportunities which will never come again, the guilt which comes with inadvertently hurting others by one's decisions (the psychopath is willing to live with dirty hands because he does not experience them as dirty). And, not having struggled, the psychopath can never experience the wholeness which comes from growth through pain.

We see that he is reacting against others rather than for himself. We see that he is a slave to his impulses, not master of his fate. From a gestalt point of view, we see that he is so hardened and defended that he does not really experience the world. He is not in touch with, or "aware" of the environment in a way that would allow him to act freely in accord with it, rather than haphazardly against it. We see that he is not only alienated from others, but almost completely alienated from his deeper self.

E. Biological Concepts

This article already notes that heritability has a strong role in the development of psychopathy, and some authors have hypothesized a biological link with such childhood disorders as attention-deficit hyperactivity disorder (ADHD). Additionally research has noted several biologically based correlates, including reduced arousal to fear-inducing stimuli, minimized startle responses, restricted affective range, inability to respond affectively to emotion-laden words, reduced conditionability, and a tendency to perseverate in terms of attention allocation. But there is more to be said. [See ATTENTION DEFICIT HYPERACTIVITY DISORDER (ADHD).]

Whereas learning and psychodynamic models emphasize the effects of parents' temperaments on children's behavior, biologically based models emphasize the effects of children's temperaments on parents' be-

havior. For example, consistent with this thinking, research has shown that because of failure to obey, antisocial children were able to elicit punitive behavior from mothers of children who had never even met them before. Psychopaths apparently elicit relatively rejecting responses from parents by being underemotional and unresponsive, by being overly active and thereby annoying, and/or by having little natural tendency to engage their parents socially.

Also, research supports the notion that some individuals (especially psychopaths) have lower baseline levels of arousal than others. In order to achieve optimal levels of arousal, these individuals require more frequent and intense environmental stimulation. It follows that in their attempts to seek out sensational experiences they would be more likely to engage in antisocial acts, i.e., low levels of conditionability and high needs for sensation-seeking combine to create high levels of antisociality and impulsivity.

IX. PROPOSED "COMMON PATH" FOR THE DEVELOPMENT OF PSYCHOPATHY

A. Pre-existing Risk Factors

1. Biological (prenatal, birth) disruption
2. Low SES
3. Family history of vocational–social–interpersonal dysfunction
4. Family history of psychopathy

B. From Birth to School Age

1. Child temperament factors
   (a) Child's lack of emotional responsiveness and lack of social interest fosters rejecting responses from parents
   (b) Child's high activity levels may cause parental annoyance and elicit punitive responses
2. Parental factors
   (a) Inconsistent parenting results in child's failing to learn behavioral contingencies
   (b) Aggressive, punitive parenting results in child's modeling aggression, experiencing hostility, becoming enured to punishing consequences, and developing a repressive defensive style (emotional "hardness")
3. Parent–child interaction
   (a) Unreliable parenting results in insecure attachment (i.e., interpersonally "avoidant" at-

tachment style); child "goes it alone" rather than risk rejection and disappointment associated with unreliable and/or abusive parents

C. School Age to Adolescence

1. Predisposing personality factors
   (a) Low baseline level of arousal (i.e., Eysenck's biological extraversion) contributes to impulsive, undercontrolled, and sensation-seeking behavior
   (b) A synergy of physiological underarousal, repressive psychodynamics, and habitual "numbness" to social contingencies results in child being insensitive to, and unable to, "condition" to environmental events; therefore, does not learn or "profit" from experience
   (c) ADHA/"soft" neurological disorder overlay may exacerbate behavior problems
2. Personality development
   (a) Peer/teacher labeling may result in self-fulfilling prophecy effects
   (b) School and social failure result in sense of inferiority and increased interpersonal hostility; child develops "moving against" interpersonal style
   (c) Initial forays into antisociality (e.g., theft, fire setting, interpersonal violence) occur; evidence for diagnosis of conduct disorder mounts

D. Adolescence

1. The young psychopath hones exploitative style in order to express hostility and "rise above" feelings of inferiority; "proves superiority" by hoodwinking and humiliating teachers, parents, peers
2. Continued antisocial behavior results in initial scrapes with the law
3. Physiological impulsivity, inability to profit from experience (exacerbated by a perseverative attentional style), and interpersonal hostility and antagonism combine to make repeated legal offenses highly probable
4. Contact with other antisocials in the context of juvenile-criminal camps or prison results in "criminal education"; increased criminality results; criminal and antisocial behavior become a lifestyle at which the psychopath can "excel"

E. Adulthood

1. Antisocial behavior escalates through the psychopath's late 20s; increasingly frequent incarceration results in increased hostility and hardened feelings
2. Unable to profit from experience, lacking in insight, and unable to form therapeutic bonds, the psychopath becomes a poor therapy-rehab risk and bad news for society
3. Antisocial behavior decreases or "burns out" in an uneven fashion beginning in the early 30s (less so with violent offenses); this may be due to lengthier incarcerations, to changes in age-related metabolic factors which formerly contributed to sensation-seeking and impulsive behavior, or perhaps to decrements in the strength and stamina required to engage in violent or felony-property crimes

X. INTERVENTION ISSUES

Nearly all significant theorists and researchers suggest that psychopaths are poor therapy candidates, and there is some evidence that the more severe, or primary, psychopaths may get worse with psychotherapy, i.e., psychotherapy may provide a "finishing school" experience for them. The treatment problem with all the personality disorders—getting the client into therapy and meaningfully involved—is acute in the antisocial personality disorder. And, to the degree the person shows primary psychopathy, the poorer are the chances for any meaningful change, no matter what treatment is used.

Most effective are (1) highly controlled settings, (2) with personnel who are firm and caring yet sophisticated in controlling manipulations, (3) and in which the antisocial client resides for a significant period of time (and these appear to be effective only while the psychopath is in residence). Any inpatient treatment program should include four major components: (1) supervision, manipulation of the environment, and provision of education by the staff to facilitate change; (2) a token economy system that requires successful participation for one to receive anything beyond the basic necessities; (3) medical-psychiatric treatments to deal with ancillary psychopathology, e.g., neurological disorders, depression; and (4) a system of necessary social cooperation to maximize conformity and encourage development of the group ethic. This last component is seldom a consideration. In such a program every task that can be found that can reasonably be performed by another and which is not essential to health should be required to be performed only by one inmate for another. This is truly an area where the psychopath is a neophyte.

Attention should also be paid to the AP's high level of stimulation-seeking. This need can be interpreted to the person with an antisocial personality disorder as similar to that of the alcoholic, in that the person will be driven to fulfill this appetite in one way or another. Therapists should attempt to work with psychopaths to develop methods, e.g., developing a consistent pattern of engagement in sports and other strenuous and/or exciting activities and jobs that provide for a high level of activity and stimulation.

Overall, a therapist would generally need to

1. As noted, expect resistance to entering therapy, and then to staying in therapy.

2. As noted, consider their proneness to boredom and their high level of stimulation-seeking.

3. Expect such clients to be deceptive about their history and present status. To the degree feasible, independently corroborate any critical questions about history or present behaviors. Contract ahead of time that if you feel it necessary, you will obtain such data from significant others, etc.

4. In line with the above, clearly confront the individual's psychopathy and any record of deviant behavior. The presentation of "objective" profiles from tests like the MMPI-2 or 16 PF can be effective here. Confront the psychopathology as a lifestyle disorder that will require treatment of a significant duration (and cost); thus, one might contract for some financial penalty for early withdrawal. At the same time, avoid the role of judge, and stay as much as possible in the role of collaborator. Maintaining a degree of adequate rapport is critical. Any exercises that help to develop empathy or social sensitivity are useful.

5. Challenge the following underlying beliefs as adapted from Beck *et al.* (1990): (a) rationalization— "My desiring something justifies whatever actions I need to take"; (b) the devaluing of others—"The attitudes and needs of others don't effect me, unless responding to them will provide me an advantage, and if they are hurt by me, I need not feel responsible for what happens to them"; (c) low-impact consequences—"My choices are inherently good. As such, I won't experience undesirable consequences or if they occur, they won't really matter to me"; (d) "I have to think of myself first; I'm entitled to what I want or feel I need, and if necessary, can use force or deception to obtain those goals"; (e) "rules constrict me from fulfilling my needs."

A. The Issue of Antisocial Burnout

Some solace may be achieved in the notion that psychopathic-antisocial behavior may diminish with age, independent of intervention. Fortunately, there is some empirical validation of this notion. Usually the downward trend begins after age 40, but unfortunately there appears to be no significant dropoff in violent crime for the true (high on Factor 1) psychopaths. And, though often at a diminished rate in nonviolent crime, more recent research suggests that more than a third of psychopath offenders remain criminally active throughout their adulthood.

XI. SUMMARY

The antisocial personality presents a murky conflux of five axioms: (1) an apparent rationality and social appropriateness; (2) an apparent inability to process experience effectively under standard social controls and punishments; (3) some evidence of behavior-determining variables, such as genetic defect and/or brain dysfunction; (4) an absence of evidence of mediating variables between these possible causes and eventual antisocial behavior; and (5) a disinterest in changing oneself, and a lack of positive response to imposed treatment methods.

However pessimistic the picture regarding treatment potential, more psychopathic treatment and outcome studies are warranted, even if they focus on only the small improvements which are made by that small percentage of psychopaths who would stay in treatment. Since psychopaths, as a relatively small percentage of the population, commit such a large percentage of violent and property crimes, even a 5–10% success rate may pay dividends in terms of overall reduction of the most severe offenses.

This article has been reprinted from the *Encyclopedia of Human Behavior, Volume 1.*

BIBLIOGRAPHY

Beck, A., and Freeman, A., *et al.* (1990). "Cognitive Therapy of the Personality Disorders." Guilford, New York.

Cleckley, H. (1955). "The Mask of Sanity." Mosby, St. Louis.

Eysenck, H., and Gudjonsson, G. (1989). "The Causes and Cures of Criminality," Plenum, New York.

Hare, R. (1991). "The Hare Psychopathy Checklist-Revised." Multi-Health Systems, Toronto.

Hare, R., Harpur, T., Hakstian, A., Forth, A., Hart, S., and Newman, J. (1990). The Revised Psychopathy Checklist: Reliability and factor structure. *Psychol. Assess.* **2,** 338–341.

Megargee, E., and Bohn, M. (1979). "Classifying Criminal Offenders." Sage, Beverly Hills.

Meyer, R. (1992). "Abnormal Behavior and the Criminal Justice System." Lexington Books, Lexington, MA.

Serin, R. (1991). Psychopathy and violence in criminals. *J. Interpersonal Violence* **6,** 423–431.

Spitzer, R., *et al.* (1967). Quantification of agreement in psychiatric diagnosis: A new approach. *Arch. Gen. Psychiatry* **17,** 83–87.

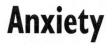

Anxiety

Nader Amir and Michael J. Kozak

Allegheny University of the Health Sciences

I. Definition
II. Theories of Anxiety
III. Measurement
IV. Epidemiology
V. Pathological Anxiety
VI. Summary

Anxiety A state that serves to mobilize an organism to escape or to avoid danger.
Fear The term fear is routinely used interchangeably with the term anxiety. However, some theorists distinguish the two, defining fear as distress about an identified threat, and anxiety as distress about a vague or unidentified threat.
Panic Sudden intense anxiety that peaks quickly and is characterized by noticeable physical reactions such as tachycardia, hyperventilation, sweating, trembling, dizziness, and so on.
Phobia Intense, persistent, and interfering anxiety about nondangerous objects or situations.

It is generally agreed that **ANXIETY** is a fundamental human emotion. Thus, our concept of anxiety is inextricably wed to our understanding of the nature of emotion itself. What is an emotion? More fundamentally, what kind of thing is emotion? If we agree that anxiety is an emotion, then anxiety is that kind of thing. Is emotion mental or physical? These questions may at first seem arcane, but their answers can help us think more clearly about more practical questions, like: (1) How can you tell if someone is anxious?

(2) Can anxiety be controlled? and (3) Should one try to control anxiety and if so should one use medication or psychotherapy?

I. DEFINITION

A. The Nature of Emotion

There has been much argument among philosophers, psychologists, and other theoreticians about the nature of emotion itself. Our approach here derives from the contemporarily influential idea that emotions are functional states. That is, emotions are states of the organism that can best be understood according to their functions. According to this idea, understanding the function of a state is a good start toward understanding whether that state is emotional in nature.

According to this conceptualization, anxiety is any state that serves a particular function or purpose. What function does anxiety serve? It has become conventional in psychology to construe anxiety as a state that serves to escape or avoid danger. Mobilization of an organism to take actions to avoid harm can be a function that enhances survivability. This is our working hypothesis about the function of anxiety. Another idea that has garnered empirical support is that the function of anxiety is to warn others about danger, particularly via facial expressions. Both of these views constitute theories of the nature of anxiety, and are subject to continuing investigation and development or decline, depending on the accumulation of relevant evidence.

Encyclopedia of Mental Health
Volume 1

129

Copyright © 1998 by Academic Press.
All rights of reproduction in any form reserved.

B. Dimensions of Emotion

Some researchers have argued that a limited number of basic emotions exist that cannot be analyzed into more fundamental emotions. These include anger, fear, sadness, disgust, and joy. Other emotions are said to be combinations of these basic emotions. For example, it has been suggested that anxiety can be conceptualized as a combination of fear, guilt, and anger.

Another approach is to analyze emotions according to their position along certain basic dimensions. Watson and Tellegan have proposed one dimension anchored by excitement/elation at one point and drowsy/dull at the other and another dimension anchored by distress/fear at one end and relaxation/calm at the other. These dimensions of positive and negative affectivity are hypothesized to encompass a variety of emotions. Particular emotions are usually depicted as points mapped onto the two-dimensional space. In this model, anxiety is characterized by excess negative affect. Another example of a dimensional approach is Mehrabian and Russell's three orthogonal axes: (1) valence (pleasant vs. unpleasant); (2) arousal (excited vs. relaxed); and (3) dominance (controlling vs. controlled).

C. Threat Meaning and Anxiety

Because our approach is to view anxiety as a state that serves to escape or avoid danger, an essential element of an anxiety state must be a perception of danger by the organism. Note that there need not be any actual danger, but only the perception of danger. The sense of danger could be very specific, like "there is a tiger about to tear out my esophagus," or rather vague, like "something seems to be wrong." We call this sense of danger "threat meaning" and think that it must be part of any state that counts as anxiety. Unless there is some perception of danger by the organism, it is hard to make sense of anxiety as a state whose function is to mobilize the organism to escape or avoid danger.

Cognitive psychology experiments have well established that there are both conscious and unconscious perceptual processes, and that perception of danger can be unconscious. Thus, a person could perceive danger but not be consciously aware of this "threat meaning." It follows that an anxious person may or may not recognize a perception of danger involved in the anxious state.

II. THEORIES OF ANXIETY

A. Conditioning

Mowrer's two-stage theory for the acquisition and maintenance of fear and avoidance behavior has greatly influenced thinking about anxiety. According to the two-stage theory, a neutral event comes to trigger anxiety if it has been experienced along with an event that itself causes anxiety. Furthermore, it is supposed that anxiety can be conditioned not only to physical events, such as snakes and spiders, but also to mental events, such as thoughts and images. This is the first stage: a process called classical conditioning whereby neutral stimuli are associated with danger cues. Once fear of a previously neutral situation is acquired in this way, methods of escape or avoidance are attempted, and successful methods are learned and maintained. This learning to escape and avoid is the second stage of the hypothesized two-stage process: instrumental, or "operant," conditioning.

It has been argued that Mowrer's theory is too simple to account for fear acquisition and maintenance. For example, it fails to account for the disproportionately high frequency of certain fears (e.g., snakes and spiders) among humans, compared to, say, phobias about electric sockets. It also does not explain the particular ease with which some fears, like taste aversions, are learned and maintained. A useful addition to the two-stage theory is the theory of biologically prepared learning, that hypothesizes that certain conditioned learning is especially easy because of evolutionary developments in the nervous system that have had survival advantages. Although preparedness theory is a plausible elaboration of two-factor theory, its experimental exploration has yielded equivocal results.

Despite the limitations of the basic two-stage theory, it maps well onto certain observations about the maintenance of phobic avoidance and escape. Specifically, it is generally consistent with the common observation that confrontation with phobic situations has been found to provoke reports of distress and elevated cardiac and electrodermal activity, and withdrawal from the situations leads to temporary relief.

Another influential theory of anxiety emphasizes the anxiogenic role of uncontrollability and unpredictability. Accordingly, unpleasant events feel much worse and have more lasting effects if they are unpredictable and uncontrollable.

B. Cognitive

These theories postulate that what people think influences how they feel. For example, Beck and his colleagues have hypothesized that unrealistic expectations and attitudes, represented as cognitive "schemas," predispose a person to emotional distress. A limitation of this sort of cognitive theory is that it does not specify what expectations and attitudes distinguish different emotions, such as fear versus anger or sadness.

Another type of cognitive theory supposes that certain styles of thinking, for example, overestimating of threat, are involved in pathological anxiety, and that the perception of threat is an important determinant of anxiety. For example, Watts and his colleagues have argued that the way people pay attention to, remember, and interpret threat-relevant information is a crucial determinant of anxiety. Furthermore, different emotions may be associated with different types of information processing bias, for example, anxiety with attentional bias, and sadness with memory bias.

C. Biological

Biological theories of anxiety emphasize the role of the nervous system in anxiety. Anxiety is routinely construed as a stress reaction, and it is generally understood that environmental stressors affect physical well-being. Hans Selye introduced the concept of a General Adaptation Syndrome (GAS) to describe physical reactions to stressors. Accordingly, there are three phases in the reaction to stress. During the first phase, the alarm reaction, the activity in the autonomic nervous system increases. In the second stage, resistance, some physiological adaptation occurs, but if the stressor persists, other physiological reactions ensue, such as ulcers and atrophy of the thymus. Finally, in the third phase, exhaustion, irreversible damage or death may result if the source of stress is not removed. [See STRESS.]

Other researchers have emphasized the importance of interpretation of events in the environment. For example, Lazarus suggests that interpretation of threat is as important as the triggering event in causing stress. For example, it has been suggested that stress occurs when a situation is appraised as exceeding the individual's adaptive resources.

The above theories of stress often refer to neuroanatomical structure that may be involved in the stress reaction. Jeffrey Gray's theory postulated that the nervous system has subsystems serving different functions, and that there is a subsystem called the "behavioral inhibition system" whose prime function is to inhibit behavior in certain situations (e.g., novel situations, aversive situations). Gray has argued that the effects of certain anti-anxiety substances such as alcohol, and of lesions of certain brain areas (e.g., septo-hippocampal system) that reduce anxiety support this theory. Furthermore, Gray suggested that individual differences in anxiety stem from differences in the activation of the behavioral inhibition system and that these differences are determined genetically.

D. Genetic and Evolutionary

As noted earlier, anxiety is believed to have survival value because it prepares the organism to avoid harm. While the avoidance of threat is essential for survival, chronic anxiety can involve hypervigilance and exaggerated perception of the number and severity of dangerous environmental stimuli. Such hypervigilance could impede, rather than enhance, the organism's survivability, by interfering with essential activities.

If this genetic advantage is passed on to one's offspring, then anxiety should be especially prevalent in relatives of anxious individuals. Genetic and family studies have found some support for this notion. For example, elevated levels of panic have been found in relatives of individuals with panic disorder. Another way of understanding genetic influence is through comparisons of identical (monozygotic) twins, who have identical genetic makeup, and dizygotic twins, who have similar upbringing but different genetic makeup. The method is to compare their concordance for anxiety, that is, to compare the number of each type of twin pair who both have anxiety. Such concordance is higher in monozygotic twins.

Together, the various genetic studies point to a component of heritability for anxiety. Notably, however, heritable vulnerability is not absolute: the concordance rate for monozygotic twins is closer to 40% rather than to 100%. This means that genetic makeup provides a limited explanation of vulnerability to anxiety disorder. Furthermore, what seems to run in families is a vulnerability to develop some kind of anxiety, rather than to develop a specific disorder. [See GENETIC CONTRIBUTORS TO MENTAL HEALTH.]

E. Diathesis-Stressor

Because of evidence that both person and environment are important in understanding anxiety, it has become commonplace to suggest that an interaction between stressors in the environment with predispositions (or diatheses) in the person cause anxiety. The predisposition could itself be environmentally caused, or it could be inherited. Hypothesized environmentally caused diatheses might be brain injury caused by prenatal hypoxia, or autonomic hyperreactivity stemming from years of child abuse or imprisonment and torture. Some theorists have suggested that individuals inherit predispositions to differing levels of anxiety and that environmental stressors are influential in determining its onset and course.

F. Animal Models

Animals experience distress in threatening situations, and this has been compared to anxiety in humans. For example, when animals are forced to make difficult choices between danger and safety signals, they show agitation, restlessness, distraction, hypersensitivity, muscle tension, and stomach ulcers. This phenomenon has been termed experimental neurosis, and can also be produced by punishment of appetitive behavior, and by long periods of restraint and monotony. There are parallels between disturbances observed in animals who are exposed to unavoidable and unpredictable stressors, and human reaction to extreme harm or threats (e.g., violent assault, physical injury). These similarities suggest that animal models can be useful for studying human reactions to extreme stress. Although animal models do not illuminate every feature of anxiety, they can probably explain some of the more prominent features.

III. MEASUREMENT

A. Indicators

Methods of assessing anxiety include interviewing, questionnaires, physiological monitoring, and obser-vations of behavior. These can be used to assess the full range of anxiety, from mild to intense. The primary technique used to assess pathological anxiety is the clinical interview addressing criterion symptoms as specified in *DSM-IV* or another diagnostic rubric. [See DSM-IV.]

An approach to anxiety advocated by Peter Lang holds that it is variously evident in three behavioral systems: semantic (what people report about themselves), physiological (e.g., heart rate, brain electrical activity), and overt behavior (e.g., avoidance), and that there is routinely some dysynchrony among the three systems. The implication of this particular view is that a thorough assessment entails measurement of the three systems.

Measurement of each system has advantages and disadvantages. Self-report indicators of anxiety require introspective description of feelings. An advantage of this indicator is that language can indicate fine nuances of meaning that are less easily accessible in other indicators. Also, self-report provides a relatively economical method of assessment, and can often be done by questionnaire. A disadvantage is that subjects are often inconsistent in their observations of themselves, and the usefulness of their report depends heavily on their limited powers of self-observation.

An advantage of direct monitoring of physiological functioning is that the data do not rely on the self-observational accuracy of the subject, but rather, on the quality of the measurement methods and monitoring equipment. There is a subspecialty of psychology: psychophysiology, which is devoted to psychological theorizing founded in physiological assessment. Disadvantages of physiological assessment are not only the technical burdens, but more fundamentally, the multiplicity of physiological determinants. To put it simply, the bodily organs do not operate just to tell us about anxiety. How much variation in a particular physiological function is irrelevant to anxiety is ambiguous, and complicates any assessment of anxiety via physiology. There is no one physiological response pattern associated with anxiety. For example, heart rate could increase or decrease in response to threat. Note also that with physiological assessment alone, one can not determine if a heart is pounding because a person is running an Olympic race, running from an assailant, or riding a roller coaster at an amusement park.

Behavioral measurement entails identifying and

quantifying overt behavior that is deemed relevant to anxiety. For example, number of errors during a 5-minute typing test could be used as a performance indicator of anxiety. Distance in feet that a person is willing to approach a dangerous object also could constitute a behavioral measure, as could frequency of eye contact in a social situation. An advantage of direct observation is that it is not subject to inaccuracies of the subject's interpretation. Disadvantages are that people act very differently in different circumstances, so it is difficult to obtain a representative sampling of behavior, and watching a person during an action often influences the target behavior, so that the observation process itself distorts the obtained behavioral sample.

B. Psychometrics

As mentioned above, individuals are often inconsistent in their observations of themselves, and the usefulness of their reports depends heavily on their limited powers of self-observation. A subfield of psychology called psychometrics concerns the technology of measurement, and includes techniques to enhance the usefulness of self-report data. These methods focus on increasing the consistency, that is, reliability, and accuracy, that is, validity of self-report data, and involve using mathematical statistics to develop self-report scales. A number of psychometrically sophisticated scales are available to measure anxiety, and many are in the form of questionnaires. Traditional psychometric approaches classify anxiety into state (transitory feelings) and trait (stable personality) attributes.

One method of evaluating the accuracy of an anxiety scale is to compare its results to other measures of anxiety, for example, interview, physiology, and observations of behavior. By assessing various aspects of anxiety, the investigator tries to gauge an emotion for which no single indicator offers a perfect yardstick.

IV. EPIDEMIOLOGY

A. Anxiety Across the Life Span

Anxiety can develop at any time in the individual's life span. However, some fears more especially characterize certain stages of development. For example, fears of heights, of loss of physical support, and of loud noises are common in infancy, but fear of strangers develops between 6 and 12 months.

Jerome Kagan and his colleagues have demonstrated that there are individual differences in the level of anxiety, inhibition, and physiological reactivity that are apparent at infancy. Furthermore, these individual differences may have long-lasting implications for individual development. [See INDIVIDUAL DIFFERENCES IN MENTAL HEALTH.]

From 1 to 3 years of age children develop other fears, including fears of darkness, injury, and animals. Kindergartners develop fears such as separation from parents, bodily harm, animals, and sleeping alone. Later, at elementary school age, common fears include test-taking anxiety, fear related to physical appearance, and illness. Fears common in adolescence include anxiety related to social interactions, physical health, sexual matters, and political and social concerns. In the general population, common fears include, snakes, spiders, heights, flying, blood, and dentists. Anxiety about physical health attains more prominence in the elderly.

B. Gender Differences

Differences exist between men and women in felt anxiety: women report more anxiety. This difference is evident in children as well as in adults. Furthermore, the objects of anxiety differ among the sexes. Environmental, agoraphobic, and animal phobias are more common among women, whereas fears of social situations, bodily injury, and illness are approximately equal among men and women. There are also sex differences in response to interpersonal threat situations, with women more likely to respond with anxiety, and men with anger. This appears related to perception of potential control of the threat by the subject. Other factors, e.g., greater cultural acceptability of reports of distress for women, probably also contribute to observed sex differences. [See GENDER DIFFERENCES IN MENTAL HEALTH.]

C. Cross-Cultural Perspective

Although anxiety is common to all cultures its expression varies. For example, as Barlow points out, the introspective interpretation of anxiety is culture dependent. For example, in China, medical treatments of emotional disorders are less successful than they are in Western cultures because of the belief that familial separation is the cause of emotional problems. Furthermore, in the third world countries, somatic symptoms appear to be the prevalent mode of anxious expression. In sum, although there are individuals in all cultures that seem anxious, the foci of anxiety and worry, and the attributions of causes of anxiety, are diverse.

V. PATHOLOGICAL ANXIETY

A. Definition

Because everyone feels anxious from time to time, it becomes useful to distinguish normal from pathological anxiety. Disabling anxiety in the absence of any actual danger is clearly pathological. As a rule, if anxiety interferes with routine functioning (e.g., work, social life, leisure) and persists when there is minimal real threat, then it is considered pathological.

B. Expression versus Suppression of Anxiety

Should anxiety be suppressed or expressed? This is a variant of the broader question of whether it is healthier to express or suppress emotions. Although a common response to unpleasant feelings is to try to control them, some theorists have proposed that attempts to suppress negative emotions can result in somatic problems, such as ulcers, asthma, arthritis, urticaria, and so on. Although there is certainly evidence for psychosomatic disease, its existence does not itself imply that emotions should always be immediately and completely expressed. Expressing intense anger at a police officer who is giving you a ticket for speeding, or at an armed combat soldier who confiscates your property, could lead to serious harm. A balanced analysis would weigh the potential disadvantages of a particular expression of anxiety against those of its suppression. An often practical alternative to either expressing or suppressing anxiety might be to identify and eliminate its source.

C. Control of Anxiety

Because anxiety can interfere with an individual's functioning it is sometimes desirable to reduce it. The most established method for reducing excessive fear is by confronting the feared situation. For example, through gradual approach, an individual who is afraid of insects can handle some insects and reduce the fear. The various components of anxiety described above, however, typically change at different rates. Although the person may be handling an insect, and so seem by his or her behavior to no longer be afraid, heartrate may still be elevated, and there may still be a suspicion that the insect is dangerous. This is an example of the often observed desynchrony among different aspects of anxiety. With more practice, the idea of threat and the physical reaction may also change.

Although it is clear that anxiety can sometimes be controlled, it is unclear to what extent vulnerability to develop anxiety can be changed. Some researchers believe that psychological and biological interventions can change vulnerability to anxiety, but this issue remains controversial.

D. Classification of Anxiety Disorders

The *Diagnostic and Statistical Manual of Mental Disorder,* Fourth Edition (*DSM-IV*), delineates seven specific anxiety disorders. This classification is based on both theoretical and practical considerations, and reflects contemporary thinking. Some theorists have argued that such classifications are too arbitrary, do not reflect "natural" categories, and should be replaced by dimensional descriptive nomenclature. The *DSM-IV* categories are: Obsessive–Compulsive Disorder, Panic Disorder, Social Phobia, Posttraumatic Stress Disorder, Generalized Anxiety Disorder, and Acute Anxiety Reaction. They differ not only according to the nature of the feared situation (e.g., social situations), but also according to the cluster of associated symptoms. [*See* OBSESSIVE-COMPULSIVE DISORDER; PANIC ATTACKS; POSTTRAUMATIC STRESS.]

C. Treatment

Treatments for anxiety disorders often mirror the underlying theories of anxiety discussed above. For example, a clinician who believes that biochemical abnormalities cause anxiety might favor pharmacotherapy with anxiolytic medicine. A clinician who believes that faulty learning or mistaken beliefs are responsible for pathological anxiety might prescribe corrective exercises, for example, facing the anxiety-provoking situation as opposed to avoiding it, or reevaluating the likelihood of danger in a given situation. Certain drug- and learning-based treatments have been studied scientifically and found helpful for various kinds of anxiety. Particular treatments have been found especially helpful for particular types of anxiety, so it is important to obtain a treatment that has been found to match the type of difficulty experienced. [*See* PSYCHOPHARMACOLOGY.]

Unfortunately, clinicians sometimes focus too much on the treatments in which they are most expert: a physician tends to prescribe medicine and a psychologist or social worker tends to prescribe psychotherapy. The kind of psychotherapy given sometimes depends more on the kind of psychotherapist (cognitive, behavioral, family, hypnosis, psychoanalytic) than on the kind of treatment that is of established efficacy for a particular type of anxiety. Ideally, a clinician should be familiar with scientific findings on the comparative efficacy of the available treatments for different anxiety problems, regardless of whether that clinician is competent with each treatment, and should guide the anxious person accordingly to choose a treatment of established efficacy. Seekers of treatments for anxiety should be cautious about treatment providers who are unwilling to explain the advantages and disadvantages of alternative treatments, including the strength of the evidence for and against each treatment. [*See* BEHAVIOR THERAPY; COGNITIVE THERAPY; FAMILY THERAPY; HYPNOSIS AND THE PSYCHOLOGICAL UNCONSCIOUS; PSYCHOANALYSIS.]

VI. SUMMARY

Anxiety is a routine part of human existence but is incompletely understood. One way of trying to understand it is by what function it serves, for example, to prepare to escape or avoid harm. Many theories about various aspects of anxiety have been proposed, but there is no generally accepted comprehensive explanation. A number of methods of assessing anxiety are available, and each has advantages and disadvantages. The incidence and expression of anxiety varies across age and culture. Anxiety merits treatment if it is severe, persistent, and disabling. Different drugs and psychotherapies have been found helpful for different types of anxiety, and careful consideration of the scientific evidence for each treatment should guide selection.

BIBLIOGRAPHY

Barlow, D. H. (1988). *Anxiety and its disorders: The Nature and treatment of anxiety and panic.* New York: Guilford Press.

Eysenck, H. (1992). *Anxiety the cognitive perspective.* Hillsdale, NJ: Lawrence Earlbaum Associates.

McNally, R. J. (1994). *Panic disorder: A critical analysis.* New York: Guilford Press.

Tuma, A. H., & Maser, J. (1985). *Anxiety and the anxiety disorders.* Hillsdale, NJ: Earlbaum.

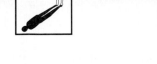

Aphasia, Alexia, and Agraphia

Rhonda B. Friedman

Georgetown University Medical Center

Guila Glosser

University of Pennsylvania

Agrammatism   Speech that is characterized by the deletion of many of the syntactic words in sentences.

Anomia   Difficulty retrieving words.

Fluency   Characterization of speech output in terms of longest number of words produced in running speech in a single phrase.

Literal (Phonemic) Paraphasia   A speech error in which one or more phonemes of the word are produced incorrectly.

Neologism   A spoken nonword that contains few phonemes in common with the target word.

Paragrammatism   Speech that is characterized by the incorrect use of the syntactic words in sentences.

Paragraphia   The incorrect production of a word in writing.

Paralexia   The incorrect production of a word in oral reading.

Paraphasia   The incorrect production of a word in speech.

Phonemes   The elemental sounds of a language.

Semantic Paraphasia   A verbal paraphasia in which the substituted word is related in meaning to the intended word.

Verbal Paraphasia   The substitution of a real word for the intended word.

APHASIA (language disorder), **ALEXIA** (reading disorder), and **AGRAPHIA** (writing disorder) refer to disorders that are acquired as a result of brain injury. The terms dysphasia, dyslexia, and dysgraphia are also used for these disorders, particularly outside of the United States. The common feature of these disorders is that they involve impairment in the comprehension, expression, or manipulation of language sounds (phonology), meanings (semantics), grammar (syntax), or written symbols (orthography). While such disorders may include a disturbance in speech, language and speech are distinct. Language refers to the code that relates certain combinations of symbols to meanings, whereas speech refers to the neuromechanical aspects of articulation and phonation.

Language disorders can also occur in association with dementing illnesses, confusional states, or syndromes of thought disorder. However, the terms aphasia, alexia, and agraphia are generally reserved for disorders of language that represent a breakdown of linguistic mechanisms caused by structural damage to aspects of the language system, resulting in characteristic language patterns and error types. The trained clinician can distinguish aphasia from the disturbed language that results from deficits in attention or confusional states.

I. INTRODUCTION: THE SYMPTOMS OF APHASIA

Anomia refers to difficulty retrieving words from one's internal lexicon. All of us experience isolated incidents of anomia, or *word-finding problems,* on occasion: you are certain that you know the word that you are trying to come up with, but you just cannot remember it at the moment. An abnormality in word finding, ranging from mild to severe, is characteristic of all patients with aphasia. Anomia can be seen in spontaneous speech, as when one is recounting an incident or telling a story. Word finding difficulties may also be encountered during the naming of pictures or objects; this is known as a *confrontation naming deficit.*

The term anomia is applied to a deficit in retrieving substantive words, that is nouns, adjectives, and verbs. This is distinguished from difficulties producing *functors,* that is, prepositions, conjunctions, pronouns, and auxiliary verbs; trouble with the latter types of words is called agrammatism (see below).

The failure to retrieve the appropriate word may result in an error of omission, in which the target word is simply deleted. Or, a circumlocution may be produced: the patient utters a sentence or phrase describing or in some way relating to the intended word (e.g., "that thing made of glass that you look out.") Another common type of error made by aphasic patients is the production of an incorrect word; this is known as a paraphasia. The production of an incorrect word in reading is called a paralexia; in writing, a paragraphia. A verbal paraphasia (or verbal paralexia, verbal paragraphia) is the substitution of a real word for the intended word. A semantic paraphasia is a type of verbal paraphasia in which the meanings of the target word and the word produced are related to one another. Thus, a patient attempting to say "window" may say "door" instead. A literal paraphasia (also called phonemic paraphasia) is an error in which the phonemes (sounds) of a word are substituted for one another (e.g., "gate" is pronounced as "kate"). When several phonemes are incorrectly produced, such that it is difficult or impossible to determine the intended output (e.g., the word "window" is pronounced as "pinmo") the patient has produced a neologism. When entire phrases or sentences consist primarily of neologisms, the patient is producing neologistic jargon.

In addition to difficulties with single words, patients with aphasia have difficulties at the sentence level as well. One pattern of output that is not uncommon is agrammatism. The patient with agrammatic speech has a tendency to delete those words that serve a largely syntactic function: the prepositions, conjunctions, pronouns, and auxiliary verbs. Affixes (e.g., *ed, ing*), which also serve a syntactic function, are also deleted or misapplied. Agrammatic speech, then, consists primarily of nouns, adjectives, and verbs. "Stay . . . hospital . . . one week" may be the attempt of an agrammatic aphasic patient to tell you that he has been in the hospital for one week.

Another pattern of sentence production seen in aphasic patients is paragrammatism. In this pattern of speech output syntactic function words are present, but they are used incorrectly. The result is often an ill-formed sentence such as "I was almost went then the hospital came to it."

Some patients with aphasia produce sentences of normal length and prosody; we say that their output is fluent. Other patients with aphasia produce pieces of sentences; the output is short and choppy, phrase length is reduced to one- or two-word phrases, and speech is halting, with many pauses. The speech of these patients is nonfluent. Fluency, then, is defined chiefly with regard to phrase length. The fluent/nonfluent distinction is an important one in characterizing aphasic speech, as it normally distinguishes between aphasias caused by lesions of the anterior portion of the cerebral language zone and those caused by posterior lesions.

Another aspect of speech production that is important in the characterization of aphasia is the ability to accurately repeat spoken words and phrases. In order to repeat spoken phrases, the patient must be able to perceive and encode the words; then, the properly encoded words must be transformed for articulatory output. Problems at any of these stages of processing may result in repetition deficits. Some aphasic patients show a striking deficit of repetition in the face of preservation of all other aspects of language. Some patients show the reverse pattern: a striking preservation of repetition in the presence of severe deficits in most other aspects of language processing. Repetition deficits are typically most pronounced for sentences that are low in predictability or contain low-frequency words such as "The barn swallow captured a plump worm." Some patients have particular difficulty repeating phrases containing many functors (grammatical words). The classic phrase used to test for this difficulty is: "No ifs, ands, or buts." Other patients can repeat these sentences, but have more difficulty repeating sentences containing many nouns, verbs, and adjectives.

In addition to language output problems, patients

with aphasia commonly experience difficulty with auditory comprehension. At the single word level, this involves an inability to access the conceptual referent of a spoken word. Careful testing may reveal access to partial information about the concept in question. Thus a patient may know the category of a word's referent, which may be reflected in a predominance of within-category errors. That is, when asked to point to the picture of the screwdriver, a patient might be more likely to point to the picture of a hammer than the picture of a comb. Word comprehension deficits may be category specific: a patient may fail to comprehend words of a particular class, such as words referring to body parts.

Patients who do not have difficulty understanding individual words may nevertheless have difficulty understanding sentences, or may be unable to follow a conversation. A very mild deficit in auditory comprehension may go unnoticed while chatting with a patient about his/her family or hobby, but may become obvious when the patient is challenged with simple passive sentences (e.g., "The girl was kicked by the boy. Which child is hurt?")

II. THE REPRESENTATION OF LANGUAGE IN THE BRAIN

Most language processing, for most people, occurs in the left hemisphere of the brain. People who are left-handed are more likely to have some language represented in the right hemisphere of the brain than people who are right-handed, but for the vast majority of left-handed people, as for right-handed people, the left side of the brain is dominant for language processing. Approximately 1 to 2% of right-handed people have language in the right hemisphere. When these people become aphasic, it is known as crossed aphasia.

The language zones within the left hemisphere lie primarily within the areas surrounding the Sylvian fissure, known as the perisylvian region. It includes a large part of the frontal, parietal, and temporal lobes, plus, when reading is involved, the occipital lobe as well. The area of the brain that appears to mediate initiation of speech is located somewhat distant from the rest of the language zone. This region, located on the medial aspect of the left frontal lobe, is known as the supplementary motor area.

Analysis of the lesions associated with aphasic defi-

cits leads to the following delineation of specific language processing regions. Phonological processing is primarily the domain of the left temporal lobe. Wernicke's area, the posterior superior temporal gyrus, is involved in the processing of the auditory patterns that make up words. This area plays an important role both in the comprehension of spoken words and in the internal generation of the pronunciation of words to be spoken.

The motor aspects of speech and language are controlled in the left frontal lobe. An area known as Broca's area, in the left posterior inferior frontal gyrus, is said to contain the codes that convert the phonological patterns of words into the articulatory codes needed to say the words. The fiber bundle known as the arcuate fasciculus connects Wernicke's area to Broca's area, allowing for the transfer to Broca's area of the phonological information that is generated in Wernicke's area. Grammatical processing is another function of the left frontal lobe.

The processing of written language begins in the primary visual cortex and subsequently the visual association areas of the occipital lobe. From there the orthographic information is transferred to the angular gyrus within the parietal lobe, which is crucially involved in the processing of written letters and words as elements of language. Thus, both reading and writing are dependent upon the angular gyrus of the left hemisphere.

III. SYNDROMES OF APHASIA

The symptoms of aphasia, described above, do not occur randomly in patients with language disturbances, but they tend to cluster in somewhat predictable patterns. This has led to the classification of patients into aphasic groups with similar constellations of symptoms. That is, patients who are classified with the same type of aphasia are likely to have similar patterns of language deficits and areas of language preservation. Such a classification system is a useful code for health care professionals, who can learn much about a patient's language just from being told his/her aphasia type. However, one should keep in mind that many aphasic patients do not fit well into any of the established categories; and that two patients who do happen to meet the criteria for the same type of aphasia will not have identical language deficits.

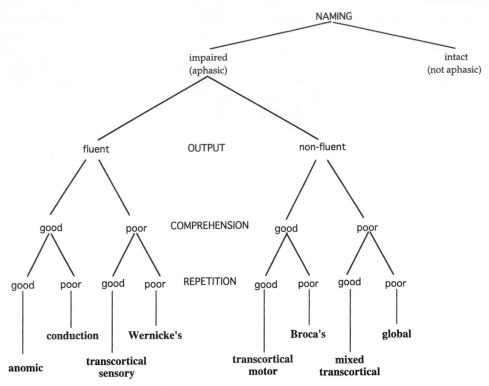

Figure 1 Eight major types of aphasia.

The eight major types of aphasia are represented in the diagram depicted in Figure 1. As mentioned above, the language impairment that is common to all aphasic patients—at least at some point during the course of their aphasia—is an abnormal difficulty in retrieving words. Aphasic patients are first classified with regard to the nature of their speech output. The feature of primary importance in this regard is fluency (see definition above). All patients with nonfluent aphasia share the characteristic of short phrase length in speech output; the speech of fluent aphasics appears facile and of normal phrase length. Among patients with fluent aphasia, some have good comprehension, others have poor comprehension. Likewise, patients with nonfluent aphasia may have good or poor comprehension. And finally, patients with fluent or nonfluent aphasia, and good or poor comprehension, may have good or poor repetition. The $2 \times 2 \times 2$ matrix formed by the features of fluency, comprehension, and repetition result in the eight types of aphasia listed at the bottom of the diagram.

A. The Fluent Aphasias

Anomic aphasia is the mildest of the aphasias. Patients with anomic aphasia have fluent speech, and no significant language impairment other than a marked deficit in word retrieval. Words representing nouns present the greatest difficulty, while the syntactic function words are typically spared. The speech of these patients sounds "empty"; nonspecific words are often used where specific words cannot be retrieved (e.g., "that thing"; "the whadayacallit"; "in that place").

Anomic aphasia may result from lesions in different parts of the language areas of the left hemisphere. The most common lesion sites for anomia are the angular gyrus of the parietal lobe and lesions of the middle or inferior temporal gyri, although occasionally the temporo-occipital cortex or the frontal lobe are implicated.

Conduction aphasia also tends to be one of the milder aphasia types, although it is more disabling than anomia. While fluency is fairly well maintained, speech is disrupted by false starts and problems in sequencing the sounds within words. Literal paraphasias are the predominant error type. Patients tend to be cognizant of their errors, and attempts at self-correction are pervasive. Compared with other aspects of language processing, repetition is the most severely impaired language function; even single words may be repeated incorrectly in some cases. Comprehension is relatively good, and is often adequate for normal conversation. However, comprehension of complex sentences may be impaired.

Lesions that result in conduction aphasia are typically found in the supramarginal gyrus, or the insula and its subcortical white matter. Conduction aphasia is often seen as the residual aphasia following recovery from a Wernicke's aphasia. As such, it may be seen with a lesion in part of the temporal lobe, including parts—but never all—of Wernicke's area.

One of the best known of aphasia types is Wernicke's aphasia, characterized by fluent, well-articulated paraphasic speech. Both literal and verbal paraphasias may be present, and in more severe cases jargon may be heard as well. Paragrammatic sentences are common. Comprehension is impaired, as is repetition. There may be a press of speech. Patients may be unaware of their deficits, particularly in the early stages.

Patients with **Wernicke's aphasia** normally have lesions that include the entire posterior superior temporal gyrus of the left hemisphere. The lesion often extends into middle temporal gyrus and nearby parietal regions as well. When parietal regions are spared, reading comprehension may be better preserved than auditory comprehension.

Patients with **transcortical sensory aphasia** have fluent speech, but speech tends to be riddled with semantic paraphasias, as well as neologisms and neologistic jargon. Literal paraphasias may be heard as well. Comprehension is impaired. In contrast to patients with conduction aphasia, patients with transcortical sensory aphasia have relatively intact repetition, often repeating long sentences without error. Another preserved ability is the production of automatized speech, that is, overlearned phrases, poems, and sequences such as the days of the week.

The lesion site for transcortical sensory aphasia is typically found in the temporo-parieto-occipital junction, posterior to the perisylvian language area. Thus it may be conceived as a disconnection of primary language areas from the posterior areas of the brain involved in other aspects of perceptual and conceptual knowledge.

B. The Nonfluent Aphasias

The form of nonfluent aphasia marked by impaired initiation of speech is known as **transcortical motor aphasia**. Patients with this form of aphasia speak very little, and tend to answer questions with one-word responses. Occasional well-formed phrases and sentences may be produced. Although speech is nonfluent, as defined by average phrase length, when speech is produced, articulation is normal. As in transcortical sensory aphasia, patients with this form of aphasia display a disproportionate preservation of repetition relative to other language deficits. This is particularly pronounced when comparing repetition of long sentences (typically produced flawlessly) with attempts at generating a sentence spontaneously or in answer to a question. Patients with transcortical motor aphasia may have a tendency to repeat back the last part of their interlocutors' utterances, a behavior known as echolalia. Comprehension is well preserved in transcortical motor aphasia.

The lesion that produces transcortical motor aphasia is found anterior or superior to Broca's area, usually deep, disconnecting the supplementary motor area (implicated in initiation of speech) from Broca's area.

Broca's aphasia is the best known of the nonfluent aphasias. Patients with Broca's aphasia have limited speech output. Their articulation is impaired to varying degrees, yet certain common overlearned phrases may be produced with normal articulation by patients who are otherwise unable to produce speech sounds. When articulation is only partially impaired, they may produce some literal and verbal paraphasias. A striking feature of their speech is agrammatism; syntactic function words are frequently absent. They tend to produce short phrases or single words. Comprehension is not perfect in Broca's aphasia, but it is often reasonably good for normal conversation. Repetition is impaired both by poor articulation and impaired syntax.

The lesion that produces Broca's aphasia includes Broca's area, but must extend deep to Broca's area, and may even include periventricular white matter.

The lesion may also include the lower portion of the motor strip. Lesions that are restricted to cortical Broca's area typically produce only a transient problem with speech production.

A nonfluent aphasia that has features of both transcortical motor aphasia and transcortical sensory aphasia is known as **mixed transcortical aphasia**, or "isolation of the speech area." As with transcortical motor aphasia, there is minimal speech output. As with transcortical sensory aphasia, comprehension is poor. As with both forms of transcortical aphasia, repetition and the recitation of automatized phrases are relatively preserved. The preservation of repetition is particularly striking in the face of the absence of any other intact language behaviors.

As might be expected, this pattern of language deficits containing features of both types of transcortical aphasia results from lesions located both anterior and posterior to the language zones, but sparing the bulk of the perisylvian language region. The lesion often involves the watershed regions between the areas perfused by the middle cerebral artery and those perfused by the anterior and posterior cerebral arteries.

As the name implies, **global aphasia** consists of impairments in all aspects of language. It is the most severe disabling form of aphasia. Speech is virtually absent, except for stereotyped phrases or interjections. As a rare example, one globally aphasic patient said nothing but "No way out of here." Expletives (e.g., "damn it!" "shit") may be produced in seemingly appropriate contexts. Comprehension is very poor, although topics of personal relevance to the patient (e.g., questions about family members) may sometimes be understood better. Repetition is virtually impossible, but the ability to produce some automatized sequences may remain.

In many instances of lasting global aphasia, left hemisphere damage is extensive, affecting most or all of the perisylvian language areas. However, permanent global aphasia may also result from relatively discrete subcortical lesions.

C. Modality-Specific Language Disturbances

Patients with aphemia (also called subcortical motor aphasia) are impaired only in the production of spoken language. These patients have a problem with articulation. The result is slow, halting, often aprosodic speech. Other aspects of language processing, including comprehension, word retrieval, grammatical sentence construction, reading, and writing remain intact. Aphemia is typically caused by a lesion of the lower motor cortex and the subcortical white matter deep to it.

Patients with pure word deafness have trouble comprehending and repeating spoken language, but comprehension of written language is not impaired. Speech and written language output are normal. Audiometric testing shows normal hearing levels, and nonlanguage sounds are recognized relatively well. The difficulty for these patients seems to lie in the recognition of auditory language patterns. The patient with pure word deafness often complains that spoken language sounds muffled, or that it sounds like a foreign language is being spoken.

Pure word deafness may be caused by bilateral temporal lobe lesions in auditory cortex, or by a unilateral lesion damaging the left auditory cortex plus pathways to it. In both cases, Wernicke's area is spared, but is cut off from auditory input.

IV. WRITTEN LANGUAGE DISORDERS

The writing and oral reading of patients with aphasia tend to parallel the characteristics of their speech production, and reading comprehension is often related to auditory comprehension. Patients whose speech is agrammatic tend to have difficulty reading the grammatical words of the sentence, while the reading of nouns and adjectives is relatively preserved. Similarly, these patients frequently have difficulty writing the grammatical function words. Patients who produce many literal paraphasias in speech will likely produce literal paralexias in oral reading, and spelling errors in writing. Likewise, patients who produce many semantic paraphasias tend to produce semantic paralexias in oral reading and may produce semantic paragraphias in writing. Patients who can repeat well, but without comprehension, may be able to read aloud, but again without comprehension. Patients with poor auditory comprehension usually exhibit poor reading comprehension as well. However, some patients with Wernicke's aphasia comprehend written language better than spoken language; these patients tend to keep a pad and pencil with them at all times.

Notwithstanding the generalizations asserted in the preceding paragraph, the correlation between type of language impairment and type of reading impairment should be considered a weak one. There is considerable variation in the nature and degree of alexia and agraphia exhibited by patients with the same type of aphasic disturbance. Although there is obviously much overlap between spoken language and written language, the visual, orthographic, and graphomotor aspects of written language have properties of their own, and hence must involve additional processing mechanisms. It is for this reason that alexic and agraphic disorders have, in recent years, been described apart from aphasia, with reference to components of orthographic processing systems and the ways that these systems break down.

A. The Alexias

Alexic disorders are characterized by the types of paralexias produced, and by the properties of words that tend to affect reading performance. These properties include letter length, orthographic regularity, part of speech, concreteness, and familiarity.

1. Pure Alexia

The best-known type of acquired alexia, described in considerable detail in the late nineteenth century, is pure alexia, also known as alexia without agraphia. As the latter name indicates, patients with this form of alexia retain the ability to write and spell. In most cases, language functions are normal, except that there is often a mild anomia present.

Although patients with pure alexia have great difficulty recognizing written words, they *can* recognize words that are spelled aloud to them. That is, the difficulty in recognizing letter strings as words is a modality-specific impairment, restricted to visually presented words. The identification of individual letters may also be impaired, particularly early in the course of the alexia. However, many patients with pure alexia recover the ability to identify and name individual letters. The ability to name letters, combined with the ability to recognize strings of named letters as familiar words, has led many patients with pure alexia to adopt a pattern of compensatory read-

ing known as letter-by-letter reading. The patient names each letter of a word, aloud or silently, in left to right order, then identifies the word on the basis of the named letters.

Patients with pure alexia show a characteristic length effect when reading written words. That is, the time needed to read words increases as the number of letters in the words increases, and more paralexias are produced for long words compared with short words. This effect of length may be a consequence of the need to identify each letter of a word individually in a serial fashion, rather than the normal rapid, automatic, parallel identification of letters within a word.

Pure alexia is caused by a lesion or combination of lesions that cuts off input to the left angular gyrus, which itself remains intact. This may result from a single lesion to the white matter adjacent to the angular gyrus, or from an infarction in the territory of the posterior cerebral artery which damages both the left occipital cortex and the splenium of the corpus callosum.

2. Surface Alexia

In normal reading, the ability to access the meaning of a word is not dependent upon first accessing its pronunciation. That is, one can determine a word's referent on the basis of its orthographic composition (the letters that it contains); the word need not be pronounced. Thus we can distinguish between the referents of *flue* (something in your fireplace), *flu* (a nasty viral illness) and *flew* (past tense of fly), despite the fact that they all share the same pronunciation. Patients with surface alexia appear to rely upon the pronunciations of written words in order to ascertain their meanings. An obvious consequence of this disorder is an inability to distinguish between *flue, flu,* and *flew*. That is, the patient with surface alexia accesses the correct pronunciation of the written word *flu,* but does not know which of the three words sharing that pronunciation is on the page before him/her. Reading comprehension is consequently impaired.

The surface alexic patient's inability to directly access a word's meaning from its orthographic composition is actually part of a larger problem in recognizing written words. Not only is the patient frequently unable to determine a word's meaning prior to ascertaining its pronunciation, but often the patient does not know whether or not it is a real word until its pronunciation is obtained. Nonwords whose pronunciations are homophonous with real words (e.g. hoam) may thus be accepted as real words.

The most salient consequence of the surface alexic patient's difficulty recognizing individual written words is the effect of orthographic regularity on reading performance. Words with regular spelling-to-sound correspondences, such as *fat,* are more likely to be read correctly than words with irregular spelling-to-sound correspondences, such as *yacht.* It appears that when the patient does not recognize a written word, and thus cannot access its pronunciation directly, the word's pronunciation is assembled using some procedure for translating subword orthographic units (letters) into phonologic units (sounds). Such a procedure, of course, favors words with predictable letter-sound correspondences (including nonwords such as *pum*) over words with novel spellings. This regularity effect is the defining feature of surface alexia.

When a spelling-to-sound translation procedure is applied to an irregular word, the result is a "regularization" error, as when the word *bear* is pronounced as "beer." However, not all errors produced by patients with surface alexia are regularization errors. In fact, it is not uncommon to see particular "*mis*applications" of spelling-to-sound conversion rules, such as the enunciation of the silent *e* in words such as home (read as "homee"). In addition, surface alexia is never absolute; all such patients do succeed in reading some irregular words correctly, especially those words that occur with great frequency in the language. And, regular words are not read with perfect accuracy.

Patients with surface alexia typically have a lesion in the temporoparietal region of the left hemisphere. Diffuse cortical atrophy is also occasionally associated with surface alexia.

3. Phonological Alexia

The reading of patients with phonological alexia may be seen as the flip side of surface alexic reading. While patients with surface alexia tend to depend upon a subword letter-to-sound translation process for reading, patients with phonological alexia are unable to read via this mechanism. This deficit is manifest in a type of familiarity effect, in which words that are known may be read well, while an unknown word or a pronounceable nonword—also called a pseudoword—cannot be read.

The advantage of real word reading over pseudoword reading—the defining feature of phonological alexia—is a *relative* advantage. That is, some simple pseudowords may be read correctly; and some real words may be misread. Real word reading errors, when they are produced, tend to occur on functors and on words with affixes. Some patients with phonological alexia also show a relative disadvantage for reading verbs compared with nouns. The relative advantage of nouns over verbs, and of nouns and verbs over functors, is known as a part-of-speech effect. In addition to a part-of-speech effect, the reading of patients with phonological alexia may exhibit a concreteness effect. Here, a word that is concrete (e.g., table) is more likely to be read correctly than a word that is abstract (e.g., idealism). Both the part-of-speech effect and the concreteness effect are suggestive of reading that is mediated by semantics, presumably because the direct route from orthography to phonology is impaired. When reading must proceed through the semantic system, it follows that words with the strongest semantic representations—concrete nouns—will be easiest to read, while words with weaker semantic representations—abstract words, functors, and so on—will be more difficult to read.

The lesions that cause phonological alexia are quite variable, within the distribution of the left middle cerebral artery. Superior temporal lobe is usually involved.

4. Deep Alexia

The defining feature of deep alexia is the production of semantic paralexias when reading aloud. A semantic paralexia is a type of reading error in which the word produced is related in meaning to the written target word. The semantic relationship may take many forms: synonyms (lawyer–attorney); antonyms (hot–cold); subordinates (bird–robin); superordinates (celery–vegetable); attributes (grass–green); associates (house–garden).

Deep alexia is known as a symptom-complex, because the presence of a significant proportion of semantic paralexias in oral reading guarantees the presence of a number of other symptoms. All patients with deep alexia have a profound disturbance in pseudoword reading. They all show a part-of-speech effect. An effect of concreteness is always present. There is difficulty reading words with affixes, and derivational paralexias are produced, in which word endings are added, deleted, or subtituted for one another.

It should be apparent that all of the features of deep

alexia, except the production of semantic paralexias, may also be seen in phonological alexia. That is, all patients with phonological alexia and all patients with deep alexia have difficulty reading pseudowords. Some patients with phonological alexia, and all patients with deep alexia, display a part-of-speech effect, a concreteness effect, and difficulty with affixed words, with the concomitant production of derivational paralexias. It appears, then, that deep alexia and phonological alexia are part of the same continuum, with deep alexia representing the most severe form of phonological alexia, in which there is an impaired direct route from orthography to phonology, plus a significant impairment in the semantic reading route.

Lesions associated with deep alexia are typically quite extensive, including much of the left frontal lobe, and extending posteriorly.

B. The Agraphias

The term agraphia is generally applied to any disorder in producing the correct spellings of words, either in written form or via some other form of output. Like the alexias, the agraphias may be described with reference to the type of underlying impairment that is causing the writing deficit. For the agraphias, the modality of output (writing vs. typing vs. block letter spelling vs. oral spelling) and the types of paragraphias are important for determining the type of writing disturbance that is present. Other relevant factors include effects of regularity, familiarity, and part of speech.

I. Lexical Agraphia

In English, and many other alphabetic languages, the correspondence between a word's pronunciation and its spelling may be of three types. In orthographically irregular words, such as *two*, the relationship between the word's sounds and its letters is unique and unpredictable. In ambiguously spelled words, such as *brain*, there are multiple ways of representing the word's sounds orthographically (e.g., brane or braine). Orthographically regular words, such as *hit*, have a single invariant correspondence between the word's sounds and its letters.

Lexical agraphia, also known as surface agraphia, refers to a relative deficit in spelling orthographically irregular words or ambiguously spelled words compared with orthographically regular words. There appears to be a loss of knowledge of the orthographic compositions of words—that is, what letters compose the word, and in what order. Note that this is not a loss of *visual* images. Orthographic information is not stored in a particular font, or case, or size; it is an abstract representation of letter identities.

The regularity effect in spelling may not be seen with words that have a high frequency of occurrence in the language. Orthographic information about high-frequency words may remain intact. It is the spellings of low-frequency irregular words that are most affected. When misspellings occur, they are frequently phonologically plausible paragraphias. That is, there appears to be an overreliance upon the pronunciation of the word in determining its spelling. Examples of such errors, obtained from patients with lexical agraphia, include the following: suede → s w a d e; clean → c l e n e. As might be expected, the spelling of homophones is particularly difficult for patients with lexical agraphia.

Patients with surface alexia always have lexical agraphia, but the reverse is not true. Lexical agraphia may be seen with surface alexia, phonological alexia, pure alexia, or no alexia.

2. Phonological Agraphia

In phonological agraphia, the spelling of unfamiliar words and of pseudowords is impaired relative to the spelling of familiar real words. The ability to convert sound sequences into letter sequences is disturbed, and spelling proceeds on the basis of the recall of stored orthographic representations of words. Consequently, spelling errors produced by patients with phonological agraphia are frequently orthographically similar to the target, that is, they contain many correct letters, but they are not phonologically plausible spellings (e.g., rinse → r i s e). There is no effect of regularity upon spelling. There may be an effect of part-of-speech, with nouns being the best-preserved words. Patients with phonological agraphia nearly always have phonological alexia; however, the relationship is not so strong in the reverse direction.

3. Deep Agraphia

The most severe form of phonological agraphia is known as deep agraphia. The syndrome of deep agraphia consists of poor spelling of pseudowords, effects of part-of-speech (functors being spelled most poorly) and concreteness, and the production of semantic paragraphias. These are errors in which the patient writes (or spells) a word that is related in meaning to the target word, but does not resemble the target word phonologically or orthographically (e.g., writing *eye* when asked to write *blink*). As with deep alexia, words with affixes also present a problem, and derivational errors (writing *speaker* for *speaking*) are produced.

4. Modality Specific Agraphias

Apractic agraphia is a modality-specific agraphia in which the patient's written output is greatly impaired, but oral spelling remains intact. Written letters are poorly formed or illegible. Writing improves when the patient is copying written words.

Because oral spelling is preserved, the deficit is localized to the final stages of the writing process, at the level of motor output. The improvement when words are copied indicates that the impairment is not one of motor weakness, but rather it is an impairment of volitional movement (praxis). Consistent with its characterization as an impairment in motor output, apractic agraphia is not associated with a specific type of alexia, and, in fact, many of these patients read normally.

Written spelling agraphia is similar to apractic agraphia in that oral spelling remains intact. However, unlike patients with apractic agraphia, patients with written spelling agraphia do produce well-formed written letters. That is, they may orally spell a given word correctly, then write a different string of (well-formed) letters. The problem for these patients is neither letter choice nor motor output, but in getting from the correct letter identity to the appropriate motor output. There is no association with any type of alexia.

V. PSYCHOLOGICAL AND SOCIAL EFFECTS OF APHASIA

Because of the crucial role that communication plays in social relations, it is common for patients with aphasia to feel isolated and lonely. A severe and lasting deficit can lead to feelings of hopelessness and depression. Expressions of anger, hostility, and frustration, including periods of crying, may be seen, particularly among patients with nonfluent aphasia. Other reac-

tions include denial, inappropriate lack of concern, and paranoia, the latter occurring most frequently in Wernicke's aphasia. [*See* ANGER; DEPRESSION.]

Not only aphasic patients, but also their spouses and caregivers may be subject to feelings of anxiety, depression, and loneliness. It is not uncommon for them to experience changes in their familial roles and in their social lives. It is important for all rehabilitation professionals, including psychologists, social workers, speech pathologists, doctors, and nurses to recognize and to attempt to deal with the psychological and social problems of aphasic patients and their families.

VI. RECOVERY AND REHABILITATION

A. Spontaneous Recovery

Spontaneous improvement in language function is most likely to be seen in the first 3 months postonset. Further recovery may occur over the next few months, though at a slower pace. The likelihood and rate of recovery from aphasia is affected by many variables, including etiology, aphasia type, initial aphasia severity, lesion size and location, and handedness.

There is as yet no consensus on the effects of age and gender on the likelihood of recovery from aphasia. While it is clear that children are far more likely to recovery from aphasia than adults, most studies of adults with aphasia have not found that the likelihood of recovery is reduced significantly with age. With regard to gender, there have been reports of better recovery of language in women than men, but other studies have failed to find such effects.

1. Etiology

Patients whose aphasia is the result of a stroke do not fare as well, with regard to language recovery, as patients who develop aphasia subsequent to a head injury. Very marked or even complete recovery from aphasia may be seen following head injury, but complete recovery is rare following stroke. On the other hand, patients with aphasia due to stroke tend to have a more circumscribed deficit confined to language function than head injury patients, who may have deficits across a range of cognitive domains (memory, attention) because of the multifocal nature of their injuries.

2. Initial Severity and Size of Lesion

The initial severity of the aphasic disturbance is predictive of outcome. Severity is highly correlated with extent of lesion. It follows that patients with larger lesions show greater initial deficits and poorer recovery rates.

3. Site of Lesion and Type of Aphasia

Apart from lesion size, the location of the lesion significantly impacts upon the course of recovery from aphasia. Site of lesion, of course, is correlated with type of aphasia. Thus, the prognosis for recovery from aphasia tends to vary with aphasia type. Conduction aphasia and anomic aphasia tend to have the best prognosis, as these syndromes are associated with smaller and more circumscribed lesions. Patients with global aphasia tend to have a wide area of cerebral pathology. Those who have not shown significant improvement within two months tend to have poor prognoses.

4. Patterns of Recovery

While language comprehension tends to improve more than expressive language across all aphasias, there are patterns of recovery that are specific to the individual aphasia types. In general, fluent aphasias evolve into milder fluent aphasias, while nonfluent aphasias tend to remain nonfluent. Global aphasia evolves towards a Broca's type aphasia. Wernicke's aphasia evolves towards conduction aphasia or anomic aphasia. Across all aphasias, spoken language shows better recovery than written language.

5. Psychological and Social Factors

As might be expected, studies have indicated that factors such as depression and anxiety can have a negative effect upon recovery from aphasia. Social factors such as educational level and occupational status have not been shown to have a significant impact upon language recovery. Many therapists believe that a well-motivated patient is essential for a successful rehabilitation program, and it is here that the support of the patient's family is crucial.

B. Aphasia Therapy

Attempts at remediation of language deficits have been in existence for a long time, but until recently there have been few efforts to validate their effectiveness. One factor making validation difficult is the fact that therapies must be tailored to each patient individually, for no two patients are alike. In recent years, research methodologies aimed at single-subject designs have been developed, and tests of treatment efficacy are now underway.

Approaches to therapy vary depending upon the theoretical assumptions guiding the therapy. One point of view is that patients with aphasia have not lost language, but have lost access to language. This approach leads to therapies designed to *stimulate* language production. Alternatively, one may consider certain language capacities to be lost, that is, no longer present, when a significant amount of brain tissue is destroyed. This point of view leads to therapies aimed at either re-teaching the lost language skills, or developing compensatory strategies.

A recent advance has been the introduction of principles of cognitive neuropsychology into the design of aphasia therapy. Language is viewed not as a single cognitive ability, but as a collection of many component abilities. Careful, detailed analyses of the patient's language deficits, guided by information processing models, are used to help pinpoint precisely which subcomponent process(es) of language are likely impaired. This information helps guide the speech therapist in targeting specific language abilities for treatment. This approach is not concerned with symptoms per se, but rather with the underlying deficit that produces the symptoms. Therefore, unlike traditional speech/language therapy, which treats all instances of a symptom (e.g., anomia) with the same therapeutic approach, a cognitively based therapist might prescribe quite different therapies for two patients whose overt symptoms look identical, if it is determined that the underlying cause of the symptoms differs in the two patients. The collaborative research efforts of speech/language pathologists and cognitive neuropsychologists hold great promise for future advances in therapy for aphasia.

BIBLIOGRAPHY

Basso, A. (1989). Spontaneous recovery and language rehabilitation. In X. Seron & G. Deloche (Eds.), *Cognitive approaches in neuropsychological rehabilitation.* Hillsdale, NJ: Lawrence Erlbaum Associates.

Friedman, R. B. (1993). Alexia. In K. M. Heilman & E. Valenstein (Eds.), *Clinical neuropsychology* (3rd ed.). New York: Oxford University Press.

Goodglass, H. (1993). *Understanding aphasia.* San Diego: Academic Press.

Goodglass, H., & Kaplan, E. (1983). *The assessment of aphasia and related disorders.* Philadelphia: Lea and Febiger.

Roeltgen, D. (1993). Agraphia. In K. M. Heilman & E. Valenstein (Eds.), *Clinical neuropsychology* (3rd ed.). New York: Oxford University Press.

Sarno, M. (Ed.) (1991). *Acquired aphasia.* San Diego: Academic Press.

Assessment of Mental Health in Older Adults

Carolyn M. Aldwin and Michael R. Levenson

University of California, Davis

Age Effects   Statistical relationships due solely to the effect of chronological age.

Cohort Effects   Statistical relationships due primarily to the effect of year of birth, for example, having lived through a particular historical era at a specific age.

Discriminant Validity   The degree to which an assessment discriminates between groups and/or shows differential patterns of correlations with different outcomes, for example, the personality trait of hostility should predict anger and resentment better than anxiety or depression.

Ecological Validity   How well an assessment applies to or reflects the experience of the particular sample under study.

Internal Reliability   The cross-item consistency of a scale, that is, whether all items in the scale assess the same construct.

Period Effects   Statistical relationships due primarily to time of measurement effects.

Predictive Validity   The degree to which an assessment predicts an outcome of some sort, generally behavior (e.g., self-reported symptoms).

Sequential Analyses   Statistical analyses which contrast age, cohort, and period effects.

ASSESSMENT OF MENTAL HEALTH processes in the elderly can be particularly challenging, in part due to the fact that many assessment instruments were developed on younger populations and may not provide as accurate a picture in older populations, who vary greatly in their levels of cognitive, sensory, and motor abilities. In addition, many physical and mental illnesses in late life can present similar symptoms, and differentiating between the two is the focus of much of the assessment research in late life. Finally, the elderly may be less likely to disclose certain types of problems, and thus special techniques may be necessary to assess sources of psychological distress, including substance abuse and life events. However, less is known about what constitutes positive mental health in late life.

I. HETEROGENEITY IN OLDER POPULATIONS

A. Age Influences on Validity and Reliability

As a developmental stage, late life encompasses more than 45 years, from roughly ages 65 to 110. Not surprisingly, there is an extraordinary amount of heterogeneity in this population. Some elders are physically and cognitively very healthy; others develop disabling chronic illnesses quite early on. Thus, it is often very difficult to make generalizations about "the elderly." Not surprisingly, gerontologists have subdivided this developmental stage into three groups: the young-old, whose ages range from 65 to 79; the old-old (80–99); and the oldest-old, or centenarians. Others differentiate between optimal aging, in which there is little decrement or even improvement in some functions; normal aging, in which there are some decrements for which the elderly can readily compensate to maintain adequate psychosocial functioning; and impaired aging, marked by declines in physical and cognitive function.

Thus, it is very important to understand the position along these continua of the elder or sample of elders to be assessed. In general, in the United States, the young-old are relatively healthy and it is likely that assessment techniques used in younger populations are quite adequate for this population. Indeed, if one attempts to use instruments developed for impaired elders in the ordinary young-old population, one rapidly runs into ceiling effects—nearly all elders will score in the top range, rendering criteria for predictive and discriminant validity nearly useless. In other words, if there is no variance on an instrument, it cannot be used to correlate with other measures or to distinguish between groups.

In contrast, for frail elders, who are more likely to be in the old-old age group, the use of standard instruments may pose a problem in both the reliability and validity of the data. Cognitively impaired elders may become confused when confronted with typical Likert scaling, and dichotomously scaled instruments may have more reliability and validity. (We have found that even elders in good condition generally dislike and mistrust the Procrustean bed of fixed response formats, and often need to be cajoled into translating their phenomenological experience into admittedly arbitrary numbers.) In addition, frail elders may have poor attention spans, requiring the administration of brief forms of standard instruments and/or multiple testing sessions over several days. Although elders in general respond as accurately on surveys as younger populations, it is unlikely that cognitively impaired elders can do so, and interviews are more likely to yield valid information.

Elders with visual impairments may have difficulty in reading questionnaires, requiring the use of larger fonts. In addition, we have found that scantron sheets which use relatively pale type faces with poor contrast (e.g., lavender script on cream-colored paper) are contraindicated with elders who have acuity problems.

Individuals with motor impairments, such as tremors associated with Parkinson's disease or severe arthritis in the hands or wrists, may have difficulty in filling out questionnaires, and will require longer periods of time to complete them. For elders with severe forms of these illnesses, scantron forms are virtually impossible. Some researchers have switched to computer presentations of instruments which can aid in overcoming such sensory and motor deficits.

In general, we have found that frail elders do best in interviews in which the required responses to questions are available in both verbal and visual forms. If Likert scales are necessary for some instruments, then response cards, written in large fonts, which elders can hold and point to responses, are very helpful. Given that cognitively impaired elders often have difficulty in switching tasks, changing response cards is a good way of signaling that one task is done and that attention needs to be refocused on another.

However, interviews conducted in home settings may pose a special problem in assessing the elderly. In our experience, it is very difficult to interview just one member of an elderly dyad, especially in long-term married couples. Such couples may learn to compensate for memory problems by consulting with each other, and typically the non-target spouse will respond to questions, making accurate assessment of the target individual problematic. Thus, we have found it necessary to physically separate couples, either by giving the non-target elder an instrument to complete in another room, or by using pairs of interviewers to conduct simultaneous interviews, again in separate rooms.

B. Cohort Influences on Validity

Gerontologists distinguish among age, cohort, and period effects. In general, age effects are those which are solely due to an individual's chronological age, cohort effects refer to historical impacts reflected in a person's birth year or events experienced by a group of peers (e.g., the Depression), and period effects refer to larger social influences at the time of measurement. Neither cross-sectional nor longitudinal designs can adequately differentiate among these three types of effects, and only sequential designs, which follow multiple cohorts over different periods, can adequately differentiate these three types of effects. For any given effect to be accurately attributed to age, one must demonstrate that individuals of a given age are more likely to exhibit a particular response, regardless of what cohort they are in or the year in which they are assessed.

Age, cohort, and period effects also have implications for the validity of assessment instruments. For example, the validity of instruments used in older populations may be affected by cohort differences in language use and expression, a problem that has received relatively little attention in the assessment literature. One must be sensitive to whether the language used in any particular inventory is appropriate to the population under study. Indeed, the language used in older instruments is often more relevant to that used by older cohorts. For example, in the MMPI, there were several items which reflected older word usage (such as playing "drop the handkerchief"). While the revised MMPI (MMPI-2) has eliminated anachronistic items, in 1991 Butcher and his colleagues found that nearly all of the age differences in the MMPI-2 still reflected either differing health statuses or cohort differences in language and experience (e.g., the use of marijuana was much less likely to be endorsed by older groups).

Many instruments commonly in use in psychology were developed on student populations, and, as such, may have poor ecological validity for the elderly. For example, a mastery or control instrument may include items about perceived fairness of grading practices or juggling work versus parenting roles. Certainly, any instruments used to assess mental health in the elderly must be sensitive to items that are more relevant to student or young adult experiences.

Less obvious sources of poor ecological validity may lie in cohort differences in reporting style. The current cohort of elders may be less willing to reveal emotional distress and/or use different terminology to refer these states. Older men in particular may be less comfortable in identifying stressors than younger men.

The possibility of response bias in the elderly has some interesting implications for the relative validity of diagnostic techniques. There is surprisingly little research available comparing the validity of self-report versus observer ratings in the elderly for specific illnesses. In general, observer ratings are thought to be more objective than self-report inventories, although there may be age-related biases in observer ratings, re-

flecting stereotypical biases about elders as more impaired, irascible, and so on.

A further problem is that clinical interviews often yield categorical classification, for example, full-blown depression versus none. To the extent that elders, even in clinical interviews, under-report symptoms, then such procedures may underestimate the existence of problems. For example, in 1992 Koenig and Blazer reviewed studies showing that the prevalence of major depression in the elderly, based upon clinical interviews, was about 1% (which is rather less than that reported for younger populations), but some 20% or more of older samples reported problems with negative affect on self-rated inventories, a figure much more comparable to younger samples. This is not to say that different criteria or cutoff points on standardized clinical assessment tools necessarily need to be developed, but rather that much more research is needed into this issue.

II. DIFFERENTIATING BETWEEN MENTAL AND PHYSICAL HEALTH PROBLEMS

Perhaps the issue which has received the most attention in the literature concerns the differentiation between mental and physical health. Many mental health scales include physical symptoms, which may be relatively uncommon in younger populations and indicative of psychological distress. However, in older populations, with their greater incidence of chronic health problems, such instruments may yield very high rates of false positives. Further, mental health problems often have physiological concomitants, and physical health problems can affect psychological states. Obviously, identifying the primary source of the symptoms is crucial in determining treatment options, although sometimes the only way in which to determine the precise etiology for a particular illness is to test different treatments. However, there are critical issues in differentiating anxiety, depression, and psychoses from a variety of physical health problems.

A. Differentiating Depression and Anxiety from Physical Health Problems

Self-report inventories of depression typically include many somatic complaints, such as fatigue, headaches, back and neck pain, constipation, and sleep disturbances. While in younger individuals these types of complaints may be indicative of depression, such symptoms are very common among the elderly. Thus, this inclusion of physical health symptoms in psychological assessment instruments may lead to Type I errors. On the other hand, there is some indication that depression in the elderly may be presented in terms of physical symptoms, and a relatively high proportion of medical visits to general practitioners by the elderly may be due to depression manifesting in physical complaints. Thus, screening for recent life events and/or changes in living conditions (see below) may be an important way for clinicians to determine whether bereavement or social isolation may be important factors underlying such visits. [*See* BEREAVEMENT; DEPRESSION.]

On the other hand, many illnesses common to the elderly, as well as prescribed medications, may have concomitant symptoms of depression and anxiety. For example, elders are at increased risk for hypothyroidism, cardiovascular disease, and chronic obstructive pulmonary disorder, which may cause fatigue, sleep disturbances, and negative affect. Other disorders, such as myocardial infarctions, vitamin deficiencies, anemia, pneumonia, and hyper- and hypothyroidism, may present with symptoms of anxiety. Further, many medications commonly prescribed in the elderly, such as antihypertensives, may also create symptoms of depression. Thus, physical, mental, and social health are often tightly intertwined in the elderly, and multipronged assessment techniques may be necessary to adequately establish the etiology of symptoms of depression and anxiety in the elderly.

B. Differentiating Depression from Dementia

Some depressive symptoms mimic cognitive impairment, especially in the elderly. In particular, psychomotor retardation and memory lapses in the elderly are usually attributed to dementing processes, but actually may reflect depression. Pseudodementias can result from a wide variety of disorders, including nutritional deficiencies, prescribed medications, alcohol and substance abuse, and surgical procedures. Thus, assessment of the occurrence of problems of this type may be an important component in elders presenting with cognitive impairment. In turn, dementia is often associated with difficulty concentrating, loss of en-

ergy, and psychomotor slowing, even in the absence of depression. A number of different screening inventories have been developed to differentiate between these types of disorders. [*See* DEMENTIA.]

In 1992, Newman and Sweet identified a number of different features which may distinguish depression from dementia. Depression often has a rapid onset while dementia often has a gradual one. In addition, there may be differences in both patient and familial awareness of the problems, with recognition greater in depression-related cognitive impairment than in problems related to dementia. Patients who are depressed may be able to provide greater detail about their impairment and to manifest subjective distress, while dementing patients may have vague, nonspecific complaints and may be more likely to conceal cognitive deficits. Depressed patients typically show poor motivation and give up easily on tasks, while dementing patients may struggle with tasks.

In addition, there are a number of differences between the two groups in both cognitive testing and neurological examination. For example, depressed patients typically have problems with both recent and long-term memory, and report poorer concentration than actual knowledge testing, whereas dementia patients typically have much worse recent than long-term memory deficits and general knowledge is worse than concentration skills. Finally, depressive patients typically demonstrate no problems with specific neurological testing, while dementing patients typically present with dyspraxias and agnosias, and show abnormal CAT scans, with increased ventricular size. In addition, the administration of antidepressive medications may be one way to distinguish depression-related pseudodementias from true dementias resulting from neurological disorders.

C. Distinguishing Schizophrenia from Dementia

While the onset of schizophrenia typically occurs in adolescence or young adulthood, schizophrenia may also occur in late life. Schizophrenia with a late life onset is often called paraphrenia, and may occur in individuals who have a history of eccentricity and are socially isolated. However, dementia can also produce hallucinations and delusions, and thus, like depression, it is important to distinguish between the two conditions.

Given that late-life onset of schizophrenia is relatively rare, very few systematic studies have been conducted. However, neuropsychological assessment studies have been done, and, in many cases, it is possible to rule out dementing processes. [*See* Schizophrenia.]

D. Assessment of Behavioral Disorders

Particularly disturbing concomitants of the cognitive and affective disorders prevalent in late life are behavioral disturbances. These disturbances, including wandering, sleep disruptions, verbal and physical aggression, and hallucinations and delusions, may have serious impacts on the quality of life for both elderly individuals and their caretakers. Patients who exhibit such behaviors may be labeled as "problems" by nursing home staff and then regularly given psychotropic medication to control their behavior, which can result in a variety of adverse physical, cognitive, and affective side effects. While there have been regulatory efforts to decrease the use of psychotropic medications in nursing homes, paradoxically, this regulation can result in increased use, as nurses are given less discretion and physicians must prescribe the use of such drugs on a regular basis.

In 1994, Teri and Logsdon reviewed the variety of scales which have been developed fairly recently to assess behavioral disturbances. These typically are observational measures, and may be administered by researchers, clinicians, nurses, or caregivers. A major purpose of these scales is to quantify the frequency and severity of such disturbances to devise appropriate treatment strategies. Detailing the exact pattern of aggressive and disruptive behavior may result in a more objective picture of the actual problems created by such patients, facilitate behavioral intervention, and result in less reliance on psychotropic medications.

III. ASSESSING FACTORS AFFECTING MENTAL AND PHYSICAL HEALTH

There are a variety of factors which can affect physical and mental health in late life. In terms of behavioral factors, alcohol and substance abuse, as well as stress, are two of the most important ones. [*See* Alcohol Problems; Substance Abuse.]

A. Assessing Alcohol and Substance Abuse in the Elderly

In the late 1960s Cahalan and his associates developed a survey assessment instrument for alcohol consumption and problems. It assessed alcohol consumption using three different scales: (1) the usual number of drinks of beer, wine, and distilled spirits consumed "nowadays," as reported in drinks per day, week, month, or year; (2) the number of drinks of beer, wine and distilled spirits consumed the day before completing the questionnaire; and (3) the regularity of alcohol consumption on specific days of the week. For example, a respondent may indicate that, in a typical week, he or she drinks one glass of wine during the evenings and two drinks each on Friday and Saturday night. Thus, this individual, on average, drinks nine drinks a week, which then usually is translated into drinks per year.

Independently of consumption, respondents indicate the frequency (e.g., never, once per week, month, or year) of experiencing alcohol problems. These items assess the frequency with which alcohol affects physical, psychological, or social functioning. In general, convictions for drunk driving and alcohol-related traffic accidents are weighted more heavily than other types of problems. Although they reflect some components of a *DSM-IV* diagnosis of alcoholism, they do not permit such a diagnosis, which requires the use of a diagnostic interview.

The shortest and simplest self report of alcohol abuse is the four-item CAGE instrument, in which a positive response to two or more of the items suggests alcohol abuse. The items assess feeling that one should drink less, being annoyed by others' criticizing one's drinking, feeling guilty about drinking, and drinking in the morning. The items have good face validity, yet this instrument does not appear to be sensitive in older populations. The Michigan Alcoholism Screening Test (MAST) for older adults is a much longer (24-item) instrument that has been validated on the hospitalized elderly but may not be practical for screening outside hospitalized populations. It should be noted that other versions of the MAST have not been equally valid in all populations tested.

The use of self-report surveys of alcohol consumption and problems may prove difficult, especially with the elderly. However, for the general population, Midanik concluded in 1988 that "the validity of self-reports is not an either/or phenomenon." There is no "gold" standard against which to compare self-reports, only a variety of "lead" standards such as collateral reports, diaries, official records, laboratory tests, or interviews. All of these methods assess over-lapping but nonisomorphic aspects of an individual's alcohol use. Sobell and Sobell noted in 1990 that the relevant issue is the extent of discrepancy among sources of information that are being used to investigate a given research question. The latter observation may be especially relevant for the elderly.

Tobacco, alcohol, and prescription drugs (usually anxiolytics) are the most abused drugs in the elderly. Indeed, alcohol consumption both reduces thiamine uptake and interacts with prescription drug use, a fact that is further complicated by the reduced capacity of elderly persons for clearing such drugs. Thus, use of both types of substances may carry a risk for health problems that increases with age. Moreover, the elderly may not recognize that their relatively nonproblematic levels of consumption at younger ages may cause problems in later life.

While drinking has been shown to decline with age, this may not be a reliable predictor of future trends since recent research has shown that changes in drinking patterns appear to be more closely associated with period rather than age effects. These considerations may render assessment of risk for problem drinking (with its attendant drug interactions) more difficult in the elderly.

In 1997, Atkinson argued that the relatively low reported rates of alcoholism in those over the age of 60 (no more than 2% in men and less than 1% in women) may underestimate the actual prevalence of problems) largely due to a failure to accurately report consumption and problems in surveys. The "discrepancy problem" may be more pertinent among the elderly than in younger populations. Thus, there may be special difficulties with self-report in the elderly, with a problem/reported problem ratio perhaps increasing with age. This is further complicated by cohort effects, with younger cohorts more willing to acknowledge problems than older ones, if such cohort differences are maintained in later life.

Excluding daily blood alcohol level testing, there are several reasonable supplements to self-report in the elderly. First, there is a pattern of cognitive deterioration associated with alcohol abuse in the elderly that

is distinct from that associated with senile dementias such as Alzheimer's and even Korsakoff's Syndrome (which involves irreversible brain damage due to long-term severe alcohol abuse). This pattern is summarized in *DSM-IV* as involving deficits in memory, language, motor functions, object recognition (without organic motor or sensory impairment), and abstract thinking and planning. Evidence has supported this diagnostic approach with an additional strong finding that name-finding was almost completely spared in alcohol-related dementias, in contrast to Alzheimer's Disease, in which dysnomia is pronounced.

Second, and perhaps most helpful, are in-home assessments. In addition to standard consumption interviews and listing the prescriptions and home remedies that the elderly use, other data and relatively unobtrusive observations can be employed. These include a history of falls, grooming, odors present in the house (also, obviously, useful for an assessment of tobacco use), bruises at the level of furniture, tremors, incontinence, and many others (many of which could be associated with non-alcohol-related dementias or depression). Naturally, such an assessment would require considerable training and would obviously be available only for that minority of the elderly who receive home care from outside agencies.

Unfortunately, there is no good way of assessing the dependence on prescription tranquilizers (principally benzodiazepines) in the elderly unless withdrawal symptoms, such as extreme anxiety and irritability, occur since dependence is not typically associated with dose increase. Such dependence is more frequent among elderly women than men. Signs of toxicity from long-term use are easily mistaken for other disorders of the elderly, such as memory loss and other cognitive impairments, as well as problems with mobility. It is likely that alcohol and drug abuse may reflect the levels of stress in elders' lives.

B. Assessing Stress and Coping in Late Life

There are several different ways of assessing stress, including traumatic events, life events, chronic role strain, and daily stressors or hassles. In the last decade, it has rapidly become apparent that both type and frequency of stressors change with age. While early studies suggested that the number of stressful life events decrease with age, perusal of the types of events typically found on early life event scales reveal that many are far more relevant to younger populations than to older ones (e.g., marriage, divorce, changing jobs, imprisonment). Several instruments are now available that assess life events that are more relevant to older populations such as caretaking for spouse and parents, institutionalization of parent or spouse, death of a child, child's divorce, problems with grandchildren, and the like. These instruments are less likely to show a decrease in stressful life events with age.

However, the number of daily stressors does decrease with age, most probably due to the decline in the number of social roles. For example, most older adults have relinquished active parenting and work roles, the source of the majority of hassles in mid-life. While there is a concomitant increase in the number of hassles associated with both health problems and avocations in retirement, for most older adults, these typically do not generate as many hassles as do work and childrearing roles.

In part, this may be due to changes in the nature of stress in late life. Stress in earlier life is more likely to be episodic in nature, such as children's crises or problems at work, whereas stressors in late life may be more likely to be chronic, for example, managing chronic illnesses or caregiving for an ill spouse. If chronic problems are successfully managed, they may not be perceived as "problems" per se. An 80-year-old with multiple health problems may well assert that he or she has had no problems in the past week, despite obvious impairments requiring careful management. Thus, among the old-old, interviews may be better assessments of stress than self-report instruments.

However, the decrease in stress reporting may also be due to age-related changes in the way individuals cope. In some ways, older people are better copers, in that they are less likely to use escapist strategies such as alcohol, drugs, or wishful thinking—or perhaps individuals who survive until late life are less likely to use escapist strategies. However, the old-old may be more likely to use denial as a coping strategy. Denial of the severity of health problems, for example, may be a palliative strategy, as long as appropriate instrumental actions are taken, such as adhering to a medical regimen. However, the old-old are often reluctant to admit problems for fear that they will be institutionalized, with all that entails, including separation from spouse and loved ones and the loss of control. Thus, they may deny and/or hide problems, even those which could be adequately treated in the home, which can lead to worse problems, greatly increasing the risk of institutionalization. Thus, accurate assessment of problems in the elderly are crucial to both their treatment and may permit successful home treatment and forestall institutionalization. [*See* COPING WITH STRESS; STRESS.]

IV. ASSESSING POSITIVE MENTAL HEALTH

Mental health is not simply the absence of symptoms, but entails positive functioning as well. Unfortunately, positive mental health has received less attention in the elderly, with the possible exception of one of its dimensions, life satisfaction.

Despite the widespread dissemination of Erikson's theory of ego development in adulthood, only a handful of scales have been developed to assess generativity and ego integrity. The most extensive scale development on positive mental health in late life has been done by Ryff and her colleagues in the 1980s. They developed measures of complexity, generativity, integrity, and interiority, as well those that assess self-acceptance, positive relations with others, autonomy, environmental mastery, purpose in life, and personal growth. Although Ryff's scales are correlated with the Big Five personality factors (neuroticism, extraversion, openness to experience, conscientiousness, and agreeableness), they correlate independently with positive affect, suggesting that they assess more than just the standard personality dimensions. It remains to be seen whether these scales will enjoy widespread use as indicators of positive mental health in the elderly.

V. SUMMARY

In summary, assessing mental health in the elderly requires attention to a number of factors, including the age and functional ability of the elder and whether or not the instrument used has adequate reliability and validity for older populations. While elders may be more or less accurate at reporting symptoms as younger groups, the crucial assessment issue appears to be differentiating between possible sources of the problems.

Further, more research needs to be done in assessing positive mental health in the elderly.

BIBLIOGRAPHY

Aldwin, C. (1994). *Stress, coping, and development: An integrative approach*. New York: Guilford.

Atkinson, R. M. (1997). Alcohol and drug abuse in the elderly. In R. Jacoby & C. Oppenheimer (Eds.), *Psychiatry in the elderly* (2nd ed., pp. 661–688). Oxford: Oxford University Press.

Garland, J. (1997). Psychological assessment and treatment. In R. Jacoby & C. Oppenheimer (Eds.), *Psychiatry in the elderly* (2nd ed., pp. 246–256). Oxford: Oxford University Press.

Howard, R., & Levy, R. (1997). Late-onset schizophrenia, late paraphrenia, and paranoid states of late life. In R. Jacoby & C. Oppenheimer (Eds.), *Psychiatry in the elderly* (2nd ed., pp. 617–631). Oxford: Oxford University Press.

Newman, P. J., & Sweet, J. J. (1992). Depressive disorders. In A. E. Puente & C. R. Reynolds (Eds.), *Handbook of neuropsycho-logical assessment: A biopsychosocial perspective* (pp. 263–308). New York: Plenum.

Pachana, N. A., Gallagher-Thompson, D., & Thompson, L. W. (1994). Assessment of depression. In M. P. Lawton & J. A. Teresi (Eds.), *Annual Review of Gerontology and Geriatrics, Vol. 14* (pp. 234–256). New York: Springer.

Rabins, P. V. (1992). Schizophrenia and psychotic states. In J. E. Birren, R. Bruce Sloane, & G. D. Cohen (Eds.), *Handbook of mental health and aging* (2nd. ed., pp. 464–479). San Diego: Academic Press.

Ritchie, K. (1997). The development and use of instruments for the psychological assessment of older patients. In R. Jacoby & C. Oppenheimer (Eds.), *Psychiatry in the elderly* (2nd ed., pp. 232–245). Oxford: Oxford University Press.

Ryff, C. D., & Essex, M. J. (1991). Psychological well-being in adulthood and old age: Descriptive markers and explanatory processes. In K. W. Schaie (Ed.), *Annual Review of Geronto-logical and Geriatrics, II,* 144–171. New York: Springer.

Sheikh, J. I. (1992). Anxiety and its disorders in old age. In J. E. Birren, R. B. Sloane, & G. D. Cohen (Eds.), *Handbook of Mental Health and Aging* (2nd ed., pp. 410–432). San Diego, CA: Academic Press.

Attachment

Lucy Robin

Indiana University

Paula R. Pietromonaco

University of Massachusetts at Amherst

Attachment Figure   A person who fulfills an individual's attachment needs, including providing comfort and security.

Attachment Style   An individual's characteristic patterns of interaction with an attachment figure.

Attachment System   A system of behaviors (e.g., seeking contact, protesting, seeking a safe haven), assumed to be biologically based, that is directed toward an attachment figure.

Internal Working Models   The sets of beliefs and expectations about the self and others that develop through interactions with attachment figures; these models are thought to guide thoughts, feelings, and behavior in social interactions.

Primary Caregiver   The attachment figure who is primarily responsible for caring for an infant or child.

Safe Haven   Attachment figures function as a safe place to which individuals can return for comfort and support in times of danger or stress.

Secure Base   Attachment figures function as a source of security from which individuals can launch explorations of their environment in times of safety.

An **ATTACHMENT** is a close, enduring social bond. The term often refers to the bond between infants and their primary caregivers, but recently it has been applied to the bond between romantic partners. This ar-

ticle will provide an overview of attachment theory, as applied to both children and adults, and it will discuss the implications of different patterns of attachment for mental health across the lifespan.

I. OVERVIEW OF ATTACHMENT THEORY

Infants form close, enduring bonds, or attachments, to their primary caregivers. This bond helps infants to survive by keeping them close to their caregiver, who can meet their physical needs as well as provide protection and safety. Attachment relationships that meet infants' needs provide a secure base from which they can explore the environment and a safe haven to which they can return when they are frightened, distressed, or in need of care. Nearly all infants form attachments, but the quality of their attachments varies depending on whether caregivers are able to satisfy their physical and emotional needs. Attachment theory focuses on why and how infants form attachments, and the mental health implications of different patterns of attachment from infancy through adulthood. Recent theorists have extended attachment theory to understand functioning in adult close relationships, and the connection between adult attachments and mental health. Evidence indicates that attachment patterns relate to key mental health variables such as self-esteem, the ability to regulate emotions, and the quality of interpersonal relationships.

A. Origins

In 1951, John Bowlby published *Maternal Care and Mental Health*. The World Health Organization had commissioned this monograph in an effort to understand the effects of the institutionalization of many children who had been separated from their parents during World War II. This pioneering work suggested that the mental health of infants required not only adequate food, shelter, and hygiene, but also a close, emotional bond with an available, responsive caregiver. In particular, Bowlby observed that young children who had been separated from their mothers experienced profound distress and anxiety.

After reaching this conclusion, Bowlby set out to explain why the infant–caregiver bond was so important, and how such bonds could influence personality development and mental health. Drawing on his training as a psychoanalyst as well as on work by ethologists on innate instincts, Bowlby observed that bonding between infants and mothers occurred across many species. This reasoning led him to propose that humans have an innate need for an attachment bond.

B. Function of the Attachment Behavioral System

Bowlby described attachment theory in a three-volume series entitled *Attachment and Loss,* published between 1969 and 1980. Bowlby proposed that infants have an inborn system of behaviors—called the attachment system—that functions to keep the infant close to the primary caregiver. Infants who feel threatened or sense that the caregiver is not accessible enough display attachment behaviors, such as signaling their needs through crying, or clinging to the caregiver. When infants feel safe and sense that the caregiver is near enough, the attachment system is not activated, and they may concentrate on play or other ways to explore the environment. In effective attachment relationships, caregivers provide a safe haven to which infants can retreat in times of danger or distress, and a secure base from which infants can venture out and explore in times of safety. Bowlby argued that the attachment system serves an adaptive function; an attachment bond promotes the survival of newborns by increasing the likelihood that their physical needs will be met and by protecting them from potential dangers.

C. Internal Working Models

Bowlby's theory also takes into account that children develop the ability to think about and form expectations of their relationships. As infants interact repeatedly with their caregivers, they build a set of expectations about their own actions and their caregiver's reactions in the relationship. Bowlby called these belief sets "internal working models" and proposed two distinct, but related, sets of working models—one set about the self and one set about significant others, and especially the primary attachment figure. Over time, children learn whether or not they are worthy and acceptable in the eyes of their attachment figure; these expectations form the core of their working models of self. Children also learn whether or not the attachment figure is readily available and responsive to their needs; these expectations form the core of their working models of a particular attachment figure. Working models are thought to exist by the end of the first year of life, and to become increasingly complex and elaborated over time. Internal working models are assumed to guide individuals' thoughts, feelings, and behavior in their interactions. Although working models can be revised or changed on the basis of new experience, such changes are thought to occur gradually and with difficulty. Working models, then, may provide a mechanism for stability in attachment patterns over time.

II. ATTACHMENT IN INFANCY AND CHILDHOOD

A. Attachment Styles

According to Bowlby, a secure attachment relationship, and accompanying positive working models, depends on whether the caregiver is available, consistent, and responsive to the infant. Children who interact with caregivers who are available, consistent, and responsive and who thus meet their emotional needs show different patterns of attachment behavior than those who have caregivers who are less able to meet their emotional needs. These characteristic patterns are called attachment styles. Researchers have identified different attachment styles, and have uncovered associations between these styles and mental health.

Pioneering work by Mary Ainsworth, a colleague of John Bowlby's, examined young children's attachment behavior in response to separation and reunion with their mother using the "Strange Situation." Ainsworth developed this laboratory procedure after observing that different infants and children in institutions reacted quite differently to reunions with their mothers after separation. The laboratory procedure allowed her to examine, under controlled conditions, whether regularities emerged in infants' responses to separation and reunion with their mothers. In the Strange Situation, young children (age 12 to 18 months) and their mothers enter an unfamiliar room containing toys and can explore and play in the presence of their mother. After a short time, a stranger comes into the room and talks with the mother. At this point, the child is briefly separated from the mother, and left with the stranger. A few minutes later, the child and mother are reunited and the stranger leaves. Research has shown that children in this situation respond in one of three ways. The majority of children (approximately 60%) show a secure attachment pattern; they cry or search for the mother when she leaves the room, but are happy to see her and are easily comforted when she returns. A sizable minority of infants show insecure attachment by displaying either an anxious–ambivalent or an avoidant pattern.

Approximately 19% of children display the anxious–ambivalent pattern. They become very distressed when the mother leaves the room, and seem inconsolable when she returns; they also show inconsistent behavior, such as wanting to be held and then angrily pushing away from the mother. About 21% of children show the avoidant pattern. These children do not appear distressed when the mother leaves the room, and do not cry or search for her. When the mother returns, these children tend to ignore her and rebuff her attempts at contact. Later research using physiological measures of distress has indicated that avoidant children may be experiencing distress that they do not show in their outward behavior. For example, the heart rates of avoidant babies increased when their mother left the room, just as those of secure and anxious–ambivalent babies did.

Further work has identified a fourth attachment style, called disorganized–disoriented or ambivalent–avoidant. These children are not classifiable using the original three patterns, because they show marked inconsistency and incoherence in their attachment behaviors, such as crying for the mother during separation, but then ignoring her on return; or, approach the mother, but with their head averted. In low-risk samples of middle-class children, only a small percentage (approximately 15%) of children are classified as disorganized. In contrast, in samples of abused or neglected children, over 50% receive a disorganized classification.

Although most insecure infants fall within the normal range of behavior, a small number of infants are diagnosed with one of two types of clinically disordered attachment, which are extreme versions of insecure attachment. Reactive attachment disorder is characterized by contradictory or ambivalent social responses in a variety of social situations, paired with such extreme emotional reactions as misery, apathy, aggression, and fearful hypervigilance. In contrast, disinhibited attachment disorder describes diffuse attachments—that is, the infant is not selective among attachment figures, and will be clingy and indiscriminately affectionate to any person who is available. Both versions of clinically disordered attachment are strongly associated with experiences of abuse (sexual and physical) and severe neglect.

B. Determinants of Attachment Style

The way caregivers respond to their infant appears to contribute to the infant's attachment style. In one study, researchers observed the behavior of mothers toward their 2-month-old infant and, when the infants were from 12 to 18 months old, determined their attachment style on the basis of behavior in the Strange Situation. Mothers of 2-month-old infants later classified as secure were more likely to cuddle their infants, to respond more promptly to crying and other vocalizations, and to respond with more tenderness and warmth in their voices than were mothers of infants later classified as insecure.

Other research examining infant–caregiver patterns in both the Strange Situation and at home has shown that mothers of secure infants are consistently available, and are able to read and respond to their infants' signals. In contrast, mothers of anxious–ambivalent infants respond inconsistently; sometimes they correctly read and respond to their child's signals, but sometimes they do not respond appropriately. Finally, mothers of avoidant infants generally are unwilling or unable to respond to their infant's signals.

Further evidence suggests that attachment patterns are linked to differences in how mothers regulate their children's behavior. In one study of mother–toddler pairs, the mother completed a questionnaire while the child was allowed to explore the empty room. Mothers of secure toddlers gave them appropriate guidance such as talking to their children and suggesting ways to pass the time. Mothers of anxious–ambivalent toddlers gave intrusive guidance, interfering with the child's ability to act independently. Mothers of avoidant toddlers provided insufficient guidance, leaving their children to fend for themselves.

Research examining infants classified as disorganized/disoriented has found that the mothers of these children are unresponsive to their cues, but also act in "frightened and frightening" ways. These mothers appear confused, fearful, and apprehensive around their child, and their intrusions into their child's behavior often evidence hostility and aggression. Thus, the disorganized, contradictory behavior of these infants reflects the conflict between their desire to use the caregiver as a safe haven who will lessen their anxiety, and the reality of the situation in which the caregiver is a source of anxiety.

C. Continuity of Attachment Style

Attachment classifications are generally stable over time. For example, in a sample of 50 infants from middle-class families, 96% of infants received the same attachment classification (i.e., secure, anxious–ambivalent, or avoidant) at 18 months as they had at 12 months. In a different sample of 101 infants from a wider range of socioeconomic backgrounds, 81% of classifications were stable from 12 to 18 months.

Longitudinal studies indicate a strong association between children's attachment classification at 12 to 18 months, determined using the Strange Situation, and their social behavior at a later age. For example, one research team examined how 2-year-old children responded to different tasks, some of which were challenging enough to require the aid of their caregiver. Children behaved differently, depending on their previous infant attachment classification. When faced with a challenging task, secure children continued to exert effort, but sought help from the caregiver and complied with her suggestions. Indeed, caregivers of these children offered many suggestions and remained highly supportive. Anxious–ambivalent children, on the other hand, became highly emotional—angry, distressed, and frustrated—in the face of this challenge. Although these children also sought and received help from their caregivers, the caregiver's suggestions were less useful in the face of a more challenging task. Avoidant children made few adjustments to the more difficult task, they did not ask for more help, and caregivers did not offer help. Caregivers of avoidant children remained minimally involved regardless of the task's difficulty.

Studies assessing attachment stability in older children have focused on cognitive and emotional processes associated with different internal working models. For example, a study of 5-year-old children assessed emotion regulation by focusing on ego control, the ability to control impulses; and ego resiliency, the ability to adapt to the demands of the situation. In this study, teachers described the ego-resiliency and ego-control of each 5-year-old. Children previously classified as secure showed high ego resiliency, and medium ego control, indicating their ability to control their impulses and respond flexibly to different situations. Children previously classified as anxious-ambivalent showed low ego-resiliency and ego-control, reflecting their difficulty in controlling impulses regardless of the situation. Finally, children previously classified as avoidant showed low ego-resiliency but high ego-control, suggesting that they had difficulty expressing wishes and desires, regardless of the situation.

Other studies examined how 6-year-old children interacted with their parent after a one-hour separation, how they drew pictures of their family, and how they talked about pictures involving separation from parents and about a family photograph. In these studies, children who had been classified as secure infants had fluid, well-balanced conversations with their parent. Children who had been classified as insecure infants held more awkward conversations with their parents; those previously classified as disorganized/disoriented infants were particularly likely to lead the conversation with their parents.

In addition, secure children drew family pictures whose figures were more individuated than insecurely classified children. Furthermore, when looking at drawings depicting a child's upcoming separation from parents, secure children described the child as feeling sad, lonely, or anxious, but also described realistic ways of dealing with such feelings. In contrast, avoidant children appeared tense in their nonverbal behavior but either denied the child's negative emotions or offered pessimistic interpretations—for example, that the parents would never come back. Children who showed different attachment styles as infants also differed in their reactions to a family photograph. Secure children showed interest in the picture, smiling and discussing it, whereas avoidant children looked away from it. Disorganized/disoriented children reacted strongly to the photograph, becoming suddenly depressed or disoriented in their behaviors.

Other studies have examined the behavior of somewhat older children. In these studies, children classified as secure during their early years were observed again at nearly 11 eleven years old. Ratings by camp counselors indicated that they were more emotionally healthy (e.g., held higher self-esteem and self-confidence), more competent, and more independent of adults than were insecure children. They spent more time with peers, as opposed to alone or with adults, and were more likely to make a friend during their camp stay than insecure children. In another study, 10-year-old secure children, compared with avoidant and anxious–ambivalent children, had more friends, interacted more appropriately with adults, and coped better with negative feelings by turning to others for support.

Although attachment patterns often remain stable, they also show change under some circumstances. Longitudinal studies of mother–child pairs have shown that changes in the mother's caregiving or in the family's life situation reduce the stability of the child's attachment style. For example, one study assessed continuity of attachment from 12 months to 4 years of age in a socioeconomically disadvantaged sample. At 4 years old, some children previously classified as insecure showed secure behavior and vice versa. Mothers of children who had become more secure reported having an easier time with their children and showed better parenting skills, possibly because of increasing maturity or other life changes. In contrast, mothers of children who had become less secure appeared to have become overwhelmed by the demands of an older child. Other studies have shown that children's attachment styles are less likely to show stability when stressful life changes occur that can influence the ability of a parent to provide care. [*See* STRESS.]

D. Attachment and Mental Health in Infancy and Childhood

In general, secure attachment appears to promote mental health, whereas insecure attachment appears to increase vulnerability to mental health problems. Longitudinal research suggests that secure infants grow into psychologically healthy children. They are more likely to take initiative in social and cognitive tasks, to be leaders and popular in social settings, to persevere in the face of failure, and to be relatively free of behavioral problems. A secure childhood attachment also can act as a buffer for maltreatment. Research investigating resiliency in abuse cases suggests that children who have a healthy relationship with their mother survive maltreatment from another adult much better than those who lack such a healthy relationship.

Anxious–ambivalent children are more likely to be the victims of bullies. Teachers view these children as needy, and often respond with extra help and patience. Anxious–ambivalent children become easily frustrated when faced with a challenging task, leading them to give up quickly. Their emotions in the face of challenge appear to overwhelm them; they "fall apart" in the face of failure.

In contrast, children with an avoidant attachment history have difficulty with their peers. They often are not socially accepted, and tend to be the bullies in the classroom. Teachers tend to have little patience with these children. Avoidant children are less likely to seek help when faced with a difficult problem, increasing their chances of experiencing failure. Avoidant children are less apt to express emotions and wishes. Nevertheless, they are more prone to outbursts of aggression. For example, one study found that, in contrast with their outwardly calm behavior in the Strange Situation, avoidant toddlers interacting at home with their mother suddenly and directly showed anger through threats of attack or outright attack (e.g., hitting or kicking).

Disorganized–disoriented children have difficulty paying attention, perform worse on some cognitive tasks, and are described as restless. In middle childhood, they may act controlling toward their own parents, exhibiting a reversal in the parent–child role. Furthermore, evidence indicates a strong link between disorganized attachment in infancy and clinically diagnosed aggressive behavioral problems in childhood. Children with a disorganized/disordered attachment history are at risk for developing oppositional defiant disorder, which is characterized by tantrums, acting out against authority figures, and argumentativeness. They also are at greater risk for the more serious diagnosis of conduct disorder, which is characterized by truancy, stealing, fighting, or even firesetting. Furthermore, children with a disorganized attachment style appear more likely to develop clinical depression. Recent preliminary evidence also suggests that these children are more likely to develop dissociative disorders, but further research is needed to confirm this link. [*See* DISSOCIATIVE DISORDERS.]

III. ATTACHMENT IN ADULT RELATIONSHIPS

Two central issues underlie most work on attachment in adult relationships. The first issue concerns whether attachment patterns during childhood influence, to some extent, attachment patterns and psychosocial functioning in adulthood. The second issue concerns whether adults show attachment patterns and processes in their close relationships that parallel those observed in infant–caregiver relationships, regardless of whether childhood patterns are carried forward into adulthood, and whether such patterns influence psychosocial functioning. Work by developmental and social psychologists has only begun to address the question of continuity in attachment from childhood to adulthood. Developmental work has focused primarily on how parents' memories of their own childhood attachment experiences contribute to their children's attachment patterns and to their own psychological functioning. Social psychological work has focused primarily on how patterns of attachment in adult close relationships, particularly romantic relationships, contribute to psychological functioning.

A. Adult Attachment to Parents

Developmental work, led by Mary Main, has examined the quality of adults' working models of attachment to their parents using the Adult Attachment Interview (AAI). During this semi-structured interview, respondents describe generally their childhood relationship with each parent, and provide specific childhood memories. Trained judges code not only the types of childhood experiences (e.g., loving and responsive vs. demanding and rejecting) mentioned by respondents, but also respondents' current state of mind about their attachment history. State of mind is indicated, for example, by whether or not respondents have resolved past difficulties with parents, have difficulty recalling specific childhood events, idealize their

parents, or still experience anger toward their parents. Particularly important is the degree to which respondents show coherence in describing their relationships with their parents. Coherent accounts evidence a realistic and balanced description of these relationships; incoherent accounts appear less realistic and include conflicting information. For example, a woman may describe her relationship with her mother as "happy" but when pressed to recall specific examples from her childhood she recalls only negative events.

The AAI has revealed several patterns of adult attachment. The autonomous–secure classification reflects secure attachment, whereas the dismissing and preoccupied classifications reflect different types of insecure attachment. Individuals who fall into any of these classifications also may receive a designation of unresolved with respect to attachment issues. Secure attachment has been associated consistently with greater mental health; conversely, insecure attachment, as indicated by any of the insecure classifications from the AAI, has been associated with greater psychopathology. The majority (50–60%) of adults in nonclinical samples fall into the autonomous–secure category; these individuals provide coherent, realistic accounts of their childhood and appear to be aware of how past experiences might affect their current lives. Although some autonomous–secure respondents describe positive childhood experiences and warm relationships with their parents, many autonomous–secure respondents are "earned secures" who have come to terms with varying degrees of unpleasant, distressing childhood experiences and are able to talk about them in a coherent, realistic fashion. These individuals appear to understand their negative experiences, and often have forgiven the problematic parent or parents. Precisely how individuals develop earned security, despite adverse attachment experiences, remains an important question for future work on the promotion of mental health.

Approximately 25 to 30% of respondents are classified as dismissing; these respondents do not wish to discuss their relationships or do not seem invested in them. The generalized statements of dismissing respondents tend to reflect idealization of their parents, yet their more specific memories often focus on negative experiences such as being neglected or rejected by a parent. This discrepancy suggests that dismissing individuals may deny their painful experiences. In one study, dismissing adults showed increased physiological responsiveness, as measured by skin conductance, at points in the attachment interview when they denied the negativity of their childhood experiences. Thus, dismissing adults experience some degree of arousal, and perhaps distress, while they are verbally denying negative experiences. These findings parallel those in which avoidant babies showed physiological arousal when separated from their mother, but did not show signs of distress in their outward behavior.

Preoccupied respondents (approximately 15%), in contrast to dismissing respondents, talk readily about their relationships, and their lengthy comments tend to be incoherent and disorganized. They often describe reversed role relationships in which the child took care of the parent. Preoccupied respondents also appear unable to move beyond their childhood issues with parents, and often express current anger toward parents or ongoing efforts to please them. The preoccupied attachment style corresponds closely to Ainsworth's anxious–ambivalent style.

Respondents who fall into one of the above three categories also can receive an additional designation, termed "unresolved," if they describe childhood trauma or loss in a way that reveals accompanying irrational thoughts (e.g., pathological beliefs, pervasive and intrusive thoughts). A majority of sexual and physical abuse survivors receive this additional designation, which suggests that it reflects psychological vulnerability.

The majority of work using the AAI has examined the link between parents' representations of their childhood attachment experiences and the attachment status of their own children. In general, the AAI classification of a parent strongly predicts (approximately 75% of the time) the attachment behavior of that parent's child in the Strange Situation. Thus, how individuals think about and organize information about their relationships with their own parents may influence their own parenting skills and, as a consequence, affect the mental health of their children. Exactly how parents transmit their working models of attachment is not yet clear. Some theorists believe that transmission occurs through parent–child communication and through behavior that reflects the parents' responsiveness and sensitivity. Other theorists suggest that temperamental characteristics, such as activity level, emotionality, and sociability, are passed from parent to child, increasing the likelihood that a child will develop a particular attachment style; thus, similar genes could account for parent–child similarity in attachment style.

Other work suggests that individuals' AAI classifications are associated with their own cognitive, emotional, and social functioning. In one study, college students classified as dismissing evidenced less ego-resilience (i.e., less ability to adapt to environmental demands) and greater hostility than those classified as secure or preoccupied; those classified as preoccupied showed greater anxiety and distress than secure or dismissing students, and less social competence than those classified as secure. In another study, mothers who showed greater preoccupation experienced more difficulty regulating emotion during conversations with their adolescent children, showed more anxiety, and were more intrusive.

Insecure AAI classifications also have been linked to psychopathology. In one sample of adults with serious psychopathology, 100% of the participants had insecure attachment styles. In other samples with varying levels and types of clinical difficulties, 84% to 98% of participants evidenced insecure attachment. Although researchers have not found many consistent associations between particular insecure attachment classifications and specific clinical disorders, recent work suggests that some differences are likely to exist in the kinds of disorders associated with dismissing versus preoccupied attachment classifications. Dismissing adolescents are more likely to be diagnosed with disorders characterized by less reported distress, such as substance abuse, conduct disorders, and antisocial personality disorder. Preoccupied adolescents and college students are more likely to be diagnosed with disorders that show high levels of distress such as depression, anxiety, or borderline personality disorders. [See ANXIETY.]

In a study comparing suicidal and nonsuicidal adolescents, all of whom were receiving psychiatric treatment, those who had attempted suicide or exhibited extreme suicidal ideation were more likely to display a preoccupied attachment style with an unresolved designation, whereas those who were nonsuicidal were more likely to display a dismissing attachment style. Work examining college women further suggests a link between preoccupied attachment and depression, and dismissing attachment and eating disorders. In addition, other research indicates that individuals with the unresolved designation may be more likely to be diagnosed with oppositional defiant disorder or borderline personality disorder, and to be hospitalized for their psychological problems.

One limitation of research using the AAI is that the way adults respond to the interview may reflect their current experiences and feelings about themselves and others rather than their childhood attachment experiences. Thus, it is not clear whether childhood experiences or current psychological status account for the link between the AAI and different outcome variables (e.g., child's attachment style, adult's psychological status). A small number of recently completed longitudinal studies suggest, however, that the AAI responses of adolescents and adults are connected to their childhood behavior in the Strange Situation. This preliminary evidence suggests that approximately 70% of adults' AAI classifications are consistent with their infant Strange Situation classifications. However, further work is needed to determine the accuracy of this estimate, and the extent of the connection between infant attachment classification and adult psychological status.

B. Adult Romantic Attachment

Although relationships with romantic partners differ from those with parents in important respects (e.g., sexuality, reciprocal caregiving), romantic partners may fulfill many of the same attachment needs for adults as parents do for their children. Adults count on their romantic partners to act as a secure base to which they can return and feel safe, and to provide a safe haven where they can obtain comfort and security in times of stress. Like childhood attachment relationships, adult attachment relationships are likely to play a role in mental health.

Pioneering work by Cindy Hazan and Phillip Shaver first examined the similarities between childhood attachment relationships and adult romantic relationships. They created descriptions of three adult attachment styles that closely paralleled Ainsworth's descriptions of infants' attachment behaviors in the Strange Situation. In their studies, adults chose the description that best characterized them. The secure description emphasized comfort with close relationships; the anxious–ambivalent (preoccupied) description emphasized a desire for greater closeness and intimacy in romantic relationships and the concern that the romantic partner might leave; the avoidant

description emphasized feeling uncomfortable with closeness and intimacy. The proportion of adults who fell into each of the three attachment styles (i.e., 56% secure, 19% anxious/ambivalent, 25% avoidant) closely paralleled the proportions found for infants in Ainsworth's research, suggesting that attachment patterns exist in adult relationships.

Does the quality of attachment in childhood relationships predict later attachment quality in adult romantic relationships? Evidence based on individuals' memories of their childhood experiences suggests that some continuity exists. In Hazan and Shaver's original studies, secure respondents reported warmer relationships with their parents than did respondents in the two insecure groups; avoidant respondents reported colder and more rejecting relationships with their mothers than did anxious–ambivalent respondents; and, anxious–ambivalent respondents reported that their parents were more unfair and intrusive. A major limitation of work relying on individuals' memories, however, is that people may not accurately recall their past experiences and their current memories may be biased by their current relationship experiences. The degree to which continuity exists will become clearer as researchers study attachment patterns in the same individuals from childhood through adulthood.

Whether or not childhood patterns are carried forward, to any extent, into adulthood, attachment processes may operate in adult relationships. A recent study of children and adolescents, ranging from 6 to 17 years old, demonstrated developmental changes in whether parents or peers met attachment functions, including proximity-seeking, safe haven, separation protest, and secure base. These attachment functions were assessed through structured interviews; respondents named the person with whom they most liked to spend time (proximity-seeking), the person they turned to for comfort when upset (safe haven), the person they missed most during separations (separation protest), and the person they felt they could most count on when needed (safe haven). Children and adolescents preferred to spend time with peers rather than parents, which contrasts with patterns observed in infants and younger children. Children aged 8 to 14 shifted their preference from parents to peers as a source of comfort and support, but they still designated parents as the people they could count on most, and the people they missed most during separations.

However, approximately 41% of those in late adolescence (ages 15–17) designated a peer (usually a romantic partner) for all four attachment functions. This work provides initial evidence that attachment processes play a role in relationships other than those with parents. Future work will need to validate these findings, and investigate the operation of attachment processes from early to late adulthood.

Over the past decade, many studies have shown that the quality of adult attachment predicts a variety of cognitive, emotional, and interpersonal consequences. Most of these studies have measured adult attachment using Hazan and Shaver's three categories. More recent work, however, has relied on Bartholomew and Horowitz's refined four-category scheme that distinguishes between two types of avoidance: dismissing versus fearful. Dismissing–avoidant adults report that they do not need close relationships and that they prefer to be self-sufficient, whereas fearful–avoidant adults report that they desire close relationships but are afraid of being rejected.

Work on the cognitive correlates of adult attachment has focused on views of self, others, and relationships, which derive from Bowlby's conception of internal working models. Adult attachment styles are connected to views of self—a central component of mental health. In studies using the three attachment categories, secure individuals consistently evidence higher self-esteem than preoccupied individuals; avoidant individuals either fall in between these two groups, or evidence lower self-esteem than secure individuals. Findings for avoidants have been clarified by studies using the four category scheme. In these studies, secure and dismissing–avoidant individuals evidence higher self-esteem, whereas preoccupied and fearful–avoidant individuals evidence lower self-esteem.

Further work has examined other aspects of self-views such as complexity and integration. One series of laboratory studies found that secure and avoidant participants showed more positive, complex views of themselves than did preoccupied participants; secure participants, however, showed greater integration (i.e., interconnections) between distinct aspects of their self-views than either insecure group. Secure individuals, in comparison to those who were insecure, also showed less discrepancies between their views of themselves as they actually are, how they ought to be, and how they would ideally like to be. Greater discrepancies between actual and ought selves have been linked to anxiety, whereas greater discrepancies between actual and ideal selves have been linked to depression. The greater discrepancies observed in the self-views of insecure people suggest that they may be more prone to anxiety, depression, or both.

Research also has investigated the link between attachment and views of others. Understanding this link is important in view of the well-established finding that people's expectations about others can influence the quality of their interactions. Some studies indicate that secure individuals hold more positive views of human nature than either anxious-ambivalent or avoidant individuals. Other work suggests that both secure and preoccupied people hold positive views of others, whereas fearful–avoidant and dismissing–avoidant individuals hold more negative views of others. Similarly, people who hold different attachment styles also hold different beliefs and expectations about romantic relationships. Anxious–ambivalent people consistently show less optimism about their relationships than secure people; they also are more likely to believe that love involves emotional extremes. Although the findings for avoidants are less consistent, their beliefs appear to differ somewhat from those of secure people; for example, they are more likely to believe that love does not last or that love is hard to find. The negative expectations held by some insecure individuals may increase the likelihood that other people will respond more negatively toward them; such interactions are likely to reinforce their negative views and limit opportunities for positive social interactions and relationships.

Studies of emotional functioning indicate that preoccupied people, in comparison with secure or avoidant people, report greater emotional extremes in their romantic relationships, and show greater emotionality and impulsiveness. In studies distinguishing between fearful versus dismissing avoidants, dismissing–avoidants often report low emotionality and interviewers rate them as less emotionally expressive than secure, preoccupied, or fearful–avoidant individuals. Recent findings indicate that preoccupied people are least able to inhibit their emotions, whereas avoidant people are most able to inhibit their emotions; secure people fall in between these two extremes. Both emotional ups and downs and emotional inhibition may make insecure people more vulnerable to affective disorders. Some findings suggest that both preoccupied and fearful–avoidant college students are more susceptible to depression.

Little research exists on the link between self-reported romantic attachment style and clinically diagnosed emotional disorders. However, one study of middle-aged married women compared those who were recovering from a clinical depression with those who had never had a clinical depression or any other psychiatric disorder. Women recovering from depression were more likely to show fearful–avoidance in their marriage than women who had never suffered a clinical depression; these recovering depressed women, however, were not more likely to show preoccupation. Further research is needed to determine whether a fearful–avoidant attachment style represents a risk factor for clinical depression. [See DEPRESSION.]

Studies of adults in dating or marital relationships have found that those with a secure attachment style report better functioning (e.g., greater satisfaction, better communication, more supportive exchanges) than either avoidant or preoccupied individuals. Some studies suggest that anxious–ambivalent attachment is associated with poorer relationship functioning in women, but avoidant attachment is associated with poorer relationship functioning in men. One three-year longitudinal study found that avoidant men and anxious–ambivalent women were remarkably likely to stay in their relationship, despite their low levels of satisfaction in the relationship. The tendency of these individuals to remain in an unhappy relationship may increase their vulnerability to mental health problems.

Another longitudinal study showed that attachment style predicted whether individuals would be involved in a romantic relationship 4 years later. Secure individuals were more likely to be married and least likely to be divorced; preoccupied people were more likely not to have a partner but to be looking for one; and avoidant people were more likely to have multiple partners or to have no partner and not be looking for one. In addition, anxious–ambivalent individuals reported more breakups but, in contrast to individuals in other attachment groups, they were more likely to break up and then reunite with the same partner. These findings are significant in view of evidence suggesting that having at least one close, confiding relationship is linked to better mental health.

IV. IMPLICATIONS OF ATTACHMENT RESEARCH FOR INTERVENTION

A number of intervention programs have begun to use knowledge derived from attachment theory, with impressive success. For example, one program designed to address behavioral problems in children incorporated attachment theory to plan discussions of attachment history with parents and children and to design workshops on changing problematic attachment and caregiving behavioral patterns. This program significantly reduced conduct disorder, oppositional defiant disorder, and attention deficit hyperactivity disorder in its clients.

Another intervention program has concentrated on the internal working models of mothers as a way of improving their relationships with their children. In this program, high-risk mothers worked with a facilitator (also a mother) who provided information on infants' needs, meaning of their signals, and developmental stages, and discussed in detail the mother's own memories and concepts of important attachment relationships in the past, and expectations for their new role as caregiver. Mothers in this program understood their infants and the infant–caregiver relationship better than mothers who did not participate in the program. They also had lower depression and anxiety scores and coped better with their daily life stress.

Adult attachment style also predicts how well patients respond to therapy. In research comparing improvement rates across attachment styles measured with the AAI, securely attached adults had high rates of compliance with treatment, and were comfortable with self-disclosure. Interestingly, the dismissing group showed the greatest improvement in response to therapy. Dismissing adults may benefit from learning to talk about relationships and relationship problems. In contrast, preoccupied adults, who characteristically spend a great deal of time considering their relationship problems, may be less likely to benefit from this aspect of the therapeutic relationship.

V. CONCLUSIONS AND FUTURE DIRECTIONS

Attachment patterns in infancy, childhood, and adulthood clearly are implicated in the promotion of mental health. Across the life span, secure attachment patterns are associated with better cognitive, emotional, and interpersonal functioning than are insecure attachment patterns. Some insecure patterns appear to increase vulnerability to clinical disorders, such as depression, anxiety, or borderline personality disorder. Although attachment patterns show a high degree of stability over time, they appear to change under some circumstances.

An important goal for future intervention and research programs will be to specify the paths to secure attachment. As part of this endeavor, researchers must pay closer attention to "earned secures" who, despite adverse conditions in childhood, show security in their adult attachments to parents and have secure children themselves. How do these individuals earn their security? What psychological or environmental factors allow them to resolve negative experiences in a healthy way? Another important issue concerns how parents transmit attachment patterns to their children. More research is needed on the precise behaviors and communication styles that promote security in children, and the interplay between genetic and environmental factors in this process.

The connection between infant attachment experiences and later adult attachment needs to be examined in studies of the same individuals over time. Do infant attachment experiences carry over into adult romantic relationships? If so, what is the nature of the transmission? Answering these questions will help to shape therapies addressing adult attachment difficulties; and provide information on how these therapies might best address infant and childhood experiences.

Further work is needed on the nature of attachment bonds in adulthood and their link to mental health. When and how do adult relationships function as at-tachment relationships? Can adults change their attachment patterns on the basis of their experiences in adult relationships? If so, what kinds of experiences lead to increased security?

Work addressing these questions will need to tackle the problem of measuring attachment. Researchers coming from different traditions rely on quite different measures (i.e., behavioral assessments, interviews, self-reports) that do not necessarily assess similar aspects of attachment. Yet, a comprehensive understanding of the contribution of attachment processes to mental health throughout the life span will require bridging the gap between these different traditions.

BIBLIOGRAPHY

Bartholomew, K., & Perlman, D. (Eds.). (1995). *Attachment processes in adulthood. Advances in personal relationships (Vol. 5).* London: Jessica Kingsley Publishers.

Belsky, J., & Nezworski, T. (Eds.). (1988). *Clinical implications of attachment.* Hillsdale, NJ: Erlbaum.

Bretherton, I., & Waters, E. (Eds.). (1985). *Growing points in attachment in theory and research. Monographs of the Society for Research in Child Development, 50* (1–2, Serial no. 209).

Greenberg, M. T., Cicchetti, D., & Cummings, E. M. (Eds.). (1990). *Attachment in the preschool years: Theory, research, and intervention.* Chicago: University of Chicago Press.

Parkes, C. M., Stevenson-Hinde, J., & Marris, P. (Eds.) (1991). *Attachment across the life cycle.* London: Tavistock/Routledge.

Sperling, M. B., & Berman, W. H. (Eds.). (1994). *Attachment in adults: Clinical and developmental perspectives.* New York: Guilford.

Waters, E., Vaughn, B. E., Posada, G., & Kondo-Ikemura, K. (Eds.) (1995). *Caregiving, cultural, and cognitive perspectives on secure-base behavior and working models: New growing points of attachment theory and research. Monographs of the Society for Research in Child Development, 60,* (2–3, Serial, No. 244).

Attention Deficit/ Hyperactivity Disorder (ADHD)

Russell A. Barkley and Gwenyth H. Edwards

University of Massachusetts Medical Center

Attention A multidimensional construct that can refer to alertness, arousal, selectivity, sustained attention, distractibility, or span of apprehension.

Contingency-Shaped Attention Continued responding in a situation or to a task as a function of the immediate consequences provided by the task or activity.

Developmental Disorder Any condition arising in childhood thought to be intrinsic to the individual that is characterized by functioning that is substantially below that expected, given the person's chronological age.

Goal-Directed Persistence The maintenance of responding that is controlled by the capacity to hold events, goals, and plans in mind and to adhere to those plans and other rules governing behavior.

Hyperactivity Characterized by increased or excessive movement of the body and its extremities. May be manifested as constant restlessness, fidgetiness, motor overactivity, or excessive talkativeness.

Impulsivity Reduced ability to resist an impulse or temptation to perform some action. Impulsive actions are those that are directed at obtaining immediate gratification without regard for the delayed consequences of the behavior.

Reinforcement The consequences of behavior that increase the probability that the behavior will occur again.

Response Inhibition The capacity to: (a) inhibit prepotent responses, or those that gain immediate reinforcement either positive or negative; (b) terminate ongoing responses as a function of feedback concerning errors or response ineffectiveness; or (c) protect ongoing self-directed and often private (cognitive) actions (i.e., thinking) from disruption by competing response patterns.

ATTENTION DEFICIT/HYPERACTIVITY DISORDER (ADHD) is a pattern of behaviors believed to be primarily of a neurodevelopmental origin that affects approximately 3 to 5% of the school-aged population. Children with ADHD experience delays relative to other children of the same age in three areas of their functioning: the ability to regulate behavior and excessive levels of activity (hyperactivity); impulse control or behavioral inhibition; and sustained attention to tasks that are not inherently interesting or rewarding. Although children diagnosed with ADHD will gradually mature and make gains in these areas as they grow older, many may always lag behind other children of the same age to a significant degree in their behavioral regulation, impulse control, and sustained attention.

I. INTRODUCTION

It is not unusual for young children to be energetic and active, or to become bored quickly and move from one activity to another as they explore their environment. A young child's desire for immediate gratification is to be expected, rather than the restraint or self-control that would be demanded of someone older. However, some children persistently display levels of activity that are far in excess of their age group. Some are unable to sustain their attention to activities, their interest in tasks assigned to them by others, or their persistence in achieving long-term goals as well as their peers.

When a child's impulse control, sustained attention, and general self-regulation lag far behind expectations for their developmental level, they are likely to be diagnosed as having ADHD. Children with ADHD have a greater probability of experiencing a number of problems in their social, academic, and emotional development and daily adaptive functioning. [*See* IMPULSE CONTROL.]

Attention Deficit/Hyperactivity Disorder (ADHD) has captured public commentary and scientific interest for more than 100 years. While the diagnostic labels for disorders of inattention, hyperactivity, and impulsiveness have changed numerous times, the actual nature of the disorder has changed little, if at all, from descriptions provided at the turn of the century. During the past century, and especially during the last 30 years, thousands of published scientific papers have focused on ADHD, making it one of the most well-studied childhood psychiatric disorders.

II. HISTORICAL CONTEXT

Serious clinical interest in children who have severe problems with inattention, hyperactivity, and poor impulse control is first found in three published lectures by the English physician, George Still, presented to the Royal Academy of Physicians in 1902. Still reported on a group of 20 children in his clinical practice whom he defined as having a deficit in "volitional

inhibition" or a "defect in moral control" over their own behavior. Still's observations described many of the associated features of ADHD that would be supported by research almost a century later, such as an overrepresentation of boys compared to girls, the greater incidence of alcoholism, criminal conduct, and depression among the biological relatives, and a familial predisposition to the disorder.

Initial interest in children with these characteristics arose in North America around the time of the great encephalitis epidemics of 1917 and 1918. Children surviving these brain infections were noted to have many behavioral problems similar to those comprising contemporary ADHD. These cases, as well as others known to have arisen from birth trauma, head injury, toxin exposure, and infections, gave rise to the concept of a "brain-injured child syndrome," often associated with mental retardation. This term was eventually applied to children without a history of brain damage or evidence of retardation but who manifested behavioral problems such as hyperactivity or poor impulse control. This concept would later evolve into that of "minimal brain damage," and eventually "minimal brain dysfunction" (MBD), as challenges were raised to the label given the lack of evidence of brain injury in many of these cases.

During the 1950s researchers became increasingly interested in hyperactivity. "Hyperkinetic impulse disorder" was attributed to cortical overstimulation resulting from ineffective filtering of stimuli entering the brain. These studies gave rise to the notion of the "hyperactive child syndrome" typified by daily motor movement that was far in excess of that seen in normal children of the same age.

By the 1970s research findings emphasized the importance of problems with sustained attention and impulse control in addition to hyperactivity in understanding the nature of the disorder. In 1983 Virginia Douglas proposed that the disorder was comprised of major deficits in four areas: (1) the investment, organization, and maintenance of attention and effort; (2) the ability to inhibit impulsive behavior; (3) the ability to modulate arousal levels to meet situational demands; and (4) an unusually strong inclination to seek immediate reinforcement. Douglas' work, along with numerous subsequent studies of attention, impulsiveness, and other cognitive factors, eventually led to renaming the disorder "Attention Deficit Disorder" (ADD) in 1980.

Just as significant as the renaming of the condition at that time was the distinction made between two types of ADD: those with hyperactivity and those without it. Little research existed at the time on the latter subtype. However, later research suggested that ADD without hyperactivity might be a separate and distinct disorder of a different component of attention (selective or focused) than was the type of inattention seen in those with ADD with hyperactivity (persistence and distractibility). Thus, rather than being related subtypes of a single disorder with a shared, common impairment in attention, future research may show these subtypes to constitute separate disorders of attention altogether.

Within a few years of the creation of the label ADD, concern was raised by Barkley in 1990 and Weiss and Hechtman in 1993 that problems with hyperactivity and impulse control were features critically important to differentiating the disorder from other conditions and to predicting later developmental risks. In 1987 the disorder was renamed Attention Deficit Hyperactivity Disorder. Diagnostic symptoms were identified from a single list of items incorporating all three constructs: hyperactivity, impulsivity, and inattention. The subtype of ADD without Hyperactivity was now renamed Undifferentiated ADD and relegated to minor diagnostic status until further research could clarify its nature and relationship to ADHD.

Around this same time (mid-1980s to 1990s) reports began to appear that challenged the notion that ADHD was primarily a disturbance in attention. Over the previous decade, researchers studying information-processing capacities in children with ADHD were having difficulty demonstrating that the problems these children had with attending to tasks were actually attentional in nature (i.e., related to the processing of incoming information). Problems in response inhibition and preparedness of the motor control system appeared to be more reliably demonstrated. Researchers, moreover, were finding that the problems with hyperactivity and impulsivity were not separate constructs but formed a single dimension of behavior. All of this led to the creation of two separate lists of symptoms for ADHD when the latest diagnostic manual for psychiatry, *The Diagnostic and Statistical Manual of Mental Disorders,* Fourth Edition (also known as the *DSM-IV*) was published by the American Psychiatric Association in 1994. In the

DSM-IV, one symptom list now existed for inattention and another for hyperactive–impulsive behavior. The inattention list once again permitted the diagnosis of a subtype of ADHD that consisted principally of problems with attention (ADHD Predominantly Inattentive Type). But two other subtypes were also identified (Predominantly Hyperactive–Impulsive and Combined Types). As of this writing, debate continues over the core deficit(s) involved in ADHD, with increasing emphasis being given to a central problem specifically with behavioral inhibition and more generally with self-regulation or executive functioning.

III. DESCRIPTION AND DIAGNOSIS:

A. The Core Symptoms

Problems with attention consist of the child's inability to sustain attention or respond to tasks or play activities as long as others of the same age or to follow through on rules and instructions as well as others. The child appears more disorganized, distracted, and forgetful than others of the same age. Parents and teachers frequently complain that these children do not seem to listen as well as they should for their age, cannot concentrate, are easily distracted, fail to finish assignments, daydream, and change activities more often than others.

Research corroborates that, when compared to normal children, ADHD children are often more "off-task," less likely to complete as much work as others, look away more from the activities they are requested to do (including television), persist less in correctly performing boring activities, and are slower and less likely to return to an activity once interrupted. Yet objective research does not find children with ADHD to be generally more distracted by most forms of extraneous events occurring during their task performance, although distractors within the task may prove more disruptive to them than to normal children. Research instead documents that ADHD children are more active than other children, are less mature in controlling motor movements, and have considerable difficulties with stopping an ongoing behavior. They frequently talk more than others and interrupt others' conversations. They are less able to resist immediate temptations and delay gratification and respond too quickly and too often when they are required to wait and watch for events to happen.

Recent research shows that the problems with behavioral or motor inhibition arise first, at age 3 to 4 years, with those related to inattention emerging somewhat later in the developmental course of ADHD, at age 5 to 7 years. Whereas the symptoms of disinhibition seem to decline with age, those of inattention remain relatively stable during the elementary grades. Yet even the inattentiveness may decline by adolescence in some cases.

A number of factors have been noted to influence the ability of children with ADHD to sustain their attention to task performance, to control their impulses to act, to regulate their activity level, and to produce work consistently. They include: time of day or fatigue; increasing task complexity where organizational strategies are required; extent of restraint demanded for the context; level of stimulation within the setting; the schedule of immediate consequences associated with the task; and the absence of adult supervision during task performance.

It has been shown that children with ADHD are most problematic in their behavior when persistence in work-related tasks is required (i.e., chores, homework, etc.) or where behavioral restraint is necessary, especially in settings involving reduced parental monitoring (i.e., in church, in restaurants, when a parent is on the phone, etc.). Such children are least likely to pose behavioral management problems during free play, when little self-control is required. Fluctuations in the severity of ADHD symptoms have also been documented across a variety of school contexts. In this case, classroom activities involving self-organization and task-directed persistence are the most problematic, with significantly fewer problems posed by contexts involving fewer performance demands (i.e., at lunch, in hallways, at recess, etc.), and even fewer problems posed during highly entertaining special events (i.e., field trips, assemblies, etc.).

B. Associated Cognitive Impairments

Although ADHD is defined by the presence of the two major symptom dimensions of inattention and disinhibition (hyperactivity–impulsivity), research indicates that these children often demonstrate deficiencies in many other abilities. These include: motor coordination and sequencing; working memory and mental computation; planning and anticipation or preparedness for action; verbal fluency and confron-

tational communication; effort allocation; applying organization strategies; the internalization of self-directed speech; adhering to restrictive instructions; the self-regulation of emotions; and self-motivation. Several studies have also demonstrated what both Still (1902) and Douglas (1983) noted anecdotally years ago—ADHD may be associated with less mature or diminished moral reasoning and the moral control of behavior.

The commonality among most or all of these seemingly disparate abilities is that all fall within the neuropsychological domain described as executive functions. The neurologist Joaquim Fuster wrote in 1989 that these executive abilities are probably mediated by the frontal cortex of the brain, and particularly the prefrontal lobes. Barkley has recently defined executive functions as being those neuropsychological processes that permit or assist with human self-regulation. Self-regulation is then defined as any self-directed form of behavior (both overt and covert) that serves to modify the probability of a subsequent behavior by the individual so as to alter the probability of a later consequence. Such behavior may even involve forgoing immediate rewards for the sake of maximizing delayed outcomes or even exposing oneself to immediate aversive circumstances for this same purpose. Self-regulatory behavior, therefore, includes thinking within this realm of private or covert self-directed behavior. By appreciating the role of the frontal lobes and the prefrontal cortex in these executive abilities, it is easy to see why researchers have repeatedly speculated that ADHD probably arises out of some disturbance or dysfunction of this brain region. [See MENTAL CONTROL ACROSS THE LIFE SPAN.]

IV. THEORETICAL FRAMEWORK

Many different hypotheses on the nature of ADHD have been proposed over the past century, such as Still's (1902) notion of defective volitional inhibition and moral regulation of behavior, and Douglas' (1983) theory of deficient attention, inhibition, arousal, and preference for immediate reward. Few of these have produced models of the disorder that were widely adopted by both scientists and clinicians or that served to drive further programmatic research initiatives. Some of these theories have suggested that ADHD is a deficit in sensitivity to reinforcement, a more general motivational disorder, or a deficit in rule-governed behavior (i.e., the control of behavior by language). Most recently, several theorists working in this area have proposed that ADHD represents a deficit behavioral inhibition; an assertion for which there is substantial evidence, at least for those subtypes that involve hyperactive-impulsive symptoms.

Consistent with these proposals, Barkley outlined a model of ADHD in 1994 that was based upon an earlier theory by Jacob Bronowski first set forth in 1966 on the evolution of the unique properties of human language and their relationship to response inhibition. Bronowski's model was subsequently combined with that of Juaquim Fuster published in 1989, which specified that the overarching role of the prefrontal cortex is the cross-temporal organization of behavior. Barkley's hybrid theoretical model of ADHD places behavioral inhibition at a central point and supportive point in relation to four other executive functions dependent upon it for their own effective execution. These functions are working memory, the self-regulation of emotion/motivation, the internalization of speech, and reconstitution (analysis and synthesis of behavioral structures in the service of goal-directed behavioral creativity). The four functions are believed to permit and subserve human self-regulation, bringing behavior progressively under the control of internally represented information, often about the future, and transferring it at least partially away from the control of behavior by more immediate consequences and external events. The executive control of behavior afforded by these functions is proposed to result in a greater capacity for predicting and controlling one's self and one's environment so as to maximize future consequences over immediate ones for the individual. And, more generally, the interaction of these executive functions permits far more organized and effective adaptive functioning.

Several assumptions are important in understanding this model as it is applied to ADHD. First, the capacity for behavioral inhibition begins to emerge first in the child's development, prior to or corresponding with the emergence of the four executive functions. Second, inhibition does not directly cause the activation of these executive functions but sets the occasion for their occurrence and is necessary for their effective performance. Third, these functions probably emerge at different times in the child's development and may have relatively independent developmental trajectories, although interactive. Fourth, the sweeping cognitive impairments that ADHD creates across these executive functions are secondary to the primary deficit in behavioral inhibition, implying that if inhibition were to be improved, these executive functions would likewise improve.

The deficit in behavioral inhibition is thought to arise principally from genetic and neurodevelopmental origins, rather than from purely social ones, although its expression is certainly influenced by a variety of social factors. The secondary deficits in the executive functions and self-regulation created by the primary deficit in inhibition feedback to contribute to further deficits in behavioral inhibition because self-regulation is required for self-restraint.

Behavioral inhibition is viewed in the model as comprising three related processes: (1) the capacity to inhibit "prepotent" responses prior to their initiation; (2) the capacity to cease ongoing response patterns once initiated such that both (1) and (2) create delays in responding to events; and (3) the protection of this delay and the self-directed (often private or cognitive) actions occurring within it from interference by competing events and their prepotent responses (interference control). Prepotent responses are defined as those for which immediate reinforcement (both positive and negative) is available for their performance or for which there is a strong history of reinforcement in this context. Through the postponement of the prepotent, automatic responses and the creation of this protected period of delay, the occasion is set for the four executive functions to act effectively in modifying the individual's eventual initial responding to events or modifying their ongoing responses to those events (creating a sensitivity to feedback or errors). The executive system described here may exist so as to achieve a net maximization of both temporally distant and immediate consequences rather than immediate consequences alone. The chain of goal-directed, future-oriented behaviors set in motion by these acts of self-regulation is then also protected from interference during its performance by this same process of inhibition (interference control). Even if disrupted, the individual retains the capacity or intention (via working memory) to return to the goal-directed actions until the outcome is successfully achieved or judged to be no longer necessary.

Space permits here only a brief description of each of the four executive components of this new model of

ADHD. The first of these involves working memory, or the capacity for prolonging and manipulating mental representations of events and using such information to control motor behavior. This particular type of memory can be thought of as remembering so as to do and serves to sustain otherwise fleeting information that will be useful in controlling subsequent responding, such as is seen in privately rehearsing a telephone number in mind so as to later dial it accurately. One component of working memory may be related to self-speech (verbal working memory), while a second component is related to perceptual imagery (visual-spatial) and probably involves self-directed sensing, as in visual imagery or covert audition. This retention of information related to past events (retrospection) gives rise to the conjecturing of future events (prospection), which sets in motion a preparedness to act in anticipation of the arrival of these future events (anticipatory set). Out of this continuous referencing or sensing of past and future probably arises the psychological sense of time. These activities taking place in working memory appear to be dependent upon behavioral inhibition. Such working memory processes have been shown to exist in rudimentary form even in young infants permitting them to successfully perform delayed response tasks to a limited degree. As the capacity for inhibition increases developmentally, it probably contributes to the further efficiency and effectiveness of working memory.

According to this model of ADHD, behavioral inhibition also sets the stage for the development of the second executive component of this model, that being the self-regulation of emotion in children. The inhibition of the initial prepotent response includes the inhibition of the initial emotional reaction that it may have elicited. It is not that the child does not experience emotion; rather, the behavioral reaction to or expression of that emotion is delayed along with any motor behavior associated with it. The delay in responding this creates allows the child time to engage in self-directed behaviors that will modify both the eventual response to the event as well as the emotional reaction that may accompany it. Because emotions are themselves forms of both motivational and arousal states, the model argues that deficits in the self-regulation of emotion should be associated with deficits in self-motivation and the self-control of arousal, particularly in the service of goal-directed behavior. [See EMOTIONAL REGULATION.]

The internalization of self-directed speech, as origi-

nally described by Vygotsky, forms the third executive component of this model of ADHD. During the early preschool years, speech, once developed, is initially employed for communication with others. As behavioral inhibition progresses, language becomes turned on the self. It now is not just a means of influencing the behavior of others but provides a means of reflection as well as a means for controlling one's own behavior (instruction).

The fourth component of this model involves the capacity to rapidly take apart and recombine units of behavior, including language. The delay in responding that behavioral inhibition permits allows time for information related to the event to be mentally prolonged and then disassembled so as to extract more information about the event that will aid in preparing a response to it. In a related fashion, previously learned response patterns can also be broken down into smaller units of behavior. This internal decomposition of information and its associated response patterns permits the complementary process to occur, that being synthesis, or the invention of novel combinations of behavioral structures, including words and ideas, in the service of goal-directed action. This gives a highly creative or generative character as well as a hierarchically organized nature to human goal-directed behavior.

Finally, the internally represented information and motivation generated by these four executive functions is used to control a separate unit within the model, that being motor behavior itself. Such information serves to program, execute, and sustain behavior directed toward goals and the future, giving human behavior an intentional or purposive quality. Task-irrelevant movement is now more effectively suppressed, goal-directed behavior better sustained, and this pattern of behavior more efficiently reengaged should disruption of the behavioral pattern occur because of the control afforded by the internal information being generated from the four executive functions.

The impairment in behavioral inhibition occurring in ADHD is hypothesized to disrupt the efficient execution of these executive functions, thereby limiting the capacity of these individuals for self-regulation. The result is an impairment in the cross-temporal organization of behavior, in the prediction and control of one's own behavior and environment, and inevitably in the maximization of long-term consequences for the individual.

How does this model account for the problems

with attention believed to exist in ADHD? According to this model, it is critical to distinguish between two forms of sustained attention that are traditionally confused in the research literature on ADHD. The first is called contingency-shaped attention. This refers to continued responding in a situation or to a task as a function of the immediate available contingencies of reinforcement provided by the task or its context. Responding that is maintained under these conditions then is directly dependent on the immediate environmental contingencies. Many factors affect this form of sustained attention or responding: the novelty of the task, the intrinsic interest the activity may hold for the individual, the immediate reinforcement it provides for responding in the task, the state of fatigue of the individual, and the presence or absence of an adult supervisor (or other stimuli which signal other consequences for performance that are outside the task itself). The model predicts that this type of sustained attention relatively unaffected by ADHD as it is behavior under the control of external events.

As children mature, however, a second form of sustained attention emerges described in the model as goal-directed persistence. This form of sustained responding arises as a direct consequence of the development of self-regulation or the control of behavior by internally represented information. Such persistence derives from the development of a progressively greater capacity by the child to hold events, goals, and plans in mind (working memory), to adhere to rules governing behavior and to formulate and follow such rules, to self-induce a motivational state supportive of the plans and goals formulated by the individual so as to maintain goal-directed behavior, and even to create novel behaviors in the service of the goal's attainment. The capacity to initiate and sustain chains of goal-directed behavior in spite of the absence of immediate environmental contingencies for their performance is predicted to be the form of sustained attention disrupted by ADHD.

Apart from this heuristically valuable distinction in forms of sustained attention, this theoretical model of ADHD makes numerous predictions about the cognitive and behavioral deficits likely to be found in those with the disorder (i.e., impaired working memory and sense of time, delayed internalization of speech, etc.), many of which have received little or no attention in research on ADHD. It also provides a framework by which to better organize and understand the numerous cognitive deficits identified in previous studies of

children with ADHD than does the current view of ADHD as being chiefly an attention deficit.

V. POTENTIAL ETIOLOGIES

The precise causes of ADHD are unknown at the present time. Numerous causes have been proposed, but evidence for many has been weak or lacking entirely. However, a number of factors have been shown to be associated with a significantly increased risk for ADHD in children.

The vast majority of the potentially causative factors associated with ADHD that are supported by empirical research seem to be biological in nature; that is, they are factors known to be related to or to have a direct effect on brain development and/or functioning. The precise causal pathways by which these factors lead to ADHD, however, are simply not known at this time.

Even so, far less evidence is available to support any purely psychosocial etiology of ADHD. In the vast majority of cases where such psychosocial risks have been found to be significantly associated with ADHD or hyperactivity, more careful analysis has shown these to be either the result of ADHD in the child or, far more often, to be related to aggression or conduct disorder rather than to ADHD. For instance, the child management methods used by parents, parenting stress, marital conflict, or parental psychopathology have now been shown to be far more strongly associated with aggressive and antisocial behavior than with ADHD. The strong hereditary influence in ADHD may also contribute to an apparent link between ADHD and poor child management by a parent—a link that may be attributable to the parent's own ADHD. The environment in which the child is raised and schooled probably plays a larger role in determining the outcomes of children with the disorder and a much lesser role in primary causation. [*See* GENETIC CONTRIBUTORS TO MENTAL HEALTH; PARENTING.]

Throughout the century, investigators have repeatedly noted the similarities between symptoms of ADHD and those produced by lesions or injuries to the frontal lobes of the brain, particularly the prefrontal cortex. Both children and adults suffering injuries to the certain regions of prefrontal cortex demonstrate deficits in sustained attention, inhibition, working memory, the regulation of emotion and motivation, and the capacity to organize behavior across time.

Numerous other lines of evidence have been suggestive of a neurological origin to the disorder. Several studies have examined cerebral blood flow in ADHD and normal children. They have consistently shown decreased blood flow to the prefrontal regions of the brain and the striatum with which these regions are richly interconnected, particularly in its anterior portion. More recently, studies using positron emission tomography (PET) to assess cerebral glucose metabolism have found diminished metabolism in adults and adolescent females with ADHD although not in adolescent males with ADHD. However, significant correlations have been noted between diminished metabolic activity in the left anterior frontal region of the brain and severity of ADHD symptoms in adolescent males with ADHD. This demonstration of an association between the metabolic activity of certain brain regions and symptoms of ADHD is critical in demonstrating a connection between the findings pertaining to brain activation and the behavior comprising ADHD.

More detailed analysis of brain structures using high resolution magnetic resonance imaging (MRI) devices has also suggested differences in some brain regions in those with ADHD. Initial studies that focused on reading-disabled children and used ADHD children as a contrast group examined the region of the left and right temporal lobes (the planum temporale). These regions are thought to be involved with auditory detection and analysis and, therefore, with certain subtypes of reading disabilities. For some time, researchers studying reading disorders have focused on these brain regions because of their connection to the rapid analysis of speech sounds. Children with ADHD and children with reading disabilities were found to have smaller right hemisphere plana temporale than the control group, while only the reading disabled children had a smaller left plana temporale. In another study, the corpus callosum was examined in subjects with ADHD. This structure assists with the interhemispheric transfer of information. Those with ADHD were found to have a smaller callosum, particularly in the area of the genu and splenium and that region just anterior to the splenium. An attempt to replicate this finding, however, failed to show any differences between ADHD and control children in the size or shape of the entire corpus callosum with the ex-

ception of the posterior portion of the splenium, which was significantly smaller in subjects with ADHD. Two additional studies examining the corpus callosum, however, documented smaller anterior (rostral) regions in children with ADHD; findings more consistent with prior studies of brain anatomy and functioning in children with ADHD. Most recently, two studies using larger samples of ADHD and normal children and MRI technology have both documented a smaller right prefrontal cortex and smaller right striatum and right basal ganglia (of which the striatum is a part) in ADHD children. Thus, despite some inconsistencies in findings across some of the earlier studies of brain morphology and functioning in ADHD, more recent studies are increasingly identifying the prefrontal regions of the brain and certain regions of the basal ganglia, such as the striatum, as probably being involved in the disorder.

None of these studies found evidence of frank brain damage in any of these structures in those with ADHD. This is consistent with past reviews of the literature conducted by Michael Rutter in 1983 suggesting that brain damage was related to less than 5% of those with hyperactivity. It is also consistent with more recent studies of twins suggesting that nonshared environmental factors, such as pre-, peri-, and postnatal neurological insults, among other factors, account for approximately 15 to 20% of the differences among individuals in the behavioral pattern associated with ADHD (inattention and hyperactive-impulsive behavior). Where differences in brain structures are found, they are probably the result of abnormalities that arise in brain development (embryology) within these particular regions, the causes of which are not known but may have to do with particular genes responsible for the construction of these brain regions.

No evidence exists to show that ADHD is the result of abnormal chromosomal structures (as in Down's Syndrome), their fragility (as in Fragile X) or transmutation, or of extra chromosomal material (as in XXY syndrome). Children with such chromosomal abnormalities may show greater problems with attention, but such abnormalities are very uncommon in children with ADHD.

By far, the preponderance of research evidence suggests that ADHD is a trait that is highly hereditary in nature, making heredity one of the most well substantiated among the potential etiologies for ADHD. Multiple lines of research support such a conclusion. For years, researchers have noted the higher prevalence of psychopathology in the parents and other relatives of children with ADHD. In particular, higher rates of ADHD, conduct problems, substance abuse, and depression have been repeatedly observed in these studies. Research such as that by Joseph Biederman and colleagues at the Harvard Medical School (Massachusetts General Hospital) shows that between 10 and 35% of the immediate family members of children with ADHD are also likely to have the disorder, with the risk to siblings of the ADHD children being approximately 32%. More recent studies even suggest that if either parent has ADHD, the risk to offspring for the disorder may be as high as 50%. [*See* CONDUCT DISORDERS; DEPRESSION; SUBSTANCE ABUSE.]

Another line of evidence for genetic involvement in ADHD has emerged from studies of adopted children, which have found higher rates of hyperactivity in the biological parents of hyperactive children than in adoptive parents of hyperactive children. Biologically related and unrelated pairs of international adoptees also identified a strong genetic component to the behavioral dimension underlying ADHD.

Studies of twins conducted in the United States, Australia, and the United Kingdom provide a third avenue of evidence for a genetic contribution to ADHD. In general, these studies suggest that if one twin is diagnosed with ADHD, the concordance for the disorder in the second twin may be as high as 81 to 92% in monozygotic twins but only 29 to 35% in dizygotic twins.

Quantitative genetic analyses of a large sample of families studied in Boston by Joseph Biederman and his colleagues suggest that a single gene may account for the expression of the disorder. The focus of research recently has been on the dopamine type 2 gene, given findings of its increased association with alcoholism, Tourette's Syndrome, and ADHD. However, difficulties have arisen in the replication of this finding. More recent studies have implicated the dopamine transporter gene as being involved in ADHD as might the D4D repeator gene, which has shown an association with novelty-seeking and risk-taking personality traits. Clearly, research into the genetic mechanisms involved in the transmission of ADHD across generations will prove an exciting and fruitful area of research endeavor over the next decade as the human genome is mapped and better understood and as more sophisticated genetic technologies arising from this project come to be applied to the study of the genetics of ADHD.

Pre-, peri-, and postnatal complications, and malnutrition, diseases, trauma, and other neurologically compromising events may occur during the development of the nervous system before and after birth. Among these various biologically compromising events, several have been repeatedly linked to risks for inattention and hyperactive behavior. Elevated body lead burden has been shown to have a small but consistent and statistically significant relationship to the symptoms comprising ADHD. However, even at relatively high levels of lead, less than 38% of these children are rated as hyperactive on teacher rating scales, implying that most lead-poisoned children do not develop symptoms of ADHD. Other types of environmental toxins found to have some relationship to inattention and hyperactivity are prenatal exposure to alcohol and tobacco smoke.

VI. EPIDEMIOLOGY OF ADHD

The prevalence of ADHD, as reviewed by Peter Szatmari in 1992, using large epidemiological studies ranges from a low of 2% to a high of 6.3%, with most falling within the range of 4.2 to 6.3%. Most studies have found similar prevalence rates in elementary school-aged children. Differences in prevalence rates are due in part to different methods of selecting these populations, to the criteria used to define a case of ADHD, and to the age range of the samples. For instance, prevalence rates may be 2 to 3% in females but 6 to 9% in males during the 6 to 12-year-old age period, but fall to 1 to 2% in females and 3 to 4.5% in males by adolescence. [*See* EPIDEMIOLOGY: PSYCHIATRIC.]

While the declining prevalence of ADHD with age may reflect real recovery from the disorder, it may also involve, at least in part, an artifact of methodology. This artifact results from the use of items in the diagnostic symptom lists across the life span that are were developed upon and chiefly applicable to young children. These items may reflect the underlying constructs of ADHD very well at younger ages but may be increasingly less appropriate for older age groups. This could create a situation where individuals remain impaired by ADHD characteristics as they mature, but outgrow the diagnostic symptom list for the disorder, resulting in an illusory decline in prevalence over development. Until more age-appropriate symptoms are studied for adolescent and adult populations, this issue remains unresolved.

Gender appears to play a significant role in determining prevalence of ADHD within a population. On average, males are between 2 and 6 times more likely than females to be diagnosed with ADHD in epidemiological samples of children, with the average being roughly 3:1. Within clinic-referred samples, the sex ratio can rise to 6:1 to 9:1, suggesting that males with ADHD are far more likely to be referred to clinics than females, especially if they have an associated oppositional or conduct disorder. It is unclear at this time why males should be more likely to have ADHD than females. This could result partly from an artifact of the relationship between male gender and more aggressive and oppositional behavior; such behavior is known to increase the probability of referral to mental health centers. Because such behavior is often associated with ADHD, clinic-referred males are also more likely to have ADHD. The greater preponderance of males might also, in part, be an artifact of applying a set of diagnostic criteria developed primarily on males to females. Using a predominantly male population to set diagnostic criteria as was done for the *DSM-IV* (see below) could create a higher threshold for diagnosis for females relative to other females than for males relative to other males. Such a circumstance argues for the eventual examination of whether separate diagnostic criteria (symptom thresholds) ought to be considered for each gender. [*See* GENDER DIFFERENCES IN MENTAL HEALTH.]

ADHD occurs across all socioeconomic levels. Where differences in prevalence rates are found across levels of social class, they may be artifacts of the source used to define the disorder or of the association of ADHD with other disorders known to be related to social class, such as aggression and conduct disorder. No one, however, has made the argument that the nature or qualitative aspects of ADHD differ across social classes. [*See* SOCIOECONOMIC STATUS.]

Hyperactivity or ADHD is present in all countries studied so far, such as New Zealand, Japan, Italy, Germany, India, and Australia. While it may not receive the same diagnostic label in each country, the behavior pattern comprising the disorder appears to be present internationally. ADHD arises also in all ethnic groups studied so far.

VII. DEVELOPMENTAL COURSE AND ADULT OUTCOME

Major follow-up studies of clinically referred hyperactive children have been ongoing during the last 25 years at five sites: Montreal, New York City, Iowa City, Los Angeles, and Milwaukee. Follow-up studies of children identified as hyperactive during epidemiological screenings of general populations have also been conducted in the United States, Australia, New Zealand, and England.

The onset of ADHD symptoms has been found to be generally in the preschool years, typically by age 3 or 4, and usually by entry into formal schooling. First to arise in many cases is the pattern of hyperactive–impulsive behavior and, in some cases, oppositional and aggressive conduct. Preschool-aged children with significant degrees of inattentive and hyperactive behavior who are difficult to manage for their parents or teachers and whose pattern of such behavior is persistent for at least a year or more are highly likely to have ADHD and to retain their symptoms into the elementary school years.

By the time ADHD children move into the age range of 6 to 12 years, the problems with hyperactive–impulsive behavior are increasingly associated with difficulties with the form of sustained attention referred to above as goal-directed persistence and distractibility (poor interference control). These symptoms of inattention appear to arise by the age of 5 to 7 years and may emerge out of the increasing difficulties ADHD children are having with self-regulation. The inattentiveness evident in children having ADD without Hyperactivity (Predominantly Inattentive Type of ADHD) may be of a qualitatively different form (focused or selective attention) and may not emerge or be impairing of the child's school performance until even later, such as mid-to-late childhood.

When ADHD is present in clinic-referred children, the likelihood is that 50 to 80% will continue to have their disorder into adolescence. Although severity levels of symptoms are declining over development, this does not mean hyperactive children are necessarily outgrowing their disorder relative to normal children; like mental retardation, the disorder of ADHD is defined by a developmentally relative deficiency, rather than an absolute one, that persists in many children over time.

The persistence of ADHD symptoms across childhood as well as into early adolescence appears to be associated with the initial degree of hyperactive/impulsive behavior in childhood, the co-existence of conduct problems or oppositional/hostile behavior, poor family relations and conflict in parent–child interactions, as well as maternal depression. These predictors have also been associated with the development and persistence of oppositional and conduct disorder into adolescence.

The Montreal follow-up study of Weiss and Hechtman reported in 1993 that at least half of their subjects were still impaired by some symptoms of the disorder in adulthood. The New York City longitudinal study by Salvatore Mannuzza and Rachel Klein suggested that 18 to 30% of hyperactive children continue to have significant symptoms of ADHD into adulthood. Most recently, the Milwaukee follow-up study by Barkley and Fischer suggests that the source of information about the symptoms may be a significant factor in establishing the persistence of the disorder into adulthood. Less than 25% of ADHD children reported having significant symptom levels of the disorder in adulthood when asked about themselves as young adults while their parents indicated that more than 60% of these subjects continued to have clinically significant degrees of the disorder as young adults. Until more studies report adult outcomes for ADHD children using clinical diagnostic criteria appropriate for adults and collecting information not only from the adult but from a parent or an immediate family member who knows them well, the true persistence of the disorder into adulthood will remain a matter of some controversy. At the very least, current research suggests it may be 30 to 50%, although the percentage may be higher among clinic-referred children followed to adulthood.

VIII. DIAGNOSTIC CRITERIA

The most recent diagnostic criteria for ADHD as defined in the *DSM-IV* (1994) are set forth in Table I. They stipulate that individuals have had their symptoms of ADHD for at least 6 months, that these symptoms exist to a degree that is developmentally deviant, and that they have developed by 7 years of age. From the Inattention item list, six of nine items must be endorsed as developmentally inappropriate. Likewise, from the Hyperactive–Impulsive item list, six of nine items must be endorsed as deviant. Depending upon whether criteria are met for either or both symptom lists will determine the type of ADHD that is to be diagnosed: Predominantly Inattentive, Predominantly Hyperactive–Impulsive, or Combined Type.

These diagnostic criteria are empirically derived and are the most rigorous ever available in the history of clinical diagnosis for this disorder. They were developed by a committee of some of the leading experts in the field, a literature review of research on ADHD, an informal survey of rating scales assessing the behavioral dimensions related to ADHD by the committee, and from statistical analyses of the results of a field trial of the items using a large sample of children from 10 different sites in North America.

Controversy continues over whether ADHD—Predominantly Inattentive Type represents a true subtype of ADHD. It is unclear if these children share a common attentional disturbance with the Combined Type and are distinguished simply by the relative absence of significant hyperactivity–impulsivity or whether they have a qualitatively different impairment in attention from that seen in the Combined Type. Several recent reviews of the literature have suggested that this is not in fact a true subtype but actually a separate, distinct disorder having a different attentional disturbance than the one present in ADHD—Combined Type. However, evidence for this subtype's existence was at least strong enough to place it within the *DSM-IV* while awaiting more research on its course and treatment responsiveness to help clarify its status. The very limited research available to date suggests that Predominantly Inattentive ADHD children have more problems in the focused or selective component of attention, appear sluggish in their speed of information processing, and may have memory retrieval problems; in contrast, those with ADHD-Combined Type have more problems with persistence and distractibility as well as with poor inhibition.

The research criteria from the International Classification of Diseases (ICD-10) for Hyperkinetic Disorders closely resemble the *DSM-IV* in stressing two lists of symptoms related to inattention and overactivity and in requiring that pervasiveness across settings be demonstrated. The specific item contents, manner of presenting these symptoms lists within the home and school setting, requirement for office observation of

Table I DSM-IV Criteria for ADHD

A. Either (1) or (2):

(1) Six (or more) of the following symptoms of *inattention* have persisted for at least 6 months to a degree that is maladaptive and inconsistent with developmental level:

Inattention

(a) Often fails to give close attention to details or makes careless mistakes in schoolwork, work, or other activities;

(b) Often has difficulty sustaining attention in tasks or play activities;

(c) Often does not seem to listen when spoken to directly;

(d) Often does not follow through on instructions and fails to finish schoolwork, chores, or duties in the work place (not due to oppositional behavior or failure to understand instructions);

(e) Often has difficulty organizing tasks and activities;

(f) Often avoids, dislikes, or is reluctant to engage in tasks that require sustained mental effort (such as schoolwork or homework);

(g) Often loses things necessary for tasks or activities (e.g., toys, school assignments, pencils, books, or tools);

(h) Is often easily distracted by extraneous stimuli;

(i) Is often forgetful in daily activities.

(2) Six (or more) of the following symptoms of *hyperactivity-impulsivity* have persisted for at least 6 months to a degree that is maladaptive and inconsistent with developmental level:

Hyperactivity

(a) Often fidgets with hands or feet or squirms in seat;

(b) Often leaves seat in classroom or in other situations in which remaining seated is expected;

(c) Often runs about or climbs excessively in situations in which it is inappropriate (in adolescents or adults, may be limited to subjective feelings of restlessness);

(d) Often has difficulty playing or engaging in leisure activities quietly;

(e) Is often "on the go" or often acts as if "driven by a motor";

(f) Often talks excessively.

Impulsivity

(g) Often blurts out answers before the questions have been completed;

(h) Often has difficulty awaiting turn;

(i) Often interrupts or intrudes on others (e.g., butts into conversations or games);

B. Some hyperactive–impulsive or inattentive symptoms that caused impairment were present before age 7 years.

C. Some impairment from the symptoms is present in two or more settings (e.g., at school [or work] and at home).

Table I *Continued*

D. There must be clear evidence of clinically significant impairment in social, academic, or occupational functioning.

E. The symptoms do not occur exclusively during the course of a Pervasive Developmental Disorder, Schizophrenia, or other Psychotic Disorder, and are not better accounted for by another mental disorder (e.g., Mood Disorder, Anxiety Disorder, Dissociative Disorder, or a Personality Disorder).

Code based on type:

314.01 **Attention-Deficit/Hyperactivity Disorder, Combined Type:** if both Criteria A1 and A2 are met for the past six months.

314.00 **Attention-Deficit/Hyperactivity Disorder, Predominantly Inattentive Type:** if Criterion A1 is met but Criterion A2 is not met for the past 6 months.

314.01 **Attention-Deficit/Hyperactivity Disorder, Predominantly Hyperactive-Impulsive Type:** if Criterion A2 is met but Criterion A1 is not met for the past six months.

Coding note: For individuals (especially adolescents and adults) who currently have symptoms that no longer meet full criteria, "In Partial Remission" should be specified.

From the fourth edition of the *Diagnostic and Statistical Manual of Mental Disorders*. Washington, DC: American Psychiatric Association, 1994. Copyright by American Psychiatric Association. Reprinted with permission.

the symptoms, and the earlier age of onset (age 6 years) clearly differs from the *DSM-IV,* as does the specification of a lower bound of IQ below which the diagnosis should not be given.

Social critics have charged that professionals have been too quick to label energetic and exuberant children as having this mental disorder and that educators also may be using these labels simply as an excuse for poor educational environments. This would imply that children who are hyperactive or are diagnosed with ADHD are actually normal but are being labelled as mentally disordered because of parent and teacher intolerance. If this were actually true, then we should find no differences of any cognitive, behavioral, or social significance between ADHD children and normal children. We should also find ADHD is not associated with any significant later risks in development for maladjustment within any domains of adaptive functioning, social, or school performance. Furthermore, research on potential etiologies for the disorder should also come up empty-handed. This is hardly the case. It should become clear from the totality of information on ADHD presented here and elsewhere in reviews such as those by Barkley in 1990 and Hinshaw in 1994 that those with ADHD have significant deficits in behavioral inhibition and associated executive functions that are critical for effective self-regulation, that these deficits are significantly associated with various biological factors, and particularly genetic and neurodevelopmental ones, and that ADHD symptoms and other associated disorders pose substantial risks for these individuals over the life span.

IX. CONCLUSION

Future research needs to address the nature of the attentional problems in ADHD given that current research seriously questions whether these problems are actually within the realm of attention at all. Most studies of ADHD point to impairment within the motor, output, or motivational systems of the brain being most closely affiliated with ADHD rather than deficiencies in the sensory processing systems where attention has been traditionally thought to reside. Even the problem with sustained attention may represent a deficiency in a more complex form of goal-directed persistence that arises out of poor self-regulation rather than representing a disturbance in the more primitive form of sustained responding that is contingency shaped. Our understanding of the very nature of the disorder of ADHD is at stake in how research comes to resolve these issues.

Key to understanding ADHD is the notion that it is actually a disorder of behavioral performance and not one of skill; of how and when one's intelligence comes to be applied in everyday effective adaptive functioning and not in that knowledge itself; of doing what one knows how to do rather than of knowing what to do. The concepts of time, timing, and timeliness are likely to prove increasingly crucial in deepening our understanding of ADHD. In particular, psychological time, how it is sensed, and how it is used in the cross-temporal organizing of complex, goal-directed behavior and in self-regulation may come to be a critical element in models of ADHD. Undoubtedly, research on brain function and structure is likely to further our understanding of the unique role of the prefrontal cortex and the midbrain structures with which it is closely associated in ADHD. But advances in theoreti-

cal models must also occur in order to better understand the nature and organization of the executive functions subserved by these brain regions and even the relationship of genetics, which builds these brain regions in embryological development, to ADHD and the deficits it produces in behavioral performance. And the current body of twin studies further suggests that while such genetic influences are important, there exists a lesser but still important role for unique (nonshared) environmental influences on the differences among individuals in symptoms of ADHD and its underlying behavioral traits. Some of these influences are no doubt social in nature while others are likely to be nongenetic pre-, peri-, and postnatal factors affecting brain development. Such studies, not only on the basic psychological nature of ADHD but also on its basic neuroanatomic and neurogenetic origins and the influence of unique social factors upon them, forebode further significant and exciting advances to come in the understanding and treatment of this fascinating developmental disorder.

BIBLIOGRAPHY

American Psychiatric Association. (1994). *Diagnostic and statistical manual of mental disorders* (4th ed.). Washington, DC: Author.

Barkley, R. A. (1997a). Behavioral inhibition, sustained attention, and executive functions: Constructing a unifying theory of ADHD. *Psychological Bulletin, 121,* 65–94.

Barkley, R. A. (1977b). *ADHD and the nature of self-control.* New York: Guilford.

Barkley, R. A. (1994). Impaired delayed responding: A unified theory of attention deficit hyperactivity disorder. In D. K. Routh (Ed.), *Disruptive behavior disorders: Essays in honor of Herbert Quay* (pp. 11–57). New York: Plenum.

Barkley, R. A. (1990). *Attention deficit hyperactivity disorder: A handbook for diagnosis and treatment.* New York: Guilford.

Biederman, J., Faraone, S. V., Keenan, K., & Tsuang, M. T. (1991). Evidence of a familial association between attention deficit disorder and major affective disorders. *Archives of General Psychiatry, 48,* 633–642.

Bronowski, J. (1977). Human and animal languages. *A sense of the future* (pp. 104–131). Cambridge, MA: MIT Press.

Denckla, M. B. (1994). Measurement of executive function. In G. R. Lyon (Ed.), *Frames of reference for the assessment of learning disabilities: New view on measurement issues* (pp. 117–142). Baltimore, MD: Paul H. Brookes.

Douglas, V. I. (1983). Attention and cognitive problems. In M. Rutter (Ed.), *Developmental neuropsychiatry* (pp. 280–329). New York: Guilford.

Fuster, J. M. (1989). *The prefrontal cortex.* New York: Raven.

Hinshaw, S. P. (1994). *Attention deficits and hyperactivity in children.* Thousand Oaks, CA: Sage.

Rutter, M. (1983). Introduction: Concepts of brain dysfunction syndromes. In M. Rutter, (Ed.), *Developmental neuropsychiatry* (pp. 1–14). New York: Guilford.

Szatmari, P. (1992). The epidemiology of ADHD. In G. Weiss (Ed.), *Child and adolescent psychiatric clinics of North America* (Vol. 1, pp. 361–372). Philadelphia: W. B. Saunders.

Weiss, G. & Hechtman, L. (1993). *Hyperactive children grown up.* New York: Guilford.

Autism and Pervasive Developmental Disorders

Deborah Fein and LeeAnne Green
University of Connecticut

Lynn Waterhouse
The College of New Jersey

Echolalia Parrot-like repetition of utterances either immediately after hearing the utterance (immediate echolalia) or at a later time (delayed echolalia).

Gaze Avoidance The tendency to avert one's eyes in order to avoid eye-to-eye contact with another.

Mainstreaming The integration, or partial integration, of a child with special needs into a classroom of typically developing children.

Metaphorical Language Idiosyncratic utterances whose meaning is clear only to those who are familiar with the child's history.

Pragmatics The social aspects of language, or the communicative uses to which language is put.

Stereotypies Repetitive and often unusual motor movements.

Stimulus Overselectivity A tendency to attend to a restricted portion of a stimulus array or a complex stimulus.

Theory of Mind An understanding or concept of the existence of mental representations, including knowledge and perspective, in others.

PERVASIVE DEVELOPMENTAL DISORDERS (PDD) is the current term for what is probably a group of related neurodevelopmental disorders characterized by similar behavioral profiles. Autistic Disorder is the most widely studied and best described of these disorders. It is characterized by deficits in social relatedness, deficits in language and communication, and stereotyped and restricted patterns of behavior, and is frequently but not always accompanied by mental retardation.

I. HISTORICAL DEVELOPMENT OF THE CONCEPT OF AUTISM

Autism was first described by Leo Kanner in 1943 and became known as Infantile Autism or Autistic Disorder. The concept has expanded since that date, and the term "Kanner autism" is sometimes used to refer to cases with symptoms similar to those of Kanner's original sample; such cases are a subset of PDD. Kanner's original description remains influential, and there is a tendency in the literature to assume that persons with "Kanner autism" represent the "nuclear" or "core" form of PDD, an assumption that may not be warranted. Kanner identified symptoms in three main groups: an autistic aloneness, a failure to use language communicatively, and an obsessive insistence on sameness in the environment; these are still the three areas of symptomatology used in current diagnostic systems. Although Kanner originally viewed the autistic aloneness as probably representing a constitutional defect, the two decades following his original work were marked by an unfortunate shift toward a psychodynamic/environmental view of the causation of autism. This served to derail any significant progress in understanding the disorder, as well as to cause a great deal of additional anguish to parents of autistic children.

Beginning with Rimland's seminal work on autism in 1964, psychology and psychiatry began to explore seriously the biological foundations of autism, and theories of autism as resulting from disturbances in attention, language, sensory integration, perceptual constancy, and other neurological functions were promulgated and tested. Beginning in the early to mid-1980s, research attention also began to focus seriously on the social and affective aspects of autism, both to clarify the range of heterogeneity in autistic children's functioning, and to posit new core deficits in these areas. Currently, researchers stressing both cognitive and social/affective deficits as primary are in agreement that the fundamental problem is a neurological, and not an environmental, one.

Differential diagnosis was a conceptual problem for early autism research. Some clinicians believed that autism was a variant of or precursor to schizophrenia. Only in the 1970s came an awareness that disorders beginning in infancy must be regarded as separate in kind from those with onset in later childhood, adolescence, or adulthood. Autistic-like disorders virtually always begin before age 3, while schizophrenic-like disorders virtually never begin before age 7. This realization revitalized interest in infantile autism as a distinct nosologic entity, leading to the development of more operationally precise diagnostic criteria and a reconceptualization of the syndrome as a pervasive developmental disorder, under which label it was incorporated by the *American Psychiatric Association* in the third edition of that body's *Diagnostic and Statistical Manual of Mental Disorders* (*DSM-III*); this conceptualization has been retained in *DSM-III-R* and *DSM-IV*. [*See* SCHIZOPHRENIA.]

II. *DSM-IV* CRITERIA

Current diagnostic practice, as reflected in the *DSM-IV*, classifies Autistic Disorder as one of four specific entities within Pervasive Developmental Disorder. Autistic Disorder is marked by the presence of symptomatology in three areas: (1) qualitative impairment in social interaction, as manifested by such behaviors as abnormal or reduced eye contact with others, failure to develop peer relationships, lack of spontaneous sharing of interests with others (e.g., showing or pointing out objects of interest to the caregiver), (2) qualitative impairment in communication, as manifested by delayed or deviant language without attempts to compensate through nonverbal communication, poor conversational skills if speech is present, and repetitive and stereotyped language and play, and (3) a restricted and repetitive repertoire of behaviors and interests, including preoccupations and rituals, or severe resistance to environmental changes.

The specific behavioral manifestations of these traits differ by degree of accompanying retardation and age. A high-functioning, older autistic individual, for example, may attempt to be social, but violate implicit rules of social behavior and be insensitive to unspoken social signals, while a low-functioning or much younger autistic individual may react to other people as if they were little different from inanimate objects. Similarly, a high-functioning, older autistic individual may have perseverative interests in such topics as constellations, train schedules, or dinosaurs, and attempt to engage others in conversations on these subjects, while a lower functioning or younger autistic individual might engage in repetitive motor rituals.

The other specific syndromes classified as Pervasive Developmental Disorders include Rett's Disorder, Asperger's Disorder, and Childhood Disintegrative Disorder. Rett's Disorder has marked behavioral commonalities with Autistic Disorder, including poor social engagement and mental retardation, but differs from Autistic Disorder in several ways: in Rett's Disorder, the retardation is more invariant and more typically severe, the disorder seems to present only in girls, it is marked by a characteristic pattern of head growth deceleration and loss of purposeful hand movements, sometimes accompanied by hand wringing behavior, following a period of normal development. Many girls with Rett syndrome also have epilepsy and other neurologic abnormalities. Asperger's Disorder is often considered a mild form of Autistic Disorder, and there is still controversy about how distinct it is from autism;

diagnostically, it can be distinguished from autism by normal development of language. Childhood Disintegrative Disorder differs from Autistic Disorder in that the former is marked by a distinctive pattern of developmental regression following at least two years of normal development. This disorder is much rarer than autism, and controversy exists here, too, about the etiological and phenomenological distinctiveness between Childhood Disintegrative Disorder and Autistic Disorder. [*See* MENTAL RETARDATION AND MENTAL HEALTH.]

III. BEHAVIORAL AND COGNITIVE CHARACTERISTICS

A. Behavioral Characteristics in Autism

1. Social Behavior

Social behavior is considered by many as the hallmark of autism. As with all features of autism, social impairment is highly heterogeneous; it varies with age, with IQ, with setting, and with interactive partner, and is modifiable by treatment.

Social impairment is generally most severe in the preschool years; it is in early childhood that genuine aloofness is seen. Older children may initiate interaction to get their needs met, or may be responsive but noninitiating to others. Older or higher-functioning autistic individuals may approach others in an idiosyncratic, intrusive, and socially insensitive way. These three general styles (aloof, passive, active-but-odd) form the basis of a social typology described by Lorna Wing, and validated by several later studies.

Highly structured settings with enforced proximity to peers may elicit the best peer interactions. Relationships with other children are almost always more impaired than the corresponding behavior with adults; other children may be ignored when adults are not.

Behavioral deficits in social interaction are varied; among the most important, especially in early life, are (1) poor spontaneous imitation of others' language and behavior, (2) gaze avoidance or other deficits in the use of eye-to-eye gaze to modulate or initiate interaction, and (3) deficits in various joint attention skills, including drawing an adult's attention to an object of interest by showing or pointing, and following an adult's attentional focus in order to share it. On the other hand, the "pervasive lack of responsiveness" described in *DSM-III* is actually uncommon; many young autistic children are selectively attached to their parents, derive comfort from their presence, and enjoy physical affection.

2. Communication and Play

Older studies were composed primarily of clinical descriptions of language features such as pronoun reversal, echolalia, and metaphorical language. More systematic studies have appeared, based on modern understanding of the separable components of language. The more severely affected autistic child may remain nonverbal or minimally verbal and poorly intelligible. In those who develop more language, phonology, syntax, and (more arguably) semantics are relatively spared, although still often at a lower level than nonverbal skills. Verbal memory, prosody, and pragmatics, on the other hand, represent areas of particular difficulty for the average autistic child. In the domain of pragmatics, it is noted that communicative functions are generally more need-oriented and less affiliative, and that violations of language use rules are common, such as violations of implicit rules concerning interpersonal distance while speaking, and the rules of turn-taking in conversational exchange, as well as word selection which is overly formal or pedantic.

Symbolic play is also often observed to be lacking in young autistic children, who sometimes prefer non-symbolic play activities such as puzzles or other manipulatives. When symbolic play develops, it can be unusually repetitive and inflexible in nature. Some recent evidence suggests that high-functioning autistic children may be not so much incapable as uninterested in engaging in frequent or complex symbolic play. [*See* PLAY.]

3. Preoccupations, Perseverations, and Resistance to Change

These constitute the third symptom group. These behaviors range from simple or complex motor stereotypies, to "self-stimulatory" sensory behaviors such as watching fans or water, to long-term perseverative interests. The resistance to change is manifested by tantrums or other extreme reactions to changes in environmental features or in routines. Despite the equal role assigned to perseverations/preoccupations and resistance to change in diagnostic criteria, some recent data suggest that resistance to change is a less common feature of autism than perseverations/preoccupations.

B. Cognitive Characteristics

Overall cognitive level, or presence of mental retardation, is an important feature of the individual autistic child, and powerfully predicts the functional outcome that can be expected for the child. Recent work by several research groups, such as the group headed by Rapin (see Bibliography) suggests that high- and low-functioning autism may be significantly different in behavioral manifestations, history, and prognosis, that approximately half of the autistic population falls into each group, and that an IQ cutoff of about 65 makes the most appropriate division between high- and low-functioning autism. Beyond studies of overall cognitive level, many investigators have examined typical cognitive profiles in autism, that is, areas of relative sparing and impairment. Some autistic children, both those with severe impairment and those who are higher functioning, display unusual gifts, especially in rote memory, calculations, and music. A majority of autistic children are known to have relative strengths in visuospatial abilities, while tasks requiring verbal reasoning, social cognition, or flexibility pose relative difficulty for the autistic child. Although this description suggests a typical cognitive profile, studies have shown that there is great heterogeneity in the autistic population, and that no single cognitive deficit is universal in autistic individuals.

1. Language

The autistic child's language profile is arguably the syndrome's most distinctive cognitive feature, which has earned it a central position in some theories of the etiology of autism. Many aspects of verbal functioning are impaired in autistic children, as many as 40 to 50% of whom are mute, although this figure is declining with the advent of aggressive early intervention. Those with speech often display echolalia, difficulties with prepositions and pronouns, and inappropriate conversational behaviors. Verbal autistic children generally are able to acquire normal grammatical morphology and syntax, although onset and development are delayed. Some autistic children learn

grapheme-phoneme correspondence, leading to early decoding of words; comprehension, however, lags far behind. Comprehension of oral language is significantly impaired relative to expression, and deficits in the semantic and pragmatic aspects of language are common. They are also deficient in interactive communication, including conversational behavior, nonverbal communication and speech prosody. In general, the more linguistic aspects of communication, including especially phonology and syntax, are spared relative to the pragmatic aspects; pragmatic deficits can be seen in the failure to use language functionally to share or request information, or perform other speech functions that serve social, rather than instrumental, functions.

2. Social Cognition

A decade of research has documented substantial deficits in autistic children's ability to understand the behavior, emotions, and cognitive states of other people. They have difficulty in matching pictures of emotional facial expressions to emotion words, to emotional situations, to similar expressions, and to vocal expressions of the same emotion.

Much recent interest has been stimulated by exploration of autistic performance on "theory of mind" tasks; in a typical theory of mind task, the subject is asked to predict behavior of a doll in a social scenario. The behavior can only be correctly predicted if the subject has a true theory of mind, that is, truly understands the concept of others' minds, with their own representational capacities, and their own limits on available knowledge. Autistic subjects have been shown to be impaired on these tasks in several studies.

A cautionary note here, however, about all of these social cognitive tasks is that many higher functioning autistic individuals do well on them; the deficits are far from universal. Furthermore, verbal IQ explains much of the variance in performance. Therefore, it remains to be demonstrated that deficits in social cognition, including theory of mind, occupy a key causal role in the syndrome; they may be more a concomitant deficit related to the overall social impairment, although opinions differ widely on this.

3. Attention

Unusual attentional processes are characteristic of autistic children. Autistic children are generally able to sustain attention in tasks adequately when given potent reinforcement or when the task is of interest to them, and higher functioning individuals are able to perform well on standard neuropsychological tests of sustained attention. In contrast, many autistic children appear to have difficulty with tasks requiring the focusing and shifting of attention. They are found to be overselective in their attention to particular parts of stimuli, and studies indicate that they may have difficulties in shifting attention between stimuli, especially across sensory modalities, perhaps contributing to the perseveration so characteristic of their behavior.

4. Memory

Memory abilities in autism have not been as fully investigated as other cognitive functions. Anecdotally, amazing feats of memory have been reported, where autistic individuals recall distant episodes with great clarity and detail; hyperdeveloped memory for stimuli such as routes, spatial arrays, schedules and calendars, and music have also been frequently reported. Tested memory for visual material in high-functioning autistic individuals is often normal. In contrast, memory for linguistic and social material is usually impaired. Autistic individuals appear not to be able to use the intrinsic semantic structure of discourse or stories to aid recall, and in this regard, are more impaired than children with specific language disorders.

5. Executive Functions

Executive functioning refers to the higher level cognitive processes of abstract conceptualization, planning, problem solving, and self-monitoring, self-correction and self-control. These processes are thought to be localized to prefrontal cortex, and are assessed with standardized neuropsychological tests developed for evaluation of frontal functions. Some autistic individuals have great difficulty with these tasks, especially in switching from incorrect strategies during tasks. Some researchers have noted similarities between certain symptoms of autism and those of patients with frontal lobe damage (e.g., perseveration, lack of inhibition), and have proposed that frontal executive system impairment causes distinct social cognitive deficits. Furthermore, some findings suggest that executive system adequacy may predict outcome for autistic adolescents better than measures of IQ.

IV. DEVELOPMENTAL COURSE AND PROGNOSIS

Autism, as a developmental disorder, cannot be fully described at a single developmental point. The typical description of the autistic child is that he or she lacks interest in relating to others and lacks communicative language. These symptoms are most characteristic of autistic children in the preschool years. Even during this period, there are often signs of increasing social relatedness, especially to caretakers. On the other hand, stereotypies and especially resistance to change, may appear in the preschool years or somewhat later. During middle childhood, autistic children often master some daily living and academic skills and make behavioral adjustments to their parents and teachers. Their behavior may come to resemble that of hyperactive and/or retarded children, or they may develop into socially motivated children, who relate in an odd or idiosyncratic way, with deficits in emotional reciprocity.

Early and middle adolescence can be particularly difficult. Besides the onset of seizures that sometimes occurs in early adolescence, a significant minority of PDD children regress behaviorally and even cognitively at this time. Some autistic adolescents show increasing interest in developing peer relationships during these years. Higher functioning individuals with PDD are prone to psychiatric problems, especially anxiety and depression, as they realize the extent of their difference from peers. On the positive side, both social and language skills often continue to improve during adolescence, and even those children who regress during early adolescence may recover and make developmental progress toward the middle or end of adolescence. Increasing interest in relating to other people can also set the stage for psychosocial interventions or behavioral skill training to be more effective.

Long-term follow-up studies indicate great variability in adult outcomes, but a generally guarded prognosis for good adjustment must be the rule. About half of all autistic adults require residential care; many of the remainder depend on relatives for daily assistance. Gainful employment and fully independent living may be achieved by about one in five. Even for the best-outcome group, social difficulties remain common, marriage or sexual relationships rare, and many social relationships revolve around work or structured activities and interests. It should be noted, however, that the generation of children who have received the benefit of modern special education and behavioral interventions have not yet reached adulthood, and their outcomes, it is hoped, will be significantly better.

Follow-up studies are consistent in demonstrating that higher IQ and communicative language by the age of 5 are strong predictors of better outcome, associated neurological signs and symptoms are predictors of poorer outcome.

V. EPIDEMIOLOGY

Prevalence rates vary according to the definition of the syndrome. Earlier and more restrictive definitions of autism yielded prevalence estimates of 2–4/10,000. Broader definitions encompassing the full PDD spectrum suggested rates three or more times greater. Recent estimates have increased. This may be attributable to improved detection, more lenient diagnoses, or actual increases in prevalence. Most recent estimates are approximately 10/10,000 for PDD disorder, including autism, and another 10/10,000 with a more broadly defined triad of deficits in social relatedness, communication, and stereotyped behavior plus mental retardation. PDD spectrum disorders are more common in males than in females, with ratios found between 2:1 and 10:1, the higher ratios applying more to the Asperger-type clinical picture. [*See* EPIDEMIOLOGY: PSYCHIATRIC.]

VI. BOUNDARY CONDITIONS AND COMORBIDITY

Specifying the boundary between autism and other PDD spectrum disorder (such as Rett's and Asperger's Disorder), mixed language disorder, or severe mental retardation can be problematic, and differential diagnoses among these conditions can be difficult. Although diagnostic definitions of autism and language disorder appear distinct, in practice, the differential diagnosis can be unclear, especially in preschool children. Studies from Rutter and colleagues in the 1970's and from Rapin's group indicate that the diagnostic groups can be distinguished not only by the presence of autism-related behaviors, but by differences in the language domain itself. The autistic children tend to have greater delays and deficits in language comprehension than the language-disordered children; in the expressive domain, delayed appearance of Wh-questions is highly discriminating. Regression of acquired language skills is also much more typical of autism, but also characterizes children with Landau-Kleffner syndrome. Landau-Kleffner syndrome, also referred to as acquired epileptic aphasia, refers to loss of language in a child in the context of clinical seizures or a frankly epileptiform EEG. There is disagreement as to whether the term should be reserved for children who have no serious associated behavior or cognitive disorders, or whether the term should be broadened so as to include those children who also develop autistic behaviors or become frankly autistic.

Autism may also have increased comorbidity with specific additional disorders. Although still controversial, some investigators present evidence that there is a greater than chance coincidence of autism and Tourette's disorder. When tics occur in autism, they tend to occur in high-functioning autism.

The relationship between autism and schizophrenia also remains a matter of debate. At one time, the two disorders were believed to be related, but different ages of onset, patterns of symptomatology, and family histories have convinced many investigators that they are unrelated. Nevertheless, reports exist of schizophrenia developing in previously autistic individuals at a greater than chance rate, and a small number of researchers believe that autism is a particularly early and severe form of childhood schizophrenia.

Autism is also related to the presence of seizure disorders. About half of autistic individuals have clinical seizures and/or abnormal EEGs. Infancy and adolescence are high-risk periods for the appearance of seizures. All types of seizures occur; generalized tonic-clonic are the most common.

VII. BIOLOGICAL FACTORS

A. Associated Biomedical Conditions and Genetic Factors

Several specific medical conditions are associated with autism, including phenylketonuria, rubella embryopathy, herpes encephalitis, fragile X syndrome, and neurocutaneous disorders such as tuberous sclerosis. Some studies estimate that between one-eighth and one-fourth of autistic children have an associated medical condition, but it is not known whether these conditions play a causal role in the development of autistic symptoms. Of possible prenatal factors, maternal rubella is most commonly associated with autism, the prevalence for which is 100 times that for the general population. Other obstetrical factors are found more frequently in autistic children than in other populations, particularly midpregnancy maternal bleeding. [*See* PRENATAL STRESS AND LIFE SPAN DEVELOPMENT.]

The fragile X genetic syndrome has been identified in an estimated 2 to 10% of the autistic population. Fragile X is a rare X-linked syndrome (most prevalent in boys) that involves intellectual impairment, attention deficits, and identifying physical features (prominent ears, long and narrow face, and macroorchidism). Within the fragile X population, it is estimated that 15 to 30% have autistic features, which are qualitatively distinct compared with those seen in the "typical" autistic child. Fragile X autistic children have been found to show perseverative speech as opposed to echolalia, and display active-but-odd social behaviors rather than aloofness. The specific route of pathology connecting fragile X to the expression of autistic symptoms is unknown.

A genetic basis for at least some forms of autism has been demonstrated by family studies. Approximately 3% of families with an autistic child will produce another child with autism, a prevalence rate which equals 50 to 100 times that of the general population. In addition, the concordance rate for autism in monozygotic twins has been found to range from 40 to 96%. Further support for genetic involvement is found in studies of characteristics in families of autistic children. Siblings of autistic children may be more likely to show superiority in visuospatial over verbal abilities (analogous to the autistic profile), cognitive difficulties such as language disorder, and social disengagement. A few studies have found that some parents of autistic children may be more likely to show unusual social behaviors. The search for specific genetic markers for autism thus far has uncovered two prospects: a marker for a gene that regulates neuron development, and abnormalities of chromosome 15. [*See* GENETIC CONTRIBUTORS TO MENTAL HEALTH.]

Taken together, studies suggest that at least a subset of autistic cases are attributable to genetic origin, either familial or mutational. The incidence of autistic symptoms in medical conditions that are not genetic, however, suggests that the PDD spectrum may represent a variety of etiologies ultimately affecting common brain systems.

B. Neuroanatomical Findings

Studies of neuroanatomical abnormalities in autistic patients have relied mainly upon postmortem neuropathology examinations and imaging techniques such as positron emission tomography (PET), computerized tomography (CT) and magnetic resonance imaging (MRI). They have generally focused on cortex, brainstem, limbic areas and cerebellum, and have found great variability in brain pathology. Gross cortical and ventricular abnormalities, for example, have been found in some cases and not others. Two structures of great interest are the amygdala and hippocampus, which are limbic structures involved in social/emotional behaviors and in memory. Abnormalities in limbic areas of the brain have been implicated in several studies, most notably in detailed postmortem examinations performed by Bauman and Kemper. These and other studies have also found abnormalities in the cerebellum, although the nature of these cerebellar abnormalities is not consistent across studies. [*See* BRAIN SCANNING/NEUROIMAGING.]

C. Neurophysiological Findings

Findings from PET studies of regional cerebral blood flow have suggested diminished temporal lobe activity, and possible delayed frontal lobe maturation in autistic children. PET studies of regional glucose metabolism, which reflects brain energy utilization, have indicated abnormal patterns of regional activation. Several others have found global glucose hypermetabolism in autistic patients, which was thought to reflect inefficient processing. This feature, however, is not unique to autism.

Studies examining brain waves and oculomotor activity in REM sleep have suggested a developmental immaturity of brain mechanisms controlling sleep and an abnormally suppressed inhibition of sensory responding in autistic children. Brainstem dysfunction has been suggested for a subgroup of autistic individuals by findings of abnormalities in brainstem ERPs, although some studies have failed to support this. Many ERP studies offer support for abnormalities of attention and information processing in autism. High-functioning autistic subjects of varying ages usually show abnormally small amplitudes for a longer latency wave of the ERP thought to reflect the detection and classification of stimuli. Deficiencies in voluntary selective attention and orientation to novel stimuli also have been shown by diminished amplitudes in waves associated with these functions. Several other neurophysiological studies relying on cerebral electrical recording have indicated disruptions in normal hemispheric lateralization in autism.

D. Neurochemical Findings

Investigations of neurotransmitter function have produced inconsistent findings. The most replicated finding among autistic patients is that of elevated blood levels of the neurotransmitter serotonin, which occurs in an estimated one-third of this population, but also is observed in other patient populations. The reason for this elevation is not yet known. Treatments with the drug fenfluramine can greatly reduce levels of serotonin, and sometimes result in improvements in stereotypies and hyperactivity. Studies of the neurotransmitter dopamine are not in agreement, despite reported improvements in many symptoms after treatments with drugs that block dopamine. Overactivity of the opiate peptide beta-endorphin has been suggested by some studies, and supported by findings that opiate blockade improves autistic symptoms in some patients. The peptide oxytocin, shown to promote affiliation in animals, also may be reduced in autistic children. It has been suggested that excess opiates may render social contact unrewarding by producing a state of intrinsic contentment, and may also serve to dysregulate oxytocin.

VIII. CLINICAL ASSESSMENT

A. Medical Assessment

If the diagnosis is made by a nonphysician and the child has not yet had a medical work-up relative to his/her autism, the following referrals should be considered. Assessment of hearing is important for successful language treatment; if behavior and cooperation are problematic, a brainstem evoked potential assessment should be done. Motor abnormalities are common;

these should be assessed by a pediatric neurologist and a pediatric OT. Some physicians believe that a full medical work-up, including EEG, genetic and chromosomal testing, CT scan, and so on, is indicated; others feel that these investigations have a low yield unless there is a specific indication for their use.

B. Neuropsychological Assessment

Children and adolescents with autism or PDD should also have periodic neuropsychological evaluations. These will describe the child's current level and profile of cognitive and language abilities, which will have implications for current education and for long-range goals. Periodic reevaluations to monitor the child's progress will help to detect any deterioration that might signal negative medical or psychological events, and will document the success of treatment and education.

C. Behavioral Assessment

Thorough behavioral description is equally important. Included in the behavioral description should be a profile of the individual's adaptive abilities and problem behaviors, including those central to the syndrome (such as social incapacity and resistance to change), those associated with the syndrome (such as self-injury and abnormal motor behaviors) and those sometimes found in association with it (such as hyperactivity, aggressiveness, and passivity). Analysis of antecedent conditions and consequences of the behaviors may clarify the role or function of the behavior for the particular autistic individual, and may dictate changes in stimulus conditions and reinforcements to ameliorate problem behaviors, as well as to foster positive behaviors.

IX. TREATMENT

A. Pharmacological Treatments

Pharmacotherapy can be an effective tool in improving the behavior of some autistic children. Serotonergic agents are often used. Fenfluramine is sometimes prescribed, and has been found to reduce hyperactivity and stereotypies in some, but not all, studies. Clomipramine has been found to enhance social relatedness and decrease obsessional behavior and aggression. Fluoxetine and other serotonin reuptake inhibitors are also used with some autistic children.

Opiate antagonists may help to diminish self-injury, and reduce social withdrawal and stereotypies. Self-injury and aggression have also reported to be improved by fluoxetine, clomipramine, buspirone and beta-blockers. Neuroleptics, such as haloperidol, and chlorpromazine, have also been found to reduce agitation, aggression and emotional lability, but most physicians are reluctant to use these agents in young children because they can produce movement disorders that may not regress even when the medication is stopped. Lithium is sometimes used to decrease aggressive, perseverative, and hyperactive behavior, and may be tried especially when a family history of bipolar disorder is present.

Other common pharmacological treatments are tricyclic antidepressants, which sometimes enhance language and social behavior. Stimulants have been administered for hyperactivity, but some autistic children experience a worsening of stereotypies or thought disorganization. Stimulants may work best in high-functioning autistic children with absent or mild stereotypies. [See Psychopharmacology.]

Natural treatments, such as dietary interventions or high-dose vitamin regimens have been advocated by some. Empirical support for the claims rests on a small number of studies, and mainstream physicians generally do not advocate their use.

B. Behavioral and Educational Treatments

Special education services and behavioral treatments are crucial in producing an optimal outcome. Recent work indicates that aggressive early intervention (as early as 15 to 18 months) can produce the best outcome. The leading proponent of intensive (ca. 40 hours/week) behavioral "drills" (O. I. Lovaas) has reported highly successful outcomes—almost half of the children being successfully included without support in a typical grade-school class. Others using his methods report results that do not replicate his degree of success, but that are nonetheless highly effective. These behavioral programs can be carried out in an educational setting or, especially for preschoolers, in the home. Other preschool programs emphasize a child-centered, developmentally oriented approach,

which attempts to stimulate the child to move along a typical developmental trajectory. Any successful program must address each of the behavioral, social, language, and cognitive needs of the children specifically. To be effective, programs should be highly structured and should teach parents behavior management techniques that can be used in the home.

Individual differences in the children partly predict outcome: higher IQ, and the presence of communicative language by the age of 5 are positive prognostic signs.

The recent trend in special education has been strongly in favor of various forms of "mainstreaming," "integration," and "inclusion," in which the child attends a class that is composed of a mixed group of special needs and typical peers, or of mainly typical peers, for part or all of the school day, sometimes with a one-on-one aide to facilitate participation. Although research has shown that exposure to normal peers can promote social behavior, the degree to which a severely autistic child can benefit from inclusion in a regular classroom remains to be demonstrated. It is clinically obvious that at least some autistic children need more intensive one-on-one teaching than is available in a mainstream setting before they can benefit from the teaching and social opportunities in a regular class.

In addition to special education or behavioral treatment, the autistic child often needs additional speech and language therapy, occupational therapy, and adapted physical education.

Clinicians must also help families to obtain other necessary services, such as respite care, extended day programs, and summer programs to prevent the behavioral and cognitive regression that can occur. They may also be able to suggest appropriate leisure activities, such as gymnastics, swimming, or play or social groups, that can provide constructive ways to spend after-school hours and opportunities for social interaction with typical children, and can promote self-esteem.

Prescription of therapies and services for the autistic individual must always include sensitivity to the often devastating effect of the disability on the family. Social support from other affected families, and keeping abreast of the latest developments in treatment and other research can help families manage their affected children and their own emotional reactions. The *Autism Society of America* (8601 Georgia Ave.,

Suite 503, Silver Spring, MD 20910) publishes a regular newsletter with much information useful to parents; another good source of information for parents and professionals on recent developments in autism is Rimland's newsletter *Autism Research Review International* (4182 Adams Ave., San Diego, CA 92116).

BIBLIOGRAPHY

Bauman, M. L., & Kemper, T. L. (Eds.). (1994). *The neurobiology of autism.* Baltimore: The Johns Hopkins University Press.

Dawson, G. (Ed.). (1989). *Autism: Nature, diagnosis and treatment.* New York: Guilford Press.

Gillberg, C., & Coleman, M. (1992). The biology of the autistic syndromes (2nd ed.). *Clinics in Developmental Medicine, 126.* London: Mac Keith Press.

Rapin, I. (Ed.). (1996). Preschool children with inadequate communication: Developmental language disorder, autism, low IQ. *Clinics in Developmental Medicine, 139.* London: Mac Keith Press.

Schopler, E., & Mesibov, G. (Eds.). (1995). *Learning and cognition in autism.* New York: Plenum Press.

Schopler, E., Van-Bourgondien, M. E., & Bristol, M. (Eds.). (1993). *Preschool issues in autism.* New York: Plenum Press.

B

Behavioral Genetics

Craig T. Nagoshi

Arizona State University

Allele   One alternate form of a gene at a particular place (locus) on a chromosome.
Dominance   The ability of one allele (the dominant) to override the phenotypic expression of another allele (the recessive).
Epistasis   Nonadditive effects of the combined actions of two or more genes, i.e., gene–gene interaction.
Gene   A segment of a chromosome (deoxyribonucleic acid or DNA) that codes for some aspect of protein synthesis.
Genotype   The genetic composition of an individual.
Heritability   The proportion of phenotypic variability that can be accounted for by genetic factors.
Inbreeding   Matings between genetically related individuals.
Linkage   The extent to which two genes near each other on the same chromosome are transmitted together instead of segregating and independently assorting.
Phenotype   The apparent, measurable characteristic or trait.
Pleiotropy   Multiple phenotypic effects of the same gene.

BEHAVIORAL GENETICS, as the name indicates, is the interdisciplinary research area concerned with determining if and how genetic factors influence any of the phenomena studied in the behavioral sciences, especially psychology. Behavioral geneticists apply the concepts and methodologies of molecular, population, and quantitative genetics to behavior as the phenotype of interest.

I. INTRODUCTION

The idea that behavior, particularly human behavior, might be determined by genetic factors has been controversial throughout human history and the history of psychology. Aristotle proposed that humans had a "human soul" possessing consciousness and free will, which was different from the biologically determined "animal soul" of other creatures. Judeo-Christian theology and Descartes' mind–body dualism emphasized that the most "human" behaviors, such as intelligence and morality, were products of a conscious mind removed from biological mechanisms. Thus, even though animal breeders had known for thousands of years that behaviors could be selected and bred for, it was still possible for behaviorism to be founded at the beginning of this century and to dominate psychological thinking, while minimizing the importance of biological/genetic processes in understanding human behavior.

Two readily apparent, related aspects of human behavior, however, make a compelling case for the need to study genetic influences. These are stability and variability.

If a behavior, e.g., scoring high on tests of intelligence, is consistently manifested by an individual across time and across many different situations, then the stability of this behavior must be due to some consistent set of physical determinants. Through consistent reinforcement and/or punishment of certain behaviors, plus generalization, a stable behavior could have been established by environmental influences on the individual. On the other hand, the behavior could be a manifestation of some consistent "hard-wired" physiological process, e.g., greater efficiency of the connections in the brain's neural network. Since all physiological/biological processes ultimately begin from some genetic code, it could be inferred that the stable behavior is the result of the individual having inherited some gene or genes for the behavior.

In turn, both the lack of variability and the presence of variability in stable behaviors also require the influence of some set of consistent physical determinants. For example, all physiologically normal humans raised among other humans acquire the ability to use language. The lack of variability in this behavior among humans, plus the absence of this behavior in this form in other animal species, is consistent with the supposition that all normal humans inherit a set of genes that code for the physiological structures that are required for language. Other stable behaviors, such as performance on intelligence tests, are characterized by great variability among humans, and this variability is maintained despite historical and social changes in the environmental factors thought to influence the behaviors. Since each individual is genetically unique, stable individual differences in behavior are also consistent with the supposition that genetic determinants may be involved.

Although behavioral genetics is concerned with establishing the genetic determinants of behavior, the discussion above makes clear that genes, in fact, do not directly cause behavior. Figure 1 reiterates the idea that genes are basically just a biochemical process for coding the synthesis of proteins which, in turn, are assembled into the physiological structures and processes of the organism. These physiological structures then become one of the determinants of behavior, and the study of this process is the realm of physiological psychology. Thus, any finding from behavioral genetics of significant genetic influences on behavior automatically implies that some physiological mechanism is the more proximal determinant.

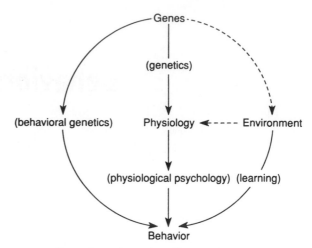

Figure 1   Relationship of genes to behavior.

Behavior can also be influenced by the environment through learning, and one dotted line in Figure 1 shows the physical monist/physiological psychology presumption that ultimately learning operates by modifying the physiology of the organism. It should thus also be noted that genetic influences always operate on physiology within the context of some set of environmental influences. The other dotted line presents the possibility (discussed below) that genetic factors can affect environmental influences.

In Figure 1, the understanding of how genetic processes are translated into physiology is noted to be the realm of genetics. Molecular genetics is concerned with the sequence and operation of biochemically defined genetic material (the DNA basepairs described below) in transcribing, transmitting, and implementing the code for the synthesis of physiological structures and processes. Quantitative genetics estimates the relative influence of genetic vs environmental influences on a variable trait by comparing differential resemblances or patterns of differential variability among individuals of different degrees of genetic relatedness. Population genetics bridges molecular and quantitative genetic approaches by seeking to relate gene frequencies and degree of genetic influence with particular traits for populations of organisms operating within particular environmental contexts.

Since behavioral genetics is basically simply the application of genetics to a special set of traits, behavior, much of this article will be an overview of genetic concepts and methodologies. Issues of particular relevance to the study of behavior will be emphasized toward the end of the article, which will also briefly describe some of the major findings from human behavioral genetics studies. We begin with a discussion of Darwin's theory of evolution by natural selection and of Mendel's work on the logic of genetic transmission.

II. EVOLUTION AND MENDELIAN GENETICS

The evolutionary theory of Charles Darwin (1809–1882) had a profound impact on Western thought. Even though it provides a basis for a unified understanding of all biological phenomena, the theory was and remains controversial. In psychology, it was integrated into the concepts of 19th century physiological psychologists, became a major inspiration for William James' school of functionalism (the school which, somewhat ironically in this context, led to John B. Watson's behaviorism) and Sigmund Freud's school of psychoanalysis, and through the work of Darwin's cousin Francis Galton, also was the starting point for the scientific study of individual differences and genetic influences on human behavior.

Darwin's theory, first published as *On the Origin of Species by Means of Natural Selection* in 1858, has three major components, each of which has important implications for the understanding of human behavior:

1. *Induction of variation* proposes that members of a species differ from each other at birth and through maturation along a multitude of different trait dimensions and that biological processes continually create these individual differences. As will soon be apparent, not only are such differences ubiquitous for any species, they are absolutely essential for the survival of the species in the face of relentless changes in environmental conditions. One obvious implication of this for psychology is that, in contrast to the ideas of several early behaviorists, individual members of a species, including humans, are biologically unique and should not be expected to respond to the same environmental influences on behavior in exactly the same way.

2. *Maintenance of variation* proposes that individual differences in the traits that vary within a species are biologically transmissible from one generation to the next. Again, this is absolutely essential for the survival of the species. This idea leads to the immediate inference that behavior must also be biologically transmissible, since stable patterns of behavior are undoubtedly essential aspects of species survival. This idea was clearly consistent with the results of thousands of years of animal breeding, noted above, when applied to non-human animals. The implications of the third component of Darwin's theory led to the controversies that still flare today.

3. *Natural selection* assumes that there are always more members of a species born at any one time than will ever survive to reproduce. Darwin proposed that environmental conditions at a particular time, e.g., availability of food, nature of predators and parasites, climate, etc., tend to give some individuals born with one set of traits an advantage in being able to survive, reproduce, and rear offspring to maturity over other individuals with different levels of these traits. Over several generations of this natural selection, more individuals with the advantageous characteristics are born with and transmit these characteristics, while there is a decreased incidence and transmission of the disadvantageous characteristics. Darwin argued that over a sufficient number of generations, particularly in response to some major change in the environment, the members of a species may now possess such different traits from the starting population that they constitute a new species.

As noted above, Darwin's theory clearly reinforces the importance of genetic transmission and biologically based individual differences as determinants of the characteristics of organisms, including behavioral characteristics. The theory also implies that all species, including humans, are biologically related on some level to every other species. The similarities and differences between and within species could be understood solely in terms of the interactions between the genetic endowments of a species and the selection pressures in the environment. Research into the determinants of behavior in other animal species in order to understand human behavior is justified, because other animals and humans have some of the same or similar physiological structures and processes that determine behavior. Other implications include the expectation that humans retain physiological structures that were once adaptive or neutral in value in natural environments, but which may be maladaptive in rapidly changing modern societies. Another implication is that even those "higher" aspects of human behavior and mental processes that supposedly differentiate us from other animals can be related to genetically transmitted physiological functions that resulted from natural selection.

Although natural selection was the most parsimonious and successful proposed mechanism for accounting for species change, at the time Darwin published his theory the way that traits were biologically transmitted was poorly understood. Darwin himself realized that the then current concept that parents gave off biological particles ("gemmules") that merged and blended in the offspring would, in fact, invalidate his principles of induction and maintenance of variation. Generations of blending traits would result in all individuals having the same averaged trait, i.e., no variation. It was only after the work of Mendel and the beginning of modern genetics that a mechanism for the maintenance of variation was established.

Gregor Mendel (1822–1884) studied the types and frequencies of plant characteristics that resulted when members of a species possessing one kind of characteristic were crossed with members having a different characteristic. For his most famous work on pea plants, such characteristics included green vs yellow pea color, smooth vs wrinkled pea form, long vs short plant stem, etc. The results of his crossbreeding studies led him to infer two principles for genetic transmission.

The *law of segregation* stated that every character (the phenotype) is determined by the combination of two elements (genes), one from each parent. These elements split off cleanly (segregate) from each other in the production of the sex cells and are transmitted intact to the offspring. Since it is possible for one form of the gene (a dominant allele) to prevent the expression of the other form (the recessive allele), a process called dominance, the same phenotype could result from different combinations of genetic elements (the genotype). For example, a green pea would result whether the genotype consisted of both alleles coding for green color (homozygous dominant) or a genotype with both green and yellow coding alleles (heterozygous), since the green allele was dominant. This was apparent when Mendel crossed "pure" green and "pure" yellow pea plants and found that the next generation all had green peas. When this second generation was crossed with each other, however, Mendel

found that one-fourth of the succeeding generation again manifested yellow peas. Thus, the yellow alleles were not blended, and the variability of the genes determining green vs yellow pea color was maintained.

The *law of independent assortment* stated that different genes determined different characteristics. These genes were randomly combined in the sex cells and, hence, independently transmitted to the offspring. Mendel found that when he looked at the results of crossing plants for two different traits, for example, green pea color/long stem with yellow pea color/short stem plants, the odds of a plant possessing green vs yellow peas were completely independent of the odds of the plant having a long vs a short stem. This was also important for Darwin's theory, since it meant that one trait could be selected for without affecting some other trait.

As it turned out, modern genetic findings have turned up several exceptions to Mendel's laws. Many traits determined by single genes (one pair of alleles) do not show dominance, such that heterozygous genotypes may result in phenotypes intermediate between phenotypes resulting from the two homozygous genotypes. Heterozygous genotypes may produce more extreme phenotypes (overdominance). Recent findings suggest that parents in a few genetic systems may be able to determine the expression of both alleles of an offspring (uniparental disomy and imprinting). With regard to independent assortment, it is now known that genes that are close to each other on the same chromosome are often transmitted together (linkage) and that single genes can have multiple phenotypic effects (pleiotropy). Nevertheless, Mendel's laws more than adequately accounted for observations of genetic transmission at the phenotypic level long before the biochemical nature of genes was understood.

Although Mendel presented his findings at a scientific meeting in 1865, they were "lost" until 1900, when several biologists rediscovered and started widely applying the laws. In the meantime, Darwin's cousin Francis Galton (1822–1911) was using the theory of evolution to establish the science of behavioral genetics.

Galton immediately inferred from Darwin's theory that all human behaviors had a biological/genetic basis and were the result of natural selection. With his book *Hereditary Genius: An Inquiry Into Its Laws and Consequences* (1869), he asserted that social eminence (reflective of intelligence) was genetically determined. He demonstrated this by showing how the incidence of eminence in the male relatives (fathers, sons, uncles, cousins, etc.) of eminent men was a strict function of the degree of biological relatedness between the probands and the relatives. He developed the idea of the twin research design, when he studied more physically similar twins vs less similar twins and asserted that the former's greater similarity on psychological traits also indicated a genetic basis for psychological as well as physical characteristics. He established laboratories for the systematic measurement of thousands of individuals on physical (height, weight, etc.) and psychological (acuity of eyesight, acuity of hearing, reaction time, etc.) traits in hopes of establishing the large data bases he knew were required to delineate genetically based distributional characteristics, social class differences, developmental trends, and familial resemblances.

Besides his enormous contributions to psychology in establishing ways of measuring psychological phenomena of all sorts, Galton's quest for ways to demonstrate genetic transmission in relatives led to the development of new statistical techniques. His student, Karl Pearson, developed the correlation coefficient to quantify familial resemblances in some standardized fashion, and genetic questions have continued to be one of the spurs for the development of statistical procedures commonly used in the social sciences (e.g., Fisher's chi-square and F tests).

Thus, much of the logic and methodologies of modern behavioral genetics had been laid down by Galton and his students by the time Mendel's ideas were rediscovered. Ironically, it took some time and controversy to reconcile Galton's ideas, that accumulations of genetic elements of some sort produce continuous, typically normal distributions of traits, such as intelligence, with Mendel's ideas about discrete traits under the control of only a few combinations of alleles. The reconciliation involved the recognition that the random combination (consistent with independent assortment) of several discrete genetic elements, all of which have some influence on the trait, would produce the continuous, normal distributions Galton saw. It is still important, though, to distinguish between traits thought to be under the control of a single gene vs those under the control of several genes.

Although Darwin's ideas were important for the school of functionalism established in the United States by William James and others at the end of the 19th century, and Galton's ideas were the starting point for trait theories of intelligence and personality, genetic explanations for behavior were largely eclipsed by behaviorism throughout the first half of this century. There was also a great amount of philosophical resistance in the general public to the idea of biological/genetic determinants of human behavior. For instance, there was considerable public controversy following the publication of Arthur Jensen's 1969 paper, from which readers inferred that, due to the high heritability of intelligence, educational programs would have only minimal effects in ameliorating race differences in IQ.

Several historical developments have led to the much greater acceptance today of behavioral genetics in both mainstream psychology and the general public. The discovery of the structure of deoxyribonucleic acid (DNA), the fundamental molecule of heredity, by Watson and Crick in 1953 spurred the vast expansion of knowledge in recent years on the biochemical characteristics and processes of what had up to then been only a hypothetical genetic mechanism. Discoveries about the biochemical workings of genes and gene products continue and will continue to be among the most exciting findings in science. The findings from physiological psychology and neuroscience have greatly expanded our understanding of the biological processes that determine behavior, while the idea of learning as the sole basis for behavior no longer has ascendancy. Meanwhile, the accumulation of findings from pedigree, twin, and adoption studies has provided compelling evidence for the significant heritability of intelligence, personality, schizophrenia, alcoholism, etc. We shall return to these findings, after an overview of molecular, population, and quantitative genetics.

III. MOLECULAR GENETICS

The DNA molecules in every living cell consist of two strands of phosphate and deoxyribose sugar groups held at a fixed distance from each other by pairs of nitrogenous compounds called bases. Each of the four bases is attached to one strand and can only pair with the corresponding base on the other strand in a particular combination: adenine with thymine and guanine with cytosine. The molecule itself is held together by its double helix structure, as discovered by

Watson and Crick. When the molecule is "unzipped," each strand thus is a mirror-image of the other strand and can be used as a template for the construction of proteins and enzymes, when 3-base ribonucleic acid (RNA) units carrying amino acids link up with the DNA strand in the order dictated by the exposed basepairs.

Through this transcription and replication mechanism, each cell programs the synthesis of the structures and chemicals needed to maintain itself, and the DNA in the cell's nucleus carries the program to create new cells. Also through this mechanism multicellular organisms transmit the program for the creation of new organisms. These strands of nuclear DNA are called chromosomes and a gene is simply a segment (locus) of the chromosome that codes for some protein or enzyme. In sexually reproducing organisms, the "blueprint" for the organism resides in one or more pairs of chromosomes (26 pairs in humans), and each parent transmits one half of each pair of chromosomes in the sex cells to the offspring. Thus, the biochemical basis for Mendel's hypothetical genes and alleles was established.

Autosomal genes are those that are on the "normal" chromosomes not involved in determining gender. When the gene (allele) from one parent pairs up with the gene from the other parent at a locus, one gene may biochemically "turn off" the transcription mechanism of the other gene. This is what Mendel observed as dominance.

Chromosomes that determine gender are often different from the other chromosomes in that both members of the pair may not be equivalent in size and, hence, amount of genetic material. In humans, normal females carry one pair of so-called X-chromosomes, while normal males carry an X-chromosome paired up with a much smaller Y-chromosome. The Y-chromosome carries almost no genetic information other than to turn on the process for altering the developmental course of the embryo to become a male. Whatever traits are coded for by genes on the X-chromosome in males (which is transmitted by the mother) will thus be expressed, including traits determined by recessive genes that might otherwise have been inactivated by a dominant gene on the other X-chromosome that females receive from the father. As will be discussed below with regard to population genetics, deleterious traits tend to be expressed by recessive genes. The results of so-called X-linkage are seen, for

example, in the higher incidence in males of the relatively common form of congenital mental retardation called the fragile-X syndrome, where a piece of the X-chromosome is "loose" or broken off and the genes on that piece are presumably inactive.

One theme that emerges from an understanding of the mechanisms of genetic transmission is the Darwinian idea of the importance of maintaining variability in a species. Sexual reproduction itself, although costly to the organism in terms of energy use, lost opportunities for food gathering, and vulnerability to predation, is clearly meant to create new genetic combinations in the offspring by combining genes from both parents. The process of splitting the chromosome pairs for the sex cells also involves recombination of genetic material, as the members of the pair cross over each other and exchange genes. Mutations that spontaneously occur as a result of transcription errors or environmental insults can alter the transmitted genes.

Another theme that emerged early on from molecular genetics was that some human behaviors and aspects of behaviors, particularly mental retardation, were clearly the result of simple genetic mechanisms (note, though, that not all instances of mental retardation have simple genetic explanations). Errors in chromosomal replication and division at times result in missing or duplicated chromosomes in the sex cells transmitted to the offspring. The offspring then end up with a missing member or piece of a member of a chromosome pair or with an extra chromosome (trisomy). These chromosomal defects are usually fatal for the fetus, when they occur on the larger chromosomes, and usually result in some degree of mental retardation when they occur on the smaller chromosomes of a viable offspring. Besides the fragile-X syndrome noted above, another common form of mental retardation is Down's syndrome, which is caused by a trisomy on chromosome 21.

Another good example of a simple genetic mechanism responsible for mental retardation is phenylketonuria, which is caused by a recessive autosomal gene that fails to code for the synthesis of an active enzyme responsible for the breakdown of the amino acid phenylalanine. The build-up of phenylalanine in the infant depresses other amino acid levels and hinders normal nervous system development. The pleiotropic effects of this genetic defect include hyperactivity, irritability, and moderate to severe mental retardation.

This syndrome is also interesting in demonstrating that genetically determined traits can be modified by the environment. Infants who are detected early with the double recessive genotype can be put on a low phenylalanine diet, and this diet has been shown to be effective in greatly reducing the deleterious effects of the gene.

A technique called linkage analysis is used to confirm that a trait is under the control of a single gene and to identify the particular chromosome the gene resides on. This involves identifying several large family pedigrees (two or more generations, with large numbers of siblings in each generation) or large numbers of sibships with a high incidence of the trait of interest (e.g., some form of mental retardation). Each individual in a pedigree is assessed for the occurrence or absence of the trait, and the pattern of transmission of the trait through the pedigree can be tested against the pattern expected by different kinds of Mendelian single-gene transmission modes, for example, autosomal dominant, X-linked recessive, etc. In addition, each individual is also tested for the co-occurrence of some other trait (a linkage marker), for example, a blood group type, known to be controlled by a single gene at an approximate locus on a particular chromosome. If the trait of interest consistently co-occurs with the linkage marker, i.e., there is a genetic correlation, then the traits are not independently assorting and must be close to each other on the same now-identified chromosome. The deviation from expected Mendelian ratios for independent assortment, indicative of linkage, is expressed as a so-called LOD (logarithmic odds) score.

Molecular genetic techniques developed over the last 20 years now allow for the possibility of identifying the exact location of a gene on a chromosome and determining not only the sequence of the gene's basepairs, but also the particular protein or enzyme synthesized by the gene. These recombinant DNA techniques include restriction enzymes for slicing the DNA strand at particular basepair sequences, polymerase chain reactions for multiplying the particular DNA segments to be studied, radioactive labeling and Southern blotting for observing variations (restriction fragment length polymorphisms (RFLP), variable number tandem repeats (VNTR)) in the DNA sliced by the restriction enzymes, restriction maps of overlapping segments of DNA sliced by different restriction enzymes to determine basepair sequences, and

cloning to insert DNA segments into cells to determine the gene products. Cloning also offers the possibility (the first such treatment studies are now under way) of correcting an individual's genetic defects by inserting active cells with the correct genes.

Linkage analyses in behavioral genetics now often involve attempts to genetically correlate behavioral traits with specific genes identified through molecular genetic techniques. For example, several groups have recently sought to demonstrate a pleiotropic relationship (by definition the most extreme form of linkage) between alcoholism and a gene that codes for one form of the neural receptor for the neurotransmitter dopamine. Current proposals for the mapping of the entire human genome will greatly facilitate such linkage analyses in the future.

IV. POPULATION GENETICS

As noted above, population genetics seeks to understand the frequencies and relative influence of genes on particular traits for a group of organisms operating within a particular environmental context. An important starting point for population genetics was the statistical derivation of the Hardy-Weinberg-Castle equilibrium, which showed that, in the absence of influences that produce disequilibrium (discussed below), the relative frequencies of alleles (dominant vs recessive, etc.) and genotypes (homozygous dominant, heterozygous, etc.) for a phenotype remain at a constant ratio over generations. This was basically just a restatement of Darwin's idea of maintenance of genetic variation, but in this case it was derived through mathematically following the logic of genetic transmission defined by Mendel.

Population geneticists have identified four major forces that can change allelic frequencies, i.e., the relative frequencies of one form of a gene vs another, in a population:

1. *Migration* can change allelic frequencies if individuals who move into or out of a population differ from the original population in their allelic frequencies. For example, it can be argued that the waves of immigrants who came to the United States throughout its history were more likely to carry genes for such traits as adventurousness, hardiness, rebelliousness, etc., compared to the populations left behind.

2. *Random genetic drift* can affect small populations, when chance causes some alleles and not others to accumulate over several generations.

3. *Mutation* is the ultimate source of inducing genetic variations, as alleles are altered by errors in genetic replication and transmission and by environmental influences. The spontaneous mutation rate, however, is thought to be quite low, and the effect of mutation on allelic frequencies in most cases is minor compared to natural selection.

4. *Natural selection* is, of course, the prime basis for genetic change described by Darwin. It should be remembered, however, that natural selection operates on the basis of the phenotypes that give an organism some advantage or disadvantage (relative fitness) in surviving to reproduce offspring who, in turn, will pass on the genes that determine the phenotype. If a trait, such as schizophrenia, is selected against by the environment, i.e., the trait reduces the reproductive success of the individual, and is determined by a dominant allele, then both homozygous dominant and heterozygous genotypes will be selected against. In this case natural selection will rapidly decrease the frequency of the dominant allele. If, however, the maladaptive trait is coded for by a recessive allele, as was the case for phenylketonuria, then only homozygous recessive genotypes will be selected against, and large numbers of heterozygotes (carriers) will continue to transmit the "bad" allele to some of their offspring. This process tends to ensure that adaptive traits are coded for by dominant alleles, while maladaptive traits are carried and maintained on recessives in populations. This picture becomes more complicated when there is not complete dominance for a gene. In the extreme case, selection may eliminate all but one form of a gene for an adaptive trait in a population or species, and this trait then becomes a species characteristic (i.e., there is no variability for the trait).

Natural selection may also act to maintain or even increase the variability of a phenotype in the population, creating a so-called balanced polymorphism. For example, sickle-cell anemia is a typically fatal medical condition in individuals of African ancestry. The disease is caused by an autosomal recessive gene; thus, homozygous recessive genotypes are selected against. Heterozygotes, however, manifest a greater resistance to malaria in malarial environments than homozygous dominants, and both alleles are maintained in the population, despite the deleterious effects of the recessive gene by itself. Predator–prey and parasite–host relationships also often manifest balanced polymorphisms, as natural selection for adaptations in one organism are constantly being compensated for by corresponding natural selection for adaptations in the other organism.

Since characteristics that increase the probability of being chosen as a mate also directly affect reproductive success, sexual selection is a special form of natural selection and can produce many of the same effects described above. On the other hand, the phenotypes chosen by mates may not be consistent with those resulting from natural selection, i.e., as a result of sexual selection, species may come to manifest traits that appear to be maladaptive.

Besides forces that change allelic frequencies, population geneticists also consider two forces, inbreeding and assortative mating, that change genotypic (but not allelic) frequencies by increasing the similarity of the genes that both parents transmit to their offspring. This is important, because such parental similarities in the genes they transmit would increase the relative frequencies of homozygous dominant and recessive genotypes, while decreasing the proportion of heterozygotes. This, in turn, typically has the effect of increasing the variability of the phenotype in the offspring generation, since there would be higher frequencies of the extreme genotypes. This increased variability might counter the reduction in variability resulting from some types of natural selection.

Inbreeding is the mating of genetically related individuals and, as described above, causes parents to be more similar in the genes they transmit to offspring. Since recessive alleles often code for deleterious traits but are not expressed, due to their being paired with a dominant, the increased incidence of homozygous recessive genotypes resulting from inbreeding often results in decreased fitness for the offspring of such matings (inbreeding depression). The counterpart to this is the increased fitness (hybrid vigor) found when more genetically unrelated individuals are mated. Some evidence for inbreeding depression effects on intelligence have been found in studies of offspring from cousin marriages, while hybrid vigor effects have been found in studies of offspring from cross-ethnic group marriages.

Assortative mating is where mates are similar in their phenotypes, whether due to mate choice or environmental factors. There are three different ways that assortative mating may occur.

In genetic similarity, mates select each other or are selected for each other on the basis of having similar genes, and the effects of this on offspring genotypic frequencies are similar to the effects for inbreeding. This phenomenon has been demonstrated in some animal species, but whether humans select mates on the basis of genetic similarity is controversial.

In phenotypic assortment, mates select each other on the basis of similarities in observable characteristics. Phenotypic assortment can only produce greater genetic similarity between the parents if there is a significant relationship between the genotype and the phenotype, i.e., if the characteristic is heritable. In fact, many human behaviors, such as intelligence, personality, attitudes, some psychopathology, etc., have been shown to produce moderate to high spouse correlations indicative of phenotypic assortment.

In social homogamy, mates are similar in their phenotypes simply because the environments in which they meet and mate only have individuals possessing certain characteristics. In a highly stratified society, social class differences can cause human mates to be highly similar in several behaviors relative to possible mates from other classes, even when there is no active phenotypic assortment at the level of individuals. Social homogamy can only produce greater parental genetic similarity if the phenotypes of interest are heritable and there is a significant gene–environment correlation (discussed below) across social classes.

One important offshoot of population genetics is sociobiology, which seeks to determine the evolutionary significance (i.e., fitness value) of behavioral systems. For example, sociobiologists are interested in the environmental conditions, physiological characteristics of the organism, and available genetically transmissible behaviors that cause one animal species to be characterized by altruistic behaviors, while other otherwise similar species are not altruistic. While behavioral geneticists generally attempt to determine the relative influence of genetic factors on variations in behavior within a species, sociobiologists thus tend to look at the influence of such factors on variations in behavior across species.

V. QUANTITATIVE GENETICS

Up until the recent widespread availability of new molecular genetic methodologies, much of behavior genetics was simply concerned with the issue dealt with by quantitative genetics, assessing the relative contribution of genetic vs environmental factors (nature vs nurture) in determining individual variations in traits within a species or population. Since only the phenotypes are measured, and the genetic bases for the familial resemblances discussed below only assumed, quantitative genetics relies heavily on various statistical techniques to arrive at its conclusions.

The starting point for quantitative genetics is variability. As discussed at the beginning of this article, stable individual differences in behavior or any other trait must be the result of genetic and/or environmental processes that are both unique for each individual and consistent in their effects across time. Heritability is defined as that proportion of the variability of a phenotype that can be accounted for by genetic factors or $h^2 = V_G/V_P$, where V_G and V_P are the genetic and phenotypic variabilities, respectively. Traits without any variability, such as the ability to use language in humans, may be entirely under genetic control, but the lack of variability for the trait precludes any statistical tests to determine the relative influence of genes and environment.

The counterpart to the assumptions about variability is that, if relatives resemble each other (i.e., do not vary) for some trait, it must be because they share the same genetic and/or environmental determinants of the variability of the trait. By comparing the relative degrees of resemblance (correlations) for the phenotype of interest across relationship types that theoretically differ in their underlying shared genetic and environmental determinants, the quantitative geneticist can infer the extent to which variability in genetic vs variability in environmental factors accounted for the variability of the phenotype.

For the commonly used study of twins reared together, first described by Galton, identical (monozygotic or MZ) twins are known to share all of their genetic variability (they literally have the same genes), as well as sharing the same family environment. Fraternal (dizygotic or DZ) twins are like non-twin siblings in only sharing half of their additive (additive vs nonadditive genetic effects are discussed below) genetic variance, but they are like MZ twins in sharing the same family environment. Hence, if MZ twins are more alike than DZ twins, it is assumed that this is because the former share twice as much genetic variability as the latter. Thus, doubling the difference between the MZ and DZ correlations should estimate the heritability. For example, MZ twins reared together typically correlate around .75 on tests of intelligence, while DZ twins reared together correlate around .50. Thus, the heritability would be $h^2 = 2(r_{MZ} - r_{DZ}) = 2(.75 - .50) = .50$, or 50% of the variability in intelligence is accounted for by genetic factors. Fifty percent heritability means that part of the MZ resemblance of .75 is still unaccounted for. This part, .25 or 25% is presumably due to the effects of shared family environment.

In fact, there are several more kinds of genetic and environmental processes that can produce resemblances among relatives. Genetic influences can be classified as additive or nonadditive. Additive effects are analogous to the idea of "gene dosage," in that for polygenetically determined traits familial resemblances are predicted from the extent of the linear accumulation of shared genes. For example, each parent shares on average 50% of the additive genetic variability for a phenotype with his or her offspring by transmitting half of the offspring's genome. Siblings share with each other on average 50% of the additive genetic variability, because for each of the two parents the probability is 25% that the same genes were transmitted to both siblings (50% to one sibling × 50% to the other). Additive genetic variability is important in that it determines the extent to which a trait can be changed in a population through natural or artificial selection.

The two types of nonadditive genetic effects, dominance and epistasis, can be thought of as being analogous to statistical interactions. The dominance effects described above for single genes are an inter-allele interaction, where the effect of one allele cannot be predicted without knowing the effect of the other allele. Thus, parents and offspring do not share any dominance genetic variability, since dominance effects require particular combinations of alleles from both parents. Siblings, on the other hand, do share 25% of dominance genetic variability, since that is the probability of both siblings receiving the exact same combination of alleles from both parents.

Epistasis is an inter-gene interaction, where the effect of one gene cannot be predicted without knowing the effect of some other gene or genes. Only identical twins share a high degree of epistatic genetic variability, since they inherit not only the same genes, but also the exact same combination and ordering of the genes. Siblings will share some epistatic genetic variability only if 2 or 3 genes are considered.

Environmental effects can be classified as shared (common), special twin, and unshared (specific). Shared environmental variability represents the assumption that individuals growing up in the same family may resemble each other because they are influenced by the same environmental determinants of the phenotype. Adoptive siblings and adoptive parents and their offspring provide strong tests of shared environmental effects, since presumably this is the only factor that would create any familial resemblances. Special twin environmental variability is a special form of shared environmental effects that assumes that twins may share more similar environments, perhaps due to being of the same age, than non-twin siblings.

Unshared environmental effects make family members different from each other. This may be due to idiosyncratic events in a person's life and differential treatment of siblings by parents. Measurement unreliability will also typically be manifested in the unshared environmental component of quantitative genetic models. Differences between identical twins reared together must be due to unshared environmental variability, since that is the only factor MZs do not have in common.

Genetic effects may also be correlated with environmental effects. Gene–environment correlations can be passive, where the child is born into a family environment in which environmental conditions created by the parents are consistent with the parents' and the offspring's genotype. They can be reactive, where the environment changes in response to the offspring's genotype, or active, where the offspring's genotype causes him or her to change the environment to make it more consistent with his or her genotype. Positive gene–environment correlations can presumably magnify genetic effects, while negative gene–environment correlations can diminish them. Gene–environment correlations also create the possibility that measures of the family environment used by psychologists, such as parents' socioeconomic status, may in fact be confounded by genetic factors.

Finally, there is the possibility of gene–environment interactions, where genetic effects cannot be predicted unless the environmental conditions are known. For example, genes determining intelligence may not have the opportunity to be expressed if a child is raised in a severely deprived environment.

Table I presents the theoretical extents to which the factors presented above can cause relatives to resemble each other across various relationship types.

Table I Components of Shared Variance for Different Familial Relationships

	Genetic			Environmental			Gene–environment	
	Additive	Dominance	Epistatic	Twin	Shared	Specific	Correlation	Interaction
Identical (MZ) twins	1.00	1.00	1.00	1.00	1.00	.00	1.00	1.00
Fraternal (DZ) twins	.50	.25	.00	1.00	1.00	.00	<.50?	<.50?
Non-twin siblings	.50	.25	.00	.00	1.00	.00	<.50?	<.50?
Parents/offspring	.50	.00	.00	.00	1.00	.00	<.50?	<.50?
Half-siblings	.25	.00	.00	.00	1.00	.00	<.25?	<.25?
Uncles–aunts/nephews–nieces	.25	.00	.00	.00	0.00?	.00	<.25?	<.25?
First cousins	.125	.00	.00	.00	0.00?	.00	<.125?	<.125?
Adoptees	.00	.00	.00	.00	1.00	.00	.00	.00

Quantitative genetic studies typically compare phenotypic resemblances across two and occasionally more relationship types, and some of the most commonly used designs will be described below. For several of these factors, the differences across relationship types are too small to reliably detect their effects. For instance, it can be seen that dominance and epistatic genetic effects are difficult to distinguish. Gene–environment correlations are confounded with pure genetic effects, and gene–environment interactions may be confounded with within-family environmental effects.

Before describing quantitative genetic designs used to estimate heritabilities for human behavior, animal behavioral genetic studies should be mentioned. To the extent that, due to evolutionary reasons, other animal species, such as drosophila (fruit flies), nematodes, mice, and rats, share with humans the same physiological processes that determine behavior, animal genetic studies have a number of advantages in providing information about the genetic determinants of human behavior. Unlike human adoption studies, in research with animals prenatal environments can be controlled by transplanting fetuses across animals with different genotypes. Rearing environments can be controlled to eliminate differences across relationship types or manipulated to test for gene–environment interactions. Inbred strains of genetically identical animals can be used to control for genetic variability. Heritabilities can be estimated by assessing the phenotypic response to selective breeding for extremes on the trait.

Family studies with humans involve obtaining parent/offspring and/or sibling correlations. As can be seen in Table I, such studies cannot disentangle the effects of genetic influences from shared environmental influences, although they can provide an "upper limit" for heritability. The extension of a family design to the examination of large pedigrees can provide evidence for the Mendelian transmission of a trait under the control of a single gene.

Comparisons of reared-together identical vs fraternal twin resemblances can provide an estimate of heritability, but cannot always disentangle additive vs nonadditive genetic effects. As can be seen in Table I, MZs may resemble each other more than DZs also due to greater shared gene–environment correlations and interactions. In addition, these comparisons assume that greater MZ than DZ resemblances for a trait are not the result of MZs being treated more alike than DZs. A few studies have validated this "equal environments" assumption for intelligence and personality, but it remains untested for other phenotypes.

Adoption studies involve some combination of comparing resemblances of biological parents with their adopted-away offspring vs the resemblances of the adoptive parents with the offspring or comparing adoptive vs nonadoptive sibling resemblances. Such designs have the advantage of theoretically separating additive genetic and shared environmental influences, although pre- and neonatal environmental effects cannot be controlled for. Attempts by adoption agencies for the sample to match adoptive parents with the biological parents (selective placement) could confound the analyses. This effect has been found to be at times appreciable in studies of intelligence (but not for personality). If the biological parents of the adopted-away offspring are tested, then selective placement can be controlled for.

In order to illustrate two other important aspects of quantitative genetic analysis, Figure 2 presents a path model for the genetic transmission of two different phenotypes (subscripts x and y) from fathers (subscript F) and mothers (subscript M) to their biological offspring (subscript O). In the model, each phenotype P is determined by a genetic factor G and an environmental factor E. The Gs of the parents are linked to the Gs of the offspring by one-half, reflecting the 50% of shared additive genetic variability of parents and offspring, which in this case is confounded by shared environment.

The first additional aspect of note are the arrows connecting the Ps at the top of the figure. These represent phenotypic assortative mating between fathers and mothers and, as can be seen, these arrows allow for greater similarity of the genetic variability transmitted by both parents to the offspring. For instance, mother's transmission of G_{Mx} to G_{Ox} is augmented by an additional path from father's G_{Fx} through the assortative mating path to G_{Mx}. This must be accounted for in estimating the heritability h^2.

The other aspect of note is the r_G arrows connecting the G_xs and G_ys. These represent the genetic correlations discussed above with regard to linkage and or pleiotropy. As can be seen in Figure 2, these genetic correlations are shared genetic effects, and they may be indicative of functional genetic relationships. For example, a significant genetic correlation between performance on tests of verbal ability and performance on tests of spatial ability would indicate some common physiological/genetic process for these abilities.

Before leaving quantitative genetics, several important caveats should be noted. Heritabilities reflect the relative influence of genetic factors on the variability of a trait for just the particular sample of individuals studied and the particular environmental conditions in which they are living. Heritability estimates may not generalize to other populations, and they may greatly change if environmental conditions change. Similarly, high heritabilities do not preclude a trait from being influenced by the environment. Another caveat refers back to the idea that high heritability is dependent on high phenotypic variability. As discussed in the section on population genetics, however, high phenotypic variability is associated with traits that have not been highly selected for, i.e., are not important for biological fitness, unless there is a balanced polymorphism. With these caveats in mind, we will now present a few thumbnail sketches of behavioral genetic findings in some domains of human behavior.

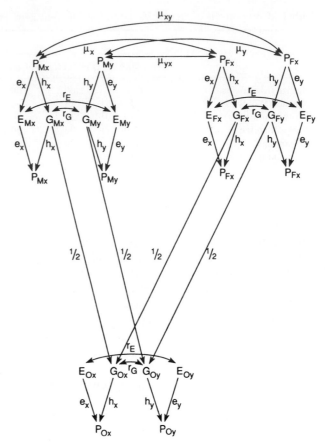

Figure 2 Path model of bivariate parent–offspring genetic transmission.

VI. BEHAVIORAL GENETIC FINDINGS

A. Intelligence

Since the work of Galton, intelligence has been the most studied phenotype in behavioral genetics. Numerous family, twin, adoption, and, more recently, separated identical twin studies have generally produced estimates of 50 to 80% heritability and about 15 to 25% shared environmental influences on performance on intelligence tests. In keeping with the caveats noted above, despite the high genetic influence on variability in intelligence, mean scores on IQ tests have risen from one-half to over one standard deviation in Western societies since World War II, a trend indicative of significant environmental influences (probably the increased availability and quality of education in these countries). [*See* INTELLIGENCE AND MENTAL HEALTH.]

B. Personality

Behavioral genetic studies of personality have been almost as numerous as those for intelligence. In general, these studies have yielded heritability estimates of around 50% for most traits, with some evidence for differential heritability for different traits and many traits showing strong nonadditive genetic effects. The most controversial finding from this domain has been the almost complete lack of shared environmental influences found in adoption studies for personality measures. Family environments appear not to make siblings alike in any way, and the importance of family environment in personality development has been questioned. This has spurred developmental research on differential treatment of offspring in families. [*See* PERSONALITY DEVELOPMENT.]

C. Schizophrenia

Schizophrenia has been the psychological disorder that has received the most behavioral genetic attention. Pedigree, family, twin, and adoption studies have all found significant heritabilities for schizophrenia, and this has been consistent with various theories about some kind of physiological basis, probably involving the dopamine system, for the disorder. On the other hand, the 20 to 50% rate of discordance (nonresemblance) between identical twins for schizophrenia indicates a significant specific environmental influence. Linkage studies have failed so far to consistently identify any single gene associated with the disorder, and the accumulated behavioral genetic evidence suggests that there are multiple genetic determinants possibly leading to multiple, etiologically distinct subtypes of schizophrenia. [*See* SCHIZOPHRENIA.]

D. Affective Disorders

Behavioral genetic studies of affective disorders have been important in making the case for the etiological separation of major depression from bipolar disorder (manic depression). Twin studies of major depression indicate a moderate heritability for the disorder and a strong shared environmental influence. The higher incidence of the disorder in women than men also indicates an environmental effect. The few behavioral genetic studies of bipolar disorder have obtained much higher heritabilities than for major depression. [*See* DEPRESSION; MOOD DISORDERS.]

E. Alcoholism

The results of large-sample adoption studies conducted in Denmark and Sweden during the 1970s convinced many researchers and the general public that alcoholism was mostly under the control of genetic determinants. This helped to spur the infusion of resources into studies of the physiological/neurochemical responses of organisms to alcohol. As discussed earlier, there have been attempts recently to identify an "alcoholism gene" by linking alcoholism to a gene known to code for a particular receptor for dopamine. The latest reports suggest that the effects of this gene are not specific for alcoholism. Meanwhile, the accumulated behavioral genetic evidence still suggests that the disorder is influenced by many different genes, as well as by significant environmental factors. [*See* ALCOHOL PROBLEMS.]

VII. BEHAVIORAL GENETICS AND PSYCHOLOGY

After a contentious start, behavioral genetics has become an accepted part of mainstream psychology. For behavioral domains whose heritability has been well-established, such as schizophrenia, future research will involve linkage analyses and molecular genetic methodologies to identify specific genes and the physiological processes associated with the genes. This holds the promise of being able to more specifically target these processes that determine a behavior. Other behavioral domains, such as attitudes, have not been well-explored by behavioral genetics, and basic heritability analyses from twin and adoption studies will continue to be important.

Finally, one theme that was apparent in the overview of behavioral genetic findings above was that behavioral genetic designs often provide important insights into environmental influences on behavior. The study of gene–environment correlations and interactions clearly will provide opportunities for the greater integration of behavioral genetics and mainstream psychology and the consequent enrichment of both.

This article has been reprinted from the *Encyclopedia of Human Behavior, Volume 1.*

BIBLIOGRAPHY

Dixon, L. K., & Johnson, R. C. (1980). "The Roots of Individuality: A Survey of Human Behavior Genetics." Brooks/Cole, Monterey, CA.

Plomin, R., DeFries, J. C., & McClearn, G. E. (1990). "Behavioral Genetics: A Primer," 2nd ed. Freeman, New York.

Plomin, R., & Rende, R. (1991). Human behavioral genetics. *Annu. Rev. Psychol.* **42**, 161.

Willerman, L. (1979). "The Psychology of Individual and Group Differences." Freeman, San Francisco.

Behavioral Medicine

Robert M. Kaplan and David N. Kerner

University of California, San Diego

Behavioral Epidemiology The study of individual behaviors and habits in relation to health outcomes.

Behavioral Medicine An interdisciplinary field concerned with the development and integration of behavioral and biomedical knowledge and techniques relevant to the understanding of health and illness.

Biopsychosocial Model A conceptualization of health and illness that considers the role of psychological, social, and physical factors in health problems. The model stands in contrast to the traditional biomedical model which focuses only on biological factors.

Cardiovascular Disease Diseases of the heart and circulatory system. These include coronary heart disease, cerebral vascular disease (stroke), and peripheral artery disease.

Cardiovascular Reactivity Changes in blood pressure in response to a stressor. Cardiovascular reactivity may be a risk factor for coronary heart disease.

Chronic Obstructive Pulmonary Disease (COPD) Diseases of airway obstruction in the lungs. COPD, which includes chronic bronchitis, emphysema, and chronic asthma affects about 11% of the adult population in the United States. The diseases are caused by or exacerbated by smoking cigarettes.

Epidemiology The study of the distribution and determinants of disease. Epidemiology seeks to identify the causes of disease in populations and determine risk factors that may be modifiable.

Health Psychology A field of study that encompasses the role of psychology in the promotion and maintenance of health and the prevention and treatment of illness.

Primary Prevention The prevention of a problem before it develops. In primary prevention the preventive effort occurs before any signs or symptoms of a disease have developed.

Psychoneuroimmunology A field of study that examines the effects of stress upon immune function and ultimately upon health and disease process.

Second Prevention Preventive efforts that begin with a population at risk. For example, secondary prevention might involve reduction of blood pressure in order to prevent a heart attack or stroke.

Tertiary Prevention Efforts to prevent an established medical condition from getting worse.

BEHAVIORAL MEDICINE is an emerging specialty. The Society of Behavioral Medicine defines the field as "the interdisciplinary field concerned with the development and integration of behavioral and biomedical science knowledge and techniques relevant to the understanding of health and illness, and the application of this knowledge and these techniques to prevention, diagnosis, treatment and rehabilitation." Several characteristics of this definition are particularly important. First, the definition recognizes the need for collaboration between physicians, biomedical scientists, and behavioral scientists. Efforts of psychologists without medical collaborators, or by physicians without behavioral collaborators, have less potential. Second, the definition stresses the application of behavioral knowledge to problems in physical health. Physical health has not traditionally been within the domain of psychology. Third, the definition excludes the more traditional topics of clinical-abnormal psychology, such as psychosis and neurosis. Although some behavioral medicine specialists study substance abuse, they tend to study traditional psychological problems only insofar as they contribute to physical health. Reflecting the view that mental and physical functioning are closely related, the *biopsychosocial* model of health and illness is endorsed by many practitioners of behavioral medicine. According to this model, health status is determined by multiple factors. The traditional medical model generally views specific biological factors as causing most health problems. Within the biopsychosocial model, psychological factors (thoughts, behaviors, feelings) and social factors are treated as equally important contributors to many health states.

I. DISTINCTIONS BETWEEN HEALTH PSYCHOLOGY, BEHAVIORAL MEDICINE, AND PSYCHOSOMATIC MEDICINE

Health psychology is the umbrella term for a variety of topics related to the interface between psychology and medicine. The Division of Health Psychology of the American Psychological Association defines its specialty as "the aggregate of the specific educational, scientific, and professional contributions of the discipline of psychology, to the promotion and maintenance of health, the prevention and treatment of illness, and the identification of the etiologic and diagnostic correlates of health, illness, and related dysfunction."

The field of behavioral medicine regards the status of medical and behavioral collaborators to be equal, with neither participant taking the dominant role. In contrast to health psychology, which emphasizes work done by psychologists, behavioral medicine emphasizes work that is collaborative between biomedical and behavioral scientists. One distinction between behavioral medicine and health psychology is that behavioral medicine is a collaboration of behavioral and

medical scientists to improve health, and health psychology is the unique contribution of psychologists to this process.

II. EXAMPLES OF BASIC RESEARCH IN BEHAVIORAL MEDICINE

Behavioral medicine encompasses a very diverse field of research. It would be impossible to review the entire domain within this short entry. Instead, we will highlight a few key research areas to provide an overview of the kinds of questions with which researchers struggle.

A. Psychoneuroimmunology, Stress, and Health

There exists a long legacy of contradictory and sometimes confused thinking regarding the relationship between mind and body. At one time, the idea that external events and stressful situations could adversely impact health was not accepted by the medical establishment. Those who believed in such a connection could offer no plausible biological mechanism. For such a relationship to be possible, the relationship between the nervous system and the immune system must be understood. These systems are known to interact through two major pathways: the autonomic nervous system and the pituitary-regulated neuroendocrine outflow. A central focus of behavioral medicine research has been to elucidate the nature of the relationship between stress and health status. The field of psychoneuroimmunology (PNI) examines the effects of stress on health and disease processes, primarily as mediated by the immune system. A number of studies have demonstrated that stress may reduce immune system functioning, in both animals and humans. [*See* PSYCHONEUROIMMUNOLOGY.]

To understand psychoneuroimmunology, it is important to understand how the immune system works. The immune system is made up of many different structures—cells (lymphocytes), tissues, and organs (e.g., thymus gland, spleen)—that communicate with each other through the bloodstream and lymphatic system. There are two major types of cells, T- and B-lymphocytes. T-cells include helper cells, which tell the immune system to "turn on" in the face of a virus or other invader, and suppressor cells, which tell the system to slow down.

Some PNI researchers ask a basic, but often elusive, question: How does the nervous system interact with the immune system at the cellular level? Recently, they have discovered that lymph nodes (which are made up of lymphocytes) receive neural input from the sympathetic nervous system. (The sympathetic nervous system is also sometimes called the "fight or flight" system.) Other researchers have found that many lymphocytes have special sites that act as receptors for neurotransmitters. Because of these and related discoveries, we now know that the nervous system exerts considerable influence on the activities of the immune system. And the reverse also seems to be true: alterations in immune functioning have been found to affect the activity of neurons in brain areas such as the hypothalamus.

A recent meta-analysis examined the literature on the relationship between stress and immunity in humans. The analysis found that increased stress is reliably associated with higher numbers of circulating white blood cells, and with lower numbers of circulating T- and B-lymphocytes. Increased stress is also linked to decreased levels of immunoglobin, another measure of immune status. Finally, stress was associated with increases in antibodies against the virus that causes herpes. [*See* STRESS.]

In one example of a stress immunity study, several immune parameters in 75 first-year medical students were assessed 1 month before final examinations and again at the start of final examinations. Immune cell activity was significantly lower at the (presumably higher stress) time of the examination than it had been a month earlier. In another study, immune status was assessed in 38 married and 38 separated or divorced women. Poor marital quality in the married group and shorter separation time in the second group were associated with poorer functioning on several immune measures.

It is important to note that there are still many unanswered questions about psychoneuroimmunology. Despite the clear relationship between stress and immune status, a solid link between stress and increased rates or duration of disease has been found with much less consistency. One reason for this shortcoming is the relatively low rate of specific poor health outcomes among a healthy population. A few studies have attempted to circumvent this incidence barrier, with some success.

One disease that is relatively easy to study is the common cold. Unlike major diseases such as cancer or heart disease, the common cold can be induced by experimenters with little risk of long-term consequences. In one intriguing study, researchers exposed 357 healthy participants to either a cold virus or a placebo. Higher rates of colds and respiratory infections were associated with higher levels of psychosocial stress.

Other studies of the psychoneuroimmunology of infectious diseases have been conducted, most notably with HIV. Although findings have been mixed, several studies have demonstrated improvement in immune parameters following behavioral or psychological interventions.

Many other issues exist in the study of psychoneuroimmunology. Debate continues, for example, on how best to define stress. Some researchers focus on objective, negative life events such as bereavement, whereas others use self-reported stress levels. Available research indicates that using objective events as the independent variable provides more consistent immunosuppressive results. Other remaining problem areas include achieving a better understanding of the immune effects of specific stressors, the role of stress duration in immune response, and the personal characteristics that make some individuals less susceptible than others to the immune effects of stress.

How people perceive stress, how they cope with stress, and how their social environment affects their reaction to stress may also explain some discrepant findings. In fact, inadequate coping in the face of marked adversity is often part of the definition of stress. According to this argument, stressful events will induce a stress response only if the organism cannot, or believes it cannot, cope with adversity. Thus, an organism's coping attempts may be an important variable in the stress–health relationship. One study found, for example, that stress with academic examinations may be more immunosuppressing among individuals who react with much more anxiety compared with those who do not. One longitudinal study of patients with metastatic breast cancer (in which the cancer has spread beyond the breast tissue) found that long-term survivors appeared to be more able to externalize their negative feelings and psychological distress through the expression of anger, hostility, anxiety, and sadness. Those who survived only a short time tended to be those individuals whose coping styles involved suppression or denial of psychological distress. [See COPING WITH STRESS.]

A relationship between suppression of emotion and poor cancer outcome has been noted with enough regularity that some researchers have identified a cancer-prone "Type C" personality that has as a main element exaggerated suppression of negative emotions like anger. In one study of women undergoing breast biopsies, women who were subsequently diagnosed with breast cancer had significantly higher levels of emotion suppression than did women who did not have cancer. Other studies have replicated these results. Because these women already had cancer, however, it was not possible to establish the causal relationship between suppression of emotion and breast cancer. [See CANCER.]

As the putative link between stress and immune functioning has gained more support, researchers have turned to interventions aimed at ameliorating the detrimental effects of stress. Relaxation training, long used in mental health contexts, was associated in one study with increased immune activity in an elderly population. Other stress control interventions, such as biofeedback and cognitive therapy, have been found in some studies to exert a beneficial influence on immune status. [See BIOFEEDBACK; COGNITIVE THERAPY; MEDITATION AND THE RELAXATION RESPONSE.]

B. Cardiovascular Reactivity

Because cardiovascular disease is a leading cause of morbidity and mortality, many behavioral medicine researchers study factors that may influence the course of this disease. Many studies focus on the effects of diet and exercise changes on cardiovascular health. Other researchers study a phenomenon known as cardiovascular reactivity. We describe some of this research in the following section.

Not all people respond to stressors in the same way. In general, being exposed to a stressor causes a rise in blood pressure. Some people react to a stressor with a relatively small rise in blood pressure, whereas for others the rise is very large. Behavioral medicine researchers have been interested in the question of whether large blood pressure increases in response to a stressor are risk factors for developing hypertension

(high blood pressure), and whether these changes predict heart attack, stroke, and death. Researchers are also attempting to determine whether individual, potentially modifiable factors such as personality are related to this hyperreactivity. Studies examining the predictive power of reactivity have had mixed results. Some studies have found that cardiovascular blood pressure reactivity in childhood predicts the development of hypertension up to 45 years later. Other studies, however, have failed to find any relationship. [See REACTIVITY.]

Researchers have examined reactivity in adulthood to predict who is most at risk for developing future vascular disease. In one well-known study, researchers attempted to identify risk factors for developing future cardiovascular disease. They found that many factors, such as resting blood pressure, smoking, and cholesterol level, were all predictive of who died from the disease 23 years later. More predictive than those variables, however, was subjects' response to a cold-presser task. The cold-presser task requires subjects to immerse a hand in ice water. Subjects are exposed for a specific time and their blood pressure is recorded. In this study, subjects who had the largest increase in blood pressure in response to the task were most likely to die from cardiovascular disease in the future.

Several factors limit our confidence in reactivity research. Notably, laboratory stressors are not the same as real-world stressors. Therefore, it has been a goal of researchers to measure blood pressure in response to stressors that individuals experience in their daily lives. Recently, the development of ambulatory blood pressure monitors has made it possible to monitor the blood pressure of an individual throughout the day. Participants can keep diaries of stressful events, and researchers can examine how blood pressure varies in response to these stressors. Clinically, this technique could eventually allow for improved risk prediction for at-risk individuals

Researchers are currently attempting to answer several puzzling questions about cardiovascular reactivity. For instance, the physiological mechanism linking hyperreactivity to undesirable health outcomes is not known. Studies have also failed to determine the cause of hyperreactivity. Is it simply a genetic phenomenon? Or are there environmental factors at work? If the cause is environmental, researchers may be able to develop treatments for hyperreactivity. Such interventions have the potential for reducing the number of people who die each year from cardiovascular disease. [*See* HEART DISEASE: PSYCHOLOGICAL PREDICTORS.]

C. Personality and Illness

Another major focus of behavioral medicine research is the relationship between personality factors and illness. Interest in this relationship dates back at least to the ancient Greeks, who classified people into one of four basic personality types (phlegmatic, melancholic, sanguine, and choleric); these personalities were presumed to be based on imbalances in bodily fluids, or humors. Early in this century, it was believed that certain diseases, such as hypertension, heart disease, cancer, asthma, ulcerative colitis, and ulcers, were "psychosomatic"—mainly caused by personality. As research data have accumulated, however, it has become clear that the association between personality and illness is much more complex than first believed. Current research examines the impact on health of psychological constructs such as motivation, self-mastery, and self-confidence, as well as the impact of alcohol and substance abuse. Related factors under study include socioeconomic status, gender, and cognitive status. [*See* INDIVIDUAL DIFFERENCES IN MENTAL HEALTH; PERSONALITY.]

Since the early 1950s, one major focus of psychosomatic research has been the relationship between the "Type A" personality and cardiovascular disease. Two cardiologists originally described a cluster of characteristics that many of their patients shared. People with Type A personalities were described as highly competitive and achievement oriented. They are also typically in a hurry and impatient; in addition, they are hostile in social interactions. [*See* TYPE A–TYPE B PERSONALITIES.]

Major longitudinal studies in the 1960s and 1970s convincingly supported the notion that the Type A personality was a major risk factor for developing cardiovascular disease. In 1981, a panel organized by the National Heart, Lung, and Blood Institute (NHLBI) concluded that Type A behavior was a risk factor for coronary heart disease (CHD). Since that time, however, several large, well-conducted studies (including the long-term follow-up to the original study which found a Type A–heart disease link) have found no association between Type A behavior and heart disease.

Researchers have proposed several possible explanations for the Type A turnabout. These include that

(1) the original findings were just a fluke; (2) the assessment of Type A may have changed over time; (3) society may have changed, making the Type A distinction anachronistic; (4) coronary heart disease population distribution has changed (changing patterns of smoking, diet, and physical activity may interact with Type A behavior in unclear ways); or (5) some aspects of Type A behavior are risk factors, but others are not. Many studies have examined this latter possibility.

In one comprehensive meta-analysis examining the effects of psychological and behavioral variables on coronary heart disease, only the anger and hostility components of Type A were found to be significant CHD risk factors. Overall, Type A was unrelated to future disease status. Other studies, using both the Type A Structured Interview and the Cook-Medley Hostility (Ho) Scale of the Minnesota Multiphasic Personality Interview (MMPI), have found that "cynical hostility" is predictive of future coronary disease morbidity and mortality. People who are cynically hostile tend to expect the worst of others and dwell on people's negative characteristics. This personality characteristic, unlike overall Type A behavior, does seem to predict future heart disease.

When considering the Type A and CHD research, it is important to note that the majority of research has been conducted with male subjects. Relatively little attention has been paid to CHD risk factors in women, despite the fact that CHD is the leading cause of death among women, killing more women than men each year. Only recently have researchers begun to examine the personality risk factors for women.

The relationship between hostility and diseases other than CHD has also been examined. A number of studies, for example, have found a link between hostility and all-cause mortality. Only one study, however, has controlled for CHD deaths in the analysis. In that study, MMPI Hostility scores correlated with 20-year, all-cause mortality rates, even when CHD-related mortality was factored out. To date, no studies have linked hostility to other major health outcomes, such as cancer.

Besides hostility, many other personal factors have been examined for their relationship to health. Notably, clinical and nonclinical depression have been related to poor health outcomes among certain disease groups. In one study of CHD and depression, clinical depression assessed in recently hospitalized post-myocardial infarction (MI; or heart attack) patients was associated with a 500% greater likelihood of 6-month mortality. In another study, 4000 hypertensive individuals were followed for 4.5 years. In this group, change in depression level (although not absolute level) predicted future cardiac events like infarctions and surgeries. [*See* DEPRESSION.]

Other studies have shown that having an optimistic, rather than pessimistic, attitude may have important health consequences. Similarly, a negatively fatalistic outlook on life and health may be a prognostic indicator of poor future health status. In one 50-month study of 74 male patients with AIDS, increased survival time was significantly associated with low levels of fatalism, which was called "realistic acceptance." Patients who had low scores on a measure of realistic acceptance had median survival times 9 months longer than patients with high levels. When potential confounds were controlled for, such as initial health status and ongoing health behaviors, the effect remained significant.

Similar findings have been obtained with other disease groups. Researchers often use all or part of the Life Orientation Test (LOT) as a measure of optimism and pessimism. In one study, a pessimistic attitude (as measured by LOT) was a significant mortality risk factor for young adults with recurrent cancer. Another study found that high LOT pessimism was associated with greater risk of MI during coronary artery bypass graft (CABG) surgery. [*See* OPTIMISM, MOTIVATION, AND MENTAL HEALTH.]

Another area of inquiry regarding personal factors and health involves recovery and adaptation after surgery. Researchers assessed a number of psychosocial variables in a population of 42 leukemia patients about to receive allogeneic bone marrow transplants. (Allogeneic transplants involve bone marrow from donors other than themselves or identical twins.) Participants who had an attitude toward cancer characterized by "anxious preoccupation" had increased mortality compared to nonanxious participants.

Finally, socioeconomic status (SES) has emerged as an important determinant of health status. Several studies have shown a clear gradient between SES and a variety of different indicators of health status. Furthermore, the association is continuous. For example, there are differences in health status between moderately poor people and those who are very poor. On the other end of the spectrum, it appears that there are differences between the very rich and those who are

moderately well off. These differences are observed in nearly all cultures, including those with universal access to health care. Thus, health care alone does not seem to explain the association between SES and health status. [*See* SOCIOECONOMIC STATUS.]

III. EXAMPLES OF BEHAVIORAL MEDICINE IN CLINICAL PRACTICE

A. Treatment of Heart Disease

Cardiovascular disease (CVD), which includes coronary heart disease, cerebrovascular disease (strokes), and peripheral artery disease, is the single most common cause of death in the United States. Caused by atherosclerosis, the buildup of fatty plaques along the inner walls of arteries, CVD causes significant disability and is a large source of health care costs. Behavioral medicine specialists have developed a number of interventions to prevent and treat CVD.

One risk factor for CVD is high blood cholesterol, or hypercholesterolemia. The diagnostic criteria for hypercholesterolemia are presented in Table I. The most prominent intervention effort aimed at treating hypercholesterolemia, initiated by the National Heart, Lung, and Blood Institute, is known as the National Cholesterol Education Program (NCEP).

If atherosclerotic buildup increases, the arteries narrow and restrict blood flow. The formation of a clot can completely stop blood flow, causing an MI or cerebral vascular accident (CVA; or stroke). Atherosclerosis is a life-long process, partially controlled by inherited genetic factors such as metabolism. Although humans have no influence over their genes, our physiological factors affecting atherosclerosis include blood cholesterol, blood pressure, and obesity. These physiological factors and CVD risk are partially

Table I National Cholesterol Education Program Guidelines for the Treatment of Hypercholesterolemia

Recommended level	200 mg/dl TC[a]	130 mg/dl LDL
Moderate risk	200–240 mg/dl TC	130–160 mg/dl LDL
High risk	>240 mg/dl TC	>160 mg/dl LDL

[a] TC, total cholesterol; LDL, low-density lipoprotein (i.e., "bad" cholesterol).

influenced by modifiable behaviors, for example, physical activity, diet, and tobacco use. Behavioral medicine practitioners are actively involved in developing effective interventions in these areas, at both the patient and caregiver level.

Regular physical activity may reduce blood pressure by reducing obesity, increasing aerobic fitness, and reducing the blood levels of certain stress-related chemicals such as adrenalin. In individuals who already have hypertension, exercise significantly reduced resting blood pressure in most studies. Other studies have examined the effect of activity interventions on individuals who do not yet have hypertension, but who are at high risk for developing it (e.g., people with "high normal" blood pressure). One such study found that increased physical activity was one factor reducing the risk of future hypertension in this population. Many other studies have found cardiovascular benefits from dietary and smoking interventions.

The benefits from these interventions, although significant, are limited. Atherosclerosis has traditionally been viewed as a unidirectional process. Therefore, behavioral and medical interventions have been aimed at slowing, rather than reversing the sclerotic process. Recently, however, the Lifestyle Heart Trial attempted to reverse atherosclerosis through behavior change. This trial was notable for its comprehensiveness. Patients with severe heart disease were randomly assigned to either a standard-treatment control group or a radical lifestyle change intervention. In the intervention group, participants were introduced to the program through a weekend retreat with their spouses. Then, participants attended 4-hour, biweekly group meetings. They were placed on an extremely low-fat vegetarian diet (fat was limited to 10% of calories, compared with a national average of about 40%). Caffeine use was eliminated, and alcohol was limited to two drinks per day. The group sessions included relaxation and yoga exercises; participants were expected to practice relaxation and meditation for 1 hour each day. Sessions also included exercise and smoking cessation instruction for participants who smoked.

The results of this intensive behavior change program were striking. Participants reduced their fat intake from 31% to 7% of total calories. They increased daily exercise from 11 minutes to 38 minutes per day. They increased their relaxation and meditation time from an average of 5 minutes per day to 82 minutes per day. As a result, participants' total cholesterol levels dropped markedly, often to below 150 mg/dl. Blood pressure also fell. They lost, on average, 22 pounds over the 1-year course of the study. Angina (chest pain) dropped by 91% in the experimental group, whereas it increased by 165% in the control group. Impressively, participants in the experimental group were almost twice as likely as control group members to show actual reductions in arterial blockage.

This study demonstrated that a behavioral intervention that includes daily exercise and relaxation, along with an extremely low-fat diet, can have an impressive impact on the clinical picture of individuals with severe heart disease. Related research focuses on the impact of behavioral interventions on individuals who do not yet have heart disease, but who may develop it in the future.

B. Adaptation to Cancer

Cancer is universally feared. According to the American Cancer Society (ACS), cancer is an umbrella term for a group of diseases "characterized by uncontrolled growth and spread of abnormal cells." Not counting some highly prevalent, rarely fatal forms of skin cancer, the most common cancers are (in order of prevalence) prostate, lung, colon/rectal, and bladder (for men); and breast, colon/rectal, lung, and uterus (for women). For both men and women, lung cancer causes the most deaths. Although it kills far fewer people than CVD, cancer is perceived as more dangerous, destructive, and deadly. In reality, the survival rate for cancer has been climbing steadily throughout this century. Taking a normal life expectancy into consideration, the ACS estimates that 50% of all people diagnosed with cancer will live at least 5 years. Nevertheless, cancer remains the second-leading cause of death and is associated with significant pain and disability.

Because behavioral factors have been implicated in the etiology of many cancers (e.g., smoking, eating a low-fiber diet, sunlight exposure), behavioral scientists have developed a large number of programs designed to help people reduce their cancer risk. In addition, behaviorists have focused on what happens to an individual after a diagnosis of cancer is made. Partly because there are so many types of cancers, the experience of cancer is highly variable. Nevertheless, there are commonalities. Most cancer treatments, such as surgery, radiation, and chemotherapy, are extremely unpleasant. Surgery often requires a great amount of recuperation, sometimes causes new physical problems, and may cause substantial disfigurement. Radiation and chemotherapy often cause significant side effects, including hair loss, sterility, even nausea and vomiting, fatigue, and diarrhea. Anticipatory anxiety, classically conditioned by these treatments, may increase the severity of many of these symptoms. In the long term, cancer patients face problems with physical, psychological, and sexual functioning, as well as family and work difficulties. Many studies have demonstrated that cancer patients exhibit increased rates of depression, and some have demonstrated increased rates of anxiety. Behaviorists working in treatment settings have attempted to help individuals with cancer cope as well as possible with these difficulties.

Health researchers have found that cancer may result in self-concept problems. In addition, one study identified four major sources of stress experienced by people with cancer: (1) loss of meaning, (2) concerns about the physical illness, (3) concerns about medical treatment, and (4) social isolation. Social isolation and reduced social activity have been observed in both children and adults with cancer. Behavioral science practitioners are developing interventions to ameliorate the psychosocial effects of cancer.

Interesting and controversial intervention studies have examined the effect of positive attitude and social support in reducing the physical effects of cancer. According to some psychoneuroimmunology studies, depressed mood may reduce immune functioning. "Wellness communities," startled by Harold Benjamin in Santa Monica, California, promote the idea that depression weakens immune response. They suggest that a positive attitude may likewise enhance it. Stronger immunity, it is argued, will lead to reduced physical manifestations of the disease.

The most well-known study of social support and cancer was undertaken with a group of 86 women diagnosed with metastatic breast cancer. (*Metastatic* means the disease has spread beyond the original organ or tissue site.) The women were randomly assigned to either a standard treatment control group or a group that included weekly support groups. The support groups were led by psychiatrists or social workers who were breast cancer survivors themselves. Women in the support group became highly involved

in helping the other participants cope with their cancer symptoms, treatment, and difficulties.

Women assigned to the support groups survived an average of 36.6 months, while those in the control group survived an average of only 18.9 months. Support group members also experienced less anxiety, depression, and pain. This study's impressive results have sparked further research into the role of social support and immune functioning, as well as the role of psychotherapy in reducing the psychosocial difficulties of the cancer experience. The study is now being replicated with a larger group of women.

Another often-cited cancer intervention study examined the effects of a 6-week intervention on patients diagnosed with a deadly form of skin cancer known as malignant melanoma. The intervention included weekly 90-minute sessions focusing on relevant education, problem-solving skills, stress management, and psychological support. Outcome data indicated both short-term and long-term effects of the intervention versus the control group. At short-term (6-week and 6-month) assessments, immune markers were significantly better in the intervention group than in the controls. When studied 6 years later, the intervention group participants had lower mortality rates and fewer recurrences than did participants in the control group.

C. Functioning in Lung Disease

Another example of behavioral medicine practice comes from studies of rehabilitation of patients with chronic obstructive pulmonary disease (COPD), which is a common ailment among smokers. It is currently the fourth leading cause of death in the United States. Chronic bronchitis, emphysema, and chronic asthma are the three diseases most commonly associated with COPD. The common denominator of these disorders is expiratory flow obstruction (difficulty exhaling air) caused by airway narrowing, although the cause of airflow obstruction is different in each. Exposure to cigarette smoke is the primary risk factor for each of these illnesses. There is no cure for COPD.

Chronic obstructive pulmonary disease has a profound effect on functioning and everyday life. Current estimates suggest that COPD affects nearly 11% of the adult population, and that the incidence is increasing, especially among women, reflecting the increase in tobacco use among women in the latter part of this century. Medicines such as bronchodilators, corticosteroids, and antibiotic therapy help symptoms, and long-term oxygen therapy has been shown to be beneficial in patients with severe hypoxemia. However, it is widely recognized that these measures cannot cure COPD. Much of the effort in the management of this condition must be directed toward preventive treatment strategies aimed at improving symptoms, patient functioning, and quality of life.

In one study, 119 COPD patients were randomly assigned to either comprehensive pulmonary rehabilitation or an education control group. Pulmonary rehabilitation consisted of 12 4-hour sessions distributed over an 8-week period. The content of the sessions was education, physical and respiratory care, psychosocial support, and supervised exercise. The education control group attended four 2-hour sessions that were scheduled twice per month, but did not include any individual instruction or exercise training. Topics included medical aspects of COPD, pharmacy use, and breathing techniques. In addition, subjects were interviewed about smoking, life events, and social support. Lectures covered pulmonary medicine, pharmacology, respiratory therapy, and nutrition. Outcome measures included lung function, exercise tolerance (maximum and endurance), perceived breathlessness, perceived fatigue, self-efficacy for walking, depression, and overall health-related quality of life.

In comparison to the educational control group, rehabilitation patients demonstrated a significant increase in exercise endurance (82% vs. 11%), maximal exercise workload (32% vs. 14%), and peak VO_2, a measure of cardiovascular fitness (8% vs. 2%). These changes in exercise performance were associated with significant improvement in symptoms of perceived breathlessness and muscle fatigue during exercise.

Traditional models of medical care are challenged by the growing number of older adults with chronic, progressively worsening illnesses such as COPD. Cognitive–behavioral interventions may help patients adapt to loss of function and, when successfully used in a comprehensive rehabilitation program that includes training in energy conservation and the use of assistive devices, may even help to increase function. As a result, behavioral interventions can improve quality of life for patients with chronic pulmonary disease.

As in our discussion of behavioral medicine research, this section on the practice of behavioral medicine has highlighted some areas of active interest. Behavioral medicine practitioners have developed successful interventions in many other areas, such as diet and physical activity, tobacco use, and pain management.

IV. BEHAVIORAL MEDICINE IN PUBLIC HEALTH

In addition to clinical contributions, behavioral medicine often takes a public health perspective. The public health perspective differs from the clinical viewpoint because of its focus on the community rather than on the individual. In public health, the emphasis is on improving the average health of an entire population rather than on the health of specific patients. Three areas where behavioral medicine intersects with public health are epidemiology, preventive medicine, and health policy.

A. Epidemiology

Epidemiology is the study of the determinants and distribution of disease. Epidemiologists measure disease and then attempt to relate the development of diseases to characteristics of people and the environments in which they live. The word *epidemiology* is derived from Greek. The Greek word *epi* translates to "among," and the Greek word *demos* translates to "people." The stem *ology* means "the study of." *Epidemiology,* then, is the study of what happens among people. For as long as there has been recorded history, people have been interested in what causes disease. It has been obvious, for example, that diseases are not equally distributed within populations of people. Some people are much more at risk for certain problems than are others.

Traditionally, most epidemiologists studied infectious diseases. For example, people who live in close contact are most likely to get similar illnesses or to be "infected" by one another. Ancient doctors also recognized that people who became ill from certain diseases, and who subsequently recovered, seldom got the same disease again. Thus, the notions of communicability of diseases and of immunity were known many years before specific microorganisms and antibodies were understood. Epidemiologic history was made by Sir John Snow who studied cholera in London in the mid-nineteenth century. Cholera is a horrible disease that causes severe diarrhea and eventually kills its victims through dehydration. Snow systematically studied those who developed cholera and those who did not. His detective-like investigation demonstrated that those who obtained their drinking water from a particular source (a well in London) were more likely to develop cholera. Thus, he was able to link a specific environmental factor to the development of the disease, and actions based on this knowledge saved many lives. This occurred many years before the specific organism that causes cholera was identified.

It is common to think of epidemics as major changes in infectious disease rates. For example, we are experiencing a serious epidemic of Acquired Immune Deficiency Syndrome (AIDS). Yet there are other epidemics that are less dramatic. For instance, we are also experiencing a major epidemic of coronary heart disease in the United States. In 1900, heart disease accounted for about 15% of all deaths, whereas infectious diseases, such as influenza and tuberculosis, accounted for nearly one quarter of all deaths. In the 1990s, cardiovascular (heart and circulatory system) diseases caused nearly half of all deaths. The days when infectious diseases were the major killers in the industrialized world appear to be over. AIDS, although rapidly increasing in incidence, still accounts for only about 1% of all deaths. Today, the major challenge is from chronic illnesses. The leading causes of death include heart disease, cancer, stroke, chronic obstructive lung disease, and diabetes. Each of these may be associated with a long period of disability. In addition, personal habits and health behaviors are associated with both the development and the maintenance of these conditions. [See HIV/AIDS.]

It is important to consider the relative importance of different risk factors and different causes of death. Heart disease is clearly the leading cause of death in the United States, with an estimated 733,867 deaths in 1993. Stroke accounted for another 145,551 deaths. Cancer accounted for 496,152 deaths in 1993. Diabetes mellitus accounted for more than 46,833 deaths, and COPD was responsible for 84,344 deaths.

B. Behavioral Epidemiology

We use *behavioral epidemiology* to describe the study of individual behaviors and habits in relation to health outcomes. Wise observers have been aware of the relationship between lifestyle and health for many centuries. This is evidenced by the following statement from Hippocrates in approximately 400 BC:

> Whoever wishes to investigate medicine properly, should proceed thus: . . . the mode in which the inhabitants live, and what are their pursuits, whether they are fond of drinking and eating to excess, and given to indolence, and are fond of exercise and labor, and not given to excess eating and drinking.

There were approximately 2,269,000 deaths in the United States in 1993 (latest CDC report). Deaths are accounted for according to major and underlying cause. The traditional biomedical model has emphasized disease-specific causes of death, and pathways to prevention have typically considered risk factors for particular diseases. For example, cigarette smoking is associated with deaths from cancer of the lung. Thus, efforts to reduce lung cancer concentrate on smoking cessation. However, most of the major causes of death are associated with a variety of different risk factors. Furthermore, many risk factors are associated with death from a variety of different causes. For example, tobacco use causes not only lung cancer, but a wide variety of other cancers, as well as heart disease, stroke, and birth complications.

Major nongenetic contributors to mortality were examined in an important analysis in 1993 by McGinnis and Foege. They identified several behaviors that account for large numbers of deaths. A summary of the estimates for actual causes of death in the United States is presented in Table II. Tobacco use is associated with more than 400,000 deaths each year, and diet and activity patterns account for an additional 300,000. These dwarf the number of deaths associated with problems that the public is generally concerned about, such as illicit drug use. The McGinnis and Foege analysis challenged society to think differently about health indicators in the United States. Only a small fraction of the trillion dollars the United States spends annually on health care is devoted to the control of the major factors that cause premature mortality in the United States. Estimates suggest that less than 5% of the total annual health care budget is

Table II Actual Causes of Death—United States, 1990[a]

Factor	Deaths	Percentage
Tobacco	400,000	19
Diet–activity patterns	300,000	14
Alcohol	100,000	5
Microbial agents	90,000	4
Toxic agents	60,000	3
Firearms	35,000	<2
Sexual behavior	30,000	1
Motor vehicles	25,000	1
Illicit use of drugs	20,000	<1
Total	1,060,000	50

[a]Source: McGinnin & Feoge, *JAMA, 270,* 2207–2212, 1993.

devoted to prevention efforts. Because behaviors are the major causes of death and disability, it is clear that behavioral scientists have an important role to play in many areas of public health and clinical medicine.

To underscore the role of behaviors in premature mortality, we consider two examples; tobacco use and physical activity.

1. Tobacco

Cigarette smoking remains the greatest single cause of preventable deaths in contemporary society. The health consequences of tobacco use have been documented in thousands of studies. Although cigarette smoking has declined in the United States and in the United Kingdom in recent years, the worldwide trend is toward increased use of tobacco products. In addition, although adult smoking has declined markedly, smoking among teens is on the rise. It is projected that worldwide there will be 10 million tobacco-related deaths per year by the year 2010. Current estimates suggest that tobacco use in the United States is responsible for 434,000 deaths each year. These include 37,000 deaths from cardiovascular disease resulting from exposure to tobacco smoke in the environment (so-called second-hand smoke). Furthermore, smoking is responsible for poor pregnancy outcomes. Between 17 and 26% of low birth weight deliveries are associated with maternal tobacco use and 5 to 6% of prenatal deaths can be attributed to maternal tobacco use. McGinnis and Foege suggest that about 25,000 deaths in the United States can be attributed to motor vehicle accidents, and about 20,000 deaths can be attributed to illicit drug use. In contrast, deaths associated with tobacco use account for more than 20 times the number associated with drug use, 16 times the number associated with auto crashes, and 15 times the number of homicides.

Financial barriers to treatment for nicotine addiction have been formidable—for the patient and for the provider. Most health insurance plans in the United States, public and private, exclude coverage for tobacco addiction treatments. This helps to explain why only 10 to 15% of the U.S. smokers who have tried to quit have ever received any formal treatment for nicotine addiction, and why low-income and disadvantaged Americans have been least likely to get help. Lack of reimbursement also helps to explain why, even today, only 50% of the nation's smokers report ever having been advised by their doctors to quit smoking. [*See* SMOKING.]

2. Physical Activity

Research shows that people who are physically active live significantly longer than those who are sedentary. These studies have documented a relationship between physical activity and all-cause mortality, CHD mortality, mortality from diabetes mellitus, and mortality associated with COPD and other lung diseases. In addition to living longer, those who engage in regular physical activity may be better able to perform activities of daily living and enjoy many aspects of life. Furthermore, those who exercise regularly have better insulin sensitivity and less abdominal obesity. Regular exercise has also been shown to improve psychological well-being for those with mood disorders. Successful programs have been developed to promote exercise for the general population. Also, specific interventions have been developed for those diagnosed with particular diseases.

Despite the benefits of exercise, few people will start an exercise program, and many of those who start do not continue to exercise. Some predictors of failure to exercise regularly include being overweight, poor, female, and a smoker. However, the most commonly reported barriers to exercise are lack of time and inaccessibility of facilities.

Studies show that exercise patterns change as people age. Children are active, but physical activity declines substantially by the late teens and early twenties. It appears that Americans are shifting toward less vigorous activity patterns, with walking becoming the most common form of exercise. Physical *inactivity* may be increasing as Americans spend more time watching television or working with computers.

Methods to enhance exercise include environmental manipulation, behavior modification, cognitive–behavior modification, and educational approaches. The behavior modification interventions use principles of learning to increase physical activity. These interventions typically control the contingencies associated with physical activity and reinforce active behaviors. Cognitive–behavior modification interventions are similar to behavior modification approaches. However, they also modify self-defeating thoughts that may turn people off to exercise. Educational interventions attempt to increase activity by teaching people about the benefits of being physically active. Statistical analysis that average results across studies (called meta-analyses) tend to show that interventions based on behavior modification principles produce the largest benefits. Interventions based on health education or health risk appraisal approaches tend not to produce consistent benefits. Cognitive–behavior modification interventions also have produced less consistent results than behavior modification approaches. Interventions that include incentives and social support increase exercise in the short term. Many of the studies show that people have difficultly maintaining their exercise programs over the course of time.

Exercise programs are now common for patients with heart, lung, and blood diseases. Cardiac rehabilitation has become a widely chosen and accepted treatment option for patients with established coronary artery disease. As recently as 1970, post-MI patients were typically hospitalized for 1 month and advised to take total bed rest. Today, the average MI patient is hospitalized for 5 to 7 days and lengths of stay continue to decline. Furthermore, the majority of patients are advised to resume physical activity relatively promptly following an MI. Exercise is the core component of the rehabilitation process. Meta-analyses of controlled studies in rehabilitation have demonstrated 20 to 25% reductions in mortality. Newer studies are beginning to demonstrate improvements in quality of life as well as life duration.

Studies of patients with COPD have also demonstrated benefits associated with exercise. Although studies tend not to show changes in lung functioning, some studies have documented improvements in exercise capacity, performance of activities in daily living, and mood. Studies have not demonstrated improvements in life expectancy.

Although there are few intervention studies, evidence suggests that physical activity also predicts survival for patients with cystic fibrosis. In one study, 83% of patients who had the highest levels of aerobic fitness survived for 8 years in comparison to 58% and 28% of patients in the middle and lowest thirds, respectively, of the distribution for aerobic fitness. [*See* EXERCISE AND MENTAL HEALTH; PHYSICAL ACTIVITY AND MENTAL HEALTH.]

C. Prevention Sciences

Behavioral medicine has a strong commitment to disease prevention. Prevention can be divided into primary and secondary. Primary prevention is the prevention of a problem before it develops. Thus, the primary prevention of heart disease starts with people who have no symptoms or characteristics of the disease and there is intervention to prevent these diseases from becoming established. In secondary prevention, we begin with a population at risk and develop efforts to prevent the condition from becoming worse. Tertiary prevention deals with the treatment of established conditions and is the main focus of clinical medicine. Table III uses the example of high blood pressure to illustrate these three approaches to prevention.

Prevention has different meanings for different

Table III Three Levels of Prevention

Level	When used	Example
Primary	For completely well people	Controlling weight to prevent high blood pressure
Secondary	For people with risks for illness (e.g., high blood pressure)	Using medicine to lower blood pressure
Tertiary	For people with developed disease (e.g., heart disease resulting from high blood pressure)	Rehabilitation to prevent the condition from getting worse

Table IV Examples of Three Types of Prevention Programs

Type of program	Description	Outcomes
Clinical preventive services	Brief counseling, referral, patient education	Difficult to institute; some evidence of success
Community-based preventive services	Changing local patterns of expected behavior, and peer pressure	Difficult to institute; better evidence of success
Social policy for prevention	Taxes, seat belt laws	Better evidence of success

people. Partners for Prevention, a nonprofit organization, emphasizes that there are at least three different components of prevention. These include clinical preventive services, community-based preventive services, and social policies for prevention. Clinical preventive services typically involve medical treatments such as immunization and screening tests. Clinical services may also include counseling and behavioral interventions. Community-based preventive services include public programs to ensure safe air, water, or food supplies, as well as behavioral interventions to change local patterns of diet, exercise, or smoking. Social policies for prevention might involve regulation of environmental exposures or exposure to hazardous materials at the work place. These social approaches also include taxes on alcohol and cigarettes and physical changes to ensure better traffic safety. Examples of these three types of prevention programs are given in Table IV.

D. Health Care Policy

The American Health Care System is perhaps the most complex in the world. The United States represents only about 5% of the world's population, but accounts for about 40% of all health care expenditures worldwide. It is difficult to describe U.S. health care as a "system." Rather, U.S. health care is a patchwork of overlapping systems of public and private insurance, with as many as 40 million persons uninsured for their medical expenses.

It is commonly argued that traditional fee-for-service medicine provides few incentives to offer behavioral medicine and preventive services. Indeed,

the higher the rates of medical service utilization the greater the profit. One attractive feature of the current move toward managed care is that there are substantial incentives to prevent illness and to reduce health care utilization. From a public health perspective, managed care organizations have responsibility for a defined population. If they can keep this population healthy by investing in prevention, they may ultimately profit by having reduced costs and higher consumer satisfaction.

There are several reasons why the potential for behavioral and disease prevention has often been overlooked by public-policy makers. Preventive services rarely make headlines or gain the same attention as high technology medical interventions. For example, transplantation of a diseased heart attracts the media and brings adulation from family and friends. A patient who survives such transplantation is thought to have benefited from the miracles of modern medical science and the surgeons are handsomely rewarded. When an illness is prevented, no one is aware that a problem has been avoided. There are no headlines because there is no news, and there are no fees for the experts who helped avoid a catastrophe. The average effect of prevention for any one person may be small, yet preventive services have the potential for a huge impact. As noted in Table II, an estimated 400,000 Americans die prematurely each year as a result of tobacco use. As many as 100,000 people die prematurely each year as a result of unnecessary injuries or illnesses related to alcohol abuse. Substantial numbers of cancer and heart disease deaths may be prevented or at least delayed through lifestyle modification.

Most of the 3 to 5% of the health care dollar used for prevention is devoted to clinical preventive services offered by physicians. For example, the great majority of expenditures on prevention relate to screening for diseases such as breast cancer, cervical cancer, and prostate cancer. The purpose of the prevention service is to detect a disease that already exists and medically treat it so that progression is retarded. The screening tests have become profitable for the providers who offer them and there is growing concern about abuses or profiteering by those who administer tests to people who do not need them. Many behavioral medicine professionals advocate a greater emphasis on prevention programs to change behaviors that are causing the most deaths.

V. SUMMARY

Behavioral medicine is a strong and growing field. It draws its strength from its comprehensive approach and interdisciplinary nature. Rather than retreating to small niches, as is so common in science today, behavioral medicine researchers and clinicians must obtain knowledge from a wide variety of disciplines relevant to their field. A behavioral medicine researcher studying CHD must know about basic cardiac functioning, personality research, and many other seemingly unrelated pieces of information. By the nature of this comprehensive approach, the behavioral medicine specialist, whether she is a nurse practitioner, psychologist, or physician, brings a much needed perspective to the science of health and behavior.

BIBLIOGRAPHY

Kaplan, R. M., Orleans, C. T., Perkins, K. A., & Pierce, J. P. (1995). Marshaling the evidence for greater regulation and control of tobacco products: A call for action. *Annals of Behavioral Medicine, 17,* 3–14.

Kaplan, R. M., Sallis, J. F., & Patterson, T. L. (1993). *Health and human behavior.* New York: McGraw-Hill.

Matarazzo, J. D. (1980). Behavioral health and behavioral medicine: Frontiers for a new health psychology. *American Psychologists, 35,* 807–817.

McGinnis, J. M., & Foege, W. H. (1993). Actual causes of death in the United States. *Journal of the American Medical Association, 270,* 2207–2212.

Peto, R., Lopez, A. D., Boreham, J., Thun, M., & Heath, Jr., C. (1992). Mortality from tobacco in developed countries: Indirect estimation from national vital statistics. *Lancet, 339*(8804), 1268–1278.

Behavior Therapy

Maxie C. Maultsby, Jr.

Howard University, College of Medicine

Mariusz Wirga

Howard University, College of Medicine

Behavior The things organisms do. There are two types: (1) *overt behavior*—observable by other people; (2) *covert behavior*—observable only by the behaving people themselves, for example, thoughts, emotional feelings, and so on.

Cognitive-Emotive Dissonance The most important stage in new learning, characterized by these two features: (1) it occurs when people first begin thinking and acting in their new, correct ways for their behavioral goal but (2) they are having the uncomfortable emotional feelings that they have when they believe they are behaving incorrectly: People usually describe this experience with "This doesn't feel right," or "This feels wrong to me." A common example of this event is: an American driver "feeling wrong" while driving correctly on the left side of the street in England. This is an unavoidable experience in psychotherapeutic or any type of change in a personal habit. In psychotherapy it is the stage of maximal therapeutic resistance. If cognitive-emotive dissonance is poorly handled in psychotherapy, patient/clients are likely to drop out or become noncompliant.

Conditioning The process of learning in which an innate behavioral response to a learned or innate stimulus becomes a new behavioral response to a formerly neutral stimulus, after that neutral stimulus has been paired a sufficient number of times with the original, learned or innate stimulus. There are two major types of conditioning: (1) Classical (Pavlovian or respondent) conditioning wherein the behavioral response being learned is an innate response for a neutral stimulus such as salivating to the sound of a bell. (2) Operant (Skinnerian or instrumental) conditioning wherein the behavior being learned is new for the subject.

Discrimination The process wherein a subject reacts appropriately to only one, of two or more similar, but different stimuli.

Drive A force that activates or impels people or animals to make a behavioral response. In behavioristic terms, drives are the results of physiologic deprivations, such as of food and water, or the result of pain or some other unpleasant stimulus.

Emotive Imagery The mental process of visualizing real or imaged events so vividly that the person reacts with the most logical emotional and/or physical response for the meaning that those mental pictures have for that person. In behavior therapy, emotive imagery is called mental practice.

Extinction The process wherein the frequency of a learned response to a conditioned stimulus decreases and ultimately disappears, due to lack of reinforcement.

Magic An imaginary but empirically nonexistent power that can exempt real events from the rule of nature that an event occurs only after its essentials for existing have been met.

Magical Thinking Thinking that describes only nonempirical illusions of realities or reality.

Punishment Any undesirable consequence of the subject's behavioral response in a specific situation that decreases (ideally to zero) the probability of that response occurring in similar future situations.

Reinforcement A process of increasing the probability (ideally to 100%) that a specific behavior will be repeated in similar future situations. The two classes are: positive and negative. (1) *Positive reinforcement* occurs when a subject receives or experiences a personally pleasant event, that is, a reward as the consequence of its specific, immediately preceding behavior. The object or experience received is a *positive reinforcer* for the behavior that preceded it. (2) *Negative reinforcement* occurs when a subject receives an unpleasant stimulus that results in a behavioral response that terminates or removes that stimulus. The unpleasant stimulus for the behavior that terminated it is a *negative reinforcer*. The unpleasant simulus is called an *aversive stimulus*. The event of termination or removal of an aversive stimulus is a positive reinforcer—also called a *secondary reinforcer*—for the behavior that immediately preceded that terminating event.

Response and Stimulus Generalization The process wherein a neutral stimulus that is similar to, but different from, a conditioned stimulus elicits the same responses that the original or conditioned stimulus elicits, without having been previously paired with either. Generalization of response is the process wherein the same response is learned to different stimuli.

Stimulus A sensory event that elicits a response from a subject. The two types of stimuli are: (1) Innate or unconditioned stimuli, which elicit only natural or innate responses from a subject such as salivation when exposed to food, and (2) learned or conditioned stimuli, which elicit the responses that innate or learned stimuli elicit, but only after having been paired several times with the real or conditioned stimulus when they elicit their normal target responses.

There are varying opinions about the best way to define **BEHAVIOR THERAPY.** However, most health professionals accept Eysenck's definition: Behavior therapy is the attempt to alter human behavior and emotions in a beneficial way according to the laws of *modern learning theory.* There is only one problem with that definition: There is no generally recognized comprehensive learning theory of human behavior.

Consequently, from a phenomenological view point, behavior therapy has the following three objective appearances. First, behavior therapy is a general field of health improvement that deals with learned, undesirable emotional and physical behavioral responses. But these undesirable responses have been practiced so much that they have become personal habits. However, the people who have these undesirable habits believe that they have little or no satisfactory control over them. That is why these habits are often the main behavioral barriers to personally satisfying lives for their owners. Second, as a field of health improvement, behavior therapy consists of a diverse collection of many different behavioral (as opposed to medicinal) regimens. Each regimen has a name and is proclaimed to be based on laws of the yet-to-be-identified modern learning theory. Without a comprehensive unifying learning theory however, behavior therapy will not soon become the genuine health science discipline that it is incorrectly assumed to already be.

Third, the behavior therapy field has a generally unrecognized or generally ignored crisis of disunity. It is quite similar to (if not the same as) the crisis of disunity that Staats recently (1990) described in psychology, the "surrogate mother" of behavior therapy. But unlike the rigidly divided field of psychology, behavior therapy has reached the threshold of identifying one unifying learning theory of human behavior that will enable it to immediately become a genuine health science discipline.

I. EARLY HISTORICAL ROOTS OF BEHAVIOR THERAPY

Attempts to help people solve behavioral problems, with maneuvers similar to those used in today's behavior therapy have a long history. Pliny the Elder, in first-century Rome tried to cure alcohol abuse by putting putrid spiders in the drinking glasses of alcohol abusers. Today that maneuver would be called *aversive conditioning.* The eighteenth-century "Wild Boy of Averyron" was taught spoken language with maneuvers that today would be called *modeling, prompting, positive reinforcement,* and/or *withholding of positive reinforcers.* A nineteenth-century equivalent of today's prison warden, Alexander Maconchi, used what today would be called a *point system* or a *token economy* as the main basis for getting inmates of a

Royal British penal colony to obey the prison rules. In the same century a French physician treated a case of obsessional thoughts with maneuvers that today would be called *thought stoppage* and/or *reciprocal inhibition*. Still, as a field of health improvement, behavior therapy is less than fifty years old.

The direct history of behavior therapy is inextricably interwoven with the history of psychology, which was its surrogate mother. Psychology resulted from the intellectual revolution of a group of scientifically minded European philosophers. They abandoned philosophy and started psychology, the science of the structure of the mind and consciousness. From their research focus came the name or their school of psychology: Structuralism. Their main research technique was structured, personal introspection. Their goal was to make psychology a "pure" natural science, on an equal "footing" with the other natural sciences. They were the first experimental psychologists; but they showed no interest in investigating human behavioral health problems.

Wilhelm Wundt started the structuralistic psychology in Germany. After training with him, Edward R. Titchener brought structuralism to America in the late nineteenth century. Passive, structured introspection of one's own mind, however, proved to be unproductive. Envy of the natural scientists soon developed among American psychologists, because unlike psychologists, the natural scientists had concrete, objectively observable constructs. Those constructs could be manipulated with satisfying predictable and reportable results. Those results could be recognized and objectively replicated, and they could produce honors and recognition for the scientists who discovered them. The charismatic Cattell, of the psychology laboratory at the prestigious Columbia University, continually made this boast. The research in his laboratory was as independent of introspection as was in the research in physics or zoology. The rapidly increasing general professional interest in doing that type of research led to the first American psychological rebellion, which occurred early in the twentieth century.

A. The Results of That Rebellion

The main result was the production of three new schools of American psychology: *Gestalt, Behavioralism, and Functionalism.* Each school had these two goals: (1) to effectively eliminate the other schools, by making their school synonymous with American psychology, plus (2) to put American psychology on as firm a scientific basis as were the natural sciences.

However, there still was no stated interest in treating behavioral health problems. That was probably due to this reality: At that time, people were usually thought of as belonging to one of only four groups: (1) normal people, that is people in everyday life situations; (2) insane people, such as inmates of those foreboding stone fortresses called insane asylums or "nut houses"; (3) criminals, such as inmates of prisons or jails; and (4) medically ill people, such as patients of physicians. There was no recognized need then for a health field devoted to behavioral health improvement.

The Functionalists seemed to have been the most well organized of the three new psychological schools. In addition, they had decided to switch their research focus from passively observing the subjective structure of a passive mind, to observing the contents of active minds at work in every day life. That interest might have led to a later psychotherapeutic focus. However, neither the Functionalist nor the other two schools attracted much attention. That was probably due largely to the aggressively attacking and rejecting stance the behaviorists took toward the other schools of psychology. The behaviorists were led by the charismatic, proselytizing behavioral psychologist named John B. Watson. He had become a strong enthusiast of the idea of making Pavlovian conditioning the basis for behavioral psychology.

II. IMPORTANT BEHAVIORISTS AND THEIR CONTRIBUTIONS

A. Ivan P. Pavlov and Classical Conditioning

Ivan P. Pavlov (1849–1936), the Russian physician and physiologist, and 1904 Nobel Prize laureate, serendipitously discovered *classical* or *respondent conditioning* in the late nineteenth century. Here is the standard procedure for producing it. First, select a neutral stimulus and an animal (human or nonhuman), for example, a dog. Animals often respond with a startle response to unusual stimuli. So, it is important to make sure that a selected stimulus is really neutral, that is, one the animal normally ignores. Common neutral stimuli used for conditioning are a light or the sound of a bell or buzzer. To ensure that it is neutral for the selected animal, the stimulus is repeatedly presented to the animal until it is consistently ignored. That maneuver is called *stimulus habituation,* or *adaptation.*

Next, select an innate, or *unconditioned stimulus*—that is, anything to which the dog has an innate response is appropriate. Common examples are food for the salivation response or electric shock for the escape response. Then, a bell or buzzer is sounded a second or two before giving the hungry dog food or before giving a satiated dog an electric shock. After several such pairings of those two stimuli, the hungry dog will salivate and the satiated dog will run away from the sound of the bell or buzzer alone. That event indicates that classical conditioning of the unconditioned stimulus' response to be a response to the formerly neutral stimulus has occurred. Then the same response will occur in response to either stimulus.

1. Drawbacks of Early Pavlovian Conditioning Theory

There were three major drawbacks in early Pavlovian Conditioning Theory: (1) Except for salivation and fear, Pavlovians ignored the other autonomic nervous system responses. That fact severely limited the variety of learned behaviors that they could study. (2) It could not explain in empirically accurate ways active and passive escape or avoidance behaviors and some of the behavioral results of punishment. Yet, those learned behaviors and the consequences of punishment are as important for survival and enjoyable living as are approach behaviors. (3) The technical aspects of Pavlovian conditioning were much more complex than those of the main competing learning theory: namely, Thorndike's reward-based, trial and error, learning-by-doing theory of behavior. Largely because of Watson's inflexible commitment to it, Pavlovian conditioning became one of the two main focuses of the behaviorists.

B. John B. Watson and Radical Behaviorism

Starting in the second decade of the twentieth century, John B. Watson (1878–1958) led American behaviorists in continual rebellion against the other schools of psychology. The behaviorists' canons were: (1) Behaviorism, a term coined by Watson, maintains that the concept of consciousness is merely an undefinable replacement of the religious concept of soul and therefore completely rejects it. (2) Behaviorism is a clean break with all of the current theories and traditional psychological terminology that do not describe directly observable responses. (3) Behavior is best explained in terms of reward and punishment learning or in terms of Pavlovian conditioning of the stimulus-response (S-R) reflexes of the subject's nervous system. Watson even believed that human language learning was best explained on the basis of spinal reflexes. On that point, Watson was more of a reflexologist than a behaviorist.

Watson was not the first one to see the positive scientific potential of focusing on Pavlov's conditioned reflexes. In his 1890 book, *Principles of Psychology,* William James wrote a chapter titled *"The Functions of the Brain."* There he described the case history of a child who had become afraid to touch a candle after having been burned by one. James' description of the child's presumed brain activity revealed a conceptual grasp of some such phenomenon as conditioning. Also, in his 1896 psychological article, *"The Reflex Arch Concept in Psychology,"* John Dewey stated his dissatisfaction about the lack of a unifying theory in psychology. He also stated his belief that Pavlov's concept of the reflex arch came closest to meeting the unifying need of psychology than any other current concept. But unlike Pavlov, who believed that activity of cerebral reflexes was important in behavioral learning, Watson rejected all reflex action that was higher in the nervous system than the spinal reflex.

Watson is best remembered for the 1920 case study of Little Albert that he and Rosalie Rayner did. They conditioned that 11-month-old infant to have an irrational fear response to furry animals. As the unconditioned stimulus they used the infantile startle response to an unexpected loud noise. That was the first confirmation of Pavlov's theory in America, using a human subject.

Little Albert spontaneously *generalized* his fear response to furry animals to other furry objects, for example, to furry articles of clothing. But he did not exhibit fear in response to nonfurry objects of clothing. It remains a mystery why that observation of *stimulus discrimination* did not lead Watson to make this insight: Little Albert could not have made the above stimulus discrimination without possessing the faculty of consciousness. Still, Watson and Rayner's work made it seem logical to assume that irrational fears could probably be eliminated by induced extinction. So with Watson's encouragement, Mary Cover Jones, one of his graduate students, successfully investigated that possibility.

To induce fear extinction, Jones subjected abnormally fearful children to a combination of behavioral conditioning maneuvers. The two most effective ones were *social imitation* (now called *modeling*) and what she called *direct conditioning*, which, 30 years later Wolpe called *counterconditioning* and *reciprocal inhibition*. For direct conditioning, Jones would gradually present to irrationally fearful children their feared object, while they were enjoying their favorite food. The effectiveness of this maneuver depended upon Jones making sure that the children always experienced stronger pleasant sensations from eating than fearful ones in response to the gradually presented, feared animal or object. For modeling, Jones would have the fearful child watch and join peers, fearlessly playing with the feared animal or object.

Watson did more to popularize behaviorism as an area of scientific study than any of his contemporary behaviorists. Still Watson's positive influence on behaviorism came more from his excellent public speaking and writing skills than from his research. Consequently, his admirer, Herrnstein, made this summary statement in his introduction to the posthumous edition of Watson's book, *Comparative Psychology*: "Watson's importance to behavioral psychology was more sociological than substantive."

C. Edward L. Thorndike: Reward Learning Theory

Edward L. Thorndike (1874–1949), was the most influential non-Pavlovian American behaviorist in the first three decades of the twentieth century. His popular 1898 book, *Animal Intelligence,* made him one of the earliest internationally renowned American psychologists. However, his subsequent work had a lasting effect on American psychology mainly because it was the professional "springboard" for the research of B. F. Skinner. Skinner was Thorndike's most famous and productive student.

Thorndike's theory was: When, by trial and error, hungry or thirsty rats behave in ways that result in them receiving food or water, the tendency to have that behavior in similar future situations is increased. Conversely, if a specific behavioral habit-reflex of a rat is punished enough with an electric shock, the ten-

dency to have that behavior is decreased and or extinguished. Or, an untrained rat will quickly learn avoidance behavior in response to those shocks.

Thorndike used a puzzle box—later called the Skinner box—in which trial and error, *reward-based learning research* was done using food- or water-deprived rats. The rats were rewarded with food or water immediately after making the appropriate behavioral responses in the experimental conditions. Thorndike also used satiated rats, to which he gave an electric shock immediately after inappropriate behavioral responses.

Unlike Pavlov, Thorndike had no interest in neuronal reflexes. For Thorndike (and later for Skinner) the stimulus-response (S-R) reflex was merely the statistical correlation of specific responses with immediately following rewards and/or punishments. Although Thorndike and Pavlov had different concepts of the behavioral stimulus-response (S-R) reflex, both theories seemed to explain approach behavior equally well. Unfortunately, each theory was equally incapable of explaining avoidance learning and some of the effects of punishment on learning in a way that accurately fit the human experience of them.

D. Burrhus F. Skinner and Operant Conditioning

Burrhus F. Skinner (1904–1990), extended, modified and perfected Thorndike's reward learning theory as *operant conditioning*. In Skinner's 1953 book with Lindsley and Solomon, the term *behavior therapy* was introduced into the psychology literature. Skinner however, had worked with nonhuman animals; so that term may have been used in reference to the past work of Mary Cover Jones. It may also have referred to the exciting new, non-Freudian hypothesis of Joseph Wolpe that neurotic fears are learned and can be efficiently treated with behavioral treatments.

Like Watson, Skinner was committed to *radical behaviorism*. He too rejected traditional psychology and all of its concepts that implied what he called *mentalism*. That meant any concept that reflected a belief in cause/effect relationships between mental entities or activities and learned behavior. In the 1966 edition of his 1928 book, *The Behavior of Organisms,* Skinner still labeled the belief that emotions are important factors in behavior a "mental fiction." He agreed with William James' assertion that "people are sorry because they cry," or that "people are afraid because they tremble." In addition, they both believed it is incorrect, or at least unscientific, to think that people cry because they are sorry or tremble because they are afraid.

To my knowledge, James' assertion has no clinical application. But, believing in that assertion is a common cause of clinical problems. For example, people who believe they are their behavior often get clinically depressed when they believe that one or two undesirable personal actions "magically change them as human beings." Such students often get depressed and quit school after 1 or 2 days of seriously thinking that they are complete failures because they failed to get the grades that they wanted. However, such thoughts and emotions cannot be directly observed; so, according to Skinnerians, to be "scientific," psychotherapists must ignore those important factors when they treat such depressions or try to get those students to stay in school. Next is the logic of their often futile treatments.

Skinner maintained that emotions are not behavioral responses; instead they are states of reflex strength, similar to drives. According to Skinner, the virtue of understanding emotions that way is that behavioral scientists can ignore them "whenever that concept loses its convenience." However, as we shall see below, Mowrer's research revealed that Skinner's ideas about emotions do not make logical sense, even for nonhuman animals. That fact is all the more interesting because Skinner's research subjects were almost all nonhuman animals—usually rats and pigeons. However, to Skinner's credit, he never advised the extrapolation of his animal research findings to human beings. As late as 1960, he warned that whether or not extrapolation of his research discoveries to people is justified cannot yet be decided. The behavioristic psychologists who introduced operant conditioning into behavior therapy were justifiably impressed by Skinner's research. But, they either did not know or ignored that nonhuman brains cannot and therefore do not process sensory input the same way that human brains process it. Therefore, even in the same stimulus situations, it is still naive to expect humans to respond exactly the way rats or pigeons respond.

I. Skinner's Most Positive and Most Negative Influences on Behavior Therapy

Probably Skinner's most positive influence on behavior therapy was his research about how different *schedules of reinforcements* significantly influence the speed of learning new behavioral habits and their resistance to extinctions. For example a fixed 1:1 ratio of an immediate reward or reinforcement for each appropriate response produces the fastest acquisition of new habits for a given, constant drive level. But those habits are most susceptible to rapid extinction if the response/reinforcer ratio increases or the reinforcers cease to appear.

If behavior therapists are skilled in managing relevant reinforcement intervals and ratios, their cooperative patients/clients will maintain high levels of motivation for therapeutic change. Also, in the world of paid work, if managers are skilled in varying reinforcement intervals and ratios, employees will maintain high morale and productivity with minimal or no increases in company budgets. *Contingency management* is the name of such goal-oriented changes in reinforcement schedules and ratios.

The sustained, high productivity that the 1:1 ratio produces is the main reason some employers prefer a piecework pay schedule over an hourly or other fixed interval pay schedule that is independent of behavioral response rate. Within the limits of a constant drive state, a variable ratio and/or variable interval reinforcement schedule produces behavioral habits that are most resistant to extinction. For example, the gambler continues to bet despite losses because reinforcement—payoff—may occur any time.

Probably the most negative influence Skinner had on behavior therapy was his empirically unjustified defense of his unreliable definition of behavior. He maintained that behavior is only what one organism observes another organism doing. Because Skinner studied nonhuman animals, he had no logical reason to be concerned about a human test of empirical common sense. Had Skinner had this concern, he might have defined behavior in a way that has a greater than 50% chance of being correct, in any specific instance.

For example, with personal observation alone, a behavior X (1) may be X and may be correctly observed and labeled as X; (2) a non-X behavior may appear not to be behavior X and be correctly observed and labeled as not being behavior X; but (3) behavior X may appear to be some other behavior, for example, Z and may be incorrectly observed and incorrectly labeled as behavior Z; (4) behavior Z can appear to be behavior X and be observed as, and incorrectly labeled as behavior X. A 50% error possibility is insufficient for scientific conclusions. Also,

Skinner's definition of behavior leads to unsuspected magical thinking.

For example, in the textbook *Contemporary Behavior Therapy* by Spiegler and Guevremont, this statement appears: "The behaviorist's model for behavior is: "People are what they do." In reality, though, only by magic can making a stupid mistake convert a human being into a stupid person, or swimming like a fish convert a human being into a fish. That is not just a matter of semantics; when one wants to describe behavior in clinically useful, scientific terms, it is all semantics. When scientists ignore that fact, they sometimes use unsuspected magical thinking to describe empirically valid research findings. As a result they misinterpret their data and formulate useless treatment procedures. That is why Mowrer's research was so important for the development of today's comprehensive behavior therapy.

E. O. Hobart Mowrer and Two-Factor Learning

More than the research and writings of any other single pioneer, behavioral psychologist, those of O. Hobart Mower made contemporary, comprehensive behavior therapy possible. He believed that to be clinically useful, any explanation of human behavior has to pass the human test of empirical common sense. Consequently, Mowrer was intrigued by this paradox: Watson was accepted as the quintessential empirical scientist. Yet the basis for Watson's behaviorist revolution against then-contemporary American psychology was mainly his unchecked belief about the concept of consciousness. He believed that consciousness is an undefinable, meaningless substitute for the ancient concept of soul.

But what if Watson had plugged Little Albert's ears (thereby eliminating his sound consciousness) prior to making the sudden loud noises to condition him to be afraid of furry objects)? That would have been the simple first step in a scientific check of his assumption. But he did not take it. The authors believe that if he had taken that simple step, instead of rejecting the concept of consciousness he might have operationally defined it (and its opposite state of being) in clinically useful terms.

Another observation that intrigued Mowrer was this: When he analyzed the research of the Skinnerians on avoidance behavior, he found their research was

carefully done and their data were valid. Their theoretical explanations of that excellent data, however, involved presumably unsuspected but definite magical thinking. That unsuspected magical thinking obscured the invalidity of the basic Skinnerian assumption that directly observable behavior itself is the only factor worthy of scientific study.

That view is called the one-factor stimulus-response (S-R) model of learned behavior. The following common conditioning experiment reveals the serious limitation of that assumption. Take, for example, a dog that has been conditioned with strong electric shocks to run away in response to the sound of a formerly neutral buzzer, which had been sounded within 2 seconds of those shocks. After four consecutive running responses occurred before the electric shock could be administered, the shocks were permanently stopped. Why then does this dog continue running away from the sound of the buzzer?

Here is the Skinnerian answer. The painful electric shock is an unconditioned aversive stimulus. The unconditioned drive states of pain and fear result from painful aversive stimuli. The dog's running responses terminated the dog's pain, and the fear that accompanied the sound or the buzzer. That freedom from those two intense stimuli is a powerful, positive reinforcer of the terminating running responses at the sound of the buzzer. But, according to Skinner, the fear (not being directly observable) could and should be ignored. The only factors worthy of scientific study were the directly observable running responses, the observable buzzer sounds and the strong, unconditioned, electric shocks.

By occurring within 2 seconds of the dog being shocked, that buzzer sound acquired an aversive property "in its own right." That acquired aversive property made the buzzer sound capable of eliciting the same running responses that the unconditioned stimulus (i.e., the electric shock) elicits. That is why the buzzer sound was then called a conditioned or secondary aversive stimulus. Also, each of the dog's running responses ended with the dog receiving the above powerful, positive reinforcements for running. That fixed 1:1 response/reinforcer schedule is the most powerful way to produce a behavioral habit and to maintain it.

That Skinnerian explanation is logical and believable; but it's also magical. Therefore, it can not pass the human test of empirical common sense. The magical component is the statement: "that buzzer sound acquired an aversive property in its own right." The empirical answer to the following question, however, reveals that that could have happened only if magic existed. What would happen if the first dog and a second, unshocked dog were to be exposed together to that buzzer sound, with its assumed "acquired aversive quality"? Unless some magical power protected the second dog, both dogs would experience and run from the "aversive quality" of the buzzer sound. In reality, though, only the first dog would run. The second dog would ignore the buzzer sound. Since magic does not exist, the only empirical explanation is that the buzzer sound had not acquired an aversive quality. Next is the evidence that supports that fact.

What would happen if the previously shocked dog were prevented from running from the buzzer sound and that dog was never shocked again? That first dog's running response would quickly extinguish and the dog would begin to ignore the buzzer, as the second, unshocked dog would have done from the beginning. Only by nonexistent magic could failure to run from a buzzer sound remove an empirically existing aversive quality of that sound. Since the concept of magic is incompatible with a scientific explanation of an event, this scientific conclusion seems obvious: The buzzer sound never acquired and never had any aversive quality.

But, it could be asked, if having been paired with electric shocks did not result in that originally neutral buzzer sound acquiring an aversive quality "in its own right," why did the first dog continue to run from it? Next is Mowrer's nonmagical, Two-Factor Learning Theory explanation of the above events and the empirically objective answer to that question.

First, it is an empirical fact that: (1) Dogs have an innate autonomic nervous system response called salivation, which is a conditionable response to associated, external sensory entities. Dogs also have autonomic nervous system responses called emotivities, which are both conditionable to associated, sensory entities and are a part of every physical behavioral response to these sensory entities. Mowrer's Two-Factor Learning Theory describes those facts this way: Stimulus, emotive response, Observable Response, or S-er-OR.

With the above shocked dog, the sensory entities were the buzzer sound, the painful electric shock, and

the emotive response, called fear. Just as hunger is an unconditioned drive for behavioral responses that terminate it, pain, via any aversive stimulus, is an unconditioned drive for behavioral responses that terminate it and its associated sensory entities. In the case of pain, the reducing and terminating behavioral response was the dog's act of running away.

The brains of normal mammals are genetically structured to include emotive responses of the autonomic nervous system in their processing of all sensory data. The innate emotive response of the autonomic nervous system to pain is fear. Fear is also an unconditioned drive for behavioral responses that terminate it. By the dog hearing a buzzer sound immediately before receiving the unconditioned pain of an electric shock, an involuntary, mental, mnemonic association resulted in that dog's brain between these sensory events: the buzzer sound, the immediately following painful electric shock, and the fear that normally accompanies pain. So, instead of the buzzer sound acquiring "an aversive property in its own right," it merely became a learned mnemonic sign or cue that fearfully alerted the dog that a painful shock was an immediately possibility.

After such a sign or cue learning experience, this happens: When the dog perceives the same or similar, future mnemonic signs or cues, part of the biolectrical component of that sensory entity stimulates its autonomic nervous system to the possibility that a fearful pain seems likely to occur. The learned buzzer cue instantly (i.e., with the speed of electricity) elicits fear, which is a drive for the old running response that had formerly protected that dog from the past electric shocks that had quickly followed past buzzer sounds. That running response still results in the same two, powerful, positive reinforcers described above.

Now, recall the second, unshocked dog mentioned earlier. Having "never been shocked," that second dog would not have learned that the buzzer sound had been associated with a painful electrical shock. Therefore, that second dog would ignore the buzzer sound, even though the first dog would continue to run from it. But, the buzzer sound itself never would have acquired any aversive property. Instead, the first dog's autonomic nervous system would have just become conditioned to instantly produce survival-related fear as a second stimulus to the pain of the electric shock as a drive for running at the perception of the learned mnemonic cue for the possibility of another electric shock.

Here is the final major difficulty that is created by assuming that the buzzer sound had acquired an aversive quality "in its own right." That assumption makes it difficult, if not impossible, to explain in a nonmagical way how natural extinction of the dog's running response occurs after the shocks permanently stop. However, Mowrer's nonmagical, Two-Factor Learning Theory easily explains it in an empirically scientific way.

An unconditioned pain drive for running occurs only when the peripheral pain fibers of the sensory area of the dog's brain are stimulated. At the same time that occurs, the dog's autonomic nervous system produces a fear drive for running away from the electric shock. Via involuntary, mnemonic association with any immediately preceding, neutral stimulus (in this case, a buzzer sound) that stimulus can become a conditioned (i.e., learned) sign or cue for the fear component of the total escape response. Afterwards, the mere perception of that sign or cue is a mnemonic stimulus for the dog's autonomic nervous system to produce that old fear drive for running.

The intensity of such fear tends to parallel the intensity of the unconditioned pain drive that precedes it. The intensity of that fear also parallels the strength of the total positive reinforcing power of the freedom from pain and fear, which reinforces the running response that terminates the fear and prevents the painful shock. Therefore, when the shocks stop, at least half of the most powerful positive reinforcement for running also instantly stops.

The physical distress and fatigue from intense running is itself an unconditioned pain event. But that discomfort, in comparison to the pain of an electric shock, is and remains trivial and ignored until the shocks stop. Then, the only drive for running is the rapidly decreasing, unsupplemented fear, cued by the buzzer sound. Now, the initially ignored physical distress and fatigue of intense running rapidly become progressively stronger punishments for continued running responses. That fact causes the decreasing, unsupplemented fear drive for running to gradually extinguish and the dog's running to stop.

In analogous ways Mowrer's Two-Factor Learning Theory also explains why and how any specific sensory stimuli (which a human or nonhuman animal mnemonically associates in appropriate sequence with painful or pleasant events) can become learned signs or cues for learned behaviors that are associated with those events. But, that explanation applies only to animals that have first had the appropriate mnemonic sign learning experience.

Humans, however, can and often do exempt themselves from that naturally occurring behavioral extinction that nonanimals normally experience. Jones' research on excessively fearful children was probably the first to reveal that fact. She noted that when re-exposure to the unconditioned aversive stimulus stopped, her human subjects' conditioned fears sometimes failed to extinguish. This indicated that nonhuman brains do not work exactly like human brains work. Modern human research on the neuro-psychophysiology of language indicates that the above difference in brain functions is probably due to these facts: Humans are the only known animals that have the faculties of self-talk (i.e., thinking about their own thinking). Humans are also the only known animals that can imagine or re-create at will mental, emotional, and physical virtual realities, independently of current or past empirical life events. That is how and why people's imagined events can be as powerful emotional and physical stimuli for habit learning as corresponding empirical life events are, or can be.

That unique human ability seems to best explain the following fact: Pavlov did not report a single dog that ever tried to eat the bell used in its conditioning experiences. Yet, humans often incorrectly call themselves and others names (such as "jackass" or "mouse") that do not refer to any real human things; then without realizing it, they condition themselves to react emotionally and physically to themselves (and to those others) as if they really are the nonexistent things to which their incorrect names refer. (See the Mouse Lady case example in the book *Rational Behavior Therapy*.) That universally popular human habit seems to be an important mental mechanism in many cases of self-mutilation and unprovoked hate crimes.

I. Mowrer's Most Important Contributions to a Unified Field of Behavior Therapy

1. Mowrer's firmly supported Two-Factor Learning Theory made this fact obvious: If consciousness and emotions had not already existed, equivalent con-

cepts would have had to be invented to serve their essential survival functions.

2. Empirical evidence that classical or respondent conditioning is the only type. In addition, during the conditioning process, the former "neutral" stimulus never acquires a new property. Instead, it becomes the subject's new, conditioned sign or cue for associated learned autonomic nervous system responses to that formerly "neutral" stimulus.

3. Empirical evidence that there are two types of behavioral learning: (1) operant or instrumental and (2) sign or cue learning. But they both are byproducts of associated, conditioned impelling emotional drives (e.g., fear, hope, anger, etc.) or other responses controlled by the brain's autonomic nervous system.

4. Empirical evidence that the main survival functions of learned behavioral signs and cues seem to be alerting the concerned subjects to possible positive or negative changes in their current situation and to help them prepare for possibly needed self-protective or other survival related actions.

5. Mowrer demonstrated that Pavlov was correct. Personally understood words are entirely real conditioned stimuli; they substitute for and elicit the same responses that are elicited by the real or imagined stimuli that they represent. Therefore, psychotherapy is word therapy, designed to change the person's internal milieu, that is, to change certain of the person's undesirable, habitual autonomic nervous system responses. That fact makes vicarious learning and extinction of behaviors possible. It also makes therapeutic imagery the main mental mechanisms by which permanent therapeutic improvement occurs.

6. Empirical evidence that via their control over their conscious thoughts, people retain executive-type controlling power over their emotional and physical behavioral responses. That insight enables empirically thinking people to instantly take these two ideally healthy, emotional actions at the same time: First, refuse to believe any longer in the universally popular, but magical and unhealthy "emotional It-monster myth." Second, stop the unsuspected, but still unhealthy emotional self-abuse that believing in that magical emotional myth causes them to experience.

The most easily recognized forms of that unhealthy emotional myth are the frequent, sincere, but irrational thoughts and accusations such as: "It or she/he made or makes me mad, sad, glad," and so on. The

empirical reality almost always is: "I made or make me mad, sad, glad, and so on, about it or what she/he is doing or did. If I want to however, I can change my belief about what they did, or are doing and thereby give myself a healthier emotional reaction to it, without using alcohol or other drugs."

III. BEHAVIOR THERAPY AT THE THRESHOLD OF IDEAL UNIFICATION

A scientific discipline cannot exist without a comprehensive, empirically valid, unifying theory. To unify the field of behavioral health improvement, a theory must be based on and/or meet at least five or the following seven sets of empirical facts and criteria.

1. The human brain is a person's main organ of survival, comfort and learned self-control.

2. The theory must make possible clinically useful explanations of both healthy and unhealthy learned behaviors, which are also based on well-established medical facts about relevant normal brain functions.

3. Human cognitive, emotional and physical behaviors interact in this hierarchical way. Coincident with the onset of correct spoken and unspoken human language, the cognitive behaviors (i.e. the brain's mental activities) instantly take executive type, control over human emotional and physical behaviors.

4. To be generally useful, a learning theory of human behavior must explain both healthy and unhealthy learned behaviors in terms of empirical, cause/effect relationships, with the cognitive activities having ultimate control of the emotional and physical behaviors.

5. Unless they are medically or psychiatrically indicated, drugs are to be excluded from the treatments of learned behavioral problems.

6. The maneuvers in behavior therapy must reflect the above-mentioned hierarchical relationships between groups of behaviors.

7. The theory must make possible accurate predictions of treatment outcomes in terms of temporary or permanent replacements of unhealthy cognitive, emotive, and physical habits with personally acceptable, healthy ones.

Space limitations in this article permit only the discussion of pioneers in the behavior therapy field whose conceptual and technical contributions reflect at least five of these seven criteria.

A. Joseph Wolpe and Systematic Desensitization

In the early 1950s, this South African psychiatrist became dissatisfied with the poor therapeutic results he was getting from treating his patients with psychoanalysis. But, at that time there was no credible alternative psychotherapy in South Africa. So, as a psychotherapeutic rebellion, Wolpe combined his medical training with his understanding of behavioral learning theory and made these two important achievements: (1) He created a medically credible, non-Freudian hypothesis of the origin of neurotic fears. (2) He formulated behavioral maneuvers for treating those neurotic fears. Wolpe's behavioral treatment maneuvers were a major contribution to the beginning of behavior therapy as a recognized field of human behavioral research and systematic, mental and emotional health improvement.

Wolpe's most popular treatment maneuver was called *systematic desensitization*. It is a combination of *deep muscular relaxation* and an effective technique of *emotive imagery*. The latter had been formulated and tested by Arnold A. Lazarus, then a psychologist, student/colleague of Wolpe and later a behavior therapist of international acclaim. A typical treatment session is an hour in which patient/clients first self-induce a state of deep muscle relaxation, followed by the therapist verbally pacing them in imagining events on a prepared list of feared objects or events. Starting with the least fearful event, patient/clients are to maintain their initial state of deep muscular relaxation as the therapist verbally paces them up the list to the target fear. If, however, the patient/client becomes noticeably anxious during the session, he or she is to terminate that imagery and focus on reestablishing their former relaxed state before resuming those images.

Wolpe quickly surprised the psychiatric field with his demonstrations of the rapid effectiveness of his behavioral treatment maneuvers. He also reported the largest number of human cases that had ever been successfully treated by one therapist. Prior to Wolpe's report behaviorists had annually reported less that three such successfully treated cases.

B. Albert Ellis and Rational Emotive Therapy

Like Wolpe (but without knowledge of his work), in the mid 1950s an internationally renowned American psychologist named Albert Ellis became discouraged because of his poor therapeutic results using psychoanalysis. Again like Wolpe, as a psychotherapeutic rebellion, Ellis developed a highly effective, authoritatively directive method of psychotherapy called Rational Emotive Therapy. The main stimulus for Ellis' new treatment method was the Greek stoic, emotional canon: "People do not get upset by things, but by the view they take of them."

Ellis saw the great psychotherapeutic relevance to that philosophical observation. So, he converted it into his internationally acclaimed, empirical, *ABC model of human emotions*. That model of human emotions has proven to be one of the most clinically useful psychotherapeutic concepts in the twentieth century. In addition, Ellis' ABC model probably made Rational Emotive Therapy the first comprehensive behavior therapy.

In the ABC model of human emotions: A is the activating event, that is, any event to which the person reacts. B is that person's personal belief about that perception. C is that person's emotional response to that A, the activating event. Ellis's ABC model reveals that people's emotional feelings are not caused by the activating events at A. Their emotional feelings are directly caused by their personal beliefs at B about their A-activating events. Ellis reasoned, therefore, that the drug-free, therapeutic way to help people most quickly behave better physically, or to most quickly feel better emotionally at C, is to get them to adopt "better personal beliefs" at B about their A perceptions.

To Ellis, "better personal beliefs" meant beliefs that seem to be the most logical ones for the person's desired new emotional and physical self-management. Ellis called such beliefs rational, and the contrary ones irrational, beliefs. Logically, therefore, Ellis' technique has always focused on getting people to recognize and eliminate their irrational belief systems. That fact probably made Ellis' technique the first cognitive therapy. In fact, Ellis is now recognized by many mental health professionals as the "father" of the cognitive therapeutic movement in behavioral psychology.

Initially, Ellis gave patients/clients and trainees little or no specific empirical guidelines for recognizing and discovering for themselves if their beliefs were rational. Still, the following two features made his method more rapidly and comprehensively effective than the other then-popular psychotherapies seemed to be. (1) Ellis' method encouraged therapists to be active, objective and firmly directive. (2) It also encouraged the effective use in talk therapy of Pavlovian-type verbal conditioning of more rational beliefs than those that seemed to have caused the patients/clients' problems. That feature enabled therapists to rapidly help patients/clients create the new emotional ABCs that produce and maintain the self-management they desired.

The inclusion of Pavlovian type conditioning in Ellis' method was sufficient for Eysenck to classify Ellis' Rational Emotive Therapy as a behavior therapy. In the 1994 revision of his original 1962 "bible" of Rational Emotive Therapy, entitled *Reason and Emotions In Psychotherapy,* Ellis changed the name of his historic therapeutic technique to Rational Emotive Behavior Therapy.

Of course there is much more to Ellis' therapeutic technique than his ABC model of human emotions. But space limitations do not permit their coverage here. However, those unmentioned features all are logically based on or related to his ABC model of human emotions.

Remarkably similar to Ellis' cognitive orientation is Aaron Beck's cognitive therapy. Beck's technique has been proved to be as effective for treating some depressive disorders as is medication. Beck's method has also proved to be more effective than medication for preventing recurrences of those depressive disorders; it therefore prevents the unhealthy medical side effects of long-term drug treatment. [*See* COGNITIVE THERAPY; DEPRESSION.]

C. Maxie C. Maultsby, Jr., and Rational Behavior Therapy (RBT)

While still a psychiatric resident, Maxie C. Maultsby, Jr., studied briefly with Joseph Wolpe in 1967 and with Ellis for the following 7 years. At the 1975 Chicago National Conference of Rational Emotive and Behavior Therapists, Maultsby described his unique method of psychotherapy called Rational Behavior Therapy, or RBT. Then RBT was (and probably still is) the only method of psychotherapy that is based on the well-established facts about the mental activities

of normal human brains that make learning and behavioral self-management possible. That fact was first noted in print by Arnold M. Ludwig, M.D., in the forward of the book *Rational Behavior Therapy.*

Rational Behavior Therapy is based on the psychosomatic learning theory of normal human behavior. Therefore, it takes the most comprehensive behavioral stance: namely that cognitive emotional and physical actions that have not been genetically determined are learned. Consequently, all three of those learned behavioral groups are the most logical, simultaneous focus of psychotherapy. This psychosomatic, human learning theory is one of the few that is based on the fact that normal human brains are genetically programmed to instantly and automatically give people the most healthy and desirable, or the most unhealthy and undesirable emotional and physical behaviors that are most logical for their beliefs and attitudes. The theory is both culture free and as universally applicable to the various learned human behavioral problems as the germ theory is to the various infections. Finally, this theory fulfills all seven sets of the essential empirical criteria (listed earlier) for being an ideal unifying theory of modern behavior therapy.

I. The Main Unique Therapeutic Constructs and Techniques in Rational Behavior Therapy

First are Maultsby's two theoretical models of habitual emotions: the AbC construct for attitude-triggered, habitual emotions, and the aBC construct for belief-triggered habitual emotions. At the neurobioelectrical level, both constructs are logical extensions of Ellis' ABC model of new or not-yet-habitual human emotions. Their two main clinical values are that the aBC belief construct reveals to patients/clients how they have unwittingly taught themselves much of their emotional problems; they will have done it via vicarious, mental practice. But most important, the aBC construct shows them why and how they can use rational beliefs and the same mental process and rapidly achieve the therapeutic success they desire. The AbC attitude construct readily reveals these two instantly helpful clinical facts: (1) How and why people's own attitudes make them instantly and automatically react in their habitual emotional and physical ways, even without initial conscious thoughts of doing it, and (2) Why it is unhealthy, incorrect, and often emotionally self-abusive to accuse "It" (some external event) or some other person of making oneself (or anyone else) have the emotional feelings one habitually has. With their silent (i.e., unspoken) AbC attitudes, people do that to themselves.

2. The Five Rules for Ideally Healthy and, Therefore, Rational Thinking

1. Rational thinking is based on obvious facts.
2. Rational thinking best helps people protect their lives and health.
3. Rational thinking best helps people achieve their own short-term and long-term goals.
4. Rational thinking best helps people avoid their most unwanted conflicts with other people.
5. Rational thinking best helps people feel emotionally the way they want to feel without using alcohol or other drugs.

For thinking (and therefore any learned behavior) to be rational, it only has to obey at least three of these five rules at the same time. Habitually thinking rationally gives people the best probabilities for being as healthy, successful, and happy as they desire to be. There are almost no life situations that cannot be handled better with ideally healthy and, therefore, rational thinking.

3. Written, Rational Self-Analysis (RSA)

This technique facilitates developing skills in instantly and automatically doing two things: (1) Deciding for oneself when it will probably be healthiest and most personally beneficial to instantly respond with positive, negative, or neutral emotional and/or physical behavioral reactions, and (2) when the opposite responses will be healthiest and most personally beneficial.

4. Rational Emotive Imagery (REI)

This technique enables patients/clients to practice at will their desired new emotional and physical behavioral responses. Thereby they decide how rapidly and successfully they achieve their therapeutic goals.

5. The Five Stages of Therapeutic Emotional and Behavioral Reeducation

Psychotherapy means word therapy, without drugs or other medical treatments. Of course, if patients/clients need medication for some existing medical or psychiatric problem, RBT therapists see that they get it. But without medication or electric shock therapy, all therapeutic change is really therapeutic emotional and behavioral reeducation. It occurs in the following five sequential stages, regardless of the type of psychotherapy being used.

First is intellectual insight, or learning what has to be practiced to achieve therapeutic success. Second is the mental and physical practice of the new therapeutic ideas that are essential for learning the desired new emotional and physical habits. Third is cognitive-emotive dissonance (see the glossary). Fourth is emotional insight; patients/clients have it when they begin to have their desired new emotional and physically responses instantly and automatically in their desired situations. Fifth is new personality trait formation. In this case, patients/clients have their desired new emotional and behavioral reactions as instantly and automatically in their desired situations as they formerly had their undesirable emotional and behavioral reactions.

There is much more to RBT than the listed therapeutic models and techniques. For more in-depth knowledge, please refer to the bibliography.

IV. BEHAVIORAL ASSESSMENT AND THE THERAPEUTIC PROCESS

Behavior therapy is designed for and meant to treat only learned behavioral problems. Sometimes, however, medical problems appear to be a learned behavioral problem; sometimes medical and a learned behavioral problems coexist. Before beginning behavior therapy, therefore, it is important for patients/clients to be evaluated to determine if they (1) have a learned behavioral problem alone, or (2) have one plus an unrelated, medical problem, or (3) have a learned behavior problem as a part of a psychosomatic disorder, or (4) have a medical problem that just appears to have been learned.

Behavioral assessment has three other goals: (1) to define the target behavioral problems; (2) to identify the cognitive habits that are maintaining those behavioral problems; and (3) to make it possible to objectively measure therapeutic progress. To best achieve the latter, behavior therapy focuses on the present manifestations of the target problems. But to ensure the most comprehensive therapeutic results, the therapist gets a detailed personal and medical history. Such historical data are easily obtained using standard personal data forms. For the target problem, however, personal interviews by the therapist are essential.

Important information about the target problem includes the following: When were patient/clients free of their problem? What has been the progression of the problem? What makes it better or worse or temporarily disappear? What desirable or undesirable personal experiences does the problem prevent or cause? What are the patient/clients' beliefs about their problem and what are their expectations for therapy? For the most immediately useful clinical understanding of a patient/client's problem, putting these data in Ellis' ABC models of human emotions is invaluable.

Effective behavior therapy produces weekly therapeutic progress. The popular self-assessment and objective behavioral monitoring forms are usually adequate for this purpose. If weekly therapeutic progress is not happening, reassess the patient/client for overlooked medical or psychiatric problems, or for problems with therapeutic involvement or misunderstanding.

V. BEHAVIORAL MEDICINE

Chronic diseases have replaced acute, infectious diseases as the leading causes of death. Those chronic diseases often have cause/effect behavioral relationships with unhealthy behavioral habits such as cigarette smoking, lack of exercise, poor eating habits, substance abuse, and so on. Those facts are the main reasons behavioral medicine is one of the most clinically valuable, recent byproducts of comprehensive behavior therapy. Behavioral medicine has already demonstrated great clinical value in preventing and treating health problems. For example, in recent decades there has been a significant decrease in the death rate for cardiovascular diseases. That decrease resulted largely from people making healthy changes in their personal habits and learning healthier techniques of emotional distress management. [See BEHAVIORAL MEDICINE.]

For more than 25 years oncologist O. Carl Simon-

ton has demonstrated the clinical advantages of treating cancer patients with behavioral techniques. His results have been confirmed in controlled prospective trials by David Spiegel at the UCLA Medical Center, even in patients with metastatic breast cancer. The patients who had received behavioral treatment plus conventional oncological treatment lived twice as long as the patients who had received conventional oncological treatment alone. [See CANCER.]

Recently, the prominent British psychologists Hans Eysenck and Ronald Grossarth-Maticek developed and reported their behavior technique, called Creative Novation Behavior Therapy. They have been using it to treat patients with cancer and cardiovascular disease. Initial treatment results indicate an additional possible potential for improved disease prevention. Further study and attempts to replicate their favorable results are in progress. However, their work is worthy of note because it is consistent with the excellent research by Robert Ader and Nicolas Cohen on conditioning healthy immune responses. The latter research has produced the newest medical subspecialty: *psychoneuroimmunology*—the descriptive label that was coined by Ader. Modern comprehensive behavior therapies have the characteristics that are needed to help psychoneuroimmunology most quickly realize its great potential for mass general health improvement and disease prevention.

BIBLIOGRAPHY

Ader, R., & Felton, D. (1990). *Psychoneuroimmunology II*. San Diego: Academic Press.

Bandura, A. (1986). *Social foundations of thought and action: A social cognitive theory*. Englewood Cliffs, NJ: Prentice-Hall.

Beck, A. T., Rush, A. J., Shaw, B. F., & Emery, G. (1979). *Cognitive therapy of depression*. New York: Guilford.

Ellis, A. (1994). *Reason and emotion in psychotherapy*. New York: Carol Publishing Group.

Masters, J. C., Burish, T. G., Hollon, S.D., & Rimm, D. C. (1987). *Behavior therapy: Techniques and empirical findings*. San Diego: Harcourt Brace Jovanovich, Inc.

Maultsby, Jr., M. C. (1984). *Rational behavior therapy*. Englewood Cliffs, NJ: Prentice-Hall, Inc. 1984.

Spiegler, M.D., & Guevremont D. C. (1993). *Contemporary behavior therapy*. Monterey, CA: Brooks/Cole Publishing Company.

Staats, A. W. (1990). *Psychology's crisis of disunity*. New York: Praeger Publishing Co.

Bereavement

M. Stroebe, W. Stroebe, H. Schut, and J. van den Bout

Utrecht University

Absent Grief A complicated form of grief characterized by the nonappearance during bereavement of overt symptoms typical of grief, coupled with the continuation of life as though the event had not occurred (note that absence of symptomatology does not always indicate mental disorder).

Bereavement The situation of a person who has recently experienced the loss of someone significant through that person's death.

Chronic Grief A complicated form of grief characterized by long-lasting presence of symptoms associated with intense grief (e.g., rumination, preoccupation with thoughts of the deceased, depression) and absence of apparent progress in coming to terms with the loss of a loved one.

Delayed Grief A complicated form of grief in which the individual shows little or no sign of grieving early on in bereavement, but does so at a later point.

Grief The primarily emotional (affective) reaction to the loss of a loved one through death, which incorporates diverse psychological (cognitive, social/behavioral) and physical (physiological/somatic) manifesta-

tions. Grief is a normal reaction to loss, not an illness or psychiatric disorder, although it is associated with higher risks of these disorders.

Grief Counseling The facilitation through counseling of the process (tasks) of normal, uncomplicated grieving to alleviate suffering and help the bereaved to reach a healthy completion within a reasonable time framework.

Grief Therapy Specialized techniques of intervention for bereaved individuals to guide an individual with an abnormal or complicated grief reaction (e.g., chronic or delayed grief) toward a normal coping process.

Grief Work The cognitive process of confronting the reality of a loss through death, of going over events that occurred before and at the time of death, and of focusing on memories and working toward detachment from the deceased.

Mourning The social expressions or acts expressive of grief, which are shaped by the practices of a given society or cultural group (e.g., mourning rituals).

Pathological Grief A deviation from the norm (i.e., that could be expected, according to the extremity of the particular bereavement event) in the time course or intensity of specific or general symptoms of grief (see also chronic, delayed and absent grief). "Complicated grief" is also frequently used to denote such deviation.

BEREAVEMENT is a life event that, while comparatively rare in childhood, sooner or later, is part of nearly everyone's experience: increasingly across the life span, people have to face the death of their parents, siblings, partners, friends, or other close loved ones. Mortality statistics underline this. According to figures compiled in the 1980s, in one single year in the United States alone, more than 2 million people can be expected to die. Infant mortality rates are estimated at 40,000 a year, while more than 16,000 children between the ages of 1 and 14 and as many as 38,000 young people between the ages of 15 and 24 lose their lives. As such, bereavement can be viewed as a normal, natural human experience, one that most people manage to come to terms with over the course of time. Nevertheless, it is associated with a period of intense suffering for the majority of people and with an increased risk of mental and physical health detriments. Adjustment can take months or even years, and is subject to substantial variation, both between individuals and between different cultural groups. Furthermore, while most people eventually recover from their grief and its accompanying symptoms, for a few, mental and physical ill health is extreme and persistent. For this reason, bereavement is a concern not only for the planning of preventive care, but one that is of clinical relevance. It has far-reaching implications too for well-being within families (e.g., potential long-term effects on mental health of losing a parent in childhood; increased frequency of divorce among parents who have lost a child) and for policy making at governmental level (e.g., economic support programs). Over the past few decades, scientific study of the symptomatology, mental and physical health consequences, and ways of coping with grief has continuously expanded. This research—in the past (although this is changing now), mainly on adults, and focused on spousal bereavement—is working toward the identification of persons early in bereavement who are likely to suffer detrimental consequences, and toward designing programs to provide preventive care for those most at risk. Headway has also been made in developing intervention programs for persons suffering from complicated forms of grief. The current state of knowledge with respect to the consequences and care of the bereaved is the focus of this article.

I. INTRODUCTION

Bereavement refers to the situation of a person who has recently experienced the loss of someone significant—notably a parent, partner, sibling, or child—

through that person's death. In everyday language, the term bereavement is used interchangeably with grief or mourning. Conceptual distinctions have, however, been made in the bereavement and emotion literatures to differentiate these terms. Thus, grief is taken to be the primarily emotional reaction to the loss of a loved one, while at the same time it is recognized as incorporating a myriad of psychological and physical reactions. Negative affect is dominant, particularly in the early days of loss, although this is balanced by more positive emotional reactions such as relief (e.g., at the end of suffering through terminal illness or strife).

Given the above description of grief, it becomes evident that grieflike reactions can follow other types of loss, such as the loss of a livelihood, loss of a job, loss of physical functioning, or divorce. Mourning, on the other hand, is specific to bereavement, referring to the social expressions or acts expressive of grief during bereavement, which are shaped by the practices of a given society or cultural group, such as funeral rites, the wearing of a specified color of clothing, or rituals bringing together family members at specified times across the duration of bereavement. It is noteworthy that the traditional psychoanalytic school defines these terms differently, using the term mourning synonomously with the way grief has been defined above. The reason for this can be found in the original German formulation: the word "*Trauer*" used by Freud and from whom psychoanalytic definitions derive, refers to both the experience as well as the expression of grief. [*See* GRIEF AND LOSS.]

II. THE SYMPTOMATOLOGY OF GRIEF

The scientific study of the impact of bereavement on mental health goes back to a classic paper written in 1917 by Freud, entitled "Mourning and Melancholia." This paper was a landmark in the analysis of distinctions between normal and complicated forms of grief. It was not until much later that a systematic analysis of the range of symptoms typically associated with bereavement was published, by Lindemann, in 1944. Current understanding still owes much to this early formulation. Thus, patterns of normal grief responses, reflected in itemizations in assessment instruments (see below) typically cover the following dimensions: Affective manifestations include depression, despair and dejection, anxiety, guilt, anger and hostility, anhedonia and loneliness. Behavioral manifestations include agitation, fatigue, crying and social withdrawal. Cognitive manifestations include preoccupation with thoughts of the deceased, lowered self-esteem, self-reproach, helplessness and hopelessness, a sense of unreality, and problems with memory and concentration. Physiological and somatic manifestations include loss of appetite, sleep disturbances, energy loss and exhaustion, somatic complaints, physical complaints similar to those that the deceased had endured, changes in drug intake, susceptibility to illness and disease.

While there is lack of evidence specifically on cross-cultural differences in these dimensions, studies from related areas, such as depression research, and clinical experience lead one to expect cultural differences in the relative frequency of symptoms across these different dimensions, for example, more somatization of grief in non-Western cultures.

Finally, while it has become familiar to talk about the "symptomatology" of grieving, following early writers in the field, it is important to remember that grief is a normal reaction to bereavement and not a physical illness or psychiatric disorder, even though it is associated with higher risks of these disorders.

III. PHASES OR STAGES OF GRIEF

Understanding of the course of grief owes much to the work of John Bowlby, whose analysis of attachment and separation processes, documented in his three-volume monograph, *Attachment and Loss*, and his observations with respect to the close relationship between manifestations of grief and time since death, led him to suggest "phases" or "stages" of grief. Phasal conceptualizations typically postulate a succession from an initial stage of shock, with associated symptoms of numbness and denial, through yearning and protest, as realization of the loss develops, to despair, accompanied by somatic and emotional upset and social withdrawal, until gradual recovery, which is marked by increasing well-being and acceptance of the loss. Durations vary, but generally the first two phases are suggested to last up to a number of weeks, and the third, intense grieving phase may last several months or even years. There is considerable cross-cultural variation in the duration of the phases across time, which has to do with mourning customs and cultural norms.

There has been wide acceptance in scientific as well as in applied fields of such phasal descriptions. However, these have been understood too literally. Almost without exception—and this certainly is the case for Bowlby's original formulation—phases have been introduced as descriptive guidelines, but have been regarded as set rules or "prescriptions" regarding where the bereaved ought to be in the "normal" grieving process. Care must also be observed in applying such labels as "resolution" or "completion" of grief, because the bereaved do not "get over it and back to normal," but rather adapt and adjust to the changed situation and generally succeed in reaching a new equilibrium.

Recently developed "task models" take more account of the richness of idiosyncratic manifestations of grief than do phasal models. Well-known, and much used in counseling and therapy, is Worden's model, in which the grief process is taken to encompass four tasks, namely, accepting the reality of loss; experiencing the pain of grief; adjusting to an environment without the deceased; and "relocating" the deceased emotionally and moving on with life. It should be emphasized that not all grieving individuals undertake these tasks and, again, they will also be dependent on cultural factors (e.g., in societies where reverence of ancestors is customary, "relocation" takes place in a very different way: the deceased is in a sense still present).

IV. NORMAL VERSUS PATHOLOGICAL GRIEF

Because grief is a normal reaction to the death of a loved one, it does not usually require the help of professional counselors or therapists. However, as noted above, a minority of bereaved people suffer from complicated forms of grief. It must be stressed that distinctions between normal and complicated grief are difficult to make, first of all, due to the lack of clarity with regard to the definition of complicated grief (or, for that matter, of normal grief to begin with). One reason for this is that categorization systems have largely been empirically, rather than theoretically, derived. Another is that complicated grief is not a single syndrome with clear diagnostic criteria. A third reason is the complexity involved in setting a cut-off point between what is "normal" in grieving and what is not (e.g., cultural patterns that view tearing one's hair as a normal symptom of grief, are not accepted in Western cultures). Fourth, perhaps most difficult is the overlap and causal sequencing of pathological grief with other mental disorders, such as affective or anxiety disorders.

These problems make any effort at definition questionable, but there are grounds enough to state that time course and intensity of symptoms are dimensions on which complicated grief can primarily be assessed. Delayed, chronic, absent, and prolonged grief, as well as unresolved, maladaptive, conflicted, distorted, neurotic, and dysfunctional grief frequently reflect these dimensions (they last too long or too short, have too little or too great an intensity, or commence too late). It is frequently the case that complications of grief manifest themselves with regard to certain symptoms, while others remain at an unproblematic level or duration.

Given the variety and richness of individual manifestations of grief, and the problem of defining even the parameters of normal grief, at the present state of knowledge the following definition appears to be useful: Pathological grief is a deviation from the (cultural) norm (i.e., that could be expected to pertain, according to the extremity of the particular bereavement event) in the time course or intensity of specific or general symptoms of grief. Subtypes of pathological grief have been distinguished in the scientific literature that are in accordance with this general definition. Thus, chronic grief is characterized by long-lasting grief, and an absence of signs that the individual is making any progress in the process of coming to terms with loss. Chronic grief is frequently associated with depression, guilt feelings, self-reproach, social withdrawal, and continued preoccupation with thoughts of the deceased. Absent grief is characterized by the nonappearance of symptoms typical of grief. The person continues with life as though nothing has happened. It is important to note that the absence of symptoms of grief does not, per se, indicate pathology. In delayed grief the bereaved person shows little or no sign of grieving at first, as in absent grief, but later on, symptoms of grief do become apparent, and indistinguishable at this later time from those of normal grieving.

V. MEASUREMENT OF GRIEF: DIAGNOSTIC INSTRUMENTS

In the last couple of decades a number of self-report questionnaires have been developed for the measure-ment of symptoms of grief. Most of these inventories have been developed for the categorization of the range of symptoms of grief in adults. Frequently used batteries include Sanders, Mauger and Strong's Grief Experience Inventory, and Faschingbauer, Zisook and DeVaul's Texas (Revised) Inventory of Grief. Over the years more specific measures have also been developed, such as Toedter, Lasker and Aldaheff's Perinatal Grief Scale, to assess grieving among parents who have suffered loss during pregnancy or the loss of a newborn baby, and Hogan's Sibling Inventory of Bereavement, designed for adolescent siblings of someone who has died.

There are limitations with respect to the application of such instruments for the assessment of grief. They are in general more appropriate for research purposes than for clinical use. Individual assessment needs to take account of variables beyond those evaluated through psychometric instruments that are based on self-reports. Furthermore, there are shortcomings with respect to the establishment of psychometric qualities and establishment of norms. Grief is also a process, and as such cannot be assessed according to normality versus deviation without taking the dimension of length of time of bereavement into account.

For the reasons outlined above, many researchers and professionals in clinical practice rely instead on diagnostic interviews to derive an assessment of the course that grieving is taking. Alternatively, many of them use general diagnostic instruments such as the Symptom Check List (SCL-90), the General Health Questionnaire (GHQ-28), or depression lists such as the Beck Depression Inventory or the Zung. In the context of traumatic bereavement, Horowitz, Wilner and Alvarez's Impact of Event Scale is frequently used for the assessment of posttraumatic stress symptomatology.

VI. HEALTH CONSEQUENCES OF BEREAVEMENT

Cases of pathological grief are comparatively rare, the overwhelming majority of bereaved persons undergoing tolerable levels of symptomatology that decline as time passes. Nevertheless, the bereaved are indeed at greater risk than the nonbereaved of suffering from a variety of mental and physical ailments and disorders, including depression, anxiety disorders, somatic complaints, and infections. Some of these ailments are most closely associated with recent bereavement, others extend over a longer time span.

How prevalent are health problems following bereavement? With respect to psychological reactions, only in a minority of cases are these so severe as to require professional intervention, or to reach levels equivalent to diagnostic criteria. To illustrate: in one study of bereaved adults in The Netherlands by Schut and his colleagues, published in 1991, although 50% reached the criteria for diagnosis of Posttraumatic Stress Disorder at one of four points of measurement within the first 2 years of bereavement, only 9% met this level at all four points. These were participants in a cohort study of bereaved people, who were not undergoing treatment. In a further small community sample study in Germany, Stroebe and Stroebe investigated the adjustment of widows and widowers under retirement age. Forty-two percent reached depression levels equal to or above a well established cut off point for mild depression on the Beck Depression Inventory, at approximately 6 months after their loss (as opposed to 10% of a comparable married group). Two years after loss, this had reduced to 27%, but as such was still significantly higher than for the married. Again, these were not treated cases. [See DEPRESSION.]

Nevertheless, large-scale statistics do show higher rates of psychiatric illnesses among bereaved as compared with nonbereaved individuals, as evidenced in general in- and outpatient admission statistics and in diagnostic-specific figures across a broad range of psychiatric categories. Some studies have found that, for widows, rates fall most frequently within the depressive disorder category (rates for widowers are, however, also highly excessive within this category), whereas widowers have the additional very high risk of succumbing to alcohol-related disorders. Although such statistics are typically available for conjugal bereavement, there are good reasons to argue that the patterns found both for mental and physical health debilities following death of a spouse are reflected in other types of losses, such as loss of a child.

Physical health detriments are also excessive among recently bereaved people compared with nonbereaved counterparts, both males and females being affected. They suffer not only from a variety of physical symptoms and illnesses, but they also have higher rates than nonbereaved individuals for disability and use of medical services, such as consultations with doctors, use of medication, and hospitalization.

The risk of mortality from many causes, notably suicide, is also higher among bereaved persons than among the nonbereaved. There is some evidence that this bereavement–mortality relationship generalizes beyond spousal loss, affecting parents, children and other family members, but more reliable and extensive statistics are available for spousal loss. Cross-sectional mortality tables showing marital status patterns from many countries of the world indicate that widowed persons in general have higher death rates than comparable married individuals, and that these excesses are greatest for younger adults and for males. This identifies younger widowers as a particularly high-risk group. While such statistics are subject to artifacts (e.g., selection), longitudinal studies have confirmed this pattern, indicating that the relative excess compared with nonbereaved, during the first year or two of bereavement, is frequently greater than 40%. Although this percentage sounds alarmingly high, it must be remembered that actual numbers of deaths per year are few, particularly in young age groups. To give a typical example, if the mortality risk of the widowed had applied to the married population of The Netherlands in the years from 1986 through 1990, then 356 more men and 123 more women per 100,000 person years would have died.

Recent research has shown biological links between grief and the increased risks of morbidity and mortality described above. Physiological theory and research have concentrated on the identification of mechanisms by which loss may affect the immune system, lead to changes in the endocrine, autonomic nervous, and cardiovascular systems, and that help to account for increased vulnerability to external agents. Recently, for example, physiological changes have been identified in the immune system following bereavement. This approach should facilitate understanding of individual differences in health outcome of bereavement: Why are some individuals more vulnerable than others? There may be predisposing risk components of a physiological nature. Another approach to answering this question has been the search for complicating and mitigating factors, which is the topic of the next section.

VII. BEREAVED PERSONS AT RISK OF POOR ADJUSTMENT

Much research effort has been put into identifying so-called "risk factors," to understand why people are affected in very different ways, and why some people (i.e., high-risk groups) suffer debilitating and/or lasting consequences while others do not. It has become clear from the above descriptions that a range of effects, including diverse psychological, physical and social functioning is involved. Thus, a "risk factor" is one that increases vulnerability across a spectrum of variables: one person may succumb to mental health problems while another may die prematurely following bereavement.

High-risk subgroups of bereaved persons have been identified and can be classified according to: sociodemographic variables, personal factors (e.g., a history of mental disturbance; personality/relationship characteristics), causes and circumstances of death (e.g., sudden death; child loss), and circumstances of bereavement (e.g., lack of social support; additional stresses). These variables have been identified by investigators—admittedly with differing levels of empirical robustness, as we will indicate below—as associated with poor bereavement outcome, at least within Western cultures. In general, one might assume intercultural similarities, although culturally specific patterns might be expected on some variables, for example, widowers may be less exceptionally vulnerable in societies with very different male–female roles/relationships.

Next, we consider what is known so far about relative risk of succumbing to detrimental effects according to the four categories of risk factors.

A. Sociodemographic Factors

Considerable attention has been paid to gender differences. Mothers have generally been found to react more overtly and for a longer period than fathers, following the death of a child. This may be related to gender differences in expressiveness and to differences in styles of coping among men and women, with men adopting the role of strong supporter for a deeply grieving partner. In the case of conjugal bereavement, there is growing evidence that widowers are relatively more vulnerable than widows to ill health, ranging from relatively higher excess rates (compared with still married counterparts) on depression, mental illness, physical symptomatology and, best established so far in the literature, from mortality.

Many investigators have concluded that there are systematic differences in health outcome according to age: younger bereaved persons have been found to be more at risk than older persons. Mortality statistics are supportive of this. A number of explanations, which are not mutually exclusive, have been put forward. For example, death for younger persons is a comparatively unexpected, often unprepared-for event, and the shock of loss is therefore all the greater. In the case of partner loss, death of a younger person is also untimely and tragic, rather than occurring "in the fullness of time." Furthermore, some of the variance may be accounted for by such factors as joint unfavorable environments or life-style, joint risk from dangerous activities such as reckless driving being more associated with younger than older age groups (what caused the death of the loved one, is a risk factor for the survivor).

Ethnic or cultural group differences in bereavement have been the topic of insufficient research to identify specific patterns of similarity versus differences with respect to health consequences. Certain general conclusions can, however, be drawn. In particular, it can be stated with some degree of certainty that grief is universal, in the sense that loss of a close, loved person causes personal upset and has been shown to affect the mental and physical health of persons in very different cultures across the world. Manifestations are, however, remarkably different (e.g., somatization in symptomatology, or continuing of bonds with and sense of presence of the deceased in cultures different from our own) and ways of coping, particularly outward expression of grieving, vary greatly and according to local norms and customs. With respect to physical morbidity and mortality, although there is also evidence of elevated risks in other cultures, comparisons between cultures are very hard to draw, given the differences in, for example, patterns of interpersonal relationships (e.g., remarriage), in health care, in diagnostic systems and in recording of national statistics. [See ETHNICITY AND MENTAL HEALTH.]

Does religion help the bereaved? Although the religious bereaved themselves frequently identify their religious and spiritual convictions as a source of strength, evidence that belief in God, in an afterlife, and in reunification with the deceased after death have not been systematically pinpointed as ameliorating the distress of bereavement: nonreligious persons have been found to be as well-adjusted as their religious counterparts in a number of studies. It seems plausible that the nonreligious turn to other sources for support and strength. For some religious people, death of a loved one shakes their faith, if, for example, God is seen as a powerful force that allowed the death to occur. [See RELIGION AND MENTAL HEALTH.]

B. Personal Factors

So far, perhaps the most striking feature to emerge consistently from empirical research is that high levels of distress in the course of bereavement are best predicted by a high level of distress early after loss. While this may reflect the mediating role of a number of different variables, such as those to do with features of the death itself, it points to individual differences in the ability of bereaved persons to come to terms with their loss. Whatever the background factors responsible, extreme distress in the early days of bereavement is a highly relevant indicator of the potential need for intervention.

The quality of the relationship with the deceased person has been found to lead to differences in the impact of bereavement. Most noticeable, ambivalence and dependence in the (marital) relationship are associated with more intense and longer lasting grief reactions. This is somewhat surprising, because one might predict that harmonious, loving, compatible relationships would be the ones most clearly identified as leading to a broken heart and dreadful loneliness. It is, of course, difficult to differentiate between close relationships in this sense of the word, and dependent ones. The outcome patterns are complex too: it does not always seem to be dependent survivors who are the ones to be more affected, for those who have adopted the care-giving role in a relationship with a more dependent partner can suffer as much as the latter during bereavement.

We have already discussed (see Section VI) that prior psychiatric debility may be a contributing factor to the development of complicated grief. In some cases, bereavement exacerbates already existing health conditions. A personal history of mental and/or physical health problems is associated with increased risk of ill health effects during bereavement. Adding to this picture, the occurrence of prior losses, possibly ones that have been multiple or occurred chronically, can put a person at very high risk.

More research needs to be conducted on the impact of personality and other individual factors on adjustment to loss, for example, the role of different styles of attachment, or of general negative affectivity. Research has, however, recently focused on the mediating role of different ways of coping in adjustment to loss. For example, analyses of the impact of confronting and working through grief on recovery did not show unequivocal support for their effectiveness in

the Tubingen Longitudinal Study. Similarly, structural analyses of the link between expression of emotions and psychological distress in the Utrecht Study by Schut and his colleagues suggested independent development of the two phenomena. These studies thus call into question the so-called grief work hypothesis that has long been accepted by the psychoanalytic and attachment theory schools (see Section VIII). Others, such as Bonanno in the United States, are currently examining the role of such coping mechanisms as denial and the presence of positive emotions in grief. The thrust of their argument is that these are not necessarily indicators of poor adjustment or signs of trouble to come, but that they may indeed be adaptive processes. [*See* INDIVIDUAL DIFFERENCES IN MENTAL HEALTH; PERSONALITY.]

C. Causes and Circumstances of Death

Some investigators have found sudden, unexpected deaths of loved ones to be associated with more intense and longer lasting grief reactions. In some studies, the difference according to expectedness of loss is not very large. It seems likely that expected deaths also carry a great burden of care giving during the final illness, leading to exhaustion and physical neglect of personal health while concentration is focused on the terminally ill loved one. This would bring high risk on bereavement.

In the study in Germany by Stroebe and Stroebe, reported above, it was also found that the type of death interacted with personal characteristics of the bereaved individual to affect good versus poor outcome. Those widowed persons who had experienced a very unexpected death of a loved one (less than a day's forewarning) and who, in addition, were persons who had low internal control beliefs (i.e., they did not think that they had control over what happened to them, or that matters in general were within their own control) were the ones who remained highly distressed over the first 2 years of bereavement. Expected death experiences had generally better recovery profiles, regardless of personal control beliefs, as had sudden death ones among persons with high internal control beliefs.

Undoubtedly, there is some confounding between the circumstances of death and its cause, in determining impact on the bereaved survivor. However, several causes have been found to be independently related to specific or more intense grief reactions. Thus, homicide is generally found to be an extremely traumatic loss, associated with Posttraumatic Stress Disorder. Death from suicide is often associated with guilt and stigma. Death from AIDS is complicated not only by stigmatization, but also by the fact that, within the gay communities where prevalence is high, such deaths are also chronically, multiply occurring and the bereaved themselves are also at high risk. Multiple losses have been found to lead to long-lasting grief reactions and depression.

Is the type of relationship with the deceased (child, spouse, parent, etc.) associated with different types and/or intensities in grief reactions? Catherine Sanders has researched this question in some detail, as described in her 1989 monograph, *Grief: The Mourning After Dealing with Adult Bereavement*. The loss of a child emerges as the most devastating of losses in industrialized societies, not only for parents, but also, some studies have shown, for grandparents. Siblings also suffer greatly from the loss of a brother or sister, not least because of difficulties arising from the fact that their parents are also grieving, and problems in communicating and understanding each other's grief —as indeed can be the case with grieving parents, whose styles of grieving may be very different. Due to preoccupation with their own grief, parents may also fail to realize the impact of loss on their surviving children. In fact, the death of a child can pose a serious threat to the marital relationship and family harmony.

The loss of a parent in childhood combined with difficult subsequent circumstances during upbringing, can trigger problems during adulthood. A renewed high-risk period could be expected after the death of another loved person at this later stage of life.

D. Concurrent Circumstances during Bereavement

Among researchers investigating the concurrent life circumstances of bereaved persons, focus has been on the impact of social support on ameliorating the effects of loss, and on the burden of additional stressors during bereavement. The general social support literature has clearly shown that those who are "buffered" from stress through the presence and help of others have fewer health problems. Thus, one would expect such

positive effects during the stress of bereavement. Subjective accounts by bereaved people also confirm that they feel helped and supported by family and friends. It is also intuitively convincing that the distress of bereavement will be ameliorated by the support and understanding of others. However, well-controlled studies have not unequivocally confirmed this. The work of Weiss (see, for example, his monograph, *Loneliness,* published in 1973) has suggested a reason why, and this has received some empirical confirmation: those grieving the loss of a loved one feel deeply lonely, even in the presence of others. While others can indeed help with certain tasks, there can be no replacement for the lost loved one, at least not early on in bereavement. As bereaved persons themselves report, they remain desperately lonely, even though they are not alone. An additional reason for the limited advantages that have been found for social support is that social interactions are frequently reported to be nonsupportive, even when intended otherwise, and that these actually serve as a supplementary source of stress. [*See* LONELINESS.]

Dominant among additional problems that add to the burden of bereavement are economic difficulties, which can lead to the need to move to a different house or to gain employment—which then, in and of themselves, create additional stress. A drop in financial resources has indeed been found to be related to poor bereavement outcome. Financial difficulties can become an additional source of stress during conjugal bereavement, where income (or comparable resources such as household care) provided by the deceased person has been lost on that person's death. Not surprisingly, given that men are still more often the main breadwinners, this is particularly a problem among widows, exacerbating their adjustment difficulties, and accounting, as some studies have shown, for part of the variance associated with poor adjustment.

In conclusion: further methodologically sophisticated research on the above risk factors, and, in particular, better understanding of mediating processes is still needed. For example, what is the impact on bereaved people of administering euthanasia to a dying loved one, or, how does the multiple occurrence of loss among communities having to deal with AIDS and accompanying stigmatization affect adjustment to bereavement? How is the grief of small children different or similar to that of adults, and what are the special risks for them?

VIII. THEORETICAL APPROACHES TO BEREAVEMENT

A. Psychoanalytic Theory

Theoretical explanations of psychological reactions and ways of coping with grief owe much to psychoanalytic theory. Freud's "Mourning and Melancholia," mentioned above, has remained influential theoretically, its impact being evident in the work of Lindemann, Bowlby, Parkes, Raphael, Jacobs, and other major figures in the field. According to psychoanalytic theory, when a loved one dies, the bereaved person is faced with the struggle to sever the ties and detach the energy invested in the deceased person. The psychological function of grief is to free the individual of his or her ties to the deceased, achieving the gradual detachment by means of a process of grief work. Grief work implies a cognitive process of confronting the reality of loss, of going over events that occurred before and at the time of the death, and focusing on memories and working toward a detachment from the deceased. Since Freud, the notion that one has to work through one's grief has been central in the major theoretical formulations on grief and in principles of counseling and therapy. The major cause of pathological grief, according to Freud, is the existence of ambivalence in the relationship with the deceased preventing the normal transference of libido from that person to a new object. [See PSYCHOANALYSIS.]

B. Attachment Theory

Bowlby's attachment theory emphasizes the biological rather than the psychological function of grieving. The biological function of grief is to regain proximity to the attachment figure, separation from which has caused anxiety. In the case of permanent loss this is not possible, and such a response is dysfunctional, in the sense that reunion cannot be achieved. However, Bowlby also argued for an active working through the loss. Like Freud, Bowlby sees the proximal cause of pathological grief in the relationship with the lost person. However the distal cause is childhood experiences with attachment figures. These experiences are assumed to have a lasting influence on later relationships. For example, frequent separation from attachment figures in childhood can lead to anxious attachment in later relationships, which results in chronic grief, a pathological reaction consisting of an indefinite prolongation of grief over the death of a partner. [See ATTACHMENT.]

C. Stress Theory

Stress theory, like attachment theory, has had a tremendous impact on bereavement research. Such an approach is reflected in the influential work of Horowitz and his colleagues, whose interest and analysis spans not only bereavement, but traumatic life events in general (see, for example, his influential 1986 book, *Stress Response Syndromes*).

The basic assumption of stress theory is that stressful life events play an important role in the etiology of various somatic and psychiatric disorders. This approach has received much impetus through the work of Lazarus & Folkman, whose volume, *Stress, Appraisal and Coping,* appeared in 1984. More specifically, it is assumed that a stressful life event may precipitate the onset of a physical or mental disorder, particularly if predisposition toward that disorder already exists. The intensity of stress created by a life event depends on the extent to which the perceived demands of the situation tax or exceed an individual's coping resources, given that failure to cope leads to important negative outcomes. Coping may either be directed at managing and altering the problem that is causing the distress (problem-focused coping) or it may be directed at managing the emotional response in order to reduce emotional distress and to help maintain one's emotional equilibrium (emotion-focused coping). Stress theory provides the theoretical underpinning for the so-called "buffering model," which suggests that high levels of social support (a coping resource) protect the individual against the deleterious impact of stress on health. Furthermore, research has identified neurophysiological mechanisms linking stress with various detrimental consequences to the immune, gastrointestinal, and cardiovascular systems. [See COPING WITH STRESS; PSYCHONEUROIMMUNOLOGY; STRESS.]

IX. INTERVENTION FOR THE BEREAVED

The distinction has been made in the literature between grief counseling and grief therapy. While, in practice, the division between the two types of intervention is hard to judge, it is nevertheless useful for the purposes of clarification of the range of support programs that are available and appropriate to assist bereaved persons through their grief process.

A. Grief Counseling

Grief counseling has been defined by Worden as "helping people facilitate uncomplicated, or normal, grief to a healthy completion of the tasks of grieving within a reasonable time frame." Emphasis is thus on general support, the offering of comfort and care, help with secondary stresses that occur, and encouragement of appropriate grief and mourning. The role in such support of the informal network is supplemented through pastoral care workers, doctors, voluntary organizations such as Widow-to-Widow or Cruse (often those who have themselves suffered a loss being involved in the counseling of recently bereaved persons), and health care professionals (e.g., social workers and psychologists).

To illustrate, one type of voluntary counseling for bereaved persons is so-called "self-help" aid as offered in Widow-to-Widow programs. Silverman was a major pioneer of this movement, and in an early paper, written in 1975 with her coauthor Cooperband, she described the principle behind self-help groups, that grieving persons may be best helped by others who have been through and mastered their bereavement themselves, as follows:

> The evidence points to another widow who has coped and accomodated as the best caregiver. Very often the first question a widow helper is asked is, "How am I going to manage?" The second question is, "How did it happen to you?" The new widow seems to be seeking a role model, someone with whom to identify. This other widow can be a friend, a neighbour, or a relative. She offers an opportunity to talk with someone who indeed really understands. She can provide perspective on feelings; she provides a role model; she can reach out as a friend and neighbour—not someone defined as concerned with abnormal or deviant behaviour.

An important aspect that was not emphasized in this description is the training of volunteers, and the availability of advice and guidance of a skilled and experienced professional to back up such voluntary aid. These days, such assistance is typically planned and organized within voluntary programs.

Is such help really effective in alleviating the pain of grief? Most participants report beneficial effects, but this does not mean, of course, that it would benefit all bereaved people. In fact, those who find no use for such a program are the most likely to have dropped out, and be lost to impact assessment figures. Clearly, too, self-reports of effectiveness are a far step from an objective evaluation of the impact of a self-help program on the course of recovery, for example, with respect to its impact on specific mental and/or physical health variables.

B. Grief Therapy

Grief therapy, also as defined by Worden, refers to "those specialized techniques . . . which are used to help people with abnormal or complicated grief reactions." Most experts see grief therapy as appropriate in cases where the grief process has "gone wrong," when grief work fails to be undertaken and completed successfully, that is, according to the late grief therapist, Ramsay, when "the 'normal' reactions of shock, despair, and recovery are . . . distorted, exaggerated, prolonged, inhibited, or delayed."

Thus, broadly speaking, while grief counselling would be appropriate for normal grief, grief therapy would be indicated for pathological grief. It is important to note that expert knowledge is necessary to evaluate whether the special techniques of therapy are necessary in a particular case, or whether the bereaved person's grief will be alleviated with the aid of counseling.

What are the goals of grief therapy? According to the grief work hypothesis, complications in the grieving process occur when the individual is unable to face up to or process the reality of the death. Avoidance of some aspect of the loss itself or of one's emotional reaction to it lies at the heart of problematic adjustment. For example, there is lack of or insufficient confrontation with emotions to do with the loss because of the fear that the intensity of these will be intolerable. Likewise, some bereaved continue to cling to, and talk about the deceased in order to remain closely bonded to him or her. This too can be interpreted as avoidance: the presence of such preoccupation serves the purpose that one does not have to face the reality of the loss. Systematic dealing with avoidance reactions is a common feature in psychotherapy programs for pathological grief.

Recently, we have drawn attention to the one-sidedness of the notion of working through grief in grief intervention. Alongside confrontation, the bereaved also have to adjust to changes in the current environment. These include the need to take on new roles, a changed identity, and the need to develop skills that are lacking due to the absence of deceased. Such so-called "restoration" tasks have so far been neglected in descriptions of therapy programs, as has the need to take "time off" from grieving.

Nevertheless, a wide variety of therapy programs have been developed to stimulate confrontation with painful associations to do with grief. These differ in the main with respect to the degree of directiveness with which confrontation is forced. Next we give brief descriptions of the major approaches.

Within behavior therapy techniques of systematic desensitization or "flooding" have been used, the intention in therapy being to break down defense mechanisms and unleash intense emotional reactions. These have proven useful, and effective for the treatment of pathological variants of grief. Cognitive (behavior) therapy and rational emotive therapy integrate behavior therapy techniques, but are directed toward certain ideas or assumptions that the bereaved have, which create additional emotional difficulties, such as perceived personal shortcomings in interacting with the terminally ill person. Therapy in such a case might be directed toward disputing the impossible demands that one places on oneself at such a harrowing, exhausting time. When the client ultimately accepts the reinterpretation, it should be possible to proceed to a stage where feelings can be expressed. [See BEHAVIOR THERAPY; COGNITIVE THERAPY.]

Psychodynamic therapy focuses on conflicts within the grieving individual. In the case of complicated grief concentration is on working through conflicts within the previous relationship, both with respect to positive and negative aspects. Psychodynamic therapy can also be oriented toward selective strengthening of the ego, which takes the form of facilitating emotions (e.g., aggression or guilt feelings).

Within the last decade, creative therapy (in combination with other forms of therapy) has also been increasingly applied to the treatment of pathological grief. This technique is particularly useful—among children and adults—when the bereaved person is unable to express his or her grief well in words. This can have to do with "inappropriate" feelings for which verbal expression might be inhibited because they are not socially acceptable, such as aggression or desire for revenge. The idea is that self-censoring is lowered

in creative therapy through the use of symbolic images, use being made of techniques such as drawing, painting, or working with clay, and also using music or photos.

Hypnotherapy is almost exclusively used in cases of traumatic loss, for example, following accidents, disasters or murder deaths. As such, what is being treated is posttraumatic stress disorder, focus being placed on the dissociation of the traumatic experience from normal consciousness. The latter process is assumed to inhibit the normal coping process. Phases in such therapy are (1) identification of the avoided traumatic memory; (2) neutralization of the trauma; and (3) therapeutic revision (this phase is not always necessary). The pain that is associated with the traumatic event is then neutralized or substituted by positive or neutral emotions or images. [See HYPNOSIS AND THE PSYCHOLOGICAL UNCONSCIOUS.]

Somewhat similar to hypnotherapy is guided imagery therapy. Again, three phases are involved: (1) reliving; (2) revising; and (3) revisiting. These phases lead to the breaking down of barriers, through which the client is able to confront the reality of the loss experience.

Certain procedures cross the barriers of different therapeutic interventions. Thus, the use of leave-taking ceremonies are frequently used in directive types of therapy. These involve rituals during which, for example, possessions of the deceased person will finally be disposed of through burning or burying the article. When carefully embedded within the context of a more general therapy program, such techniques can be enormously helpful. Likewise, bibliotherapy, the reading of selected publications can be effective in the treatment of pathological grief. Reading and discussing (auto)biographies can be very facilitating, in that they show how normal certain grief reactions are. The bereaved remember similar feelings of their own and recognize that these are common to bereavement.

Also common to all therapy forms is the assumption that the client will ultimately come to the (cognitive and emotional) realization that loss is irrevocable, and that leave must be taken from the deceased. This does not mean that the deceased is forgotten or banished from one's thoughts, but rather than the deceased is displaced, in the sense of finding a new place, in the bereaved's existence. And, most of all, it means the revival of personal experiencing without the continued presence of the deceased loved one.

Finally, we need to consider the effectiveness of therapy programs in general. Few methodologically sound research projects have been conducted to evaluate interventions for pathological grief. Those that are available in the literature indicate that behavior therapy, cognitive therapy, hypnotherapy, and psychodynamic in general all have postive outcomes with respect to guiding pathological forms toward normal ways of grieving. More research is needed to assess the relative effectiveness of the different forms of therapy.

X. SUMMARY AND CONCLUSIONS

There is no doubt that the loss of a loved person causes deep suffering and that the costs to health can be extreme. These consequences are reason enough for bereavement to have become the subject of considerable scientific study. Much is now known about typical manifestations of grief, and about factors that complicate the course of grieving over time. Progress has also been made in the planning and implementation of services for recently bereaved individuals, and for those whose grieving process runs a complicated course. Much can be done within the community and through health care professionals to promote adjustment to bereavement and prevent the development of pathological forms of grief. For the comparatively small number of persons for whom grief takes a complicated course, specific intervention programs have been designed that help to reduce extreme consequences and restore grieving to a normal course that will, eventually, result in adjustment to life without the loved person.

BIBLIOGRAPHY

Corr, C. A., & Balk, D. E. (Eds.). (1996). *Handbook of adolescent death and bereavement.* New York: Springer Publishing Company.

DeSpelder, L. A., & Strickland, A. L. (Eds.). (1995). *The path ahead: Readings in death and dying.* Mountain View, CA: Mayfield Publishing Co.

Fulton, R., & Bendiksen, R. (Eds.). (1994). *Death and identity.* Philadelphia: The Charles Press.

Jacobs, S. (1993). *Pathologic grief: Maladaptation to loss.* Washington, DC: American Psychiatric Press.

Klass, D., Silverman, P. R., & Nickman, S. L. (Eds.). (1996). *Continuing bonds: New understandings of grief.* (3rd ed.). Washington, DC: Taylor & Francis.

Parkes, C. M. (1996). *Bereavement: Studies of grief in adult life.* Harmondsworth, UK: Penguin.

Sanders, C. M. (1989). *Grief: The mourning after dealing with adult bereavement.* New York: Wiley.

Stroebe, W., & Stroebe, M. (1987). *Bereavement and health: The psychological and physical consequences of partner loss.* New York: Cambridge University Press.

Stroebe, M., Stroebe, W., & Hansson, R. O. (1993). *Handbook of bereavement: Theory, research and intervention.* New York: Cambridge University Press.

Worden, J. W. (1991). *Grief counseling and grief therapy: A handbook for the mental health practitioner.* New York: Springer Publishing Co.

Biofeedback

Elise E. Labbé

University of South Alabama

Autonomic Nervous System   The peripheral nervous system that includes neurons outside the bony enclosure of the spinal cord and skull; comprised of the sympathetic nervous system and the parasympathetic nervous system.

Electroencephalograph   Instrumentation that monitors brain waves.

Electromyograph   Instrumentation that monitors muscle activity.

Operant Conditioning   A behavioral principle that states when behavior is reinforced it will increase and when punished or not reinforced will decrease.

Parasympathetic Nervous System   Originates in the cranial and sacral regions of the spinal cord and plays a role in conserving energy and is often associated with a relaxed state.

Psychobiology   A field of study that considers the interaction of psychological and biological variables in behavior and physical and mental health.

Psychophysiological Disorders   Physical disorders in which there are no evident physiological causes and etiological factors may be of a psychological nature. Examples are migraine headache and ulcers.

Self-Regulation   The process in which an individual regulates internal physiological responses, as well as emotional, behavioral, and cognitive responses.

Stress Management   Psychotherapy focused on helping people cope with stressful events more effectively and reduce anxiety, depression, and sympathetic nervous system responses.

Sympathetic Nervous System   Originates within the thoracic and lumbar regions of the spinal cord and is associated with bodily responses that mobilize the organism and is referred to as the "flight or fight" response.

BIOFEEDBACK is a methodology as well as a clinical tool that provides information about an individual's physiological functioning in relation to her cognitive, emotional, and behavioral responses. This article will present a psychobiological approach in discussing the development of biofeedback, theoretical models, types of biofeedback, current research status, and applications of biofeedback.

I. INTRODUCTION TO BIOFEEDBACK

A. Definition of Biofeedback

Biofeedback is any process in which an external device generates information to an individual about his or her physiological responses and that allows the individual to then regulate these responses and receive feedback on changes in the physiological responses. The physiological responses may be any responses that can be measured by an external device. The most common responses measured are muscle tension, heart rate, skin-temperature, and galvanic skin response. The feedback may be in a variety of forms, the most common being visual and auditory. The feedback may be continuous, intermittent, or provided once a threshold is crossed.

Biofeedback can also be considered a methodology used in studying psychophysiological processes. The methodology includes a baseline measurement of the physiological response(s), then feedback is given to an individual with some sort of instruction to manipulate the physiological response(s). The physiological response is measured during feedback and compared to the baseline measurement. Inferences are then drawn as to the relationship between the physiological response and the individual's response to the biofeedback.

B. Historical Survey of Biofeedback Development

Psychophysiology is the scientific study of the interrelationships between cognitive, emotional, behavioral, and physiological processes. Biofeedback techniques and applications grew out of the research in psychophysiology. Biofeedback research became widespread in the 1960s, when studies reported that a variety of presumable nonvoluntary responses could be brought under operant control. Many studies using electroencephalographic feedback were reported which indicated that alpha brain activity could be brought under voluntary control. As these studies gained the attention of clinicians, soon biofeedback was applied to treating various disorders such as migraine headache and hypertension. The growing body of research on stress also provided support for the use of biofeedback as a research tool as well as a treatment approach. Research on the effects of relaxation, meditation, and hypnosis in producing the relaxation response to counteract the effects of stress provided further support for the concept of self-regulation using biofeedback. Advancing technology provided more efficient, reliable, and sophisticated instrumentation that has allowed for greater in-depth study and validation of applied biofeedback. Researchers also became interested in evaluating the various theories being proposed regarding how and why biofeedback works.

Biofeedback experimentation and methodology represents a major advance in the scientific evaluation of the relationships between behavior, environment, and the regulation of physiological processes. Some

historians suggest that it is the single most significant development to occur in the area of psychophysiology. Biofeedback methodology has widened the scope and increased the capability of behavioral models of experimentation and analyses in research on physiological functioning and self-regulation. It has stimulated interest in behavioral models of etiology and treatment of psychophysiological disorders. Biofeedback experimentation has provided evidence for new approaches to the alteration of emotional states and the study of consciousness.

II. THEORETICAL MODELS OF BIOFEEDBACK

Over the years several models have been proposed that attempt to describe what processes and principles allow biofeedback to work. Four of the more popular models will be briefly described: these are the operant conditioning framework, the informational processing model, the skills learning model and the psychobiological model of self-regulation.

A. Operant Conditioning Model

The operant conditioning model is basically atheoretical. This approach emphasizes the use of reinforcement, positive, negative, and punishment, that are made contingent on selected ongoing physiological responses, and the learning that follows the application of reinforcement. Research in this area has focused on a variety of conditioning principles, physiological responses, and human and animal behavior. The emphasis has been on examining similarities and differences between conditioning of skeletal motor and visceral or neural processes within the individual. Systematic exploration of operant techniques has not occurred and there needs to be a more consistent examination on the effects of the environment on physiological regulation. Examples are evaluating the effects of combining different schedules and types of reinforcement with the feedback on a person's ability to learn to change a physiological response.

B. Information Processing Model

In defining biofeedback training, the concept that the individual is "fed" "back" information about biological responses that he or she is not aware of is important. This information provides a sensory analog of the currently occurring physiological responses. Information is provided to the individual at the same instant that the physiological activity is occurring or after a very brief delay. Therefore, some part of the output of a process is now introduced into the input of a process so as to alter the information processing. According to the information processing model, biofeedback stimuli can be conceived of as a symbolic representation of the physiological event, and the individual engages in a response to either reduce or enhance the biofeedback stimuli, resulting in changes in the physiological responses themselves. Research in this area may evaluate different types of feedback stimuli to determine the best display of information. This may include examining the differences between auditory and visual feedback.

C. Theory of Voluntary Control

The theory of voluntary control proposed by Brener emphasizes discrimination and awareness of internal bodily responses and processes. Biofeedback is thought to aid the individual in the learning process and increase awareness of sensations related to physiological responses, or to sensitize the individual to other motor responses as a means of mediating voluntary control over the physiological changes. Thus, emphasis is given to learned physiological control as a form of complex human learning of motor skills.

D. Psychobiological Model

All three of the theories discussed thus far have been supported by some empirical data. There are a number of studies that attempt to isolate and differentiate the effects of the hypothesized variables. At this stage of knowledge, there is no strong empirical evidence to support one viewpoint over another. The psychobiological model integrates these concepts by emphasizing the interrelationships between psychological processes and biological processes. The psychobiological model supports the view that biofeedback helps the self-regulation of the individual's total functioning. The concepts from the information modeling approach provide a way to explain how needed feedback is provided that will allow for better self-regulation. The concepts from the operant approach

are used to emphasize the individual differences in effectiveness of various types of feedback and schedules of reinforcement, and the importance of considering environmental influences in self-regulation. Finally, the theory of voluntary control helps explain how individuals can adjust their current motor responses to impact on processes that they are not aware of.

III. THE BIOFEEDBACK LABORATORY

A. Components of the Biofeedback Laboratory

The biofeedback laboratory should be a quiet room free from visual distractions. A recliner chair allows the subject to rest comfortably. The laboratory equipment can vary depending on the goals of the clinician and purposes for which the biofeedback will be used. With the advances in technology, most biofeedback systems are quite compact and attractive. Some of these systems are integrated with a computer screen and will allow for printing of and/or computer display of the feedback. A computer system is advisable so that the results of the biofeedback session can be stored for future reference. Biofeedback instruments monitor physiological responses of interest and allow for measurement of these responses. The instrumentation then presents it in a way that the individual can use and manipulate the information.

Electrodes and transducers convert responses from the skin's surface that are transformed to electrical impulses that go to a preamplifier and then to an amplifier. The amplified signal then drives an output device such as an audio signal or visual display. Electrodes are used to detect electrical currents from one electrode to the next. Transducers come in a variety of forms. A thermistor is one type of transducer used to detect heat. A photoplethysmograph is a transducer used to detect changes in density of the skin as a result of changes in blood volume. And a strain gauge is a transducer that measures mechanical changes, such as the movement of some part of the body.

B. Establishing a Biofeedback Laboratory

A minimum requirement would be to establish a large enough area that could hold a recliner, a chair for the individual conducting the biofeedback session, the biofeedback equipment, a personal computer, and lighting that can be dimmed. After space is established for the laboratory then the practitioner would begin searching for the type of equipment that would serve the goals of the practitioner. There are several nationwide companies that can be contacted to provide bids on biofeedback equipment. Some individuals prefer to buy individual biofeedback components for each response, often called "stand alone" modules. Another approach would be to purchase the preamplifier/amplifier components that various transducers and electrodes could be plugged into. In order to connect the biofeedback equipment to a computer a component called an analog-to-digital converter needs to be purchased.

C. Safety Considerations

There is a small chance of electrical safety problems when using biomedical instrumentation. In order to minimize risks Schwartz and associates in 1987 suggested that each power line piece of auxiliary equipment be evaluated periodically for electrical safety; all individuals should be kept out of arm's reach of all metal parts; and equipment should be properly grounded.

IV. TYPES OF BIOFEEDBACK

A. Electromyographic Biofeedback

Electromyographic (EMG) biofeedback is the most widely used biofeedback technique with both children and adults. EMG biofeedback provides information about the individual's striate muscle tension in the area where the electrodes are attached. As the muscle constricts it generates an electrical current between one motor neuron and the next. The EMG sensors pick up the intensity of that electrical current. Typically, there is one reference electrode that is used and two active electrodes. It is important to place the electrodes lengthwise over the muscle of interest so that the electrodes are picking up the electrical current as it moves from one motor neuron to the next within the same muscle. If the electrodes are placed on two different muscles, then the information obtained reflects the electrical difference between two different muscles. The muscles most commonly monitored are the frontalis, masseter and trapezius muscles. The frontalis is the forehead muscle that tenses when an individual is worried or under pressure. Some clinicians believe the tension in the frontalis area is one of the best indicators of overall body tension. The masseter muscle is connected to the jaw bone and contracts when an individual is tense or angry. The trapezius muscle contracts the shoulders when an individual is alarmed or chronically anxious. These muscles are often the focus in biofeedback training because they typically respond to stress and can be measured without much interference from other muscles. They can be a good starting point from which muscle relaxation training can be generalized.

B. Skin Temperature Biofeedback

Skin temperature feedback monitors fluctuations in surface body temperature. These are most often measured by monitoring finger, hand, or foot temperatures. A sensor is usually attached to the index finger of the hand. The sensor, a thermistor, is a heat-sensitive semiconductor in an epoxy bead.

Skin temperature monitoring is useful because skin temperature tends to become cooler as one experiences greater sympathetic nervous system (SNS) arousal and stress. Peripheral vasoconstriction and reduced blood flow to the tiny capillaries in the skin are what causes the skin temperature to decrease. During SNS arousal, changes in blood flow takes blood from the skin and sends it to the skeletal muscles, allowing large muscles to respond to the flight or fight challenge. This response in turn protects the peripheral parts of the body, by reducing blood flow to the hands or feet in order to reduce bleeding if these body parts were injured. Thus, it is suspected that when the person experiences greater parasympathetic nervous system arousal, changes in blood flow return the blood to the skin and smooth muscles. Increased blood flow to the skin causes increases in skin temperature, and this may reflect relaxation.

C. Galvanic Skin Response Biofeedback

A feedback dermograph measures the electrical conductance or electrical potential in the individual's skin. The galvanic skin response (GSR) biofeedback machine can monitor minute changes in the concentration of salt and water in sweat gland ducts. The natural metabolism of cells produces a slight voltage that varies as sweat gland activity changes. The lower the measurable voltage, in millivolts, the less there is of sweat gland activity. With skin conductance techniques an imperceptible electric current is passed through the skin. As the sweat glands become more active, the monitor registers the skin's increased ability to conduct electricity. The reverse of this procedure is called skin resistance.

The GSR has been used in lie detectors as a measure of emotional arousal. The sympathetic branch of the autonomic nervous system controls sweating. GSR biofeedback helps the individual gain control of the arousal produced by the autonomic nervous system. Two sensors or electrodes are usually placed on the ends of two fingers. Many clinicians prefer not to use GSR responses because they change rapidly and often respond to irrelevant stimuli.

D. Electroencephalographic Biofeedback

Electroencephalographic (EEG) biofeedback is another frequently used biofeedback training method with children and adults. EEG biofeedback gives information about the brain's electrical activity. Brain waves have been classified into four states: beta, which occurs when the individual is wide awake and thinking; alpha, which is associated with a state of calm relaxation; theta, which reflects a deep reverie or light sleep; and delta, which is associated with deep sleep.

In the typical procedure the subject is provided with feedback about the presence or absence of some specified amplitude and/or frequency of brain electrical activity. Often the goal of EEG biofeedback is to produce alpha waves because they are associated with relaxation.

E. Heart Rate, Blood Pressure, Pulse, and Volume Biofeedback

The heart rate monitor uses electrodes to measure the action of the heart muscle. Heart rate biofeedback usually involves measuring heart beats per minute. In general, greater SNS arousal is associated with a faster heart rate, and a relaxed state is associated with decreased heart rate. Blood pressure biofeedback monitors the diastolic and the systolic pressure of the cardiovascular system. Increases in blood pressure reflect greater SNS arousal; thus, in most cases the goal of blood pressure biofeedback is to reduce the pressure.

Blood pressure is difficult to monitor as one has to use a blood pressure cuff that must be inflated and deflated to measure the changes in pressure. It is has been shown that the inflating and deflating of the cuff actually alters the blood pressure response. Newer technologies have been developed to overcome this problem; however, they are more expensive.

Blood pulse and volume are measured using a photoplethysmograph. A photoplethysmograph generates a small amount of infrared light that is monitored with a light sensor. As blood volume increases the density of the skin increases and less light passes through the skin and is reflected back and is registered by the light sensor. Blood volume feedback helps the individual constrict or dilate the blood vessels or artery being monitored. Blood pulse is also measured with a photoplethysmograph and is often used as an indirect measure of heart rate.

F. Sexual Response Biofeedback

Sexual arousal in males is usually measured by penile tumescence. A strain gauge is used and it measures the physical changes of the penis as arousal increases and decreases. Female sexual arousal is measured with a thermistor or photoplethysmograph that is placed near the clitoris. Sexual response biofeedback may be used in the treatment of sexual deviations as well as sexual dysfunctions.

G. Gastrointestinal Biofeedback

Measuring the activity of the gastrointestinal system can be accomplished by measuring the electrical activity on the surface of the skin where the stomach is. Muscular activity is screened out. Greater electrical activity is related to greater stomach motility. This type of biofeedback may be useful in treating stomach disorders that are affected by stress and anxiety.

V. CURRENT RESEARCH FINDINGS IN BIOFEEDBACK

A. Research on the Best Methods of Biofeedback

Studies indicate that initially feedback should be salient to the individual, continuous and given when small changes are made. As the individual begins learning to manipulate the response, then feedback can be contingent on greater change and may be given intermittently. The clinician can experiment with a variety of forms of feedback, many people prefer audio feedback as they can close their eyes while trying to relax.

It is important to include segments of "self-control" training in which the feedback is turned off and the individual is instructed to continue to manipulate the response without feedback. Research also indicates that home practice is necessary for lasting changes to occur. Practicing self-control of the physiological response for 10 to 20 minutes several times a week is recommended. It appears that it is best to have the patient plan out the practice schedule ahead of time and to practice earlier in the day. If the patient waits until right before they go to sleep they may fall asleep during the practice. As the patient gets better at controlling the response, he or she should be encouraged to do this while continuing normal activities.

Studies indicate that changes in symptoms come slowly with most changes occurring four to six weeks after biofeedback therapy has begun. It is important to explain to the patient that biofeedback does not work like most medication and that changes occur slowly and often accompany a real change in the person's behavior and attitude about the problem and how to cope with it. Also, biofeedback may not eliminate the symptoms but it may reduce the intensity, frequency, and/or medication usage.

B. Research Investigations on how Biofeedback Works

In the late 1970s and early 1980s research in biofeedback was focused on evaluating the different models of biofeedback discussed above. Many interesting findings were reported, but more questions were raised than were answered as to how biofeedback works. Much of the recent research on biofeedback has focused on evaluating the clinical efficacy of biofeedback, and little systematic work is now being done on discovering how it works. In order to address the question of how it works some researchers have attempted to design false feedback studies. Results of these studies have been mixed, with some studies reporting that even when false feedback is given subjects alter their response as instructed. Some researchers have compared

biofeedback training with relaxation only and found that in both conditions, decreases in ANS arousal can be achieved. Other researchers are now examining the role of cognitions in the biofeedback process. The bottom line is that we are not sure how it works but studying this question allows for a fascinating journey into the mind-body research arena.

C. Research on Differences between Children's and Adults' Responses to Biofeedback

In general children are more open and responsive to biofeedback than adults. Children are usually fascinated with the equipment, and motivation and curiosity are high. Research on nonclinical populations response to biofeedback indicate that children between the ages of 8 and 12 are able to achieve greater changes in physiological responses using biofeedback than any other age group. For clinical groups biofeedback may be a good alternative to medication if the medical treatment has potentially negative short- and long-term consequences for the developing child. Research evaluating the effectiveness of biofeedback with children who have headaches indicates that more children improve and to a greater degree than do adults.

Besides play therapy, behavior modification, and some of the newly developed cognitive strategies, there are only a few individual therapy techniques to be used directly with children. Most interventions involve changing or teaching parenting skills, or manipulating the child's environment. Biofeedback offers the therapist a mode to teach the child concepts of self-control, stress management, and an opportunity to begin talking about feelings and stressors and how these may affect physical health. Most children have an external health locus of control in which powerful others have responsibility for their health. Biofeedback may help the child gain an internalized view that acknowledges one's own role in maintaining good health.

Although children may be more responsive in the therapy setting, they may have greater difficulty than adults in remembering to practice outside of the therapeutic settings and to record changes in their symptoms. Often a parent is recruited to gently remind the child to practice and record symptoms.

VI. CLINICAL USE OF BIOFEEDBACK

A. How and Why Biofeedback Is Used in Clinical Settings

A major use of biofeedback is to teach relaxation skills. A second use of biofeedback is to alter patho-physiological processes such as blood flow or SNS arousal for migraine headache patients, to decrease the flow of gastric juices for ulcer patients, to decrease muscle tension and increase proper posture for the chronic back-pain patient. Biofeedback should be considered as a therapeutic tool that can help introduce the client to therapy in a concrete and nonthreatening manner. It can be especially useful for the patient who focuses on physical problems or insists his problems are not physiological. Biofeedback can also be used to increase feelings of self-efficacy and self-control. The client learns quickly the connection between emotions, thoughts, and physiological responses. [See EMOTIONAL REGULATION.]

Biofeedback may be used when there are no viable medical alternatives, or when the physician determines that medication should not be used. Sometimes patients do not want to take medication and biofeedback may be a treatment alternative. For example, a chronic back-pain patient may have to use pain medication to control the pain for the rest of her life because there are no other medical treatments to reduce the pain. The patient may choose to try biofeedback to help cope and reduce the pain instead of taking pain medication, which is addictive and may have undesirable side effects. [See PAIN.]

Biofeedback has also been used in modifying behavioral problems. Two examples are hyperactivity that is associated with attention deficit disorder and maladaptive behaviors that are associated with mental retardation. Motor responses may be monitored using biofeedback; the child is rewarded as the problem behavior decreases. [See ATTENTION DEFICIT HYPERACTIVITY DISORDER (ADHD).]

Biofeedback should be used clinically only after a competent medical diagnosis has been made and the examining physician has decided that biofeedback may be valuable. Patients coming directly to psychologists for biofeedback or other behavioral treatments of physical disorders should be referred first to a medical specialist for a thorough medical examination. The need for medical consultation in any bio-feedback case is both an ethical and legal responsibility of the psychological practitioner.

B. Biofeedback, Relaxation Training, and *Stress Management*

The question has been raised as to the difference in effectiveness of outcome between biofeedback and relaxation training in reducing stress. This has been a controversial question as many clinicians and researchers argue that you can get the same benefits from relaxation strategies as from biofeedback for most problems. Furthermore, they point out that the relaxation strategies are not as costly nor do they require knowledge of complicated equipment. Only a few large-scale controlled outcome studies on the efficacy of biofeedback as compared to other behavioral techniques in the management of physiological disorders have been reported. Most of these do not find that biofeedback provides a distinct advantage over other behavioral procedures. The selectivity of physiological control often achieved by biofeedback methods would suggest that the methods would have a unique advantage in disorders in which the symptom is quite specific, for example, cardiac arrhythmias, seizure disorders, and various neuromuscular disorders. However, at the present time there is not enough research evidence to discount the idea that biofeedback may be better for some disorders, and that some people may respond better to biofeedback than relaxation therapy. As technology advances equipment is becoming less expensive and more user "friendly." Biofeedback may be particularly useful for children as cognitively they can understand concrete examples of what is happening in their bodies as compared to relaxation training that may be more abstract. In a culture that provides video games, robots, computers, and other high-tech games and toys for children, they are usually attracted and eager to participate in the biofeedback session. [See STRESS.]

C. Clinical Issues in Using Biofeedback

Biofeedback can be abused if it used outside of the context of therapy. It cannot be used in the same manner that one would administer medication. *Individual differences* must be noted and addressed using an individualized protocol before biofeedback can be successful. Also, the individual should be closely monitored and changes recommended if problems arise. Biofeedback may be successful in the clinic, but patients may not be able to modify their responses in the natural environment without biofeedback. Thus the development of self-control should be included in the protocol.

Sometimes a person's baseline physiological responses are normal, but the individual may experience exaggeration of SNS responses when stressed. Biofeedback should be focused on helping these individuals decrease SNS arousal during stressful situations. Thus, in biofeedback therapy it is important to teach biofeedback skills in a variety of situations and intensities of stimuli.

Biofeedback allows for discrete control of a response system. For example, one component of autonomic nervous system (ANS) activity can be modified without other ANS systems being called into play. Specific EEG patterns can be modified and discrete muscle groups as small as a single motor unit can be trained independently with the use of feedback. However, for the ANS it appears that increases in arousal-like activity are easier to obtain than decreases in arousal-like activity. Thus, researchers have more consistently demonstrated voluntary blood pressure and heart rate increases and skin temperature decreases than the opposite processes. This indicates that biofeedback may be more useful in lowering high levels of arousal such as those associated with clinical stress conditions or pathological states than normal or healthy states

The specific form and structure of the biofeedback training must depend largely on the individual characteristics of the patient, the physiological symptoms in question, the particular physiological system for which feedback is to be given, the nature of the disorder itself, and the goals of treatment. Through an accumulation of knowledge gained through basic and clinical research, including systematic case studies, certain generalizations may be possible. However, at this time generalization are made with caution. The biofeedback clinician must choose a specific procedure on the basis of all the facts in the case and his or her own understanding of the current technology and state of research knowledge. The astute clinician can proceed in a systematic manner through trial, error, and close observation of clinical outcomes as they occur for a given patient.

Compliance to the biofeedback practice may be difficult at times as positive effects usually do not always happen instantaneously. The patient must be prepared to expect that decreases in symptoms may not occur for several weeks. Patient motivation may be low because for some disorders there are no short-term aversive consequences such as in hypertension. Another motivation reducer is that the symptom itself may be reinforced in the natural environment. The patient may experience secondary gain. For example, a patient may use talking about her problem in social situations to gain attention. What will she do in social situations if she does not have a problem to discuss? The patient may also be a candidate for social skills training, so that as the symptom is reduced she will have acquired other skills to help her cope in social situations. Another possible area of motivational difficulty may arise from other behaviors strongly entrenched in the patient's repertoire that are in conflict with the aim of therapy. An example is a young man who has overextended himself in extracurricular activities and has poor time-management skills. This young man is quite able to learn the biofeedback skills but cannot find time to practice at home. This issue must be addressed by the therapist if treatment is to be successful.

If the patient is on medication that may effect the response that is being manipulated, consult with the patient's physician to determine if the medication can be kept at a constant level while biofeedback therapy is occurring. If during the biofeedback training the patient or physician wants to decrease or increase medication intake, ask that this be reported so that this information can be used to evaluate the success of the biofeedback therapy.

VII. OPPORTUNITIES IN AND FUTURE OF BIOFEEDBACK

A. Professional and Research Opportunities

Reports on studies of biofeedback have steadily declined over the past 10 years. This is unfortunate as there are still so many unanswered questions regarding how and why biofeedback works. The area of biofeedback research provides a wealth of opportunities, particularly as technology improves and instrumentation becomes more reliable and valid. There are now more training opportunities to learn biofeedback instrumentation and methodology. The Biofeedback Society of America encourages continued scientific investigations of biofeedback, and there are numerous high-quality scientific journals that publish biofeedback research, including *Psychophysiology; Biofeedback and Self-Regulation;* and *Biofeedback and Behavioral Medicine.*

On the professional level biofeedback techniques and therapy have become more widely accepted as a method of treatment for numerous mental and physical problems. Those interested in developing a profession in biofeedback can contact the two national societies, the Biofeedback Society of America and the American Association of Biofeedback Clinicians. There are also many state and regional biofeedback societies that provide training and scientific meetings.

B. Future Directions in Research, Clinical Practice, and Biofeedback Technology

Biofeedback is alive and well as there continues to be a steady output of high-quality research, greater acceptance of biofeedback as a clinical tool, and improvements in technology. Although biofeedback has been used to treat problems, it may have advantages in helping individuals develop self-regulation skills to prevent mental and physical health problems. For example, a study was reported in which children with no clinical problems were taught skin-temperature bio-

feedback. These children learned to relax and incorporated this in their daily schedule. They also demonstrated decreases in anxiety and depression scores, even though these scores were in the normal range. Biofeedback may have helped them achieve a greater degree of psychological health.

With the advent of greater access to personal computers people may be able to purchase inexpensive biofeedback devices that they can use at home to teach themselves self-regulation skills. Of course, as with all self-help approaches, misunderstanding of instructions, the problem, or proper follow-through may diminish the effectiveness of self-help biofeedback. However, combining home devices with some therapist assistance may be as effective as time-intensive, outpatient biofeedback training. These are just some of the future directions to be explored.

BIBLIOGRAPHY

Andrasik, F. (1994). Twenty-five years in progress: Twenty-five more? *Biofeedback and Self-Regulation, 19,* 311–324.

Miller, L. (1994). Biofeedback and behavioral medicine: treating the symptom, the syndrome, or the person? *Psychotherapy, 31,* 161–169.

Schwartz, M. S. (1987). *Biofeedback: A practitioner's guide.* New York: Guilford.

Shapiro, D. (1977). A monologue on biofeedback and psychophysiology. *Psychophysiology, 14,* 213–227.

Surwillo, W. W. (1990). *Psychophysiology for clinical psychologists.* Norwood, NJ: Ablex.

Body Image

Todd F. Heatherton and Michelle R. Hebl

Dartmouth College

Body Dysmorphic Disorder A clinical preoccupation with a trivial or imagined defect in one's appearance.

Body Image Self-perception of appearance that includes both perceptual experience and subjective evaluation.

Body Image Distortion The extent to which individuals inaccurately perceive their body size.

Body Image Satisfaction The extent to which individuals positively evaluate the shape or size of their bodies.

Restrained Eating Individuals who frequently or chronically diet and who vacillate between restricting caloric intake and engaging in bouts of disinhibited eating.

Stigma A mark or feature that brands individuals as being undesirably different or abnormal in some way and makes them susceptible to prejudice and discrimination.

BODY IMAGE is a multifaceted construct composed of the perceptions, thoughts, and feelings that individuals hold about their physical being. This article presents a review of the factors that influence the development and maintenance of body image. It also summarizes the disorders associated with body image deficits.

I. MEASUREMENT ISSUES

Body image refers to perceptions, thoughts, and feelings about one's physical appearance. It involves a self-perception that consists of both perceptual experience and subjective evaluation, based in part on the reactions of others. Despite its long history, the construct of body image is poorly understood, probably because of its multifaceted and complex nature.

The measurement of body image typically focuses on either perceptual estimation or on affective reactions to self-evaluation. Perceptual assessment techniques examine the accuracy of judgments about physical size. For instance, participants might be asked to estimate the width of their waist, hips, and thighs by adjusting the width of light beams onto a dark surface to match their judgment of the relative width of those body parts. Body image is then measured by comparing perceptual estimates with actual body widths, and the resulting difference indicates whether individuals under- or overestimate their bodies.

Whole-body procedures typically present participants with a visual representation (through photographs, silhouette selection, video image, or mirror image) that has been distorted by the researcher to be larger or smaller than the participant's actual image. Participants then modify or adjust the distorted image so that it matches their estimation of their correct physical size. Again, the difference between perceived and actual body size is used as an indicator of body image.

The usefulness of perceptual estimates for assessing body image has yet to be reliably demonstrated. Body image distortions are common and occur with equal frequency across many diverse subject populations, including those with eating disorders, those who are obese, and those who are of average weight. These distortions are also unrelated to body image satisfaction, they do not indicate any pathological condition, and they have little diagnostic utility for identifying disordered eating. Moreover, the various body size assessment techniques tend not to be highly correlated with each other, and there are serious concerns about whether any of them have adequate reliability or validity.

There are a number of conceptual reasons to believe that the accuracy of size estimation is a poor indicator of self-perception of physical appearance. Disparities between estimated and actual body size may be influenced by experience, motivation, subjective evaluation, and context. For example, most people have limited experience with estimating the size of their bodies. Examining video or still pictures of one's body is of little use for estimating size; after all, such images are usually quite a bit smaller than actual size. Similarly, the reflection of physical image depends on the optical properties of the reflective surface, and it is possible that estimations of physical size are based on mirrors that distort the physical image. The physical context in which one experiences or evaluates physical size may also bias body size estimation. One basic psychological principle is known as perceptual contrast—sticking one's hand in a bucket of cold water after having it in a bucket of warm water will make the water feel especially cold. In an analogous way, judgment of one's own physical size will be influenced by the physical characteristics of others in proximity. For example, a person may feel particularly heavy after he or she has been around thinner people, or particularly thin after being around heavier people. It is not clear, therefore, that people should be expected to have a particularly accurate appraisal of their physical size. In short, the use of perceptual estimation techniques cannot be recommended at this time.

The second major method of assessing body image is through subjective evaluation, as measured by affective, cognitive, or behavioral reactions to one's physical appearance. These various measures indicate the extent to which individuals are satisfied or dissatisfied with their bodies. For instance, one widely used technique has subjects view a number of silhouettes that depict a range of body figures from underweight to overweight. Individuals choose the silhouette that best represents their current body size, as well as the silhouette that best represents their ideal body size, and the discrepancy between these two indicates level of body image satisfaction. Note that although this requires some degree of perceptual estimation, it is the subjective discrepancy between current and ideal that is relevant to body image; whether people's estimates of their current size are accurate is usually not of interest to those who use this method. Other common techniques for assessing body image evaluation include self-ratings of physical attractiveness; ratings of specific body part satisfaction (i.e., hips, thighs, nose, and chest); self-ratings of weight, size, or shape satisfaction; and affective reactions (such as anxiety or depression) to thoughts about the body. A wide assortment of rating scales exist that are suitable for evaluating body image.

Although the majority of people are relatively satisfied with their bodies, evaluative measures of body image indicate that many individuals, both men and women, from young to old, are dissatisfied with their bodies. Current North American society has been described as being obsessed and preoccupied with the body, and national surveys indicate that at least one third of men and more than one third of women are dissatisfied with certain aspects of their bodies. Moreover, nearly half of all men and the vast majority of women report wanting to lose at least a modest amount of body weight. Perhaps surprisingly, body image dissatisfaction is also relatively common among the elderly and among very young children, some of whom starve themselves to the point of stunted physical growth in order to avoid being fat.

The measurement of body image satisfaction is not without conceptual, definitional, and psychometric problems. For instance, some measures of body image dissatisfaction may reflect general negative affect (such as low self-esteem or depression) rather than specific unhappiness with one's body, and it is unclear whether negative affect is the cause, consequence, or mere correlate of body image dissatisfaction. The precise manner by which physical appearance affects global self-esteem has not yet been determined. Some conceptual models of self-esteem treat physical appearance (including the body) as one facet of self-concept that contributes to global self-esteem, whereas other theories treat body image as only tangentially related to global self-esteem, which is based more on self-efficacy and positive regard from significant others.

In addition, the vast assortment of different methods for assessing body image satisfaction has led to some conceptual ambiguity. A desire to lose weight, for example, might indicate body image dissatisfaction or it could indicate a desire to lead a healthier lifestyle. Although more than three quarters of women report wanting to lose at least 10 pounds, the majority of women are generally more positive about their bodies than they are negative. A great deal of evidence indicates that most people (both men and women) are ambivalent about their bodies rather than totally dissatisfied or satisfied. That is, people typically are happy with some of their physical features but are quite unhappy with other features. Although it is generally true that disliking multiple physical features is linked with increased overall body dissatisfaction, the structural properties of the body image construct (i.e., how the various parts contribute to the whole) have yet to be precisely determined.

In summary, there is little consensus about the best methods for measuring body image. Although it is clear that evaluative measures are more useful than perceptual measures, the particular evaluative measure chosen should be based both on the specific goals of the evaluation or research and on the psychometric properties (i.e., reliability and validity) of the specific instrument.

II. PHYSICAL AND PHYSIOLOGICAL INFLUENCES

Almost every physical characteristic plays *some* role in determining body image (e.g., genetic hair loss, facial acne, pregnancy, wrinkles, pubertal changes). Four characteristics in particular, however, are central to the development and maintenance of body image.

The first of these factors is body weight. Individuals who are objectively or subjectively overweight tend to hold a negative body image. Such dissatisfaction is especially likely to occur among those who were

(or are) overweight as adolescents. Note, however, that there are only slight negative correlations between body weight per se and global self-esteem or psychological well-being. That is, body weight is only modestly related to satisfaction with other aspects of the self-concept (such as academic achievement or social skills). However, believing oneself to be overweight, whether one is or not, is closely related to body image dissatisfaction. Thus, body image mediates the relation between body weight and self-esteem. [*See* SELF-ESTEEM.]

A second factor that influences body image is gender. Across the life span, women tend to have lower body image satisfaction than men. Women are more likely than men to evaluate specific body features negatively, to attempt weight loss, to report anxiety about the evaluation of their physical appearance, and to have cosmetic surgery. Body image dissatisfaction among women is almost invariably related to self-perceptions of overweight, whereas dissatisfaction among men is equally divided between worries about being overweight and worries about being underweight. Being physically large may have benefits for men because of the association between size and power. Men who are physically large are viewed as more powerful than men who are physically slight, and a significant number of men engage in compensatory behaviors to increase physical size or musculature. Thus, very thin men are much more likely than very thin women to experience body image dissatisfaction.

The link between mass and power in men also illustrates the importance that a third physical factor, body height, has on determining body image, particularly for men. Whereas most women are satisfied with their height, many men have a desire to be taller and tend to overreport their height. This is not surprising, given the well-documented link between men's height and positive social outcomes such as leadership, power, income, and perceptions of attractiveness. Many short men report dissatisfaction with their stature and some evidence suggests that they are more likely to experience decreased self-esteem and more negative body image relative to their taller male counterparts. For women, the importance of height is less clear, although a relatively tall stature appears to be a desirable trait for most women. Height may be an important component of a positive body image only to the extent that it allows women to appear thinner and leggier. However, women who are particularly tall sometimes report decreased body image satisfaction, in part because their height makes it difficult to satisfy the societal injunction that the male be taller than his female partner.

A fourth factor that contributes to one's body image is physical attractiveness. Physical attractiveness refers to specific facial and body features that are valued by members of a society. The specific attributes that are prized differ depending on gender. For women, facial features that indicate youthfulness (e.g., large eyes, small nose, big lips) and body features that are petite and thin (e.g., long legs, flat stomach) tend to be desirable. For men, facial features that imply maturity (e.g., square jaw, visible cheekbones) and body features that indicate mass and largeness (e.g., height, mesomorph build) tend to be desirable. Some evidence indicates that average rather than unusual features are viewed as most attractive. For instance, some research on this topic uses computer programs to average facial features from many different faces. The composite averages are typically viewed as being more attractive than the individual faces. Of course, it is important to note that it is personal beliefs about attractiveness that influence body image. Most studies have found only a modest association between objectively rated physical attractiveness (i.e., ratings made by independent observers) and body image. However, subjective ratings of physical attractiveness (i.e., personal beliefs) are closely linked to body image satisfaction.

The four components of body image are determined primarily by physiological and genetic factors. Height, gender, and physical appearance are typically immutable, except through surgical modification. Genetic influences also play a prominent role in body weight, although public perception is that body weight is much more mutable than other physical characteristics. Most people grossly underestimate the physiological influences on body weight and perceive it to be a matter of individual control and willpower. Believing that body weight, especially one's own body weight, is controllable contributes to body dissatisfaction.

III. CULTURAL INFLUENCES

Throughout history, cultural influences have played significant roles in determining body image. For instance, the Greeks revered the male body, the Romans prized thinness, and people from the Middle Ages showed a preference for larger, rounder female body types, as later epitomized in Rubenesque art. Modern American society places an emphasis on individuality and self-definition, whereas individuals in previous eras tended to rely less on themselves and more on the structure of society to define aspects of their selves. Thus, the meaning and definition of body image change over time as a function of cultural and societal influences.

Although a limited number of physical attributes deemed to be attractive have remained stable over time and across cultures (e.g., fleshiness rather than flabbiness, cleanliness, and symmetry in one's body), most evaluative aspects of physical appearance are culturally bound—what is beautiful in one culture is not necessarily beautiful in another. For instance, styles of clothing, hair, and makeup vary greatly. Individuals will also go to great lengths in an attempt to conform to cultural standards of physical attractiveness. Extreme examples of this include the Burmese tradition of women affixing brass rings around their necks to stretch their necks to lengths of up to 15 inches; women in Victorian England wearing corsets so tight that the corsets distorted internal organs and damaged the ribcage; the East Indies tradition of filing teeth down to the gums; the South American (Abipone) tradition of inflicting deep wounds on the face, breasts, and arms; the Chinese tradition of binding women's feet to the point of crippling and deforming them; and the recent proliferation of Americans piercing and tattooing various body parts.

Within a single culture, mandates for what is beautiful and desirable also undergo substantial variation across time, particularly for women. For instance, during the 1820s, some women drank vinegar to lose weight and stayed up all night to look pale and fragile; in the mid-nineteenth century, a big, voluptuous figure was in vogue and women often worried about appearing too thin; in the early twentieth century, a more slender but very sturdy physique was desirable. After World War I, flat chests became desirable as did a new trend of applying makeup to one's face. Although the preference for body size has fluctuated over the last century, Americans have been obsessed with thinness for at least the last 30 years. Indeed, the 1990s saw a return to prizing the thin, pale, and fragile appearance of the 1820s (i.e., the waif, Kate Moss or Gwyneth Paltrow).

Even within the same time frame, there can be substantial heterogeneity in what is perceived as ideal. For instance, throughout the 1940s and 1950s, a voluptuous ideal (i.e., Marilyn Monroe) shared center stage with a thin ideal (i.e., Audrey Hepburn). In the 1980s, a muscular, healthy physique (i.e., Jane Fonda) gained prominence at the same time that a softer, more feminine physique (i.e., Dolly Parton) was also thought to be attractive.

Although beauty is conceived of in many heterogeneous ways, there is a clear message to women in our society that beautiful physical appearance is a must for happiness and success. There are consistent media messages targeted at women that portray the notion that "what is beautiful and thin is good." Severely underweight women are overrepresented in glamour magazines, on television programs, and in the movies. The typical woman presented in the glamour industry is 5 feet 11 inches tall and weighs approximately 110 pounds, which is 7 inches taller and 30 pounds lighter than the average woman in our country. This portrayal of an ideal that is 20% below the average creates and reinforces the stigma of the large body size.

A. Obesity

Possessing a stigma, a strongly undesirable physical or dispositional characteristic, typically has negative repercussions on many aspects of one's life. It has adverse effects on factors such as interactions with nonstigmatized individuals and on many aspects of the self-concept, including body image. The stigma of obesity is particularly detrimental because it involves the perception of a deformation in the body as well as characterological weakness. Thus, obesity evokes immediate negative responses from observers not only because of its displeasing aesthetic qualities but also because obese individuals are held personally responsible for their condition. For instance, people are 40 times more likely to hold obese individuals responsible for their condition than they are to hold blind individuals responsible. Obese individuals who offer some medical reason for their weight problem (e.g., a thyroid condition) or provide evidence that they are on a diet to lose weight are less likely to be stigmatized. However, obese individuals who do not offer such information are typically derogated and held in contempt for their apparent lack of control and insufficient willpower.

Not all members of North American society equally stigmatize the obese. Black individuals appear to stigmatize obesity much less than do White individuals. For instance, Black men are more likely than White men to find bigger and heavier women attractive and desirable. Black women are much less likely to consider themselves obese and are much more satisfied with their weight than are White women, despite the fact that Black women are twice as likely to be obese. Black women also rate large Black body shapes much more positively than do White women rating large White body shapes. The lack of obesity stigma among Black women may, in part, reflect the impressive number of role models who are large Black women (e.g., Oprah Winfrey, Aretha Franklin, Toni Morrison, Jocelyn Elders, and Maya Angelou). In summary, a variety of evidence demonstrates that being overweight is much more stigmatizing for White women than for Black women.

Recent research indicates that the stigma of obesity varies greatly across cultures. For example, Fijians, Kenyans, Samoans, Mexicans, and Israelis stigmatize obesity less than do Americans, Canadians, and the British. These differences may partially reflect cultural ideology, especially in terms of the value placed on self-reliance and self-determination. For instance, American college students tend to believe that obesity is self-determined and therefore are more likely than Mexican college students to believe that the poor treatment of the obese is deserved. Similarly, children in Israel hold relatively positive views of the obese, possibly because they are raised in a society that tends not to view the obese as personally responsible for their large body size.

The stigma of obesity has a number of negative consequences for those who are overweight. In particular, those who are perceived to be obese are subject to public rejection and ridicule. Obese children and adults are less liked than their slimmer peers and are often excluded from clubs, friendships, dates, and marriages. Perhaps surprisingly, research shows that formerly obese individuals continue to be stigmatized for having been obese even after they obtain a normal body weight. This can be taken as further evidence that the stigma of obesity is as much about character as it is about physical appearance.

Obesity takes its toll not only on psychological well-being, but also on socioeconomic status, possibly through overt discrimination. For instance, colleges admit proportionately fewer obese individuals, and especially obese women, than average-weight individuals, despite similar interests in attending college and similar high school ranks, IQ scores, and PSAT and SAT test scores. This discrimination is especially likely to occur among prestigious colleges that interview applicants. Indeed, although at least 20% of young American adults are obese, the percentage of obese students in the Ivy League is less than 2%. An additional limiting factor that interferes with obese women attaining higher education is that their parents are significantly less likely to assist them financially in their education than are parents of nonobese daughters (even after controlling for the parents' socioeconomic status).

There is considerable evidence for widespread discrimination against those who are obese. Many employers are reluctant to hire obese individuals and some occupations openly discriminate against overweight workers, despite a lack of evidence documenting any relation between body weight and occupational ability. Although some occupations require high levels of physical fitness among its workers (e.g., firefighters, police officers), exclusions are sometimes made on the basis of appearance rather than on the basis of tests of physical ability or fitness (e.g., flight attendants, retail sales clerks). It is unclear why a flight attendant who weighs 175 pounds is any less capable than one who weighs 115 pounds.

Obese women tend to achieve a lower socioeconomic status than average-weight and underweight women. Unlike their slimmer peers, heavy women are less likely to achieve a higher status than that held by their parents. The weights of female (but not male) adolescents have been found to influence future earnings such that women who were obese at 11 and 16 years of age earned significantly less at age 23 (regardless of whether they maintained their obesity) when compared with women who were not obese at 11 and 16. Multiple explanations exist for why there is a strong negative correlation between women's body weight and socioeconomic status (SES), but serious consideration must be given to the possibility that the stigma of obesity is responsible for this pattern. It is interesting to note that although low SES is associated with obesity in developed countries, high SES is associated with obesity in developing countries.

In summary, body image is influenced by current cultural fads, fashions, and preferences, all of which are subject to change. Those who possess physical characteristics that are valued within a culture will likely have a positive body image, whereas those who possess culturally devalued characteristics are often stigmatized and will most likely experience poor body image. [See OBESITY.]

B. Disability and Body Image

Physical disability or disfigurement may have a profound impact on body image, depending on the type and severity of the disabling condition. For instance, permanent damage to major portions of the body (i.e., paraplegia, quadriplegia, major limb amputation) are more predictive of body image dissatisfaction than are less severe physical disabilities.

The degree to which physical disability influences body image is also determined by factors such as onset timing, visibility of the condition, and the cause of the disability. First, disabilities that originate early in life (e.g., congenital blindness) have less impact than do disabilities that arise after childhood. When disabilities occur after childhood, individuals have to deal not only with their physical disability, but they must also cope with the loss of their former nonstigmatized identity. Second, if the disability can be hidden (e.g., a prosthetic device), body image is less likely to be disrupted than if the disability cannot be hidden (e.g., wheelchair). Third, believing that the disability was caused by factors under personal control may preclude full acceptance of the disability, especially if the person dwells on their former nonstigmatized self and continually engages in counterfactual thinking (e.g., "if I hadn't been injured, I would be happier").

Physically disabled individuals' body images are also threatened by the reactions that they receive from nonstigmatized others. Specifically, attitudinal research reveals that individuals often hold negative attitudes toward physical disability and disfigurement. These attitudes may be displayed overtly or covertly. Research examining social exchanges between physically disabled and nondisabled individuals reveals that nondisabled individuals exhibit a number of nervous and avoidant behaviors (e.g., they are more physiologically aroused, terminate the interaction sooner, stand at greater speaking distances, and show more behavioral inhibition) when interacting with a physically disabled person than a nondisabled person. Such verbal and nonverbal gestures likely have a negative influence on body image.

The self-perception that one is being stigmatized

may have a negative impact on body image even if the supposed stigmatizer is unaware of the target's stigmatizing condition. In a series of clever studies, a fake scar was applied to a subject's face and the subject then interacted with another person. Unbeknownst to the subject, the experimenter had actually removed the scar before the social interaction. In this situation, those who believed that they had a scar (even though they did not) believed that they were the targets of stigmatization. This self-fulfilling prophecy shows that the self-perception of being the target of discrimination is an important component of body image.

IV. DEVELOPMENT OF BODY IMAGE

Physical appearance is an omnipresent feature of self that has important implications for body image throughout the life span. As early as infancy, attractive babies are responded to with more positive attention (e.g., increased smiling, eye contact, greater expectations for intelligence) than are unattractive babies. In addition, mothers of attractive babies are more affectionate and play with their babies more than mothers of unattractive babies. This differential treatment of attractive and unattractive individuals continues into preschool and school-age years. Adults rate attractive children as possessing more positive personality traits, having greater academic ability, being more intelligent, and being more likely to be successful than unattractive children, and such ratings are made solely on the basis of appearance. These differential evaluative reactions may have a strong and detrimental impact on the self-esteem and body image of unattractive or overweight children.

Adolescence is a critical period during which maturational changes in body size and shape influence body image. During puberty, most girls gain approximately 25 pounds. This weight gain is not evenly distributed across the body, but rather the added weight predominantly settles in the breast, hip, and thigh regions. This pattern of weight gain is particularly displeasing to many adolescent girls because it conflicts with the cultural ideal of a thin, tall, and fat-free female figure. Adolescence is also a time of increased self-reflection and self-attention, such that many girls become obsessed with body image issues.

Heightened concern with body weight is probably responsible for the initiation of chronic dieting and its commonly related disordered eating. By the ninth grade, nearly all female adolescents report having at some point dieted in an attempt to lose weight. The societal emphasis on female thinness may explain why women are more concerned with eating, weight, and appearance across the life span than men, and why they feel stigmatized in ways that men do not as a result of being slightly (as little as 5 to 10 pounds) over their ideal body weight.

White girls who come from upper or upper-middle class families are the most likely to worry about their weight, show the greatest decreases in self-esteem during adolescence, and are at the greatest risk for developing eating disorders. One possible explanation is that cultural expectations for these girls are more rigid and demanding than for girls of other ethnic and socioeconomic backgrounds, which may lead to feelings of perfectionism and inadequacy. These girls are expected to be thin, beautiful, and smart, and to marry well.

In addition to cultural pressures, body image is also influenced by parents and peers. Family dysfunction and parental conflict relate to a variety of psychological problems, including body image dissatisfaction and disordered eating. Research has demonstrated that eating disorders and poor body image may be especially likely among girls whose parents are perfectionistic, critical, or overcontrolling, and who make comments about their daughter's weight or physical appearance. Similarly, the children of parents who themselves are preoccupied with body weight issues and dieting, or who have symptoms of disordered eating are at a greater risk for developing body image dissatisfaction.

Negative comments from peers, particularly in the form of teasing, are important predictors of body image dissatisfaction. Unattractive and obese individuals are liked less, are excluded from clubs and social events, and are viewed by their peers as possessing more negative traits (e.g., lazy, sloppy) than their slimmer and more attractive peers. This social exclusion may promote a self-fulfilling prophecy, in that ostracized individuals have fewer opportunities to acquire social skills (because of their limited social opportunities) and, in turn, their diminished social skills reinforce people's avoidance of them.

Body image dissatisfaction tends to remain fairly stable during adulthood. As individuals mature into adulthood and begin to focus on family and career issues, some individuals may even show increased body image satisfaction. This is especially likely to occur when individuals enter long-term committed relationships with supportive and nurturing partners. Individuals who gain large amounts of weight during adulthood may experience some body image dissatisfaction as a result of their increased corpulence. Excessive weight gain in adulthood is common in the United States and carries a number of potentially serious health consequences. Preventive health care workers and physicians emphasize body image issues in order to promote weight loss among those whose health is at risk. Thus, body image dissatisfaction may motivate efforts to have a healthful life style. Conversely, body image dissatisfaction may, and often does, lead to dangerous dieting practices and unhealthful weight cycling.

Finally, changes in appearance and physical stamina that accompany old age may have a negative influence on body image. The adage that men view body as a tool and women view body as decoration may explain why many elderly individuals experience some degree of body image dissatisfaction. Older men may feel a decline in their body satisfaction because of their declining physical abilities. Women, however, may be more concerned about excess weight as well as their wrinkling skin and hair loss. Both men and women may also be concerned about being too thin, as being frail may serve as a constant reminder of the inevitability of death. Although there are insufficient data to examine such issues, it seems plausible that individuals who have the greatest degree of body image dissatisfaction during early adulthood will continue to have the greatest body image dissatisfaction during old age, even if the precise factors influencing body image change.

V. BODY IMAGE DISORDERS

Severe body image problems motivate a number of potentially unhealthy behaviors, including chronic dieting, disordered eating, compulsive exercise, or excessive use of cosmetic surgery. Beginning in early adolescence, and continuing thereafter into adulthood, individuals compare their body shape and weight with a perceived cultural ideal. Those who perceive minimal discrepancy between cultural ideals and personal standing are likely to show body image satisfaction. A discrepancy between self-evaluation of current shape and ideal body shape often motivates people to undertake dieting in order to achieve a more attractive body size. Unfortunately, dieting is rarely successful, with fewer than 1% of individuals who lose weight being able to maintain weight loss over 5 years. One of the primary causes of diet failure is occasional bouts of overeating. Such overeating is often precipitated by emotional distress. That is, those who chronically diet (restrained eaters) become disinhibited by emotional distress, eating much more when they are upset than they do when they are happy and calm. Difficulties coping with emotional upset may be one of the primary reasons that most diets are doomed to fail. [See DIETING.]

When dieters fail to achieve weight loss, they commonly blame their failure on a lack of willpower, vowing to try harder on the next diet. Continued dietary failures may have harmful and permanent physiological and psychological implications. Physiologically, weight loss and weight gain cycles ("yo-yo-ing") alter metabolism and may make future weight loss more difficult. Psychologically, repeated failures are likely to diminish body image satisfaction and may damage self-esteem. Over time, repeated dietary failures may induce a particularly negative view of self that includes feelings of helplessness, hopelessness, and anxiousness. In essence, a downward spiral occurs in which dietary failure increases the perceived need for additional dieting but reduces the likelihood of future success. That is, negative affect interferes with successful dietary self-regulation, and yet each failure also increases negative affect. Over time, many dieters eventually engage in more extreme behaviors to lose weight, such as fasting, excessive exercise, or purging. For individuals who are vulnerable, chronic dieting may promote the development of a clinical eating disorder.

The two most common eating disorders are anorexia nervosa and bulimia nervosa. Individuals with anorexia nervosa typically have an excessive fear of becoming fat and as a result, they refuse to eat. Their self-imposed starvation initially draws favorable comments from friends and relatives, although the anorexic is still quite displeased with her body size. As the anorexic approaches her emaciated ideal, family and friends may become quite concerned and medical attention may be required to prevent death from starvation. [See ANOREXIA NERVOSA AND BULIMIA NERVOSA.]

Individuals with bulimia nervosa tend to alternate between fasting and binge eating. Bulimics tend to be average weight, or even slightly overweight women who regularly binge eat, feel that their eating is out of control, have excessive worries about body weight issues, and most often engage in one or more compensatory behaviors, such as self-induced vomiting, vigorous exercise, or the use of laxatives. Unlike anorexia nervosa, many cases of bulimia go undetected by family or friends. Bulimic individuals typically are quite secretive when it comes to eating, particularly with respect to bingeing and purging.

It is commonly believed that individuals with anorexia or bulimia have unusually distorted body images. However, the evidence collected using perceptual techniques indicate that although some individuals with eating disorders overestimate their body size, they apparently do not do so to a greater extent than normal-weight control subjects. That is, body size estimation appears to be as inaccurate among those with eating disorders as it is in the general population. However, those with eating disorders do consistently report greater body image dissatisfaction than those without eating disorders. They report low physical appearance self-esteem, they report wanting to lose weight, they describe discrepancies between current size and ideal size, and in general are quite unhappy with their self-perceived physical appearance. Thus, body image disturbance for those with eating disorders refers to dissatisfaction rather than distorted perception.

Body image dissatisfaction may promote an unhealthy obsession with attempts to change physical appearance through cosmetic surgery. Cosmetic surgery is performed not only to change a specific feature of physical appearance, but also to enhance psychological well-being and improve body image. Approximately 700,000 cosmetic surgeries are performed yearly by plastic surgeons, with more than three quarters performed on women. The most common types of surgeries involve liposuction, breast augmentation, eyelid surgery, nose surgery, and facelifts.

There exist a wide array of motivations for seeking cosmetic surgery, from correcting some genuine cosmetic deformity (e.g., cleft palate) to an unwarranted preoccupation with and desire to change some physical feature that is judged as deficient only by the possessor or that is viewed as falling short of some aesthetic ideal (e.g., an imperfect nose or modestly sized breasts). The cosmetic surgeon is in a unique position to observe and facilitate body image change. Such changes typically involve perceptual, affective, and cognitive components. Many individuals who undergo cosmetic surgery report being temporarily disturbed by the change in physical appearance (e.g., sleeplessness, reduced body sensation), although the majority of these individuals adjust well to the change with the passage of time.

Although many individuals who undergo cosmetic surgery are satisfied with the outcome, a significant number report moderate to extreme dissatisfaction. Often surgical patients feel satisfied with their altered features but become dissatisfied and preoccupied with other perceived physical deficiencies. They may subsequently have frequent surgeries to correct or improve multiple physical features. Some of these individuals have a clinical preoccupation with trivial or imagined defects in their appearance. Such a preoccupation is called *body dysmorphic disorder*, which is a pathological disturbance in body image in which individuals feel extreme distress about minor flaws in some part of the body, such as the size or shape of the ears, eyebrows, mouth, hands, feet, fingers, or buttocks. Individuals with this disorder describe their preoccupations as tormenting, extremely painful, and devastating, and thoughts about their "defect" dominate their lives. In some cases, disturbed thoughts are so intrusive that individuals avoid work and public places, going out only at night when they cannot be seen. Those who have body dysmorphic disorder often undergo cosmetic surgery, but unfortunately for some, the surgery fails to alleviate body image dissatisfaction. Indeed, in some cases it increases their concerns as a doctor's willingness to provide surgery validates their views of abnormality, which may give rise to intensified or new preoccupations.

For the majority of those undergoing cosmetic surgery (i.e., correcting an obvious disfigurement or perceived aberration), physical changes enhance body image. However, surgery will likely be insufficient for improving body image among those with clinical preoccupations of self-perceived physical inadequacies.

VI. IMPROVING BODY IMAGE

Anecdotal and clinical evidence suggest that the key to reducing body image dissatisfaction is through increasing self-acceptance. Although this goal is itself difficult to attain, progress toward self-acceptance can be accomplished in a number of ways. For instance, those who believe they are overweight should be encouraged to exercise and to eat a nutritionally balanced diet rather than go on a strict calorie reducing diet. The goal is therefore one of health rather than one of improved physical appearance. Individuals need to learn to accept and perhaps even value their physical appearance with techniques such as positive self-statements and careful self-examination in front of mirrors, as well as questioning the basis for their desire to lose weight (i.e., the reasons that they want to lose weight or why they believe they are overweight). Sometimes people benefit from education about the determinants of physical characteristics, such as genetic influences on body weight and anatomical discussions of bone structure. Moreover, it is often useful for people to be told that a certain degree of body image dissatisfaction is common, even among those who are objectively highly attractive (and who possess all of the physical attributes that most people desire).

Because body image dissatisfaction arises in part out of fear of social evaluation, increasing social skills and assertiveness may be especially useful for alleviating body image dissatisfaction. Stigmatized individuals may have limited opportunities to develop and refine social interaction skills, and therefore interventions that focus on increasing conversational skills, controlling nonverbal behaviors, and increasing assertiveness might increase positive social interactions, which in turn might diminish some aspects of body image dissatisfaction.

Particularly intense body image dissatisfaction might require some form of counseling or therapy. Treatment is indicated when body image dissatisfaction interferes with normal activities, becomes an obsession that involves unwanted or disturbing thoughts, or when it prevents people from coming into social contact with others. A therapeutic environment might assist individuals in coping with family conflict, social anxiety, or disordered cognitions. Group sessions in which individuals are allowed to decry the social importance placed on the superficial and simplistic criteria of body weight and shape, and to meet others in similar situations, work toward increasing self-satisfaction and providing a social support context for positive body image change. Cognitive–behavioral approaches to improving body image have shown some success in diminishing body image dissatisfaction. Programs that emphasize coping strategies and social skills may be the most beneficial for moderate body image dissatisfaction. Appropriately treating individuals for depression, whether through psychotherapy or medication, may also be an effective strategy for increasing body image satisfaction.

BIBLIOGRAPHY

Cash, T. F., & Pruzinsky, T. (1990). *Body images: Development, deviance, and change.* New York: Guilford Press.

Fallon, A. (1990). Culture in the mirror: Sociocultural determinants of body image. In T. F. Cash & T. Pruzinsky (Eds.). *Body images: Development, deviance, and change.* New York: Guilford Press.

Goffman, E. (1963). *Stigma: Notes on the management of spoiled identity.* New York: Prentice Hall.

Jones, E. E., Farina, A., Hastorf, A. H., Markus, H., Miller, D. T., & Scott, R. A. (1984). *Social stigma: The psychology of marked relationships.* New York: W. H. Freeman.

Polivy, J., Herman, C. P., & Pliner, P. (1990). Perception and evaluation of body image: The meaning of body size and shape. In J. Olson and M. Zanna (Eds.), *Self-inference processes.* Hillsdale, NJ: Lawrence Erlbaum.

Seid, R. P. (1989). *Never too thin: Why women are at war with their bodies.* New York: Prentice Hall Press.

Body Rhythms/Body Clocks

Jose C. Florez*, Lisa D. Wilsbacher, and Joseph S. Takahashi

Howard Hughes Medical Institute and Northwestern University

Circadian Rhythm Biological rhythm that oscillateswith a periodicity approaching, but not exactly, 24 hours; in the organism's natural conditions, it is synchronized to the 24-hour light/dark cycle.

Entrainment Synchronization of a biological rhythm to an external oscillation.

Oscillator Biological structure that exhibits self-sustaining periodical cycles in the state of a given variable under constant environmental conditions.

Pacemaker Oscillator capable of driving other physiological rhythms.

Period Time interval between recurrences of a defined phase of the oscillation.

Phase-Response Curve Plot that indicates how the amplitude and direction of a phase shift induced by a single stimulus depends on the circadian time at which the stimulus was administered.

Phase Shift Displacement of the timing of an oscillation with respect to the original time frame.

Suprachiasmatic Nucleus Area of the hypothalamus responsible for the generation of circadian rhythms in mammals; the anatomical site of the mammalian circadian pacemaker.

Transgene Exogenous DNA coding for a particular gene which is injected into the fertilized oocyte pronucleus and integrates with endogenous DNA.

BIOLOGICAL RHYTHMICITY is a cardinal feature of living organisms. Circadian (~24-hour; see glossary) rhythms are the subset of biological rhythms that keep an organism synchronized to the 24-hour environment. Disorders of circadian rhythmicity can have serious consequences for the health and well-being of affected individuals. This article discusses the theoretical framework underlying circadian rhythms, the physiological systems involved in their generation, the molecular mechanisms by which they are regulated, and the significance of circadian rhythms for human health and disease.

I. BIOLOGICAL RHYTHMICITY

The biological functions performed by a living organism in order to sustain itself can be classified into one of two categories according to their time course of activity. Those that must be carried out at all times are called constitutive processes, while those that cycle between the active and inactive states are called biological rhythms. Cellular respiration is an example of a constitutive process in biological organisms. A cell must always take up oxygen, convert oxygen's energy into ATP (or other high-energy phosphates), and dispose of carbon dioxide waste; failure to do so quickly leads to death of the cell. Biological rhythms

---

*Jose C. Florez is presently at Massachusetts General Hospital, Boston, MA.

exist in all forms of life; prominent examples in humans include the heartbeat and the breathing pattern (high frequency), daily hormonal surges (moderate frequency), and the menstrual cycle (low frequency). At the level of the whole organism, these rhythms coordinate biological processes with internal or external variables and thus allow for temporal compartmentalization when spatial separation is not viable or beneficial. The hallmarks of biological rhythmicity include predictability, relative sensitivity to changes in the external environment, and ability to profoundly affect an organism when disrupted.

Circadian (~24-hour) rhythms are an important class of biological rhythms that evolved in response to the 24-hour cycle of light and darkness caused by the earth's rotation. The fundamental properties and the molecular organization of circadian rhythms are the focus of the first sections of this article. In later sections, we illustrate how disruption of the circadian system can lead to detrimental consequences in the overall well-being of the individual.

II. CIRCADIAN RHYTHMS

A. Why Did Circadian Rhythms Evolve?

The daily rhythm of light and darkness is a powerful environmental stimulus. Organisms that could use the light/dark cycle and related cycle of temperature to measure the time of day could then reliably coordinate physiological processes with these environmental rhythms. Furthermore, because daylength changes with season, species which could sense the progressive lengthening of one of the phases of the light/dark cycle could also optimally adapt their behavior to the changing climate. The emergence of an endogenous pacemaker that can oscillate with a periodicity approaching 24 hours and that can be entrained or synchronized by external lighting cues allowed organisms to incorporate a temporal dimension into the maintenance of internal homeostasis.

Circadian rhythms are ubiquitous in nature. They exist in every eukaryotic and some prokaryotic species examined to date and directly regulate functions such as bioluminescence, activity, body temperature, hormonal secretion and the sleep-wake cycle. The circadian pacemaker also gates specific biological processes, such as the ovulatory surge in female rodents, to allow their expression only at specific times of the day. The defining characteristic of circadian rhythms is their persistence for several cycles in constant environmental conditions devoid of time cues (Fig. 1). The basic features of circadian rhythms are outlined in the next section.

B. Fundamental Properties

Circadian rhythms share several fundamental properties:

- They are generated by a self-sustaining endogenous pacemaker and oscillate with a period approximating 24 hours in constant conditions;
- They can be entrained by certain environmental signals, and a single stimulus by one of these signals can permanently shift the phase of the oscillation;

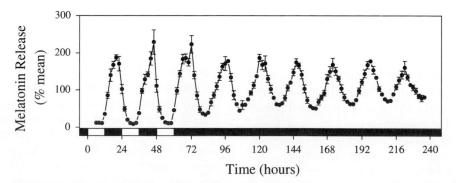

Figure 1 Circadian oscillation of melatonin output in dissociated chick pineal cell cultures. Chick pineal cells contain a circadian oscillator, as expressed by the rhythmic production of melatonin with a period approximating 24 hours. The rhythm persists in constant darkness for several cycles. (Figure courtesy of Dr. Keith Barrett.)

- Their period remains relatively constant over a wide range of temperatures;
- They are genetically determined, not learned.

1. The Pacemaker and Periodicity

If circadian rhythms can persist in the absence of superimposed environmental oscillations, they must be generated by an internal pacemaking system. This endogenous pacemaker serves as an internal *circadian clock* that tells the organism the approximate time of day. Its localization to a particular organ by the laboratories of R. Y. Moore and I. Zucker constituted one of the early achievements of circadian anatomists; experimental lesion studies have shown that destruction of the anatomical structure that contains the circadian pacemaker—which varies depending on the species—induces loss of circadian rhythms.

Period length of the circadian rhythms generated by the endogenous pacemaker varies from species to species. In most cases, the endogenous circadian pacemaker exhibits a period close to, but not exactly equal to, 24 hours. The slight discrepancy between circadian period and environmental period forces an organism to readjust its clock each day.

2. Entrainment and Phase-Shifting

The circadian clock can be *entrained,* or synchronized, to oscillations of relevant external variables known as *Zeitgebers.* The light/dark cycle appears to be the dominant *Zeitgeber* in most species, as sectioning of the specific visual pathway that conveys light information to the mammalian pacemaker (see below) weakens or abolishes circadian rhythmicity. As shown by J. Aschoff and others, other factors such as temperature, food and water availability, and social cues can also serve as entraining agents. In order to entrain an organism, information from the environment must reach the circadian clock and alter its oscillation. Circadian systems across species appear to follow a common conceptual design (Fig. 2): external stimuli reach the pacemaker via an input pathway, and the pacemaker in turn sends an output signal that drives the overt rhythms of the organism.

As mentioned above, an organism must readjust its circadian clock each day to match the 24-hour light/dark cycle. The effect of the *Zeitgeber* on synchronizing the circadian clock is known as *phase shifting.* Under experimental conditions, it has been shown that a single stimulus of light can phase shift the circadian

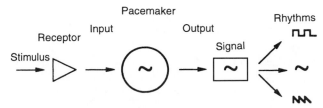

Figure 2 Schematic diagram of the main components of the circadian system. An entraining stimulus activates a receptor, which relays this message to the oscillator via an **input** pathway. The **pacemaker** generates oscillations (even in the absence of entraining information) relaying an **output** signal which in turn drives various overt rhythms. (Reprinted from Florez, J. C. and Takahashi, J. S. (1995). The circadian clock: from molecules to behaviour. *Ann. Med., 27,* 481–490. Copyright © 1995 by Blackwell Science.)

oscillator permanently, such that the pacemaker retains its new phase for every cycle subsequent to the initial stimulus. Furthermore, the direction and magnitude of the phase shift depends on the time at which the stimulus was administered, such that the same stimulus will cause phase advances or phase delays depending on the point along the circadian cycle at which the oscillator finds itself. If a complete circadian oscillation under constant conditions (i.e. when the oscillator is free-running) is considered as a *circadian day,* a light pulse given in the subjective dawn will phase advance the clock, whereas a pulse of the same intensity and duration given in the subjective dusk will phase delay it. For example, in the days leading to the summer solstice a diurnal animal's activity onset occurs earlier as the sun rises earlier, whereas a nocturnal animal delays activity onset as the sun sets later. This is accomplished by the pacemaker's response to light: when the animal is exposed to light in the early morning, the circadian oscillator is *phase advanced;* when it is exposed to light shortly before the onset of darkness, it is *phase delayed.* The *phase-response curve* exhibits the magnitude and direction of a phase shift in response to an environmental pulse stimulus at any *circadian time* (Fig. 3). Both the shape of the phase-response curve and the endogenous period are thought to constitute internal properties of the pacemaker itself. Manipulations of either property affect the oscillator itself, not just its input or output pathways.

3. Temperature Compensation

Most biological reactions are temperature-sensitive; as the temperature is raised, the rate of the reaction

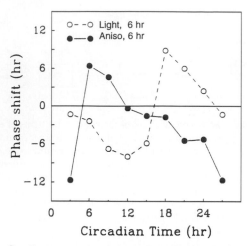

Figure 3 Phase-response curves of the melatonin rhythm in cultured chick pineal induced by two different phase-shifting stimuli. Dotted curve with open circles, 6-hour light pulses; solid curve with filled circles, 6-hour pulses of the protein synthesis inhibitor anisomycin. (Reprinted from Takahashi, J. S., et al. (1989). The avian pineal, a vertebrate model system of the circadian oscillator: cellular regulation of circadian rhythms by light, second messengers, and macromolecular synthesis. *Recent Progr. Horm. Res.*, 45, 279–352. Copyright © 1989 Academic Press.)

increases. However, as shown in seminal experiments by Pittendrigh, circadian rhythmicity is temperature-compensated: the period of the rhythm is held relatively constant across a broad temperature range. Temperature compensation is essential for maintaining circadian rhythm stability: in this way, poikilotherms preserve a constant circadian period throughout climactic changes, and homeotherms retain appropriate rhythms during specialized temperature changes such as fever.

4. Genetics

The argument could be made that circadian rhythmicity is a learned behavior rather than an inborn property. The isolation of circadian rhythm mutants in *Drosophila* by Konopka and Benzer in 1971 demonstrated the heritable nature of circadian rhythmicity: mutant flies with a long period or short period passed that trait on to their offspring in a semidominant fashion. These studies led to the cloning of the first circadian rhythm gene, *period* (see below). In the 25 years following this discovery, much progress has been made in determining the genetic basis of circadian rhythmicity. Additional circadian rhythm mutants have been discovered or experimentally induced

in *Drosophila*, the mold *Neurospora*, the plant *Arabidopsis*, the cyanobacterium *Synechococcus*, the hamster, and the mouse. Identification of other circadian rhythm genes should allow the elucidation of all genetic components of the circadian clock.

III. THE SUPRACHIASMATIC NUCLEUS, THE MAMMALIAN CIRCADIAN CLOCK

As elegantly described by Moore and others, the *suprachiasmatic nucleus* (SCN) of the anterior hypothalamus is a distinct, bilaterally paired cluster of ~10,000 neurons located dorsal to the optic chiasm and immediately lateral to the third ventricle. Several lines of evidence implicate the SCN as the anatomical substrate of the mammalian circadian clock: (i) destruction of the SCN by experimental lesions abolishes circadian rhythmicity; (ii) transplantation of fetal SCN tissue into a lesioned host restores the circadian rhythm of locomotor activity; (iii) the SCN shows circadian rhythms in 2-deoxyglucose uptake and neuronal firing; (iv) when surgically isolated from surrounding tissue, a suprachiasmatic "island" still maintains a circadian rhythm in electrical activity; (v) dispersed SCN neurons cultured on a multielectrode array plate show circadian electrical activity with an intrinsic period for several cycles; (vi) the SCN receives direct photoreceptive input from the retina via the *retinohypothalamic tract* (RHT); and (vii) transplantation of SCN tissue from mutant hamsters who have a short free-running period into SCN-lesioned wild-type hosts restores circadian rhythms of locomotor activity with the period determined by the donor's mutant phenotype.

Although the SCN can be readily identified by conventional histological stains in the rodent brain, in humans its borders are less precise and more subject to interindividual variation. Recent immunocytochemical studies have delineated its cytoarchitecture and outlined the differences between the human SCN and that of other species. The SCN—with the periventricular nucleus—is the most rostral hypothalamic nucleus in the human brain, first identified around the antero-lateral margin of the optic recess dorsal to the optic chiasm (Fig. 4). The human SCN is sexually dimorphic: it is more elongated in the dorsoventral axis in women and more spherical in men. It is composed of heterogeneous groups of neurons which stain vari-

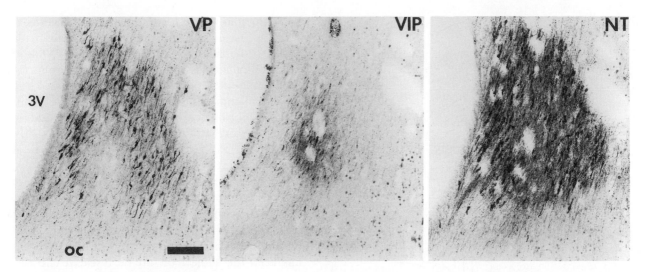

Figure 4 Photomicrographs of coronal sections through the human suprachiasmatic nucleus (SCN) prepared to show three different neuronal populations. The SCN lies above the optic chiasm (OC) and immediately lateral to the third ventricle (3V). VP, stained with an antiserum to vasopressin. VIP, stained with an antiserum to vasoactive intestinal polypeptide. NT, stained with an antiserum to neurotensin. Scale bar = 200 mm. (Figure courtesy of Dr. Robert Y. Moore.)

ably for the neuropeptides vasopressin (VP), vasoactive intestinal polypeptide (VIP), neuropeptide Y (NPY) and neurotensin (NT). On the basis of animal studies, it appears that the central subdivision of the human SCN (containing VIP neurons) receives retinal input. The class of neurons responsible for the generation of circadian rhythmicity has not yet been elucidated in either humans or animal models.

The rodent SCN has been more thoroughly investigated. For example, in the rat most or all of the SCN neurons also express the inhibitory neurotransmitter GABA. Regarding the input pathways, it appears that the neurotransmitter employed by the RHT in transmitting photic information to the SCN is an excitatory amino acid (glutamate), although its identity has not yet been conclusively demonstrated. In addition, light input also reaches the SCN through the intergeniculate leaflet of the thalamus, which sends NPY-containing and GABAergic projections to the SCN via the geniculohypothalamic tract. Whether these features are preserved in the human circadian system awaits further work.

The rodent SCN projects to a variety of other brain structures, including several hypothalamic nuclei, the thalamus, and the basal forebrain. Which specific anatomical projection is associated with particular circadian rhythms is still under investigation. The pathway to the pineal gland, however, has been well described. In mammals, the pineal gland is not a site of the circadian clock; it receives an output signal from the SCN via a multisynaptic pathway to synthesize melatonin at the appropriate time of day. Fibers from the SCN innervate the paraventricular nucleus of the hypothalamus (PVN); the PVN sends projections to the intermediolateral column of the thoracic spinal cord, where they synapse on preganglionic sympathetic neurons; and these in turn project to the superior cervical ganglion, which sends postganglionic sympathetic fibers to the pineal gland (Fig. 5). At night, activity from SCN neurons results in the secretion of norepinephrine by postganglionic sympathetic terminals in the pineal gland, which leads to an increase in intracellular cyclic AMP levels and a dramatic rise in melatonin production.

How does the SCN generate a rhythmic signal? The rhythmic output produced by the SCN could be the end result of the complex interaction of a neuronal network, difficult to characterize physiologically and to replicate experimentally. Conversely, circadian rhythmicity could be an intrinsic cellular property, such that isolated cells could maintain the expression of a circadian signal and entrain to the environment provided the appropriate synchronizing stimulus was made available. The question of whether circadian rhythmicity can be generated by single cells has been addressed in nonmammalian systems by G. D. Block,

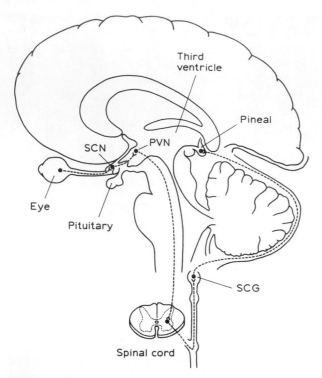

Figure 5 Diagram of the human brain (mid-sagittal section) showing the regulation of the pineal gland melatonin rhythm by the suprachiasmatic nucleus via a multisynaptic pathway. See text for details. Abbreviations: SCN, suprachiasmatic nucleus; PVN, paraventricular nucleus; SCG, superior cervical ganglion. (Reprinted with permission from Hofman, M. A., and Swaab, D. F., The human hypothalamus: comparative morphometry and photoperiodic influences, *Progress in Brain Research, 93,* 133–149. Copyright © 1992 with kind permission of Elsevier Science–NL, Sara Burgertstraat 25, 1055 KV Amsterdam, The Netherlands.)

G. E. Pickard, and others: isolated neurons of the eye of the mollusk *Bulla gouldiana* express a circadian rhythm in membrane conductance, and single pineal cells in lower vertebrates synthesize melatonin in a circadian fashion. The recent recording of single-cell electrophysiological rhythms in dispersed SCN cell cultures in the laboratory of S. M. Reppert suggests that cell autonomy is a property of mammalian pacemaking organs as well.

Experiments in the hamster recently showed that a second circadian clock, independent of the SCN, exists in the mammalian retina. These experiments, performed in the Menaker laboratory, demonstrated a circadian rhythm of melatonin produced by isolated hamster retinas in constant darkness. Multiple sites of circadian pacemakers exist in lower vertebrates (the

SCN, the pineal gland, and the retina); however, this was the first definitive demonstration of a circadian oscillator outside the SCN in a mammal. While this retinal oscillator is not likely to directly affect the broad range of physiological rhythms regulated by the SCN in mammals, it does suggest that some rhythms may be coordinated by separate clocks. In addition, the retinal oscillator may indirectly affect SCN-driven rhythms by gating photic input through the retinohypothalamic tract.

If circadian rhythmicity can be generated by single cells, endogenous biochemical mechanisms must exist that give rise to a cyclical signal in the absence of external input. The elucidation of the biochemical pathway involved in the production of circadian rhythms has been the subject of intense research efforts for more than two decades. Genetic analyses of the circadian system indicate that this pathway involves cyclic gene expression and regulation. Because these mutations were first uncovered in simple organisms, they provide models for the organization of circadian rhythmicity at the cellular level, as explained in the next section. The recent discovery of circadian mutations in mammals may soon illustrate whether such mechanisms are preserved in higher vertebrates.

IV. MOLECULAR ORGANIZATION OF CIRCADIAN RHYTHMS

The experimental generation of circadian mutants in the mold *Neurospora* and the fruitfly *Drosophila* have allowed the identification of key molecular components of the circadian clock in both species. The *period* and *timeless* genes in *Drosophila* and the *frequency* gene in *Neurospora* are defined by mutant alleles that alter period length or disrupt circadian rhythms. A common theme emerging from this line of work is their functioning through negative feedback loops which include transcriptional and translational steps. The salient features of both systems are reviewed here as a way to introduce a model that is likely to be conserved in mammals.

In *Drosophila,* the period gene (*per*) regulates circadian rhythms of pupal eclosion and locomotor activity. Extensive work performed in the laboratories of M. Rosbash, J. C. Hall, M. W. Young, and others has shown that different mutations in this gene can cause changes in period length or loss of rhythmicity. Oscillations of both *per* mRNA and PER protein have been demonstrated in adult flies, and the rhythm persists in constant darkness with an endogenous period that correlates with the fly genotype. Arrhythmic *per* null mutants can be rescued by germline transformation (a type of transgenic manipulation) with wild-type *per* DNA, which restores both circadian behavior and endogenous *per* RNA cycles. Transient induction of a *per* transgene regulated by a heat-shock promoter results in behavioral phase shifts. Taken together, these results suggest that PER protein regulates *per* RNA cycling via negative feedback, possibly at the level of transcription.

In addition to *per,* the gene *timeless* (*tim*) also shows a similar circadian fluctuation in its mRNA levels and is required for the expression of circadian rhythms in *Drosophila* flies. *Tim* null mutants fail to express both locomotor activity rhythms and *per* RNA oscillations. Furthermore, the TIM and PER proteins have been shown to bind to each other, and the presence of TIM is necessary for the translocation of PER to the nucleus. Pulses of light lead to the rapid degradation of TIM protein. When these pulses are administered in the early subjective night (when TIM protein is being actively synthesized), they delay the accumulation of TIM protein and the translocation of the PER-TIM complex to the nucleus, thus resulting in slower transcriptional activation or repression of presumptive circadian genes and behavioral phase delays; in contrast, when the pulses are given in the late subjective night (when *tim* transcription has already been suppressed after PER-TIM nuclear entry), the rapid degradation of TIM protein leads to an early disappearance of PER and phase advances both in the molecular cycling of circadian transcripts and in the expression of behavioral rhythms. In this manner, a unidirectional signal (a single pulse of light) results in bidirectional behavioral effects (phase advances or delays), providing a molecular answer to a long-standing unresolved question in the circadian field. A working model of the circadian system incorporating some of the above findings is presented in Fig. 6.

In *Neurospora,* the *frequency* (*frq*) gene product has been recently shown by J. C. Dunlap, J. Loros, and co-workers to be a central component of the *Neurospora* circadian oscillator. This pivotal role is substantiated by the observations that the amount of *frq* mRNA oscillates with a circadian period, *frq* mutants have mRNA oscillations of a different periodicity,

in null mutants both circadian rhythmicity and *frq* mRNA oscillations are abolished, high constitutive expression of a *frq* transgene in a wild-type background abolishes circadian rhythmicity and depresses endogenous *frq* transcript levels, and the phase of the overt rhythm can be reset by step reductions in the concentration of the inducer used to express the *frq* transgene. In addition, light induces the expression of *frq* mRNA and protein. Taken together, these results conclusively show that the *frq* gene product regulates the *Neurospora* circadian oscillator by exercising negative feedback on its own transcription.

Similar genetic experiments are difficult to replicate in mammalian species, where longer generation times and smaller litter sizes limit the power of genetic analysis. The fortuitous discovery by Ralph and Menaker of a circadian mutation in the hamster, *tau,* has been an effective aid in providing some answers to key questions regarding the mechanisms of circadian rhythmicity in mammals. The *tau* mutation is an autosomal, semidominant mutation that shortens the circadian period to about 22 hours in heterozygotes and 20 hours in homozygotes. Studies with *tau* mutant hamsters helped to confirm the genetic heritability of circadian features in mammals and to demonstrate the pacemaking role of the mammalian SCN, as SCN-lesioned wild-type hamsters recovered short-period phenotypes after receiving a *tau* SCN transplant. The hamster retinal clock is also affected by genotype: the period of the melatonin rhythm from isolated retinas is about 23.8 hours in wild-type animals but about 21.2 hours in *tau* homozygous mutant hamsters. Nevertheless, the paucity of information available on the hamster genome has hampered efforts to map and clone the *tau* gene.

Therefore, in order to uncover the molecular components of the mammalian circadian clock, a circadian clock mutation had to be produced or discovered in an organism with a better potential for genetic analysis. Rather than screening for spontaneous mutants, a high-efficiency germline mutation method has recently been used by our laboratory to produce the first circadian mutation in the mouse. This mutation, called *Clock,* is defined by a single-gene, autosomal semidominant locus that results in the lengthening of the free-running period by about 1 hour in heterozygous mice. Homozygotes express extremely long periods in the first few days of constant darkness (27–28 hours), which soon degenerate into arrhythmicity

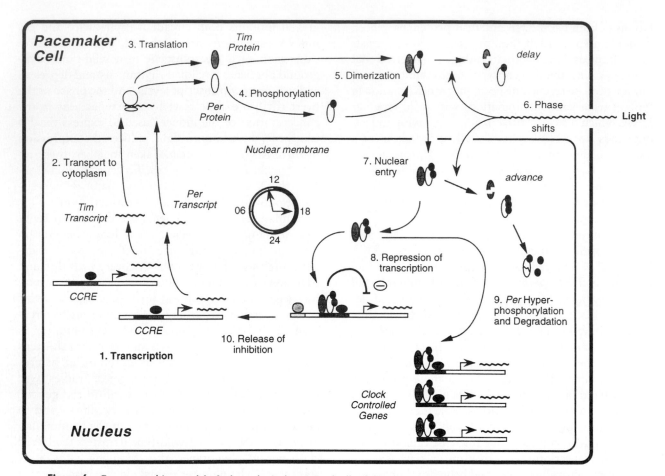

Figure 6 Current working model of a hypothetical negative feedback loop generating circadian oscillations, which incorporates various elements of both the *per* and *frq* systems. All circadian functions are confined to a single pacemaker cell and involve transcriptional and translational processes (the figure flows *clockwise*): Transcription of *clock transcripts* (*per* and *tim* in this case) is regulated via circadian clock-response elements or CCREs (1). The clock transcripts are processed and transported to the cytoplasm (2), where they are translated into PER and TIM proteins (3). PER protein undergoes post-translational phosphorylation (4), and after a lag period PER and TIM dimerize (5) which enables their translocation to the nucleus (7). TIM protein is subject to rapid degradation in response to a light signal; the timing of this event determines whether the light stimulus will cause advances or delays (6). In the nucleus, the protein dimer (possibly in conjunction with other factors) may bind DNA, repress its own transcription (8) and regulate the transcription of various *clock-controlled genes*. After degradation of PER protein (9), transcriptional inhibition is released and the cycle resumes (10). (Modified from Florez, J. C., and Takahashi, J. S. (1995). The circadian clock: from molecules to behaviour. *Ann. Med., 27,* 481–490.)

with no obvious circadian components (Fig. 7). Using mapping crosses, the *Clock* gene was mapped to the midportion of mouse chromosome 5 in a region with conserved synteny to human chromosome 4. The molecular nature of the *Clock* gene was determined by positional cloning and transgenic approaches. In order to prove that a particular segment of DNA coded for *Clock*, small portions of wild-type DNA from the region to which *Clock* maps were injected into fertil-

ized mouse oocytes. These transgenic animals were bred with *Clock* mutant mice; progeny mice that were determined by molecular analysis to contain both the mutant *Clock* gene (in heterozygous or homozygous state) and one particular transgene expressed a wild-type circadian period in constant darkness. This "rescue" of the mutant phenotype proved that this transgene contained *Clock*. The DNA sequence of that region indicated that *Clock* is a basic-helix-loop-helix-PAS domain transcription factor, where the PAS domain, named after the first three proteins shown to contain this motif (PER, ARNT, and SIM), is involved in protein dimerization. Sequence analysis of the mutant *Clock* gene showed a single A → T point mutation, which alters a splice donor site (Fig. 7). This discovery provides the first molecular handle with which to analyze the role of gene transcription in generating circadian rhythms in mammals. In addition, new genetic screens and the identification of genes that interact with *Clock* in defining different circadian phenotypes is expected to begin the elucidation of the molecular mechanisms that generate mammalian circadian oscillations.

V. HUMAN CIRCADIAN RHYTHMS

Human beings have also organized their behavior around the 24-hour light/dark cycle. The sleep/wake pattern, meal schedules and social or professional habits follow the periodicity imposed by the natural oscillation in light and darkness. More interestingly, physiological processes over which we have little control also undergo daily fluctuations. For example, body temperature follows a diurnal rhythm that peaks in the evening and falls to a minimum in the early morning (about 2–3 hours before awakening), with almost a 1°C difference between the two. It could be argued that the dawn-dusk difference in body temperature is the direct result of increased voluntary activity during the day, likely to generate a certain amount of body heat; however, this is only partially correct, since the circadian rhythm in body temperature (as well as rhythms in various hormones such as cortisol, thyroid-stimulating hormone, melatonin, prolactin, and growth hormone) can be demonstrated when subjects follow a constant routine. In this protocol, designed to abolish masking influences (i.e., effects on circadian rhythms by variables other than the circadian pacemaker), experimental subjects remain in conditions of constant bedrest, enforced wakefulness, dim indoor light and constant caloric intake for 30 to 50 hours, and show circadian fluctuations in multiple physiological variables (Fig. 8). As shown in Fig. 8, the rise of a rhythmic parameter at the beginning of the second day of constant routine occurs spontaneously at the expected time in the absence

Wild-type

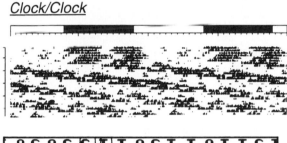

Clock/Clock

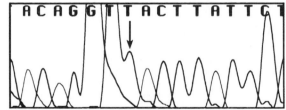

Figure 7 Identification of the *Clock* mutation. Wheel-running activity records and DNA sequence data from both a wild-type mouse and a *Clock/Clock* mutant mouse are shown. Wheel-running activity is indicated by black marks on the record; the X axis denotes a 48-hour period, with successive days plotted both to the right of and below each 24-hour record. Animals were entrained to a 12:12 light/dark cycle for the first 8 days (as shown by the black and white bar at the top of the figure) and then transferred to constant darkness for the remainder of the record. DNA sequence analysis shows a single A → T transversion (marked by the arrow) at the intron-exon splice junction 3′ to exon 19. This mutation causes skipping of exon 19 during mRNA processing and results in the deletion of a 51-amino acid segment in the C-terminal end of CLOCK. (Reprinted from King, D. P., et al. (1997). Positional cloning of the mouse circadian *Clock* gene. *Cell, 89,* 641–653. Copyright © 1997 by Cell Press.)

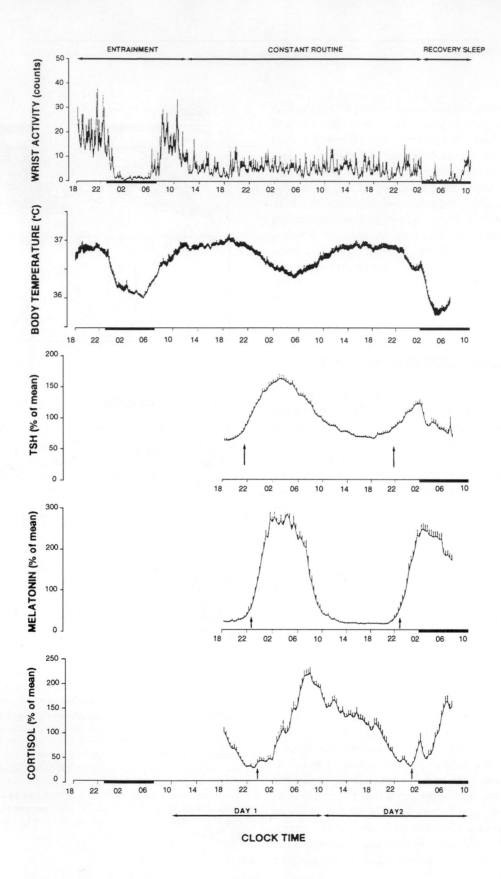

of any time cues. In addition, the oscillations of different rhythms that regulate disparate physiological functions appear to be temporally coordinated, in that they all maintain the same periodicity.

The above results indicate that human beings are also endowed with an endogenous pacemaker that coordinates circadian rhythms. It is perhaps significant that parameters such as body temperature and the hormones mentioned above are regulated by hypothalamic nuclei, in close anatomical proximity to the SCN. Whether the SCN sends direct neural input to subservient circadian oscillators needs to be resolved, but it is not required; as outlined in Section III, the rhythmic output of the hormone melatonin by the pineal gland is driven by the SCN via a multisynaptic pathway through several relay neuronal stations.

Other behavioral functions are subject to regulation by the circadian clock. For instance, the sleep/wake cycle is gated by the circadian pacemaker, such that the duration of sleep, the subjective feeling of sleepiness, the propensity to enter a particular phase of sleep and sleep tendency are all determined by the circadian phase of the oscillator. In addition, there are specific circadian times at which it is very difficult to initiate sleep, even after sleep deprivation. Human beings also appear to experience circadian rhythmicity in subjective alertness, mood, and performance efficiency.

Like all circadian pacemakers, the human circadian clock can be entrained by external signals. Human beings in a constant routine experience phase shifts in the rhythms of both body temperature and melatonin production by single pulses of light. As in other species, light is a powerful entraining agent; even moderate amounts of lighting at the appropriate circadian times can significantly affect the human circadian oscillator. However, human beings often modify their environment by voluntary actions, which in turn directly affect their physiology: thus, other entraining agents that can reset the human circadian clock include social cues, meal schedules, and the level of activity. Nevertheless, there is a limit to the degree of advance or delay imposed on the circadian clock from one cycle to the next. When the human circadian system is stretched too far in any one direction, one encounters the disorders of circadian rhythmicity that are the focus of the next section.

VI. DERANGEMENTS OF CIRCADIAN FUNCTION

A. Classification and Treatment

Disorders of circadian rhythmicity can be divided into two classes: those that result from noncircadian artificial conditions (i.e. *exogenous*) and those that are caused by pathological aberrations in the circadian system itself (i.e. *endogenous*). Two separate categories will also be considered in this section: the changes in the circadian system observed with normal *aging,* and the direct influence of circadian parameters on the psychiatric condition known as *seasonal affective disorder.*

I. Exogenous Alterations in Circadian Rhythmicity

As mentioned at the end of the previous section, human beings can voluntarily impose changes in their circadian behavior. Other animals and all plants, if left undisturbed, will follow the circadian program dictated by their physiology and entrained by the external light/dark cycle. Perturbations of this program, for example by light pulses or bouts of forced activity at unexpected times, will shift the circadian oscillation in a predictable direction.

Human beings, however, have created artificial environments that either modify the person's perception

Figure 8 Example of a constant routine protocol. Patients are maintained in a forcibly awake recumbent position in dim light, fed with regular light snacks and isolated from time cues. Wrist activity, body temperature, and various hormonal rhythms are monitored. The stable level in wrist activity after 1200 hours on day 1 indicates that masking influences have been eliminated by the constant routine protocol; the rise in different hormonal markers on day 2 provides evidence of circadian rhythmicity in humans. Curves indicate mean profiles; vertical bars show standard error; horizontal black bars denote recovery sleep periods. (Reprinted with permission from Van Cauter, E., et al. (1994). Demonstration of rapid light-induced advances and delays of the human circadian clock using hormonal phase markers. *Am. J. Physiol., 266,* E953–E963. Copyright © 1994 by the American Physiological Society.)

of external diurnal cycles or enforce patterns of activity on the individual that are outside the circadian frequency. The first case can be found in people subjected to constant environmental conditions for an extended period of time, such as patients in an intensive care unit (ICU) or a newborn nursery. The second case is common among the millions of workers engaged in activities that require different shifts throughout the day that rotate among the available personnel from week to week. It is perhaps ironic that one of the societal groups which most blatantly disregards the organism's preference for a circadian routine is that of health care professionals.

Shift work entails the voluntary subjection of the body to contradictory entraining signals, where sleep, wakefulness, artificial lighting, and professional cues suggest one circadian pattern whereas natural lighting, social cues, and meal schedules might suggest another. The complex interaction of varied entraining signals might direct the pacemaker to generate an undesired oscillation (e.g., with propensity to sleep peaking during working hours), support circadian rhythms out of phase with one another, and/or cause continuous phase shifts in the circadian pacemaker. All of these effects can lead to internal temporal disorganization.

The unattractive notion of a permanent shirt-work schedule out of phase with general societal patterns led to the concept of rotating shifts among employees, such that each employee is only required to work during out-of-phase (nocturnal or "graveyard") shifts for alternating periods. Although in theory the circadian system would then only be subjected to external stresses on half or one-third of the time, in reality this practice introduced the added strain of requiring large phase shifts on change-of-shift days. The effect of such phase shifts on the individual, which are usually on the order of 8 hours, is similar to that experienced by travelers who cross multiple time zones in rapid fashion, popularly known as "jet lag." The body requires several days to adjust to the new schedule, because some rhythms can only be advanced or delayed by about 2 to 3 hours per day. The effect is compounded when workers change shifts frequently (e.g., weekly), such that half of the days in each shift are spent adjusting to the new schedule. Consequently, individuals who choose or are required to work in this fashion spend periods in which they cannot function at peak performance due to physiological constraints.

The long-term effects of continuous exposure to temporally disorganizing stimuli on human health have not been studied; some of the practices leading to such behavior are only relatively recent. Similarly, the correlation between the number of on-the-job accidents and the circadian status of the individuals involved has not been analyzed systematically in a large population. Even less forthcoming is information on the direct cost to industry incurred by accidents induced by circadian dysfunction, in numbers of days of work lost or the amount of worker compensation claims. Such studies are necessary both for the epidemiological understanding of this problem and to provide solid evidence that might motivate management to introduce appropriate changes. An interesting report made use of statistics on U.S. professional sports teams: this study showed that baseball teams traveling from the west to the east coast of the United States had a worse performance on the day following rapid transmeridian travel than those traveling westward, regardless of whether they were playing at home or at an away location.

Despite the dearth of published reports on this issue, a large amount of anecdotal evidence exists on the subjective discomfort experienced by individuals under such circadian stresses. In addition, animal studies from the last several decades have provided a basis for recommendations to ensure optimal performance by circadian pacemaker: (i) it appears to be easier to delay the human clock than to advance it, or to travel westward than to travel eastward; therefore, work shifts might be designed such that people delay the time they begin sleep, rather than advance it (i.e., from day shift to night shift to graveyard shift); (ii) if possible, shifts should be designed so that they impose no more than a 4-hour change from the previous shift; (iii) workers should remain in the same shift for longer than 1 week (especially if the previous recommendation cannot be implemented) and attempt to conform their whole life-style to the schedule imposed by the professional shift; (iv) the work environment should be well illuminated, and the sleep environment totally dark and free of noise and interruptions; and (v) a regular time for rising and retiring should be maintained as much as possible, even on weekends.

Some additional points can be made about sleep hygiene, or habits designed to ensure that good quality sleep is obtained. Besides keeping the bedroom completely dark during sleep time and observing a regular time for getting up and going to bed, stimulants (e.g. caffeine or nicotine) should not be used near bedtime, irregular naps during the day should be avoided, and enough time should be scheduled for sleep. If sleepiness persists during the day or a bed partner complains of excessive snoring, frequent movements, or prolonged episodes of not breathing during sleep, a sleep specialist should be consulted. Daytime sleepiness may be a symptom of an underlying sleep disorder, a subset of which includes intrinsic derangements of circadian function. [*See* SLEEP.]

2. Endogenous Alterations in Circadian Rhythmicity

As mentioned in Section IV, there exist examples in the animal kingdom of individuals whose circadian system is profoundly altered as a result of a genetic mutation. In the two mammalian species reported to date, one of them was spontaneously induced (the *tau* mutation in the hamster) and the other was generated with a mutating agent (the *Clock* mutation in the mouse). *Tau* homozygous hamsters show a shorter free-running period (about 20 hours), whereas *Clock* homozygous mice show a long free-running rhythm (about 27 hours) when initially released into constant darkness (soon followed by total arrhythmicity). Since many genes show sequence conversation across mammalian species, the recent cloning of mouse *Clock* should soon lead to the identification of human *Clock*. The expected cloning of human *Clock* and related genes will undoubtedly lead to a better understanding of the mechanisms that underlie the human circadian pacemaker. In addition, it is very likely that mutations in the human circadian system exist that render an individual less susceptible to entrainment to an external agent or even unable to conform to the societal diurnal norms.

Clinical experience suggests that this is the case. Patients with *delayed sleep phase syndrome* (DSPS) have a very difficult time falling asleep at conventional times and are only able to doze off several hours after going to bed; similarly, they get up hours after being roused. Such patterns are not explained on the basis of temporary circumstances: they are persistent, exaggerated, and apparently unmodifiable, despite great efforts on the part of the affected individual to conform to social requirements. When these patients are tested in a sleep laboratory, where they are subject to strict entraining conditions, they show an abnormal

relationship between their sleep/wake cycle and the endogenous circadian pacemaker, as measured by the melatonin rise and/or the body temperature rhythm. Such an effect may be caused by defects in the entrainment pathway, by an abnormal endogenous circadian period, or by a preceding history of voluntary postponement of sleep at appropriate circadian times.

The converse occurs with its pathological counterpart, *advanced sleep phase syndrome*. Patients with this disorder go to sleep much earlier than usual and get up hours before average people in their same environment. As with DSPS, these symptoms continue over an extended period time with extreme alterations in one's schedule and resistance to change, and an abnormal phase relationship between sleep onset and endogenous markers of circadian rhythmicity can also be documented. Both disorders are difficult to diagnose because they require an environment free of masking influences; this can usually only be obtained in a specialized sleep laboratory with a constant routine protocol and a strict set of lifestyle guidelines prior to the test, which can only be carried out in a handful of specialized facilities. Treatment for both disorders includes exposure to bright light at appropriate times: early in the night to produce phase delays and late in the night (early in the morning) to produce phase advances.

Blind people who cannot perceive the external light/dark cycle receive a weaker entraining input and thus have to use social cues to attempt to synchronize their circadian pacemaker to the external environment. Their entrainment pathway is impaired, but their circadian oscillator is presumably intact. A more serious disorder, *non-24-hour sleep/wake syndrome,* has been documented in some blind children who also have other neurological abnormalities. Patients with this disorder show complete arrhythmicity that persists beyond the years of infancy, and they can never adapt to their parents' conventional schedule. Because the endogenous melatonin rise signals the onset of darkness, exogenous melatonin administered at bedtime has been used successfully as an entraining agent in these patients. In addition, a recent report showing successful entrainment to light and the suppression of melatonin by light pulses in some blind subjects indicates that the visual pathway regulating circadian rhythmicity may have been preserved in some sightless patients. The use of melatonin to alleviate other derangements of circadian function, such as jet lag, is only experimental and has not been substantiated by large clinical trials; whether the beneficial response of this drug in some individuals is due to a resetting of their biological clock or to the restoring effects of sleep caused by the well known sleep-inducing properties of melatonin awaits further experimentation.

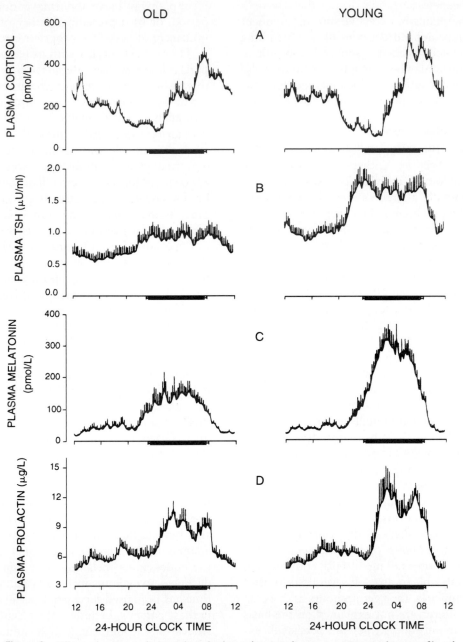

Figure 9   Effects of aging on the circadian rhythms of various hormones. Mean 24-hour profiles of plasma cortisol (A), thyroid-stimulating hormone (TSH; B), melatonin (C), prolactin (D) and growth hormone (GH; E), as well as levels and distribution of slow wave (SW; F) and rapid-eye-movement (REM; G) stages of sleep in young and old men. Vertical lines represent standard errors, and black horizontal bars correspond to mean sleep period. (Reprinted with permission from Van Coevorden, A., et al. (1991). Neuroendocrine rhythms and sleep in aging men. *Am. J. Physiol, 260,* E651–E661. Copyright © 1991 by the American Physiological Society.)

There exists an initial suggestion that a genetic component plays a role at least in DSPS; in the years ahead, the genetic basis of this familial subtype may be established through the construction of appropriate informative pedigrees. Similarly, enhanced screening in sleep and/or chronobiology clinical facilities is likely to discover new human circadian mutations. In addition, parallel progress in isolating and cloning circadian genes in other mammalian species may serve to identify their human homologues by conventional molecular biology techniques. Identification of genes involved in the control of the human circadian pacemaker will not only contribute to our understanding of the molecular organization of this important physiological mechanism but will also provide avenues for the therapeutic manipulation of the clock when required by exogenous or endogenous circumstances.

C. Aging

Several changes take place in the circadian system as a person ages. The amplitude of several hormonal rhythms is decreased in older individuals (Fig. 9). The varied nature and number of different rhythms affected suggest that this reduced amplitude may reflect a damped oscillation in the pacemaker itself. In addition, older people show about a 90-minute phase advance in their sleep/wake and body temperature rhythms with respect to younger individuals. This altered phase relationship often leads to early morning awakening and complaints of insomnia in the aged. Changes in sleep architecture, increased frequency of napping, and an altered need for sleep have all been reported, although whether these are organic changes due to aging or the effect of environmental modifica-

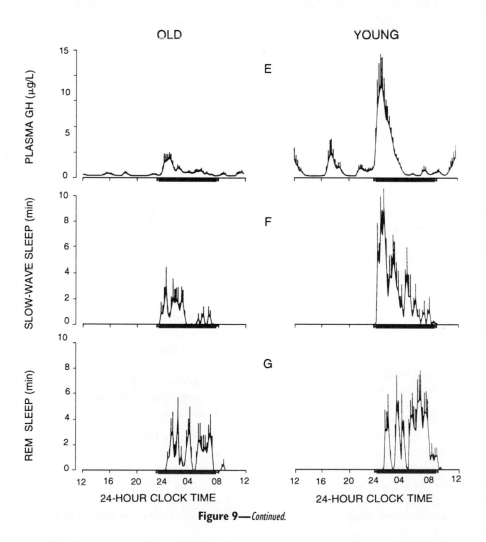

Figure 9—*Continued.*

tions in living conditions has not been clearly determined. Experimental approaches in animal models and selected human populations are currently underway to evaluate the precise nature of the age-related changes in the circadian system as well as their accessibility to environmental manipulation. As a general principle, it appears that taking measures that lead to an increased amplitude in circadian oscillations (e.g., by exposure to bright light in individuals who might seldom venture outdoors during the course of the day) leads to improved subjective comfort and increased level of alertness during waking hours.

D. Seasonal Affective Disorder

Some individuals experience bouts of diagnosable depression that follow striking seasonal patterns. During the winter months they feel lethargic, apathetic, unmotivated, and have the propensity to gain weight; these symptoms disappear with the coming of spring. They recur on a yearly basis, and their severity and persistence is beyond what would be explainable by the effects of the weather on a person's mood. They are more common in people who live in temperate climates or higher latitudes. Together they define a psychiatric syndrome known as *seasonal affective disorder* or SAD.

Current theories postulate the involvement of the circadian system in SAD. It is well known that animals who follow seasonal cycles for certain behaviors use their circadian system to perceive the progression of seasons by measuring changes in day length. Thus, the physiological changes induced by seasonality can be reproduced in the laboratory by merely altering the light/dark pattern to which the animals are exposed. Similarly, it is thought that in humans with SAD the gradual shortening of days as winter approaches is sensed by the circadian system and this signals the onset of winter depression.

Under this model, it would be expected that exposure to light in patterns that mimic the long days of summer should alleviate the depressive symptoms in affected individuals. Indeed, exposure to bright light for several hours has been shown to eliminate most symptoms of depressive mood in these patients; the timing of exposure, however, does not seem to be important. Therefore, it appears that a general treatment of increased light exposure rather than an exact reproduction of summer lighting conditions is the only required therapeutic intervention; whether such an ef-

fect is achieved via the circadian system remains to be determined. [*See* DEPRESSION.]

VII. THE CIRCADIAN COMPONENT IN DISEASE

Besides disorders of intrinsic circadian dysfunction, there exist human disease states that are significantly affected by the circadian system. Similarly, the efficacy of pharmacological therapies used to treat certain illnesses can vary greatly depending on the time of administration. The recognition of both of these effects has given rise to the two incipient clinical disciplines of *chronopathology* and *chronopharmacology*. Both of them embrace the concept of selective temporal vulnerability: some pathophysiological events are more likely to occur during specific circadian windows, because the temporal conditions in the organism are more propitious to their development; similarly, affected tissues may be more amenable to the pharmacological action of certain drugs at specific times of the day.

The following are but a few examples that illustrate the concept of selective temporal vulnerability, collected from the growing body of literature on the subject:

- There exists a well-documented circadian pattern in the incidence of myocardial infarction, which is three times more likely to occur in the early morning than in the evening;
- Similarly, there exists a morning peak and a nocturnal trough in the risk of onset of thrombotic cerebrovascular accidents;
- Both of the above correlate with an increase in the propensity of platelets to aggregate in the early morning as well as a decreased effectiveness in anticoagulation measures by constant heparin infusion at that time of the day;
- Asthmatic patients also report a greater propensity to airway compromise in the early morning, which is accompanied by reduced pulmonary expiratory flow values.

From the therapeutic perspective, we have already seen how plasma values of certain hormones will differ markedly depending on the time of the day at which the sample is drawn. Similarly, it seems obvious that circadian rhythms in renal and hepatic function are likely to lead to differences in the clearance of certain drugs, which affects the levels of their concentration in plasma in a diurnal manner. This effect has been most studied in reference to cancer chemotherapeutic agents. In animal studies, injections of a chemotherapeutic agent resulted in a 87.5% mortality for animals treated in regular 3-hour intervals, versus a 20% mortality in those receiving the same doses in a circadian schedule. This difference in toxicity when treatments are administered at a particular time of the day has also been documented in humans receiving chemotherapy for ovarian cancer. In the example shown in Fig. 10, rats or patients receiving a particular type of drug showed reduced toxicity and en-

hanced tolerance of higher doses when the drug was infused in a circadian manner.

Thus, from both standpoints of prevention and cure, health care professionals need to take the circadian variable into account. Large epidemiological studies should be carried out to uncover a circadian propensity in other common diseases; similarly, clinical trials must be undertaken to evaluate the efficacy of particular drugs at different times of the day, and appropriate recommendations on therapeutic protocols which maximize clinical outcome ought to be implemented. As the pervasive influence of the circadian system in human health and disease receives greater

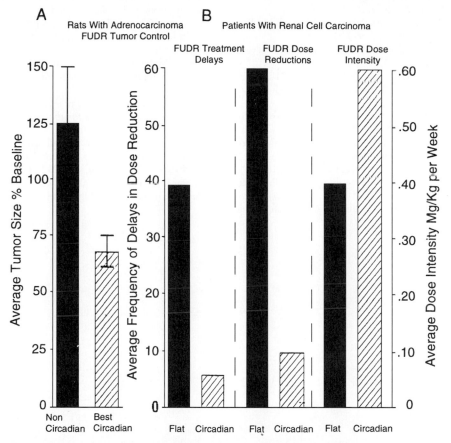

Figure 10 (A) The circadian schedule-dependency of floxuridine (FUDR)-induced tumor control in a rat tumor model system is contrasted with (B) the circadian schedule-dependency of FUDR toxicity in human patients. (A) Rats or (B) patients received continuous constant-rate FUDR infusion (solid bars) or infusions peaking at the interface of usual daily activity and sleep (hatched bars). In the rat, toxicity of FUDR was affected by the circadian shape of the infusion (data not shown) and tumor shrinkage was similarly enhanced by the same optimal circadian FUDR infusion shape. (B) In cancer patients, all measures of toxicity and dose-intensity were markedly diminished by optimal drug timing. (Reprinted with permission from Hrushesky, W. J. M., and Bjarnason, G. A. (1993). Circadian cancer therapy. *J. Clin. Oncol., 11,* 1403–1417. Copyright © 1993 by W. B. Saunders Company.)

recognition, our present conceptual framework of human biology may be significantly altered. At the beginning of the century the theory of relativity modified the dominant physics paradigm by introducing the fourth dimension of time; we can envision how as this century draws to a close our present static anatomical model based on spatial dimensions is being enriched by the dynamic component of circadian rhythmicity.

BIBLIOGRAPHY

Czeisler, C. A. (1995). The effect of light on the human circadian pacemaker. *Ciba Found. Symp., 183,* 254–290.

Dunlap, J. C. (1996). Genetic and molecular analysis of circadian rhythms. *Annu. Rev. Genet. 30,* 579–601.

Florez, J. C., & Takahashi, J. S. (1995). The circadian clock: From molecules to behaviour. *Ann. Med. 27,* 481–490.

Klein, D. C., Moore, R. Y., & Reppert, S. M. (Eds.) (1991). *Suprachiasmatic nucleus: The mind's clock.* New York: Oxford University Press.

Hall, J. C. (1995). Tripping along the trail to the molecular mechanisms of biological clocks. *TINS 18,* 230–240.

Hrushesky, W. J. M., & Bjarnason, G. A. (1993). Circadian cancer therapy. *J. Clin. Oncol. 11,* 1403–1417.

Hrushesky, W. J. M., Langer, R., & Theeuwes, F. (Eds.). (1991). *Temporal control of drug delivery.* New York: Annals of the New York Academy of Sciences.

Menaker, M., & Tosini, G. (1996). The evolution of vertebrate circadian systems. In K.-I. Honma and S. Honma (Eds.), *Circadian organization and oscillatory coupling,* pp. 39–52. Sapporo: Hokkaido University Press.

Moore, R. Y. (1996). Entrainment pathways and the functional organization of the circadian system. In R. M. Buijs et al. (Eds.), *Hypothalamic integration of circadian rhythms. Progr. Brain Res., 111,* 103–119. Amsterdam: Elsevier Science.

Moore-Ede, M. C., Sulzman, F. M., & Fuller, C. A. (1982). *The clocks that time us.* Cambridge, MA: Harvard University Press.

Pittendrigh, C. S. (1960). Circadian rhythms and the circadian organization of living systems. *Cold Spring Harbor Symp. Quant. Biol., 25,* 159–184.

Rosbash, M., Allada, R., Dembinska, M., Guo, W. Q., Le, M., Marrus, S., Qian, Z., Rutila, J. E., Yaglom, J., & Zeng, H. (1996). A *Drosophila* circadian clock. *Cold Spring Harbor Symp. Quant. Biol, LXI,* 265–278.

Sack, R. L., & Lewy, A. J. (1993). Human circadian rhythms: Lessons from the blind. *Ann. Med., 25,* 303–305.

Schwartz, W. J. (1993). A clinician's primer on the circadian clock: Its localization, function, and resetting. *Adv. Intern. Med., 38,* 81–106.

Takahashi, J. S. (1995). Molecular neurobiology and genetics of circadian rhythms in mammals. *Annu. Rev. Neurosci., 18,* 531–553.

U.S. Congress, Office of Technology Assessment (1991). *Biological Rhythms: Implications for the Worker.* Washington, DC: U.S. Government Printing Office.

Wehr, T. A. (1996). A 'clock for all seasons' in the human brain. In R. M. Buijs et al. (Eds.), *Hypothalamic integration of circadian rhythms. Progr. Brain Res., 111,* 321–342, Amsterdam: Elsevier Science.

Wetterberg, L. (1994). Light and biological rhythms. *J. Intern. Med., 235,* 5–19.

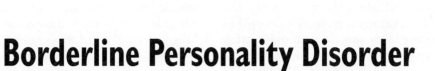

Borderline Personality Disorder

Jerome Kroll

University of Minnesota Medical School

As-If Personality   A type of personality lacking a stable core identity, which then takes on characteristics of persons in the environment.
Cluster B   The grouping of four personality disorders (narcissistic, borderline, histrionic, and antisocial) in Axis II of DSM-III-R.
Dissociation   An altered state of consciousness that appears split off from one's ongoing sense of awareness and self-consciousness.
Rejection-Sensitive Dysphoria   A transient form of depressed mood brought on by perception of rejection by others.

BORDERLINE PERSONALITY DISORDER is a term that identifies a heterogenous group of patients with serious character pathology and behavioral disturbances. The main features of this disorder are behavior that is impulsive, dramatic, and often self-destructive; moods that are labile and reactive to life circumstances; interpersonal relationships that are stormy; and a sense of self-identity that is fragile and contradictory.

I. HISTORICAL DEVELOPMENT OF THE CONCEPT

More than one decade after the development and publication of *DSM-III*, borderline personality disorder (BPD) remains the most controversial category in the nomenclature. Disagreement persists regarding the term itself, the particular diagnostic criteria established for BPD by *DSM-III* and *DSM-IV*, the scope of applicability, and the extent of overlap with Axis I and other Axis II disorders. Ultimately, this degree and intensity of dispute reflect both the range of difficulties in identifying and working with those persons designated as borderline, as well as the more basic question of validity: whether the BPD construct describes a meaningful unitary syndrome that corresponds to an actually existing state of affairs. While this latter question can certainly be asked of any of the personality (Axis II) disorders, something about the borderline concept seems to have engendered the strongest controversy.

At least one major reason for the ongoing disputes is the fact that the very concept of borderline was born out of attempts to explain the clinical observation that certain patients seemed to do very poorly in psychodynamic psychotherapy. Thus, from the very first, this category was used to describe a disparate group of patients who had two things in common: they responded to psychotherapy by developing transient psychotic symptoms and they did not meet classical definitions of schizophrenia. It is not that they did not necessarily improve; many obsessional patients, for example, did not improve with psychotherapy. Rather, it is that these patients worsened in psychotherapy with a fairly specific pattern of acting out that showed up most dramatically in the development of severe transference problems. The difficulty confronting the predominantly psychoanalytic theoreticians and skilled therapists was how to fathom the nature of these patients who gave promise of being good psychotherapeutic cases, yet deteriorated during the course of a psychotherapy. Thus, the very origins of the borderline concept arose in the context of a clinical puzzle.

The solution to the puzzle, keeping in mind that American psychiatry held a much more encompassing concept of schizophrenia in the 1940s and 1950s than at present, was to conceptualize these patients who became worse in psychotherapy as having a schizophrenic core underlying the neurotic facade. This notion was given concrete expression in a paper by Hoch and Polatin in 1949 describing the new category of pseudoneurotic schizophrenia. The construct fit neatly into a psychoanalytic model that postulated a spectrum of psychopathology based upon increasing primitiveness of defense mechanisms, extending in an unbroken chain from mild neurotics at one end to deteriorated schizophrenics at the other. The pseudoneurotic patient served as the missing link, bridging neurosis and psychosis, and thus serving as visible proof of the continuity connecting mild and severe psychiatric disorders. [See DEFENSE MECHANISMS; SCHIZOPHRENIA.]

The problem with the pseudoneurotic schizophrenia construct was that the patients did not go on to develop the more classical symptoms of hallucinations and delusions nor the deteriorating course that is the usual outcome of schizophrenia. Nevertheless, the observation that there existed a group of patients who appeared neurotic, but worsened with intensive psychotherapy, was a valid finding that outlived the misleading label attached to it. The focus of what might be wrong with these difficult-to-treat patients shifted away from schizophrenia to consideration of severe character pathology, described as borderline states by Knight in 1953 and as the psychotic character by Frosch in 1964. In addition, the joint U.S.–U.K. diagnostic studies carried out in the mid-to-late 1960s demonstrated convincingly that many patients diagnosed as schizophrenic by American psychiatrists fit much better with manic–depressive and personality disorder symptoms and outcome. This diagnostic realignment tightened the diagnostic criteria for schizophrenia, thereby further emphasizing the differences between borderline conditions and schizophrenia.

In 1968, Grinker and colleagues published the results of their study of 58 hospitalized patients who fell into a broadly defined notion of borderline syndrome. These patients had difficulties in interpersonal relationships, transient losses of reality testing under stress, angry and depressive affects, and deficient self-identities. Cluster analyses of the data, primarily of measurements of ego functions, produced four major clusters. There was a "core" borderline group, two groups defined as bordering upon the psychoses and neuroses, and a fourth group embodying certain "as-if" features, most notably absence of a core self-identity. Grinker's study, the first to utilize psychometric instruments and statistical analyses, moved the borderline concept away from the realm of schizophrenic spectrum disorders and provided the basis for future empirical studies that continued the attempt to define the still vague borderline syndrome.

It is instructive that in the next series of studies carried out by Gunderson and Singer in 1975, the primary diagnostic concern was still to demonstrate that borderlines were different than schizophrenics. At the same time that empirical studies were focusing on narrowing the construct of borderline, Kernberg developed a broader notion of borderline, based upon a fusion of ego psychology and object relations theory, to designate a form of personality organization that was characterized by the use of primitive ego defenses (denial, splitting, projective identification), intact reality testing (with transient regressions under stress), and identity diffusion. Kernberg's construct of borderline personality organization includes the milder as well as the more severe forms of character pathology, and, in essence, encompasses most of the patients presently grouped under the Cluster B (dramatic, unstable) personality disorders: histrionic, narcissistic, borderline, and antisocial.

This was the state of affairs while the *DSM-IV* committee developed inclusion and exclusion criteria for the personality disorders. There were four competing and overlapping concepts of borderline, and the final result represented some degree of compromise between the various groups. Since ideological and economic considerations, in addition to empirical studies and clinical lore, influenced the final product, it is important to define these considerations in some detail. The four overlapping concepts of borderline were as follows: (1) A residual model based upon the schizophrenic spectrum concept, using the term borderline to designate those persons, usually relatives of schizophrenics, who displayed odd, eccentric thinking and schizoid interpersonal relationships; this group was given the term schizotypal personality disorder. (2) An affective disorder model, which considered BPD as an affective spectrum illness displaying prominent features of mood instability with a predominance of depression, anger, and preoccupations with suicide. (3) An empirically derived model based primarily on the research of Gunderson, with diagnostic symptoms placed into five major groupings: impulse/action patterns (including self-destructive behaviors); ego-dystonic, transient psychotic episodes; mood instability with primarily negative affects; disturbed but intense interpersonal relationships; and an unstable sense of self. (4) A psychoanalytic concept based primarily on the work of Kernberg, but encompassing theoretical formulations by Mahler relating to difficulties in the separation/individuation phase of child development.

The final configuration of BPD adopted was most influenced by Gunderson's work, but nevertheless showed the strains inherent in a compromise between points of view that are ideologically very divergent. The results were the creation of several new personality disorders within Axis II, not based upon empirical studies, but with each reflecting to some extent components that were once loosely connected to the borderline concept. Essentially, in dividing the broad territory of the borderline syndrome, as this concept evolved during a 40-year span, the cognitive disturbances that had long been noticed were placed in the schizotypal personality disorder, the milder dramatic and attention-seeking traits were placed into the histrionic personality disorder, self-centeredness and entitlement became the core of the narcissistic personality disorder, and the affective symptoms of mood instability and negative affectivity (depression, anger, anxiety), along with impulsivity, were given prominence in the borderline personality disorder.

Borderline personality disorder was defined by *DSM-III-R* as a condition marked by a pervasive pattern of instability of mood, interpersonal relationships, and self-image, beginning by early adulthood and present in a variety of contexts, as indicated by at least five of the following:

1. A pattern of unstable and intense interpersonal relationships characterized by alternating between extremes of overidealization and devaluation.
2. Impulsiveness in at least two areas that are potentially self-damaging, e.g., spending, sex, substance use, shoplifting, reckless driving, binge eating.
3. Affective instability: marked shifts from baseline mood to depression, irritability, or anxiety, usually lasting a few hours and only rarely more than a few days.
4. Inappropriate, intense anger or lack of control of anger, e.g., frequent displays of temper, constant anger, physical fights.
5. Recurrent suicidal threats, gestures, or behavior, or self-mutilating behavior.
6. Marked and persistent identity disturbance manifested by uncertainty about at least two of the following: self-image, sexual orientation, long-term goals or career choice, type of friends desired, preferred values.
7. Chronic feeling of emptiness or boredom.
8. Frantic efforts to avoid real or imagined abandonment.

The revision of *DSM-III-R* into *DSM-IV* was completed by late 1993. Although the BPD construct did not undergo any major alterations, several changes were instituted which served to correct the overemphasis in *DSM-III* on the close relationship between BPD and the affective disorders and the omission of cognitive deficits. Criterion 3 (Criterion 6 in *DSM-IV*), which outlined the affective symptoms seen in BPD was changed to reflect reactivity of mood; this serves to emphasize the difference between the mood disturbances seen in BPD and the relatively situation-independent mood disturbances characteristic of the endogenous affective disorders (major depression and manic–depressive illnesses). Complementing this more accurate delineation of the type of mood disorder seen in BPD was the inclusion of a new criterion to reflect the specific cognitive disturbances of BPD. The *DSM-IV* calls for a ninth criterion as follows: Transient stress-related paranoid ideation or severe dissociative symptoms. There were a few additional changes to the original eight criteria, but these are relatively minor, either reflecting grammatical alterations in the interest of clarity or the result of low sensitivity/specificity ratings for a few items on further field testing. Thus, the description of the identity disturbance in Criterion 6 was reworded and the construct "boredom" was dropped from Criterion 7.

II. CORE SYMPTOMS AND CHARACTER STYLE

The clinical description of a psychiatric disorder does not correspond exactly to that disorder's diagnostic criteria in *DSM-III*. The main reason for this is that a clinical description needs to be a full and rich portrayal of the condition under question, whereas the requirements for diagnostic criteria are vastly different. Diagnostic criteria must aim for those characteristics of an illness that capture a few of its core symptoms while avoiding overlap with neighboring conditions. For example, as indicated above, while boredom may very well be a characteristic mental state in BPD, it was also found in histrionic and narcissistic personality disorders and therefore was of little specific diagnostic value. It did not help discriminate between BPD and other Cluster B personality disorders. In addition, diagnostic criteria must have acceptable validity and reliability. The issue of validity of psychiatric disorders, especially of personality disorders, is a troublesome one, since there are not external validators. The construction of *DSM-III* had paid major attention, some would say excessively so, to reliability issues. For example, certain factors that most workers would agree are characteristic of a disorder, such as the psychological defense of splitting in BPD, were not included in the diagnostic criteria because of a preference for behavioral rather than psychological phenomena, presumably because assessment of behaviors permits greater agreement as to whether they are present or not as compared to psychological constructs.

As indicated at the beginning of this article, there remains considerable controversy about the core characteristics and boundaries of BPD. Workers in the field have tended to bring to the evaluation of BPD their own theoretical and clinical perspectives in the evaluation of borderlines. In addition, some of the

core characteristics of BPD, such as an increase in dissociative phenomena, appear to be changing in the past decade, a possibility that raises the question of the cultural influences and even faddish quality of some of the symptoms.

Most workers would agree that BPD is a relatively severe personality disorder, seen primarily in young adults, that presents with a characteristic cognitive style, mood disturbances, problematic interpersonal relationships, negative and deficient sense of self, and a variety of dramatic and impulsive behaviors usually of a self-injurious nature. These diagnostic features represent points distributed on a continuum of personality traits with somewhat arbitrary use of social norms to determine cut-off scores separating normal from pathological. Because of this, some workers in the field have advocated use of a dimensional rather than categorical model for the personality disorders, but a categorical model has always been adopted because it is easier to use in clinical work.

The cognitive style seen in borderline individuals encompasses three overlapping features. First, borderlines tend to have altered states of consciousness; these are usually referred to as dissociative states, and vary in intensity, density, and duration. They run the gamut from brief periods of self-absorption to fugue states lasting hours. The person may be partially or fully amnestic for some of the dissociative episodes. Second, borderlines tend to split their universe into good and bad, black and white. They have difficulty conceptualizing a person, including themselves, or an event, as encompassing positive and negative features. They tend to swing between the opposite poles of idealization and devaluation in their affections toward others. Third, borderlines tend to have impressionistic and global rather than precise and focused perceptions. They tend to be intolerant of unpleasant thoughts and images and to interrupt these processes with impulsive action, dissociation, and drug and alcohol use. There is a tendency toward imprecision and exaggeration, with a loss of salient detail. All of these disturbances are increased under conditions of stress.

The affective disturbances are characteristically mood instability or lability. Mood is typically reactive to environmental circumstances, but this must be taken to include the borderline's own thought processes too. Negative affects, such as sadness, anger, and anxiety predominate the emotional landscape, but too literal adherence to this description would belie the positive affects and interpersonal warmth that borderlines can exhibit.

Problematic interpersonal relationships are a hallmark of borderlines. Their relationships are characteristically intense, stormy, and conflictual. Dependency needs, power struggles, and the idealization/devaluation swings described earlier tend to complicate most meaningful relationships. Victimization and entitlement themes in which the borderline alternates between being exploited by others and demanding reparations from others for damages incurred are frequent patterns seen in this disorder.

Borderline individuals tend to have a deficient sense of self, and what enduring image of themselves they may have is usually negative. A deficient sense of self refers to the absence of a stable sense of core identity, of knowing who you are. A certain degree of this is expected in adolescents and young adults in Western culture, but the borderline problem with identity, by definition, must go beyond the norm for this age group. Borderlines will take on different roles and personality characteristics, depending upon the dominant features of the group they are associating with. This has been referred to as the "as-if" personality, first described by Helene Deutsch in 1942. When not caught up in a persuasive group identity, borderlines tend to have very negative notions about themselves, ranging from dislike to contemptuous loathing.

Finally, borderlines characteristically are dramatic and impulsive in their actions. The patterns of impulsivity include directly self-injurious behaviors as well as an assortment of either ill-considered or risk-taking behaviors that also may be seen as self-destructive. Alcohol and drug abuse, bulimic eating disorders, promiscuity, and attraction to predatory partners are among the impulsive actions seen in borderlines. As with the other core features of borderlines, the self-injurious behaviors range from infrequent and mild delicate cutting of the wrists to deep cutting of the limbs, torso, and genitals, as well as occasional ingenious use of cigarettes, lighters, caustic solutions, and hot irons to burn themselves. Suicide threats and attempts are also hallmarks of borderlines, most frequently but not exclusively with prescription as well as nonprescription medication overdoses. There are many more threats and gestures than serious attempts, leading to the use of the term "para-suicide" to describe these provocative actions of borderlines, but often the differentiation between manipulative and serious attempts is not at all clear.

III. DEMOGRAPHIC AND DATA-BASED STUDIES

There are no accurate measures of the prevalence of BPD in the community. Most estimates range from 0.5 to 1%, but may go higher as a broader concept of borderline, such as that used by Kernberg, is applied. The prevalence of the disorder in clinical settings is influenced by the type of clinical population under consideration. An average across studies indicates that the general prevalence of BPD is 10–15%, in inpatient settings about 20%, among outpatients with a personality disorder 30–35%, and among inpatients with a personality disorder 60–65%. Prevalence figures alone may be deceptive; it is possible that borderlines in an inpatient setting may have little similarity to outpatients who have never needed hospitalization. In most studies, excepting those done in VA and prison settings, 60–75% of BPD are women.

Although *DSM-III* diagnostic rules do not permit differential weighting of the different criteria, most studies have demonstrated that several items contribute disproportionately to diagnostic efficiency. The presence of two, or at most three, specific criteria (impulsivity, unstable–intense interpersonal relationships, and self-injurious behaviors) predict most strongly the diagnosis of BPD, although once again, the type of clinical setting (inpatient or outpatient) will influence this finding.

There is considerable overlap (20–60%) between BPD and the other personality disorders, especially those of Cluster B, as well as schizotypal and dependent personality disorders. This finding continues to raise the question of whether personality disorders are discrete entities truly different from each other or reflect points on a continuum of serious character pathology. There are several Axis I disorders that have substantial overlap with BPD. These are alcohol and substance abuse disorders, bulimia, and the mood disorders, primarily dysthymia and major depression. To some extent, this finding reflects overlapping criteria (e.g., substance abuse is listed as a criterion for BPD), the heterogeneity of the BPD concept, and the fact that traits such as impulsivity and mood lability do express themselves in a wide array of behaviors. [*See* PERSONALITY DISORDERS.]

IV. ETIOLOGY AND RELATIONSHIP TO OTHER DISORDERS

Since it appears that BPD is not a unitary disorder, and since diagnostic threshold can be met in a polythetic system by fulfilling any five of eight (or nine, under *DSM-IV*) criteria, it is highly unlikely that a unitary etiology will be found for this or other Cluster B personality disorders. Theories about the etiology of BPD tend to follow major trends of interest in the behavioral sciences in general. Thus, the predominance of psychoanalytic constructs as explanatory hypotheses of human health and illness has given way to a variety of biological–genetic models in the past decade. Even the recent robust correlations between childhood sexual abuse and adult BPD symptoms are increasingly explained more in terms of long-lasting neurophysiological alterations of stress–response systems rather than in terms of psychodynamic mechanisms. The major theories of the etiology of BPD are as follow:

A. Psychoanalytic model of stage-specific difficulties
  1. Deficit model (Masterson; Adler)
  2. Conflict model (Kernberg)
B. BPD as an affective spectrum model
C. BPD as post-traumatic stress disorder secondary to childhood sexual and physical abuse
D. BPD as an impulse spectrum disorder

A. Psychoanalytic Hypotheses

Based upon Mahler's theories of the importance of successful resolution of the rapprochment subphase of the separation/individuation processes in toddlerhood (ages 15–30 months), several overlapping psychodynamic hypotheses were advanced to explain those BPD features that were thought to represent the consequences of rapprochment failure. These features were the mental operation and defense of splitting, identity diffusion, and deficiencies in object constancy and object relationships. Differences of opinion and emphasis exist between various psychodynamic theories: Masterson has suggested that the mother of the borderline is herself borderline and establishes emotionally impossible conditions for the toddler to

achieve age-appropriate separation and individuation, thereby resulting in the development of a borderline personality in the child. Adler has emphasized the borderline child's inability, under circumstances similar to those described by Masterson, to form internalized soothing, holding introjects, such that the borderline child (and adult) lacks basic ego functions such as frustration tolerance, stable self-object relationships, and methods for calming itself during periods of stress. Kernberg has postulated the likelihood of an excessive aggressive drive in the infant that interferes with the fusion of sexual and aggressive drives; Kernberg's model therefore sees borderline pathogenesis as the result of a complex interaction between infant and caregiver rather than as unilaterally caused by a "not-good-enough" mother.

The basic problem with the psychoanalytic hypotheses regarding etiology of BPD is shared by psychodynamic explanations of behavior in general: first, difficulty in operationalizing and thereby in testing various theories and second, a lack of specificity whereby certain postulated mechanisms at best appear to be general risk factors (e.g., parental psychopathology) rather than the specific and inevitable cause of a particular outcome. This latter problem, of course, applies to all unitary theories of etiology. Finally, the nature of the psychodynamic hypotheses are such that supportive evidence comes primarily from retrospective rather than prospective studies, and from individual case studies in which the investigator testing the hypothesis is also the therapist commited to the hypothesis.

B. BPD as an Affective Spectrum Disorder

The observation that borderline patients are frequently depressed, and the prominence of mood instability in the symptom picture, have led to the hypothesis that an affective disorder underlies the borderline condition. Attempts to validate this hypothesis examined a variety of biological markers, familial patterns, follow-up data, and pharmacological responses. The initial findings, varying somewhat from study to study, were that from 20 to 60% of borderline patients met diagnostic criteria for an affective disorder, usually major depressive episode. This was not particularly surprising since the diagnostic criteria for BPD were slanted toward affective type symptoms. The studies have shown that patients with depression and borderline patients who were concurrently depressed resembled each other in regard to several biological markers of depression, such as the dexamethasone suppression test, REM latency time, and thyroid stimulating hormone response to thyrotropin, but the resemblances fell away with "pure" borderline patients, i.e., borderline patients who were not depressed. [See DEPRESSION.]

Similar results were found in the family pedigrees of borderline patients. Borderline patients with concurrent depressions had a greater prevalence of relatives with affective disorders. However, this finding is true for most of the Axis II disorders, namely, that there is a higher prevalence of depressed persons in the families of patients with any personality disorder and depression. On the other hand, borderline patients without depression tend to have increased familial linkages to other disorders, namely, borderline and antisocial personality disorders, and alcoholism and drug abuse. Studies of pharmacological efficacy with borderlines have demonstrated minimal benefit from antidepressants, even with depressed borderlines, except for some amelioration of depressive symptoms. Lithium therapy has not proven valuable in treating BPD. There have been some indications that monoamine oxidase inhibitors are effective in reducing core borderline symptoms, thereby supporting the atypical depression model of BPD, but these findings have never been sufficiently replicated to be more than suggestive. Finally, the long-term follow-up studies have shown that most borderline patients do not go on to develop depressive syndromes, again arguing against a causal linkage between BPD and affective disorders.

Despite the fairly clear evidence that BPD is not a variant of affective disorders, most studies do show that a certain percentage of borderline patients have a recurrent affective disorder (either depressive or bipolar type II, i.e., depressions and hypomanias) and evolve into a typical affective disorder pattern after the dramatic borderline symptoms recede in the 30s. Thus, it seems likely that a subclass of borderlines has a primary affective disturbance.

C. BPD as Posttraumatic Stress Disorder Secondary to Childhood Sexual and Physical Abuse

There has been an increasing awareness of the frequency of childhood sexual abuse in the life history of many psychiatric patients. This awareness has paralleled a growing public consciousness of domestic violence of many types. The question remains unresolved as to whether child abuse and other forms of violence have indeed become more common recently, reaching epidemic proportions, or whether the social taboos that maintained silence over such assaults have been lifted, with the result of greater casefinding and reporting of such episodes. Among psychiatric patients, rates of childhood sexual abuse range between 25 and 80%, depending on the population surveyed and the survey methods. Surveys from such varied locations as state hospitals, community hospitals, outpatient clinics, and emergency rooms have been consistent in these findings. Reported rates are highest for borderline personality disorder, in the order of 50–80%. In the borderline population, there also appears to be a correlation between severity of certain types of symptoms, such as self-injurious behaviors and dissociative episodes, and the severity of the childhood sexual abuse experiences, as judged by age of first abuse, frequency and duration of abuse, degree of force and violence employed, and absence of ameliorative factors in the life of the child. The correlations between abuse and borderline symptomatology have been robust enough to lead several workers to hypothesize that most patients who have been diagnosed BPD are really suffering from PTSD and that this latter diagnosis makes better scientific and social sense, removing the stigma that has been attached to a BPD label. The case is strengthened by the logic of borderline symptoms, such as dissociation, as a learned response of the abused child to the horrors of the abuse experience, a response that was once adaptive, but has now become generalized as a response to all emotional flooding. In a similar way, self-injurious behavior seems to make sense as an expression of the self-hatred that the abuse victim directs inwardly. [See CHILD SEXUAL ABUSE; POSTTRAUMATIC STRESS.]

There are several obvious problems to the linear causal chain that links childhood abuse to borderline symptomatology. The major problems relate to specificity between abuse and outcome. Patients with many psychiatric diagnoses, as well as many persons who do not have psychiatric symptoms have histories of childhood sexual abuse. Only a percentage of abused persons develop the BPD or PTSD picture. Conversely, not everyone with BPD has a history of childhood abuse. In addition, the abused child was most likely raised in a chaotic home with many other disturbing features, such that it is not valid to single out the experience of sexual abuse as the cause of adult problems. There are also considerable methodological problems related to the very sensitive nature of the topic and the fact that most of the research and clinical work are based upon retrospective reports of abuse in childhood. The methodological problems slice both ways; there are persons who have been abused and who deny it, and there are patients who may distort, exaggerate or invent abuse histories. There is no easy resolution to these issues, but, in general, the detailed reports by patients about their abuse appear to have credibility and are accepted by most researchers and health care workers. The particular diagnostic question discussed here about the overlap of BPD and PTSD, however, is less an issue of data than definition of causal relationships in human behavior. Thus, it appears that childhood sexual abuse and the disturbed environment in which the abuse occurred function as general risk factors predisposing to increased severity of many types of psychiatric and physical illnesses. Within the BPD population, there does appear to be a large subgroup whose symptoms and personality styles were profoundly affected by the experiences of childhood sexual abuse and whose symptoms can be understood as a form of PTSD. It needs to be kept in mind that PTSD is still a fairly vague concept encompassing many types of traumas and responses, and that most persons suffering from PTSD do not show borderline symptoms.

D. BPD as an Impulse Spectrum Disorder

Although it sounds tautological to say that a syndrome characterized by impulsivity may be an impulse spectrum disorder, more is implied in the statement than meets the eye. Essentially, such a hypothesis raises the question of whether there is a group of disorders that share some common features in addition to impulsivity, such as familial linkage, associated psychiatric disorders, and underlying neurophysiological mechanisms. Family studies have shown an increased rate of alcoholism, substance abuse, and antisocial personality in the relatives of borderline personality. Other disorders considered related to problems with impulsivity include compulsive gambling, bulimia, intermittent explosive disorder, and the other Axis II personality disorders within Cluster B (histrionic and narcissistic). Studies are presently under way to investigate serotonergic and dopaminergic mechanisms that may have some linkage to impulsive behaviors.

It is well recognized that the notion of "impulsivity" is very vague, such that the various conditions being considered as impulse disorders may turn out to have very little in common beyond surface appearances. Conceptual clarification concerning what the terms "impulsive" and "compulsive" mean, and how these relate to the notion of "addiction," will be necessary if the hypothesis regarding impulse spectrum disorder is to be of any practical use.

V. COURSE OF BORDERLINE PERSONALITY DISORDER

The initial delineation of borderlines as encompassing a group of difficult treatment cases combined with the finding of a poor outcome on short-term follow-up led to a fairly pessimistic outlook for patients with this diagnosis. Patients who were diagnosed in their late teens or early 20s as borderline were still doing poorly 2 to 5 years later, with ongoing self-injurious behavior and suicide attempts leading to multiple hospitalizations. It was not until the late 1980s that follow-up studies covered the 10- to 20-year period after initial hospitalization. Surprisingly, the outcome was much more favorable than the early studies indicated. In several independent studies from different parts of the country, it became clear that between 50 and 60% of BPD patients were doing fairly well as they moved into their 30s. Another 30–40% of patients showed varying levels of disability. Suicide rates ranged from 8 to 15% on 10-year follow-up. The largest follow-up series of patients was reported by Stone, who traced 502 of 550 patients (of whom 193 met *DSM-III* criteria for BPD) who had been hospitalized on an intensive long-term psychotherapy ward at New York State Psychiatric Institute during the years 1963–1976. As judged by Global Outcome Scores (GAS), 63% of the BPD patients were in the good to recovered categories, another 16% had made a fair adjustment, 12% were doing poorly, and 9% suicided. Less favorable outcome was correlated with the presence of major affective disorder, antisocial personality, and a pattern of alcohol and drug abuse. Poor outcome was not correlated with self-mutilative behaviors in the early years of the illness. Patients with a history of childhood neglect or sexual abuse tended to do less well than patients without these histories. Finally, there was not a good overall correlation between outcome and psychiatric treatment; some patients with very good outcomes had minimal treatment following index hospitalization and some patients with extensive treatment had poor outcomes. It is possible that averaging the outcome data washes out a treatment effect, but this remains to be demonstrated.

VI. TREATMENT OF BPD

Three has been as much controversy about the treatment of BPD as there has been about the diagnosis. To a large extent and with some overlap, treatment modalities have tended to follow etiological hypotheses. As one might expect with a condition that drew its initial delineation from a group of difficult-to-treat patients, no single modality has yet demonstrated clearcut superiority or even effectiveness. Studies designed to evaluate treatment of BPD have been plagued by the usual problems of therapy outcome research: differing characteristics of the patient population, despite use of *DSM-III* criteria; difficulty in determining what constitutes evidence of improvement; difficulty in establishing control groups.

Psychodynamic psychotherapy has been the standard and accepted form of treatment of BPD, despite the many problems that arise in this form of treatment. In a sense, the BPD population, comprising primarily young verbal adults who are dysfunctional but nonpsychotic, have appeared to be the obvious if not ideal candidates for psychotherapy. Close to 50% of psychotherapy patients seen in private practice and at most outpatient clinics will have a diagnosis of BPD or a related Axis II Cluster B (narcissistic or histrionic) disorder. While there has been no canon defining a specific therapeutic protocol for BPD (or any other disorder), the work of Kernberg has been most influential in guiding the theory and practice of psychotherapy with borderlines. The therapy has tended to be a mix of supportive and exploratory work, with special attention paid to avoiding becoming enmeshed in ill-advised rescue attempts and other acting out features that are the hallmarks of borderline patients. The outcome results of the Menninger psychotherapy project reported by Wallerstein and Stone's follow-up study suggest that it is impossible to predict, from patient characteristics alone, which patients would bene-

fit most from supportive and which from exploratory psychotherapy, nor is there evidence that ultimate outcome is better with exploratory than supportive psychotherapy. A single study by Stevenson and Meares employing a 12-month psychotherapy regimen that utilized a written protocol based upon self-psychology demonstrated significant improvements across a broad range of measurements. Patients served as their own controls (pre- and post-treatment measures); a separate control group of patients was not used. [*See* Psychoanalysis.]

There has been increasing interest in cognitive–behavioral treatment (CBT) modalities for BPD. The essence of these modalities is a focus on recognizing and eliminating the factors that reinforce self-injurious behaviors, and learning and practicing new behaviors that will enhance the quality of life of the patient. Therapy is not directed toward underlying psychodynamic causes, since the assumption of CBT is that self-injurious behavior is a learned behavior that has become relatively independent of the specific causes that originally inspired it. CBT is done individually and in groups. Techniques that are taught and practiced include behavioral skill training, contingency management, cognitive restructuring, exposure to emotional cues, distress tolerance, interpersonal skills, and emotional regulation. Linehan and colleagues reported significant improvement in self-injurious and parasuicidal behaviors in a group of SIB borderlines in CBT compared to a group receiving treatment as usual. The improvements were not accompanied by changes in severity of reported depression, suicidal ideation, or reasons for living. [*See* Behavior Therapy; Cognitive Therapy.]

The relationship of BPD to PTSD in those borderlines who experienced sexual abuse in childhood suggests that a PTSD-oriented treatment program should be helpful. To date, this has not been the case, most likely because no overall effective program for the treatment of PTSD has been demonstrated. The treatment of PTSD usually includes group therapy, desensitization techniques, and pharmacological agents. There has been a proliferation of incest and sexual abuse treatment groups, some of which seem to be very helpful and some of which have a deleterious effect on some group members. No controlled studies have been reported. Pharmacological treatment of PTSD is in its infancy; different medications have been reported to be effective with particular components of PTSD, especially the sleep disturbance and depressions that accompany PTSD, but no agents appear to interrupt the flashbacks and intrusive imagery that form the hallmark of this disorder.

The pharmacological treatment of PBD is widely used, but relatively disappointing. Tricyclic antidepressants are effective only in alleviating depressive symptoms in those borderlines who are also depressed. Monoamine oxidase inhibitors have been reported to reduce the target symptom of rejection-sensitive dysphoria, but a controlled study is still wanting. There have not been controlled studies of the efficacy of the specific serotonin reuptake blockers to date. Lithium has not appeared to be of special benefit. There are mixed reports on the benzodiazepine anti-anxiety agents; there may be some benefit to the anti-anxiety properties, but several studies have reported a worsening of impulsive behaviors in BPDs taking these agents. In addition, long-term use of benzodiazepines would not be indicated in patients with significant alcohol or drug abuse histories. The single class of medications that has demonstrated significant short-term effectiveness in several key borderline symptoms has been low-dose anti-psychotics, but here the benefits must be weighed against the serious long-term side effects of these agents. A study of Soloff and associates in 1993 failed to replicate the positive findings of their earlier study reporting improvement in borderline patients with the use of antipsychotic medications.

There has been a recent trend away from long hospitalizations for borderline patients. While much of the driving force toward brief hospitalizations in all medical fields has been concern about rising medical costs, there has also been growing awareness of the deleterious rather than helpful effect of prolonged hospitalization of borderlines. Although there are undoubtedly some patients who benefit from a controlled hospital environment that prevents major self-destructiveness, the general experience has been that borderline patients continue their self-injurious behaviors in the hospital. This behavior sets up major conflicts with staff regarding proper responses to pa-

tients who challenge staff to prevent them from hurting themselves. Placing patients on one-to-one or constant observation has seemed to encourage rather than discourage self-injurious acts. The broad, but not unanimous consensus recently is that hospitalizations should be kept as brief as possible within the boundaries of responsible patient care, with the option of brief rehospitalizations seen as preferable to lengthy hospital stays.

This article has been reprinted from the *Encyclopedia of Human Behavior, Volume 1.*

BIBLIOGRAPHY

Druck, A. (1989). "Four Therapeutic Approaches to the Borderline Patient." Jason Aronson, Northvale, NJ.

Gunderson, J. G. (1984). "Borderline Personality Disorder." American Psychiatric Press, Washington, DC.

Herman, J. L. (1992). "Trauma and Recovery." Basic Books, New York.

Kernberg, O. (1984). "Severe Personality Disorders." Yale University Press, New Haven, CT.

Kroll, J. (1988). "The Challenge of the Borderline Patient." WW Norton, New York.

Kroll, J. (1993). "PTSD/Borderlines in Therapy: Finding the Balance," Norton, New York.

Linehan, M. M., Armstrong, H. E., Suarez, A., Allmon, D., and Heard, H. L. (1991). Cognitive-behavioral treatment of chronically parasuicidal borderline patients. *Arch. Gen. Psychiatry* **48**, 1060–1064.

Links, P. S. (1990). "Family Environment and Borderline Personality Disorder." American Psychiatric Press, Washington, DC.

Paris, J. (1992). "Borderline Personality Disorder: Etiology and Treatment." American Psychiatric Press, Washington, DC.

Soloff, P. H., Cornelius, J., George, A., Nathan, S., Perel, J. M., and Ulrich, R. F. (1993). Efficacy of phenelzine and haloperidol in borderline personality disorder. *Arch. Gen. Psychiatry* **50**, 377–385.

Stevenson, J., and Meares, R. (1992). An outcome study of psychotherapy for patients with borderline personality disorder. *Am. J. Psychiatry* **149**, 358–362.

Stone, M. (1990). "The Fate of Borderline Patients." Guilford, New York.

Wallerstein, R. S. (1986). "Forty-Two Lives in Treatment." Guilford, New York.

Brain

Bryan Kolb and Ian Q. Whishaw

University of Lethbridge, Canada

Jan Cioe

Okanagan University-College, Canada

Action Potential   Brief electrical impulse by which information is conducted along an axon. It results from short-lived changes in the membrane's permeability to sodium.

Amnesia   Partial or total loss of memory.

Aphasia   Defect or loss of power of expression by speech, writing, or signs, or of comprehending spoken or written language caused by injury or disease of the brain.

Cerebral Cortex   Layer of gray matter on the surface of the cerebral hemispheres composed of neurons and their synaptic connections that form four to six sublayers.

Hippocampus   Primitive cortical structure lying in the medial region of the temporal lobe; named after its shape, which is similar to a sea horse, or hippocampus.

Neuron   Basic unit of the nervous system; the nerve cell. Its function is to transmit and store information; it includes the cell body (*soma*), many processes called *dendrites*, and an *axon*.

Neurotransmitter   Chemical released from a synapse in response to an action potential and acting on postsynaptic receptors to change the resting potential of the receiving cell; chemically transmits information from one neuron to another.

The **BRAIN** is that part of the central nervous system that is contained in the skull. It weighs approximately 1450 g at maturity and is composed of brain cells (neurons), as well as support cells, that are organized into hundreds of functionally distinct regions. Neurons communicate both chemically and electrically so that different brain regions form functional systems to control behavior. Measurement of brain structure, activity, and behavior has allowed neuroscientists to reach inferences regarding the mechanisms of the basic functions, which include (1) the body's interactions with the environment through the sensory systems (e.g., vision, audition, touch) and motor systems, (2) internal activities of the body (e.g., breathing, temperature, blood pressure), and (3) mental activities (e.g., thought, language, affect). By studying people with brain injuries it is possible to propose brain circuits that underlie human behavior.

I. ANATOMICAL AND PHYSIOLOGICAL ORGANIZATION OF THE HUMAN BRAIN

A. Cellular Composition

The brain is composed of two general classes of cells: neurons and glial cells. Neurons are the functional units of the nervous system, whereas glial cells are support cells. Estimates of the numbers of cells in the human brain usually run around 10^{10} neurons and 10^{12} glial cells, although the numbers could be even higher. Only about 2–3 million cells (motor neurons) send their connections out of the brain to animate muscle fibers, leaving an enormous number of cells with other functions.

There are numerous types of neurons (e.g., pyramidal, granule, Purkinje, Golgi I, motoneurons), but they share several features in common. First, they have a cell body, which like most cells contains a variety of substances that determine the function of the cell. Second, they have processes called *dendrites,* which function primarily to increase the surface area on which a cell can receive information from other cells. Third, they have a process called an *axon,* which normally

originates in the cell body and transmits information to other cells (Fig. 1). Different types of neurons are morphologically distinct, reflecting differences in function. These various types are distributed differentially to the many regions of the brain reflecting regional differences in brain function.

Neurons are connected with one another via their axons; any given neuron may have as many as 15,000 connections with other neurons. These connections are highly organized so that certain regions of the brain are more closely connected to one another than they are to others. As a result, these closely associated

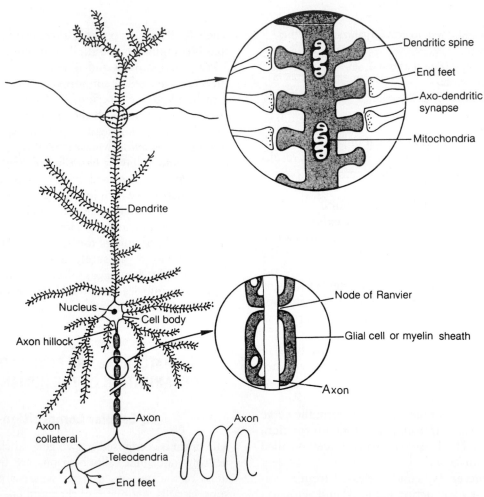

Figure I   Summary of the major parts of a stylized neuron. Enlargement at the top right shows the gross structure of the synapse between axons and the spines on dendrites. Enlargement on the bottom right shows the myelin sheath that surrounds the axon and acts as insulation. [From Kolb, B., and Whishaw, I. Q. (1990). "Fundamentals of Human Neuropsychology," 3rd ed. Freeman, New York.]

regions form functional systems in the brain, which control certain types of behavior.

B. Gross Anatomical Organization of the Brain

The most obvious feature of the human brain is that there are two large hemispheres which sit on a stem (i.e., the brainstem). Both structures are composed of hundreds of regions; nearly all of them are found bilaterally. Traditionally, the brain is described by the gross divisions observed phylogenetically and embryologically as summarized in Table I. The most primitive region is the hindbrain, whose principal structures include the cerebellum, pons, and medulla. The cerebellum was originally specialized for sensory-motor coordination, which remains its major function. The pons and medulla also contribute to equilibrium, balance, and the control of gross movements (including breathing). The midbrain consists of two main structures, the tectum and the tegmentum. The midbrain consists primarily of two sets of nuclei, the superior and inferior colliculi, which mediate whole body movements to visual and auditory stimuli, respectively. The tegmentum contains various structures including regions associated with (1) the nerves of the head

Table I Divisions of the Central Nervous System

Primitive divisions	Mammalian divisions	Major structures
Prosencephalon (forebrain)	Telencephalon (endbrain)	Neocortex Basal ganglia Limbic system Olfactory bulb Lateral ventricles
	Diencephalon (between brain)	Thalamus Hypothalamus Epithalamus Third ventricle
Mesencephalon (midbrain)	Mesencephalon (midbrain)	Tectum Tegmentum Cerebral aqueduct
Rhombencephalon (hindbrain)	Metencephalon (across brain)	Cerebellum Pons Fourth ventricle
	Myelencephalon (spinal brain)	Medulla oblongata Fourth ventricle

(the so-called cranial nerves), (2) sensory nerves from the body, (3) connections from higher structures that function to control movement, and (4) a number of structures involved in movement (substantia nigra, red nucleus), as well as a region known as the reticular formation. The latter system plays a major role in the control of sleep and waking.

The forebrain is conventionally divided into five anatomical areas: (1) the neocortex, (2) the basal ganglia, (3) the limbic system, (4) the thalamus, and (5) the olfactory bulbs and tract. Each of these regions can be dissociated into numerous smaller regions on the basis of neuronal type, physiological and chemical properties, and connections with other brain regions.

The neocortex (usually called the *cortex*) is composed of approximately six layers—each of which has distinct neuronal populations. It comprises 80% of the human forebrain by volume and is grossly divided into four regions, which are named by the cranial bones lying above them (Fig. 2). It is wrinkled, which is nature's solution to the problem of confining a large surface area into a shell that is still small enough to pass through the birth canal. The cortex has a thickness of only 1.5–3.0 mm but has a total area of about 2500 cm². The cortex can be subdivided into dozens of subregions on the basis of the distribution of neuron types, their chemical and physiological characteristics, and their connections. These subregions can be shown to be functionally distinct.

The basal ganglia are a collection of nuclei lying beneath the cortex. They include the putamen, caudate nucleus, globus pallidus, and amygdala. These nuclei have intimate connections with the neocortex as well as having major connections with midbrain structures. The basal ganglia have principally a motor function, as damage to different regions can produce changes in posture or muscle tone and abnormal movements such as twitches, jerks, and tremors.

The limbic system is not really a unitary system but refers to a number of structures that were once believed to function together to produce emotion. These include the hippocampus, septum, cingulate cortex, and hypothalamus, each of which have different functions (Fig. 3). [*See* LIMBIC SYSTEM.]

The thalamus provides the major route of information to the neocortex, and different neocortical regions are associated with inputs from distinct thalamic regions connected with the neocortex. The dif-

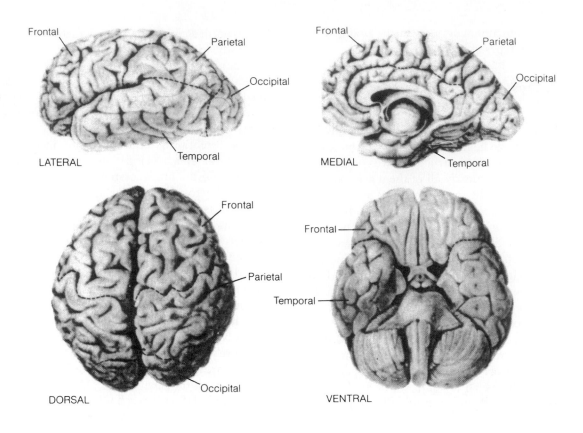

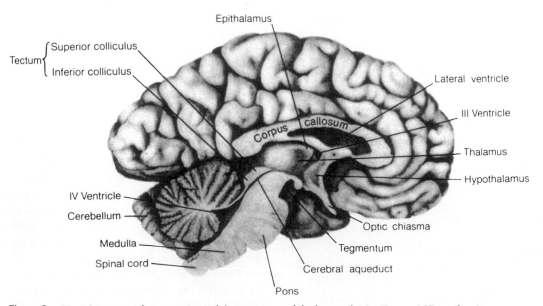

Figure 2 (Top) Summary of gross regions of the neocortex of the human brain. (Bottom) View of major structures of the brain. [From Kolb, B., and Whishaw, I. Q. (1990). "Fundamentals of Human Neuropsychology," 3rd ed. Freeman, New York.]

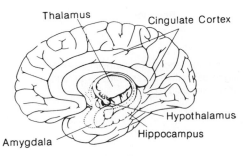

Figure 3 Medial view of the right hemisphere illustrating positions of limbic structures. Anterior is to the left.

ferent thalamic areas receive information from sensory and motor regions in the brainstem as well as the limbic system.

C. Physiological Organization of the Brain

Like other cells in the body, the neuron has an electrical voltage (potential) across its membrane, which results from the differential distribution of various ions on the two sides of the membrane. In contrast to other body cells, however, this electrical potential is used to transmit information from one neuron to another in the nervous system, which is accomplished in the following way. Neurons have a resting potential across the membrane of the dendrites, cell body, and axon, which remains relatively constant at about −70 mV. If the membrane permeability for different ions changes, the electrical potential will also change. If it becomes more negative the cell is said to be hyperpolarized, and if it becomes less negative (i.e., more positive) it is said to be depolarized. When the membrane of a neuron is perturbed by the signals coming from other neurons or by certain external agents (e.g., chemicals), the voltage across the membrane changes, becoming either hyperpolarized or depolarized. These changes are normally restricted to the area of membrane stimulated, but if there are numerous signals through many synapses to the same cell, they will summate, altering the membrane potential of a larger region of the cell. If the excitation is sufficient to reduce the membrane potential to about −50 mV, the membrane permeability for positive Na$^+$ ions changes. The influx of ions raises the potential until it becomes positive (e.g., +40 mV). This change in membrane potential spreads across the cell and if it reaches the axon, it travels down the axon, producing a self-propagating signal.

This change in permeability is quickly reversed by the cell in about 0.5 msec, allowing the cell to send repeated signals during a short period of time. The signal that travels down the axon is known as an action potential (or nerve impulse), and when it occurs, the cell is said to have fired. The rate at which the impulse travels along the axon varies from 1 to 100 m/sec and can occur as frequently as 1000 times/sec, depending on the diameter of the axon; the most common rate is about 100/sec.

D. Chemical Organization

Once the nerve impulse reaches the end of the axon (the axon terminal), it initiates biochemical changes that result in the release of a chemical known as a neurotransmitter into the synapse. Although the action of transmitters is complex, their effect is either to raise or to lower the membrane potential of the postsynaptic cell, with the effect of making it more or less likely to transmit a nerve impulse.

Dozens of chemicals are known to be neurotransmitters, including a variety of amino acids [e.g., glutamic acid, glycine, aspartate, and gammaaminobutyric acid (GABA)], monoamines (e.g., dopamine, norepinephrine, serotonin), and peptides [e.g., substance P, β-endorphin, corticotrophin (ACTH)]. Any neuron can receive signals from neurotransmitters through different synapses. The distribution of the various transmitters is not homogeneous in the brain as different regions are dominated by different types. Because drugs that affect the brain act by either mimicking certain transmitters or interfering with the normal function of particular transmitters, different drugs alter different regions of the brain and subsequently have different behavioral effects.

II. FUNCTIONAL ORGANIZATION OF THE BRAIN

A. Principles of Brain Organization

The fundamental principle of brain organization is that it is organized hierarchically such that the same behavior is represented at several levels in the nervous system. The function of each level can be inferred from studies in which the outer levels have been removed, as is summarized in Figure 4. The principal

Brain

| Anatomy | Preparation | Behaviors |

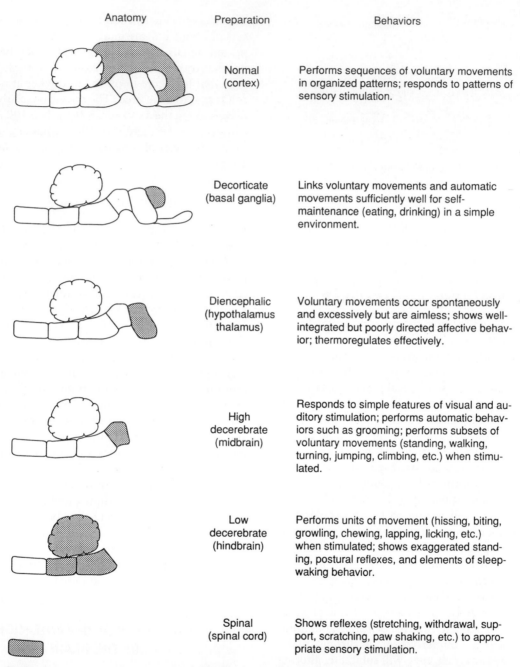

| | Normal (cortex) | Performs sequences of voluntary movements in organized patterns; responds to patterns of sensory stimulation. |

| | Decorticate (basal ganglia) | Links voluntary movements and automatic movements sufficiently well for self-maintenance (eating, drinking) in a simple environment. |

| | Diencephalic (hypothalamus thalamus) | Voluntary movements occur spontaneously and excessively but are aimless; shows well-integrated but poorly directed affective behavior; thermoregulates effectively. |

| | High decerebrate (midbrain) | Responds to simple features of visual and auditory stimulation; performs automatic behaviors such as grooming; performs subsets of voluntary movements (standing, walking, turning, jumping, climbing, etc.) when stimulated. |

| | Low decerebrate (hindbrain) | Performs units of movement (hissing, biting, growling, chewing, lapping, licking, etc.) when stimulated; shows exaggerated standing, postural reflexes, and elements of sleep-waking behavior. |

| | Spinal (spinal cord) | Shows reflexes (stretching, withdrawal, support, scratching, paw shaking, etc.) to appropriate sensory stimulation. |

Figure 4 Summary of the behavior that can be supported by different levels of the nervous system. Shading indicates highest remaining functional area in each preparation.

idea is that the basic units of behavior are produced by the lowest level, the spinal cord, and at each successive level there is the addition of greater control over these simple behavioral units. At the highest level, the neocortex allows the addition of flexibility to the relatively stereotyped movement sequences gen-

erated by lower levels, as well as allowing greater control of behavior by incorporating complex concepts such as space and time. Although new abilities are added at each level in the hierarchy, it remains difficult to localize any process to a particular level because any behavior requires the activity of all regions for its successful execution. Nonetheless, brain injury at different levels will produce different symptoms, depending on what functions are added at that level.

B. Principles of Neocortical Organization

The cortex can be divided into three general types of areas: (1) sensory areas, (2) motor areas, and (3) association areas. The sensory areas are the regions that function to identify and to interpret information coming from the receptor structures in the eyes, ears, nose, mouth, and skin. The motor complex is the region involved in the direct control of movement. The association cortex is the cortex that is not ascribed specific sensory or motor functions.

Distinct regions of the sensory cortex are associated with each of these sensory systems, and each region is made up of numerous subregions which function to process a specific type of sensory information. For example, in the visual system separate regions are devoted to the analysis of form, color, size, movement, etc. Damage to each of these regions will produce a distinct loss of sensory experience. In each system there is a region of sensory cortex that produces an apparent inability to detect sensory information such that a person will, for instance, appear to be blind, unable to taste, or have numbness of the skin, etc. In each case, however, it can be shown that other aspects of sensory function are intact. Thus, a person who is unable to "see" an object may be able to indicate its color and position! Similarly, patients may be able to locate a place on the body where they were touched while being unable to "feel" the touch. Regions of sensory cortex producing such symptoms are referred to as primary sensory cortex. The other regions are known as unimodal association regions, and damage to them is associated with various other symptoms. Thus, in every sensory system there are regions of cortex that, when damaged, result in an inability to understand the significance of sensory events. Such symptoms are known as agnosias. For example, although able to perceive an object (e.g., toothbrush) and to pick it up, a person may be unable to name it or to identify its use. Similarly, a person may be able to perceive a sound (e.g., that of an insect) but be unable to indicate what the sound is from. Some agnosias are relatively specific (e.g., an inability to recognize faces or colors).

The motor cortex represents a relatively small region of the cortex that controls all voluntary movements and is specialized to produce fine movements such as independent finger movements and complex tongue movements. Damage to this region prevents certain movements (e.g., of the fingers), although others (e.g., arm and body movements) may be relatively normal. Although the motor cortex is a relatively small region of the cortex, a much larger region contributes to motor functions, including some of the sensory regions as well as the association cortex. For example, a person may be unable to organize behaviors such as those required for dressing or for using objects as a result of damage to this larger region. Such disorders are known as apraxias, which refers to the inability to make voluntary movements in the absence of any damage to the motor cortex.

The regions of the neocortex not specialized as sensory or motor regions are referred to as association cortex. This cortex receives information from one or more of the sensory systems and functions to organize complex behaviors such as the three-dimensional control of movement, the comprehension of written language, and the making of plans of action. The principal regions of association cortex include the prefrontal cortex in the frontal lobe, the posterior parietal cortex, and regions of the temporal cortex. Although not neocortex, it is convenient to consider the medial temporal structures, including the hippocampus, amygdala, and associated cortical regions, as a type of association cortex. Taken together, damage to the association regions causes a puzzling array of behavioral symptoms that include changes in affect and personality, memory, and language.

III. CEREBRAL ASYMMETRY

One of the most distinctive features of the human brain is that the two cerebral hemispheres are both anatomically and functionally different, a property referred to as cerebral asymmetry.

A. Functional Asymmetry

The clearest functional difference between the two sides of the brain is that structures of the left hemisphere are involved in language functions and those of the right hemisphere are involved in nonlanguage functions such as the control of spatial abilities. This asymmetry can be demonstrated in each of the sensory systems, with differences in left-handed and right-handed persons. We will first consider the common case of the right-handed individual. In the visual system the left hemisphere is specialized to recognize printed words or numbers, whereas the right hemisphere is specialized to process complex nonverbal material such as is seen in geometric figures, faces, route maps, etc. Similarly, in the auditory system the left hemisphere analyzes words, whereas the right hemisphere analyzes tone of voice (prosody) and certain aspects of music. Asymmetrical functions go beyond sensation, however, to include movement, memory, and affect. In the control of movement, the left hemisphere is specialized for the production of certain types of complex movement sequences, as in meaningful gestures (e.g., salute, wave) or writing. The right hemisphere has a complementary role in the production of other movements such as in drawing, dressing, or constructing objects. Similarly, the left hemisphere has a favored role in memory functions related to language (e.g., written and spoken words), whereas the right hemisphere plays a major role in the memory of places and nonverbal information such as music and faces. With respect to affect, the right hemisphere is superior to the left for recognizing emotional aspects of stimuli and seems to play an important role in the comprehension of humor.

B. Anatomical Asymmetry

The functional asymmetry of the human brain is correlated with various asymmetries in gross brain morphology, cell structure, neurochemical distribution, and blood flow. Differences in gross morphology and cell structure are most easily seen in the regions specialized for language, including the anterior (Broca's) and posterior speech areas (Fig. 5). For example, one region in the posterior speech area, the planum temporale, is twice as large on the left hemisphere in most brains, whereas a region involved in the processing of musical notes, Heschl's gyrus, is larger in the right temporal lobe than in the left.

C. Variations in Cerebral Asymmetry: Handedness and Sex

There is considerable variation in the details of both functional and anatomical asymmetry in different people. Two factors, handedness and sex, appear to account for much of this variation. First, left-handers

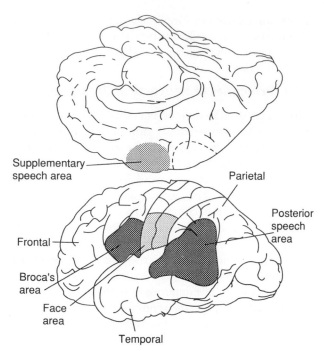

Figure 5 Schematic diagram showing the anterior speech area (Broca's area) in the frontal lobe, the posterior speech area (including Wernicke's area) in posterior temporal and parietal regions. Shaded region between speech areas is the motor and sensory cortex controlling the face and tongue. [From Kolb, B., and Whishaw, I. Q. (1990). "Fundamentals of Human Neuropsychology," 3rd ed. Freeman, New York.]

have a different pattern of anatomical organization than do right-handers. For example, left-handers appear to have a larger bundle of fibers connecting the two cerebral hemispheres, the corpus callosum, which implies that the nature of hemispheric interaction differs in left- and right-handers. Similarly, left-handers are less likely to show the large asymmetries in the structure of the language-related areas than are right-handers. Functionally, the organization of the left-handed brain shows considerable variation: Language is located primarily in the left hemisphere in about two-thirds of left-handers, in the right hemisphere in about one-sixth, and in both hemispheres in about one-sixth. Left-handers with different speech organization than right-handers do not simply have reversal of brain organization, however, although the nature of their cerebral organization is still poorly understood. Second, males and females also differ in functional and structural organization. For example, the corpus callosum of females is larger relative to brain size than that of males, and females are less likely to show gross asymmetries or to have reversed asymmetries. Animal studies have shown a clear relation between anatomical organization and the presence of the perinatal gonadal hormones present at about the time of birth, suggesting that these hormones differentially organize the brain of males and females. Functionally, the effect of brain damage in males and females differs as well, although in complex ways that are poorly understood. It does appear, however, that frontal lobe injuries in both human and nonhuman subjects have differential effects in the two sexes, with larger behavioral effects of frontal lobe injury observed in females. Other factors are also believed to influence the nature of cerebral asymmetry, especially experience, interacting with both sex and handedness.

IV. ORGANIZATION OF HIGHER FUNCTIONS

Complex functions such as memory or emotion are not easily localized in the brain, as the circuits involved include vast areas of both the cerebral hemispheres and other forebrain structures. Part of the difficulty in localizing such functions is that they are not unitary things but are inferred from behavior, which in turn results from numerous processes. Nonetheless, it is possible to reach some generalizations regarding such functions.

A. Memory

Memory is an inferred process that results in a relatively permanent change in behavior, which presumably results from a change in the brain. Psychologists distinguish many types of memory, each of which may have a distinct neural basis. These include, among others, (1) long-term memory, which is the recall of information over hours, days, weeks, years, etc.; (2) short-term memory, which is the recall of information over seconds or minutes; (3) declarative memory, which is the recall of facts that are accessible to conscious recollection; (4) procedural memory, which is the ability to perform skills that are "automatic" and that are not stored with respect to specific times or places (e.g., the movements required to drive); (5) verbal memory, which is memory of language-related material; and (6) spatial memory, which is the recall of places or locations.

The neural basis of human memory can be considered at two levels: cellular and neural location. Thus, changes in cell activity and structure are associated with processes like memory, which may occur extremely rapidly in the brain, possibly in the order of seconds or at least minutes. Further, there is a variety of candidate regions for memory processes, the region varying with the nature of memory process. One structure that plays a major role in various forms of memory is the hippocampus. Bilateral damage to this structure leads to a condition of anterograde amnesia, which refers to the inability to recall, after a few minutes, any new material that is experienced after the damage. There is only a brief period of retrograde amnesia, which refers to the inability to recall material before the injury. The relatively selective effects of hippocampal injuries in producing anterograde but not retrograde amnesia suggest that different brain regions are involved in the initial learning of information and its later retrieval from memory. As a generalization, it appears that the temporal lobe is involved in various types of long-term memory processes, whereas the frontal and parietal lobes play a role in certain short-term memory processes. Damage to these regions thus produces different forms of memory loss, which are further complicated by whether the injury is to the left or right hemisphere. [*See* AMNESIA.]

B. Language

Damage to either of the major speech areas (Broca's or the posterior speech zone, which is sometimes referred to as Wernicke's area) will produce a variety of dissociable syndromes, including aphasia (an inability to comprehend language), alexia (an inability to read), and agraphia (an inability to write). There are various forms of each of these syndromes that relate to the precise details of the brain injury. A number of other forms of language disturbance result from damage outside the speech areas, including changes in speech fluency [i.e., the ability to generate words according to certain criteria (e.g., write down words starting with "D"; give the name of objects)], spontaneous talking in conversation, the ability to categorize words (e.g., apple and banana are fruits), and so on. It appears that nearly any left hemisphere injury will affect some aspect of these language functions, as does damage to some regions of the right hemisphere. [*See* APHASIA, ALEXIA, AND AGRAPHIA.]

C. Emotional Processes

Like memory processes, emotional processes are inferred from behavior and include many different functions including autonomic nervous system activity, "feeling," facial expression, and tone of voice. Certain subcortical regions (hypothalamus, amygdala) play a major role in the generation of affective behaviors, especially the autonomic components such as blood pressure, respiration, and heart rate. In addition, damage nearly anywhere in the cortex will alter some aspect of cognitive function, which in turn will alter personality and emotional behavior, but damage to the right hemisphere produces a greater effect on emotional behavior than similar damage to the left. Moreover, the frontal lobe plays a special role as well, possibly because it has direct control of autonomic function as well as of spontaneous facial expression and other nonverbal aspects of personality. Thus, damage to the right hemisphere, or the frontal lobe of either hemisphere, is likely to lead to complaints from relatives regarding a change in "personality" or "affect." The control of emotional behavior may not only be relatively localized to different regions of the brain, but also related to specific neurotransmitter systems in the brain. For example, one dominant theory of the cause of schizophrenia proposes that there is an overactivity of the dopaminergic neurons (i.e., neurons that use dopamine as a neurotransmitter) in the forebrain, likely in the frontal cortex (hence, the dopamine hypothesis of schizophrenia). Similarly, the dominant theory of depression is that it is related to low activity in systems that employ norepinephrine or serotonin as neurotransmitters. Because there are asymmetries in the cerebral distribution of these transmitters, it is reasonable to expect that depression may be more related to the right than left hemisphere, which is consistent with the dominant role of the right hemisphere in emotion. [See DEPRESSION; SCHIZOPHRENIA.]

D. Space

The concept of space has many different interpretations, which are not equivalent. Objects (and bodies) occupy space, move through space, and interact with other things in space; we can form mental representations of space, and we have memories for the location of things. It is difficult, therefore, to define space or to know how the brain codes spatial information. Damage to different parts of the cerebral hemispheres can produce a wide variety of spatial disturbances including the inability to appreciate the location of one's body, or even the location of one's body parts relative to one another. It is generally accepted that the right hemisphere plays the major role in spatial behavior, but there can also be spatial disruptions from left hemisphere damage, especially if the behavior involves verbalizing space. The major region in the control of spatial behavior is the parietal cortex, although the hippocampus is also involved.

E. Conclusions

One of the key features of the brain is the localization of function. We have seen that certain brain structures are critical for a number of the higher human functions and that damage in specific locations on one particular side of the brain can result in the loss of behaviors which are not seen when the other side is injured. This localization of function results from the unique inputs and outputs of the subregions of the brain. Nevertheless, the hierarchical organization of the brain guarantees that control of a specific behavior is seldom restricted to a single area. There are multiple representations of the different cognitive functions in the different levels of neural organization but they are not simply backup circuits. Each level adds its own unique contribution which ultimately produces a degree of complexity that makes it possible for humans to behave flexibly in a changing environment.

This article has been reprinted from the *Encyclopedia of Human Behavior, Volume 1.*

BIBLIOGRAPHY

Kolb, B., & Whishaw, I. Q. (1990). "Fundamentals of Human Neuropsychology," 3rd ed. Freeman, New York.

Nauta, W. J. H., & Feirtage, M. (1986). "Fundamental Neuroanatomy." Freeman, New York.

Brain Development and Plasticity

John H. Ashe and V. Bessie Aramakis

University of California, Riverside

Cell Adhesion Molecules Integral cell membrane glycoproteins that promote cell-to-cell adhesion by the interaction of the same molecular species on opposing surfaces of interacting cells.

Down-Regulation A decrease in cellular metabolic activity that can lead to decreased gene expression, decreased neurotransmitter release, or decreased responsiveness to receptor activation.

Long-Term Potentiation A long-lasting increase in the effectiveness in synaptic communication between neurons that is often elicited by high-frequency stimulation of afferent fibers.

Neurotrophins Proteins that belong to a larger family of neurotrophic factors and support the growth, differentiation, and survival of neurons in the developing nervous system.

Pathfinding A term used to describe the mechanisms and cues that provide axons with precise guidance to their targets in the developing nervous system.

Plasticity The ability of the nervous system to make physiological adaptations to changing environmental influences during development and in adulthood.

Receptor An integral or membrane-bound protein specialized to recognize a particular neurotransmitter, hormone, or biologically active agent. Engagement of a receptor by such a substance will result in activation of a particular cellular effector system to produce a physiological response.

Up-Regulation An increase in cellular metabolic activity, which can lead to increased gene expression, increased neurotransmitter release, or increased responsiveness to receptor activation.

PLASTICITY is a general term that refers to the ability of the nervous system to make adaptations to changing environmental influences. This entry examines the importance of plasticity in development and how mechanisms of plasticity that operate during development are retained and function in the mature brain. We describe some basic processes in the development of the mammalian nervous system, with particular emphasis on development of the brain and neocortex. To this end we discus the role and potential effects of specific molecules characterized as neurotrophic factors on plasticity in the developing and mature nervous systems.

I. INTRODUCTION

The functional organization of the mammalian brain is the end product of a complex interaction between its basic genetic substrate and individual experience. The central nervous system (CNS), consisting of billions of cells, is typically regarded as the most complex and highly organized form of matter known. These cells vary vastly in both size and shape and are interconnected by means of immensely complex synaptic networks. The principal cell types that comprise the nervous system, that is, neurons and neuroglial cells, are interrelated to effect complex information processing and decision making. Neurons appear to be especially adapted for this task. The roles for neuroglia in the development and function of the mature nervous system appear increasingly diversified and include cell proliferation and uptake and release of neurotransmitters. Current research is rapidly clarifying the nature of the chemical and electrical signals that are used to accomplish cellular communication and information processing, but there is still much to learn about both the signaling process and reception and decoding of these signals.

Throughout a lifetime, synaptic circuits are continuously changing, strengthening and weakening in influence, in response to a continuously changing environment. The detailed structural and physiological rules that govern continual change in the nervous system are not known; however, these mechanisms can operate only within genetically determined boundaries. Plasticity is a general property of the nervous system that refers to the findings that neurons adjust their information-processing and communicative properties under a broad range of conditions. Historically, hypotheses about plasticity, particularly learning and memory, proposed that underlying mechanisms might be similar in adulthood to those mechanisms that led to the formation of the nervous system during development. Thus, mechanisms of change, growth, and strengthening that operate during development may extend, in their essence, to plasticity in the mature nervous system. As a more restrictive example, morphological and physiological modifications, which reflect synapse formation and synapse strengthening, occur in neurons in both developing and mature nervous systems. It is from this viewpoint that development and plasticity within the nervous system are often considered together.

We cannot here hope to summarize comprehensively the entire fund of current knowledge of CNS development and plasticity. However, there are many detailed and excellent reviews of the literature, which we have listed in the bibliography. Our intention is to provide the reader with a balanced mix of some of the fundamental findings and directions of current research that in our view are especially interesting and likely to be particularly fruitful.

II. GASTRULATION AND NEURAL TUBE FORMATION

The nervous system of all vertebrates begins as a longitudinal strip of neuroectoderm which appears on the dorsal surface of the early developing embryo. The neuroectoderm is a product of an early stage of embryonic development, gastrulation. Gastrulation marks a stage in embryonic development that is characterized by development of the germ layers—ectoderm, mesoderm, and endoderm—that serve as the basis of further growth and development.

The neuroectoderm, a derivative of surface layer ectoderm, thickens and its central portion sinks beneath the surface of the embryo to form the neural plate. This invaginated neural plate together with its surrounding walls forms a deep gutter-like structure, the neural groove. Eventually, the walls of the neural groove role together and fuse to form a distinctive structure, the neural tube, which extends the length, from head to tail, of the developing embryo. It is from the neural tube that the fundamental divisions of the central nervous system begin to form. The most rostral part of the tube will generate the brain, and the more caudal portion will generate the spinal cord and much of the peripheral nervous system (PNS).

III. PRINCIPLES FROM PERIPHERAL NERVOUS SYSTEM DEVELOPMENT

The PNS is that portion of the nervous system outside the brain and spinal cord, that is, outside of the CNS. It has two main divisions, somatic and the autonomic. The somatic division of the PNS innervates the skin, skeletal muscles, and joints. The autonomic division can itself be divided into two major subdivisions, sympathetic and parasympathetic. Together, the sympathetic and parasympathetic subdivisions comprise the motor system for smooth muscles, internal organs, and glands. The PNS and CNS are two clearly identifiable major anatomical components of the nervous system; however, they are functionally interconnected to act as an entity in the production and coordination of behavior.

A. Neural Crest

During the closing and fusing of the neural tube, a portion of cells extending longitudinally along the lateral aspect of the neural tube move out onto the dorsal surface. This band of cells forms the neural crest. These cells begin to disperse from the neural crest, laterally and ventrally throughout the embryo, to accumulate in defined regions. Descendants of the neural crest cells differentiate into a wide variety of neuronal and nonneuronal cell types in the PNS, including neurons located in peripheral ganglia and Schwann-type neuroglia cells.

B. Axonal Pathfinding

Neural processes destined to become mature axons and dendrites are termed neurites. Neurites grow and extend by means of growth cones. Growth cones are knob-looking structures with finger-like extensions that form at the ends of neurites. Growth cones only form when the neurite is in contact with an appropriate substratum and they are in constant motion, moving outward and retracting back, moving to the right and to the left, reminiscent of searching motions. Once the peripheral ganglia (and other neuronal aggregates) have formed, neurons within them sprout neurites that slowly increase their length to make eventual contact with their targets. This process entails a high degree of specificity. For the axon, the process by which the neurite of a developing neuron projects to and identifies an appropriate target cell is called axonal pathfinding. As might be expected, axonal pathfinding is complex and utilizes several cellular strategies and molecular mechanisms to establish precise contact with the appropriate destination. Although the mechanisms are not fully understood, it appears that the growing tips of axons are guided along a particular pathway by at least two mechanisms, growth along a chemical gradient and by contact guidance. Some evidence suggests that for innervation of distant targets, the initial growth may be guided by substrata contact; whereas chemical gradients guide growth when axon terminals are in close proximity to the target. Thus, it appears that axonal pathfinding requires directional growth guided by specific molecules found on cell surfaces and within the extracellular matrix.

Growth cones show a clear preference for some substrate molecules over other substrate constituents.

Molecules that mediate such cell-to-cell and cell-to-substrate adhesion in growth cone guidance are members of a protein superfamily (immunoglobulins, structural glycoproteins involved in neuronal cell adhesion) that includes neural cell adhesion molecule (N-CAM) and neuroglia cell adhesion molecule. N-CAM is an integral cell membrane protein that promotes cell-to-cell adhesion through interaction with comparable proteins on opposing surfaces of interacting cells. It is through these types of molecular interactions that N-CAM promotes the aggregation of nerve cells, the extension of neurites, and the binding together of growing axons into bundles. However, because of its homogeneous nature in tissue of the developing nervous system, it is unlikely that N-CAM plays a primary role in directional guidance, but rather only a permissive role in axon outgrowth. Cell adhesion molecules have also been implicated in neuronal plasticity and in mechanisms of learning and memory in the adult. With regard to directional outgrowth of neurites, a variety of other extracellular matrix adhesion molecules are important. These molecules are less widely distributed than N-CAM and their subtle concentration gradients are thought to be critical in guiding the ultimate direction of neurite growth.

IV. DEVELOPMENT OF THE CENTRAL NERVOUS SYSTEM

A. Origin of Brain Regions

As indicated, the CNS derives from the neural tube. Cells of the rostral portion of the neural tube proliferate, regionalize, and develop into the three primary brain divisions: the prosencephalon (embryonic forebrain), mesencephalon (midbrain), and the rhombencephalon (embryonic hindbrain) (Figure 1; Table I). Continued growth and differentiation of the prosencephalon gives rise to the telencephalon (anterior portion) and diencephalon (posterior portion). The mesencephalon does not develop additional divisions. The rhombencephalon gives rise to two secondary divisions, the metencephalon (anterior portion) and the myelencephalon (posterior portion). Thus, the mature brain consists of five major divisions: telencephalon, diencephalon, mesencephalon, metencephalon, and myelencephalon. The posterior end of the neural tube generates the spinal cord.

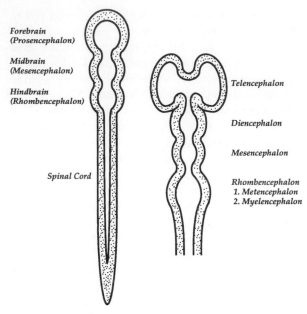

Figure 1 Principle divisions of the developing vertebrate brain. The nervous system begins as the neural plate that folds into a neural tube. The major subdivisions of the CNS develop gradually from enlargements in the rostral aspect of the tube. To the left is that portion of the neural tube, at an early stage, that will become the brain. There are initially three relatively distinct regions: forebrain, midbrain, and hindbrain. With continued development, the forebrain forms the telencephalon and diencephalon, and the hindbrain forms the metencephalon and myelencephalon. These five regions constitute the general organization of the adult brain.

Table 1 Major Subdivisions of the Embryonic and Adult Brain

Three-division stage	Five-division stage	Major mature structures
Forebrain (Prosencephalon)	Telencephalon	Cerebral hemispheres: Cerebral cortex Basal ganglia Hippocampal formation Amygdala
	Diencephalon	Thalamus Hypothalamus Retina
Midbrain (Mesencephalon)	Mesencephalon	Inferior colliculus Superior colliculus Red nucleus Substantia nigra
Hindbrain (Rhombencephalon)	Metencephalon	Pons Cerebellum
	Myelencephalon	Medulla

The telencephalon is that region of the embryonic forebrain in the neural tube that gives rise to the cerebral hemispheres and its components, the cerebral cortex, the hippocampal formation, the basal ganglia (i.e., caudate nucleus, putamen, and globus pallidus), and the amygdala. These regions are concerned with higher-order processing and integrative functions, including cognitive processing, integration of cognitive processing with emotional state, and refined motor function.

The diencephalon is that region in the embryonic forebrain in the neural tube that gives rise to the thalamus, hypothalamus, and retina. The thalamus consists of a number of relatively discreet subregions (nuclei) that are classified as either specific nuclei or nonspecific nuclei. The specific nuclei are so termed because they rapidly receive and process information from the major sensory receptors, that is, visual, auditory, gustatory, and somatosensory, and then relay this processed information onward to well-defined areas of the neocortex. The receiving areas of the specific thalamic nuclei are neocortical regions that are primarily concerned with processing information regarding the same sensory modality. For example, the medial geniculate nucleus (i.e., auditory thalamus), lateral geniculate nucleus (i.e., visual thalamus), and ventral posterolateral nucleus (i.e., somatosensory thalamus) project to auditory, visual, and somatosensory cortex, respectively. The nonspecific thalamic nuclei receive input from several sensory modalities and send major projections to cortical association areas. Thalamic nuclei also receive reciprocal input from the neocortex and have regions devoted to processing information concerning motor functions. The hypothalamus, although relatively small in size, is large in functional importance. Its major function is in maintaining physiological homeostasis by means of close interaction with the autonomic nervous and endocrine systems. It is important in the organization of general life-sustaining and motivational functions such as feeding, fleeing from danger, defensive and aggressive fighting, and hormonal and behavioral aspects of mating.

The mesencephalon is often called the midbrain and is the midportion of the rostral neural tube. It gives rise to the colliculi (inferior colliculus and superior colliculus), red nucleus, and substantia nigra. The inferior colliculus is part of the auditory pathway and receives acoustic information from the cochlea and forwards it, rostrally, to the medial geniculate nucleus of the thalamus. The superior colliculus integrates visual, auditory, and somatosensory information and also functions in regulation of involuntary eye movements. It projects to specific visual and also to nonvisual nuclei of the thalamus. The red nucleus and substantia nigra function to regulate movement.

The metencephalon is that region in the embryonic hindbrain in the neural tube that gives rise to the pons and cerebellum. The cerebellum functions in the fine coordination of skeletal muscles to produce smooth motor activity and may also be significantly involved with the learning of motor skills. The cerebellum is also associated with another structure in the metencephalon, the pons. The pons contains axons coursing to and from the cerebellum and to other parts of the brain and spinal cord.

The myelencephalon is that region in the embryonic hindbrain in the neural tube that gives rise to the medulla. It is the rostral extension of the spinal cord moving into the brain. The medulla includes several centers responsible for autonomic functions that are essential for life, such as breathing, control of heart rate, and control of body temperature.

B. Cell Migration in the CNS: Development of Cortical Layers

The central portion of the neural tube constitutes the embryonic ventricular system, and most neurons (and nonneuronal cells) arise from divisions of precursor cells near the ventricular wall (Figure 2). In many laminated structures of the brain, such as the neocortex, early generated neurons usually remain in the vicinity

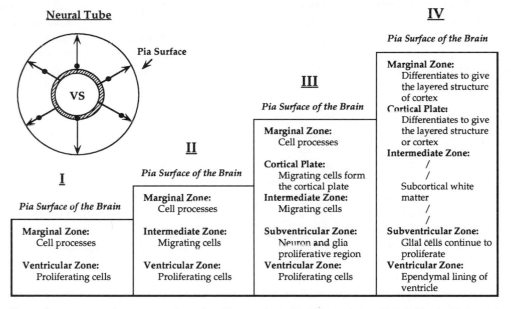

Figure 2 Origins and migration of neurons. The vertebrate CNS originates as a longitudinal strip located on the dorsal surface of the early embryo. This strip of cells sinks inward and rolls up to form the neural tube. Once the neural tube has formed, there is rapid neuronal proliferative activity along the medial wall of the ventricular system (VS). Neurons (solid circles) migrate radially outward from the medial wall through the proliferative zone (shaded area) toward the pia surface of the brain. Neuronal migration requires neuron–glial cell interactions. Radial glial cells (arrows), whose cell bodies line the ventricular surface of the neural tube have processes that are distributed radially to the pia. The radial processes of these glial cells form the substrate to which the neurons adhere, and move along until they reach their final destination. In the original zone of proliferation (stage I), there are two layers, the ventricular zone, in which neurons continue to proliferate, and the marginal zone, in which the outermost processes of developing neurons are located. Neurons migrate upward from the ventricular zone to form the intermediate zone (stage II). Regions that will eventually laminate and form cortical zones, neurons, pass through the intermediate zone and continue to migrate upward to form the cortical plate (stage III). The cerebral cortex derives from the original marginal zone and the cortical plate, which ultimately differentiates to give the typical layered structure of neocortex (stage IV).

of the ventricular wall, necessitating the neurons generated later to migrate past the earlier neurons until they arrive at their final destination at positions further away from the ventricles. Radial migration from the ventricular zone is not haphazard, but is supported and guided by a special type of nonneuronal cell, the radial glial cell. These are glial cells with elongated, radially oriented processes that extend across the distance between the inner and outer surfaces of the neural tube and that provide the substrate for radial migration of cells from the ventricular zone. This process is schematically illustrated in Figure 2. Briefly, the wall of the neural tube at an early stage consists of two layers: a ventricular zone, which contains proliferating neurons moving through the mitotic cycle, and a marginal zone, into which processes of ventricular zone immature neurons extend. In the human fetus, the proliferation of neurons is, for the most part, occurring during the first 4 to 4½ months after conception. In the brain, after completion of cell division, the newly "born" neurons, under the guidance of radial glia, migrate away from the ventricular zone toward the outer, or pia, surface of the neural tube. The first cells to begin their outward migration move from the ventricular zone to form an intermediate zone. In the forebrain region, neurons that begin migration later pass through the intermediate zone to form an additional zone called the cortical plate. The cortical plate undergoes later differentiation to contribute to the typical three-layered structure of the hippocampal cortex and six-layered structure of the neocortex. The final mature structure of the neocortex is derived from neurons of the marginal zone plus the cortical plate. The intermediate zone below the cortical plate becomes the subcortical white matter. It is from this stage that these still immature neurons begin to develop the morphological and physiological characteristics of mature neurons. Dendrites develop their extensive and elaborate branching patterns which provide the major receptive portion of the neuron. Axons, with the help of neurotrophic factors, begin to find their correct destinations, and synaptic contacts and neurotransmitter identity are established.

V. DEVELOPMENTAL INTERACTION WITH EARLY EXPERIENCE

Early environmental experience can have a profound influence on the developing brain. This in and of itself is not surprising; however, in some instances, there are well-defined periods in which developing brain circuitry and physiology are particularly susceptible to environmental influences. These periods are referred to as critical periods and they present challenging examples of the interactions that occur between genetic endowment and environment during development. Critical periods exist during the course of development of many normal behaviors, such as imprinting, binocular vision, and social interaction in humans and other primates.

A useful example for understanding the relevant neuronal mechanisms operating during critical periods comes from studies of the critical period for the development of neurons with binocular responses in the visual cortex of kittens. When deprived of visual experience, there is a permanent alteration of the visual system if deprivation occurs during a critical period during development. Different effects occur depending on whether deprivation is monocular or binocular. The essential findings are that elimination of visual information from one retina, by temporary eye closure, results in weakened responsiveness (response strength and orientation specificity) of visual cortical neurons to afferent input after the reversal of eyelid closure. In this type of experiment (monocular deprivation), cortical responses elicited by stimulation to the closed eye are compared to those elicited by stimulation to the unclosed eye. Thus, the reduction of visual information to one eye, with the consequent reduction of neuronal afferent activity to the visual system from that eye, results in the loss of influence of that eye in higher neuronal processing. Monocular deprivation does not result in the failure to form essential synaptic connections within the visual system, because in the kitten, these connections are present at birth. Thus it appears that already established connections are, in some way, disrupted.

With binocular, rather than monocular, eyelid closure, the result is strikingly different. The deficits following binocular closure are much less pronounced than those that follow monocular closure. This unexpected result indicates that closure of one eye has a more pronounced effect on normal developmental processes than does closure of both eyes. Thus it appears that the important factor is not disuse of the synaptic connections from the deprived eye, but rather that normal development of visual cortical cell physiology requires interaction between afferent synaptic activity from both eyes. In other words, binocular experiments show that normal function does not depend only on the absolute amount of afferent impulse activity because there is much less visual input when both eyes are closed; rather, there appears to be a competitive relationship between activity in the two sets of afferents. For kittens, the nervous system is susceptible to the influence of visual deprivation and to disruption of competitive balance between afferents during roughly the second and third postnatal months. The interrelation between genetically programmed developmental processes and environmental factors becomes apparent with the finding that visual deprivation terminated before the second month or begun after the third month has no detrimental effects on visual system development. Thus, there are mechanisms that operate differently, qualitatively or quantitatively, during the critical period between the second and third postnatal months compared with their operation either before or after that period. These mechanisms include those that govern competitive interactions and those, perhaps including a role for neurotrophic factors, that contribute to the eventual stability of the nervous system. Comparable effects have been found in macaque monkeys, but with a different critical period. Understanding critical periods in development is highly significant for understanding many aspects of mature behavior. Uncovering the underlying mechanisms may lead to a broader depth of understanding of the ongoing sculpturing of the brain that results in enduring and effective changes in behavior.

VI. NEUROTROPHIC CONCEPT

The preceding sections gave an abbreviated review of mammalian nervous system development, with emphasis on neocortical development. This section provides a brief account of chemical substances and mechanisms that may participate in plasticity and may provide the link that spans across development to full maturity.

Trophic agents can be defined as chemical substances that cause a long-term increase in metabolic activity, survival, or differentiation of nerve cells. The idea of neurotrophic factors stems from early studies of Viktor Hamburger and his colleagues Rita Levi-Montalcini and Stanley Cohen on the interaction between developing neural regions (later to become cell aggregates such as sympathetic ganglia) and their tar-

gets of innervation. The basic finding indicated that the size of a neural region was positively correlated with the size of the target tissue innervated. Thus, if a developing target organ (e.g., an extremity) was experimentally reduced in size, there was a corresponding reduction in the size of the neuronal cell aggregate sending processes to that target. Similarly, an increase in target size was associated with an increase in the neuronal cell aggregate. Another important and illuminating discovery was that cell death occurred during neuronal development and that the reduced size of neuronal aggregates, after target reduction, was associated with increased degeneration of neurons that would normally innervate the target tissue. These findings, and others, eventually lead to the hypothesis that necessary factors regulating the survival and growth of neurons are released from target tissues. In the early 1950s, the survival and growth-promoting factor released from target tissue of major neural crest-derived neurons, that is, sympathetic and peripheral sensory neurons, was identified. As it turns out, this growth factor was a specific peptide, now called nerve growth factor (NGF). Thus the hypothesis evolved that once a developing neuron extends its processes to its target, there is a competition with other developing neurons for a limited amount of a neurotrophic factor released by the target tissue. Once released by target tissue, the trophic signal is transported retrogradely from the terminals of neuronal processes to the cell bodies to promote events resulting in survival and growth. Developing neurons that successfully acquire sufficient amount of neurotrophic factors survive. Developing neurons that are unsuccessful competitors for neurotrophic factors die. This view has been elaborated over the years and research has provided much supporting data. In 1986, Levi-Montalcini and Cohen were awarded the Nobel Prize in Physiology and Medicine for their discoveries of growth factors.

A. Neurotrophins

Neurotrophins are proteins that belong to a larger family of neurotrophic factors that support the growth, differentiation, and survival of neurons in the developing nervous system. Nerve growth factor was the first of this family of proteins to be identified and is the prototypical neurotrophin. Among the other known neurotrophins are brain-derived neurotrophic factor (BDNF), neurotrophin-3 (NT-3), neurotrophin-4 (NT-4), and neurotrophin-5 (NT-5). All of these are distinct from, but have some functional overlap with NGF. As its name suggests, BDNF was first isolated from brain; NT-3, NT-4, and NT-5 are named sequentially according to their date of discovery.

Important questions are the following: Is each neuron responsive to one and only one of the neurotrophins or is an individual neuron, or class of neurons, affected by more than one neurotrophin? If so, is this action simultaneous or sequential? Are all of the known neurotrophins target-derived factors as is NGF? Does the target produce one or several neurotrophic factors for each innervating population of cells? These and other related questions are at the cutting edge of current research.

B. Neurotrophin Receptors

The neurotrophins produce their effects by binding to and activating specific cell surface receptors localized on neurons or neuronal processes that are susceptible to the influence of any particular neurotrophin. The neurotrophins bind to Trk tyrosine kinases receptors. The term Trk is pronounced "track" and stands for tropomyosin-receptor-kinase. The members of the Trk family are TrkA, TrkB, and TrkC, and each is a receptor tyrosine kinase. Tyrosine kinase receptors mediate the transduction and processing of many extra- and intracellular signals. Nerve growth factor is a potent activator of TrkA, BDNF and NT-4/5 activate TrkB, and NT-3 activates TrkC. Once activated, tyrosine kinase receptors initiate a cascade of intracellular events, which ultimately leads to changes in gene expression that support growth, differentiation, and survival of neurons in the developing nervous system.

C. Neurotrophins in the CNS

In addition to actions in the PNS, neurotrophins and their receptors are expressed in several regions of the CNS. Of particular interest has been the basal forebrain acetylcholinergic neurons and the neurotrophins. These acetylcholine (ACh)-releasing neurons send their axons to innervate cortical regions, especially the neocortex and hippocampus, and have been implicated as having an important role in higher cognitive functions. Nerve growth factor and BDNF are produced in the hippocampus and neocortex. They

are likely target-derived factors acting on in-growing axons of developing basal forebrain cholinergic neurons to enhance gene expression and cellular differentiation of these neurons. Genetic expression of key proteins such as TrkA, the major receptor for NGF, and choline acetyltransferase, the synthetic enzyme for ACh, as well as increase in cell size, all begin at about the same time that cortical levels of NGF begin to rise.

In humans, Alzheimer's disease is associated with degeneration of basal forebrain acetylcholine neurons with a corresponding loss of cortical cholinergic markers such as choline acetyltransferase. These degenerative effects parallel the degree of cognitive dysfunction experienced by these individuals. Also, deficits of cortical ACh in experimental animals impair performance on specific behavioral tasks. Conversely, the discharge rates of basal forebrain ACh neurons is closely related to the expectation of reward, and their level of activity increases during the acquisition of learned behaviors. It is now apparent that NGF and other neurotrophins can act on mature neurons in the CNS and thus may have important functions in the mature brain. These encompass modifiable functions, including synaptic plasticity, learning and memory, aging, and response to disease and injury.

D. Activity-Dependent Regulation of Neurotrophin Synthesis

In the CNS, one important means of regulating neurotrophin synthesis is by neuronal discharge activity resulting in the release of neurotransmitters (Figure 3). The neurotransmitters glutamate, γ-aminobutyric acid (GABA), and ACh all have a subtle role in regulating the production and release of neurotrophins. The evidence appears to favor the involvement of BDNF with activation of glutamate receptors, and NGF with activation of muscarinic ACh receptors. One of the general rules of nervous system function is that any given neurotransmitter can act on several structurally distinct receptors. Indeed, the consequences of transmitter release are dependent on the receptors to which it binds rather than on the nature of the transmitter *per se*. Glutamate, ACh, and GABA all act on unique families of receptors. That is, glutamate binds predominantly to N-methyl-D-aspartate (NMDA) and non-NMDA receptors; ACh binds to several types of nicotinic or to several types of mus-

A

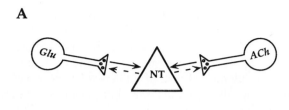

B

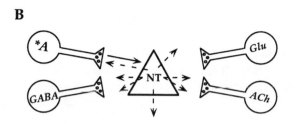

C

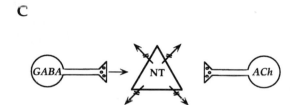

Figure 3 Activity- and neurotransmitter-dependent regulation of neurotrophin-containing neurons. A. Neurotransmitters, by acting on appropriate receptors, regulate the synthesis and release of neurotrophins. The neurotransmitters ACh and glutamate (Glu), after release by stimulation, can act on neurotrophin (NT)-containing neurons (solid lines). The effect of either of these transmitters is to increase the rate of NT synthesis (up-regulate) and increase the amount of NT release. A general pattern, if not rule, is that glutamate is most effective in up-regulation and release of brain-derived neurotrophic factor; whereas ACh is most effective in up-regulation and release of NGF. This general scheme does not rule out the release of other neurotrophic factors by theses transmitters, or the involvement of other types of neurotransmitters in regulating neurotrophic factors. The released factors have the potential for positive feedback onto the cholinergic and/or glutamatergic neurons to enhance the release of these neurotransmitters (dashed arrows). B. In concept, the activity-dependent NT release, initiated by either Glu or ACh secretion from an activated neuron (*A; solid line) can feedback on that active axon terminal and additionally diffuse to effect initially inactive terminals (dashed arrows). The latter effect of diffusion would include GABA-releasing terminals (inhibitory) in the local area to enhance their synaptic strength in response to subsequent activation. C. In contrast to the actions of either ACh or Glu, activity of GABA-containing neurons down-regulates the levels and decreases subsequent secretion of NT.

carinic receptors; and GABA binds to $GABA_A$ and $GABA_B$ receptors. Each subtype of these receptors, that is, subtypes belonging to the family of receptors responsive to glutamate, ACh, or GABA, can be thought of as a special gate to particular functional pathways within the receptive neuron. Recent evidence indicates that the amounts of BDNF and NGF are regulated by these three neurotransmitters. Glutamate and ACh both up-regulate the levels of these neurotrophins, whereas GABA down-regulates their levels. Up-regulation by glutamate is by way of either NMDA or non-NMDA receptors, and up-regulation by ACh occurs through muscarinic receptors. At this juncture it is important to note that muscarinic actions of ACh and NMDA actions of glutamate are central to neural mechanisms of synaptic plasticity and the higher level, but related, functions of learning and memory. It may well be that the strengthening and weakening of selective synapses in the neocortex depend, to some extent, on neurotrophic effects that are regulated by these neurotransmitters.

Information processing at the level of the cortex, including hippocampus and neocortex, occurs predominantly but not exclusively by the neurotransmitters glutamate, GABA, and ACh. A current major issue concerns the identification of the synaptic interactions that function in neocortical information processing and plasticity. For example, in auditory neocortex there are five synaptic potentials that occur in pyramidal neurons. Pyramidal neurons are the principal neurons of neocortical circuitry, serve as the major input to one another, and are the exclusive output neuron of the cortex. These five synaptic potentials differ with respect to the eliciting neurotransmitter and/or the nature of the receptors engaged (Table II).

Table II Cortical Neurotransmitters, Receptors, and Synaptic Potentials

Neurotransmitter	Receptor	Synaptic potential
Glutamate	AMPA/kainate	Fast-EPSP
	NMDA	Slow-EPSP
	Metabotropic (Quisqualate)	?
GABA	$GABA_A$	Fast-IPSP
	$GABA_B$	Slow-IPSP
Acetylcholine	Nicotinic	? (likely fast)
	Muscarinic	Very slow-EPSP

Four of these potentials are mediated by amino acids and the fifth is mediated by ACh. The excitatory amino acid synaptic potentials consist of an early-EPSP that is mediated by glutamate acting at (α-amino-3-hydroxy-5-methylisoxazole-4-propionic acid/kainate (AMPA/kainate) receptors, and a late-EPSP mediated by glutamate at NMDA receptors. Inhibitory amino acid synaptic potentials consist of an early- and late-IPSP and are produced by GABA binding to $GABA_A$ and $GABA_B$ receptors, respectively. The ACh-elicited synaptic potential is a long-lasting EPSP that requires repetitive stimulation for its appearance and occurs by binding of ACh to muscarinic-type receptors. This complex of excitatory and inhibitory synaptic potentials that occurs in auditory cortex is similar in most respects to synaptic potentials described for other sensory neocortical areas.

The NMDA-type receptors mediate excitatory neurotransmission in the brain, and are important in learning and memory and in some neurodegenerative disorders. Thus, it is of considerable interest to note that one of the major functions of GABA and ACh in neocortex is to regulate neural transmission mediated by NMDA receptors. In general, NMDA-mediated synaptic responses are unable to respond to repetitive stimulation and thus remain an unimportant player in cortical information processing unless this unresponsive state is alleviated. However, the ability of NMDA receptors to respond to repetitive stimulation is controlled by GABA. Under reduced influence of GABA inhibitory synaptic potentials, NMDA transmission is facilitated. Thus, NMDA receptor-mediated potentials will be elicited by input to the cortex that is of insufficient strength to activate inhibition or by a pattern of input that results in reduced inhibition.

As indicated earlier, ACh has been repeatedly implicated in higher cognitive processes and the supply to the neocortex arises predominantly from large neurons within the basal forebrain. However, until recently, there has been very little direct evidence concerning how ACh might interact with ongoing cortical processing to modify function, although the action of ACh is usually described as subtle and neuromodulatory. Recent research indicates that ACh interacts with ongoing cortical processing in several ways.

Whereas the likelihood of NMDA-mediated response occurring is regulated by the strength of GABA transmission, ACh, acting at muscarinic receptors, facilitates the amplitude of the NMDA synaptic potential, thereby increasing the likelihood that the response will elicit cell firing. Additionally, and in general, ACh regulates the activation and excitability state of the cortex. An appropriate activation level readies the cortex for its fundamental task of higher-order information processing, and increased excitability ensures that even weak signals will be received with high resolution. Consequently, ACh facilitates the transfer of information from subcortical brain regions to the neocortex and increases the reaction to that information by cortical neurons. Regulation of the activation state of cortical neurons contributes to the formation and maintenance of the networks in which they functionally participate. It appears that ACh-mediated changes also underlie systematic modifications of neuronal receptive fields. This constitutes a direct indication of plasticity in information processing. In the auditory cortex, this plasticity is an alteration of the frequency tuning of cortical cells. Overall, it appears the ACh has a critical role in the establishment of new information. All of these actions of ACh occur by engaging muscarinic receptors leading to subsequent metabolic changes in the receptive neurons.

The important summarizing point is that there is a rich, and precise, synaptic organization of neocortex that provides the substrate for intricate processing of environmental information. Clearly, this processing involves glutamate, GABA, and ACh, along with their multiple receptor subtypes at the decision-making level (i.e., synaptic level). These three neurotransmitters are principal regulators of neurotrophin activity. It is interesting to note that the appearance and strength of the NMDA-mediated late-EPSP is controlled by the GABA-mediated IPSPs, and that the levels of BDNF and NGF, in some neurons, is also regulated by a balance between activity at glutamate and GABA receptors.

E. Neurotrophins and Plasticity

Neurotrophins, especially BDNF and NGF, have been implicated in neuronal modifications that have important functional and theoretical significance, such as long-term potentiation (LTP), spatial memory, and structuring of visual receptive fields, to name a few.

The phenomenon of LTP provides a useful example of the role of neurotrophins in plasticity, because the underlying mechanisms of LTP are beginning to be fairly well understood. Long-term potentiation is a form of electrically induced synaptic plasticity in which appropriate stimulation of incoming axons (i.e., afferents) results in a long-lasting increase in the synaptic efficacy of their connections with postsynaptic cells. This type of synaptic plasticity has been studied intensively in two cortical regions involved in learning and memory, the hippocampus (archicortex; three-layered) and the neocortex (six-layered), and has yielded important candidate mechanisms as a synaptic model of memory. The mechanism for the induction of at least one form of this type of plasticity requires glutamate to bind to NMDA receptors, that is, NMDA-dependent plasticity.

Recent evidence suggests that BDNF may participate in NMDA-receptor mediated LTP. In the hippocampus, stimulation of glutamate receptors in a manner that induces LTP results in expression of BDNF messenger ribonucleic acid (mRNA) in these neurons, and this implies subsequent elevation of BDNF levels. The participation of NMDA receptors in expression of BDNF is strengthened by the finding that levels of BDNF mRNA do not increase if glutamate is prevented from binding to NMDA receptors by specific pharmacologic agents. Evidence also suggests that BDNF is elevated in rats raised in an enriched environment characterized by abundant sensory stimulation. These animals also have improved performance on spatial memory tasks.

As mentioned earlier, there is a close interaction between activity of ACh-releasing neurons and NGF. The study of this relationship has benefited greatly by development of experimental means to target specifically and render inactive, cholinergic neurons of the basal forebrain. The immunotoxin 192 IgG-saporin consists of an antibody (192 IgG) against the NGF receptor that is conjugated to saporin, a ribosome-inactivating compound. The 192 IgG-saporin, when injected into the brains of experimental animals, is taken up specifically by basal forebrain cholinergic neurons and inactivates these neurons by disruption of their ribosomes. This is an especially valuable tool, because the role of basal forebrain cholinergic neurons during development and maturity can then be determined.

Depletion of basal forebrain ACh neurons and, consequently, NGF receptors in developing or adult animals results in a loss of ACh innervation to cortical regions. This loss is reported to be accompanied by deficits in spatial memory and passive avoidance.

These results are highly promising; however, detailed electrophysiological studies to pinpoint the changes in synaptic physiology and network dynamics, after immunotoxic lesion, remain to be done.

Overall, these data indicate that neuronal activity can result in elevation of BDNF and NGF in cortical areas. In the CNS, the target of target-derived neurotrophic agent appears to be other neurons. The immediate effect of appropriate neuronal activity is to release glutamate and ACh which act on glutamate (especially NMDA-type) and ACh receptors, respectively. Receptor activation leads to the synthesis and release of neurotrophins. Interestingly, both BDNF and NGF enhance the release of glutamate and ACh. Thus, there is positive feedback on transmitter release. Enhanced transmitter release strengthens synaptic transfer of information. Thus, a reasonable hypothesis is that neurotrophins function in plasticity as retrograde factors that contribute to the strengthening and stabilizing of synaptic contacts. Strengthening of synaptic transmission is the central factor of LTP, and is widely held to be a primary factor in behavioral learning.

VII. CONCLUSION

The nervous system is capable of extremely complex information processing and decision making. Part of this ability requires precise communication among its principal cell type, the neurons. Effective communication requires appropriate spatial relationships and contacts between neurons. This is established, under the guidance of the genome, during embryonic and early postnatal periods. However, as we noted at the outset, development of the nervous system is not completely predetermined. A considerable amount of the fine detail of connectivity and physiology is the result of environmental shaping. This neuronal plasticity occurs, and has been studied, in many of the brain's systems. Through the course of evolution, a large number of elegant mechanisms have become specialized to ensure the appropriate connectivity and physiology during development. Some of these mechanisms have been mentioned in the current discussion. Evidence from a variety of sources, using a variety of approaches, leaves one with the conclusion that similar or identical mechanisms that operate during developmental stages may function in plastic adjustment in the mature brain. That is to say, that mechanisms of synaptic and behavioral plasticity that occur in the immature brain may continue to operate, in similar fashion, in the mature brain. If we can begin to understand how the brain develops, and the plasticity revealed by the effects of early experience, we shall be in a better position to understand plasticity in the young mature and mature brain. Mechanisms that strengthen synapses and neurotransmitter release initiated by neurotrophic factors are of particular interest given the role of synaptic modification in higher level cognitive functions, disease conditions, and response to CNS damage. The functioning of neurotrophins and the strengthening of anatomical and physiological contacts now requires consideration not only in brain development but also in higher cognitive function and in the cellular/molecular basis of learning and memory.

BIBLIOGRAPHY

Cowan, W. M. (1979). The development of the brain. *Scientific American, 241,* 113–133.

Holtzman, D. M., & Mobley, W. C. (1994). Neurotrophic factors and neurologic disease. *Western Journal of Medicine,* **161,** 246–254.

Jacobson, M. (1979). *Developmental neurobiology* (2nd ed.). New York: Plenum Press.

Kandel, E. R. (1985). Early experience, critical periods, and developmental fine-tuning of brain architecture. In E. R. Kandel and J. H. Schwartz (Eds.), *Principles of neural science* (pp. 757–770). New York: Elsevier.

Nauta, W. J. H., and Feirtag, M. (1979). The organization of the brain. *Scientific American,* **241,** 88–111.

Thoenen, H. (1995). Neurotrophins and neuronal plasticity. *Science,* **270,** 593–598.

Brain Scanning/Neuroimaging

Richard J. Haier

University of California, Irvine

Co-Registration When one image is aligned, scaled and superimposed over another image so both fit the same space.

EEG Electroencephalogram

fMRI Functional Magnetic Resonance Imaging

MEG Magnetoencephalogram

MRI Magnetic Resonance Imaging

PET Position Emission Tomography

Pixel The smallest unit of an image; each pixel is quantified.

Radiotracer A radioactive substance that imaging devices measure to show where the tracer goes.

Region-of-Interest (ROI) Any brain area defined and located anatomically or mathematically.

SPECT Single-Photon Emission Computed Tomography

Stereotactic A method of defining brain area location using coordinates of a standard brain.

Tomography Process of making a mathematical picture.

A variety of **MEDICAL IMAGING TECHNOLOGIES** show the brain in ways not possible previously. Functional imaging is especially useful for identifying brain areas involved in specific cognitive tasks and states. Each imaging method has different strengths and weaknesses. There are several core issues concerning image analysis that must be considered by researchers and clinicians. The combination of advanced imaging technology with sophisticated psychological experiments is a powerful tool for helping understand the normal and abnormal brain.

I. BASIC CONCEPTS

A. Structural and Functional Imaging

Through the 1970s researchers had access to the living human brain mostly through the study of blood, urine, and spinal fluid. Only electroencephalograph (EEG) methods and occasional probing during brain surgery provided direct data on human brain functioning. Computed Axial Tomography (CAT) scans and early Magnetic Resonance Imaging (MRI) showed brain structures in considerable detail (see Fig. 1) but provided no functional information. That is to say, CAT and MRI scans may show tumors, strokes, and other forms of structural brain damage but they do not show brain activity during learning, memory, language processing, emotion, sleep, and other brain states. In fact, structural imaging may show the brain in fine anatomic detail but whether the patient is alive or dead is not apparent in the images. Functional brain imaging is designed to reveal regional brain activity while the person is engaged in a psychological task chosen to maintain the brain in a specific mode during the imaging procedure. Functional images, therefore, change in a person depending on the task performed or the state of

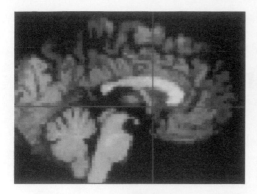
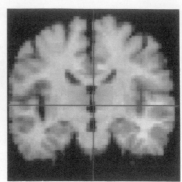
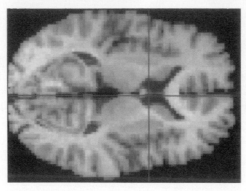

Figure I Image orientations. The upper left image shows an MRI slice in sagittal or side orientation; the front of the brain is on the right. The upper right image shows a coronal or cross section orientation looking through from the front of the brain. The bottom image shows an axial or top down view; the front of the brain is on the right.

the brain (awake, asleep, at rest, problem solving, etc.) whereas in structural imaging, the pictures look the same irrespective of the brain's work or state. For CAT scans and MRI, it does not matter if the person is performing a task of attention or memory, or whether the person is awake or asleep, or eyes open or closed. The structural image is the same and the tumor or stroke is revealed just as well. Structural imaging has been of great importance in making clinical evaluations regarding the extent and location of brain damage in individual patients. Researchers have also used structural imaging to compare anatomic measurements of brain size and volume among groups of interest. These data augment earlier autopsy studies and, in many instances, are more accurately assessed in the living brain undamaged by death and brain fixation procedures.

As dramatic as structural brain images can be, however, functional images have captured the imagination of many clinicians and researchers. These images show the brain responding to activation by cognitive tasks. Functional brain imaging techniques now available include Positron Emission Tomography (PET), Single Photon Emission Computed Tomography (SPECT), functional MRI (fMRI), topographic EEG, and Magnetoencephalogram (MEG, also known as Superconducting Quantum Interference Device or SQUID). The older methods of acquiring blood flow images with xenon gas are no longer used much in activation studies, although pioneering work was done with these techniques. Functional images show the brain at work and often reveal complex relationships between activation or deactivation in well-defined anatomic areas and specific cognitive processes. The interpretation of functional images depends on the psychological task or brain state engaged during the imaging and the sophistication of the task is a major factor to be considered.

B. Key Role of Psychological Tasks and Brain States

Functional imaging shows the brain "at work." The type and amount of work are specified in a task performed by the subject during the scanning procedure. Scans during two or more task conditions or states can be compared to show the brain areas that differ in activity between the conditions. Task condition is critical for functional imaging. During the early years of PET, many subjects were studied at rest with eyes closed and ears plugged; no task was used. These studies compared brain function during this "resting" state in one group of subjects to another group. The resting condition, however, is not particularly well controlled because subjects are free to engage in any cognitive activity to pass the time during the scan procedure. Moreover, even when a specific task condition is compared to a resting condition, the same problem remains. The choice of a control task, therefore, is often more complex than choosing a "resting" state. As cognitive psychologists and neuropsychologists have engaged in functional imaging experiments, the choice of tasks has become more sophisticated. Many tasks are chosen to maximize elemental cognitive processes and to minimize individual differences in performance and learning (habituation). These studies tend to focus on localizing brain areas involved in various aspects of cognition. Many a priori hypotheses from a cognitive neuropsychology perspective have been tested by comparing such tasks as generating words, listening to words, and speaking words. Other tasks are chosen to maximize performance differences among individuals to help identify relationships between brain activation and performance. These studies address questions concerning task difficulty, mental effort, and other parameters of performance. For example, one may use a test of reasoning to identify salient brain areas and then use easy and hard versions of the reasoning task to help identify relationships between mental effort and regional brain activation. The more complex the task, the more difficult it is to interpret the results in terms of elemental cognitive processes. Nonetheless, complex tasks can be used to examine performance differences and the functional relationships among brain areas. Because the manipulation of brain engagement and state are critical in functional imaging, these techniques are fundamentally psychological.

C. Standard Images and Types of Image Analyses

Empirical analyses of structural and functional neuroimaging data have evolved dramatically from 2D stereotactic based regions-of-interest to 3D anatomi-

cally precise localization. Much neuroimaging now uses structural MRI as the basis for individual or group data and superimposes (coregistration) functional data. MRI thus provides an accurate anatomical template for functional data. PET, SPECT, EEG, MEG and fMRI data all can be displayed on MRI images in 2 dimensions or 3 dimensions (see Fig. 2). A typical analysis begins by taking each image slice (from different brain levels) from each subject and averaging them into a group brain image. Individual brains vary enormously in size and shape, especially in cortex; internal features and regions-of-interest also vary considerably. This variation presents a problem for averaging individuals into a group image. Each person's image must be fit to a standard brain where shape and size are fixed. Each person's image is then pushed and pulled and stretched to fit the standard (see Fig. 3). There are many ways to define the standard and many ways to accomplish the fitting to it. For example, a standard brain outline can be derived from stereotactic atlases and internal areas can be located according to a grid system. Because the most popular atlases used for this purpose are based on only one person's brain, generalizations are limited. An alternative method is based on averaging a large number of brain images (e.g., MRI scans) and deriving an average outline, although there are a number of

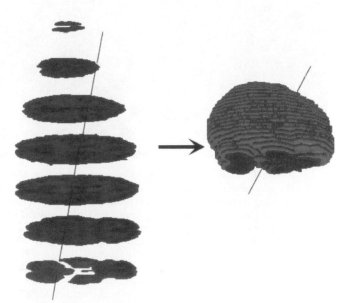

Figure 2 3-dimensional reconstruction. Shows how a series of axial slices from any imaging modality can be stacked to construct a 3-dimensional image.

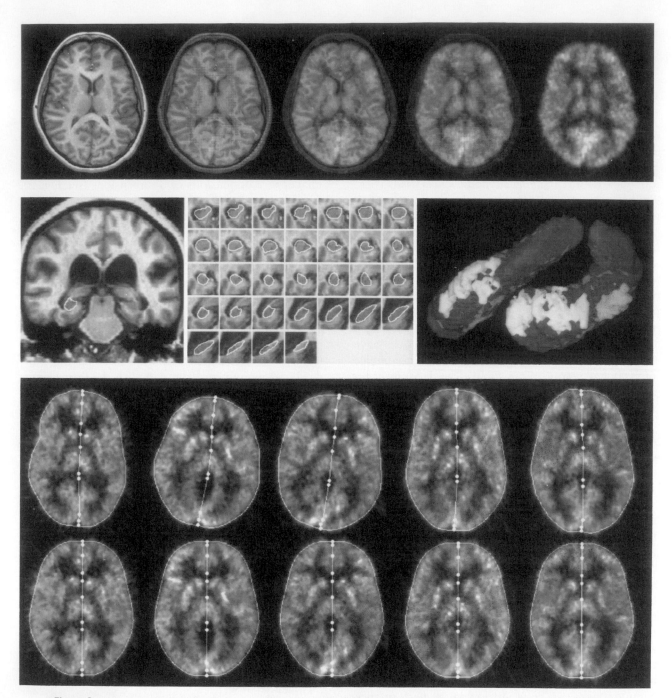

Figure 3 Top row: Gradient from structure to function. MRI (left) provides anatomical information about the brain showing the gray matter where cell bodies and dendritic connections are made, the white matter which is composed of the cell axons coursing between gray matter areas, and the cerebrospinal fluid filled spaces shown in black. PET (right) reveals the metabolic rate of glucose, the main energy source for brain activity. The images were formed by aligning the axial MRI and PET scans from the same person and then calculating images composed of pixel values drawn 100% from MRI, 75% MRI and 25% PET, 50% MRI and 50% PET, 25% MRI and 75% PET, and 100% PET. Subject is performing a memory task involving viewing words on a screen so visual cortex is activated (bottom of PET images on right). Middle row: Visualization of the hippocampus in 3 dimensions. Left: The hippocampus can be traced on MRI anatomical images cut in coronal sections. Middle: Each successive tracing of the 3D object is assembled. Right: 3D reconstruction of the successive surfaces for left and right hippocampus showing glucose metabolic activity (white) from aligned PET scan. Bottom row: Warping individual brains for comparison. Top shows the individual variation in size and shape among five normal subjects' PET scans (one slice each). Midline landmarks and brain edge identified on MRI scans matched to the PET are used to warp all images to the same configuration (bottom) so that individuals can be compared directly using statistical parametric mapping techniques. (Courtesy of Dr. Monte Buchsbaum.)

ways of doing this as well. Once the average outline is established, each person's image can be stretched, pulled, warped, or morphed to the standard using the brain outline or internal landmarks. Although there have been some attempts to standardize this process, no clear advantage of any method over others has been compelling to date.

Once standard images are created for a group of subjects, various statistical analyses are possible. A common analysis for functional data is based on a subtraction procedure. For example, each pixel value (e.g., glucose metabolism) in one group image is subtracted from the value of the corresponding pixel in a second group (see Fig. 4). Each of the thousands of resulting subtractions can be expressed statistically (e.g., as *t*-tests) and the value of each statistical comparison can be displayed pixel by pixel. Usually this is done for a significance level of probability so the resulting image shows at a glance, the brain areas where there is a statistically significant difference between the groups. Within a group, subtractions can be made between task conditions. This is one of the most frequently used analysis for group or condition analyses. Because of the very large number of tests, often thousands per slice, statistical corrections for multiple comparisons can be applied. A number of corrections have been proposed using multivariate methods, Monte Carlo simulations, resampling, and other techniques. All require assumptions that are more or less applicable to particular research circumstances and no

single approach has been adopted as a standard. Because of high per-scan costs (due largely to hardware investment), most imaging studies report small sample sizes, further compounding the statistical problems. Replication of results, in combination with a priori hypotheses, is regarded by many researchers as the most effective way to overcome the statistical difficulties inherent in this kind of work.

In addition to subtraction of means, some data and research designs allow analyses based on individual differences. Correlations, for example, can be computed between task performance and functional data pixel-by-pixel or brain area-by-brain area. The subtraction analyses may identify a brain region activated by a task; whereas, the correlation analysis shows the correspondence between task performance and activation of specific areas. For instance, researchers can ask if brain activity increases more or less in a salient area in those people who have the best task performance. Correlations can also be computed among brain areas, even pixel-by-pixel, to reveal functional relationships throughout the brain. For example, the statistically significant correlations between one brain area, say the superior frontal lobe, with all other brain areas can be shown for a specific condition or in a specific group. The pattern of correlations can then be compared for other conditions or groups. Other statistical approaches like path analysis can be used to help identify functional neurocircuity.

It is also possible to display an individual brain im-

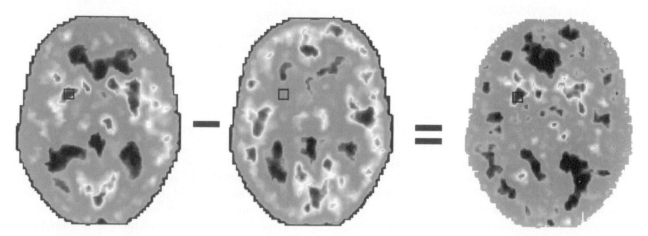

Figure 4 The image subtraction concept. After being warped to a standard, one image can be subtracted from another pixel by pixel. Here the middle image is subtracted from the left image and the resulting image is shown on the right. The box is 7 × 7 pixels and shows the subtraction in the left caudate area. The resulting image can be displayed as a significance probability map where the subtraction for each pixel is statistically summarized.

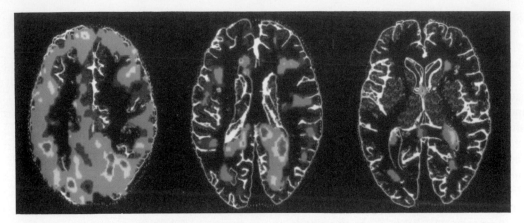

Figure 5 Standard score display. Shows three axial PET slices from a subject with Down Syndrome warped to a standard shape. Each pixel is displayed as a standard score for this subject based on the mean and standard deviation for each pixel measured in a control group. In these images, gray shows areas where the standard scores are greater than 2. (Courtesy of Dr. Richard Haier.)

age where each pixel is a standard score based on a group mean and standard deviation. For functional images, this allows a person's unique pattern of brain activity to be shown relative to a comparison group or task condition (see Fig. 5). Standard score images may be most useful for clinical applications including diagnostic classification and treatment strategies.

Specific examples of these analyses from several areas will be discussed after a review of the major brain/neuroimaging techniques.

II. POSITRON EMISSION TOMOGRAPHY (PET)

A. Methodology for Glucose Metabolic Rate (GMR)

PET is a functional imaging technique based on the use of positron emitting radiotracers. A number of positron emitters can be used for PET but the two most commonly used for brain imaging are fluorine (18) and oxygen (15). F18, for example, can be attached to an analog of glucose, 2-deoxyglucose, to form fluorodeoxyglucose (FDG). When FDG is injected into a person's blood stream, the deoxyglucose part enters the glucose pool and is used by neurons for energy. The more a neuron fires, the more deoxyglu-

cose it uses and the more the neuron is labeled with F18. Thus, the harder a brain area works during a task, the more FDG it takes up. Following the injection of FDG, it takes about 32 minutes for the brain to use most of it. Therefore, whatever the brain is doing for the 32 minutes following the injection determines the pattern of glucose use. When FDG is used, the scanning begins only after the 32 minute labeling period. The person is not even in the scanner during this time. The person does perform a psychological task and the brain areas most active use the most FDG, resulting in regional patterns of GMR. At the end of the 32-minute task, the brain is labeled with F18; the more neuronal firing in any area, the more F18. As each positron decays spontaneously (as it strikes a free electron), two gamma rays are emitted at a 180° angle to each other. When the head is placed in the center of the scanner and surrounded by a ring of many detectors, a computer determines each time a pair of gamma rays 180° apart is detected. These coincident events are reconstructed mathematically showing the origin of each pair of gamma rays; the more positrons in an area, the more pairs of gamma rays are emitted. The resulting images show the pattern of accumulated brain activity over the 32-minute period—not the activity while the person lies in the scanner, because by this time there is no more FDG to be taken up by the brain. Even if the person suddenly died as the scanning begins, a colorful image can be made showing what the brain had been doing during the prior 32-minute labeling period. By contrast, if the person dies as the FDG is being injected, the subsequent scanning will show no image because the dead brain had no metabolism and took up none of the FDG. If a second task is to be studied in the same person, at least 10 hours (5 half-lives) must pass before a second injection of FDG can label the new activity. Most FDG studies use a between scan interval of 2 to 7 days, a logistical disadvantage compared to blood flow techniques. FDG studies have the advantage of quantification as glucose metabolic rate (GMR) following the method of Sokoloff and associates. Spatial resolution can range from about 3.5 mm in plane for the newest scanners to about 8mm for older models. Spatial resolution for PET is usually measured as Full Width Half Maximum (FWHM), a complex measure suggesting the smallest distance that can be resolved between two small points.

B. Methodology for Blood Flow

The use of O15 for PET requires a different procedure although positrons decaying into gamma rays detected by the same scanner are still the basis for the image. O15 is attached to water molecules. The radioactive water, emitting positrons, is injected or inhaled into the bloodstream and for the next 60 seconds, while a task is performed, the distribution of the water can be followed in blood flow. For this method, the person must be in the scanner during the 60-second uptake time of the O15 during which a task is performed. The images show blood flow patterns during the 60-second task performance; brain areas that are activated show increased blood flow. The half life of O15 is only about 2 minutes compared to about 2 hours for F18. Thus, for blood flow PET studies using O15, the person can be injected with a second dose after a 10 minute period (5 half-lives) and a different task can be studied. Often several tasks are studied in the same person over a session; each task is studied for 60 seconds and 10 minutes pass between tasks. This is advantageous for subtraction procedures. Spatial resolution for O15 images may not be as good as for F18 since the 32-minute uptake period produces more gamma ray detections than the 60-second period. While O15 PET studies have the advantage of providing several 60-second experiments in one session, 60 seconds is far too long a period for most psychological studies of cognitive processes best studied in milliseconds. For some psychological studies, FDG has the advantage of a relatively strong signal-to-noise ratio in a 32-minute experiment with hundreds of stimuli. Functional MRI, described below, also determines blood flow with a time resolution on the order of 2 seconds or better. Spatial resolution is also better and no radioactive injection is required. Therefore, most researchers using blood flow PET techniques are switching to fMRI (see below).

C. L-Dopa and Other Tracers

PET can also be used with other radiolabels so that receptor binding sites can be imaged. For example, F18 can be attached to L-dopa, a drug that binds to dopamine receptors. This fluorinated L-dopa can then be used to make images of dopamine system function. Such images have been used to study Parkinson's Disease, a disease of dopamine deficiency, and schizophrenia, a brain disorder treated with dopamine acting drugs. This kind of neuroimaging research has potential for predicting drug response of individual patients. For example, Buchsbaum and colleagues reported that schizophrenics with low GMR in some dopamine-rich brain areas (i.e., the basal ganglia) may show a good clinical response to a dopamine acting drug whereas a similar patient without low basal ganglia GMR will not respond to the same drug. In other studies, fluorinated cocaine has been used to image drug abusers to help understand the mechanism of addiction and, possibly, vulnerability to addiction. Many other positron-emitting receptor labels available for use in PET can image aspects of the serotonin, benzodiazapine, NMDA, and other neurotransmitter systems. This diversity for specific brain system imaging is an advantage over other imaging techniques, especially for the study of psychopathology.

D. SPECT (Single-Photon Emission Computed Tomography)

This is similar to PET in principle. However, the radioactive sources used to emit gamma rays do not produce pairs of gamma rays at 180° and they are not metabolically active so full quantification is not available. The sources are, however, very long lived so a local cyclotron is not necessary. Spatial resolution is not generally as good as PET but SPECT, because it is cheaper hardware and does not require short-lived isotopes, is more available than PET.

III. MAGNETIC RESONANCE IMAGING (MRI)

A. Methodology

MRI was first used as a structural imaging technique that had better spatial resolution than CAT scans for many organs without any radiation exposure. Originally called nuclear magnetic resonance (NMR), MRI uses a strong magnetic field to align spinning protons in hydrogen atoms throughout the body into a north/ south orientation. The stronger the magnet, the greater number of protons are aligned. There is no subjective feeling of this alignment taking place while the person lies in the MRI scanner tube, surrounded by the powerful magnetic field. Radio frequencies are pulsed into the magnetic field very rapidly; each pulse briefly throws protons out of the magnetic north/south alignment but because the body is always in the magnetic field during the procedure, the protons realign immediately. As the protons lose and then regain alignment in the magnetic gradient, different radio frequencies that contain spatial information are produced. These frequencies are detected by antenna-like coils within the MRI scanner and provide the basic data for the mathematical reconstruction that produces the images. Because hydrogen is especially sensitive to the magnetic/radio frequency alternations, water is particularly well imaged so organs like the brain with high water content can be imaged in exquisite spatial detail, often about a millimeter or less (see Fig. 6).

By increasing the speed of acquiring enough information to make an image (under 50 milliseconds in some cases using the echoplanar technique), fast MRI now allows functional information to be collected as changes from one image to the next can be measured. These changes are related to blood flow and they can be imaged with fMRI (functional MRI). The hardware is basically the same as for structural MRI but advanced software and special magnetic coils allow the rapid scanning sequences that can show small changes in blood flow when the magnetic/radio frequency signals in one task condition are subtracted

from another condition pixel-by-pixel, much like the routine subtraction procedures used in PET. These signal changes are then superimposed (coregistered) as colored areas on the person's structural MRI (see Fig. 7), typically acquired in the same session.

At this point in development, there is some controversy over whether the fMRI signal changes show actual blood flow or hemoglobin parameters related to oxygenation of the blood. The time resolution of fMRI is also difficult to determine because the images can be generated in much less than a second using very powerful magnets but it is not clear whether blood flow changes in response to a cognitive task occur in less than a second or two. These problems aside, fMRI is used for many cognitive studies. It has the appeal of wide availability because there are more than 5000 MRI units in the United State alone (PET is limited to about 50 centers) and it has no associated risks so that it can be used repeatedly in adults and in children.

IV. EEG AND MAGNETOENCEPHALOGRAM (MEG)

A. EEG

EEG recordings provide functional brain information. EEG was first used to make functional brain images of cortical electrical signals in the 1970s when computers allowed the integration of simultaneous EEG recordings from multiple electrode sites and interpolation among sites. Early EEG images displayed EEG parameters (e.g., alpha, beta, theta waves) interpolated across the surface of the cortex using from 8 to 16 electrode sites. The placement of the electrodes was standard, using head landmarks, and each person's data was fit to a standard brain outline, pioneering many of the techniques subsequently applied to PET and MRI. The pattern of EEG activity over the cortical surface could be displayed from task to task, millisecond by millisecond and, as computers became more powerful, these displays even could be shown in real time. Evoked potentials (EP), a special EEG technique that averages EEG to specific stimuli over many trials, also can be displayed as an image using the same interpolation methods. One of a number of early methods to display such images was Brain Electric Activity Mapping (BEAM). Spatial resolution for EEG and

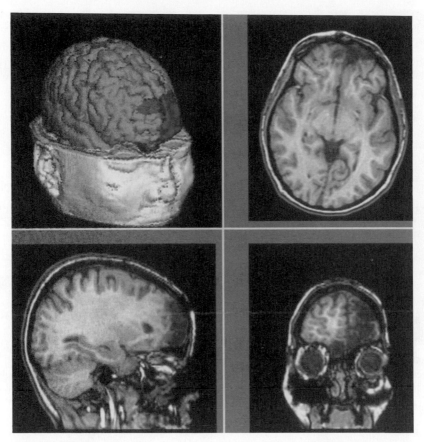

Figure 6 Structural MRI. Reconstructions are shown in one head injury patient with brain damage (dark areas) to the frontal lobe, especially in the right hemisphere. The upper left shows a 3-dimensional view, the upper right shows an axial view, the lower left shows a sagittal view and the lower right shows a coronal view. (Courtesy of Dr. Erin Bigler.)

EP images depend on the number of electrode sites. The more sites, the more accurate the interpolations among sites. Arrays of more than 100 electrodes currently provide the best spatial resolution. Time resolution is millisecond by millisecond, essentially real time, and far exceeds all other functional imaging techniques. EEG and EP also are relatively inexpensive and logistically easy to use. There is no restriction for repeated testing in adults or children. The spatial resolution with more than 100 electrode sites is similar to PET but only the cortical surface is shown most accurately. There are advances in computing the possible deep brain sources for cortical signals. Gevins and colleagues have pushed EEG and EP methods to their limits for describing complex temporal topographic patterns of electrical activity during sensory, motor, and cognitive tasks (see Fig. 8).

B. MEG

MEG uses supercooled detectors (SQUID—superconducting quantum interface device) to measure the extremely weak magnetic fields produced by the electrical activity in the brain that results from neurons firing. MEG can localize the source of these fields and provide functional images showing these sources as they change from one task or state to another. As an adjunct to EEG and EP mapping, MEG gets below the cortical surface and can map the entire brain, although best results come from cortical areas. Like fMRI, MEG results are typically coregistered on structural MRIs. Currently, MEG is limited to only a few centers worldwide; it is expensive and difficult to use. Hari and colleagues have published extensively on MEG and sensory activations.

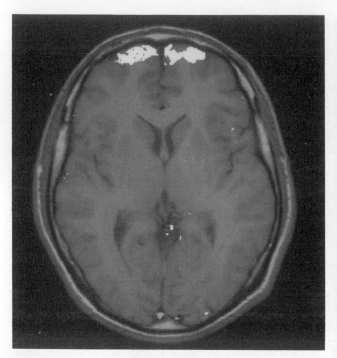

Figure 7   Functional MRI. The white areas show blood flow increases when this subject counted backward by 2s compared to resting. The functional information is superimposed on a structural MRI.

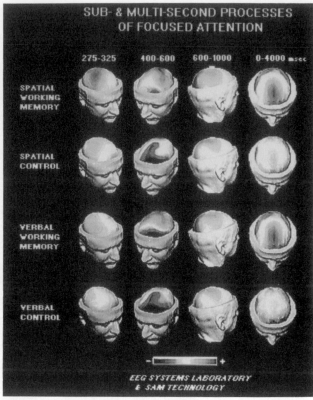

Figure 8   EEG measures from multiple electrode sites in four time ranges during four psychological tasks are displayed as cortical regional patterns of activity. This demonstrates the millisecond time resolution of this imaging technique. (Courtesy of Dr. Alan Gevins.)

V. NEUROIMAGING FINDINGS
AND NORMAL BRAIN FUNCTION

Xenon blood flow, EEG, and CAT scan images have been used to characterize normal and abnormal brains for more than 30 years. PET research on normal brain function began about 1980 when controls were studied for comparisons to various brain disorders like schizophrenia and Alzheimer's Disease. For the last 10 years, many PET studies have studied only normal subjects performing a variety of tasks for the purpose of understanding normal cognition. Functional MRI has been used for this purpose only in the last few years but the use of fMRI is growing dramatically as more and more psychologists and neuroscientists gain access to study language processing, attention, reasoning, personality, emotion, learning and memory. Currently, many cognitive researchers and neuropsychologists favor fMRI or PET over topographic EEG, mostly because the latter is more limited to cortex assessment rather than whole brain, despite the temporal resolu-

tion superiority. MEG is the least available to researchers. Although the study of normal and abnormal cognition with neuroimaging complement each other, the focus of this review is on a relatively few recent findings in normals to give the flavor of how brain imaging is advancing our knowledge of cognition in key areas.

A. Language

One of the first cognitive areas studied with PET in normals was language processing. Researchers at Washington University, St. Louis, reported a number of subtraction comparisons between elemental language processing tasks and regional cerebral blood flow using the O15 method. In a classic study by Petersen and colleagues in 1989, normal subjects were imaged while viewing words, listening to words, speaking words, and generating words. Using the pixel-to-pixel subtraction technique, cerebral blood flow during each of these conditions was compared (e.g., listening minus viewing, speaking minus listening, generating minus speaking). Each task activated a distinct set of brain areas, demonstrating both that elemental cognitive tasks are somewhat localized and that the salient brain areas are organized into networks that underlie specific mental operations. One major goal of current research is to establish further the nature of these networks. Another goal is to understand disorders of language, especially in children. The radioactivity used in PET has limited functional imaging research in children but fMRI can be used without this concern.

B. Learning

Some PET studies in normal volunteers suggest that GMR decreases after learning a complex task, suggesting that the brain becomes more efficient, perhaps in learning what areas not to use for good performance. Other PET studies show a shift in the pattern of GMR use after learning, suggesting that different brain areas become involved. Some fMRI studies suggest that learning increases the size of the cortical brain area used during a task, suggesting that adjacent neurons are recruited to the effort. At this point, brain imaging studies of learning are preliminary and not completely consistent. Children with learning disabilities or attention deficit disorder have not been studied extensively, although a number of fMRI projects are underway. Even at this early stage of research, the results indicate the enormous potential for further work to help understand brain mechanisms of learning.

C. Memory

A large number of recent studies with PET and fMRI are providing evidence that, just as for language processing, memory involves localized areas organized into networks for specific functions. Imaging studies of normals show that some memory tasks activate the hippocampus, a part of the temporal lobe known to be important for various memory functions. PET studies of Alzheimer's Disease confirm lower activity in temporal lobe/hippocampal areas. In combination with genetic testing, functional imaging of these areas may have potential as an early screening for Alzheimer's Disease. Other memory studies address frontal lobe involvement. For example, Tulving and associates have advanced the idea that functional imaging results indicate that the left prefrontal cortex is more related to retrieval of semantic information and encoding novel aspects of it into episodic memory; the right prefrontal cortex is more related to retrieval of episodic memory. Other work by Cahill and colleagues published in 1996 has reported correlations between GMR in the amygdala while subjects watch an emotional video and recall of the emotional information three weeks later. Interestingly, in this study, there was no mean difference in amygdala GMR between the emotional and neutral conditions, but the correlation technique showed significant correlations between amygdala GMR and subsequent memory in only the emotional condition. In general, memory research, like language processing research, benefits from an extensive empirical literature that is the basis for sophisticated theories which support testing explicit hypotheses about the brain with neuroimaging. This allows relatively rapid progress on basic issues as well as generating new hypotheses.

D. Reasoning/Intelligence

Brain theories about the basis of high level reasoning and problem solving are not so advanced. Neuroimaging studies in this area are more exploratory. For example, in 1988 Haier and colleagues published a PET study of GMR in normal volunteers while they performed a difficult test of abstract reasoning, the Raven's Advanced Progressive Matrices (RAPM). The RAPM is a standard test that requires the subject to solve 36 problems, each one comprised of a series of nine symbols arranged in a pattern. One symbol, however, is always missing from the pattern. Once the subject understands the pattern, the missing symbol can be selected from eight possible choices. Scores on the RAPM are highly correlated with IQ. Surprisingly, this study found an inverse relationship between RAPM scores and brain GMR. The subjects with high RAPM scores (i.e., good performance) had lower GMR, especially in the temporal lobe. This was interpreted as evidence that the efficiency of brain energy use was more important for good cognitive performance on this complex task than the level of GMR. Whether brain efficiency involves task strategy, mental effort, characteristics of individual neurons, or other parameters has yet to be determined. Other PET research also reports inverse relationships between performance on

complex tasks and brain function. A study of mild retardation and Down Syndrome reported by Haier and
colleagues in 1995 showed higher brain GMR in both
groups compared to matched controls. They speculated that a failure of normal developmental neural
pruning could be the basis for a person having too
many synaptic connections and redundant brain circuitry resulting in inefficient problem solving, low IQ,
and high GMR. Standard score images for each retarded subject revealed considerable heterogeneity of
GMR patterns. In the same study, MRI was used to
measure brain volume. For the combined samples of
mildly retarded, Down Syndrome, and controls, there
was an inverse relationship between GMR and IQ and
an inverse relationship between GMR and brain volume. There also was a positive relationship between
brain size measured by MRI and IQ, consistent with
many other studies. Clearly, the use of brain imaging to
study complex reasoning in humans has potential for
elucidating the biological basis of problem solving
and individual differences in intelligence. At this stage,
sophisticated theoretical formulations for hypothesis
testing are awaiting the accumulation of additional
empirical observations. [See INTELLIGENCE AND MEN-
TAL HEALTH; MENTAL RETARDATION AND MENTAL
HEALTH.]

E. Sleep and Consciousness

Several PET studies have addressed patterns of GMR
changes during REM and non-REM sleep. During
dreaming, GMR is about the same as during the
awake state but during deep non-REM sleep, whole
brain GMR is down about 40% compared to the
awake state. Other PET studies by Alkire and colleagues of anesthetic agents show even larger whole
brain decreases during unconsciousness induced by
propofol and by isoflurane. Moreover, the pattern of
regional GMR decreases in propofol anesthesia suggests the biggest decreases are in brain areas rich in
GABA receptors. This is an example of using neuroimaging to help discover possible mechanisms of action for specific drugs. Moreover, these data tenta-
tively support a theory relating whole brain GMR reduction to loss of consciousness rather than a theory
of a specific consciousness control center. Further im-
aging/anesthesia studies hold great promise for helping to establish the neural basis for consciousness and
unconsciousness. [See SLEEP.]

F. Aging

Chugani and colleagues have published several PET
studies of children and young adults that show that
GMR increases in most brain areas from birth to ages 3
to 5 years and then slowly decreases through about age
20. This pattern parallels the pattern of changes in synaptic density previously demonstrated in autopsy studies. Other imaging studies suggest continued small
decreases in whole brain GMR with increasing age beyond 20 years but these data are not consistent among
all studies. Grady and colleagues used PET blood flow
imaging and reported in 1996 that normal aging appears associated with shifting or compensatory activation in various brain systems for some specific cognitive tasks. For example, during a face-matching task
where young and old subjects performed the same,
older subjects had more activation in frontal cortex
and other areas than younger subjects. Whether this
pattern is related to regional brain atrophy or other
structural parameters is not yet known. Imaging studies with very large sample sizes are required to examine the various aspects of aging, cognition, and brain
function.

G. Sex Differences

A number of brain structural differences have been
noted between men and women in studies using structural imaging. Recent functional imaging with PET has
yielded inconsistent results with some studies showing
women having slightly higher brain metabolic rates
than men but other studies showing no differences.
Most of the studies addressing this issue were done in a
resting condition. Task activation imaging studies published in 1995 show some intriguing male/female differences. For example, Shaywitz and colleagues studied language processing using fMRI. They found blood
flow increases in specific frontal lobe areas during
phonological processing in males; but in females, areas
of increased activation were more diffuse. Haier and
Benbow matched men and women for average or high
mathematical reasoning ability in a PET study. Mean
GMR did not differ much between any of the four
groups but there were significant correlations between
temporal lobe GMR bilaterally and mathematical reasoning scores in the men; there were no GMR/math
score correlations in the women for any cortex area.
More studies with large samples and a variety of tasks
need to be done.

VI. CONCLUSIONS

A. Interpretation Issues

Even these brief descriptions of a few neuroimaging studies demonstrate the potential for new understandings of the brain. Brain images of structure and function are compelling glimpses into complex relationships. The most sophisticated neuroimaging techniques, however, are no more sophisticated than the research designs and methods that make use of them. High-resolution functional brain imaging is only as good as the psychological tasks used to probe or stimulate brain areas. A simple approach of finding brain areas activated by a simple task is a good start but is still simple. Tasks can also deactivate areas or circuits. Brain activation may also indicate excitatory or inhibitory activity. That is, when inhibitory cells are activated, GMR or blood flow will increase in that brain area although the effect of the increased inhibitory firing is decreased activity somewhere along the circuit. Moreover, the functional relationships among brain areas may be more important than specific areas alone. Even the range of activity within a brain area may be related to the range of task performance during which the activity was measured. This recognition of individual differences may produce additional surprising results when incorporated into research designs to augment standard group comparisons.

B. Future Advances

New neuroimaging studies can use increasingly sophisticated research designs incorporating levels of cognitive ability (e.g., bright and average subjects), task strategy alternatives (e.g., chunking or not chunking memorized items into categories), easy and hard versions of tasks (i.e., low and high mental effort), and a variety of tasks to probe specific brain areas and systems. The combination of neuroimaging techniques in the same subjects, even simultaneously, also promises to advance research. Structural MRI, for example, now is essentially necessary for exact anatomical localization irrespective of the functional technique used. Functional MRI and MEG results routinely are displayed on structural MRIs. In the future, neurosurgeons and researchers may use virtual brains created from a variety of imaging procedures to explore the re-lationships between structure and function as computer models of cognition generate responses to test stimuli. In the near future, human PET studies using different radiolabels and using drugs to manipulate brain state during task conditions will help discover which neurotransmitter systems are related to specific sensory, motor, and cognitive performance. Neuroimaging studies have already begun to bridge the gap between animal experiments and human studies because animal studies can provide specific hypotheses for human testing. Neuroimaging technology will likely advance our abilities to test hypotheses in ways beyond the scope of our current theories. These abilities will drive new theories of how the brain works normally and how it fails when it is broken.

BIBLIOGRAPHY

Alkire, M. T., Haier, R. J., Barker, S. J., Shah, N. K., Wu, J., & Kao, J. (1995). Cerebral metabolism during propofol anesthesia in humans studied with PET. *Anesthesiology, 82:* 393–403.

Bigler, E., Yeo, R., & Turkheimer, E. (Eds.). (1989). *Neuropsychological function and brain imaging.* New York: Plenum Press.

Buchsbaum, M. S. (1996). Neuroimaging: PET and the averaging of brain images. *American Journal of Psychiatry, 153*(4), 456.

Cahill, L., et al. (1996). Amygdala activity at encoding correlated with long-term, free recall of emotional information. *Proceedings of the National Academy of Sciences, vol. 93,* 8016–8021.

Gevins, A., Leong, H., Smith, M. E., Le, J., & Du, R. (1995). Mapping cognitive brain function with modern high-resolution electroencephalography. *Trends in Neurosciences, 18*(10), 427–461.

Haier, R. J. (1993) Cerebral glucose metabolism and intelligence. In P. A. Vernon (Ed.), *Biological approaches to the study of human intelligence.* Norwood, NJ: Ablex Publishing Co.

Haier, R. J., et al. (in press). Brain imaging and classification of mental retardation. In Soraci & McIlvane (Eds.), *Perspectives on fundamental processes in intellectual functioning.* Norwood, NJ: Ablex Publishing Co.

Petersen, S. E., Fox, P.T., Posner, M., Mintun, M., & Raichle, M. (1989). PET studies of the processing of single words. *Journal of Cognitive Neuroscience, 1*(2): 153–170.

Phelps, M. E., Mazziotta, J.C., & Schelbert, H. R. (1986). *Positron emission tomography and audoradiography.* New York: Raven Press.

Posner, M., & Raichle, M. (1994). *Images of mind.* Scientific American Library. New York: W. H. Freeman & Company.

Roland, P. E. (1993). *Brain activation.* New York: Wiley-Liss. John Wiley & Sons, Inc.

Shaywitz, B. A., et al. (1995). Sex differences in the functional organization of the brain for language. *Nature, 373,* 607–609.

Brainwashing and Totalitarian Influence

Dick Anthony*

Graduate Theological Union

Thomas Robbins

Santa Barbara Center for Humanistic Studies

Brainwashing A pattern of interrogation and indoctrination to which Western prisoners of war were exposed during the Korean War; more generally, a coercive style of persuasion which allegedly radically alters beliefs against the will of the individual through the induction of primitive states of consciousness in which the person is powerless to resist new ideas.

Thought Reform The historical process of indoctrination in totalitarian ideology utilized for the coercive re-education of non-Communists by the Chinese; more generally, refers to the attempt to transform personal identities through intensive or stressful indoctrination in the context of a totalistic ideology.

Totalism An all-encompassing ideology which interprets the world in terms of a comprehensive set of polarized, black versus white categories, typically designed to legitimate a totalitarian state. The term also refers to the pattern of psychological characteristics that predisposes individuals to enthusiastically submit to totalitarian ideologies, social movements, and governments.

Totalitarianism A comprehensive organization of a nation state and total society in terms of a militant totalist ideology.

---

*Dick Anthony is presently in private practice in forensic psychology.

BRAINWASHING has been used to denote the actual historical experience of the indoctrination of Western prisoners of war in Korea and the methods of influence employed by their Communist captors. More generally the term denotes an extreme mode of indoctrination which allegedly is qualitatively different from normal social influence and other modes of indoctrination in that it is supposedly derived from scientific research and capable of overwhelming free will.

Brainwashing supposedly undermines subjects' true political and religious beliefs and the sense of identity based upon them. It is alleged to coercively substitute sharply contrasting beliefs and a false self. The variables which determine the efficacy of influence are assumed to be esoteric and technical, such as the use of drugs, hypnosis, and distinctive conditioning procedures based upon scientific research. These factors allegedly involve the creation of a distinctive, altered state of consciousness within which the subject is highly suggestible and in which alternative beliefs and an alternative identity are coercively implanted. The predisposing characteristics of subjects are not considered salient. Physical coercion is not considered essential to the process.

An alternative perspective, which focused on personality and motivational factors determining the attraction of persons to totalitarian ideologies and groups, emerged at roughly the same time that the notion of brainwashing developed. This perspective emerged from within a general interdisciplinary analysis of totalitarianism, and was used to interpret the indoctrination of Westerners within Communist prison of war camps and prisons by, among others, Edgar Schein and Robert Lifton.

The latter approach, which we will refer to in this paper as the analysis of totalitarian influence, found that such influence was not capable of causing the involuntary substitution of false beliefs for true ones, nor of supplanting a person's real self with an inauthentic one. The appearance of involuntary alteration of beliefs and identities, according to this perspective, was created primarily by prisoners' simple behavioral compliance to their captors' wishes because of extreme physical coercion, resulting in no real change in belief. The small amount of real change in belief by Westerners in Communist prisons, on the other hand, was based upon characterological and ideological predispositions and did not result from novel or distinctive techniques of influence.

I. EMERGENCE OF THE BRAINWASHING MODEL

The "brainwashing" idea developed during World War II when both Nazi and American intelligence services became interested in developing techniques to more effectively interrogate prisoners and, optimally, to transform enemy prisoners and internal subversives into "deployable agents" who would be enthusiastic converts to general political attitudes diametrically opposed to the ones which their interrogators found objectionable. The intelligence services had in mind a variety of uses for such converts, such as using them as secret agents who, because of their pasts, would be more likely to escape detection than more conventional agents. Additional goals for the brainwashing process included improving the capacity of soldiers to resist hostile interrogation and developing more effective wartime propaganda techniques.

The feasibility of "brainwashing" or the radical psycho-political re-education of persons whose will was to be overwhelmed was suggested to German and American intelligence services by the Moscow show trials in the late 1930s. At these trials high Soviet officials confessed implausible crimes relating to allegedly counterrevolutionary activities. The Stalinists were at that time presumed by many journalists, social scientists, and Western public officials to have discovered the key to the scientific conquest of the human will.

Most informed scholars now believe that physically coerced behavioral *compliance* and not some mode of inner *conversion* was operative in both the Moscow show trials of the 1930s and later Communist trials in Eastern Europe, such as that of Cardinal Mindzenty,

who made a sensational confession. However, in the 1940s and 1950s the brainwashing explanation of such confessions was taken very seriously by German and American officials, and both countries funded ambitious research programs to develop brainwashing techniques. The German program was conducted by the S.S. and the Gestapo, and the American program was conducted by the Office of Strategic Services [OSS], the World War II predecessor of the Central Intelligence Agency, and later by the CIA itself.

Most of the CIA funded research was carried out under the auspices of two supposedly independent philanthropic foundations which served as front organizations disguising the CIA origin of the funding. The research was conducted by American and Canadian psychiatrists, psychologists, and other social scientists, many of them very prominent. (Some may have remained ignorant of the CIA sponsorship of these projects.)

In many attempts to replicate the apparent overwhelming of the wills of Stalin's victims, the scientists working on the issue assumed that an essential prerequisite to authentic brainwashing was a *deconditioning* process to eradicate subjects' prior mental patterns. This was in part the rationale for the use of powerful psychedelic drugs such as Mescaline and LSD which were viewed as potent deconditioning agents. Scientists believed that once a person's mind was wiped clean by such drugs, or by other deconditioning agents such as sensory deprivation or electroshock therapy, new political attitudes and a new sense of self could then easily be implanted by conditioning techniques or by hypnosis. The American research program, which eventually became heavily involved in experiments with LSD, was influenced by earlier Nazi work with Mescaline. In general, the key elements of government research programs were (1) drugs, (2) sensory deprivation and isolation, (3) hypnosis, (4) conditioning procedures, and (5) physical debilitation. Electric shock, psychosurgery, and insulin shock were occasionally employed.

The Nazi research program, which was less ethically inhibited than the American program, had a significant death rate among subjects, although CIA sponsored research in the United States and Canada also produced casualties in terms of mental breakdown and disorientation. Civilian psychologists and psychiatrists who collaborated in these programs were also concerned with finding methods of curing mental illness which were more effective and less time consuming than Freudian talk therapy. Thus, the research, which was not successful in terms of its original goals, nevertheless impacted psychotherapy in terms of drug therapy, behavioral conditioning, and electroconvulsive therapy.

It is important to note that intelligence officials regarded traditional methods involving physical coercion and threat as having some serious limitations. It was difficult to discern whether persons who were compliant out of fear were being truthful when they answered questions or expressed beliefs. Advanced scientific techniques were regarded as promising to improve upon crudely coercive tactics and prolonged incarceration in this respect.

To some degree *deception* was regarded as the basic alternative to physical constraint: subjects were sometimes told they were simply being treated for emotional and mental problems, and they were not aware of the nature of the drugs they imbibed, nor of the coercively indoctrinational intent of the conditioning procedures that were applied to them. In some cases subjects were administered strong psychedelic drugs without even being informed that they were being given any drugs at all.

Despite the scope and ambitiousness of these German and American mind control research programs (the American research program went on for over 25 years), in terms of their original goals of improving interrogation and coercive indoctrination tactics beyond that obtainable with physical coercion or other traditional methods, they were complete failures. The German program produced many deaths but no reliable alternatives to extreme brutality and terror in interrogation and indoctrination procedures and was never able to convert enemies into deployable agents.

The American program also had some serious casualties. For instance, the covert administration of psychedelic substances caused some psychotic episodes and on at least one occasion led to the suicide of a subject. In addition, one large project, which involved a combination of drugs, electroshock, conditioning procedures, and sensory deprivation resulted in (1) the mental breakdown and disorientation of some subjects; (2) over 60% of its subjects suffering severe memory problems for up to 10 years; (3) some cases of permanent brain damage.

As we have indicated, despite the intensity and severity of these methods the American program never

learned how to change people's minds about their political orientations or to force them to reveal deeply held secrets. The most that could be said for the methods evaluated is that they could drive people crazy or make them mentally defective, but even such casualties became no more sympathetic to political opinions with which they disagreed, and would have been too disabled to be useful even if they had. After 25 years of dedicated effort and the involvement of the cream of American psychiatry and psychology, the American CIA had become no more capable of coercively creating deployable agents than it had at the beginning.

II. IMPACT OF CHINESE POW CAMPS

Some of the CIA sponsored research we have referred to actually was conducted in the 1950s during or after the Korean War. During this period the notion of "brainwashing" had become popular with the public largely because it seemed relevant to explaining the grim experiences of American soldiers in Communist prison camps in Korea. Although few if any soldiers were converted to Communism, some American POW's were induced by their captors to make statements critical of American policy and supportive of Communist allegations that American forces were employing germ warfare. These performances troubled many Americans but stimulated writers and movie makers, who presented an extreme scenario of traumatically induced psychosis and mind control, the movie *The Manchurian Candidate* being the best known entertainment product.

The research supported by the CIA on how to achieve mind control described above was not actually influenced by the POW ordeals. Knowledgeable researchers and officials were aware that the Chinese were not employing advanced scientific methods or attempting systematic radical deconditioning and the transformation of thought patterns. However, the agency conducted a disinformation campaign aimed at exploiting the brainwashing idea to reassure Americans that germ warfare allegations made by POW's were not true, that captured American soldiers were not traitors or weak, and that no competent (i.e., unbrainwashed) person could voluntarily accept Communist ideology, which was assumed to be inherently implausible to a rational person.

Central to this effort was the publication by Edward Hunter, a propaganda expert employed by the CIA who worked undercover as an American journalist, of *Brainwashing in Red China*. This volume explained the apparent success of the Chinese thought reform programs in terms of sinister but advanced science-based techniques much like the ones which the CIA-sponsored research program in the United States had so far been unsuccessful in creating. Hunter coined the term brainwashing in this volume because of its sinister overtones of overpowered human will and falsely claimed that the term was a translation of a Chinese term for thought reform. Thus, not only the process of brainwashing but also the very term itself was a sham constructed for propaganda purposes.

The Communist thought reform programs, Hunter claimed in a later volume, were capable of transforming a person into a "puppet" or "human robot" and of inserting new beliefs and thought processes into a captive body. Hunter formalized what we will term the "robot" or "brainwashing" model of psychologically coercive social influence. As portrayed by Hunter and those writers whom he influenced, brainwashing is a sinister psycho-technology assumed to be highly effective in overpowering human will through means of deception, induced hypnotic states, and Pavlovian conditioning, which undermine resistance to persuasion. Initial individual dispositions are simply overwhelmed and are thus not major factors in predicting who will be influenced by the process.

The "robot" mind control paradigm was expressed in various works by writers such as Hunter, William Sargent, Joost Van Meerloo, Aldous Huxley, Farber *et al.,* and others. Several of these works credited the Russian scientist I. Pavlov, working with dogs, with discovering a way of inducing a primitive mental state in which both animals and humans exhibit an enhanced susceptibility to conditioning. A primitive trance state of high suggestibility could thus, it was thought, be induced by various means, e.g., hypnosis, in which individuals could more easily be programmed by scientific conditioning procedures.

Some writers maintained that this primitive state of consciousness was rare in the United States where reason and education prevailed, but was the normal state of consciousness in other, especially Oriental and preliterate cultures, and was moreover associated with religious rituals, including, in one formulation, early Methodist revivals. The connection between the brain-

washing model and religion thus did not begin with recent "cults."

With respect to totalitarian societies also, the robot perspective was frequently expanded from the analysis of coercive indoctrination in prison situations to a general model of totalitarian control of whole societies. According to authors utilizing this paradigm, the general public within totalitarian societies were controlled by technical innovations in communication techniques, such as hypnosis and conditioning which allegedly operated by means of mass rallies and propaganda. As with the analysis of interrogation situations, the robot perspectives focused upon supposedly irresistible techniques that overwhelm free will and downplayed the fear of the coercive apparatus of the state or the voluntary acceptance of totalitarian ideologies by people who were attracted to them for their own reasons.

At least with respect to coercive indoctrination and interrogation situations, the available data on approximately 7000 Korean War American POW's does not support the robot model. More than 30% of the prisoners died but approximately 4500 were ultimately repatriated. Of these only 21 POW's refused repatriation, and of these 10 subsequently changed their minds. Thus, only 11 out of 4500 persons, approximately one-fifth of 1% of those who survived imprisonment, arguably accepted anti-American perspectives.

Comparison with turncoat rates of American POW's in former wars indicates that the rate during the Korean War was the lowest in our history. Thus, these data indicate that the alleged overpowering brainwashing techniques of the Chinese and Korean Communists not only were completely ineffective, but if anything they actually encouraged continued allegiance to American ideology and policies.

Despite the lack of effectiveness of Chinese indoctrination techniques revealed by these statistics, the government nevertheless hired researchers to study returning POW's and to evaluate the nature of Communist brainwashing. Edgar Schein, Robert Lifton, and Albert Biderman each headed projects on POW brainwashing funded by the armed forces and given armed forces cooperation. The reports of their research on Communist POW's by Lifton and by Schein foreshadowed their later, more ambitious research studies on the nature and effect of the attempted Chinese Communist thought reform of Western civilian prisoners in China.

The CIA appointed Cornell University psychiatrists Lawrence Hinkle and Harold Wolff to conduct its own secret study of all the different varieties of alleged Communist brainwashing, e.g., Russian show trials, Chinese Communist thought reform of their own countrymen as well as of imprisoned Westerners in China, and of Korean War POW's. The Hinkle and Wolff project was given access to all the CIA secret files and they conducted interviews which the CIA arranged with former Communist interrogators and prisoners alike.

A declassified version of the Hinkle and Wolff CIA sponsored study was eventually published and was considered by other experts to be the definitive U.S. government work on the subject of Communist brainwashing. In addition to Hinkle and Wolff's own research, this report summarized the results of the government funded research on Korean War brainwashing by Schein, Lifton, Biderman, and others. In general, according to Hinkle and Wolff, the Maoist techniques were not novel or extraordinary or based on advanced science. There was no evidence of the use of hypnotic processes or induced altered states of consciousness.

Compared to Soviet methods, the Chinese Communists did innovate in their emphasis on fervently propagandizing military captives. Constant propaganda was combined with the alternation of long isolation with peer group pressures, severe debility, torture, and extreme threat and total uncertainty about the future. In re-educating dissidents and deviants, the Chinese departed from the Soviet preference for one on one, interrogator–interogatee interaction (the "Darkness at Noon" model) to emphasize peer group dynamics and a managed interpersonal environment.

With respect to the effectiveness of Communist methods, Hinkle and Wolff confirmed the impression conveyed by the failure of the CIA's own brainwashing research projects. That is, no known brainwashing techniques, whether German, Communist, or American, have been capable of indoctrinating people with political or social attitudes conflicting with ones to which they are naturally attracted. Specifically, Hinkle and Wolff argued that the Communists have not been successful in converting Americans to Communist doctrine in either of the two well-known situations—

American POW's in Korea or American civilians imprisoned in Communist China—in which brainwashing theorists such as Hunter argued that coerced conversions had occurred.

In addition to the fact that very few American POW's refused repatriation, Hinkle and Wolff pointed out that even those few who did refuse did so for reasons other than conversion to Communism, e.g., fear of punishment for collaborative activities that they had engaged in for practical rather than ideological reasons. With respect to Western civilians imprisoned in China who upon their release issued statements to the press which sounded sympathetic to Communism, Hinkle and Wolff's repudiation of a brainwashing explanation was, if anything, even more unequivocal.

According to Hinkle and Wolff, who claimed to have access to intensive research on a number of American civilians allegedly brainwashed in China, all of those studied were sympathetic to Chinese Communism and antipathetic to American values *before* their imprisonment by the Chinese. Consequently, the Communist values that they expressed upon their release were little different from the ones that they had long been committed to before the thought reform experience. Contrary to the sensationalistic accounts of their supposedly brainwashed viewpoints by the American press and by authors such as Hunter, Sargent, and Meerloo, no substantial change in their viewpoints had occurred under the impact of brainwashing.

The Chinese thought reform methods were also demystified by Edgar Schein, a social psychologist, whose well-known volume, *Coercive Persuasion*, pronounced the attempted thought reform of Western civilian prisoners by the Chinese to have been a relative failure. Only one or two of Schein's 15 subjects who had undergone Chinese thought reform showed any substantial degree of positive attitude change toward Communism, and even in these isolated instances such change stopped well short of conversion to Communism. The rest of his subjects showed only behavioral compliance to the demands of their captors, without significant ideological change. Schein also criticized the elements of brainwashing analyses which emphasized dissociative states, conditioning, suggestibility, and defective thinking. Schein found that such altered states and exotic techniques were not at all characteristic of Chinese thought reform.

Schein emphasized that rather than such alleged brainwashing techniques, the physically coercive setting and methods of Chinese thought reform define Communist coercive persuasion, which involves a setting from which there is no escape. On the other hand, Schein affirms the presence of the purely psychological, i.e., nonphysical, elements of coercive persuasion in conventional American institutions such as reputable religious orders, fraternities and sororities, rehabilitation organizations, etc.

Furthermore, according to Schein, the purely psychological techniques used in Communist coercive persuasion, and in many normal American institutions as well, are not inherently objectionable. Such techniques should be judged, he claims, according to the nature of the values which they are intended to promote, not because they, when judged simply as methods of influence, are inherently inimical to human freedom.

III. INVESTIGATING THE "PSYCHOLOGY OF TOTALISM"

An alternative to the "Robot Model" of extremist indoctrination emerged out of the concern of many intellectuals and scholars about proliferating totalitarian movements and governments and their interest in the kinds of persons who are attracted to totalitarianism.

Although the Mussolini regime began in the 1920s to use the term "totalitarianism" in a positive sense to denote monolithic national unity, many intellectuals were troubled by the rise of Fascism and dedicated themselves to the study of totalitarian states, parties, and ideologies. This intellectual phenomenon became the basis for a large and multi-faceted genre of "totalitarian studies," a part of which dealt with the psychology of totalitarian movements. Initially in the 1930s such studies focused primarily upon the analysis of developments in Fascist states, e.g., Italy, Germany, and in some interpretations Spain, Japan, and Rumania. After the Second World War, Communist states such as the Soviet Union and Communist China were also generally included in most analyses.

The most influential general analyses of totalitarianism as a uniquely modern political phenomenon appeared in books by Hannah Arendt (1950) and Carl Friedrich and Zbigniew Brzezinski (1956). These books synthesized more specialized studies by other scholars of totalitarianism into overall interpretations of the phenomenon. In addition, a seminal conference on the nature of totalitarianism was held by the American Academy of Arts and Sciences in Boston in 1953. The committee planning the conference was chaired by Carl Friedrich and those attending included the creme of scholars in totalitarian studies including Arendt, Alex Inkeles, Else Frenkel-Brunswick, Erik Erikson, George F. Kennan, and many others. The papers delivered at the conference were published in a book edited by Carl Friedrich.

These general analyses by Arendt and by Friedrich and Brzezinski, and most of the papers in the conference volume, shared a common framework of assumptions about totalitarianism which had developed in the previous 20 years of scholarship, and were, especially Arendt's, immensely influential with other scholars as well as the educated general public.

The books by Arendt and by Friedrich and Brzezinski, as well as most other general analyses within totalitarian studies, include the following criteria as characteristic of totalitarianism as a mode of ideological societal reconstruction: (1) Totalitarian *ideology* is apocalyptic and millenarian and identifies a holy remnant or vanguard elite that will lead the world into a utopian new age. Totalitarian ideology is basically Manichean, i.e., it poses absolute black and white alternatives for human kind, society, and the individual. The state is identified as the key agent of a purposive, revolutionary historical process. (2) A thorough *structural reorganization of society* is implemented to reshape all significant social institutions in terms of the messianic ideology and the state assumes an unprecedented degree of control over all social institutions. (3) The state maintains a monopoly over all media of communication and all communication must conform to ideological tenets. (4) The systematic use of *terror* and extreme physical coercion serves as the essential device to maintain social control. (5) Certain social groups are designated as the carriers of evil and are considered to be beyond redemption. No limits are imposed upon the measures which should be taken in combatting and destroying such internal and external enemies. (6) Totalitarian societies have unlimited expansionist intentions, i.e., they intend to use force to establish worldwide domination of other societies.

This view of totalitarianism does not involve the theory that commitment to totalitarian ideologies and practices are involuntary except in the mundane sense that behavioral conformity is coercively enforced by harsh physical means. A certain percentage of the population is viewed as being sincerely committed to a totalitarian view of the world, but such people have converted to the millenarian viewpoint because of their own inner motives. Another segment of the population are opposed to totalitarian beliefs, but are coerced into behavioral compliance through physical force. Many people are intermediate between these two extremes, being neither clearly in favor of nor clearly opposed to the goals and beliefs of the revolution, but they conform to its demands because of a mixture of fear of the consequences of disobedience and sincere but half-hearted belief in its possible value. Contrary to the brainwashing paradigm, none of these groups have lost their inner free will in any novel ways that are unique to totalitarian societies.

A. Pre-existing Motives for Conversion to Totalitarian Social Movements

Fascist and Communist social movements existed within the societies they eventually came to control prior to the point at which such control was achieved. Members of such movements, or people like them, become the segment of the population in totalitarian societies who are "true believers" once totalitarian domination has been achieved.

Research shows that motivational predispositions to join totalitarian social movements exist prior to any actual contact with such movements. The determination of who actually joins such movements results from the interaction of individual totalitarian, or authoritarian, motives with the extreme dualistic absolutism and apocalypticism of the totalist ideology which satisfies such yearnings.

A distinctive "totalist" psychology, that is the psychological dimension of totalitarian societies, ideologies, and individuals, was described by Robert Lifton in his book *Chinese Thought Reform and the Psychology of Totalism.* Lifton's book reported the results of an interview study of people who had undergone the thought reform process in China, the process that Hunter and other brainwashing theorists considered to be the most clear-cut example of brain-

washing. Lifton explicitly attempted to evaluate the brainwashing concept in his study, and finished by repudiating both the brainwashing term and the concept of overwhelmed will which it signified.

Lifton replaced the brainwashing concept with the concept of "totalism" in describing the thought reform process. Both the term and the concept of totalism were originally defined by Erik Erikson in a 1953 article (Wholeness and Totality—A Psychiatric Contribution) which constituted his contribution to the volume of papers resulting from the historically important 1953 conference on totalitarianism sponsored by the American Academy of Arts and Sciences that we described above.

Erikson later expanded on the totalism concept in his 1958 book *Young Man Luther,* in which he also further developed the concepts of "negative identity" and "negative conscience" which are constituent elements of totalism as he defines it. Lifton draws upon both of these discussions of totalism in his use of Erikson's concept in his book, and upon related passages in Erikson's other books and articles as well.

In the article in which he originated the concept of totalism, Erikson maintained that persons with certain personality characteristics are particularly attracted to movements, governments, and ideologies which manifest a characteristically totalitarian ideological and persuasive style. He defined totalism as "man's inclination, under certain conditions to undergo . . . that sudden total realignment and, as it were, co-alignment which accompanies conversion to the totalitarian conviction that the state may and must have absolute power over the minds as well as the lives and the fortunes of its citizens." (p. 159).

Both Erikson and Lifton are psychoanalysts, and the concept of totalism involves an application of psychoanalytic conceptions of child development to the issue of the types of persons who are attracted to totalitarianism. Erikson's formulation of the psychology of totalism was strongly influenced by a tradition of the psychoanalytic analysis of totalitarian influence which originated in the study of the types of persons attracted to Fascist political orientations. Leading authors in this tradition include Wilhelm Reich, Eric Fromm, and the co-authors of the landmark study *The Authoritarian Personality,* Theodore Adorno, Daniel Levin, Else Frenkel-Brunswick, and Nevitt Sanford.

According to this tradition of thought, people attracted to Fascism are also ethnocentric, i.e., prejudiced against cultural, religious, and racial groups different from their own. Such people are also strongly attracted to hierarchically organized social systems which rigidly control the lives of those caught up in them. According to the authors of *The Authoritarian Personality,* these tendencies result from being reared in circumstances in which children are rigidly controlled and forbidden to express aggression towards their parents.

People reared in these circumstances, according to authors in this tradition, tend to have a polarized self-sense in which a precariously maintained, unrealistically positive self-concept is always on the verge of being overthrown by a powerful but largely unconscious negative self-image. Such a child becomes "extra-punitive," i.e., always on the lookout for someone else to blame when things go wrong.

Totalitarian ideologies appeal to such people because they rigidly divide the world into the saved and the damned, and thus support the maintenance of unrealistically positive self-concepts by encouraging the projection onto scapegoats of unconscious negative self-images. Totalitarian social systems also reproduce on a larger scale the rigidly hierarchical structure characteristic of authoritarian family systems and thus appeal to people who have difficulty functioning in circumstances that require more individual creativity and personal responsibility than they are used to.

Although Erikson's concept of totalism was influenced by this tradition of thought, and shares its key assumptions, Erikson himself had earlier strongly influenced the theory of authoritarianism described in *The Authoritarian Personality.* Early in the Second World War, Erikson published a now classic article upon the development of Hitler's own authoritarianism and the general cultural and familial circumstances that created widespread authoritarianism in Germany. The conception of the relationship between authoritarian child-rearing practices and the development of an authoritarian personality expressed in the book *The Authoritarian Personality* owes much to Erikson's earlier article.

Erikson's later concept of totalism broadens the concept of authoritarianism from Fascist to Communist types of totalitarianism, and to other types of totalitarian influence as well. Erikson's thought on the relationship between personality formation and attraction to totalitarianism both contributed to and

drew from the larger psychoanalytic tradition concerned with these issues. Neither Lifton's nor Erikson's use of the totalism concept can be properly understood outside of its relationship to this larger tradition of thought and research.

As indicated above, Lifton's book interpreted the experiences of his subjects, who had undergone Communist thought reform, in terms of Erikson's concept of totalism. (He extensively interviewed 25 Westerners and 15 Chinese who were subjected to Chinese Thought Reform. The Westerners were imprisoned during the process.) Following Erikson, Lifton stated "By this ungainly phrase [ideological totalism] I mean to suggest the coming together of immoderate ideology with equally immoderate individual [totalist] character traits—an extremist meeting ground between people and ideas." (p. 419)

In analyzing influence within the thought reform environment as resulting from an interaction between individual predispositions toward totalitarianism and the characteristics of totalitarian ideology, both Erikson and Lifton locate the psychology of totalism approach squarely within the perspective of general totalitarian studies. By showing that Erikson's concept of individual totalism as a characterological gestalt accounts for the variation in responsiveness to totalitarian ideology, even within thought reform prisons, Lifton persuasively repudiates the brainwashing theory that thought reform consists of specialized communication techniques that convert people to totalitarian ideology against their will or their intrinsic predispositions.

Parenthetically, Schein, in his book *Coercive Persuasion,* which described his research upon the thought reform of Western civilians in China, was also influenced by the theoretical tradition concerned with discovering the inner motives for conversion to totalitarianism, of which Erikson's concept of totalism was a part, as well as by general totalitarian studies. He discusses the views of Fromm, Erikson, Adorno *et al.,* and Hoffer upon predispositions to totalitarianism in a chapter of Coercive Persuasion entitled "A Passion For Unanimity," wherein he also discusses more general analyses of totalitarianism such as that of Friedrich and Brzezinski. (The title of this chapter is probably taken from a chapter subsection from the Brzezinski book entitled "The Terror and the Passion for Unanimity.") Psychological predispositions to totalitarianism are also discussed by Schein in his chapters "The Special Role of Guilt in Coercive Persuasion" and "A Socio-Psychological Analysis of Coercive Persuasion."

Insofar as Lifton's book involves a description of conversion to totalitarian ideology, it is more a speculative application of Erikson's concept of totalism than it is an empirically grounded scientific study. Only 2 of Lifton's 25 Western subjects and none of his Chinese subjects substantially changed their political and social opinions and attitudes as a result of their thought reform experience. (Neither of the 2 subjects who were influenced converted to Communism, but they did become somewhat more sympathetic to Chinese Communism than they had been at the beginning of their thought reform experience.) Lifton could scarcely have generated a description of the general characteristics of the psychology of totalitarianism based upon the experiences of only 2 subjects, neither of whom actually converted to Communism.

Insofar as it was actually an empirical study at all, then, Lifton's project was more a demonstration of the failure of thought reform to influence the 38 of his 40 subjects who did not appreciably change their attitudes, than it was of the nature of conversion to totalitarianism. Lifton thus confirmed earlier studies, e.g., Hinkle and Wolff, as well as the failure of the American research to create deployable agents, which had also indicated little or no evidence that people substantially change their political opinions primarily as a result of attempted brainwashing.

Moreover, as we have indicated, Lifton found that each of his two subjects who were influenced by thought reform had strong totalistic predispositions prior to their experience. In this respect, also, Lifton's results confirm the results of early studies, e.g., Hinkle and Wolff's, which indicated that those who emerge from thought reform sympathetic to Communism already have totalistic characteristics prior to their participation in the process. Lifton's overall results thus confirm the results of earlier studies which indicated that the Communists possessed no capacity to convert people against their will to Communist ideology.

In the years since the publication of Lifton's book, his phenomenological description of the eight psychological themes that constitute totalistic ideological influence is sometimes treated, particularly in a popular or journalistic context, as equivalent to a general formulation of the characteristics of brainwashing, that is as characterizing a process that coercively changes people's political or religious opinions against their will. The misinterpretation of Lifton's description of the general features of totalitarian influence as being equivalent to a brainwashing explanation of involuntary political or religious conversion has probably been partly due to the cold war anti-communist climate which prevailed when his work was published. The misinterpretation also probably owes something to the cultural ubiquity and dominance of the robot or Manchurian Candidate view of the nature of totalitarian influence that emerged after the Korean War.

However it developed, the interpretation of Lifton's analysis of the general features of ideological totalism as equivalent to an endorsement of the concept of involuntary brainwashing is clearly mistaken. Lifton uses the term "brainwashing" in several places, yet he tries to demystify the term, which, in his view, has acquired a misleading connotation of "an all-powerful, irresistible, unfathomable and magical method of achieving total control over the human mind." Such usage "makes the word a rallying point for fear, resentment, urges for submission, justification for failure, irresponsible accusation, and for a wide gamut of emotional extremism."

By the end of the 1960s, then, two different models of extreme social influence and manipulative indoctrination associated with totalistic groups had emerged, the robot/brainwashing model on the one hand and the totalitarian influence model on the other. The two models have distinctly different emphases in terms of four partly interrelated issues.

1. The brainwashing process as sought after by Nazi and American government researchers and as described by Edward Hunter and others with regard to Korean POW's, Chinese thought reform, and Soviet show trials is viewed by its proponents as a very effective psycho-technology which overrides the will of helpless, passive victims. This conceptualization is not borne out by the studies of Schein, Lifton, Hinkle, and Wolff, and others who found that Communist indoctrination was ineffective in coercively altering the political and social opinions of people opposed to Communist ideology.

2. Adherents of the totalitarian influence approach tended to see extreme physical coercion as intrinsic to Communist social control in general and to the thought reform process in particular. From this point of view, physical coercion is the sole means by which

Communist societies and the thought reform process produce involuntary compliance. Brainwashing approaches on the other hand maintain that Communist societies and the thought reform process produce involuntary compliance primarily through the involuntary alteration of political opinions and identities. From the brainwashing perspective, physical coercion is not essential to producing involuntary compliance in Communist societies.

3. From the standpoint of brainwashing theory, the inescapable potency of this psycho-technology renders individual predilections irrelevant. Scholars within the totalitarian influence tradition, on the other hand, contend that those who convert to totalitarian ideologies and movements are predisposed to do so because of pre-existing personality characteristics and ideological preferences.

4. Finally, the robot brainwashing model draws a sharp line between indoctrinated totalists and the rest of the population, particularly freedom-loving Americans. The latter are viewed as being innately opposed to totalism but as unable to resist it if they encounter brainwashers because of their omnipotent technology of mind control. In contrast, Fromm, Adorno, Erikson, Lifton, Schein, and others do not sharply differentiate between indoctrinated cadres and members of a Western culture which is itself permeated by proto-totalist themes, as are many of its social groups.

From the point of view of Adorno *et al.,* Erikson, Lifton, and the other theorists of the totalitarian influence approach, individuals in Western culture experience in varying degrees the tensions which fuel totalist movements, and most participate in conformist social groups, e.g., religions, college fraternities, the armed services, dysfunctional families, which are totalistic to one degree or another. This prophetic critique of conventional society is an intrinsic part of the totalitarian influence approach to explaining totalistic conversion, and it tends to blur the boundary between pervasive authoritarian conformism in the culture and the totalitarianism of extremist groups.

IV. CONTROVERSIES OVER CULTS

After the Korean War and the furor over the treatment of POW's subsided, popular media and even scholarly interest in brainwashing declined. There was a resur-

gence in the mid-1970s, which was initially associated with the criminal career and trial of Patricia Hearst.

Beginning in the middle 1970s, an intensive anticult movement began to form which adopted the brainwashing argument as a central dimension of its ideology. This movement worked to oppose the apparent popularity of esoteric religious or religio-therapy movements ("cults") such as The Church of Scientology, The Unification Church, Hare Krishna, or The Children of God, which had initially at least gained most of their converts from the 1960s counterculture. According to anticult ideology, such counterculture religions employ brainwashing techniques to beguile and enslave participants and to enable the latter to be ruthlessly exploited.

Initially the primary social practice adopted by the anticult movement for combatting alleged cultic brainwashing was "deprogramming." Deprogramming is an intensive influence practice whereby individuals are removed from residence in religious groups and subjected to counterindoctrination. Deprogramming usually transpires under conditions of forcible restraint following a kidnapping, sometimes involves legally mandated incarceration imposed under conservatorship laws, and occasionally occurs through the voluntary agreement of the convert.

Deprogramming was designed to free converts from the alleged psychic imprisonment caused by cultic brainwashing. Sometimes it was successful in convincing people to withdraw from the religious group, sometimes not. When it was not successful litigation often ensued, either kidnapping charges or disputes over the use of conservatorship laws in support of deprogramming.

Although litigation over deprogramming persists, by the early 1980s, legal reverses had led to less reliance upon coercive deprogramming as the primary anticult tactic. The anticult movement had switched its emphasis to civil actions against cults for fraud, infliction of emotional distress, false imprisonment, and other legal causes of action. These claims are buttressed in court by testimony about the effects of psychologically coercive cultic conditioning in radically undermining the personal autonomy and responsibility of participants and disorienting and psychologically damaging the latter. Similar claims have arisen in a variety of other legal areas including child custody cases, prosecutions against members or leaders of certain groups for various crimes (e.g., child abuse), and prosecutions of former members who seek to base defenses of insanity or diminished capacity on claims about mind control and disorienting trauma.

Throughout the 1980s, litigants' legal briefs and supportive expert testimony and depositions tended to refer to "brainwashing," "coercive persuasion," and "thought reform" and often to the "foundational" work in this area by Edgar Schein, Robert Lifton, and Hinkle and Wolff. Margaret Singer, a clinical psychologist, and Richard Ofshe, a sociologist, were the most active anticult witnesses, and they also co-authored articles formulating their version of anticult brainwashing theory. Singer and Ofshe also played leadership roles in the anticult movement itself, serving on the boards of anticult organizations and publications, and giving talks at their conferences.

Although anticult witnesses claim to be using the theories of totalitarian influence developed by Schein, Lifton, and Hinkle and Wolff, their actual testimony bears the hallmarks of the brainwashing arguments developed by Hunter, Sargent, Farber *et al.*, and others. Anticult witnesses claim that cultic brainwashing regularly produces involuntary acceptance of ideologies and memberships which bear no relationship to converts predisposing motives and true beliefs. In some cases, the identity displayed by converts is described as, in effect, a dissociated false self while the true self is allegedly suppressed by cultic manipulations.

Anticult witnesses typically allege that such mental enslavement is produced by "hypnotic" processes, which are allegedly constituted by normal religious activities, e.g., meditation, repetitive chanting, guided imagery or boring lectures, as well as practices which allegedly induce "primitive" states of consciousness through other means such as pseudo-psychotherapeutic emotional arousal or physiological debilitation supposedly resulting from poor diet or too little sleep.

Anticult witnesses testify that such altered states of consciousness constitute a primitive condition of mind in which suggestibility is enhanced and in which the "conditioning" procedures of cults are more effective. They insist that physical coercion is not an essential factor in totalitarian influence. They also insist that there is a clear dividing line other than physical coercion between the influence tactics of totalitarian groups and cults, on the one hand, and those of conventional institutions such as the Catholic Church, the army, college fraternities, mental hospitals, and so on. (They have considerable difficulty articulating what

that dividing line consists of, however. The only criteria that they have come up with are exceedingly imprecise, e.g., the alleged "intensity and pervasiveness of cultic conditioning procedures.")

In several important cases, the robot brainwashing paradigm of Farber, Harlow, and West was explicitly used as the framework for describing the conditioning of the former cultic allegiances and attitudes of the plaintiffs. The altered states allegedly induced by cultic rituals are said to produce intense sensations which gurus and prophets falsely interpret in persuasive terms which manipulate the practitioners to submit to the group and its leadership.

Richard Delgado, in a series of law review articles, has articulated the basic legal rationale for heightened control of religious movements by the government, e.g., civil suits such as those described above, laws regulating religious practices, and conservatorships for the purposes of involuntary deprogramming. Delgado's analysis is designed to explain why the constitutional protection of freedom of religion does not apply where cults are concerned. Basically what his argument boils down to is that if conversion to a religion is involuntary, then prohibitions against governmental regulation of religion do not really apply.

Delgado argues that state intervention is legitimate when a person joins a group under conditions in which consensuality (or voluntariness) is not present. Delgado's formulation of what such involuntariness or loss of free will at the hands of cults actually consists of is heavily dependent upon robot brainwashing conceptions, however. He avoids citing any of the methodologically superior studies on conversion to new religious movements that have failed to confirm the brainwashing analyses.

Delgado's formulation, which has influenced a number of appellate court outcomes, treats deception as a functional equivalent of physical coercion in terms of bringing the indoctrinee onto the premises and keeping him or her there pending application of the high powered brainwashing psycho-technology. In 1988, a California Supreme Court decision influenced by Delgado's point of view abridged the constitutional protection which would otherwise be accorded even to religious speech acts constituting "coercive persuasion" in the special case in which a group has concealed its identity. The legal strategy of those making claims of destructive psychological manipulation against cults is to expand the boundary condition of concealment of the identity of the organization to include conduct such as not warning recruits of controversial anticult allegations that group practices and rituals such as medication or chanting produce dangerous dissociative states and heightened suggestibility.

The anticult strategy of basing civil suits upon robot brainwashing testimony was initially, in the late 1970s and early to middle 1980s, very effective. Juries were almost without exception responsive to this line of testimony and were for the most part not persuaded by contrary testimony put on by defense experts which pointed out the scholarly deficiencies of brainwashing analyses. Survey evidence indicates that the general public widely accepts the accuracy of cultic brainwashing analyses, and the widespread acceptance of such theories is apparently too deeply ingrained for scientific witnesses for the defense to be able to penetrate it.

Several cases resulted in judgments for the plaintiffs in the 20 to 30 million dollar range. One of these judgments required a number of state organizations of the Hare Krishna movement to go into receivership and put the continued existence of this movement in the American context in peril. Some knowledgeable observers contended that as a result of these events the separation of church and state in the United States was in greater doubt than it had ever been.

Recently, i.e., from 1985 until the present, the legal pendulum seems to be swinging the other way, primarily because of the judicial application of rules with respect to the necessity that expert testimony must meet general scientific standards of acceptability before it can be presented to a jury. Several important decisions have been overturned on appeal on the grounds that the robot brainwashing paradigm is not generally accepted as valid in the relevant scientific community, i.e., in psychology and sociology, and therefore should not be used as a basis for the circumvention of governmental guarantees of freedom of religion. (Margaret Singer was the primary witness in two of these cases.)

Moreover, several courts have held in advance of the actual trials in anticult brainwashing cases that anticult brainwashing witnesses could not testify because their theories were not generally accepted in the academic world. In two of these cases, Margaret Singer's and Richard Ofshe's testimony was specifically excluded upon the grounds of its lack of scientific

acceptance, and also because their testimony did not represent an accurate interpretation of its claimed theoretical foundation, i.e., Lifton's and Schein's theories of totalitarian influence.

A. Scientific Problems with Anticult Brainwashing Testimony

For the most part, crude and sensational robot/brainwashing, "Manchurian Candidate" theories such as flourished in the 1950s and early 1960s are currently not taken seriously in the academic world, although they appear in popular volumes with evocations of cultists "snapping" in and out of states of mind control. As we have indicated, models which are utilized in claims of psychological coercion made against cults tend to veer in the "robot" direction, particularly in the form in which such theories are presented in court testimony and depositions.

Formulations that veer in the robot direction tend to have the following characteristics. (1) Cultist mind control is seen as very effective. (2) Predisposing motivational factors are either denied or are trivialized as mere buttons pushed by manipulative indoctrinators. Predisposing factors are definitely not viewed as evidence that participation in cults is voluntary. (3) Dissociative states, hypnotic processes, and altered states of consciousness are emphasized, as well as consequent patterns of defective or impaired thinking. (4) Indoctrinees are presumed to thoroughly lose their capacity to make decisions, i.e., there is a definite loss of free will. (5) "Mind controlling" organizations are regarded as utilizing techniques of influence which are qualitatively distinct from those used in mainstream institutions. These five emphases are attributes of robot brainwashing arguments which are contradicted by the theories of totalitarian influence developed by Lifton, Schein, Erikson, Adorno *et al.*, and others.

In addition to the incompatibility of robot brainwashing testimony with its claimed theoretical foundation, it also is generally incompatible with almost all of the research upon the question of brainwashing in cults which has been published in mainstream scientific journals. There has been abundant research upon "new religions" or "cults" in recent decades. A number of trends have emerged in these findings which appear to be incompatible with brainwashing models but may be more consistent with a theory of interaction between motivational factors and the properties of totalitarianism.

1. Research has indicated that there is considerable interest in exotic religious groups among young persons that is not explainable in terms of coercive influence. Many students indicate that they would be interested in associations with alternative groups even before they have ever had actual contact with one. It is not, therefore, a matter of initially hostile persons (such as POW's) who may subsequently face an overriding of their will and radical alteration of their ideas through thought reform. There is a pool of preconverts with pre-existing orientations compatible with involvement in some esoteric or controversial groups.

2. A number of studies have examined the process of induction into controversial and stigmatized movements such as the Unification Church ("Moonies"). Such conversion usually consists of several stages of increasingly more intensive involvement occurring over several weeks or months, rather than being a simple all or nothing decision. It is apparent from such studies that only a small percentage of persons who go through each stage of influence actually go on to the next stage of the process.

Those who actually complete the process and become full-fledged members are a very small fraction of those who are initially contacted by the movement. The process, therefore, cannot reasonably be portrayed as overwhelmingly effective in overriding individual predilections. Moreover, questionnaires and interviews administered at each stage of the process indicate that the people who continue at each stage are being persuaded by theological arguments and symbols rather than being mindlessly responsive to suggestion because of being in a primitive state of consciousness.

A careful study of the Unification influence process by Eileen Barker, an English sociologist, rejected the notion that an overwhelming external stimulus from the influence procedures themselves accounted for the (few) conversions which were affected. Her book reporting this study won an award for distinguished scientific achievement by the leading professional association in the sociology and psychology of religion.

3. Numerous studies have indicated that most converts do not remain long in high-demand, marginal religious groups, particularly highly stigmatized communal groups such as the Unification Church. Such high-demand groups appear to be somewhat like "revolving doors," with persons continually coming and going. The average length of membership in the Unification Church, for instance, is 2 years.

Moreover, most people leave such groups voluntarily rather than through involuntary deprogramming or through other contact with the anticult movement. This pattern of sporadic affiliation and disaffiliation seems more consistent with the typical voluntary, bidirectional influence process between individuals and groups in a pluralistic society than it does with a totally unidirectional process in which an individual is a helpless captive of overwhelmingly external influence.

On the other hand, groups such as the Meher Baba movement, which are not totalistic, not communal, and which are compatible with other social involvements and normal career tracks appear to keep their members over a longer period. The latter type of groups do not generally tend to be controversial or to attract allegations of brainwashing.

4. There are a number of clinical studies that indicate that involvement in certain demanding and controversial groups produces a sense of well-being or "relief from neurotic distress" on the part of many converts. This is quite consistent with the psychology of totalism approach, which has shown that totalitarian or authoritarian movements tend to reduce conscious emotional pain resulting from pre-existing identity confusion or negative identities. The findings that alternative religions reduce neurotic distress are incompatible with brainwashing analyses, on the other hand, which insist that such involvements have a uniformly negative impact upon mental health.

Other clinical studies have indicated an absence of serious psychopathology in some highly stigmatized groups, although depth psychological factors such as those intrinsic to totalitarian influence approaches such as those of Fromm, Adorno *et al.*, Erikson, etc., have usually not been dealt with in these studies.

5. A number of studies have indicated that ex-devotees are much more likely to attest that they had been "brainwashed" by and to strongly recriminate against a group if they had been forcibly removed from the group and if they had substantial subsequent contact with "anticult" networks which conduct de-

programming and other "rehabilitation" programs, e.g., "exit counseling," ex-member support groups, etc. The vast majority of ex-members, on the other hand, who leave groups voluntarily and have no substantial contact with the anticult movement tend to view their experiences with these groups much more favorably and do not see themselves as having been brainwashed.

Authors of these studies tend to interpret these findings as indicating that the brainwashing view of cultic membership results from indoctrination by the anticult movement, which itself has some of the characteristics of a totalistic social movement, rather than being an objective empirical description of the experience.

6. There are a number of well-designed studies indicating cognitive competence among devotees of certain controversial groups. This would seem to disconfirm the more lurid robot brainwashing analyses which maintain that members of totalistic groups subsist during their tenures in such groups in primitive, dissociated states of consciousness.

7. Some research has evaluated the existence of personality factors predisposing individuals to join totalistic religious movements. Anthony and Robbins conducted participant observation studies of the Unification Church and reported some qualitative impressions and phenomenological analyses of the conversion process in terms of the conversion of negative to contrast identities along the lines described by Erikson and Lifton. Another researcher published a study which interpreted the conversion process in a Jesus movement commune in terms of a totalistic conversion process. Anthony and his research team at the Graduate Theological Union, one of whom was Nevitt Sanford, one of the co-authors of *The Authoritarian Personality,* evaluated the incidence of authoritarianism in a variety of alternative religious movements. They administered an updated version of the F scale, which is designed to measure the personality syndrome underlying attraction to authoritarian movements. The average scale score did vary widely from movement to movement, indicating that variation in individual totalism may indeed be a factor in explaining why people join specific movements and are not attracted to others. In the typology of new religious movements published in the book *Spiritual Choices,* Anthony and Ecker report that one group of alternative religions,

which includes the People's Temple and Synanon, is characterized by authoritarianism and contrast identities among their members.

In addition to these few studies on psychological totalitarianism in alternative religions, considerable research has been done over a period of 40 years indicating that some traditionally conservative religious groups attract people who score highly on various measures of totalitarianism, e.g., the F scale or Rokeach's Dogmatism scale. Such people also tend to score highly upon measures of ethnocentrism. (Some of the most important research of this sort is reported in the books upon "right-ring authoritarianism" by Bob Altemeyer.)

It seems likely that these results upon certain Christian groups would generalize to alternative religious movements or cults, as many of them have theological and social beliefs that seem similar to those in some fundamentalist denominations. These results are also compatible with Lifton's insistence that fundamentalist religious movements are totalistic, and with the few studies specifically evaluating totalism in new religions. In general, then, there is some intriguing evidence supporting a totalitarian influence explanation of conversion to alternative religions, and this would seem to be a fruitful direction for further exploration. The same research tends to contradict brainwashing explanations for conversion, however, because proponents of the latter paradigm insist that people who join cults do so only because of external influence and not because of personality characteristics that predate contact with the group.

In the legal arena the outcomes of claims pressed about cults in various kinds of cases have been mixed. Nevertheless, in recent years those critics of cults who employ a brainwashing model have consistently experienced key setbacks. Certain legal weaknesses of the model have emerged: (1) Brainwashing theories have been seen to challenge the authenticity and truth of devotees' faith in a manner which elicits the constraints of the first amendment. Attempts to explicitly legalize the coercive deprogramming of adult converts through guardianships or conservatorships issued to parents fell afoul of this objection. (2) Absent the objective standard of physical restraint or threat, experts wanting to testify about cultic thought reform have had difficulty in credibly "drawing the line" between influence procedures which allegedly are and those which are not so overwhelmingly coercive as to incapacitate converts such that their commitment becomes involuntary.

Given some degree of emotional intensity, group solidarity, and experiential ritual behavior such as meditation, almost any group can be accused of using psychological coercion by virtue of alleged hypnotic trance states, emotional manipulation, and pressure for group conformity. Physical constraint or threat, which might provide some objective criteria for line drawing, has been explicitly rejected by cultic brainwashing theorists since the groups being considered clearly do not use physical coercion as a characteristic mechanism of social control or indoctrination.

Decisions in a series of cases have found that Lifton's theory of thought reform may not be used as the basis for brainwashing testimony in the absence of extreme physical coercion. Several courts have found that in the absence of scientifically credible criteria for drawing the line between groups that brainwash and those that do not, brainwashing testimony expresses a constitutionally impermissible attempt to restrict the freedom of religious belief.

The lack of scientific criteria for drawing the line was one reason why in 1990 a federal judge barred the testimony of Margaret Singer and Richard Ofshe about alleged brainwashing in support of a diminished capacity defense of an ex-Scientologist being prosecuted for mail fraud.

Some courts making procedural rulings to bar testimony about psychological coercion in cults were explicitly influenced by the action of the American Psychological Association in rejecting a report which had been authored by a task force appointed by the APA to report on alleged coercive persuasion in cults and other groups. Originally appointed by the APA, and chaired by Margaret Singer who was the senior author of its report, the task force was composed primarily of scholars and clinicians who are active in advocacy against cults and in court cases. After receiving evaluations of the task force's report by several outside reviewers, the APA rejected the report and declined to issue it as an official APA document because it did not meet the APA's standards of scientific acceptability. The rejection of the report was cited as proof that the anticult brainwashing theory is not generally accepted in the relevant scientific community in

procedural rulings in the two cases in which Margaret Singer's and Richard Ofshe's testimony was forbidden in advance of the trial.

In the light of the sequence of cases in which anticult brainwashing testimony has been excluded as unscientific, and/or unconstitutional, it seems likely that judges will no longer permit such testimony in most courtrooms. The proposed use of thought reform research as a basis of testimony with respect to cults makes it likely that a witness will not be allowed to testify at all, or will have his testimony severely limited. Consequently, such experts are seeking other theoretical grounds for criticizing allegedly coercive conversion processes in new religious or therapeutic movements.

Recently a number of "experts," including Richard Ofshe in several cases, who were testifying or proposing to testify about psychological pressure in religious or therapeutic groups, specifically denied that their testimony would be based upon research with respect to brainwashing, coercive persuasion, or thought reform, or to POW research and the work of Schein and Lifton, etc.

V. VIOLENCE AND VOLATILITY

It is conceivable that in the aftermath of the shocking apparent collective suicide of members of a "cult" in Waco, Texas, in April of 1993, the robot/brainwashing model, which has suffered legal setbacks, may recover some of its prestige. It is ironic that tragic events such as Waco and the 1978 mass suicides in Jonestown should be popularly viewed as supportive of brainwashing perspectives. Sympathetic discussions of such theories as applied to cults often appear to depict cult leaders as motivated by selfish and material interests. Why then should such "con men" consider suicide to be in their interest? A more promising avenue of inquiry might consider Erikson's notion of the relationship between "negative identity" and totalism. Individuals with polarized identities find in apocalyptic sects a meaning system which can alleviate emotional distress by projecting negativity onto scapegoats and demonic outsiders while constructing a "purified self" for the leader as well as the members. But such resolutions are always precarious such that the group and its individual members may be highly volatile. Threats to the "boundary" of the group are met with paranoia and militant defensiveness.

The raid on the Davidian Waco compound by federal agents in February of 1993 apparently appeared to confirm leader David Koresh's violent apocalyptic visions, but on another level it threatened to disconfirm his beliefs, i.e., if he were captured or gave himself up peacefully and the world went on as before, his totalist system of psycho-ideological reconstruction would collapse. What Robert Lifton has called "revolutionary immortality" was imperiled, and consequently revolutionary suicide provided a way out.

The tragedy which ensued in Waco in April of 1993 may be more explicable in terms of the psychology of totalism rather than brainwashing theory. The further development and application of the former analytical perspective might ultimately be conducive to the development of *strategies of mediation* which might be more effective than the confrontational tactics sometimes favored by those persons influenced by brainwashing notions.

This article has been reprinted from the *Encyclopedia of Human Behavior, Volume 1.*

BIBLIOGRAPHY

Adorno, T., Frenkel-Brunswick, E., Levinson, D., and Sanford, N. (1950). "The Authoritarian Personality." Norton, New York.

Anthony, D. (1990). Religious movements and brainwashing litigation. In "In Gods We Trust" (T. Robbins and D. Anthony, Eds.), 2d ed. Transaction, New Brunswick, NJ.

Anthony, D., and Robbins, T. (1991). Law, social science and the "brainwashing" exception to the first amendment. *Behav. Sci. Law* 10 (1), 5.

Arendt, H. (1979). "The Origins of Totalitarianism." Harcourt Brace Jovanovich, San Diego.

Barker, E. (1984). "The Making of a Moonie: Choice or Brainwashing?" Blackwell, Oxford.

Bromley, D., and Richardson, J. (1983). "The Brainwashing–Deprogramming Controversy." Edwin Mellen, New York/Toronto.

Bromley, D., and Hadden, J. (Eds.) (1993). "Handbook of Cults and Sects in America," Vols. 3–4. J.A.I. Press, Greenwich, CT.

Erikson, E. (1942). Hitler's imagery and German youth. *Psychiatry* 5, 475–493.

Erikson, E. (1953). Wholeness and totality—a psychiatric contribution. In "Totalitarianism: Proceedings of a Conference Held at the American Academy of Arts and Sciences." Harvard University Press, Cambridge MA.

Friedrich, C., and Brzezinski, Z. (1956). "Totalitarian Dictatorship & Autocracy." Praeger, New York.

Hinkle, L. E., Jr., and Wolff, H. E. (1956). Communist interrogation and the indoctrination of "enemies of the states." *A.M.A. Arch. Neurol. Psych.* 76, 117.

Hunter, E. (1951). "Brainwashing in Red China." Vanguard, New York.

Lifton, R. (1989). "Chinese Thought Reform and the Psychology of Totalism." University of North Carolina Press, Chapel Hill.

Marks, J. (1980). "The Search for the Manchurian Candidate." Random House, New York.

Singer, M., and Ofshe, R. (1992). Thought reform programs and the production of psychiatric casualties. *Psychiatric Ann.* 20 (4), 188.

Burnout

Michael P. Leiter

Acadia University

Christina Maslach

University of California, Berkeley

Burnout   A syndrome of emotional exhaustion, depersonalization, and reduced personal accomplishment that is a particular risk for individuals who work with other people in some capacity.

Cynicism   A state of psychological distance from one's work, usually associated with doubts about its significance.

Depersonalization   A negative, callous, or excessively detached response to other people (often the recipients of one's service or care).

Emotional Exhaustion   Feelings of being emotionally overextended and depleted of one's emotional resources.

Engagement with Work   An energetic state of involvement with personally fulfilling activities that enhance one's sense of professional efficacy.

Organizational Health   An organizational design that balances work demands with resources in a manner that facilitates individual health.

Personal Accomplishment   Feelings of competence and successful achievement in work.

Professional Community   A network of collegial affiliations, including the sharing of technical expertise, emotional attachment, and a professional service ethic (commitment to service quality).

Professional Efficacy   The expectation based upon experience that one can have an intentional impact through one's occupation.

BURNOUT is a type of prolonged response to chronic emotional and interpersonal stressors on the job. It has been long recognized as a serious problem for people who work in interpersonally oriented occupations, such as the human services. This article will present a multidimensional model of burnout and its healthy alternative, work engagement. It will analyze the causes and consequences of burnout, as well as summarize various strategies for prevention and remediation of this syndrome.

I. INTRODUCTION

Burnout is a psychological syndrome of emotional exhaustion, depersonalization, and reduced personal accomplishment, which is a special risk for individuals who work with other people in some capacity. It is considered to be an individual stress experience embedded in a context of complex social relationships, and it involves the person's conception of both self and others.

A. Burnout Components

This three-component conceptualization of burnout stands in contrast to most unidimensional models of stress. Emotional exhaustion refers to feelings of being emotionally overextended and depleted of one's emotional resources. Depersonalization refers to a negative, callous, or excessively detached response to other people (often the recipients of one's service or care). Reduced personal accomplishment refers to a decline in feelings of competence and successful achievement in one's work.

Recent work has extended the burnout concept to occupations other than the human services by recasting the burnout components in relation to work that is highly involving, rather than just to work with service recipients. In this conceptual extension, the three burnout components are considered to be exhaustion, cynicism, and reduced professional efficacy. The new exhaustion construct does not make exclusive reference to emotional issues, while the new professional efficacy refers to personal feelings of effectiveness independent of work that has an impact on people. The cynicism factor differs to the greatest extent from its corresponding human service factor, depersonalization. It includes doubts about the importance of work and feelings of indifference toward it, while depersonalization describes a distant, cold view of service recipients.

The principal measure of burnout is the Maslach Burnout Inventory (MBI), which provides distinct assessments of the three burnout components. Different forms of the MBI have been developed for different types of occupations: the human services survey (MBI–HSS), the educators survey (MBI–ES), and the general survey (MBI–GS). As a result of international interest in burnout research, the MBI has been translated into many languages.

B. The Burnout Experience

The costs of burnout are evident in staff members' physical and mental well-being, career development, and work behaviors.

1. Health Symptoms

Physical consequences of the exhaustion of burnout include headaches, gastrointestinal illness, high blood pressure, muscle tension, and chronic fatigue. Symptoms of associated mental distress include anxiety, depression, and sleep disturbances. There are important distinctions between burnout and depression. Depression is a clinical syndrome whereas burnout describes a crisis in one's relationship with work, especially therapeutic relationships with service recipients or creative involvement with a task. Depression is global, pervading every aspect of a person's life, whereas burnout is specific to the job. As a clinical syndrome, depression is a quality of an individual, whereas burnout is more a personal reaction to the social environment of an organization. People experiencing severe depression may be incapacitated in all domains of their life. A person experiencing burnout may be functioning well outside of the occupational context. As such, burnout and depression are distinct psychological concepts. A close examination supports the idea that burnout is not a clinical syndrome, but a cognitive and emotional state that is responsive to the social and organizational environment in which people work. [See DEPRESSION.]

2. Job Behaviors

Burnout has been associated with absenteeism and intention to quit jobs. There is anecdotal evidence of individuals who ended a career in nursing or mental health work as a consequence of significant burnout crises. These changes occur at great cost to individuals who walk away from careers to which they have committed time, effort, and money in training and experience. Whether in human service work or other fields, burnout is primarily a hazard for people who deeply care about their work. Leaving behind a career to which one has made such a commitment may have a devastating impact.

For people who do not leave a career, burnout is inconsistent with productivity and fulfillment at work. Exhaustion and distance from people and work are incompatible with the extra effort and focus necessary to produce work of exceptional quality. There is evidence that the presence of some individuals experiencing burnout in a work setting influences their colleagues' relationship with their work: burnout tends to perpetuate itself through informal interactions on the job. While the primary impact of burnout is at work, it also has an impact on family life.

Burnout is associated with decreased commitment to a job or an organization. That is, people experiencing exhaustion and low levels of accomplishment are less enthusiastic about the organization with which they work and less willing to exert effort to help it to meet its goals. They are less likely to believe that they share basic values with their organization when experiencing burnout. A similar pattern is evident in regard to job satisfaction: the reduction in a sense of accomplishment or effectiveness that is a central component of the experience of burnout diminishes opportunities for satisfying experiences at work. This relationship may be somewhat circular in that dissatisfaction with work may aggravate subsequent experiences of burnout.

II. A PROCESS MODEL OF BURNOUT

There is an established body of evidence that burnout is related to the organizational environments in which people work. In general, the emotional exhaustion and depersonalization components of the syndrome arise from demands and conflicts confronting workers, while personal accomplishment is influenced by the availability of social support and opportunities to develop professionally. The complex relationships among various aspects of organizational environments with the three components of burnout have encouraged the development of structural models in much of burnout research. This approach permits researchers to examine the contribution of many potential influences and consequences simultaneously, separating unique contributors to the development of burnout from those that are redundant with one another. Figure 1 displays a process model of burnout that summarizes major research findings.

In the center of Figure 1 are the three components of burnout: exhaustion, depersonalization (or cynicism), and personal accomplishment (or efficacy). The relationship from exhaustion to depersonalization is the most reliable aspect of the process model. Exhaustion is not only strongly related to depersonalization, but it mediates the relationship of organizational factors with depersonalization. For example, work overload does not have a direct impact on depersonalization, but only on exhaustion. Staff members depersonalize only to the extent to which organizational demands are experienced as exhausting. In contrast, the relationship of accomplishment with the other two components of burnout does not necessarily signify direct causal paths between them. Various aspects of organizational environments can aggravate exhaustion and diminish personal accomplishment or effectiveness simultaneously. These aspects of the work environment have a direct impact on staff members' sense of accomplishment: they are not mediated through ex-

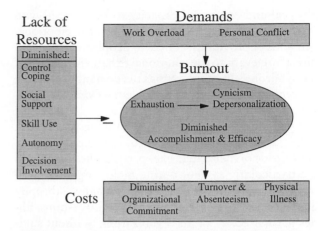

Figure 1 General model of burnout, with major antecedents and consequences. From Maslach, C., Jackson, S. E., & Leiter, M. P. (1996). *Maslach burnout inventory manual* (3rd ed.). Palo Alto, CA: Consulting Psychologists Press. Modified and reproduced by special permission of the Publisher, Consulting Psychologists Press, Inc., Palo Alto, CA 94303 from the *Maslach Burnout Inventory Manual* by Christina Maslach, Susan E. Jackson, and Michael P. Leiter. Copyright 1996 by Consulting Psychologists Press, Inc. All rights reserved. Further reproduction is prohibited without the Publisher's written consent.

haustion, although they may be experienced as exhausting as well as diminishing a staff member's sense of accomplishment. This sense of discouragement may occur in work that is not necessarily exhausting. In fact, work that is not at all challenging may undermine a staff member's sense of accomplishment or effectiveness over time.

A. Contributing Factors to Burnout

1. Job Characteristics

The primary antecedents of exhaustion are work overload and personal conflict at work. Demands to do too much work in too little time deplete staff members' capacity to be involved energetically and emotionally in their work. Human service providers are concerned with excessive caseloads that interfere with their capacity to address the personal, emotionally charged issues confronting their clientele. They find the pressures of excessive caseloads to be incompatible with their ideals. In their attempts to provide high-quality services they overextend themselves through long hours that invade their personal time or through an unsustainable level of intensity at work. Exhaustion occurs when they are unable to replenish their physical and emotional capacity to be engaged with their work. In human service settings, the emotional demands of providing services to people in distress are directly relevant to the emotional exhaustion aspect of the syndrome. In other settings the demands of intense concentration and creative problem solving are a major cause of exhaustion.

Qualitative work overload is an issue when work demands require staff members to accept responsibilities outside of their range of expertise. These problems are particularly evident during major organizational transitions when work roles may change abruptly due to downsizing or realignments of job responsibilities across sectors of an organization. Without sufficient support from colleagues or through training programs, an opportunity to expand work responsibilities may become an unsustainable burden. Qualitative work overload is evident when service providers lack sufficient resources to address persistent problems of their clients. Service providers who interpret clients' problems as arising from endemic poverty, social isolation, or racism may be overwhelmed by the difficulties in effecting meaningful change. People in management positions often encounter abrupt expansions of their job responsibilities with little preparation. Although they may be highly motivated to expand their range of activity, they are vulnerable to the exhausting demands of working outside their range of experience.

Personal conflict is the second major contributor to exhaustion. Conflict with colleagues, supervisors, subordinates, or service recipients undermines staff members' confidence in their worksetting. The frequency of conflict as well as its intensity make demands upon the emotional energy of staff members. In addition to the direct experience of conflict, witnessing personal conflict among others contributes to strain. Conflict has an impact on exhaustion both through its demands on the emotional energy of individuals as well as through its weakening of staff members' confidence in the social environment of the organization. Conflict in an organizational environment is indicative of distinct and incompatible values among members of an organization or between these members and their constituents. Together, conflict and work overload constitute ongoing demands on staff members that imply substantial problems with the social environment of the organization.

Staff members' capacity to manage these demands depends to a large extent upon the resources they have available to them. Among the most central resources that have been a focus of burnout research are collegiality, skill development, control, and cooperative interactions with service recipients. Collegiality includes both supportive relationships with supervisor as well as coworkers. Although both types of support are of general relevance to burnout, level of supervisor support is more apt to be negatively related to exhaustion while coworker support is more closely related to personal accomplishment. Supervisors are not only sources of potential praise or recognition, they also have control over many of the demands faced by staff members. An antagonistic relationship with a supervisor implies a lack of control over work responsibilities and access to necessary resources. Coworker support has fewer implications for control over workload, and therefore less impact on exhaustion, but has more implications for staff members' evaluations of their accomplishments or effectiveness. Staff members often consider recognition and support from coworkers as reflecting a deeper understanding of the actual demands that they confront in a job. Often this recognition is more personally satisfying, although recognition from people in authority may have more of an impact on practical aspects of work. In contrast to the contradictory values implied by enduring conflict, active expressions of support suggest that colleagues share fundamental values and perspectives within the organization. This implicit agreement builds staff members' sense of accomplishment and professional efficacy.

Among human service professions, client cooperation is an important component of social support at work. In many service sectors cooperation or active appreciation from recipients are unusual. When they are not directly evident, service providers are more dependent on the other aspects of the organizational context—supervisors and coworkers—for validation and support. The direct response of an appreciative service recipient on whom a staff member has had a noticeable impact is a powerful confirmation of the value of work. On the other extreme, interacting with service recipients who resent receiving services and who actively resist whatever assistance is provided undermines staff members' sense of personal accomplishment. [*See* SOCIAL SUPPORT.]

In addition to these predictors of burnout that arise from the conduct of the central tasks of an organization, opportunities for professional development influence the manner in which burnout develops. The use and development of sophisticated occupational skills are consistent with a strong sense of accomplishment and effectiveness and thus contrary to the experience of burnout. Skill use and development confirm the value of the staff member to the organization and confirm a consistency between individual and group values. When in conflict they aggravate exhaustion through repetitive tedium in the work and a lack of career direction.

Another relevant area of organizational life is the opportunity for staff members to participate in decisions that affect their work and to exercise autonomy over their contributions. Participation in decision making may occur in a variety of ways, all of which imply a sharing of power among members of an organization. Group decision making may occur because of an individual initiative of a manager or as part of an organizational policy assigning prerogatives to organizational entities. Participation may range from serving an advisory role prior to major decisions through voting privileges to a full consensus model of unit management. Full participation in shared decision making provides a means through which staff members may enact their values through their work.

2. Personal Characteristics

Although the research on burnout has focused primarily on the organizational context in which people work, it has also considered a range of personal qualities. One of the most promising areas has been that of coping styles. Burnout is consistent with a escape-oriented coping style in which people avoid thinking about difficulties at work and avoid demanding situations that arise during the workday. In contrast, people who use a control-oriented coping pattern experience less burnout. This pattern includes cognitive strategies, such as clarifying goals and managing time, as well as actions, such as discussing problems directly with supervisors and coworkers. Further, burnout is consistent with self-defeating symptom management. In fact, depersonalization or cynicism itself is an ineffective attempt to cope with excessive exhaustion that undermines a staff member's effectiveness. By putting distance between themselves and their jobs or their service recipients, staff have less opportunity for self-fulfilling work. As a consequence, high levels of de-

personalization or cynicism are inevitably associated with high levels of exhaustion: there is no evidence that distancing oneself from work reduces exhaustion.

Although thought of as a personal characteristic, coping patterns are not entirely independent of the work context. Some organizational settings are tolerant or even supportive of active coping on the part of staff members. In other settings people in authority react punitively to staff members' attempts to take control of the problems they confront in their work, and colleagues disparage their actions. Although control coping is associated with reduced burnout, it is also related to greater supervisor support and the presence of open organizational decision making processes. The work environment is a powerful social environment that shapes a wide range of experiences and behaviors. [See COPING WITH STRESS.]

Research on other personality variables, such as Type A behavior pattern or locus of control, has produced inconsistent results. Some research suggests that people with Type A behavior pattern are more prone to burnout, but other research has identified situations under which the reverse appears to be true. As with coping styles, it remains unclear how much of what is being defined as personality characteristics are functions of long-term development or of the ongoing work context.

There are few consistent relationships of burnout with demographic characteristics. Although weak associations with gender, age, or years of experience are reported in the literature, the only widely reported pattern is a tendency for men to score slightly higher on depersonalization. These weak demographic relationships are congruent with the view that the work environment is of greater significance than personal characteristics in the development of burnout.

B. Engagement with Work

At the opposite end of the scale from burnout is a productive and fulfilling state of engagement with work, which is an energetic experience of involvement with personally fulfilling activities that enhance a staff member's sense of professional efficacy. This state is distinct from established constructs in organizational psychology of organizational commitment, job involvement, or job satisfaction. It is characterized by an energetic, intense focus on work associated with feelings of effectiveness that are based upon experiences of enacting values through work. The extensive research on burnout has consistently found linear relationships of workplace conditions across the full range of the MBI subscales. Just as high levels of personal conflict are associated with high levels of emotional exhaustion, low levels of conflict are strong predictors of low exhaustion. Conversely, high personal accomplishment is associated with supportive personal relationships, the enhancement of sophisticated skills at work, and active participation in shared decision making. These patterns indicate that the opposite of burnout is not a neutral state, but a definite state of mental health within the occupational domain. While the burnout concept describes a syndrome of distress that may arise from enduring problems with work, engagement describes a positive state of fulfillment.

III. THE ORGANIZATIONAL CONTEXT OF BURNOUT AND ENGAGEMENT

Figure 2 summarizes the relationship of organizational environments with the continuum of burnout through engagement. Many aspects of the social environment of organizations are related to the experience of burnout. Burnout arises from strained interactions with a variety of people at work, and has its principal manifestations in problematic interactions with service recipients. There remains considerable research to be done to specify the precise relationships

between specific aspects of an organizational environment with a single component of burnout. Although the evidence is conclusive that interpersonal conflict of any sort is strongly related to emotional exhaustion, the relationship between control coping and burnout is less consistent across organizations. In some settings control coping styles both alleviate exhaustion and enhance personal accomplishment or effectiveness.

A newly developed model of the burnout–engagement continuum may provide greater insight into the relationship between the organizational environment and people's experiences of burnout. This model focuses on the match, or fit, between the worker and the workplace. It proposes that the greater the match, the greater the likelihood of engagement; conversely, the greater the mismatch, the greater the likelihood of burnout. This framework builds on prior theories of job–person fit, but its unique contribution is the specification of six areas in which this match or mismatch can take place: workload, control, reward, community, fairness, and values. This model focuses attention on the relationship between the person and the social environment, rather than either one or the other in isolation. It provides a new way of identifying the sources of burnout and engagement in any particular job context, and of designing interventions that will actually incorporate situational changes along with personal ones. Furthermore, the recognition of six areas of job–person mismatch expands the range of options for intervention. Confirmatory research has yet to be done, but this approach is very promising for dealing with individual burnout in its organizational context.

A. Organizational Health

Viewing the opposite end from burnout as a state of engagement has direct implications for health. In the first place it defines health at work in terms of relationships. In human service work, burnout focuses on service relationships themselves, not solely in terms of their emotional demands, but their potential for meaningful accomplishment as well. Service relationships occur within the context of myriad organizational relationships with colleagues, supervisors, distant management, and subordinates. The role of these other relationships in generating demands on staff members and providing resources for coping with service de-

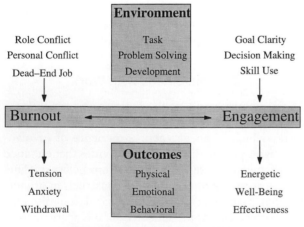

Figure 2   Burnout and engagement.

mands has been the focus of studies of burnout. They are relevant to staff members in a diverse range of organizations within the human services or in other occupational domains.

Burnout provides a perspective on individual mental health that reflects the health of the organizations in which people work. From this perspective health is not limited to the physical or emotional well-being of individuals, but is evident in enduring patterns of social interactions among people. This is similar to the position of family therapists that it is often more productive to recast difficulties in a trouble family as a breakdown of a social system rather than as the problems of an individual whom the family has identified as the patient. A family problem is one for which each member shares a responsibility. The family regains health by all members changing the way in which they interact with one another. In an organizational setting some problems, such as burnout, are more readily cast as difficulties of the social context of work than as failings of individual employees.

Organizational health is evident through the social context in which people work. As with individuals, organizational health requires a reasonable balance of demands with appropriate coping resources. Periods of extreme demand that prompt an organization to work at peak levels are balanced with periods of rest and recuperation within an ongoing context of a readily manageable pace of activity. When this balance is exceeded for a prolonged period, members of the organization experience the strain on the organizational systems: a stressed organization creates strain for its members. This resolution is contrary to the long-term viability and productivity of the organization in a manner similar to a breakdown of an individual's health: the whole individual suffers when any bodily system is under excessive strain. In contrast, engagement with work is associated with a sense of well-being for both individuals and organizations. [See ORGANIZATIONAL AND OCCUPATIONAL PSYCHIATRY.]

IV. IMPLICATIONS FOR INTERVENTIONS

Preventing burnout is synonymous with developing and supporting engagement with work. Strategies for developing engagement with work involve enhancing energy, involvement, and professional efficacy. Interventions may emphasize treatment of burnout after it has occurred or its prevention through building a worksetting that is conducive to productive engagement with work.

Considerable personal and organizational costs provide compelling reasons for preventing or alleviating burnout. The three-component structure of the burnout syndrome gives a valuable framework for setting goals to guide interventions and for generating strategies to reach these objectives. Intervention may focus on the individual, workgroup, or an entire organization. At each level, the number of people affected by an intervention and the potential for enduring change increases. Following on Figure 1, various approaches to interventions are described.

A. Focusing on the Individual

The structure of the burnout syndrome and research into its development provide direction for treatment and prevention strategies. The first approach to maintaining emotional and creative energy is to address severe acute fatigue that can be the basis for the chronic exhaustion of burnout. Individual strategies include pacing involvement in demanding tasks, especially during times of peak demand or emergencies, as there are rarely adequate opportunities for recovery in a chronically demanding workplace. Goal setting and time management strategies can increase an individual's control over demands. Simply enduring chronic exhaustion is rarely effective.

I. Coping with Work Demands

The occupational demands that are of most direct relevance to burnout in human service professions are those arising from emotionally charged interactions with clients. Maintaining an optimal degree of involvement with clients is one of the primary challenges of these careers. An engaging participation with this work involves sensitivity to service recipients' distress and a capacity to respond in a manner that acknowledges their feelings without exhausting emotional resources. Successfully meeting that challenge is essential to avoiding burnout. Sustaining this involvement over the long term requires that staff members replenish emotional and creative energy.

Alleviating burnout once it occurs requires an immediate response to the problems people are experiencing. Exhaustion and diminished accomplishment are distressing to staff members. Further, staff members experiencing exhaustion do not have the energy to devote to intense, demanding intervention programs, while diminished accomplishment reduces their confidence in the potential success of interventions. Feelings of depersonalization or cynicism reduce staff members' enthusiasm for any major undertaking at work. The ideal intervention for intense burnout avoids introducing new demands on individuals while providing opportunities for success that will revive staff members' engagement in their work.

2. Reducing Personal Conflict

Interpersonal problem solving or negotiation skills can be valuable resources for managing life within a workplace. The consistent and strong relationship of emotional exhaustion with personal conflict on the job indicate the potential contribution of interpersonal skills to controlling this aspect of burnout. Building staff members' conflict resolution skills and their capacity to communicate effectively and clearly are interventions that can contribute to the reduction of personal conflict at work.

3. Control Coping

Control-coping interventions focus on enhancing an individual's capacity to manage challenges at work in a manner that prevents exhaustion. Individuals may cope with demands more effectively through active cognitive strategies, such as time management, or behavioral strategies, such as negotiating with colleagues or supervisors. In contrast, escape coping strategies, such as ignoring occupational problems or overusing sick days, are ineffective to the point of aggravating burnout in some circumstances. In general, control-oriented coping is consistent with a responsible and effective approach to work. While escape strategies can be effective in the short term, giving relief from excessive demands, they do not provide a means of gaining control over the demands themselves.

A major part of control coping is the development of resources. Exhaustion arises as much from inadequate resources as from excessive demands. A diverse range of resources can contribute to reducing exhaustion. These include developing professional skills and redesigning the workplace. Staff members draw from their range of professional skills to address demands that arise at work; a wider range of skills provides more options for actions. Often a deeper understanding of organizational dynamics can help to alleviate exhaustion. Anxiety about impending organizational change can be exhausting to staff members who lack a conceptual framework for making sense of developments.

4. Impact of Reducing Exhaustion

To a considerable extent depersonalization and cynicism reduce as staff members alleviate their exhaustion. The direct relations between these two aspects of burnout indicates that they will both respond to similar aspects of interventions. In addition to reducing exhaustion, cognitive interventions are appropriate to reducing depersonalization and cynicism. Focusing on the enjoyable and fulfilling aspects of a job can reduce the tendency to become distant from work when experiencing exhaustion and can direct staff members toward more constructive ways of coping.

B. Focusing on the Workgroup

Workgroup interventions may evolve from occupational health programs aimed at developing productive life-styles or from team-building interventions. In the former instance, members of a workgroup develop a shared understanding of the demands confronting the group and the resources available to address them. They may develop scheduled breaks from work routine, manage more flexible work hours, or serve as a support group for encouraging regular exercise programs to manage tension. Team-building interventions help members of a workgroup to identify points of congruence between their individual values and those of the group. These interventions help to reduce role conflict and interpersonal conflict that are major contributors to exhaustion.

1. Reducing Conflict

Individual approaches to treating burnout are limited by the inherent interdependency among coworkers. Job responsibilities are more often assigned than chosen. Coworkers depend upon one another to perform at a certain rate for a certain time at an expected level of quality. An individual coping strategy that disrupts the interactions among coworkers may generate problems for other members of the workgroup. Without explicit cooperation among coworkers, individual coping with burnout is too often limited to the individuals' prerogative to leave the workplace or profession entirely. Interactions with colleagues may also be sources of enduring personal conflict that aggravate exhaustion. Interventions that focus directly upon the day-to-day experiences of a workgroup have both a broader impact and a greater potential for enduring change.

2. Building Social Support

Social support at work encompasses both emotional exchange among friends and instrumental assistance of colleagues furthering shared objectives. More effective teamwork among colleagues increases the availability of occupational resources from other people, increasing team members' access to knowledge, skills, and abilities beyond their personal resources. While individual social skills make a contribution, team-building initiatives that actively involve the larger group enhance a team's functioning more directly. With adequate resources readily shared among members of a workgroup, demanding situations constitute rewarding challenges rather than occasions for exhaustion. Further, a supportive environment within a workgroup permits staff members to use individual coping responses more effectively.

A reduced sense of accomplishment may reflect inadequate support systems or unrealistic expectations of a job. When the job is at odds with expectations, staff members may change their expectations or modify the worksetting to be more in line with their expectations. People generally adapt their expectations as they learn about a new situation, or as significant changes unfold in a setting with which they are familiar. They resist changing expectations that reflect deeply held, emotionally charged values about a job. When they do relinquish their expectations and develop no meaningful substitutes, they cannot maintain a sense of accomplishment and effectiveness. A team-building process that assists a group to clarify its values can be effective at alleviating and preventing burnout.

A clear understanding of career goals, especially as they pertain to involvement with service recipients, contributes to a human service worker's capacity to maintain engagement with work. Advanced training programs have recognized this need in their provision of seminars that consider professional and ethical issues of practice. These perspectives make a greater contribution when individuals reflect upon their rele-

vance to their personal career values. A review of these issues at the level of the workgroup furthers the impact of this learning in day-to-day work by building a shared sense of purpose among colleagues.

Enhancing access to organizational resources and support systems enhances personal accomplishment and effectiveness while it reduces exhaustion. More frequent experiences of success and greater recognition by colleagues and supervisors are effective even in situations of continuing demand. Both direct experiences of effectiveness and collegial recognition of success contribute to staff members' feelings of personal accomplishment. Developing a systematic and credible means of recognition within a workgroup may have a significant impact on personal accomplishment or professional efficacy.

C. Changing the Organization

Some individuals will survive or even thrive in demanding, unsupportive environments. Most will not. Creating supportive, developing professional communities will contribute to the health of people in diverse occupations. Although they have a much broader impact than individually oriented approaches, workgroup interventions occur within a larger organization that may limit their impact. Often, control over work demands rests primarily with senior management within the organization, or with government or corporate entities beyond. These sectors may overrule a workgroup's attempts to manage its demands and access to resources, and thereby undermine its attempts to alleviate burnout.

Interventions on the organizational level are potentially the most effective for addressing burnout as a reaction to a strained work environment, but they are also the most difficult to implement. They are more effective because any change is more enduring when it is embedded in the ongoing procedures and structures of an organization. They are more difficult to implement because effective interventions require broad-based cooperative efforts throughout the various sectors of an organization. They require effective communication networks within and between these sectors to enhance their responsiveness to the diverse perspectives that the organization encompasses.

The challenge to management is to define a work context in which people may maintain an energetic engagement in their work. The structure of the burnout syndrome and its relationship to organizational environments provide direction for management interventions to prevent the development of burnout. Often management interventions function through the support they provide to individuals and workgroups.

1. Autonomy

Control over the way in which a job is performed is a serious consideration for people who do engaging work. Although some aspects of autonomy depend upon the personal initiative and beliefs of individuals, organizational policies are of greater consequence. Rigid decision rules constrain staff members within predefined courses of action, reducing their sense of personal accomplishment and increasing their distance from their work. Rules increase the potential for role conflict when they conflict with one another or with the values of staff members. Initiatives that devolve responsibility and authority to frontline staff members build engagement with work. However, they require planning and discussion to assure that the necessary support services and training are in place to facilitate the expansion of occupational roles.

2. Decision-Making Involvement

Closely related to professional autonomy are staff members' decision-making prerogatives. Increasing participation in decisions depends upon initiatives at the organizational level. Informed decisions require open communication networks to keep people throughout the organization aware of current issues and to provide relevant background to consequential actions. Staff members often require training or coaching to enhance their decision-making skills, especially their capacity to manage collaborative decision making with their colleagues. Most importantly, increasing staff members' capacity to make consequential decisions changes the power structure of an organization.

3. Building a Professional Community

A professional community is a network of collegial affiliations, including the sharing of technical expertise, emotional attachment, and a professional service ethic (for example, commitment to service quality). Strong professional communities within a large organization or across associated organizations enhance the impact of workgroup interventions in a manner similar to the support that workgroups provide to individual coping initiatives. Building the mutually beneficial relationships involved in a professional community is an undertaking by individuals, workgroups, and their organizations. A shared vision is required for the organization to fulfill its mission.

A professional community, especially one that is an active force in a staff member's day-to-day work, makes a significant contribution to supporting engagement with work. The contribution of colleagues in terms of expertise and emotional support helps to maintain energy. It is a resource upon which they may draw during times of peak demand. It is a source of support during prolonged tedium. In both of these ways membership in a professional community reduces exhaustion and maintains energetic involvement.

The idealism and focus on ethical issues that are fundamental to a professional community are incompatible with depersonalization or cynicism. Clearly articulated principles giving priority to client needs and emphasizing the validity of their perspectives encourage service relationships that are personal and considerate. The ongoing support and scrutiny of colleagues keep this perspective salient and help to prevent depersonalization during times of emotional demand. Similarly, in other occupations an active professional community reduces excessive distance from work; the shared concern with contributing to a high-quality product or service maintains a close engagement with work.

The community maintains professional efficacy and experiences of personal accomplishment by providing valuable peer recognition. The exchange of skills, support, and expertise among members of a professional community increases the chance of successful outcomes, and provides confirmation of success when it occurs. The opportunity to support colleagues extends a staff member's potential to have a significant impact on the organizational task and on the welfare of colleagues.

D. Intervention and Treatment

The structure of the burnout syndrome and its complementary state, engagement with work, provide direction for both treatment interventions and for prevention programs designed to build a more supportive and effective workplace. The central quality of burnout is a chronic experience of exhaustion, distance, and discouragement. These occupational hazards are prevalent and they have a serious detrimental impact on staff members. Gaining control over them in an enduring fashion is to design a better place to work.

Preventing burnout is based upon sound human resource management policies. Maintaining high quality, intense professional performance requires a recognition of personal limits of individuals, the strains and resources inherent in a workgroup, and an acknowledgment of the organization's role in supporting purposeful work. In many worksettings, demands expand faster than support systems develop, leaving individuals and groups to draw more heavily on their personal resources. This sequence increases the potential for exhaustion and for reduced accomplishment or efficacy as individuals encounter difficulties in their new roles. Supporting engagement with work requires clear policies on the organizational level to maintain clear communication and to take effective action.

V. CONCLUSION

The concept of burnout and its opposite pole, engagement with work, provide a valuable and distinctive perspective on health. Organizations constitute stable settings that shape the behavior and subjective experience of their staff members. Reactions to these environments range from intense involvement and satisfaction through indifference to the exhausted, distant, discouraged state of burnout.

An enduring productive relationship with work makes a considerable contribution to psychological health. First, it is indicative of the fulfillment of personal needs for achievement. The work domain is the setting in which people most often explore the limits of their capabilities and go farthest toward realizing their potential for sophisticated action. A worksetting that encourages the thorough and effective use of abilities while providing recognition, assistance, and resources necessary to support these efforts is indicative of a healthy organization.

Engagement with work also promotes productive participation in the social environment of an organization. This includes interactions with service recipients, which have been a central concern from the initial development of the burnout concept. Staff members who provide services to people in distress are vulnerable to being overwhelmed by the emotional demands of their work. To remain productively engaged, rather than being overwhelmed, staff members must achieve a resolution in which they can pace the rate and intensity of their involvement with service recipients while replenishing their energy through supportive interactions. Even when the organization's task does not involve emotionally demanding interactions with service recipients, sustaining the energy and concentration necessary for high quality work requires sufficient control for self-pacing and support from colleagues.

Formal employment is a significant domain of life in terms of its time commitments, its demands on sophisticated skills, and its potential for fulfilling human needs related to achievement. Burnout is a reliably identifiable syndrome that undermines staff members' capacity to make a meaningful contribution through their work and it impairs the quality of their lives. Alleviating burnout and building more engaging workplaces are important steps toward developing healthier life-styles. The social focus of burnout, the solid research basis concerning the syndrome, and its specific ties to the work domain make a distinct and valuable contribution to understanding health and well-being.

BIBLIOGRAPHY

Cherniss, C. (1980). *Professional burnout in human service organizations.* New York: Praeger.

Cordes, C. L., & Dougherty, T. W. (1993). A review and integration of research on job burnout. *Academy of Management Review, 18,* 621–656.

Golembiewski, R. T., & Munzenrider, R. (1988). *Phases of burnout: Developments in concepts and applications.* New York: Praeger.

Kahill, S. (1988). Symptoms of professional burnout: A review of empirical evidence. *Canadian Psychology, 29,* 284–297.

Leiter, M. P. (1991). The dream denied: Professional burnout and the constraints of service organizations. *Canadian Psychology, 32,* 547–558.

Maslach, C., Jackson, S. E., & Leiter, M. P. (1996). *Maslach Burnout Inventory Manual* (3rd ed.). Palo Alto, CA: Consulting Psychologists Press.

Maslach, C., & Leiter, M. P. (1997). *The truth about burnout.* San Francisco: Jossey-Bass.

Schaufeli, W., Maslach, C., & Marek, T. (Eds.) (1993). *Professional burnout: Recent developments in theory and research.* Washington, DC: Taylor & Francis.

C

Caffeine: Psychosocial Effects

Joseph P. Blount

Widener University

W. Miles Cox

North Chicago Veterans Affairs Medical Center
The Chicago Medical School

Caffeinism The official diagnostic category for excessive caffeine consumption to a point of intoxication.

Double Blind A type of research design in which neither the subject nor the experimenter (but only some third party) knows whether the subject has received a drug (e.g., caffeinated coffee) or an inert substance (e.g., decaffeinated coffee). The advantage of this design is that it allows the investigator to isolate the pharmacological effects of the drug from the psychological effects.

DSM-IV The current diagnostic manual of the American Psychiatric Association.

Ergogenic Aid A substance that helps an athlete generate increased force or endurance.

State-Dependent Learning A drug-induced effect on memory that occurs when information that is learned in one drug state is later more accurately recalled when the individual is in the same drug state rather than a different one.

Statistical Significance The assurance, through a statistical test, that an observed data pattern is genuine rather than having occured by chance.

Theobromine A xanthine closely related to caffeine that is found especially in cacao beans and chocolate.

Theophylline A xanthine closely related to caffeine that is found in tea leaves.

Withdrawal Symptoms Symptoms that occur when a person suddenly stops taking a drug that he or she is accustomed to taking. Headache and fatigue are the most common symptoms associated with withdrawal from caffeine.

CAFFEINE is a psychoactive drug that occurs naturally in many foods and beverages (e.g., coffee, tea, cocoa) and is added to many commercial products (e.g., soft drinks, analgesics). Caffeine is closely related chemically to theophylline and theobromine; all three compounds are methylated xanthines. Coffee contains caffeine, tea contains both caffeine and theophylline, and cocoa contains both caffeine and theobromine. Caffeine is used very widely, often in high doses, and it has been the subject of much research. Four major questions have been raised regarding caffeine and its effects: (1) What are its physical and mental benefits? (2) What are the possible harmful effects of caffeine from single doses or chronic use? (3) Is caffeine consumption a social problem? (4) What are the short- and long-term mechanisms that cause its physiological and behavioral effects? Scientific studies have given us considerable understanding of the mechanisms by which caffeine has its effects and have clarified much of the speculation about potential health risks. Biomedical results are not discussed in detail here, but a summary (Blount and Cox, 1991) and an evaluative review (James, 1991) are listed in the references. Research results on psychological well-being and behavioral effects of caffeine have greatly increased our understanding of the complex ways in which caffeine can produce beneficial effects in one individual but harmful effects in another, or different effects in the same individual at different times. Given the current state of knowledge, mild caution about excessive use of caffeine is prudent for the general population, reduced intake is indicated for certain clinical populations, and further research is needed in particular areas.

I. INTRODUCTION

According to more than one legend, caffeine was introduced to humans through divine intervention. The existence of such legends indicates the important role caffeine has had in society throughout the ages. One of the more interesting legends appears geographically correct. An Arabian goatherd noticed that the beans made his goats energetic and unable to sleep, and he decided to try some himself. He became happy, danced and whirled and leaped and rolled about on the ground. In today's terminology this might be called the first coffee trip. A holy man joined the goatherd's orgy and took instructions from Mohammed to boil the beans and have monks drink the liquid to stay awake longer and continue their prayers.

In the 10th century A.D., an Arabian medical book suggested that coffee was a cure for almost everything including measles and excessive lust. By the 15th century, coffee plants were being cultivated and transported, and coffee consumption spread in the Islamic world. In the 17th century, Dutch cultivation spread coffee to Europe (in greenhouses), to the East Indies, and eventually to the more favorable climate in Latin America. Coffeehouses and coffee consumption and the method of using ground beans spread rapidly in England and France.

The women in England reacted with a petition against coffee, calling it an enfeebling liquor. The real problem was not reducing lust, but social change: The coffeehouses were a place to relax, do business, or learn the news of the day, and people were spending a lot of time there. Old social patterns were being challenged. In Mecca, this activity was seen as competing with attendance at mosques. Coffee bean supplies were burned, and the use of coffee was outlawed. Of course, illegal coffee channels grew up, and soon the prohibition was lifted. In England, Charles II feared

seditious plots would originate in coffeehouses; therefore, he outlawed them—only to have to withdraw his ruling 11 days later. By the 18th century, coffeehouses were functioning as "penny universities" where anyone could learn from great literary and political figures. The famous insurance company, Lloyd's of London, began in Edward Lloyd's coffeehouse around this time.

Caffeine consumption has always been closely intertwined with financial issues. In 17th century France there was competition between coffee establishments and wine establishments. In the English colonies in the new world, tea at first served as a cheaper and more readily available alternative to coffee. However, a British tea tax reduced some of this economic advantage and was credited with contributing to political separation and with shifting the new nation's habits from tea to coffee. Technological improvements and marketing seem to have contributed to industrial growth across the 19th century. Roasting of coffee beans improves the flavor of the drink and commercial roasting increased convenience by eliminating the necessity for home roasting. At the turn of the century, vacuum packing permitted indefinite storage of commercially roasted and ground coffee. In 1892, the first commercial combination of different beans was introduced. The success of Maxwell House was probably not due to "superior" flavor or association with a famous hotel. Rather, the blend introduced a new level of consistency in taste for which preferences could be developed and brand loyalty cultivated.

Societal factors outside the coffee industry seem to have had large impacts on coffee consumption. When alcohol prohibition was imposed in the United States in 1920 coffee consumption increased 40% in 1 year alone and fears were expressed that it had reached a threshold of abuse. Coffee did not seem to be serving merely as a social substitute for alcohol. When prohibition was repealed, coffee consumption continued to rise. During World War II, consumption reached a peak about double its prohibition level; perhaps the war effort and work schedules created the need to use coffee for its stimulating effects. Consumption then declined during the 1950s (no war effort, price increases in coffee), 1960s (competition from soft drinks), and 1970s (health-consciousness and changes in lifestyle).

Empirical research has shown a logical association between beliefs and consumption: those who "always" or "usually" select noncaffeinated beverages believe that such beverages are habit forming, increase nervousness, and contribute to medical conditions such as ulcers, high blood pressure, and cancer. Those who "rarely" or "never" select noncaffeinated beverages believe the beverages give people more energy, help them to relax, and help them to feel better. The coffee industry has responded as if beliefs are important determinants of caffeine consumption, in part with increased marketing of decaffeinated coffees and in part by sponsoring research to show that caffeine has only benign effects (Dews, 1984). Industry support of scholarly research is to be commended; however, selective reporting and interpretation of results in ways favorable to the industry are to be condemned and guarded against. Industry fears of a net loss of markets have not occurred: the decline has leveled off and consumption has remained constant across the 1980s and early 1990s. Current per capita consumption is higher than what it was just before Prohibition. It is difficult to ascertain how much of this leveling is due to new marketing techniques, such as the promotion of drip grinds, gourmet blends, espresso methods of preparation, and iced coffees. The fear is that users of decaffeinated products will temporarily maintain consumption but then drink fewer cups per day because decaffeinated products lack caffeine's taste-enhancing action and tendency to produce physical dependence (see below). The level of concern in the industry is represented by a multi-component marketing technique used in Australia. Caffeine is added to flavored milk so that milk's healthy image will overcome caffeine's negative one. The beverage is targeted at children in the hope that they will become life-long consumers of caffeine. The advertisements try to capitalize on the allure of the drug counterculture and on the public's new awareness of the psychoactive properties of caffeine by inviting consumers to obtain "the maximum hit." Coffee is an important worldwide commodity of trade second only to oil. Hence, even a small reduction in consumption could have a sizable impact on international relations, capital investments, and job dislocations.

In a 1984 sociological analysis, Troyer and Markle compared coffee drinking to cigarette smoking. They suggested that coffee drinking was an emerging social problem and that society's future attitude toward the problem would be largely decided by biomedical experts. Like smoking, health risks could lead to societal constraints against the industry and consumers' behavior. One danger is that certain organizations could bias the experts by emphasizing ill effects, or others by portraying the caffeine as safe. The debate over what caffeine-related conditions to include in the American Psychiatric Association's revised version of the *Diagnostic and Statistical Manual of Mental Disorders* takes on many of the characteristics that Troyer and Markle pointed out (see Addiction below). Another danger is that scientists would be deterred from working with caffeine for fear of media-fanned public outcry about results that went against established patterns of behavior. Although individual scientists have expressed discomfort at organizational, media, or public pressures, in the last 9 years, there has been a wealth, not a lack, of research. Because the objective results have remained mixed, the medical community has not yet put caffeine in the same category as alcohol and nicotine. The remainder of this article summarizes the current state of the field with regard to caffeine and human behavior.

II. PSYCHOPHARMACOLOGY

Caffeine is an alkaline compound in the family of naturally occurring derivatives of xanthine. Although most other alkaloids are insoluble in water, caffeine is slightly soluble and becomes still more so in the form of complex double salts. After oral ingestion in humans, caffeine is rapidly absorbed in the gastrointestinal tract and distributed into all parts of the body, including in the case of pregnant women, the mother's milk and her fetus. Peak blood plasma levels of caffeine are reached within about 30 minutes after ingestion of tea or coffee, and within about 1 hour for Coca Cola (and presumably other soft drinks). That rates of caffeine absorption are slower for soft drinks than for coffee is a surprising finding because of the fact that the rate of absorption of alcohol is increased by carbonation.

Caffeine primarily acts as a central nervous system stimulant. Moderate doses of 200 mg (about two cups of coffee taken close together) activate the cortex; higher doses activate the spinal cord or autonomic nervous system. Single caffeine doses decrease heart rate during the first hour after administration and increase heart rate and cardiac output during the following 2 hours. Caffeine dilates systemic blood vessels, but constricts cerebral blood vessels. Caffeine causes a slight increase in basal metabolic rate (10%). Caffeine increases the secretion of stomach acids, increases the respiratory rate, and slightly increases the production of urine. It acts as a bronchodilator by relaxing the smooth muscles. On the other hand, caffeine strengthens the contraction of skeletal muscles.

About 95% of a dose of caffeine is metabolized by the liver into other products and excreted by the kidneys. Very small portions may be excreted in pure form or through other channels, such as in saliva, semen, or breast milk. About 97% of a dose of caffeine is eliminated in 15 to 30 hours. Many factors may cause the rate of clearance to vary. For example, clearance is much slower among smokers, persons with liver disease, women who are pregnant or use oral contraceptives, and infants (because infants lack certain enzymes). When a chronic adult user abruptly discontinues all use of caffeine, complete removal of caffeine from the body can take up to 7 days.

III. PREVALENCE OF CAFFEINE CONSUMPTION

Caffeine intake can be calculated as the product of a person's consumption of food, beverages, or other products containing caffeine times the caffeine content of these products. Such data can be obtained by having people keep diaries of what they consume or retrospectively report what they remember consuming or by having a third party record what they consume. There is substantial agreement among these different methods of collecting data. Furthermore, there is close agreement between these methods and certain measures of caffeine production, such as the amount of coffee imported per capita. These intake data reveal interesting patterns. For instance, the most prominent source of caffeine in Britain is tea, but in the United States, it is coffee. The shift in preference from tea to coffee in the United States has been attributed to the British tax on tea in the 1700s. The U.S. peak of more than three cups of coffee per day per capita in 1962 fell to less than two cups in 1983, a shift that has been variously attributed to poor advertising and/or a decline in the quality of coffees in the 1960s. Currently in the United States, females drink more coffee than males, and the younger generation gets its caffeine primarily from soft drinks. Caffeine consuming habits also change with age. For example, those 35–64 years old drink more coffee than younger or older age groups. On the other hand, tea consumption shows no difference across ages, and soft drink consumption declines.

The second factor necessary to calculate caffeine intake is the amount of caffeine in a source. The amount of caffeine depends on both methods of commercial production and personal methods of preparation. Tea is especially variable, ranging from 8 to 91 mg per serving. Due to such variation and to differences in the definitions of serving size (and sometimes definitions are not reported), various authors report different data on caffeine content. Nonetheless, it is useful to have representative values for the caffeine content of major dietary sources, and these are given in Tables I and II. Many people believe that the dark color of soft drinks indicates which ones contain caffeine. In actuality, caffeine forms a white powder, a yellow residue (caffeine is a xanthine and xanthine is the Greek word for "yellow"), or a clear solution.

Table I Levels of Caffeine in Common Foods and Beverages

Beverage/food	Serving size (oz)	Approximate mg caffeine/serving
Coffee		
Drip	5	150
Percolated	5	110
Instant, regular	5	50–100
Instant, flavored mix	5	25–75
Decaffeinated coffee	5	1–6
Tea		
Black		
1-min brew	5	20–35
3-min brew	5	35–45
5-min brew	5	40–50
Green		
1-min brew	5	10–20
3-min brew	5	20–35
5-min brew	5	25–35
Instant	5	30–60
Cocoa beverage	5	2–20
Soft drinks		
Jolt	12	70
Caffeinated cola drinks	12	30–65
Mountain Dew, Mello Yello, Sunkist Orange	12	40–50
7-Up, Sprite, RC-100, Fanta Orange, Hires Root Beer	12	0
Chocolate		
Cake	1/16 of 9-inch cake	14
Ice cream	2/3 cup	5
Mr. Goodbar	1.65	6
Special Dark, Hershey	1.02	23

Table II Levels of Caffeine in Common Drugs

Drugs	Standard adult dose	Approximate mg caffeine/std. dose
Prescription painkillers		
Darvon compound capsule	1	32
Cafergot tablet (migraine)	1	100
Nonprescription (over-the-counter)		
Painkillers		
Anacin, Midol, Vanquish	2	65
Plain aspirin	2	0
Cold/allergy		
Dristan	2	30
Coryban-D, Sinarest, Triaminicin	1	30
Stimulants		
No-Doz	2	200
Vivarin	1	200

Note that root beer is dark and contains no caffeine, whereas Mountain Dew is clear and contains caffeine.

Despite this variability, a number of authors have used the figures for caffeine content to calculate the average person's daily caffeine intake. For American adults (consumers and nonconsumers) a representative average including all sources, not just coffee, is 200 mg (3 mg/kg body weight) per day. Adults who are considered heavy consumers ingest 500 mg (7 mg/kg) per day or more. A 27-kg child who consumes three soft drinks and two chocolate bars would have equivalent body levels of caffeine and could therefore also be considered a heavy consumer! Some adults who consume 2000 mg/day have sought professional help to reduce their intake. Note that laborers consume more caffeine than others; college students consume more caffeine when preparing for examinations than at other times. Several segments of society consume less than these figures: Pregnant women appear to consume about 2.1 mg/kg, although the data are limited and pregnancy-related weight gains have not always been taken into account. Children under 18 (both consumers and nonconsumers) ingest about 37 mg (1 mg/kg) per day. The health code of the Mormons, as well as that of certain other religious groups, prohibits all use of stimulants.

IV. COGNITIVE TASKS

The popularity of caffeine is probably due to its stimulant action. Many people report that caffeine in-

creases their mental arousal, and it is widely believed to improve actual performance. Researchers have attempted to objectively assess the effects of caffeine on attention, speed of reaction, memory, and/or the flow of thoughts.

At the perceptual level, acute caffeine ingestion lowers visual luminance threshold, and improves auditory vigilance. On visual vigilance tasks, caffeine increases alertness and speeds up responding while reducing attention to detail. Chronic caffeine users show enhanced sensitivity (d'), but increased errors on visual vigilance tasks. Regarding reaction time, small to moderate amounts of caffeine (i.e., 32 to 200 mg) help speed reactions to simple, routinized tasks, such as indicating whether an even or odd digit was presented, pressing buttons corresponding to bulbs lit in a circular pattern, or watching for strings of three even numbers. Conversely, when habitual caffeine users abstain for 2 days, their reactions are slowed and their attention is impaired. (The physical indicator of impaired attention is less anticipatory heart-rate deceleration.) For novel or slightly more complex tasks, it is difficult to predict whether caffeine will improve or impair performance. For example, whereas visual reaction times are often improved by caffeine, caffeine seriously impairs performance on the Stroop test. The Stroop test involves naming a color of ink while ignoring an incompatibly spelled color (e.g., the word "red" printed in green ink). The impairment is understandable if one realizes that the drug cannot selectively speed one kind of processing. By enhancing both word reading and color naming, the interference between them is increased and performance impaired.

Because to a large extent driving a car is routinized, the improvements in auditory vigilance and visual reaction time would seem to imply benefits for late-night driving—if not counteracted by loss of fine motor coordination (see effects on physical performance below). No researcher seems to have carefully tested the net effects of caffeine on driving performance. It is noteworthy, though, that several researchers have used laboratory tasks to test the common belief that caffeine counteracts the effects of alcohol, and have found that coffee further impairs rather than improves performance. For example, a person who has consumed enough alcohol to be close to the legal level of intoxication and then drinks a cup and a half of coffee (150 mg of caffeine) has even slower reaction times than if only the alcohol had been consumed. In short, consuming coffee after consuming alcohol may make one more prone to accidents rather than less so. On the other hand, more recent research has found some indication that caffeine may counteract the effects of alcohol, but the amount of "antagonism" is surprisingly small. The practical importance of this issue calls for careful research that uses doses of caffeine typical of social use (instead of using only excessive doses), pairing wider ranges of alcohol and caffeine doses, adjusting both kinds of doses to subjects' body weights, taking into account subjects' typical patterns of alcohol and caffeine use, and including as part of the experiment a demonstration that caffeine alone actually improves performance.

Many people believe that arousal produced by caffeine is beneficial to learning and retention. At the simplest level of habituation (e.g., to an aversive noise or to the demands of a visual vigilance task), acute caffeine ingestion reduces the rate of habituation. Chronic caffeine users seem to have a modified habituation process. At the level of learning and memory, some research has, in fact, shown beneficial effects. However, many studies involving short-term memory have shown no effect or impaired performance due to caffeine. It has been proposed and partially demonstrated that this lack of consistency can be resolved by disentangling the complex interactions among personality type (extrovert/introvert and/or high/low impulsivity), diurnal rhythm of arousal, task requirements (e.g., sustained information transfer, short-term memory), dosages matched to body weights, and the curvilinear relationship with arousal level (moderate arousal enhances performance, whereas excessive arousal hinders it). For example, coffee may improve an extrovert's performance on a particular task in the morning, but impair the same person's performance on the same task in the afternoon. Conversely, coffee may hinder an introvert in the morning, but facilitate that person in the afternoon.

Another kind of drug-induced effect on memory is state-dependent learning. It occurs when information learned in one drug state is later recalled better when the individual is in the same drug state rather than a different one. An example of state-dependent learning is the alcohol drinker who while sober forgets what he or she did while intoxicated, but recalls it again when next intoxicated. In the experimental laboratory, state-dependent learning with alcohol has been demonstrated with social drinkers. However, several attempts to demonstrate state-dependent learning in the laboratory with caffeine have been unsuccessful. One possible cause for the latter negative results is that the "drug" and "nondrug" states that were supposed to be different actually were not. The experimenters assumed that the drug state involved a high level of arousal because caffeine was consumed, and that the other state involved a low level of arousal because a placebo (i.e., no caffeine) was consumed. However, subjects in the latter condition may have also been aroused, because, for example, they had been challenged to perform well on the experimental task, or they were excited by being in an unfamiliar setting and in the presence of a stranger. The first explanation is especially plausible because many people find that having to take any kind of a test causes them to be anxious. Assuming that alcohol reduces test anxiety would account for the state-dependent learning that was found in one study that, from the learning to the test phase of the experiment, shifted subjects from a combined alcohol/caffeine state to (a) the same state (which produced no decrement in performance), (b) an alcohol-only state (which produced a performance decrement), (c) a caffeine-only state (which produced small decrement), or (d) a no-drug state (which produced maximal decrement). In short, at the present time, it is not entirely clear whether caffeine does or does not produce state-dependent learning. It seems that there is a good chance that caffeine does produce state-dependent learning, but that this effect will be difficult to isolate.

Many people report that caffeine helps them think more clearly and creatively. In the public stereotype, creative persons use drugs to excess. Survey research has shown that, contrary to the stereotype, writers, artists, and musicians do not use drugs, not even caffeine, to excess. In fact, most creative people say they learned early in their career that drugs interfere with the creativity process. When they do use caffeine, it is only to counteract the effects of lack of sleep.

Whether ordinary people's more mundane cognitive performance improves while they are under the influence of common levels of caffeine has been tested using a variety of tasks, ranging from simple subtraction, to identifying errors in written passages, to taking the Graduate Record Examination (among many others). A very wide range of positive results have been found. In a number of cases, the results have been replicated. However, a large number of inconsistent findings have also turned up. One explanation for the inconsistencies was that caffeine cannot enhance performance in normal situations, but can merely restore degraded performance in situations of fatigue or boredom. In response to these suggestions, a number of researchers took fatigue-based results, tested them in nonfatigue contexts, and found true caffeine enhancement. A second attempt to explain the inconsistencies was a model of arousal that involved personality characteristics of the subjects and the time of day that they were tested (see the discussion of memory above). This approach seemed especially promising because there were a wide variety of supportive results. However, recently there have been a number of findings inconsistent with this model and alternative theoretical accounts have focused on "postlunch dip" rather than diurnal rhythm. A third attempt to explain the inconsistencies was to examine the information processing components of the task. This was done in the case of the Stroop test discussed earlier above. Humphreys and Revelle have analyzed tasks in terms of information transfer versus short-term memory functions. The problem is that there is no agreed upon set of principles by which to analyze the processing components of a given task. In summary, the problems described here are a classic example of the complex contextual nature of social science research in contrast to the searches for simple, universal laws that are common in the physical sciences.

An important criticism of many of the positive findings is that they used doses of caffeine much larger than those common in everyday life. Only a few studies have directly compared such dose sizes. Often, these studies have found statistically significant effects with large doses but weak or nonexistent effects with everyday doses. If this pattern of results can be interpreted as a threshold effect, then moderate consumption can be recommended. However, if this pattern is interpreted as a linear dose–response relationship, then complex tradeoffs must be considered in deciding how much caffeine a given individual should consume.

One particularly interesting inconsistent result is a study that reported high caffeine intake among college students was associated with *low* academic grades. It is impossible to conclude from this association that coffee drinking is the cause of the low grades. It could be that low grades cause coffee drinking or that a third variable causes both. Because this report is frequently cited, it should be replicated and cause and effect relationships should be investigated. Furthermore, it

would be important to have more studies of other "real-world" forms of thinking, such as reading comprehension and problem solving. Studies that compared fatigued or bored subjects with alert ones would help resolve the issue of whether caffeine actually improves performance generally or is largely confined to restorative effects. Do the benefits of caffeine occur at the expense of impaired performance later in the day? Is the period of increased stimulation/metabolism followed by a restorative period of decreased stimulation/metabolism? Researchers do not seem to have addressed these simple, practical questions.

V. PHYSICAL PERFORMANCE

In addition to mental arousal, people report that caffeine increases their physiological arousal. Assuming these subjective impressions reflect underlying physiological changes, one would expect effects on fine motor coordination, spontaneous gross motor activity, and athletic endurance. In fact, hand steadiness has been shown to be about 25% worse after consuming 200 mg of caffeine (about two cups of strong coffee). Furthermore, there have been a number of empirical reports of caffeine impairing motor skills which involve delicate muscular coordination and accurate timing. Unlike the cognitive measures discussed above, hand steadiness is a very sensitive measure and there is great consistency in the findings. For these reasons, it should be included in all studies as a standardized index of the behavioral effects of the doses used.

Animal studies have consistently found that caffeine increases activity without producing the "locomotor stereotypy" or persistent repetitive movements produced by amphetamine. There are only a few studies with humans; those using high dosages have found increases in gross motor activity for both children and adults. Some studies have found no increases in activity, but only decreases for high consumers who abstain in order to take part in the study and then are in a no-caffeine condition. Careful naturalistic observation studies with doses the size of two-thirds of a soft drink have failed to find any changes in activity for 5 year olds.

Many people believe that caffeine is an ergogenic aid, a substance that helps an athlete generate increased force or endurance. Witness the coffee drinking rituals preceding marathons or the use of coffee to get through the daily grind of training. Empirical studies have shown improved work production in trained cyclists, runners, and cross-country skiers, for example, extending mean cycling time to exhaustion by 20% when cycling at 80% of maximal capacity. Such ergogenic effects occur only during prolonged work and not during short-term work episodes. When the work conditions have been varied or when dosage or caffeine habits are not sufficiently accounted for, effects have been equivocal (although none have been in the reverse direction). Caffeine seems to delay deterioration in performance due to fatigue through both psychological and physical effects. It decreases perceived exertion, perception of fatigue, and drowsiness. It increases self-reported alertness and motivation.

An athlete concerned about the use of caffeine should realize that there is a great range of variability in responses to caffeine. For example, in contrast to others, more sensitive individuals may become overstimulated and show performance decrements. To obtain a beneficial effect while avoiding acquiring tolerance, the athlete might consider abstaining from caffeine for several days before a major event and then consume a moderate serving of coffee (e.g., two cups) 1 hour before competition. For some activities, the diuretic effects of caffeine may be a problem if maintaining hydration is important and difficult. Regular, heavy use throughout training may reduce benefits during competitive performance and may increase blood cholesterol and the risk of heart attack or other medical problems. Finally, the athlete should realize that the International Olympic Committee has banned caffeine when its values are greater than 15 μg/ml in a urine test.

VI. MOOD

One of the most frequent things people report about caffeine is that it affects their mood, and the great majority of research supports these claims. How these mood changes are described depends upon the wording of the questionnaire the researcher uses. In general, consuming moderate quantities of caffeine increases self-reports of alertness, vigor, contentedness, clarity of mind, energy, and efficiency. What counts as a moderate quantity depends on one's personality, habits, and current blood plasma level of caffeine. Higher doses increase reports of nervousness, anxiety, anger, and tenseness, while reducing relaxation or boredom. Finally, it sould be noted that the subjective effects are not as strong in the elderly. These subjective effects seem related to the reinforcing properties of caffeine. For example, when given a choice between color-coded capsules without being told which contains caffeine, those who choose the caffeine capsules are those who report positive mood changes. Those who do not are those who report negative mood changes.

VII. PERCEPTION

Can consumers of a caffeinated beverage perceive the presence or absence of caffeine in the beverage based on immediate sensory qualities at the time of consumption? Apparently they cannot at normal levels of concentration in colas, tea, or coffee; however, when concentration reaches 200 mg per cup of coffee, the presence of caffeine can be reliably detected. At medium and high concentrations, elderly women (67–77 years old) are less sensitive (have larger Weber ratios) to caffeine than younger women (18–25 years old). Ability to rate the intensity of caffeine is unrelated to ability to taste thiourea. Neither acute nor chronic caffeine ingestion appreciably affects other taste thresholds.

One rationale for adding caffeine to foodstuffs is that it enhances flavor. Experimental results have failed to show any enhancement for a variety of substances, even when "whole mouth" procedures are used. In a mixture with sucrose, taste suppression is the most common finding.

Caffeine has been reported to reduce the kinesthetic after-effect in highly impulsive subjects. Higher caffeine users who also use oral contraceptives show poorer color discrimination than nonusers of oral contraceptives for the yellow-through-blue portions of the color spectrum. According to anecdotal reports, caffeine increases synesthesia. Olfactory hallucinations triggered by 500 mg injections have been reported.

Can a person who ingests a caffeine or placebo capsule perceive the presence or absence of caffeine later (30 minutes to 2 hours has been tested in various studies) on the basis of pharmacological effects? Various researchers have found that untrained observers can make this discrimination reliably at 300, 200, or 100 mg. With training, most people can make the discrimination at 56 mg, a fraction at 18 mg, and only a few at 10 mg. That physiological and subjective effects are present at these low doses is noteworthy. In these studies, different people rely upon different cues, and there are wide individual differences in sensitivity to caffeine. It is not clear to what extent the discrimination is controlled by direct effects of caffeine versus suppression of withdrawal effects.

VIII. ADDICTION

Is caffeine really an addictive drug? By the criteria used in the 1970s, a drug of addiction must have psychoactive properties, must have reinforcing properties, and must result in withdrawal symptoms when its use is abruptly discontinued. Caffeine is psychoactive: witness the stimulating effects people report. Caffeine is reinforcing according to people's reports as well as carefully controlled experimental studies. Does removing caffeine produce withdrawal symptoms? The adverse effects are well documented. When caffeine users abstain, they experience such sumptoms as dysphoria, drowsiness, yawning, poor concentration, disinterest in work, runny nose, facial flushing, headache, fatigue, irritability, and anxiety. The symptoms typically begin between 12 and 24 hours after the person discontinues use of caffeine. The symptoms vary from individual to individual; they can be mild to extreme, peak within 20 to 48 hours, and last for a week. Headache, for example, is reported by about one-fourth of the heavy users who abstain. In a few cases, the symptoms have been reported to appear when caffeine intake was gradually reduced over several weeks rather than abruptly. Even someone who is a relatively light user, habitually consuming as little as 200 mg of caffeine per day, may experience some withdrawal symptoms. Nonusers can become quickly addicted—within as little as 6 to 15 days, if high doses are consumed. Drugs of addiction tend to upset the homeostasis of the body. Addicts would, in fact, be in constant disequilibrium except for the fact that they develop compensatory responses, i.e., physiological changes the opposite of those induced by the drug. Furthermore, these compensatory responses become conditioned to the cues that precede drug use. In short, the body prepares itself for the drug assault. Caffeine users, like users of other addictive drugs, develop compensatory responses that become conditioned to the stimulus cues associated with caffeine consumption. For example, the sight of coffee inhibits salivation in chronic users of caffeine, a response that compensates for the increase in salivation produced by caffeine. Note that decaffeinated coffee provides the same visual and gustatory cues as caffeinated coffee, thereby also inhibiting salivation. Clearly, then, caffeine is a drug of addiction by these standards. [*See* SUBSTANCE ABUSE.]

More recent discussions of the "abuse liability" of drugs emphasize drug use properties that maintain self-administration despite other drug-use properties that interfere with fulfilling life's responsibilities or with healthy bodily functions. Additional clinical criteria include unsuccessful efforts to control use, continued use despite knowledge of a problem caused by use, and tolerance to the behavioral effects of the drug. With regards to these criteria, caffeine has not maintained self-administration behavior as reliably as classic drugs of abuse such as cocaine or *d*-amphetamine. One study found 100- or 200-mg caffeine capsules acted as positive reinforcers and maintained self-administration, but that study gave subjects an unusual kind of additional support: when the subjects chose between capsules, the experimenters reminded them of their own subjective responses to each kind of capsule during past administrations. In this study, 400- and 600-mg doses acted as punishers. Other studies have varied the caffeine content of available capsules or coffee to see if self-administration varies. There is some evidence for daily regulation of caffeine intake, but compensation is very imperfect. There are some intriguing initial results that show one respect in which caffeine is stronger than alcohol: placebo responses to caffeine include motor and cognitive behavior, not just social and affective behaviors. Because caffeine generally has weaker functions or has effects only in more limited situations, some authors have suggested (reasonably) that it has less dependence potential than, say, *d*-amphetamine. Others have gone further to suggest that caffeine withdrawal but not caffeine abuse be included in a newly revised *Diagnostic and Statistical Manual of Mental Disorders*. Others have (unreasonbly) suggested that caffeine is not capable of promoting dependence.

A. Tolerance

When an individual has developed tolerance to a drug, larger dosages are required than previously to achieve a given effect. This pattern of decreasing effects can cause drug users to increase dosages in order to compensate for the decrease. With chronic caffeine use, it takes larger dosages to achieve the same (mild) diuretic and salivary effects. Caffeine users show smaller blood pressure increases than nonusers with the same caffeine dosage. There is some evidence to suggest that these different levels of tolerance develop only a few days of chronic use and are lost within a day, although one would like to see this research replicated. On the other hand, less tolerance seems to develop for the stimulating effects of caffeine on the central nervous system. Furthermore, for many individuals, increases in caffeine dosage would be self-limiting because higher doses exacerbate undesirable symptoms (nervousness, anxiety, restlessness, insomnia, tremors, gastrointestinal disturbances, and feelings of uneasiness).

B. Toxicity

In contrast to the high toxicity of theophylline, caffeine is not very toxic. Nevertheless, caffeine can produce symptoms that require medical consultation. For example, sudden increases in consumption have been associated with a variety of adverse effects, such as delirium, abdominal cramps, vomiting, high levels of anxiety and hostility, and psychosis. More gradual increases may not show toxicity because tolerance develops. Higher doses of caffeine can cause convulsions and still higher doses can cause death from respiratory failure. A lethal dose in adults appears to be 5 to 10 g, the amount of caffeine in approximately 200 cola beverages. There is little concern that death could occur from beverage consumption because gastric distress and vomiting would prevent concentrations from reaching life-threatening levels. Although similar principles would seem to apply to over-the-counter caffeinated drugs, at least seven deaths from ingested caffeinated medications were reported between 1959 and 1980. One death after injection of 3.2 g has also been reported.

IX. PSYCHOPATHOLOGY

Many years ago, the well-known psychologist Harry Stack Sullivan observed "incipient depression and neurasthenic states" in a client after "unwitting denial of the accustomed caffeine dosage." He surmised that "there might be times when a cup of coffee would delay the outcropping of a mental disorder." Recent concerns reflect the opposite point of view, namely, that consumption of caffeine might lead to caffeine intoxication, that it might exacerbate other psychological disorders, or that its symptoms might be misdiagnosed as another disorder.

A. Caffeinism

Caffeine consumption to the point of clinical manifestations is termed "caffeinism" or "caffeine intoxication." The *Diagnostic and Statistical Manual* (*DMS-IV*) defines three diagnostic criteria: (1) recent consumption in excess of 250 mg (2 to 4 cups of strong coffee), (2) at least five somatic symptoms, and (3) no diagnosis of another covering physical or mental disorder. Because health professionals have traditionally ignored patterns of caffeine consumption (cf. the anecdote about Sullivan above), this diagnostic category performs the useful function of drawing attention to caffeine and helping prevent misdiagnosis. Nonetheless, all of the criteria are open to criticism. The 250-mg threshold may be too low in that the majority of the population exceed this level on any given day. The 12 candidates for somatic symptoms is an imprecise collection troubled by subjective terms, duplications, omissions, and overlap. The third criterion provides no way to eliminate competing hypotheses.

B. Anxiety Disorders

The relationship between caffeine and emotional health has been most often studied in terms of generalized anxiety disorder (GAD) and panic disorder (PD). Several biologically plausible mechanisms for anxiogenic (anxiety-producing) effects of caffeine have been studied, but definitive results have not yet been obtained.

The idea that caffeine consumption should correlate positively with anxiety level is too simplistic. Population studies have found positive, null, and negative correlations. The most persuasive studies have shown moderate *negative* (about −.25) correlations between caffeine consumption and anxiety. One explanation is that anxious people avoid caffeine because of its stimulant effects. Note that this explanation depends on the original presumption that acute caffeine doses cause increases in anxiety; furthermore, this explanation makes it impossible to predict even the direction of a population correlation. That direction depends upon what proportion of the people recognize the link between caffeine and anxiety and self-regulate their intake.

In laboratory studies that use low doses, some healthy people interpret the stimulation provided by caffeine as a pleasant, general elevation in mood, whereas others find it unpleasant. After consuming moderate amounts of caffeine (200 mg), many people report increased feelings of restlessness, tension, and anxiety. Larger doses (300 mg) can lead to further anxiety, hostility, and depression. Similar induction of anxiety has been found in animals. Although the human data indicating these effects were obtained from self-reports, they have been corroborated by objective observers. In double-blind experiments, observers were able to reliably see the increased restlessness and "drug effect" of caffeine on users. In even larger doses, the symptoms may be indistinguishable from anxiety disorders. Reductions in daily caffeine level can reduce anxiety, although sudden withdrawal can increase it.

Most laboratory studies have shown that caffeine increases anxiety for normals and that patients with panic disorders are particularly sensitive to the anxiogenic effects of caffeine. In addition to the usual symptoms, they show palpitations, nervousness, fear, nausea, and tremors. They show clear dose-response effects. A 480-mg dose is enough to create a panic attack in these patients, although a much larger dose would be required to create similar panic in a normal person. In contrast to these studies, one study found caffeine injections of 250 mg increased state anxiety for normals but not for GAD or PD patients. This "failure" may have been due to overshadowing effects from the injection procedure, the paper and pencil dependent measure, or the small dose size. In summary, additional studies are needed to establish the true physiological mechanism by which caffeine affects anxiety and to corroborate the interpretations of the behavioral data proposed above. In the meantime, all the available data strongly reinforce the clinical wisdom that patients with anxiety disorders should avoid caffeine-containing foods and beverages. [*See* Anxiety; Panic Attacks.]

C. Depressive Disorders

One theory is that caffeine interferes with the hypothalamic-pituitary-adrenal axis and thus plays a role in major depression. At present, there is no physiological evidence for this. A contrasting theory is that during depressive episodes, patients self-medicate with caffeine to raise themselves out of their depression. Either theory implies a positive correlation between level of depression and level of caffeine consumption. One population study found such a positive correlation, but a weak one. Some laboratory studies have found that caffeine increases feelings of depression and exacerbates manic-depressive symptoms; furthermore, reducing daily caffeine intake can improve mood. Caution must be used in applying this finding clinically. For example, in two cases of bipolar affective disorder who were on lithium treatment, reduction of caffeine intake increased lithium tremors.

In contrast to the studies with positive results, several have found null results. At this time, the relationship between caffeine and depression, if any, is unclear.

The role of low-dose oral or i.v. caffeine in electroconvulsive therapy (ECT) presents a much clearer picture. When ECT is indicated for major depression patients, it is often difficult to achieve desired seizure duration and to hold settings within desired ranges. Pretreatment with doses from 100 to 125 mg of caffeine can maintain duration and settings and achieve equivalent therapeutic outcome with no cardiac complications, cognitive side effects, or additional complications. One note of caution: patients can respond differently on different trials; hence careful monitoring on every trial is necessary. As chemists invent new xanthine derivatives, there is some chance that they will find one without unwanted side effects and with more selectivity for adenosine receptors thus allowing more circumscript pharmacological intervention. [*See* Depression.]

D. Schizophrenic Disorders

Schizophrenic patients have been observed to drink 20 cups of coffee a day, wear coffee-brown "mustaches," and snort instant-coffee crystals. Populations studies have shown that they chronically consume more caffeine than the general public (although some studies have failed to find this difference). Caffeine ingestion has been shown to exacerbate schizophrenic syndromes as evidenced in paper-and-pencil self-reports as well as in nurses' observations. Both case studies and hospital floor studies have shown that caffeine removal reduces schizophrenic symptoms, in particular, aggression. One of these studies on aggression is difficult to interpret because in the same time period, a nearby state hospital showed the same decline in aggressive patient acts without any change in caffeine consumption! Other studies have failed to find any effect of caffeine removal. Some authors have tried to explain seemingly contradictory results by saying the effects occur for only certain subgroups of schizophrenic patients (those who are impulsive and those who are hypersensitive to caffeine). Different proportions of these subgroups could account for different outcomes. [See SCHIZOPHRENIA.]

Note that while chronic caffeine consumption is associated with increased aggression, acute consumption decreases aggression. There is a plausible physiological mechanism for acute effects: benzodiazepine elicits maternal-like aggression in virgin rats and causes disinhibition in humans; caffeine is a benzodiazepine antagonist and hence should decrease aggression. Laboratory data with both rats and humans show this decrease in overt aggressive behaviors. Just as with anxiety, the opposite relationships for acute and chronic consumption should not be viewed as a paradox. Rather, different complex sets of factors contribute to the difference in relationships.

E. Clinical Precautions and Conclusions

Two issues are important for their practical implications, although there has not been a lot of research related to them. (1) Clinicians working with anorexics may want to monitor their patients' caffeine intake. In their striving to be thin, anorexics have been observed to consume large quantities of diet colas or coffee, apparently because these beverages have few calories but suppress the appetite. (2) Clinicians working with patients who are taking psychotropic medication should be aware of potential drug–caffeine interactions. Diazepam has antagonistic and synergistic interactions with caffeine, although the exact nature of these interactions is controversial. Presumably other benzodiazepines have similar interactions. Coffee and phenylpropanolamine have been reported to produce manic psychosis. Coffee and tea both form flaky, insoluble precipitates with antipsychotic drugs. One case study reported caffeine consumption increased step by step with increased medication. Conversely, with caffeine abstinence, the symptoms disappeared and so did the need for medication.

The relationship between caffeine and psychopathology is an important but confusing area. Intoxication among inpatients is probably much more common than has been realized; therefore, routine assessment of patterns of consumption is advisable. The use of "coffee groups" in therapy needs to be considered carefully, case by case. The results reported above and the simplicity of restricting caffeine recommend trying the restriction in many cases. Nonetheless, blanket condemnation of caffeine intake is unwarranted. What is detrimental for some appears beneficial for others. Furthermore, restricting one intoxicant (e.g., caffeine intoxication) may lead to others (e.g., water intoxication).

X. OTHER ISSUES

A. Sleep Disturbance

It is commonly believed that the ingestion of caffeine, particularly in the form of drinking coffee close to bedtime, interferes with sleep. Indeed, there is evidence (both in the form of questionnaire and experimental studies) that caffeine has adverse effects on sleep. Caffeine can interfere with both the quantity of sleep (e.g., a delay in sleep onset) and quality of sleep (e.g., adverse effects on the depth of sleep). However, definitive conclusions are difficult to draw, because the effects of caffeine on sleep can be modified by such factors as the time when caffeine is ingested, an individual's habitual pattern of caffeine intake, and individual differences in sensitivity to caffeine. Moreover, caffeine can have adverse consequences on sleep without the individual being aware of such effects. [See SLEEP.]

B. Heritability

To what extent is caffeine consumption influenced by genetic factors? During the 1980s and early 1990s, the media reported "astonishing successes" in the field of behavior genetics in identifying genes underlying such crippling diseases as cystic fibrosis or Huntington's disease, and more complex traits, such as manic–depressive disorder and alcoholism. The influence of genetics has been sought even for such seemingly personal choices as cigarette smoking and coffee drinking. One common research technique is to look for stronger patterns of inheritance in twins than in brothers and sisters or in adopted siblings. The calculated heritability is the degree to which the trait stems from genetic factors. Studies of male twins have reported an unadjusted heritability estimate for coffee drinking of 46% that drops to 36% when the confounding factor of cigarette smoking is adjusted for. That the heritability estimate remains sizable and highly statistically significant supports the conclusion that coffee drinking is, in part, genetically determined. However, this result must be interpreted cautiously. These estimates are confounded by other sources of variance in the data, such as age and sex, that have not been adjusted for. The estimates are based on self-reports that may not be as reliable as desired, and involve substance use, not addiction or caffeinism that may have different estimates. Causal interpretations cannot be made directly from the heritability estimate. For example, viral diseases may show the same patterns of incidence in families—not because the virus is inherited, but because susceptibility is.

C. Premenstrual Syndrome

The media have given what appears to be premature coverage to a purported link between caffeine consumption and severity of premenstrual syndrome. Only one researcher has reported a connection, and that in poorly controlled studies. Another researcher has failed to find a connection. [*See* PREMENSTRUAL SYNDROME (PMS).]

D. Headache and Migraine

There is a debate over whether caffeine has independent analgesic effects equivalent to acetaminophen. Several researchers have found promising indications that sumatriptan relieves migraine headaches more quickly, effectively, and with fewer side-effects than caffeine compounds (or aspirin compounds). There is one interesting report that shows the relevance of personality variables to biomedical research: for introverts, caffeine in combination with analgesics may potentiate pain stimulation.

E. Treatment for Obesity

Although neither caffeine alone nor ephedrine alone leads to effective weight loss, the compound seems effective through anorexia (75%, diminished appetite) and increased thermogenesis (25%, heat produc-

tion). Newer selective β-agonists should be compared against this reference.

XI. CONCLUSIONS

Because caffeine consumption involves both pharmacological effects and behavior, both behavioral and biomedical science are needed to fully understand its impact on health. The research to date has discounted some but not all of the potential concerns about negative health consequences. Caffeine has both beneficial and adverse effects on physical and mental performance, but these are not well-established because of the intricacies of the research methodology. There is much more to be learned about the mechanisms by which caffeine produces its effects. Researchers have come to opposite conclusions on many of the issues, and in the process have revealed extraneous variables that must be taken into account. It is important that there be future research to resolve these issues, and that the studies be well-designed and well-controlled, taking these new variables into account.

Some organizations have used the research on caffeine to advocate that caffeine consumption be considered a social problem. This level of alarm is inappropriate; however, more education of the general public regarding caffeine is warranted. Educational efforts should cover known and probable health risks, misconceptions that caffeine counteracts the effects of alcohol, misconceptions about sources of caffeine, becoming aware of one's actual intake, and ways to reduce one's intake. Those who want to reduce or eliminate caffeine intake may do so on their own by reducing the concentration of caffeine in the foods or beverages that they consume (e.g., by steeping tea 1 minute instead of 5, mixing caffeinated and decaffeinated coffee), substituting noncaffeinated products for caffeinated ones (e.g., carob for chocolate, drinking fruit juice during coffee breaks, noncaffeinated for caffeinated over-the-counter medications), gradually eliminating occasions on which caffeine is consumed (e.g., coffee with the evening meal), and by organizing a support group of friends or co-workers. Some individuals may find it hard to reduce their intake of caffeine because they lack motivation, because of social pressure to consume, or because they do not want to give up the stimulating effects of caffeine. Such individuals may want to seek the help of health-care professionals who use systemic multi-component interventions that have been shown to be successful. In short, in order for individuals to decide to continue or change their caffeine habits, they must be informed.

This article has been reprinted from the *Encyclopedia of Human Behavior, Volume 1.*

BIBLIOGRAPHY

American Psychiatric Association. (1994). *DSM-IV: Diagnostic and Statistical Manual of Mental Disorders,* 4th ed. American Psychiatric Association, Washington, DC.

Benowitz, N. L. (1990). Clinical pharmacology of caffeine. In "Annual Review of Medicine: Selected Topics in the Clinical Sciences" (W. P. Creger, C. H. Coggins, and E. W. Hancock, Eds.), Vol. 41. Annual Reviews, Inc., Palo Alto, CA.

Blount, J. P., and Cox, W. M. (1991). Caffeine. In "Encyclopedia of Human Biology" (R. Dulbecco, Ed.), Vol. II. Academic Press, San Diego.

Blount, J. P., and Cox, W. M. (1985). Perception of caffeine and its effects: Laboratory and everyday abilities. *Percept. Psychophys.* **38,** 55–62.

Bruce, M. S., and Lader, M. H. (1986). Caffeine: Clinical and experimental effects in humans. *Hum. Psychopharmacol.* **1,** 63–82.

Dews, P. B. (Ed.) (1984). "Caffeine: Perspectives from Recent Research." Springer-Verlag, Berlin.

Griffiths, R. R., and Woodson, P. P. (1988). Caffeine physical dependence: A review of human and laboratory animal studies. *Psychopharmacology* **94,** 437–451.

Fudin, R., and Nicastro, R. (1988). Can caffeine antagonize alcohol-induced performance decrements in humans? *Perceptual and Motor Skills* **67,** 375–391.

Hughes, J. R., Oliveto, A. H., Helzer, J. E., Higgins, S. T., and Bickeal, W. K. (1992). Should caffeine abuse, dependence or withdrawal be added to DSM-IV and ICD-10? *Am. J. Psych.* **149,** 33–40.

Humphreys, M. S., and Revelle, W. (1984). Personality, motivation, and performance: A theory of the relationship between individual differences and information processing. *Psychol. Rev.* **91,** 153–184.

James, J. E. (1991). "Caffeine & Health." Academic Press, San Diego.

Revelle, W., Humphreys, M. S., Simon, L., and Gilliland, K. (1980). The interactive effect of personality, time of day, and caffeine: A test of the arousal model. *J. Exp. Psychol. Gen.* **109,** 1–31.

Troyer, R. J., and Markle, G. E. (1984). Coffee drinking: An emerging social problem? *Soc. Problems* **31,** 403–416.

Watson, R. R. (1988). Caffeine: Is it dangerous to health? *Am. J. Health Promot.* **2**(4), 13–22.

Cancer

Barbara L. Andersen

The Ohio State University

Biobehavioral Model A theory of the interaction of psychological, behavioral, and biological factors for understanding the relationships among these variables and cancer progression.

Natural Killer Cell Leukocytes that play a role in nonspecific immunity by the specific lysis (killing) of cancer cells.

Stress An interaction between a person and the environment that includes the individual's appraisal of the event(s) and the available coping resources, in addition to his/her psychological and physiological responses to the event(s).

CANCER is a major health problem. The psychological adjustment to the disease and treatments can be difficult, and data suggest that such stress may be related to important biologic effects, such as downward regulation of the immune system. A biobehavioral model of adjustment to the stresses of cancer is discussed, including the mechanisms by which psychological and behavioral responses may influence biological processes and disease outcomes.

I. THE MAGNITUDE OF THE PROBLEM

Cancers vary in their prevalence, gender distribution, and mortality. Tables I and II display data from the United States on the incidence and death rates by specific sites and genders. These data indicate, for example, that women are most commonly diagnosed with breast cancer and men with prostate cancer, but that lung cancer is the number one killer of both sexes; in fact, the American Cancer Society reports that over the last 30 years lung cancer death rates have increased 94% in men and 433% in women. In examining death rates worldwide, the top killers of women include breast, colon and rectum, lung, and uterine cancers. For men, lung, colon and rectum, prostate, and stomach cancers are the common cancer killers.

II. THE BIOBEHAVIORAL MODEL

The mental health community emphasizes the need to reduce stress and prevent deteriorations in quality of life for those with cancer. The importance of such efforts is underscored by three contextual factors. One, the stability of many cancer mortality rates, particularly those with the highest incidence such as lung and breast, makes it imperative that new, innovative treatments be developed to improve survival rates. Two, research has demonstrated that psychological interventions result in significant improvements in quality of life. Three, both qualitative and quantitative summaries of the psychoneuroimmunology (PNI) literature conclude that psychological distress and stressors (i.e., negative life events, both acute and chronic) are reliably associated with changes—downregulation—in immunity. Thus, addressing the mental health needs of those with cancer will have impor-

Table I Cancer Incidence (New Cases) by Site and Gender—1996 Estimates[a]

	Cancer incidence		
Male (Total est. 764,300)		Female (Total est. 594,850)	
Site	Number (%)	Site	Number (%)
Prostate	317,100 (41%)	Breast	184,300 (31%)
Lung	98,900 (13%)	Lung	78,100 (13%)
Colon &		Colon &	
Rectum	47,600 (9%)	Rectum	65,900 (11%)
Bladder	38,300 (5%)	Uterus	49,700 (5%)
Lymphoma	29,900 (4%)	Ovary	26,700 (4%)
Oral	20,100 (3%)	Lymphoma	22,800 (4%)
Melanoma		Melanoma	
of Skin	21,800 (3%)	of Skin	16,500 (3%)
Kidney	18,500 (2%)	Pancreas	13,900 (2%)
Leukemia	15,300 (2%)	Bladder	14,600 (2%)
Stomach	14,000 (2%)	Leukemia	12,300 (2%)
Pancreas	12,400 (2%)	Kidney	12,100 (2%)
Larynx	9,200 (2%)	Oral	9,390 (2%)

[a] Adapted from Cancer Facts & Figures–1996. (1996). American Cancer Society, Inc.

tant quality of life benefits and the possibility is raised of positive biologic (or health) consequences as well. [*See* PSYCHONEUROIMMUNOLOGY.]

Table II Cancer Deaths by Site and Gender—1996 Estimates Cancer Deaths[a]

	Cancer deaths		
Male (Total est. 292,300)		Female (Total est. 262,440)	
Site	Number (%)	Site	Number (%)
Lung	94,400 (32%)	Lung	64,300 (25%)
Prostate	41,400 (14%)	Breast	44,300 (17%)
Colon &		Colon &	
Rectum	22,700 (9%)	Rectum	23,700 (10%)
Pancreas	13,600 (5%)	Ovary	14,800 (6%)
Lymphoma	12,400 (4%)	Pancreas	14,200 (5%)
Leukemia	11,600 (4%)	Lymphoma	10,900 (4%)
Stomach	8,300 (3%)	Uterus	10,900 (4%)
Esophagus	8,500 (3%)	Leukemia	9,400 (4%)
Liver	8,400 (3%)	Liver	6,800 (3%)
Bladder	7,800 (3%)	Brain	6,100 (2%)
Brain	7,200 (2%)	Stomach	5,700 (2%)
Kidney	7,300 (2%)	Multiple	
		Myeloma	5,100 (2%)

[a] Adapted from Cancer Facts & Figures–1996. (1996). American Cancer Society, Inc.

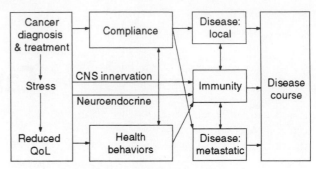

Figure I A biobehavioral model of the psychological (stress and QoL), behavioral (compliance and health behaviors), and biologic pathways from cancer stressors to disease course. (CNS = Central Nervous System). From Andersen, Kiecolt-Glaser, & Glaser (1994). Copyright © 1994 by the American Psychological Association. Reprinted with permission.

Figure 1 provides a conceptual model of the psychological and behavioral factors and biologic mechanisms by which disease or health outcomes might be influenced. The majority of the paths move in one causal direction.

A. Stress and Quality of Life

The model first considers the potential for stress and lowered quality of life that comes with the diagnosis and treatments. These are objective, negative events. Although negative events do not always produce stress and lowered quality of life, data from many studies document severe, *acute* stress at diagnosis. However, it is also clear that lengthy cancer treatments and disruptions in major life areas occur, producing *chronic stress*. Emotional distress, in combination with the other life disruptions, can result in a stable but lower quality of life. For example, in a study of Hodgkin's Disease survivors, men reported lowered motivation for interpersonal intimacy, increased avoidant thinking about illness (which is characteristic of posttraumatic stress), illness-related concerns, and difficulty in returning to predisease employment status long after treatment had ended. Other permanent sequelae, such as sexual problems and/or sterility, may impact intimate relationships and social support. Unemployment, underemployment, job discrimination, and difficulty in obtaining health insurance can also become chronic stressors. [*See* STRESS.]

B. Health Behaviors

There are also important health behavior sequelae (see arrow from cancer stress and lowered QoL to health behaviors in Fig. 1), specifically an increase in negative behaviors and/or a decrease in positive ones. There may be many examples of negative health behaviors. For example, individuals who are depressed and/or anxious are more likely to self-medicate with alcohol and other drugs, and, in addition, alcohol abuse can potentiate distress. Distressed individuals often have *appetite disturbances* or dietary changes that are manifest by eating less often or eating meals of lower nutritional value. While there are individual differences in behavior changes of this type, women may be at risk, and women who have undergone changes in their eating habits (e.g., restriction due to cancer treatments) may have even greater vulnerability. Distressed individuals may report *sleep disturbances,* such as early morning awakening, sleep onset insomnia, and middle-night insomnia. *Cigarette smoking and caffeine use,* which often increase during periods of stress, can intensify the physiologic effects of psychosocial stress, such as increasing catecholamine release. [*See* Alcohol Problems; Anxiety; Depression; Sleep; Smoking.]

Conversely, individuals who are stressed may not begin or abandon previous positive health behaviors, such as regular *physical activity.* There is a positive relationship between physical activity or fitness and psychological health. In the case of breast cancer patients, positive mood effects as well as increased functional capacity were found for women receiving chemotherapy but also participating in a program of aerobic interval training. [*See* Exercise and Mental Health.]

The model suggests that health behaviors may, in turn, effect immunity (see arrow from health behaviors to immunity in Fig. 1). The covariation of immunity and the health behaviors noted above has been found. Also, some problematic health behaviors interact to produce detrimental immune consequences. For example, substance abuse has direct effects on immunity as well as indirect effects via alterations in nutrition, and poor nutrition is associated with a variety of immunological impairments. Conversely, there is growing evidence that physical activity may have positive consequences for both the immune and endocrine systems, even among individuals with chronic diseases. In summary, these lines of data suggest that distressed individuals tend toward negative health behaviors that may potentiate their stress and, concurrently, affect their immunologic functioning; positive health behaviors, such as exercise, may have the converse effect.

The model suggests that health behaviors may be directly related to disease progression (see arrow from health behaviors to disease: metastatic in Fig. 1). Considering all the health behaviors noted above, the strongest case can be made for the importance of nutrition and diet in breast cancer. A variety of data link nutrition/dietary factors and risk for breast cancer, such as epidemiologic data of varied cancer rates corresponding with population differences in body fat, animal models linking high-fat diets and tumor growth, and correlations between rates of obesity and the increase of breast cancer incidence. More germane to the model are data suggesting that increased fat intake, obesity at diagnosis, and weight gain may be related to recurrence and survival. Alternatively, some suggest that fiber, rather than fat, is the critical dietary factor, in that fiber is postulated to modify serum estrogen levels by increased fecal excretion of estrogens. Taken together, these data suggest that behavioral factors relevant to nutrition, fat/fiber balance, and energy expenditure (vis-a-vis weight gain) may be relevant to disease progression in breast cancer. [*See* Food, Nutrition, and Mental Health; Obesity.]

C. Compliance

The second behavioral factor noted in the model is *treatment (non)compliance* as the available data suggest that psychological factors may be important (see arrow from stress/QoL to compliance in Fig. 1). Compliance problems cross a wide range of diseases, therapies, and individual patient characteristics. In cancer, some patients become discouraged and fail to complete treatment. A general implication of such behaviors is the invalidation of clinical trials, but a specific implication for the individual patient is that his/her survival may be compromised if an inadequate dosage of therapy is received. That is, dosage reductions can compromise one's survival if a lower intensity of cancer therapy results in differential (i.e., lower) survival rates. The model presumes that a range of compliance behaviors may be relevant as different treatment regimen characteristics may produce different behavioral difficulties. The model suggest that poor compliance can effect either local or metastatic control of the disease or both, and which route is selected depends on the treatment regimen as well as the characteristics of an individual's noncompliance.

D. The Interaction of Health Behaviors and Compliance

The model specifies that the processes governing compliance and health behaviors may interact (see double-headed arrow between compliance and health behaviors in Fig. 1) or even be synergistic. That is, those who are compliant may expect better health outcomes and, thus, comply with diet, exercise, sleep, and so on, or other behaviors indicative of "good health." Despite their importance, health behavior and compliance variables have been understudied in psychological intervention studies, including those with immune outcomes and those without. It is also noteworthy that changes in health behaviors and/or compliance have been offered as post hoc explanations for some of the most notable intervention findings such as the survival difference in the 1989 report by Spiegel, Bloom, Kraemer, and Gottheil (see discussion below).

E. Biological Pathways

Stress sets into motion important biological effects involving the autonomic, endocrine, and immune system. Stress may be routed to the immune system by the central nervous system (CNS) via activation of the sympathetic nervous system or through neuroendocrine-immune pathways (i.e., the release of hormones; see Fig. 1). In the latter case, a variety of hormones released under stress have been implicated in immune modulation (e.g., catecholamines, cortisol, prolactin, and growth hormone).

Without any stress pathway (effect) to immunity, there is evidence for the importance of the immune responses in host resistance against cancer progression, and hence the arrows going in both directions from immunity to local and metastatic disease. Experts in the immunology/cancer area cite the following important findings with regards to the specific importance of NK (natural killer) cell activity: (1) patients with a variety of solid malignancies and large tumor burdens have diminished NK cell activity in the blood; (2) low NK cell activity in cancer patients is significantly associated with the development of distant metastases; and, (3) in patients treated for metastatic disease, the survival time without metastasis correlates with NK cell activity.

In considering these mechanisms, a central issue is whether an immune response can be effected by stress.

Of some relevance is the fact that both qualitative and quantitative summaries of the psychoneuroimmunology literature conclude that psychological distress and stressors (i.e., negative life events, both acute and chronic) are reliably associated with immune down-regulation in noncancer populations. Both *time limited (acute) stressors* can produce immunologic changes in relatively healthy individuals, as well as *chronic stressors*. Some of the largest NK cell effects are found for lengthy stressors and/or ones which have interpersonal components. Many of the qualities of chronic stressors [continued emotional distress, disrupted life tasks (e.g., employment) and social relationships] occur with the decrements in quality of life found in studies of cancer patients, and so it may be possible that stress in the context of cancer may also lead to immune down-regulation. In studies with cancer patients, the data are generally in line with data from healthy individuals with "positive" indicators of QoL (e.g., social adjustment) predicting higher NK cell lysis and "negative/distress" indicators (e.g., emotional distress) predicting lower.

F. Disease Course

Are there adverse health (illness) consequences of stress? There are few data on this important issue. One of the more compelling studies, however, came from Cohen, et al.'s 1991 experiment with healthy volunteers. Subjects participating in an experiment focused on the development of the common cold were inoculated with either a cold virus or a placebo. Analyses revealed that rates of both respiratory infection and clinical colds increased in a dose-response manner with increases in psychological stress across five different strains of cold viruses. Data from the Kiecolt-Glaser/Glaser laboratories show that Alzheimer care givers had slower healing of a wound (punch biopsy) than matched community controls. Thus, experimental data from stressed but otherwise healthy samples suggest covariation of stress and selected health outcomes.

III. PSYCHOLOGICAL INTERVENTIONS

Current psychological interventions for cancer patients emphasize relaxation, coping, social support, and disease-specific components. Interventions typically are offered within weeks or months of the diagnosis, with the attempt to reduce the crisislike distress that can occur early in the process. In contrast, there has been little attention to the maintenance of change. If one intent of interventions is to produce a biologic response (immune enhancement) in concert with improved quality of life, then the *maintenance* of psychological and behavioral changes becomes essential. Thus, interventions might be designed to yield immediate (acute) psychological posttreatment changes, but also include elements to ensure that change continues.

Few studies have examined immune or health consequences, but there are three notable exceptions. The most comprehensive study is that of Fawzy, Cousins, Kemeny, and colleagues in 1990. They studied newly treated Stage I or II melanoma patients randomized to no intervention or a structured short term (10 sessions) group support intervention. Significant psychological and coping outcomes for the intervention subjects were evident by 6 months posttreatment; additionally, there were increases in the percentage of large granular lymphocytes, the NK cell phenotype, and interferon alpha-augmented NK cell activity. Importantly, the magnitude of the NK changes was frequently greater than 25%. The correlation data was also supportive: interferon-augmented NK cytotoxic activity increased with concomitant reductions in anxiety ($-.37$) and depression ($-.33$). Fawzy and colleagues found that 6-year follow-up data on disease endpoints indicate significant group differences on disease progression, with 29% of controls and 9% of experimental subjects dying in the 6-year interval. Post hoc analyses indicate that from baseline to the 6-month assessment, the survivors reported significant decreases in affective distress, increases in active behavioral coping, and increases in CD16 NK cells and interferon alpha augmented NK cell activity (i.e., immune up-regulation). In contrast, those who died showed no significant changes on any of these variables, that is, no QoL improvement or immune enhancement.

Data from a relaxation intervention study provide confirmatory evidence as well. Gruber, et al. studied 13 stage I, node negative breast cancer patients who received EMG biofeedback assisted relaxation training. Assessments during the 9-week intervention indicated significant immune differences between the treatment and control groups in the expected direction.

Other relevant data come from studies with poor prognosis patients—women with recurrent breast cancer and lung cancer patients. Spiegel, Bloom, and colleagues randomized women with metastatic breast disease to no treatment or a group treatment that met weekly for at least one year. The intervention group reported significantly lower emotional distress (POMS) and fewer maladaptive coping responses than the controls. A 10-year follow-up by Spiegel and colleagues in 1989 found a striking survival difference between the groups, 18.9 months for the control subjects and 36.6 months for the intervention subjects from study entry until death. Contrary data comes from Linn, Linn, and Harris who offered a supportive death and dying intervention program to male cancer patients (46% had lung cancer). Despite favorable QoL outcomes for the intervention subjects there were no survival differences. Aside from the many methodology differences of the two studies, a disease factor accounting for the discrepancy might be the shorter survival "window" for metastatic lung cancer in contrast to metastatic breast cancer (Five-year survival rates are 18% and 76%, respectively, for initial Stage III disease and 2% and 20%, respectively, for initial Stage IV disease), and the fact that hormonal factors may be important for breast cancer whereas that is not the case for lung cancer. Also of note is the duration of the intervention in the Spiegel study—one year—which may have ensured the continuation and maintenance of psychological gains.

IV. CONCLUSION

The biobehavioral model offers that stress, QoL, health behaviors, and compliance are the major factors in a conceptual model of adjustment to the cancer stressor. Also part of the model is the physiological system—the immune system—which may be one of the more important ones for moderating the effects of stress on disease processes. The literature confirms that QoL benefits accrue from psychological interventions. In contrast, health behaviors and compliance have rarely been an intervention target, although data suggest that such a broadened approach would be effective and would provide added benefits. This model provides a testable conceptualization for the mental health and health implications of cancer, and it provides a framework for testing specific biologic or health consequences of psychological/behavioral interventions.

BIBLIOGRAPHY

Andersen, B. L. (1992). Psychological interventions for cancer patients to enhance the quality of life. *Journal of Consulting and Clinical Psychology, 60,* 552–568.

Andersen, B. L., Kiecolt-Glaser, J. K., & Glaser, R. (1994). A biobehavioral model of cancer stress and disease course. *American Psychologist, 49,* 389–404.

Cohen, S., Tyrrell, D. A., & Smith, A. P. (1991). Psychological stress in humans and susceptibility to the common cold. *New England Journal of Medicine, 325,* 606–612.

Fawzy, F. I., et al. (1990a). A structured psychiatric intervention for cancer patients. *Archives of General Psychiatry, 47,* 729–735.

Fawzy, F. I., et al. (1990b). A structured psychiatric intervention for cancer patients: I. Changes over time in immunological measures. *Archives of General Psychiatry, 47,* 729–735.

Fawzy, F. I., Fawzy, N. W., Hyun, C. S., Elashoff, R., Gutherie, D., & Fahey, J. L., et al. (1993). Malignant melanoma: Effects of a structured psychiatric intervention, coping, affective state, and immune parameters on recurrence and survival six years later. *Archives of General Psychiatry, 50,* 681–689.

Gruber, B. L., Hersh, S. P., et al. (1993). Immunological responses of breast cancer patients to behavioral interventions. *Biofeedback and Self-Regulation, 18,* 1–22.

Herbert, T. B., & Cohen, S. (1993a). Depression and immunity: A meta-analytic review. *Psychological Bulletin, 113,* 472–486.

Herbert, T. B., & Cohen, S. (1993b). Stress and immunity in humans: A meta-analytic review. *Psychosomatic Medicine, 55,* 364–379.

Kiecolt-Glaser, J. K., Marucha, P. T., Malarkey, W. B., Mercado, A. M., & Glaser, R. (1995). Slowing of wound healing by psychological stress. *Lancet, 346,* 1194–1196.

Linn, M. W., et al. (1982). Effects of counseling for late stage cancer patients. *Cancer, 49,* 1048–1055.

MacVicar, M., Winningham, M., & Nickel, J. (1989). Effects of aerobic interval training on cancer patients' functional capacity. *Nursing Research, 38,* 348–351.

Maier, S. F., Watkins, L. R., & Fleshner, M. (1994). Psychoneuroimmunology: The interface between behavior, brain, and immunity. *American Psychologist, 49,* 1004–1017.

Parker, S. L., Tong, T., Bolden, S., & Wingo, P. A. (1996). Cancer statistics, 1996. *CA—A Cancer Journal for Clinicians, 46*(1), 5–27.

Spiegel, D., & Bloom, J. R. (1983). Group therapy and hypnosis reduce metastatic breast carcinoma pain. *Psychosomatic Medicine, 45,* 333–339.

Spiegel, D., Bloom, J. R., & Yalom, I. (1981). Group support for patients with metastatic cancer: A randomized outcome study. *Archives of General Psychiatry, 38,* 527–533.

Spiegel, D., Bloom, H. C., Kraemer, J. R., & Gottheil, E. (1989). Effect of psychosocial treatment on survival of patients with metastatic breast cancer. *Lancet,* 888–901.

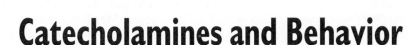

Catecholamines and Behavior

Arnold J. Friedhoff and Raul Silva

New York University Medical Center

Antidepressant Drugs These medications are used to treat a variety of conditions such as depression, panic attacks, and obsessive-compulsive disorder. Generally speaking there are three different groups: the tricyclic antidepressants, which include imipramine and related agents, amitriptyline, and nortriptyline; the monoamine oxidase inhibitors (MAO inhibitors) such as tranylcypromine and phenelzine; and the newest group, the serotonin reuptake blockers, which include clomipramine, fluoxetine, sertraline, and paroxetine.

Antipsychotic Drugs These medications are also used in a variety of conditions. The name is derived from the improvement they produce in certain psychotic behaviors such as delusions and hallucinations. The first such agent, chlorpromazine, was synthesized circa 1950. Examples of the classical antipsychotic agents are haloperidol and chlorpromazine. New atypical agents include clozapine and risperidone. These medications are also called neuroleptics.

Catecholamines There are three endogenously produced substances (epinephrine, norepinephrine, and dopamine) called catecholamines. These compounds serve as neurotransmitters.

Limbic System These are a group of structures located in the brain that are involved in regulating emotion and its association with behavioral and mental functioning.

Neurotransmitters These are compounds that are released into interneuronal junctions called synapses. They are released from the axon of a presynaptic neuron and impact on the receptors of the postsynaptic neuron, the nerve cell on the other side of the synapse. This is the chemical means by which the transfer of information occurs in the brain.

CATECHOLAMINES are powerful chemicals that can be found in neurons throughout the body. The effects of these compounds are responsible for the functioning of the brain even during the early fetal stages of life. They help regulate an endless number of functions ranging from thinking and mood to motor control. In this article we review the structure, the anatomical distribution, and the role these substances have in functioning and behavior.

I. NATURE OF THE CATECHOLAMINERGIC SYSTEMS

A. Introduction

Catecholamines are relatively small organic molecules that function in the brain and elsewhere in the body, primarily in a regulatory or modulating role, to keep various systems functioning smoothly in response to demands of the internal and external environment. The most familiar of the three natural catecholamines is adrenaline, or epinephrine. Its effects have been experienced by all of us, in response to a frightening experience, for example. Its release from the adrenal gland and from nerve cells or neurons regulating heart rate and blood pressure help to put us into a readiness state for fight or flight. Norepinephrine, the closest chemical relative of epinephrine, is more prominently localized in the brain than epinephrine, but is also found in so-called peripheral neurons (those neurons found outside of the brain). In the brain norepinephrine regulates mood and level of emotional arousal and alertness. Dopamine, the third catecholamine, is prominently involved in regulating motor or movement functions, and also in the coordination of associative thinking and integration of sensory motor function. Thus, key volitional acts such as movement and thinking are fine-tuned, integrated, and given emotional coloration through the actions of the three catecholamines.

Understanding the role of catecholamines in normal and pathological behavior is important in understanding the structural organization and functional aspects of this system in the brain. The relationship of the catecholaminergic system to behavior has been deduced largely by using drugs to alter the function of various components of the neural networks that make up the system.

B. Neurotransmission

Information transfer in the brain is carried on mainly by synaptic transmission, or the passage of a message across synapses or gaps between communicating cells. This occurs through a combination of electrical transmissions which take place within a neuron and the release of a chemical or neurotransmitter which crosses the synaptic gap and then acts on a postsynaptic neuron via specialized detection sites called "receptors"; however, there are some exceptions to this general model. For example, some neurons, not catecholaminergic, relate to each other entirely by change in electrical potential. In many cases involving the catecholaminergic system, other substances are co-released with the neurotransmitter which modify or modulate its effect. The nature of the effector response can vary depending on the type of receptor, location of the membrane and nature of the neuromodulators. For example, the stimulation of β-3-adrenergic receptors located in adipose tissues will stimulate the breakdown of fats (lipolysis). This can be contrasted with the stimulation of different α-2-adrenergic receptors,

one of which may inhibit the release of certain neurotransmitters at the presynaptic level of adrenergic nerve cells thereby causing inhibition of norepinephrine release. Meanwhile, stimulation of another α-2-adrenergic receptor located on the membranes of the β cells of the pancreas will cause a decrease in insulin secretion.

The synapse is an important locus for the action of drugs that modify behavior. By blocking reuptake of transmitters the effect of the transmitter can be enhanced or exaggerated. Conversely by blocking receptors on postsynaptic cells, transmitter effect can be reduced. A third possibility, which has been exploited pharmacologically, is the modification of the ion exchange involved in electrical transmission. This too can have effects on motor and mental activity.

C. Biosynthesis of Catecholamines

The starting point for the synthesis of all the catecholamines is L-tyrosine, which is a nonessential amino acid that can be found in the diet. L-Tyrosine is hydroxylated (gains an OH group) to form dihydroxy-L-phenylalanine, which is also known as levodopa or L-dopa. The enzyme responsible for this transformation is tyrosine hydroxylase. In dopaminergic neurons, L-dopa is metabolized to dopamine by means of the enzyme dopa decarboxylase. This enzymatic process occurs in the cytoplasmic component of neurons. In noradrenergic nerve cells and in the adrenal medulla, dopamine is transformed to norepinephrine. It has been estimated that approximately 50% of the dopamine synthesized in neuronal cytoplasm of noradrenergic cells is metabolized to norepinephrine. Norepinephrine can then be transformed to epinephrine by the addition of a methyl group ($CH3$) to its amino group, through the action of the enzyme phenethanolamine-N-methyltransferase. This last step occurs in certain neurons of the brain and in the adrenal medulla (graphic and schematic representations of the biosynthesis and breakdown of catecholamines can be found in mnay of the references listed at the end of the article). In general the enzymes described in this section are produced in the neuronal cell bodies and are then transported via axoplasmic flow and stored in nerve endings. Therefore, the process of catecholamine biosynthesis takes place within these terminals. The catecholamines synthesized are then taken up and stored in vesicles (chromafin granules) of the nerve terminals which are located near the cell membrane. During neural transmission catecholamines are released from these vesicles into the synaptic cleft. Although certain precursors of catecholamines (such as L-dopa) penetrate the blood brain barrier the catecholamines do not. Thus, all of the catecholamines found in the brain are produced there.

The amount of catecholamines that exist within the adrenal medulla and the sympathetic nervous system is generally constant. Initial changes that occur in the synthesis of these substances in response to changes occur in minutes, while slower adaptational changes occur over much longer periods, even days in some cases. Catecholamines in the body are maintained at constant levels by a highly efficient process that modulates its biosynthesis, release, and subsequent inactivation.

When an appropriate signal is received by a catecholaminergic neuron it is transmitted down the axon to the presynaptic terminal where it initiates the release of quanta of neurotransmitter into the synaptic cleft. The transmitter acts on receptors in follower cells, resulting in the activation or inhibition of these cells.

D. Inactivation of Catecholamines

There are two major means for catecholamine inactivation; reuptake and enzymatic degradation. The reuptake system is fast and highly efficient. It operates through a rapid reuptake of released transmitters back into the presynaptic terminal. The involved transporter reuptake protein has two functions: (1) it rapidly inactivates transmission by removing transmitter from the synapse and (2) it conserves transmitter by restoring that which is not used in signal transmission. Catecholamines made in the neuron but not stored in terminal vesicles are catabolized by a series of isoenzymes known as monoamine oxidases (MAO) which are located in most living tissues. Another enzyme important in the breakdown of catecholamines released into the synapse is catechol-O-methyltransferase. Discussion of all of the metabolic steps in degradation of catecholamines is beyond the scope of this chapter; however, it is important to note that drugs that increase catecholamine levels in the synapse, particularly norepinephrine, are successful antidepressant medications. The concentration of norepinephrine can be altered by two types of drugs: reuptake blockers which prolong the life of norepinephrine in the synapse by

preventing its re-entry into the presynaptic neuron and monoamine oxidase inhibitors which interfere with breakdown by monoamine oxidase.

From observations of the action of these drugs it has been proposed that depression is the result of low levels of norepinephrine in the brain; however, direct evidence for this proposal has not been found. In support of the proposal, the antihypertensive drug reserpine, which depletes norepinephrine and the other catecholamines, sometimes causes serious depression. Curiously, drugs that increase levels of serotonin, a noncatecholamine found in the brain, are also antidepressants. [*See* DEPRESSION.]

Norepinephrine and epinephrine also act as hormones when released from the adrenal medulla. Epinephrine is the principal catecholaminergic hormone produced in the medulla. Norepinephrine is the primary neurotransmitter in all postganglionic sympathetic neurons except for those that supply the vasodilator blood vessels of the skeletal muscular system and the sweat glands. The sympathetic nervous system, along with the parasympathetic nervous system, makes up the autonomic nervous system which helps regulate the visceral functions of the body. The autonomic nervous system has control centers which are located in the spinal cord, hypothalamus, the reticular formation of the medulla oblongata, and other regions of the brain stem. The centers located in the spinal cord and in the brain stem are regulated by the hypothalamus which also communicates with the pituitary and cerebral cortex. This interconnection enables the complex orchestration of multiple somatic, visceral, and endocrinological functions.

The noradrenergic system has two major areas of origin in the brain: the locus coerulus and the lateral tegmental nucleus. The projections of this system extend to all regions of the brain. As explained earlier, dopamine is the precursor in the synthesis of norepinephrine and epinephrine. In addition to this, dopamine has its own complex system and specialized function. The dopamine system is composed of three subdividions. These are the mesocortical, mesolimbic, and nigrostriatal systems. The mesocortical system extends from ventral tegmentum to a variety of areas such as the olfactory tubercles, the accumbens, and the prefrontal cortex. The neurons of the mesolimbic system orginate in the substantia nigra and the ventral tegmentum, and project to the accumbens, amygdala, and olfactory tubercle. It is believed that the limbic system is probably more involved in regulating certain mental processes. The nigrostriatal system extends from the substantia nigra to the neostriatal regions. In addition to other functions, the nigrostriatal system is involved in motor movement. Disturbances of vital structures in this area are related to illnesses such as Parkinsonism. [*See* LIMBIC SYSTEM.]

E. Catecholaminergic Receptor Sites

Catecholamine receptors are proteins imbedded in the plasma membrane of a neuron. Activation of these receptors by catecholamines can produce excitatory and/or inhibitory responses. Receptor number, in many cases, is increased or decreased as an adaptive response. For example, blockage of dopamine receptors by antipsychotic drugs, which are dopamine receptor antagonists, often results in a compensatory increase in the number of receptors. There are a number of types of catecholamine receptors which respond to one of three catecholamines, dopamine, norepinephrine, or epinephrine.

1. Dopaminergic Receptors

Five types of dopamine receptors have been identified. They are all called dopamine receptors because they all respond to dopamine and are relatively homologous in structure; however, two types, D1 and D2, can be discriminated pharmacologically by both agonists and antagonists. It is very likely that drugs selective for the other three types will also be found. The ability to selectively activate or inactivate different aspects of the dopaminergic system with drugs that act on one receptor type has made it possible to explore the role the D1 and D2 dopaminergic system plays in behavior.

1. D1 receptors are found in the caudate nucleus and cortex. There are a variety of extraneural sites where these receptors are located, including the vascular structures of the brain, heart, renal, and mesenteric systems.

2. D2 receptors have been identified in the putamen, caudate nucleus, striatum, as well as in limbic structures and in low density in the cortex. There have been two subtypes of D2 receptors identified (D2a and D2b) but differences in anatomical location and physiological properties have not been worked out.

3. D3 receptors have been identified in the limbic system.

4. D4 receptors have been recently identified in the frontal cortex, basal ganglia, medulla, midbrain, and the amygdala.

5. D5 receptors have also recently been identified in the caudate, putamen, olfactory bulb, and tubercle as well as in the nucleus accumbens.

2. Adrenergic Receptors

There are two types with subdivisions within each.

a. α-Adrenergic Receptors

1. α-1-Adrenergic receptors are located on postsynaptic effector cells such as those on the smooth muscles of the vascular, genitourinary, intestinal, and cardiac systems. Additionally, in humans these receptors are located within the liver.

2. α-2-Adrenergic receptors inhibit the release of certain neurotransmitters. For example, at the presynaptic level in certain adrenergic nerve cells these receptors inhibit norepinephrine release, while in cholinergic neurons they are responsible for inhibiting acetylcholine release. α-2-Adrenergic receptors are also located in postjunctional sites such as the β cells of the pancreas, in platelets, and in vascular smooth muscle. Although there are at least two subtypes of both α-1 and 2-adrenergic receptors, the details concerning the actions and localization that would differentiate these particular subtypes have not been worked out.

b. β-Adrenergic Receptors

1. β-1-Adrenergic receptors have been located in the heart, the juxtaglomerular cells of the kidney, and the parathyroid gland.

2. β-2-Adrenergic receptors have been identified in the smooth muscles of the vascular, gastrointestinal, genitourinary, and bronchial structures. Additionally, β-2-adrenergic receptors have been located in skeletal muscle and in the liver as well as on the α cells of the pancreas which are responsible for glucagon production.

3. β-3-Adrenergic receptors are reported to be located in adipose tissue.

F. Plasma Catecholamines

The three catecholamines, when found intact in plasma, do not come from the brain because they cannot cross the blood–brain barrier; however, their metabolites can. Thus, metabolites in plasma originate both in brain and in peripheral tissues. Study of these metabolites has provided certain insights into the role catecholamines play in behavior. However, direct study of catecholamines in living human brain tissue has not been possible. Fortunately, the new imaging technologies such as PET scanning, NMR, and SPECT open up possibilities for visualizing catecholaminergic function in live conscious human subjects during waking hours. There are a variety of methods available for measuring catecholamines in plasma.

II. IMPACT OF CATECHOLAMINES ON BEHAVIOR

Most of the information that is available concerning the functions of catecholamines in regulating human behavior directly results from the use of a group of medications often called psychotropic drugs, and antidepressant medications called thymoleptics. Other medications include psychostimulant medication such as the dextroamphetamines, methylphenidate (most commonly known by its trade name, Ritalin), and L-dopa (which has been used to treat Parkinsonism) as well as a medication that was intially used to treat high blood pressure, reserpine. Most of these drugs impact on more than one system (for example dopaminergic, noradrenergic, or serotonergic systems). Catecholamines have been proposed as mediators of most psychiatric illnesses including schizophrenia, Tourette's syndrome, depression, autism, pervasive developmental disorders, attention deficit hyperactivity disorder, stereotypic movements, and tremors. Unfortunately, to date no definitive evidence for their role in any of these has been forthcoming. What is definite, however, is the role catecholamines play in mediating the action of mood-altering, mind-altering, and other types of psychotropic drugs. Antipsychotic drugs that block dopamine receptors reduce the more classical psychotic symptoms (delusions and hallucinations). There is some speculation about which dopamine receptors these agents block in order to produce improvement, but the prevailing view is that the more traditional agents block D2 receptors while the newer atypical agents (such as clozapine) may also block D4

receptors. The fact that agents that block dopamine receptors produce improvement in schizophrenia has led to the proposal that schizophrenia is caused by overactivity of the dopaminergic system. In support of this so called "dopamine hypothesis," at least one group has reported an increased density of D2 receptors in brains of schizophrenic patients using a relatively new imaging technology called positron emission tomography (or PET scanning). Increased density of these receptors in postmortem brain tissue from patients with schizophrenia has also been reported. Most patients, however, have received neuroleptic treatment which, itself, can cause these changes. Thus, it is not clear whether this increased density is an effect of the pathophysiology or the result of treatment. It is well established that reducing dopaminergic activity with neuroleptics inhibits hallucinatory activity and normalizes delusional or paranoid thinking. It seems probable that the dopaminergic system, particularly the D2 system, has a physiological role in keeping thinking and level of suspiciousness in bounds. Curiously, patients who respond well to antipsychotic medication have a decrease in plasma HVA, the principal metabolite of dopamine, during treatment, whereas nonresponders do not. What is odd about these findings is that most plasma HVA does not come from the central nervous system.

Antipsychotics improve certain other symptoms associated with schizophrenia such as impaired thought processes and attentional problems. Thus, it seems that the dopaminergic system may also regulate associative processing and attention. Drugs that improve psychotic symptoms have one more important effect. They product emotional blunting or so called "flat affect." Inasmuch as these drugs reduce dopaminergic activity, it seems that dopamine may play a role in affect regulation.

Another illness that may illuminate the role of dopamine in regulation of behavior is Tourette's syndrome. This is an illness with onset usually between 4 and 8 years of age; however, it can occur at any time. It is characterized by rapid, repetitive movements known as motor tics, which can be as simple as eye blinking or as complex as assuming contorted body positions. In addition to these movements, vocal tics occur—ranging from repetitive coughing and throat clearing to shouting obscene words. These utterances can be a great source of embarrassment to the affected individuals. Both the vocalizations and the motor tics respond to antipsychotic drugs which are, of course, dopamine receptor blockers. This effect on Tourette's symptoms occurs even though the patients are not psychotic. Although dopamine is known to play a role in integrating motor movements, there is a distinct possibility it may also inhibit socially undesirable movements and vocalizations.

It seems that Tourette's syndrome is in some way related to obsessive–compulsive disorder (this latter illness being particularly prevalent in families of Tourette patients). Obsessive–compulsive disorder is often responsive to drugs that increase serotonergic activity. Thus, there appears to be a complex interaction between the serotonergic and dopaminergic systems in the regulation of psychomotor activity. [*See* OBSESSIVE–COMPULSIVE DISORDER.]

The study of psychological depression and its treatment can also help to illuminate the role of catecholamines in the regulation of behavior. Drugs like the tricyclic antidepressants and the monoamine oxidase inhibitors, both of which increase norepinephrine in the synapse, are useful in treating depressed patients. As a result of those observations it was first concluded that depression resulted from abnormally low activity of the noradrenergic system. It now appears, however, that increasing norepinephrine levels via drug treatment serves to compensate for unknown pathology in depression. Additionally, all of the drugs useful in treating depression affect other transmitters besides norepinephrine.

These observations are, nevertheless, informative. It seems probable that norepinephrine, by regulating its own activity, in concert with other transmitters, plays a role in the relief and prevention of depression if not in the cause of depression. Norepinephrine may regulate mood, level of emotional arousal, sleep/wakefulness states, and appetite (all of which are often disturbed by depression).

Autism is a serious psychiatric condition that begins in infancy or early childhood. It is characterized by a qualitative impairment in interaction and socialization. Autistic children appear to be oblivious to their surroundings but, ironically, can react with a temper tantrum if a single toy is moved from its usual location. They are often lacking verbal and nonverbal communication skills. Speech may be limited to repeating a word over and over, and they may not even point to something they want in order to obtain it. Autistic individuals exhibit a restriction of activities and engage in a variety of odd behaviors such as sniffing, twirling, and spinning, and inordinate interest in the single function of an object (i.e., staring at a wheel spinning on a toy car for hours). They also sometimes present with violent or self-injurious behavior and temper tantrums. Some of these patients may possess striking talents beyond their apparent cognitive capacity (often referred to as savant-like traits). A few can masterfully play the piano without ever receiving instruction or memorize an entire city's bus routes. [*See* AUTISM AND PERVASIVE DEVELOPMENTAL DISORDER.]

The pervasive developmental disorders are illnesses that may vary in presentation. They may present with only one feature of autism or most of the features (but by definition not all). Though elevated serotonin levels in whole blood seem to be the most consistent finding in autism, there have been reports of increased norepinephrine levels in the plasma of these children when compared to normal control groups. Additionally, the effectiveness of dopamine-blocking neuroleptics on attention and improvement of certain behaviors in autistic children cannot be ignored. One investigation of biological markers in children with pervasive developmental disorder reported that the group that responded to treatment had lower initial plasma levels of HVA (the principal metabolite of dopamine.)

Attention deficit hyperactivity disorder, or ADHD, is characterized by overactivity, fidgetiness, impulsivity, and distractibility. It is more frequently seen in males and there is usually a family history of the disorder. The illness begins early in life but often is not diagnosed until the child is in school, as its pathology becomes more evident when more controlled behavior is required. There is strong evidence for involvement of the catecholaminergic systems in this illness. Prevailing theories propose a decrease in turnover of both dopamine and norepinephrine. Findings include decreased norepinephrine metabolites in the plasma of these individuals and treatment involves the use of drugs that have norepinephrine-like effects. Oddly, increases in noradrenergic activity in the activating systems of the brain produces emotional arousal and many of the attendant symptoms of ADHD. In addition, adults given the psychostimulants used to treat ADHD in children have the expected activating effects. Perhaps then the function of the noradrenergic system may be developmentally regulated. [*See* ATTENTION DEFICIT HYPERACTIVITY DISORDER (ADHD).]

III. CONCLUSIONS

Catecholamines in the brain act at the highest levels of mental function. Although their role in specific mental disorders is not entirely clear, there is little doubt that they modulate, if not mediate, functions like processing of associations, integration of thought processes with movement and speech, emotional tone or affect, mood, appetite, arousal, and sleep/wakefulness state. Most of these functions have not been successfully modeled in non-human species, leaving their study to be carried out in living humans. This limitation has made more than inferential conclusions as to behavioral and mental function impossible.

New technological advances in functional brain imaging and in studies of gene expression in accessible human cells have opened new windows into the brain, but definitive studies await further advances.

This article has been reprinted from the *Encyclopedia of Human Behavior, Volume 1*.

BIBLIOGRAPHY

Axelrod, J. (1987). Catecholamines. In "Encyclopedia of Neuroscience" (G. Adelman, Ed.) Vol. I, 1st ed. Birkhauser, Boston.

Davis, K. L., Khan, R. S., Ko, G., & Davidson, M. (1991). Dopamine in schizophrenia: A review and reconceptualization. *Am J. Psych.* **148**(11), 1474–1486.

Friedhoff, A. J. (1991). Catecholamines and Behavior. In "Encyclopedia of Human Biology" (R. Dulbecco, Ed.), Vol. II. Academic Press, San Diego.

Friedhoff, A. J. (Ed.) (1975). "Catecholamines and Behavior." Vols. I & II. Plenum, New York.

Gilman, A. G., Rall, T. W., Nies, A. S., & Taylor, P. (Eds.) (1990). Goodman & Gilman's: "The Pharmacological Basis of Therapeutics," 8th ed. Pergamon, New York.

Kaplan, H. I., & Sadock, B. J. (Eds.) (1989). "Comprehensive Textbook of Psychiatry/V," 5th ed. Williams & Wilkins, Baltimore.

Silva, R. R., & Friedhoff, A. J. (1993). Recent advances in research into Tourette's Syndrome. In "Handbook of Tourette Syndrome and Related Tic and Behavioral Disorders" (R. Kurlan, Ed.). Marcel Dekker, New York.

Wilson, J. D., Braunwald, E., Isselbacher, K. J., Petersdore, R. G., Martin, J. B., Fauchi, A. S., & Rood, R. K. (Eds.) (1991). "Principles of Internal Medicine." McGraw-Hill, New York.

Charisma

Ronald E. Riggio

Claremont McKenna College

Charisma   The ability to arouse or inspire others via skilled, emotional communication.

Emotional Contagion   The process by which emotion is transmitted and vicariously experienced by others; believed to be related to the charismatic person's ability to emotionally "infect" others.

Emotional Control   Ability to regulate or control emotional communication.

Emotional Expressivity   The ability to convey emotions and feelings; the most visible component of charisma.

Emotional Sensitivity   Skill in receiving and interpreting the emotional messages of others; related to emotional empathy.

Referent Power   The base of power most associated with charismatic leaders, it consists of the power derived from the fact that one is admired by others.

Social Control   Skill in social self-presentation and role-playing ability; related to notions of social competence.

Social Expressivity   Verbal speaking skill and the ability to engage others in conversation.

Social Sensitivity   Ability to decode verbal communication and knowledge of social norms.

CHARISMA, a widely discussed topic in the fields of psychology, leadership, political science, sociology, and communication, is a very elusive construct. The term "charisma" itself means a "divine gift of grace." Yet, most modern researchers of charisma do not believe that charisma is an inherited, inborn quality. Moreover, few psychologically oriented theorists would argue that charisma is something that is bestowed on an individual. Instead, charisma is best approached as a constellation of personal characteristics that cause an individual to have impact on others—to inspire them, lead them, influence them, or in some other way affect their feelings and behaviors.

I. INTRODUCTION

This chapter focuses on the construct of charisma from a psychological and mental health perspective. From this orientation, charisma is defined as a constellation of basic communication and social skills. Critical to the possession of personal charisma is skill in emotional communication, particularly emotional expressiveness. Research on charisma and social skills indicates that charisma plays an important role in social effectiveness, in leadership, in interpersonal relationships, and in fostering psychosocial well-being. By improving communication and social skills one can enhance personal charisma and improve interpersonal effectiveness.

II. HISTORY AND THEORIES OF CHARISMA

The roots of the concept of charisma, and of charismatic leadership, are in religious writings. Religious prophets, such as Moses or Mohammed, were said to possess special characteristics that allowed them to captivate and inspire followers. Although it is unclear exactly what these characteristics consisted of, religious charisma was often associated with magical or divine powers. For example, charismatic persons were those who were believed to have the power to perform miracles, to foresee the future, or to heal others.

Social scientists became seriously interested in charisma following the work of German sociologist Max Weber. Charismatic individuals, according to Weber, possessed some "extraordinary quality" that captivated others. Drawing heavily on religious notions of charisma, Weber believed that the key to a leader's charisma lay in the relationship between the leader's qualities and the follower's belief in and devotion to the charismatic leader. Weber's conceptualization of charisma provoked a great deal of interest by sociologists and political scientists into the charisma of notable political and national leaders. To this day, Weber's notion that a leader's charisma lies in the leader–follower relationship is quite popular and has influenced theories of general leadership and research on leadership in the workplace.

Another theory of charisma and charismatic leadership is the psychoanalytic approach championed by Irvine Schiffer and others. According to the psychoanalytic theory of charisma, followers project their needs onto a chosen leader and imbue the leader with great qualities, much in the same way that a young child might look up to and idolize a parent. From the psychoanalytic approach, charisma lies more in the followers and their deeply rooted psychological needs than in any particular qualities of the charismatic leader. The psychoanalytic theorists do, however, point out that certain characteristics of the potential leader such as attractiveness, an air of mystery, or some other quality that draws attention to the potential leader (e.g., a foreign accent, a physical flaw), allows certain individuals to be more likely candidates for charismatic leadership. [*See* PSYCHO-ANALYSIS.]

Another recent theory of charisma, proposed by Charles Lindholm, also emphasizes the role of the follower in charisma. For Lindholm, there are a number of qualities that can make a leader charismatic, but it is the followers' reaction to the leader that constitutes charisma. According to Lindholm, the masses of followers look to charismatic leaders as a means of escaping from their mundane everyday existence. Like the psychoanalytic theorists, this approach emphasizes some sort of deficiency in followers that motivates them to seek out persons who offer some sort of promise of salvation, change, or a better life. Yet, the one element overlooked by all of these theories concerns the qualities that allow only a certain few individuals to emerge as charismatic.

Leadership researcher Jay Conger defines charisma as a constellation of behavioral traits that induce perceptions of charisma in others. These behavioral traits associated with charismatic leaders include the ability to detect unexploited opportunities, sensitivity to followers' needs, the ability to formulate and communicate visionary goals, the building of trust in followers, and the ability to motivate followers to achieve the leader's vision. According to Conger, the likelihood of followers perceiving a leader as charismatic depends on the *number* of charismatic behaviors the leader exhibits, the *intensity* of those behaviors, and the *relevance* of the behaviors to the situation. While Conger's notion of charisma emphasizes the behaviors emitted by charismatic leaders, many of these behaviors are situationally based. That is, they are behaviors that center on the particular leadership situation and on the relationship between the charismatic leader and followers.

Although these various theories of charisma are quite different, they contain common elements. One common theme is the charismatic person's ability to draw attention. Ability to communicate, to capture the attention of potential followers, could constitute this attention-getting device. Also implicit in the various charisma theories is the notion that charismatic individuals have the ability to "touch" others at some deep, emotional level. Many of the theories also denote some sort of "attractiveness" that draws others to the charismatic person. Finally, some charisma theories, such as the psychoanalytic approach, and to a certain extent Weber's conceptualization of charisma, also emphasize the "mystical" or "mysterious" qualities that add to an individual's charisma.

II. AN EMOTIONAL AND SOCIAL SKILLS APPROACH TO UNDERSTANDING CHARISMA

In the 1980s, in an effort to better understand the personal characteristics associated with charisma and charismatic leadership, a new approach to charisma was developed that focused on the role that emotional communication and social skills play in determining charisma. Rather than viewing charisma solely from a leadership context, this new approach to charisma emphasized personal characteristics that can cause any individual to appear to others to be "charismatic." This approach focuses on an individual's "personal charisma," rather than on any situationally determined charisma that might stem from the relationship between leaders and followers.

Personal charisma lies in an individual's ability to communicate. From this perspective, charisma is defined as a combination of highly developed basic communication and social skills. Although charisma is a constellation of several types of communication skills, particularly important for charisma are skills in emotional communication—the ability to express emotions, the ability to "read" the emotions of others, and the ability to control one's own emotional communication. Also important in determining personal charisma are basic social skills, including verbal speaking skill, the ability to engage others in conversation, knowledge of social norms, and the ability to adopt various social roles. [See EMOTIONAL REGULATION.]

There are three classes of basic communication skills that underlie charisma. These three classes of skills are skills in sending (termed expressive skills), skills in receiving (referred to as skills in sensitivity), and skills in regulating, or controlling, communication. Furthermore, these three basic classes of skill operate in two areas: in the domain of emotional communication, and in the social domain. Thus, there are 6 basic social/communication skills: emotional expressivity, emotional sensitivity, emotional control, social expressivity, social sensitivity, and social control. Definitions of each of these basic social/communication skills are presented in Table I.

In order to quickly measure an individual's personal charisma, a multidimensional instrument has been developed to assess the basic communication skill components that are hypothesized to underlie charisma. The Social Skills Inventory (SSI) is a 90-item, self-report measure designed to assess these 6 basic social/communication skills. Separate 15-item scales were designed to measure each of the basic communication skills. The total score on the SSI has been used as an indicator of charisma potential, although research suggests that possession of social skills, as as-

Table I Emotional and Social Skill Components of Charisma

Emotional Expressivity The ability to convey felt emotional messages and feelings. Persons who are emotionally expressive are animated, emotionally charged, and are able to arouse or inspire others because of their ability to transmit feelings. Emotional expressivity is a key ingredient of charisma and its most "visible" component.

Emotional Sensitivity Skill in receiving and interpreting the emotional messages of others. Persons who are emotionally sensitive are empathic and responsive to the feelings of others. Individuals who are extremely emotionally sensitive may be more susceptible to emotional contagion—empathically experiencing others' emotional states.

Emotional Control The ability to regulate and control emotional and nonverbal displays. Emotional control also includes the ability to convey particular emotions on cue and to stifle felt emotions and present a different emotional "mask"—such as laughing appropriately at a joke or putting on a cheerful face to hide felt sorrow. Control over emotional displays is a critical skill for charismatic persons.

Social Expressivity Verbal speaking skill and the ability to engage others in social discourse. Persons skilled in social expressivity are verbally fluent, appear outgoing and gregarious, and are good conversationalists. Social expressivity is a critical component for charismatic leaders.

Social Sensitivity A complex skill that includes the ability to interpret the verbal communications of others, and attentiveness to the social behavior of others and oneself. Social sensitivity also involves an awareness and understanding of the norms governing appropriate social behavior.

Social Control Skill in social self-presentation and social role playing. Persons skilled in social control are adept, tactful, and self-confident in social situations and can adjust to just about any type of social situation. Social control is the charisma component that is most closely associated with conceptions of social competence or social intelligence.

sessed by the SSI, can also be used to measure basic social competence or social intelligence. The Social Skills Inventory is, in many ways an extension and elaboration on another measure of charisma potential, the Affective Communication Test (ACT). The ACT focuses more directly on assessing nonverbal expressiveness—the most visible of the various social skills that combine to form true charisma. Because the ACT correlates quite highly with total score on the SSI, the ACT is a good predictor of personal charisma.

Possession of high levels of each of these basic social/communication skills, without any particular "imbalances" among the skill dimensions, is what, according to this model, constitutes an individual's "charisma potential." Research evidence indicates that such charismatic, socially skilled individuals make more positive first impressions on others, are evaluated more favorably in social interactions, are more likely to be viewed as leadership "material," have greater numbers of friends, have greater social networks and receive more social support, and are better adjusted than persons who are lacking in basic social/communication skills. Moreover, it seems that individuals who are exceptionally high in basic communication skills are "qualitatively" different than those who are low or moderate in communication skills. Thus, it appears that the components of what is commonly labeled "charisma" are highly developed social/communication skills.

A. Charisma, Emotions, and Nonverbal Communication

There is little doubt that an important component of charisma is the ability to communicate emotions. Charismatic leaders, for example, are typically characterized by their ability to arouse, inspire, or affect others at an emotional level. Early research on charisma from the communication skill perspective focused on nonverbal emotional expressiveness as the key element of charisma. It was found, for example, that emotionally expressive persons made more favorable initial impressions, were better liked, and that they were more likely to hold elected offices and jobs that involved interacting with people than were individuals lacking in emotional expressiveness.

Emotional expressiveness involves the ability to nonverbally convey affect through facial expression, gestures, and tone of voice. Nonverbal expressiveness

may also involve, however, the nonverbal communication of attitudes or projecting cues of status and dominance. A great deal of research has shown that emotionally expressive individuals are indeed more skilled senders, or encoders, of basic emotions such as happiness, anger, fear, or sadness. Emotionally expressive people are also distinguished by distinctive and frequent changes in their facial expressions and by variations in their tone of voice. [See NONVERBAL COMMUNICATION.]

An interesting study demonstrated that charismatic individuals appear to use their emotional expressiveness as a means for inspiring or influencing others. In this laboratory experiment, participants who had been previously measured for emotional expressiveness were assembled into groups of three in a "waiting room." Participants were chosen so that there would be one individual in the group of three who was exceptionally high on emotional expressiveness. Immediately upon entering the waiting room, participants completed a scale designed to assess their moods. They were then instructed that they would have to wait for a few minutes while the apparatus for an experiment was set up. Participants were instructed that they were not to talk to each other during this waiting period. A few minutes later, participants were again given the same mood scale. Analysis of the mood scales demonstrated that the mood of the expressive individuals influenced the mood of the other participants. That is, regardless of the expressive person's initial or final mood, the other two participants' moods tended to gravitate toward the mood of the expressive individual. What is most striking about this study was that there was no intent on the part of the expressive person to influence the moods of the others. Yet, the emotionally expressive individual was able to affect the moods of the other participants totally through nonverbal channels of communication (i.e., facial expressions, gestures) in just a few short minutes. This process, which is labeled "emotional contagion," suggests that a charismatic person uses emotional expressiveness to arouse emotions in others. In fact, it is likely emotional expressiveness that people associate with charismatic persons upon first meeting them. Charismatic persons are characterized as being "emotionally charged" and instantly able to "light up a room," reflecting emotional expressiveness.

Although a key element, emotional expressiveness

alone does not constitute charisma. Persons who are emotionally expressive may have an advantage in initial encounters, but if they are unable to regulate their emotionally expressive behavior, the initial positive impression may wear off as these individuals are viewed as emotionally "out of control." Thus, control over emotional expression is another important component of charisma. A charismatic leader, for example, needs to emotionally inspire others, but it is not advantageous to always "wear one's heart on one's sleeve." At times, it is necessary to stifle the expression of felt emotions and to use another emotional expression as a mask. It is skill in emotional control that allows a charismatic leader to continue to emotionally inspire followers despite the fact that the leader may be personally experiencing some negative affect.

Emotional control, combined with emotional expressiveness, is what makes charismatic individuals superb emotional "actors." That is, charismatic persons are able to successfully enact emotions on cue, in order to influence or inspire others. A classic example of a charismatic leader's emotional acting occurred during the 1980 U.S. Presidential campaign, when then-candidate Ronald Reagan met other Republican presidential candidate hopefuls for a televised debate in a New England high school gymnasium. When the debate moderator tried to limit candidate Reagan's speaking by turning off his microphone, Reagan angrily leaped to his feet, grabbed the microphone and exhorted, "I paid for this show. I'm paying for this microphone." The crowd cheered, and the image of Reagan, the indignant citizen-candidate defending his rights, seemed to have important impact on his campaign. Later, it was learned that Reagan and his campaign advisors had planned to use just such a controlled emotional outburst if the situation presented itself. As one political analyst noted, it was Ronald Reagan's "outburst of vivid yet controlled emotion" that helped him win the Republican nomination.

In addition to emotional expressiveness and control over emotions, a truly charismatic individual must also possess the ability to recognize the emotional needs of others. The charismatic leader, for example, must be able to read the emotions of the crowd of followers in order to be responsive to them. Some theories of work place leadership reflect this by emphasizing that an effective leader must be "empathic." Nearly all theories of charisma stress the requirement that a charismatic leader be responsive to the needs of followers. There-fore, emotional sensitivity is another basic component of charisma.

Studies of well-known charismatic leaders show evidence that emotional sensitivity is indeed linked to a leader's charisma. For example, Martin Luther King, Jr., and President John Kennedy were both characterized as very good at reading the emotional needs of persons with whom they interacted. Eleanor Roosevelt (herself a charismatic figure) characterized John Kennedy as "totally intentive . . ." and "a superb listener."

Skills in nonverbal and emotional communication are critically important components of charisma. Emotional expressiveness is the one characteristic, however, that is most commonly associated with charisma because of its "visibility." It is the charismatic person's expressiveness that captures the attention and imagination of others. Yet, a truly charismatic individual must also be emotionally sensitive—able to read the subtle nonverbal cues of others—and the charismatic person must also be in control of his or her emotional and nonverbal messages.

B. Charisma and Social Skills

Skills in nonverbal/emotional communication are not the only components of charisma. True charisma also involves well-developed verbal communication skills. There are three basic dimensions of social skill that are elements of personal charisma. These are termed social expressivity, social sensitivity, and social control. Although these social skill dimensions illustrate the charismatic individual's ability to communicate verbally, they are much broader constructs than their names imply, involving knowledge of social norms and rules, social role playing, and the ability to initiate and maintain social ties with others.

The charisma component labeled social expressivity consists of verbal speaking skill and the ability to engage others in social interaction. Social expressivity complements emotional expressiveness. While emotional expressivity involves the spontaneous expression of feelings, social expressivity is related to the spontaneous translation of thoughts into words and actions. Socially expressive persons are "good talkers"—able to speak easily on just about any topic. However, if the socially expressive individual lacks emotional expressivity, the conversation will appear dull and lifeless, even though the dialogue might be interesting and thought-provoking. Most charismatic public figures are quite socially expressive since much of their public persona involves speaking extemporaneously.

Social sensitivity is another charisma component that involves a complex social skill. Although social sensitivity consists of one's ability to decode and understand verbal messages, it is also strongly related to the charismatic person's knowledge of social rules and conventions. It is skill in social sensitivity that allows a charismatic person to "read" the demands of various social situations. While social sensitivity is a critical skill for a charismatic individual, contributing to his or her ability to be sensitive to situational constraints and analyze social situations, social sensitivity is also related to an individual's sense of social anxiety. In other words, possession of high levels of social sensitivity, without also being socially expressive and without possessing the third critical social skill of social control, can lead to high levels of social anxiety and actually inhibit social performance. One way to look at social sensitivity is that it is important to be socially aware—to be concerned about and cognizant of whether one's social behavior is appropriate and that one is adhering to social norms and conventions. However, if an individual becomes overly sensitive to social situations, it can lead to social withdrawal. The charismatic individual thus needs just the right amount of social sensitivity.

The third social skill component of charisma is labeled social control, but is more complex than the name implies. Social control is basic social role playing skill. Persons who possess high levels of social control are good social actors, able to adopt a variety of social roles, and easily able to fit into any type of social situation. Social control is the one basic communication skill that is most strongly related to common conceptions of social competence. In part, it is social control that contributes to the confidence exuded by charismatic individuals. The awareness that one has the ability to perform well in a variety of social situations leads to the development of a form of social self-confidence, or social self-efficacy. The importance of the skill of social control to role playing success was demonstrated in a study of soon-to-be college graduates who were participating in a mock hiring interview prior to actual on-campus interviews. Social control was found to be a good predictor of successful hiring interview performance as judged by experienced evaluators. More recently, social control was a consistent predictor of assessment center performance of individuals engaged in a variety of role playing situations, including exercises requiring participants to engage in a leaderless group discussion, give a prepared speech, and perform in a mock hiring interview.

It is important to emphasize that charisma is the combination of the three basic skills in emotional/nonverbal communication and the three skills in social/verbal communication. Moreover, truly charismatic individuals possess high levels of each of these six basic skill dimensions, while the levels of skill are relatively balanced. A good analogy to this emotional and social skill conceptualization of charisma is found in theories of intelligence. Many models of intelligence view it as multidimensional, with general intelligence composed of verbal skills, mathematical abilities, analytical reasoning, and so on. While high levels of these various intelligence dimensions combine to create a highly intelligent individual—a "genius"—high levels of basic social/communication skills combine to create a person who is "charismatic."

IV. CHARISMA AND SOCIAL EFFECTIVENESS

As has already been noted, charismatic individuals, because of their expressiveness, are particularly effective at making positive first impressions on others. In fact, people will often make quick judgments of another's charisma from relatively brief initial encounters, from watching a prepared speech, or even from brief television sound bites.

Another important aspect of the charismatic person's social effectiveness apparently lies in the ability of charismatic individuals to appear credible to others. In a study focusing on ability to deceive and detect deception, participants were given the Social Skills Inventory to measure their social skills and charisma potential weeks before they were scheduled to participate in a videotaped experiment. At the earlier point, their attitudes on a wide variety of sociopolitical topics were assessed. At the later date, participants had to make brief, prepared pro- or counterattitudinal speeches, along with some speeches on which their feelings were "neutral." Ratings were made on how much each participant "truly believed in what he or she was saying." Although charismatic individuals were not more successful at deception (defined as being judged truthful when lying) than were noncharismatic participants, charismatic individuals were judged as more truthful overall—regardless of whether they were truth-telling, deceiving, or felt neutral about the topic. This tendency for individuals to appear honest/credible or deceptive regardless of what they are saying is referred to as a "demeanor bias." Charismatic persons simply look more honest than noncharismatic persons.

Why are socially skilled, charismatic persons more honest-appearing and more persuasive? Detailed content analyses of participants' behaviors in these tasks—tallying nearly two dozen verbal and nonverbal behaviors from the videotapes—revealed that charismatic persons spoke faster and more fluently, were more emotionally expressive (more smiles and changes in facial expressions), exhibited more cues of immediacy (i.e., more eye contact, greater use of "inclusive" pronouns such as "we," and more outwardly directed gestures), and fewer stereotypic cues of nervousness (e.g., scratching oneself, shifting posture) than did noncharismatic speakers.

A well-known illustration of the perceived credibility of charismatic and noncharismatic individuals can be seen in the 1960 U.S. presidential debates. In these televised debates, John Kennedy's charisma projected an image of poise, confidence and credibility. On the other hand, Richard Nixon (who is frequently mentioned in lists of "noncharismatic" leaders) appeared nervous and ill-at-ease—exhibiting many of the nonverbal cues (shifty eyes, nervous mannerisms) that are often associated with a "dishonest" demeanor bias. Interestingly, by his own admission, Richard Nixon was shy, introverted, and lacking in some of the basic social/communication skill dimensions that make up charisma.

By definition, then, charismatic persons possess the basic social and emotional skills that cause them to be effective in a wide range of social situations. The social effectiveness of charisma, however, is best illustrated in the leadership situation, where charismatic leaders inspire groups of followers to achieve goals.

A. Charisma and Leadership

By far, the greatest research interest in the area of charisma focuses on charismatic leadership. The Weberian notion that charismatic leadership lies in the relationship between the leader's exceptional qualities and the follower's devotion to the leader has already been discussed, as has Conger's theory that focuses on charismatic leader behaviors. An additional theory

of charismatic leadership is championed by psychologist Robert House and his colleagues. According to House, charismatic leaders have the ability to communicate shared group goals, and they convey confidence in their own abilities and in the abilities of their followers. House believes that charismatic leaders do particularly well in situations that are ambiguous—where the groups' goals are unclear and where environmental conditions are uncertain or unstable. Charismatic leaders are effective in these ambiguous situations because they are able to articulate a vision of where the group should be headed.

A very interesting study by House and his colleagues applied his charismatic leadership theory to the effectiveness of U.S. presidents. Using historical documents, the charisma of all presidents from Washington to Reagan were rated. Results indicated that the more charismatic the president, the more effective he was in dealing with the economy and with domestic affairs—the areas of government that most directly impact the followers. Thus, charismatic presidents seemed to be responding to the most immediate needs of followers.

Most theories of charismatic leadership, from Weber forward, emphasize the importance of situational elements in determining the charismatic leader's effectiveness. For Weber, the situation must be "ripe" and the followers must show acceptance of and devotion to the leader for him or her to become a charismatic leader. For Conger, the effective charismatic leader must exhibit charismatic behaviors, but those behaviors must be relevant to the particular leadership situation. In House's model, the leader inspires the group toward the attainment of goals by using charisma to articulate a vision and to assist followers in making sense out of an ambiguous situation. The emotional and social skill approach to charisma does not ignore the situational influences on a charismatic leader, but leaders who possess the basic social skills required for charisma are able to read the demands of the social situation (as well as the needs of the followers) to adapt his or her leadership behaviors to the situational requirements. Thus, the truly charismatic, socially skilled leader is "flexible" or adaptable, and can be effective across a range of leadership situations.

B. Charisma and the Role of the Follower

Although there has been almost no research directly focusing on the followers of charismatic leaders, followers play an important role in the leader's charisma. First, it is the strong devotion of followers that attracts additional attention to the charismatic leader. Research on power and influence refers to this as the leader's referent power. Followers are willing to be persuaded by the leader because of the attraction they feel for the leader and because they strongly identify with the leader. In some instances, a leader himself or herself may go relatively unnoticed by the general public, while it is the apparent "blind devotion" of followers that first catches the public's eye. Adolf Hitler would be a good example. Hitler was not considered to be "leadership material," and certainly was not the type of person one would instantly label "charismatic." It was the behavior of his ardent followers that first drew attention. Later, the focus shifted to Hitler's apparent charisma. From the emotional and social skill perspective, Hitler did indeed possess amazing expressive skills and he was an adept social performer.

Followers also play an important part in distinguishing charismatic from noncharismatic leaders. It may be that charismatic individuals attract a certain type of follower. Research on the emotional contagion process that is believed to be important in the charismatic leader's ability to emotionally affect others indicates that certain individuals may be more susceptible to others' emotions. In a like manner, some people may be more "persuadable" than others. It is likely that many followers of charismatic leaders are persons who are simply more susceptible to the powerful emotional and verbal messages that skilled charismatic leaders transmit. Another, related possibility is that followers of charismatic leaders see in the charismatic individual characteristics that they themselves lack. Identification with the charismatic leader may then be some form of psychological compensation for the followers' real or imagined deficiencies.

C. Charisma and Physical Attractiveness

Many of the various theories of charisma, including the political and psychoanalytic theories of charisma, emphasize the attractiveness of the charismatic leader. Early research on charisma from the emotional and social skill approach also found that emotionally expressive individuals were found to be more attractive than their nonexpressive counterparts. In later studies, it was determined that socially skilled, charismatic individuals were also viewed as more attractive in initial interactions than persons low in social skills.

Ratings revealed that these expressive and charismatic persons were viewed as more "likable," more "positive," and more "attractive as a potential friend" or "attractive as a potential dating partner" than were persons lacking in the emotional and social skill dimensions that make up charisma. Yet, the "attractiveness" of these charismatic persons was not necessarily caused by static physical characteristics that made these individuals beautiful or handsome (e.g., attractive faces or bodies). In fact, when the effects of static physical attractiveness (i.e., beauty) were taken into account, charismatic persons were found to still be more attractive than their noncharismatic counterparts. Charismatic individuals thus possessed what was termed "dynamic attractiveness"—a way of communicating and presenting themselves that made them more attractive to others.

This notion of the charismatic individual's dynamic attractiveness can readily be seen with famous charismatic leaders. Although many famous charismatic leaders are physically attractive, beautiful people, such as John Kennedy or Eva Peron, other charismatic leaders were not classically handsome or beautiful, such as Winston Churchill, Eleanor Roosevelt, or Mahatma Gandhi. Yet, these charismatic persons still had the ability to draw people toward them via the dynamic attractiveness derived from their expressiveness and high levels of communication and social skills. In fact, some theorists of charisma have discussed the curious "attractiveness" and appeal of infamous charismatic leaders who would not necessarily be described as classic beauties—Adolf Hitler, Charles Manson, Rasputin. In all likelihood, what these authors see as the physical attractiveness of these evil charismatic leaders is the dynamic attractiveness caused by their communicative powers rather than any static physical beauty.

D. Charisma, Shyness and Related Constructs

On the surface, the relationship between charisma and characteristics such as shyness, social anxiety, or feelings of loneliness and social isolation is straightforward. The research evidence consistently finds a negative relationship between possession of these attributes and the emotional and social skills that underlie charisma. For the most part, charismatic individuals are much less likely to experience shyness or loneliness than are persons who lack charisma. Yet, the relationships between some aspects of social anxiety and charisma are not necessarily straightforward. For example, successful charismatic individuals need to be aware of how their own behavior impacts others. Therefore, charismatic, socially skilled individuals must possess some social awareness or a form of "social anxiety" that helps them to anticipate how their behavior is perceived by others. In the emotional and social skill framework, this form of "positive" social anxiety is part of the skill labeled social sensitivity. It is skill in social sensitivity that enables the charismatic person to realize and anticipate how others are reacting to what he or she is saying or doing in a social interaction. In addition, social sensitivity prevents the charismatic individual from violating important social norms or behaving in ways that might prove embarrassing.

Interestingly, research on shyness by Dr. Philip Zimbardo and others has indicated that several famous charismatic people have described themselves as "shy." Entertainers Johnny Carson, Carol Burnett, and charismatic political leaders Gandhi and Robert Kennedy all admit to being basically shy persons (although most charismatic leaders in business and the entertainment industry tend not to be shy). It is likely that the feelings of shyness that these famous charismatic people experience derives from their social sensitivity—their concern with the appropriateness of their own social behavior and the impact their behavior has on others in social situations. [See SHYNESS.]

IV. CHARISMA AND WELL-BEING

A final stream of research on charisma from the emotional and social skill approach has focused on the relationship between possession of the various communication skills underlying charisma and psychological adjustment and well-being. There is a substantial amount of evidence that charismatic, socially skilled individuals are indeed better adjusted than persons lacking charisma. For instance, in a study of college student dormitory residents, socially skilled, charismatic students were less lonely, more self-confident, more satisfied with their lives, more satisfied with their college experience, and more active in extracurricular activities than their noncharismatic counterparts (although charismatic students did not do better in school, as indicated by their grade-point averages). A study of elderly couples also found that older charismatic persons are less lonely and more satisfied with their lives than older persons lacking charisma.

The notion that the communication and social skills that underlie charisma are related to psychological adjustment is not new. Several clinical researchers have noted the relationship between social skill deficiencies and psychopathology. It has been suggested that a lack of social skills may play a part in the etiology of some forms of mental illness, and therapeutic interventions that promote the development of social and communication skills have been a successful form of treatment for some disorders.

Charisma also seems to be effective in helping people cope with the stresses of everyday life. For example, socially skilled, charismatic persons report having larger and more supportive social networks than persons lacking the emotional and social skill dimensions underlying charisma. Presumably, these social support networks help charismatic individuals deal with stress more effectively. There is also some evidence that charismatic, socially skilled persons use more diverse coping strategies than do noncharismatic individuals. This greater repertoire of coping strategies may also enable the charismatic person to cope more successfully with stress. [See COPING WITH STRESS; SOCIAL SUPPORT; STRESS.]

VI. INCREASING CHARISMA AND SOCIAL SKILLS

Because charisma is derived from exceptional abilities to communicate with others, to inspire, motivate, and arouse others to action, charisma can indeed be developed and learned. Programs that are designed to make people more effective communicators, such as Dale Carnegie-type courses, courses in public speaking, interpersonal/social skill training programs and programs that are labeled "charisma training," do appear to be somewhat effective in improving the social effectiveness and communication skills of participants. Yet, there has been little systematic research evaluating the effectiveness of programs designed to train people to be more charismatic.

One of the few systematic attempts to increase charisma used college student participants, and was quite successful. This program focused primarily on improving participants' emotional and nonverbal sending (encoding) and receiving (decoding) skills, although participants also engaged in exercises to improve their more general social-communication skills. For several weeks, participants attended training session in which they engaged in various communication skill training exercises. For example, they studied the facial expressions of emotion, their meaning, and how to enact them. They were taught to recognize nonverbal cues, and they participated in a number of role playing exercises. Importantly, participants in this charisma training program were given homework assignments that involved practicing what they had learned on friends and family members. Pretraining and posttraining videotaped interviews of participants revealed startling differences in comparison to a nontrained control group. Charisma trained individuals were more animated, persuasive and were generally better communicators after the training session. Moreover, participants reported increased feelings of confidence and reported improved communication with friends which they attributed directly to the training program. Researchers who have implemented similar social skill training programs report comparable results.

VII. CONCLUSION

Charisma is indeed an elusive and understudied construct, yet it is one that has important implications for mental health and psychological adjustment. Evidence from the emotional and social skill approach to charisma defines it as possession of highly developed skills in both emotional/nonverbal and verbal/social communication. Research indicates that emotionally and socially skilled persons are more socially effective, are better adjusted, and that they have important leadership qualities. Moreover, there is evidence that people can increase their personal charisma by improving their communication skills.

BIBLIOGRAPHY

Conger, J. A. (1989). *The charismatic leader: Behind the mystique of exceptional leadership*. San Francisco: Jossey-Bass.

Friedman, H. S., Riggio, R. E., & Casella, D. (1988). Nonverbal skill, personal charisma, and initial attraction. *Personality and Social Psychology bulletin, 14,* 203–211.

House, R. J. (1977). A 1976 theory of charismatic leadership. In J. G. Hunt & L. L. Larsen (Eds.), *Leadership: The cutting edge.* (pp. 189–207). Carbondale, IL: Southern Illinois University Press.

Lindholm, C. (1990). *Charisma*. Cambridge, MA: Basil Blackwell.

Riggio, R. E. (1986). Assessment of basic social skills. *Journal of Personality and Social Psychology, 51,* 649–660.

Riggio, R. E. (1987). *The charisma quotient*. New York: Dodd, Mead.

Riggio, R. E. (1989). *Manual for the Social Skills Inventory*. Palo Alto, CA: Consulting Psychologists Press.

Shiffer, I. (1973). *Charisma: A psychoanalytic look at mass society*. Toronto: University of Toronto Press.

Child Care Providers

Alice M. Atkinson

The University of Iowa

Center Based Care   Care for a group of children in a nonresidential setting for all or part of the day.

Child Care   Supplemental care for children provided by persons other than the parents.

Developmentally Appropriate Practices   Guidelines developed through the National Association for the Education of Young Children to help establish care that is sensitive to the abilities of children of a given age as well as to the interests and abilities of individual children.

Family Child Care   The care provided for a small number of children in the caregiver's home.

Young Children   Children between birth and age eight.

The term *CHILD CARE* refers to the supplemental care of dependent children by persons other than parents. Most research and concern has focused on the care used by parents while they are employed outside the home. However, programs that provide specific intervention and support for children at risk and programs designed to generally enrich childrens' experiences are also important types of supplemental care. Family child care, in which providers care for a small number of children in a private home, is an important part of the day care services available to parents.

I. CHILD CARE IN THE UNITED STATES

The growth in the number of employed mothers with young children has been a major change in the American labor force. As most parents work outside their home today, day care meets a critical need in providing care and education for children. Parents use a variety of methods to care for children. Some employed mothers use no supplemental care as they work at home or work hours that allow their spouses to share in providing child care, or they allow the children to care for themselves. Three major categories of supplemental care and education can be found; center-based care, home-based care, and care by relatives, babysitters, or other individual caregivers. Significant differences exist within these categories as to the reasons these services have developed, the population served, and the type of services provided.

Center-based child care programs usually provide full-day care and may range in size from 15 to more than 100 children. They are usually required to be licensed by the state, although regulations vary greatly. Day care centers have primarily evolved from early child welfare programs created to provide care for children from poor families when mothers were employed outside the home. A primary goal of these full-day programs was to improve the health of children and remedy perceived deficits in the children's homes. In contrast, nursery schools were created to provide education and enrichment for children from middle- and upper-class homes and often were part-day programs. Parent education was an important part of these programs and parents often served as assistants to professionally trained teachers. Today, the distinction between these two types of center-based care has lessened as day care centers commonly have an educational component and many nursery schools have longer hours to fit parental needs.

Before- and after-school programs have been created to provide care when schools are in session but school time does not match parental hours of employment. These programs are often housed in schools. The caregivers in these programs supervise homework and provide a safe place for children to be with their friends until their parents finish work. Other less common types of center-based care include those organized on a volunteer basis (such as Mother's Day Out programs) or as cooperative care programs managed by parents without professional staff.

Family child care refers to the care of a small number of children (often 6 or fewer) in a private home. All states have some type of regulation for family child care but the specific regulations vary between states, and many homes operate legally without licensing or registration. Typically, home care providers have lower levels of education and training than caregivers in center-based care but with a smaller group of children they can provide more one-on-one care. A small number of family child care homes are organized under the sponsorship of administrative agencies that supply providers with services and referrals. Family child care centers are licensed to care for larger groups of children. These larger groups often require the help of at least one additional person over the age of 14 years.

A variety of individual caregivers also provide significant amounts of care for young children. There is little regulation of this type of care and it is often used for recreation and leisure, errands and appointments, as well as for employment. A great deal of the care of young children is provided by grandparents or other relatives such as aunts, sisters, and sisters-in-law. Often this care is provided without charge or at a low cost. Nannies are often employed by parents with rela-

tively high income to provide full-time care in the child's home. In some cases nannies live in the child's home. A final category is baby-sitting care that is arranged informally. Baby-sitters include friends and teenagers, and care for children is in the child's own home, often on an irregular basis.

Many children spend a majority of their waking hours in day care during the week as parents need care for a 40-hour work week plus transportation time. This may mean care is needed from 6:00 in the morning or earlier to 5:30 in the evening or later. Care is most commonly available from Monday through Friday, with limited care available during the evening hours, overnight, and on weekends. Care is often difficult to find when parents have irregular hours or rotating shifts. Parents need also back-up care arrangements for times when the baby-sitter or provider is unavailable due to bad weather, holidays, or illness. Many families must use several caregivers in order to meet the different needs of each child in the family. Care for children who are ill or recovering from an illness is difficult to find. Many parents must make difficult choices when they have to take extended amounts of time away from their work for child care, especially when children have frequent illnesses or care is unreliable.

A final type of "care" is self-care. This is a more common solution for child care needs as children grow older. The suitability of self-care depends on a number of variables such as the child's level of comfort with this arrangement, maturity and skill levels, the safety of the neighborhood, and whether the parent or other adult is available by telephone. The number of children caring for themselves is unknown with wide variation in the number estimated.

More than 12 million children under the age of 5 are estimated to spend at least some time on a regular basis in the care of someone other than their parents. Slightly over half of the preschool children are cared for by someone other than relatives. Thirty percent of these children are cared for in center-based care while 17% are cared for in family child care settings and 5% are cared for by in-home baby-sitters. Other children are cared for by fathers (16%) and other relatives (26%) or by the mother at work (6%). Older children attend kindergarten and primary classes, located in public schools. By the early 1990s, a majority of children had attended a center-based program before entering kindergarten.

II. CHILD CARE AS A RESOURCE FOR CHILDREN

Child care provides care for children while parents are employed, but supplemental child care also provides children with increased opportunities for education, enrichment, and socialization. Much of the available research has focused on trying to identify the positive and negative consequences of day care attendance. An initial assumption held by many researchers and policymakers was that children would suffer negative consequences if cared for by anyone other than the mother. Experiences during World War II and in orphanages often showed negative results as children did not develop strong emotional relationships to adults and many were greatly delayed in their general development when they were separated from parents. However, there are significant differences in the complete separation of children and parents under traumatic circumstances, and the daily separation and reunion of children and parents who have an on-going relationship. Most controversy today revolves around the care of infants and toddlers by nonfamily caregivers and the impact this may have on the development of a strong and secure attachment between parents and children. Important variables may be the responsiveness and stability of the supplemental caregiver, the quality of the program, the ability of the child to adapt to new situations and the timing of changes in caregivers.

Children enrolled in day care gain experience in how to successfully interact with both peers and adults. Daily interaction with other children helps a child learn how to negotiate with peers, become a member of a group, and learn expected patterns of behavior of their society. This experience is especially valuable when trained teachers are available to help children develop skills and to guide social interaction. Children in group care programs develop friendships with peers from a relatively early age that may serve as a source of information and social support, especially in times of change or stress.

Studies of the cognitive development of children have shown that children participating in early intervention programs such as Head Start show increased levels of intellectual performance. However, as noted by critics, the gains measured by standardized IQ and achievement scores tend to decline in elementary school. Analysis of the long-term results of early intervention preschool programs have shown other benefits such as reduced placement in special education, and less grade retention, teenage pregnancy, delinquency, and welfare. This may result in a significant benefit–cost ratio for the expenses of early intervention programs.

Child care can also provide an environment that gives children an increased opportunity to learn during the critical early years of learning. Typically, there is a greater variety of equipment and more activities available in child care as well as a wider variety of play opportunities than a single home can provide. Caring adults who have different experiences and knowledge than parents may extend learning opportunities for children in a nuclear family. These programs and adults may also provide critical support and protection for children who live in high-risk families and neighborhoods.

Child care has generally been found to provide a safe place for children with relatively few reports of accidental injury or child abuse, although many of the studies have been done with laboratory centers associated with universities. The support and guidance of federal programs has encouraged many centers and homes to provide children with nutritious meals and snacks. This is critically important when much of the child's daily diet is eaten in day care. Infectious diseases are a concern in groups of children as illnesses are easily "shared" by other children and staff alike. Good sanitation and hand-washing practices are essential to minimize the spread of diseases.

The suitability of infant day care has been widely debated. Initial reports indicated that the separation of infants and parents may result in a less-secure attachment. However, later research has not supported these findings. Critical aspects for infant and toddler care appear to be similar to child care in general and include the physical environment, the number of children and adults and the relationship between children and adults.

III. CHILD CARE QUALITY

The quality of child care is an important factor influencing children's development. The widely used concept of "developmentally appropriate practices" refers to guidelines created with the input and feedback of many early childhood practitioners with the guidance of a professional organization, the National Association for the Education of Young Children. The goal of this document has been to establish guidelines for good-quality child care by considering the appropriateness of activities for children. Consideration is made of care practices that are both age-appropriate for children within the normal sequence of growth as well as individually appropriate activities that consider the abilities and interests of individual children. Although these guidelines have been criticized as being shaped by cultural expectations, they do provide a tangible guide in the task of creating environments that are appropriate for children.

The determinants of quality in family child care may differ somewhat from the characteristics identified in center-based care. Research has indicated that the relationships between caregiver characteristics such as education, training, and experience, and the quality of care may not be as strong in family day care as it is in center-based care. Home child care providers who provide high-quality care have been found to care for more children part-time and to be more likely to care for their own children. The development of children varied primarily according to their family background and the quality of the family child care rather than characteristics of the caregiver or the conditions of caregiving.

Staffing has been found to be an important variable in creating high-quality child care. Continuity of employment of caregivers is an important aspect of good-quality care and stability is linked to working conditions of staff. The National Child Staffing Study reported that teacher salaries were the best predictor of classroom environments and effective teaching. However, average salaries for child care workers are low, especially considering the high level of skill needed to work successfully with children.

The degree of congruence in values and the relationship between the family and the day care setting may be an additional important variable. Work is being conducted to better understand specific populations of children, including children living in minority cultures, children living in different family structures, child care in rural areas, children at risk for not succeeding in school, children with special needs or who are delayed in their development, and children without a permanent home. Mothers' attitudes concerning the desirability of employment and child care may also influence the child's experience in day care.

IV. THE ECOLOGY OF CHILD CARE: CHILDREN AND PARENTS

Initial research in day care conceptualized a simple relationship between attendance in day care and the child's development. Much effort was spent in trying to show the impact of various types of curriculum on the child's socioemotional and cognitive development. Today, greater emphasis is placed on identifying relationships among providers/teachers, children, and families, and the influence of employers, community support, and public policies on day care.

A. Children

The complex effect of child care on children is shaped by the characteristics of the care, the children, and their families. A growing body of research has identified at least some of the variables that comprise "quality" care. A clean, safe, and stimulating physical environment appears to be an important factor. Structural variables that include the ratio of children to adults, the number of children in the group, and the education and training of the caregivers are typically identified. In general, care with a small group size, small child to adult ratio, and well-educated and trained staff with a low staff turnover is found to be a high-quality child care. Process variables, the interactions between staff and children and between children, are also important in establishing warm, nurturing, and sensitive relationships within the day care. Often research has found that "good things go together." A small group of children with a skilled caregiver in a safe and stimulating environment often leads to the creation of positive relationships between the caregiver and the child.

Many characteristics of an individual child may interact to influence children's experiences in day care. Temperament, children's characteristic emotional responses to life, appear to be important in structuring the child's experience. Children with an "easy" temperament can adjust to new events in their lives much better than those with a "difficult" temperament. Highly active children, who tend to be negative in their reactions and are irregular in their needs will have a different experience than a child who is more calm, positive, and predictable. The age of the child will also make a difference. Very young children in the process of developing emotional attachments to adults find it more difficult to make changes in caregivers than older children with a better developed conception of his or her world. Some research has suggested that boys may show more negative consequences in day care than girls.

B. Parents

Almost all studies show that the selection of good quality and appropriate child care is primarily the responsibility of parents. Parents typically give a positive evaluation of the care they are using and report that they are very satisfied. Most mothers indicate that if they had to decide all over again in regards to selecting a provider they would make the same choice and would recommend their provider to a friend.

Often mothers select a provider because they feel comfortable with the individual and have trust in their personality and experience. Many mothers prefer to use a family member or at least someone that they have known previously. This often seems to be more important than the providers' formal credentials such as education or licensure. Parents generally agree on the importance of the child's safety in day care, the providers' and parents' communication and agreement about the child, and a warm and responsive relationship between the provider and the child.

There does not appear to be a strong relationship between maternal satisfaction with day care and a high rating of quality as measured by outside observers. There may be several reasons. The criteria used to identify satisfactory care may differ between parents and child care professionals. Some parents may lack the knowledge, time, or energy to find good child care, they may be able to only afford poor-quality care or they may have no other alternatives. They may report satisfaction as the care they are using is the best they can find or afford. Their sources of child care information such as relatives or friends may lack knowledge about the characteristics of high-quality child care. Research indicates that the children who may be in need of high-quality child care may be less likely to be enrolled in this care.

Women have traditionally been considered to be responsible for the care of young children. However, fathers are also concerned and involved with child care, although their participation may take a somewhat different pattern. Fathers report significant involvement in helping children get ready for day care and in transporting them to the day care setting. They may also provide a significant amount of care in emergencies and for sick children. Although mothers appear to retain primary responsibility for selecting and evaluating child care, fathers are also involved in this decision. Within a day care setting, fathers may provide support for the teaching and activities of the children or be actively involved in teaching. At a societal level, fathers actively shape the information gathered about day care and children and create political policies that influence children. The actions of political leaders, who often are fathers, shape the national agenda for child care.

Fathers' involvement in the care of their children may range in duration from a few minutes a day to all-day interaction, and in intensity from a distant to a highly involved relationship. One influence on fathers' role in the family may be the family structure. Fathers in two-career families may differ from sole breadwinners in that they may spend more time in direct interaction with children and they may be more accessible to them. The involvement of fathers who are house husbands, single parents, or stepparents may differ in unknown ways.

Several factors may discourage fathers' participation in child care. Employed fathers (as well as mothers) may have to sacrifice or delay some of their career goals if they invest significant time and energy in the care of their children. Other men may criticize them for the time spent caring for children, considering child care to be an easy escape from traditional male responsibilities. Some mothers may not support father's participation in child care, either believing fathers to be incompetent or preferring to retain authority in this realm. Institutional policies may also discourage fathers' participation in day care with limits on the flexibility and amount of time that can be spent away from work. [*See* FATHERS.]

V. FAMILY CHILD CARE

Family child care refers to the care of a limited number of young children in the home of an individual who may or may not be related to the child. The number of children allowed before the home is required to be licensed or registered differs among states. Variables used for classification are usually the number of children (often 6 or fewer), whether the families and the caregiver are related, and/or the number of families receiving care. Many family child care homes are exempt from state regulations because they care for few children or children who are related. However, a large number of homes that should be registered or licensed operate illegally.

The position of a family child care provider is a unique occupation. The work is conducted in the provider's home with little professional structure and regulation. Usually there are no other colleagues in the home and the content of the job often allows the inclusion of mother's regular child care and housework responsibilities.

A sole provider has an advantage in being able to be more flexible in setting policies for hours of care, cost of services, and the children served than caregivers in center-based care. Some home day care providers care for children during evening hours, overnight, or on weekends. In many communities, this may be the only type of care that is available to shift workers, individuals on rotating shifts or who work different hours each week, or workers employed on weekends. Family child care may be important for school-age children who need care for limited hours before and after school, care in the summers, and on days when school is not in session. The small group size of family day care is widely valued for the care of infants and toddlers.

Family child care is less expensive on average than center-based care or in-home baby-sitters. Fees for family child care may include no-cost or reduced-cost care from relatives, a trade of services with relatives and friends, or minimal charges by untrained caregivers, to charges as high or higher as those in center-based care. Cost may be a particularly important factor in deciding care for families with low incomes and limited financial resources.

A. Family Child Care Providers

Many home-based providers are women who have young children of their own. If they do not have skills that allow them to make a profit when child care expenses are subtracted, work in the home allows them to earn an income while caring for their own children. Given the high cost of child care and the stress of transporting children, working at home makes a great deal of economic sense. Many women are married to husbands who also earn limited income. Both hus-

bands and wives may hold traditional values for a life-style in which the husband is considered the primary family breadwinner. Family child care again fits these values by allowing a traditional life-style with the husband as the major breadwinner and masking the fact that the woman is employed.

Other family child care providers are older women with limited job skills that can be used in employment outside the home. In some cases, these caregivers may be related to the children and provide care for a parent unable to afford care or who cannot find other child care. A small group of family child care providers includes younger women without children. Finally, a small percentage of providers are men, often fathers who chose to stay home with their children. Little is known of these providers.

Family child care in general is not a well-paying profession. Research indicates that on average, family child care provides approximately one-third of the family income. Most providers would not be able to support their family on their income from child care alone, but their income does provide a significant supplement to their husband's income. Work as a family child care provider does not include any type of benefits such as social security, health care, or sick leave time. A few providers are able to negotiate yearly vacations or even a day off weekly with their parent users.

Several contradictions have been found in the structure of family child care. Family child care providers who work longer hours have been found to have higher job satisfaction, commitment, and greater stability than other providers. This appears to stem from greater commitment to child care as a profession. However, caring for many children is more complex, demanding, and stressful. Caring for one's own children while running a small business may be satisfying and a benefit of home day care, yet job satisfaction and commitment may be lower when the provider's own children are present.

Providers must provide consistent care for client families but may find parents to be inconsistent in the time they need child care services. Parents may unexpectedly reduce the number of hours that service is needed by taking children out of care temporarily or permanently because they lose their jobs, or they may request additional child care time such as overnight or weekend care. Although each parent may be employed for a standard 40-hour week, their work hours may be staggered so that their provider must offer her services for much longer than 40 hours. Clients' time for transportation to their work place also adds hours to families' need for day care and parents may arrive late to pick up children.

Providers often identify their relationship with parents as one of the most difficult aspects of home day care. Parents may consider providers as a "mother at home" rather than a professional or business owner and may not pay fees or pick up children on time. Many providers work on a friendship rather than a business basis and do not have written contracts specifying hours of service, consequences for late payment, or other terms of service. Parents may also make requests for special services that providers find difficult to fill, such as the frequency of diaper changes or the amount of time spent reading to children. Since providers do many of the tasks that parents also do, and have traditionally been done for no income, little respect may be given for the providers' needs or professional status.

The care of a dependent child is closely shared between two families in family child care. This shared responsibility often leads to a provider becoming attached to the children she cares for. Relationships between providers and their clients are often personal in nature. These relationships may enhance communication between parents and provider and allow them to establish similar routines in the two care environments. Having shared common experiences may also result in a bond of friendship that helps reduce isolation for the provider. However, it may also make it more difficult for the provider to enforce or impose rules, or to increase fees for a friend who is experiencing difficulties. Some providers refuse to provide care for relatives for this reason.

As in the parenting role, the provider must constantly be alert and focused on the safety and well-being of each child. Because children vary greatly in their needs it may be difficult for the provider to plan what she can accomplish during the day. Infants and toddlers may have relatively unpredictable schedules and little tolerance of waiting. Some groups of children may "fit" and play together well some days but not others, while other children require constant close supervision. As a result, providers may have the advantage of not punching a time clock, but yet have little ability to control the activities of their day with any certainty.

A growing number of studies have detailed sources of stress for providers. Comparison of stress levels reported by providers who were mothers of young children, unemployed mothers with young children at home, and mothers of young children who were employed outside their home, showed that providers reported significantly higher levels of stress. A variety of reasons may account for providers' higher stress level. Children are an intrusive element in the home as the provider must be aware of their safety and well-being at all times of the day. Providers are often isolated from other adults and lack the social support that may be found in other occupations. Since the work of providers is similar to the tasks of mothers who are usually not considered professionals, there is generally little recognition of their expertise or professionalism. Parents may take advantage of providers' hours of care assuming that they will not mind since they are already at home. The provider may end up with both the disadvantages of employment plus the disadvantages of being a parent at home with children. [*See* STRESS.]

Providers may also experience stress in their limited authority for the well-being of the child. Although they can provide a safe and nurturing environment for the child during the time he/she is in their care, the provider cannot control the type of care that the child receives from parents. In addition, children receive care from the provider for a relatively short period of time, rather than the lifetime care provided by parents. Providers who have a child leaving their care must deal with a sense of loss if they have cared for the child for a significant period of time and he/she has become part of the family. Provides must create a balance between being an objective business owner and at the same time be sensitive to the needs, language, and habits of the child in order to provide responsive care. This relationship must be accomplished with the backdrop of recognizing that the child will eventually leave.

The questions as to what factors predict provider job satisfaction and reduce burnout and turnover are critically important, as 30% to 50% of providers are estimated to leave child care per year on a national level. Providers enter family child care for many reasons and their expectations for success vary widely. Providers' difficulties in maintaining a balance between mothering tasks and the occupational role as a caregiver may lead to burnout. Variables such as their education and training and the financial return may make a significant differences in the job satisfaction and length of time as a provider. Providers are most likely to leave child care at two points: during their first year of providing care and when their last child enters school. Further research is needed to understand how providers' education, training and expectations, the presence of their own children, and the degree of social and emotional support may be related to their degree of professionalism. [*See* BURNOUT.]

B. Impact of Family Child Care on the Providers' Family

Because the child care is provided in the home, the presence of children from other families may have an impact on spouses (usually husbands) and the children of the provider. Spouses may become annoyed with the additional mess, noise, and "stuff" associated with the day care children. The activities of additional children may also damage the family home beyond the normal wear and tear of family living. Changes may be needed in the home to meet the needs of the family day care children, such as additional space for storage, room for nap times, eating, and play, and extra equipment and play materials. Family members may not volunteer to help the provider with the housework, assuming that she has been home all day. However, the provider usually has extra work in preparing for and cleaning up after the day care children so she may end up with double duty on house work.

Husbands may still expect the same services from their wife with little recognition that even though she has been in the home all day, she also has been working in a stressful occupation. They may resent finding the house a mess and active noisy children present when they return home from their work. Husbands who interact with other adults at work during the day may want peace and quiet at home while providers who care for children all day may crave discussion with an adult. Although a positive relationship has often been found between husbands' contribution to house work and the wife's income, this relationship may not hold for providers. Providers' husbands often spend less time with children than the husbands in other situations. The result is often a high demand on providers based on the number of children, husbands' income, and time spent with children and family resources.

There may be significant problems with the provider's own children feeling jealous of the family day care children. Family children may not want to share their toys and their rooms with the day care children especially if the other children handle their toys roughly and break them. Children may be confused if the accepted norms for their behavior changes from when only family members are present to when the day care children arrive. In homes with sufficient space the children's bedrooms can be made "off-limits" while families living in smaller homes must use all available space for the day care children. Providers vary in how they deal with this problem. Some providers indicate that they treat all children equally, while others give special privileges to their own children. This may include allowing the children privacy in their own rooms, special toys, or extra attention. The adjustment of their own child may be an important influence in determining how long the mother remains a provider.

On the positive side, family children often find the day care children to be good companions and become bored on the weekends when the children are not there. Providers comment that their children learn to take turns and become more responsible for others because the other children are present. Mothers may initiate more educational activities because of the day care children. In families with older children, husbands may enjoy having young children around again with the added benefit of not being responsible for them all the time. They may help with the care of children, often through playing and disciplining them, and they may provide respite care for the provider.

Providers use a variety of methods to control the impact of nonfamily persons entering their household. Providers generally recruit through informal networks of friends rather than list openings through newspapers and other blind advertisements. This creates a way to screen potential families based on the knowledge and recommendations of friends who have similar experiences and values. Providers may refuse to care for a child when they feel the child will be too great a burden, the relationship will involve too great an emotional commitment, or that they will not be able to develop a positive relationship with the child or parents. Another screening device is the use of information forms. The information requested from parents often includes general health and permission forms, but it may also include information about the child and serve to clarify parental expectations about the family day care services and policies.

Providers may attempt to reduce stress by separating their own family life from the day care. Often providers create a separate space for the day care children by restricting the family day care children to certain areas in the house. Other providers create special places for storage to keep the children's belongings separate from those of family members. Although children often have access to the entire home, many providers would prefer to have more space and consider a separate area for day care an ideal solution. Providers also control their time of operation as another method of separating day care and family life. Time limits may be enforced by financial penalties.

C. Relationships between Parents and Family Child Care Providers

Parents and providers have a similar general goal of creating an environment where children are safe, well cared for, and where they can comfortably grow and learn. However, specific concerns of parents and providers may differ because of the differences in the relationship that parents and providers have with children. Parents have a life-long interest in their own child, beginning with the birth of the child and extending into dreams for the child's future. Parents have a deep emotional relationship with the child, and its well-being is a prime concern. Providers also develop personal relationships with children but the time in which they care for the child is much shorter and limited to the time that the child is in their care. Providers' concerns and expectations of children are usually based on their knowledge of children in general.

As a result of differences in parents' and providers' relationships with children, they may differ in their evaluations and criteria for good quality child care. Professionals generally identify the educational training and licensure of a caregiver as a measure of quality. Parents, on the other hand, tend to select someone they feel they can trust to provide a good experience for their child and provide care similar to their own, including ethnic background and income level. Parents must also consider their own situation based on their employment, including the time care is needed, the cost, and the location of the care when selecting child care. When the availability of care is limited, parents have to compromise their preferences. Parents

may also make choices in care based on the age of the child and their perceptions of the child's needs. Parents with very young children may look for more family-like care, while parents of older children may prefer a more educationally based program.

When parents and providers come from different cultures and experiences, they may find they have significant differences in child care values and how daily routines are to be structured. Some differences are minor and can be negotiated while other differences are more basic. For example, the proper role of a mother may be seen differently between parents and providers. Providers who care for their own children are more likely to have negative attitudes toward mothers who are employed, and they may be critical of employed mothers who leave their children in the care of another person. Interestingly, mothers who hold more traditional views of motherhood and who feel guilty about working are more likely to choose care in a home rather than in a center. Parents' demands for how their child is to be cared for reinforces the fact that the provider is not the final authority in raising the child.

Relationships with parents are also important in providers' satisfaction as a care provider. Positive parent–provider relations are often associated with higher job satisfaction, and providers may be an important emotional support for employed parents. Providers may receive a great deal of satisfaction in knowing that they are providing good child care and that they are an important link in a family's ability to succeed.

VI. RELATIVES AS PROVIDERS

Most available research on family day care has focused on providers who are not related to the children in their care. However, relatives including grandparents, sisters or sisters-in-law, and aunts of the children are another significant group of providers. The percentage of care by relatives has decreased over time as more parents select center-based care; however, relatives are still an important group of providers, especially for infants and toddlers. One reason that relatives provide less child care may be that relatives are also employed, limiting the time they are available for child care. In spite of this, many relatives continue to provide care when their work hours allow them to do so.

Mothers' motivations for using relatives may vary. Care by relatives is often free or low cost with less than half of relatives receiving cash payments. Not surprisingly, low-income families are more likely to use relatives for care than are high income families. Black and Hispanic mothers rely on relatives for care more frequently than White mothers, and this may be closely tied to income. Families who receive welfare benefits are more likely to depend on relatives for care. Some mothers prefer using a relative for care with the assumption that there will be a closer match of values and methods of child care. For other mothers, relatives are the only available alternative for care. Mothers working evening or night shifts are more likely to use relatives than mothers working part-time.

Care by relatives has been assumed to provide a greater certainty of emotional warmth and attachment than care by adults not related to the child. Certainly, relatives are more likely to know the child as an individual, to have shared past experiences with the child, and to anticipate a life-long future relationship. Some research however, has indicated that relatives may not always have a more secure relationship with children. In situations where relatives are socially stressed and live an isolated life of poverty, the provider may not be able to provide a warm and nurturing home environment for the child. They may provide care solely because there is no alternative for the parents and they may have a limited commitment to their role as a caregiver. The quality of child care in these situations may be low and the child may not develop a secure attachment to the relative. Unlike subsidized care in centers, the home-based care and relative care used by low-income families is often of lower quality than the care used by high-income families.

VII. RURAL CHILD CARE

Approximately one-fourth of the population of the United States lives in rural areas, defined as the open countryside and places with fewer than 2500 inhabitants. In the past, relatively few rural women were employed outside the home, but currently a majority of rural women over the age of 15 are in the labor force. Rural children live in poverty at rates equal to that of children in central cities. Some of the poverty is due to changes in employment but another part is thought to be due to an increased rate of female-headed families. Minority rural families are more likely to live in poverty.

Rural mothers have been found to be significantly more likely than urban mothers to use child care by relatives than nonrelated caregivers or center-based care. When center-based care is available, it is likely to be subsidized care for low income families. Rural mothers may use child care less than urban mothers and use significantly fewer caregivers but for more hours of care. As with urban families, most rural relatives do not charge for their care. Rural as well as urban mothers select care on the basis of a previous relationship with the caregiver, as well as practical reasons such as availability, cost or location of care. Fathers assume an important role in child care with a majority of fathers providing some child care during the week.

Rural mothers are more likely to identify care through information from friends rather than information and referral services. A majority of the care for children under the age of two is provided by relatives outside the child's home. Rural family day care providers may be less qualified as they tend to be less well educated, less likely to have specialized training, and to have higher adult–child ratios. Families without family resources for providing child care may have an especially difficult time finding suitable child care. The evidence suggests that there is a shortage of caregivers in rural communities, especially a lack of group care facilities due to the less dense population.

VIII. PUBLIC AND PRIVATE SUPPORT FOR CHILD CARE PROGRAMS

Supplemental child care in the United States has become a major expenditure as the combined payments by parents, local, state and federal governments, and the private sector reaches nearly $40 billion a year to purchase and subsidize child care services for children of all ages. Families provide most of the cost of child care and researchers have estimated that in 1990 consumer expenditures made up about 70% to 75% of all expenditures for child care. The proportion of this expense varies greatly according to family income. For families with incomes under $15,000 a year, child care expenses may be one-fourth or more of their income. Parents with salaries greater than $54,000 will likely require only 6% or less of their family income to be able to purchase child care.

Federal, state, and local governments fund subsidies to child care with most funds provided by the federal government in two programs, Head Start and the Child and Dependent Care Tax Credit Program. Head Start programs are federally funded with a 25% match required from the local community. It is primarily targeted for children from low-income families with 3- and 4-year-old children. The programs include child development, early education, social, health, and nutrition services and they typically are part-day and part-year. Although of good quality, the programs have not been funded at a level to allow all eligible children to attend. As a result, low-income families whose children attend subsidized care and high-income families who can afford centers with a high level of resources may have the highest levels of quality of care. The children of low- to middle-income families are often only able to attend programs with low resources and quality of care.

The Child and Dependent Care Tax Credit program is a primary source of public assistance for child care with the benefits from this program primarily received by middle- and upper-income tax payers. A parent who has earned income and pays someone else to care for their child under the age of 13 while working (or looking for work) can qualify for credit on their federal income tax return. A maximum credit is allowed and the parent must provide documentation of the care on their tax return. States also provide tax-based subsidies.

The Child and Adult Care Food Program provides federal funding and nutrition education for licensed and registered child care centers and family child care homes. When children eat most of their meals away from home, the nutritional quality of meals and snacks becomes a critical issue. The future of this program is currently unknown. Although public funds available for preschool programs such as Head Start and public school programs such as Title I and Goals 2000 have been increased, they are not sufficient to meet the needs of all children eligible for these programs.

Child care is increasingly being recognized as an important part of family welfare reform as welfare-to-work initiatives mean that increasing numbers of low-income mothers must work or attend job-training pro-

grams. In 1996, several federal funding programs for child care (Aid to Families with Dependent Children, Transitional Child Care and At-Risk Child Care) were replaced with a single Child Care and Development Block Grant. States and localities will now have greater responsibility for many human services, including child care. Many questions remain as to how a sufficient amount of good quality child care will be provided for parents with low income who are required to be employed full-time.

An increasing body of evidence indicates that good child care can increase the productivity of employees, although a minority of businesses and corporations provide financial support for child care. Examples of care includes providing child care space on the premises or collaborating with other employers to establish child care centers. Other companies support child care resource and referral programs or provide vouchers for subsidized child care. Flexible benefit packages on a pretax basis allow parents to select what supports are most needed for dependent care. Some parents have maternity leave provided but not all parents can afford to take extended periods of leave without pay. Finding sick and emergency care remains a stress point for many families as it is an irregular need and can be quite expensive.

Private organizations such as United Way, a network of community-wide organizations that support local human service agencies, provide funds for child care programs, often programs that serve low-income families. A variety of private foundations provide one-time assistance in start-up funds for new programs or to upgrade existing programs. Many organizations also provide direct or in-kind support of child care programs through donated services and supplies. Finally, the most important hidden subsidy may be that provided by the caregivers themselves who earn significantly less as a child care worker than they could in other occupations.

Professional organizations provide information and education regarding child care issues, and provide support and opportunities for providers to network. These organizations identify common problems and provide leadership in finding ways to solve them. Many states and local agencies have developed training programs in a variety of aspects of child care such as good business practices, safety and health issues, curriculum and program planning, and discipline.

Many of these programs have been effective in improving the quality of available child care.

IX. SUMMARY

The changes that have occurred in the patterns and the location of work for mothers and fathers have had profound implications for the care of children. As a majority of parents are now employed outside the home, the need for supplemental care for young children has increased. Although there have been and continue to be serious concerns about the quality and suitability of nonfamily care, there are also positive consequences for children and families.

Research is beginning to be able to carefully define the elements of care that are needed to create environments that are supportive to children and their families. Although center-based care has been the initial focus of research, family child care is also an important source of child care. The role of provider holds many contradictions in expectations and demands that if unresolved, lead to caregiver stress and burnout. However, most providers find their work with children a satisfying and rewarding experience.

The complexity of child care as a system with many participants is slowly being understood. The characteristics and perceptions of the direct participants of children, parents, and caregivers are important variables. Their actions are further influenced by factors outside the family such as cultural values, employment policies, the economy, and governmental programs. The recognition of the needs and influence of all participants is an important and major undertaking that is necessary in creating a new and high quality system of child care.

BIBLIOGRAPHY

Atkinson, A. M. (1992). Stress levels of family day care providers, mothers employed outside the home and mothers at home. *Journal of Marriage and the Family, 54,* 379–386.

Atkinson, A. M. (1994). Rural and urban families' use of child care. *Family Relations, 43,* 16–22.

Behrman, R. E. (1996). Financing child care. *The future of children,* Vol. 6, No. 2 (Summer/Fall). Los Altos, CA: Center for the Future of Children, the David and Lucille Packard Foundation.

Bredekamp, S. (1987). *Developmentally appropriate practice in early child programs serving children birth through age eight.* Washington DC: National Association for the Education of Young Children.

Casper, L. M. (1995) What does it cost to mind our preschoolers? *Current Population Reports,* U.S. Department of Commerce, P70–52, Census Bureau.

Craven, H. (1993). *Before Head Start.* Chapel Hill: The University of North Carolina Press.

Deery-Schmitt, D., & Todd, C. (1995). A conceptual model for studying turnover among family child care providers. *Early Childhood Research Quarterly, 10,* 121–143.

Galinsky, E., Howes, C., Kontos, S., & Shinn, M. (1994). *The study of children in family child care and relative care: Highlights of findings.* New York: Families and Work Institute.

Kontos, S. (1992). *Family day care: Out of the shadows and into the limelight* (NAEYC Research Monograph Series). Washington, DC: National Association for the Education of Young Children.

Kontos, S. (1994). The ecology of family day care. *Early Childhood Research Quarterly, 9,* 87–110.

Mallory, B., & New, R. (Eds.). (1994). *Diversity and developmentally appropriate practices.* New York: Teachers College Press.

Moss, P., & Pence, A. (Eds.). (1994). *Valuing quality in early children services: New approaches to defining quality.* New York: Teachers College Press.

Nelson, M. (1990). *Negotiated care: The experiences of family day care providers.* Philadelphia: Temple University Press.

Peters, D., & Pence A. (Eds.). (1992). *Family day care: Current research for informed public policy.* New York: Teachers College Press.

Childhood Stress

Barbara G. Melamed and Bonnie Floyd

Albert Einstein College of Medicine and
Ferkauf Graduate School of Psychology
Yeshiva University

Attachment The strong, affectional tie felt toward special persons leading to pleasure during interaction and comfort during stressful periods.

Concrete Operational Stage Piaget's third stage of cognitive development in which thought becomes logical, flexible, and organized in its application to concrete information.

Encopresis Soiling in one's pants due to faulty toilet training or regression.

Formal Operational Stage Piaget's final stage of cognitive development in which adolescents develop the capacity for abstract, scientific thinking.

Learned Optimism Seligman's concept about learning to develop high expectations for success in the face of challenging tasks.

Modeling Imitation or observational learning that involves copying the behavior of others.

Self-Efficacy Beliefs about personal abilities and characteristics which guide responses to situations.

Time-Out The process by which the child is excluded from social and other reinforcers for a brief period of time.

Transactional Theory Lazarus' cognitive-emotional theory of stress which highlights the appraisal of environmental demands as overwhelming coping abilities.

CHILDHOOD STRESS and coping are processes that vary with developmental skills and the nature of the stressor. We define the problems of measurement, discuss theoretical approaches, provide an age-related taxonomy of situations that produce stress, and describe various aspects of prevention and treatment of problems. This approach stresses the importance of family influences and vulnerability factors such as childhood illness and uncontrollability and unpredictability of the stressor, and takes into account the importance of understanding the normal developmental skills used in problem-solving.

I. DEFINITION OF STRESS AND COPING

A. Stress

One of the difficulties in studying stress and coping has been the multiple definitions of "stress." Some refer to stress as an external event; others define stress as the response to such events. Seyle's General Adaptation Syndrome (GAS) postulates a systemic response to stress that enhances the arousal level. This is described as a three-stage sequence of adjustment to stress: alarm reaction (increased autonomic excitability, adrenalin), resistance (the body's attempt to meet this through adaptive responses), and exhaustion (if prolonged stress, adaptation mechanisms fail). In contrast, Holmes and Rahe defined stress as a stimulus (strain referred to an individual's response). More recent definitions have highlighted the importance of an individual's appraisal of events as a predictor of stress. Lazarus conceived of stress as a transaction involving the perception of environmental demands as exceeding individual coping abilities.

Stress has been measured in diverse ways. Physiologic variables and paper-and-pencil assessments have been used to quantify individuals' stress levels. Measures include heart rate, blood pressure, galvanic skin response, and cortisol and catecholamine levels (i.e., epinephrine and norepinephrine). Standardized assessments include the Holmes and Rahe Social Readjustment Rating Scale, Sarason's Schedule of Recent Events, and Lazarus' Hassles and Uplifts Scale.

The majority of assessments, however, have been developed to measure stress in adult populations. Although several childhood-specific measures of stress have been put forth (e.g., Children's Hassles), little validation across varying ages or different situations has occurred. It is necessary to quantify the degree of stress experienced during normal developmental periods, acute stressors, and chronically stressful conditions. It is important to distinguish between children's normal reactions to stressful developmental transitions and abnormal reactions to normal periods of change. Children's behavior as well as what they report should be evaluated to understand the intensity of their reactions to acute and chronic forms of stress.

Instruments often rely on parents' ratings of childhood stressors and caregivers' or teachers' perceptions. Depending on how observable the stressor is and how quantifiable is the reaction to it, often these ratings do not match the children's accounts of stressful situations. Assessments need to be developed that specifically target children's perspectives of stressful events.

Stress research has revealed that other individuals in the environment can influence both positively and negatively how much stress the child exhibits. Social support protects against the damaging effects of stress by offering emotional, tangible, informational, and network forms of assistance. Parents, teachers, and other adults may be directly responsible for providing children with the resources believed to moderate the effects of stress. They may also provide direct guidance or reinforcements as the child approaches a

stressful situation. Research in childhood stress, therefore, should include age-sensitive measures and an indicant of the degree of concordance between stressful situations and adults' capabilities to buffer their children's stress in these situations. [See SOCIAL SUPPORT; STRESS.]

B. Coping

Similar to the concept of stress, coping has been defined in a variety of ways. Folkman and Larazus delineated emotion-focused and problem-focused means of coping. Coping has also been divided into trait and state dimensions. Some researchers believe that individuals cope with a variety of stressors in similar ways (i.e., trait coping). Others have conceptualized coping as being dependent on the specific aspects of a given situation (i.e., state coping).

Children, like adults, differ widely in their interpretations of external events. Coping methods follow from children's perceptions of stressful situations and their ability to call up previously successful coping responses or to develop additional strategies. Thus, if children believe that they do not have coping skills they may look toward others to help them solve the problem situation. It is important to remember that children's perceptions of how stressful events are may be heavily influenced by their parents' reactions and ability to cope. Influential adults, including parents and teachers, model both appropriate and unsuccessful methods of coping. Younger children are heavily dependent on adults' emotional and tangible resources in order to cope with stressful life events. Adults' modeling of reactions have a critical role in shaping children's patterns of coping with a wide variety of situations. Therefore, a parent's anxiety may serve to inhibit a child from approaching certain settings. When discrepancies exist between children's and parents' perceptions, children may be tempted to doubt the validity of their personal interpretation of situations.

Children's patterns of coping are also influenced by a variety of factors such as age, gender, physical health, academic abilities, peer networks, family financial resources, and community involvement. Although the characteristics of stressful events influence children's coping, it is critical to note that children with adequate internal and environmental resources often display resilience in stressful situations. Children may develop response styles such as defensive repression or seeking information to deal with the impending stress. Unfortunately, few investigators have looked at the stability of these cognitive styles across the age span. It is also critical to see whether the mechanisms used are sufficient to deal with the task. Children who are flexible and who have multiple coping strategies are less likely to experience stress when coping with novel or threatening experiences. There are at least 140 specific scales in use with children to measure coping success across different situations. It is likely that age-related normative data should guide the choice of any particular scale. Table I lists some of the most widely used scales to measure coping. Lazarus, as early as 1974, stated that for coping strategy categories to be useful they must be mutually exhaustive and have all subcategories capture the universe of responses. They should be theoretically driven and be able to account for the individual behavior. Here, we address theories of child development as they impact on the concepts of stress and coping and try to synthesize the data that exist in prescribing approaches to measurement and intervention. [*See* COPING WITH STRESS.]

II. THEORETICAL CONTRIBUTIONS TO UNDERSTANDING CHILDHOOD STRESS

A variety of theoretical contributions to child development are reviewed to get a better understanding of childhood stress. These theories may be applied to different developmental periods: preschool, elementary school, and the transition to middle school. It is important to recognize the strengths and limitations of each theory. They are presented in alphabetical order so as not to judge the importance of a single approach. The most useful strategy for understanding childhood stress may represent a synthesis of different theoretical orientations.

Theoretical contributions to child development, nevertheless, need to be balanced with children's resources for addressing the demands of varied stressful situations. Unlike adults, children may be heavily influenced by their parents' strategies for coping with stress. Children's coping styles may not be observed consistently, because they are often in formative stages of development. Earlier methods of confronting stress may

evolve into well-established means of managing subsequent demands.

A. Ainsworth's Attachment Theory: Preschool Period

Ainsworth delineated categories of attachment in child–caregiver dyads. Secure, avoidant, and ambivalent categories of attachment may affect children's development of resources for coping with stress.

Securely attached infants may develop into children who view stressors as challenges rather than as threats. Attachment also enables children to learn about the strengths of others so that they begin to discover who can be trusted to give help when it is needed and how to obtain it. Avoidantly attached infants may eventually mature into children who withdraw from healthy social relationships with their peers. Ambivalently attached infants may develop into children who are the least prepared to face stressful challenges. Individuals with few "available attachments" are at special risk of developing neurotic symptoms under adversity.

It is important to recognize that this quality of child–caregiver attachment, along a security–insecurity continuum, may influence subsequent coping processes. In fact, there are data suggesting that the insecurity and ambivalent attachment to the mother in early childhood predicts an adolescent's tendency to act out in socially inappropriate ways. Overprotective forms of attachment may foster the development of less adaptive coping behaviors. Girls who are excessively protected may tend to withdraw from situations that are perceived as challenging or stressful; boys may exhibit greater levels of passivity and dependency in response to stressful situations. [*See* ATTACHMENT.]

B. Bandura's Social Learning Theory: School Age Period

Bandura's social learning theory explains child development in terms of how behavioral responses are acquired. His theory emphasizes the importance of self-efficacy, or the perception that one will be successful if persistent, as a predictor of optimal coping strategies.

Younger children's selection of coping strategies may be heavily influenced by their parents' own coping behaviors. Parents shape children's perceptions of effective coping strategies when they effectively model appropriate reactions to stressful situations. In contrast, parents may adversely affect the development of adaptive coping strategies when they exhibit ineffective responses to challenging situations. Siblings may also influence children's responses to stressful situations. As children mature (especially between 5 and 12 years of age), peers become important sources for modeling coping strategies. Coping techniques may be primarily selected because they are modeled by children who have achieved relatively greater social status. Unfortunately, aggressive children are often imitated because of their dominance in children's hierarchies. Likability is also a determining factor. Children do not only cope individually, but they may also join gangs if they feel they need protection from others and a group identity.

C. Erickson's Psychosocial Theory

Erickson regarded development as the result of environmental demands that shape children's personalities in order to promote the acquisition of attitudes and skills that contribute to effective social functioning. He delineates the basic conflicts between varying developmental periods. Children's responses to basic psychosocial conflicts determine whether healthy or maladaptive outcomes are achieved.

During the preschool period, children must resolve the challenges of two stages: basic trust versus mistrust, and autonomy versus shame and doubt. Parents' responses help foster the development of autonomy when they do not force or shame their children. Children's subsequent coping responses may reflect their degree of success in dealing with early situations that involve decision-making skills.

Before entering school, children enter the psychosocial stage of initiative versus guilt. By supporting children's sense of responsibility, parents promote the development of initiative. Guilt results when caregivers demand too much self-control from children; stress levels may be excessive when parents have excessive expectations for children's self-control abilities.

During middle childhood, children enter the industry versus inferiority psychosocial stage. School experiences allow children to obtain skills in working and cooperating with others. Childhood stress may be enhanced if educators fail to develop age-appropriate tasks. During this stage, children are exposed to how their peers respond to the same educational demands.

A sense of inferiority may develop when negative school, home, or peer experiences produce feelings of incompetence. Although children's abilities to succeed in traditional academic tasks remain important in assessing childhood stress, recent attention has begun to focus on alternative definitions of intelligence. The concept of emotional intelligence has been proposed to describe the adaptive regulation of emotion. Teaching components of emotional intelligence may allow children to obtain additional resources for buffering the effects of stressful experiences. [*See* OPTIMAL DEVELOPMENT FROM AN ERIKSONIAN PERSPECTIVE.]

D. Lazarus' Appraisal Theory

Lazarus' cognitive appraisal theory of adaptation, discussed earlier, has led to the development of effective intervention strategies. As children develop more sophistication in coping choices as a result of previous successful and unsuccessful attempts at coping, they develop more active coping strategies. Thus, many therapies involve giving the child a success experience, whether through behavioral rehearsal, guided imagery, or other cognitive skill training programs.

E. Seligman's Learned Optimism Theory: Developing Stress Resistance

Seligman's seminal contributions to the role of learned helplessness in the development and maintainance of depression have shaped current understandings of childhood stress. More recently, Seligman has stressed the importance of optimism as a protective factor against the development of childhood depression.

Children display a wide range of individual differences along an optimism–pessimism continuum. These differences interact with characteristics of external stressors to affect children's unique coping strategies. Children who are more optimistic are more likely to confront stressful situations as temporary, and therefore surmountable, forms of setbacks. In contrast, pessimistic children are more likely to interpret the same stressful situations as pervasive and permanent impediments to success. Optimism has been postulated as the most salient predictor of cognitive–behavioral therapy's success in treating depression; therefore, it is important to consider how optimism may affect children's coping strategies during periods of affective distress. Snyder developed a Children's Hope Scale which explores both the coping strategy adopted and children's sense of optimism. Kazdin developed a Hopefulness Scale for children, and there is a well-established children's version of the Locus of Control Scale, which also relates to persistence and optimism (see Table I).

F. Vygotsky's Sociocultural Theory

Vygotsky's sociocultural theory stresses that child development results from a combination of maturational processes and social interactions with more knowledgeable members of society. His theory highlights the importance of culture—the values, beliefs, customs, and skills of a social group—in shaping adaptive skills. It also focuses on how cultural components are passed along to the next generation. Previous theories have tended to underestimate the importance of cultural differences in children's responses to stressful situations.

A sociocultural emphasis helps explain the varied coping processes children exhibit in response to stressful circumstances. Vygotsky's theory provides additional information about the wide variation in cognitive skills across diverse cultures. Cultures may not have specific labels for conveying such concepts as aggression or peacefulness; children's coping strategies, therefore, should not be assumed to mirror those exhibited in cultures that provide these labels. Differences in cognitive skills, in turn, may influence children's selections of coping strategies across a variety of stressful situations. There has been inadequate research and clinical attention to the transcultural factors that affect children's conceptualizations of stress.

III. FACTORS PREDICTING VULNERABILITY TO STRESS

A. Age of Child

Young children are less experienced in generating stress solutions, and they also have fewer previously successful experiences. As children develop cognitive structures that allow reasoned choices; they are less likely to avoid or deny the stressful event. In preparing children for surgical procedures, Melamed and her colleagues found that younger children should have less time to think about the event, whereas older children can plan ahead about actions they might consider depending on the similarity to previous situations.

B. Predictability of the Stressor

The predictability of the stressor (i.e., when and where it will occur and who will be present to assist) may reduce the amount of anticipatory anxiety. When an aversive situation is expected, the amount of time it will last often influences the child's choice of action.

C. Controllable or Uncontrollable Stressors

If the actual stressor cannot be avoided (i.e., immunization, preschool experience), then children usually cope by emotion-focused means, expressing their fear and how they will try to get through it. If, however, the child can control the amount of time he or she must deal with a stressor, he or she is more likely to formulate a plan to modulate the experience. Thoughtful planning does involve higher cognitive levels of problem solving.

D. Social Support Networks

The presence of a parent, older sibling, teacher, or caregiver is often found to buffer the experience of stress, providing the child with helpful options and rewarding his or her successful attempts. [See SOCIAL NETWORKS.]

E. Personality and Coping Styles

Children may have temperamental differences, either through genetic endowment or early childhood shaping, which leads them toward stereotyped solutions to stress. For instance, a so-called "difficult" child may find it hard to appraise a situation accurately and may withdraw from problematic or novel situations. Children who are shy and dependent may require the intervention of adults to initiate coping skills. Aggressive children may overuse aggression—threats or actual physical or verbal abuse—when faced with frustration or interpersonal stress. Children who learn optimism from those around them are less likely to give up easily when stressed and more likely to persist in coping efforts. The age and gender of the child may also determine socially acceptable coping responses. Younger children tend to use concrete efforts such as distraction or play, whereas older children may seek information about impending events and rehearse how they might

Table I   Taxonomy of Children's Coping Strategies[a,b]

Category	Definition	Children's scales
Aggressive act	Verbal or motor activities that may be hurtful to persons, animals, or objects	Novaco Anger Training
Behavioral avoidance	Behavior other than isolating that is an attempt to keep away from the stressor	Procedural Behavior Rating Scale (Katz and Kellerman)
Behavioral distraction	Behavior other than isolating or avoidant that delays the need to deal with a stressor	
Cognitive avoidance (Blunting)	Deliberate cognitive attempts to avoid acknowledging the existence of a stressor	Miller Behavior Style Scale
Cognitive distraction	Deliberate attempts to keep thoughts away from a stressor	
Cognitive problem-solving	Thoughts focused on ways to modify or prevent the problem	Ways of Coping for Children Nowicki Locus of Control
Cognitive restructuring	Thoughts that alter one's perception of characteristics of the stressor	Irrational Belief Scale—Ellis
Emotional expression	Behavior other than aggressive motor and verbal activities that express emotion	Child Depression Inventory Anxiety Disorders Inventory Scale for Children
Endurance (self-esteem)	Behavior that causes one to face the stressor and accept its consequences	Rosenberg's Self-Control Scale Hopefulness Scale
Information seeking (Monitoring)	Behavior that involves obtaining information about the stressor	Miller Behavioral Style Scale
Isolating activities	Behavior that separates the individual from the presence of others	Index of Peer Relations
Self-controlling activities	Behavior that separates the individual from the presence of others	Impulsivity, Relaxation Training Scale
Social support	Nonaggressive behavior that involves seeking the presence of others	Index of Peer Relations
Spiritual support	Behavior that suggests appealing to a higher being	Religious beliefs and attitudes
Stressor modification	Noncognitive behavior that eliminates the stressor or modifies the characteristics of the stressor	Reframing lists

[a] This list was adapted from "A Taxonomy of Children's Coping Strategies" by Nancy Ryan-Wenger, 1992, *American Journal of Orthopsychiatry, 62*, Many of these scales are available from HaPI—a CDROM entitled: Health and Psychosocial Adjustment. An excellent source is in Corcoran and Fischer *Measures for Clinical Practice.* Cal., Free Press.

[b] General coping inventories include Coping Strategies Test (Asaranow), KIDCOPE (Spirito), and Behavioral Strategies Coping Scale.

handle these situations. [*See* AGGRESSION; PERSONALITY; SHYNESS.]

F. Stress Taxonomy by Age

Table II describes the types of situations that may trigger distress. Childrens' stressors are different from adult stressors. Often, children cannot change some of the situations themselves; these include such factors as

social class, poverty, the school system, and/or parental mental health.

G. Coping Taxonomy by Age

An attempt to form a taxonomy of mutually exclusive coping strategies, representing research findings of examplars of actual strategies used by children in stressful situations and those that may predict likely choices

Table II Developmental Stressor and Treatment

Grade/developmental age	Normal concerns/skills available	Therapy approaches

Preschool—1st grade
  Social: separation fear, parallel play
  Cognitive: concrete thinking
  Physical: fine motor movements begin
    to develop
	Daycare, sibling rivalry, emergency
	  room, immunizations, fear of noises,
	  dark, small animals, injuries
	Toileting, eating
		Graded exposure, information provided,
		  systematic desensitization, doll or
		  group play

Elem.-middle school
  Social
  Cognitive
  Physical
	Peer group influences, fear of rejection,
	  fear of academic performance
	Concrete thinking, impulsivity
	Can use fine motor skills, not always
	  coordinated
		Social skills training, behavioral re-
		  hearsal operant, reinforcement, token
		  economic rewards after a period of
		  work or success
		Recreational activities, exercise

Preteen–adolescence
  Social
  Cognitive
  Physical
	Fears of rejection, being different,
	  conforming to peer values, sexual
	  concerns
	Abstract reasoning, ability to delay
	  gratification
	Performs coordinated tasks
		Social skills training, problem solving
		  behavioral rehearsal, sex education
		
		Sports activities, music lessons, soccer,
		  karate, exercise

and outcomes in future situations, was undertaken by Ryan-Wenger in 1992 and is illustrated in Table II.

IV. STRESSORS IN EARLY CHILDHOOD: PRESCHOOL TO FIRST GRADE

A. Chronic Illness

It is often found that during a critical period from about 6 months to 3 years of age, children separated from a parent because of death, illness, divorce, abandonment, and so on, may suffer from attachment problems. This is particularly likely if the children are sick themselves and are in a hospital or other institution with a low staff-to-child ratio for extended periods.

Adaptation to chronic illness is influenced by the rate at which improvements are being made in medical research. For example, adjustment to childhood cancer previously meant providing assistance to families who were anticipating a child's inevitable death. Better survival rates for certain childhood chronic illnesses, including cancer, cystic fibrosis, and AIDS, necessitate new models of adjustment to long-term changes in health status.

Despite significant medical advances, chronic illnesses still need to be conceptualized as long-term sources of stress for both children and their families.

Long-term health disturbances involve repeated hospitalizations, discomfort, uncertain outcomes, multiple diagnostic procedures, and periodic medical evaluations. Financial resources may be severely strained in families with a chronically ill child, diverting funds from other pursuits. Childhood stress, in turn, may be increased without the additional resources for pursuing special-needs educational programs and recreational activities.

Siblings may resent parents' increased attention toward a chronically ill child, especially as sibling conflicts tend to increase during middle childhood. Conflicts are affected by a combination of children's temperaments and parental behavior. Illness changes functioning and roles within the family. [See CHRONIC ILLNESS.]

B. Death or Divorce

The loss of a parent because of illness, death, or divorce can cause problems in children, particularly in those who are just beginning to identify strongly with the parent. Children learn about gender role modeling through their interactions with parents of the opposite sex as well as with their primary caretaker. Young boys often become aggressive in trying to fill an absent father's role. Girls have more problems with sexual identity the older they are. In any case, additional stressors may also include depression and ineffective parenting in the remaining parent, changes in financial status, moving to a more affordable living situation, sharing living quarters with grandparents, and changing schools. Bowlby states that among conditions necessary for a favorable outcome are the child continuing to have a secure attachment, either to the surviving parent or to a substitute, and being fully informed about the death or absence and given ample and repeated opportunities to discuss its implications.

C. Developmental Delays

Children who are slow to learn motor and speech expression, whether due to a birth incident, genetic defect, or other physical insults, have trouble fitting in with their peer group. The lack of communication may inhibit social play and lead to isolation from others. In addition, parental concerns about permanence and guilt or conflict over the cause of these problems are likely to be communicated to the young child, especially in parents who deny the problem and fail to seek rehabilitative and medical services. Many parents continue to "doctor shop" until they find a professional who will dispute the diagnosis.

D. Emotional Development

Children learn reciprocal behaviors by interacting first with their mother and then with others. To develop appropriate emotions, they must learn to imitate, recognize, and empathize with the emotional responses of others. Kagan has pointed out that children at first do not differentiate more than happy and sad affect. They respond primarily with crying and smiling depending on their state of hunger, warmth, dryness, or physical contact. At around age 9 months, children usually recognize their own mother and begin to show fears around strangers. At first, much of emotional responding is tied into reflex activity, for example, pulling hand off hot stove, startling at sudden or loud noises, and fearing sudden change in position. In institutionalized children (e.g., orphans), the disruption of bonding leads to serious attachment problems. Even in these youngsters, as physical maturation takes place, so does the ability to recognize and differentiate more complex emotions. The child can inhibit crying if no one is present, or show frustration and anger by movements of arms and legs. Emotional learning also involves gender differences, with girls developing a wider repertoire at an early stage. Goleman suggests that this is related to intelligence and adaptability to stress. [See EMOTIONAL REGULATION.]

E. Eating Problems

Children may have colicky behaviors from an accumulation of gas or from difficulty digesting milk or solid foods. Some children have more serious lactose intolerance and must consume soybean products in place of milk. Children in their second to third year are expected to develop habits of good nutrition. Unfortunately, many struggles between parent and child as to what good nutrition is can make children vulnerable to more serious eating disturbances such as anorexia or obesity. It is thought that children develop most of their fat cells during this early period. Evidence supports the risk of coronary disease in children who produce plaque in their arteries as a result of high fat intake in childhood. [See FOOD, NUTRITION, AND MENTAL HEALTH; OBESITY.]

F. Separation Disorders

Some children develop attachment disorders if they do not learn to associate their mother or caretaker with a sense of security. If children are weaned too early from the breast they may also feel frustration in this relationship. The parent who may have a psychiatric disorder, such as depression or anxiety, may not be capable of handling separation issues in a developmentally appropriate way. School phobias may result more from the parent's inability to "let go" of his or her child.

G. Sibling Rivalry

Sibling rivalry is a normal phase of development; children close in age often compete for parental attention. It may be exacerbated if one sibling has a chronic disease which may make the healthy sibling feel guilty or deprived of attention.

H. Sleep Disorders

Children rarely have more than transient sleep disturbances because of anxiety or lack of ritual in bedtime activities. Children may have nightmares in which they are feeling attacked by some animal or person. The children who have night terrors may experience sleepwalking (somnambulism) and other more serious problems, such as sleep apnea, which may require medical or psychological attention. Most phobias concerning darkness and ghosts are developmental and transient. It is only when the fear is excessive or out of proportion to the danger, causing the child to avoid people or situations, that a professional needs to be consulted. [*See* SLEEP.]

I. Soiling (Encopresis)

Soiling may be the result of inadequate toilet training or regressive loss of bowel control due to a trauma, such as parental loss or divorce. If it continues and occurs in the elementary school-aged child, it may lead to social isolation, teasing, and avoidance of school or social activities. After the pediatrician has ruled out sphincter or other physical causes, the child should first be treated for any accompanying constipation or diarrhea and then a behavior modification program should be developed with a specialist. The longer this problem exists, the more likely it is to be accompanied by a more serious personality disorder.

J. Traumatic Events

Children who have been repeatedly abused or sexually molested by a member of the family or extended network will appear shy, withdrawn, and often have sleeping problems. These stressors, when identified, need to be immediately attended to, because if they are not, the child may learn inappropriate social behavior or turn to drugs or alcohol to hide his or her feelings.

Accidents are actually a leading cause of death in young children. Burns may leave children vulnerable to infections, physical deformity and ridicule, and exposure to painful debridement procedures. Automobile and bicycle accidents may result in fearful responses and may need therapies such as reframing and building up confidence. Systematic desensitization and guided participant modeling which use gradual reexposure to elements associated with the accident are widely used. Basically, parents need to establish or reestablish safety principles and clearly communicate these to their children.

V. DEVELOPMENTAL CHALLENGES IN MANAGING STRESS IN SCHOOL-AGED CHILDREN

Elementary school-aged children, as well as those experiencing the transition from primary to middle school, face several developmental and situational stressors that will challenge their coping resources. Outcomes are determined by the interplay between children's and family's resources, in addition to the specific characteristics of the stressors themselves. Older children have different conflicts to face. Peer acceptance and achievement motivation are examples of the typical demands children face during development. Some children may also face the stresses associated with unique childhood experiences. These may include chronic illness, eating disorders, or the issues related to divorce (e.g., custody arrangements, remarriage).

A. Peer Acceptance

As children master important early childhood developmental changes, they begin to experience developments in their peer networks. Although children's parents and siblings remain important influences, peers begin to affect children in a variety of important ways. It is important to recognize that peers may influence children in both socially desirable and undesirable ways. As children mature, the influence of peers may be restrained by an increasing emphasis on the need to respect others' opinions.

Childhood aggression has been assessed for its influence on peer acceptability. All aggressive children do not experience peer rejection, nor are all rejected children aggressive. Nevertheless, the single most influential reason for peer rejection is aggressive behavior.

Children may define friendships as relationships among small groups who share similar interests, rather than as relationships between only two individuals. Children with more extensive peer networks, and who have a strong close friend, have additional resources during stressful periods. If they experience a conflict with one of their friends, the availability of additional friends provides a valuable buffer against stressful situations. A wider peer network also provides children with increased access to valuable information. For example, academic stress may be buffered by having several peers with whom to study before an examination.

B. Achievement Motivation

Children's advancing cognitive capacities exert an important influence on their academic motivation. Developmentally appropriate cognitive tasks provide children with adequate levels of cognitive stimulation, whereas inappropriate assignments may create additional sources of childhood stress. During elementary school, children experience the cognitive developments associated with Piaget's concrete operational stage. Children's thoughts begin to display logical, flexible, and organizational characteristics. For example, children are able to understand the principle of conservation. They recognize that the physical characteristics of objects do not change when their outward appearances are altered; children understand that a pile of pennies that has spilled onto the floor contains the same number of pennies if arranged as a row on a table.

As children experience the transition from elementary to middle school, they experience the beginnings of formal operational thought. At this point, children begin to consider hypothetical factors influencing the outcome of a situation, in addition to its concrete characteristics. Children's cognitive development allows for flexibility in problem-solving strategies; when children are able to think in abstract terms, they are able to entertain numerous approaches to resolving the same problem.

Children may experience heightened levels of stress if they are subject to external demands that exceed their cognitive abilities. Parents may communicate approval through their children's attainment of academic success. High parental levels of achievement expectations may be overtly transmitted to children. Even children who possess exceptional academic capabilities may suffer from unrealistic internal demands for success.

Although children's abilities to succeed in traditional academic tasks remain important in assessing childhood stress, recent attention has focused on alternative definitions of intelligence. The concept of emotional intelligence has been proposed to describe the adaptive regulation of emotion. A child in control of emotional outbursts is more likely to engage friends in the problem solving of frustrating tasks. Empathy for the emotions of others is a prerequisite for developing prosocial behaviors such as sharing and altruism.

C. Beliefs about Chronic Illness

Childhood chronic illnesses differ widely with regard to their complexity of medical management. Juvenile diabetes, for example, involves daily adherence to dietary restrictions, blood glucose testing, and insulin injections. Diseases such as juvenile rheumatoid arthritis and juvenile diabetes may cause heightened levels of discomfort. A child may suffer in terms of feeling

different from others, which is especially painful in middle childhood.

With their advancing cognitive abilities, children develop more sophisticated notions of cause-and-effect processes in illness development. The cause of illness shifts from being viewed as an external person or action to an event located within the body. As children's cognitive development matures to include concrete operational thinking, illness representations are altered. Illness beliefs refer to lay understandings of how disease processes develop. Children between ages 7 and 10 are initially likely to conceive illness in terms of contamination; this implies that an external person, object, or action is responsible for producing illness. Later, children begin to explain illness in terms of internalization. Children, however, have only vague understandings of disease processes at this point.

Additional advances in cognitive development introduce new understandings of how illness develops. At approximately age 11, children begin to understand how internal physiological processes are altered to produce disease. The cause of illness shifts from being viewed as an external person or action to an event located within the body.

D. Divorce/Custody Arrangements/Remarriage

Marital separation, divorce, and remarriage occur under a variety of circumstances; these transitions may occur earlier or later in the course of a family's development. Therefore, childhood responses that have been typically presumed to reflect adjustment to marital dissolution may actually reflect the family's previous level of disruption.

Several factors are related to children's adjustment to divorce: age, temperament, and gender. Younger children are more likely to blame themselves for a parental breakup; they may show more intense levels of separation anxiety. Older children, particularly boys, may act out with frequent displays of disruptive behavior. It is important to emphasize that divorce is not a static event for children; it involves a series of ongoing changes for family members. Children's adjustment to divorce must take into account the developmental stage at the time of divorce and whether the adjustment will be to a single parent or consist of remarried households and step-siblings. Earlier conceptions of divorce as a short-term event have given way to a more sober appraisal of its long-term effects for children.

Parental disagreements also influence children's responses to altered living arrangements; children may initially experience relief if divorce results in a less volatile living arrangement. Childhood stressors may increase in conjunction with parents' own adjustment concerns. Caregivers, most notably mothers, may sometimes display less sensitivity to their children's needs when they face increased financial demands or sink into depression. Stress levels may rise as a result of separation from one parent, as well as from emotional changes in the primary caregiver. Childhood stress may increase when parents are less attentive to needs, display increased irritability, and exhibit less consistent parenting.

Disputes regarding child visitation place children under increased levels of stress. Child custody arrangements may be voluntary or forced, producing vastly different consequences for children. It is important for parents to avoid engaging in power struggles after a divorce. Children may experience heightened adjustment difficulties if they feel as though they must remain loyal to only one parent. Parental transitions, including remarriage, may affect child custody arrangements. Research suggests that children are exposed to the greatest levels of stress when they experience inconsistent parenting styles. Variations in parenting may occur with a primary caregiver, as well as with the noncustodial parent.

Despite its initially positive portrayal, joint custody arrangements may create additional childhood stress. Children may have to make multiple adjustments when they maintain contact with both parents. Additional sources of stress include changes in children's peer networks and friendships during periods of changed living arrangements.

Remarriage introduces additional adjustments for children. Heatherington's research has shown that mothers and daughters display the highest levels of conflict during the initial phase of remarriage. Boys, in contrast, seem to benefit from the introduction of a male role figure. In nonremarried families, in contrast, mothers and daughters continued to experience closer relationships than mothers and sons. [*See* DIVORCE.]

E. Eating Disorders

Eating disorders represent extreme adaptational responses to childhood stress. Cultural expectations for ideal attractiveness, including a pervasive societal emphasis on unrealistic levels of thinness, may interact to promote the development of an eating disorder. Body image disturbances interact with preoccupations with being thin in children who develop eating disorders. Although problems in managing stress may promote the development of an eating disorder, it is important to recognize that these disorders also introduce additional forms of stress, including medical complications. [*See* BODY IMAGE.]

Middle childhood may introduce stressors that influence the development of eating disorders. These include anorexia nervosa, a disorder in which individuals starve themselves because of an irrational fear of becoming fat. Anorexia may result in death for 5% of those with this disorder. Bulimia, an eating disorder characterized by periodic eating binges followed by induced vomiting, may also develop. Anorexia nervosa and bulimia represent disorders along a spectrum of two basic components: fear of gaining weight and fear of losing control over eating. Gender differences are very pronounced in eating disorders; the vast majority of individuals developing these problems are female. Girls who mature early and those who pursue dancing, athletic, or modeling avocations are at the greatest risk for developing anorexia. Many anorexics are perfectionists with extremely high standards for their academic performance. They may not be viewed as vulnerable to stress because of their typical presentation as ideal daughters. Childhood stressors and poor attachments to the mother may influence the progression from adopting healthy lifestyle behaviors, including a concern with maintaining ideal body weight and being physically active, to becoming excessively concerned with thinness. [*See* ANOREXIA NERVOSA AND BULIMIA NERVOSA.]

VI. CONCLUSIONS

Despite advances in understanding childhood stress, this area is a critically important field in need of continued research and clinical attention. Definitions of stress and coping need to be specifically tailored to address the unique aspects of adaptation to stressors during childhood. Measures of coping need to be age-relevant and situationally specific. Previous research in this area has primarily extrapolated from models of adults' reactions to stress, rather than focusing on the unique developmental characteristics that affect reactions to childhood stress.

Several theoretical models may be used to provide

a framework for understanding children's responses to stress during different developmental periods: preschool, elementary school, and the transition from primary to middle school. These include Ainsworth's attachment, Bandura's social learning, Erickson's psychosocial theories, Lazarus' appraisal, Seligman's learned optimism, and Vigotsky's sociocultural theory. Rather than being mutually exclusive, these models may be used in combination to understand how children cope with specific stressors during varying developmental periods.

Conceptualizations of childhood stress must include a balanced perspective of the dual effects of protective and risk factors. It is inadequate to consider the qualitative and quantitative aspects of stressors without an awareness of children's intrinsic personality traits and environmental characteristics. Reactions to stressors reflect a complex interaction of child, family, and environmental resources and demands. While not denying the effects of stressful life experiences, children's resilience to stressful circumstances should also be emphasized.

Childhood stressors include normative developmental transitions, such as the increasing importance of peer acceptance and achievement motivation. Stressors may also include adaptations to specific life events, such as chronic illness or divorce. The effects of both types of stressors depend on the complex interplay between children's and families' unique vulnerabilities and resources.

Understanding children's responses to childhood stress provides the foundation for the development and implementation of effective interventions for normative and unique stressors. The most important benefits of addressing childhood stress may be reflected in preventing developmental transitions and situational challenges from evolving into more prolonged adjustment disorders.

The most serious shortcoming in the research literature is the tendency for investigators to "control for age" without understanding the influence in terms of a particular child's developmental and cognitive capacities. Measures of coping should be standardized by defining ranges of children's resources, both physical and cognitive. Interventions must be developed to teach children to cope more effectively depending on the situational and interpersonal context in which the stressor occurs. Whether or not the stress is controllable, predictable, and similar to other successfully handled situations can modulate the intervention strategy. Children may develop different abilities to cope and enhance self-efficacy. Flexibility in applying these strategies in appropriate situations is as important as which strategy is used. There are no good or bad coping strategies. One needs to evaluate whether what one does actually keeps the task within the resources one has to bring to the situation. Learning by facing frustration and stress is accepted by both psychodynamic and social learning theorists as a necessary prerequisite for developing effective coping.

ACKNOWLEDGMENT

We gratefully acknowledge the Beker Family Foundation Fellowship provided to Bonnie Floyd.

BIBLIOGRAPHY

Bandura, A., & Walters, R. H. (1963). *Social learning and personality development*. New York: Holt Rinehart & Winston.

Baumrind, D. (1989). Rearing competent children. In W. Damon (Ed.), *Child development today and tomorrow* (pp. 349–378). San Francisco: Jossey-Bass.

Berk, L. E. (1994). *Child development* (3rd ed.). Boston: Allyn & Bacon.

Berndt, T. (1989). Friendships in childhood and adolescence. In W. Damon (Ed.), *Child development today and tomorrow* (pp. 332–346). San Francisco: Jossey-Bass.

Goleman, D. (1997). *Emotional intelligence*. New York: Bantam.

Hobbs, N., Perrin, J., & Ireys, H. (1985). *Clinically ill children and their families*. San Francisco: Jossey-Bass.

Kagan, J. (1988). Development of emotions. In J. Kagan (Ed.), *The development of the child*. San Francisco: Jossey-Bass.

Lazarus, R. (1991). *Emotion and adaptation*. New York: Oxford University Press.

Ryan-Wenger, N. (1992). A taxonomy of children's coping strategies. *American Journal of Orthopsychiatry, 62,* 256–263.

Sroufe, L., & Waters, E. (1977). Attachment as an organizational construct. *Child Development, 48,* 1184–1199.

Wallerstein, J. S. (1991). The long-term effects of divorce on children: A review. *Journal of the American Academy of Child and Adolescent Psychiatry, 30,* 349–360.

Child Maltreatment

Raymond H. Starr, Jr.

University of Maryland Baltimore County

Child Protective Services (CPS) A branch, typically of the Department of Social Services, with responsibility for protecting children, including investigating maltreatment allegations, treating substantiated cases, coordinating case management with other agencies, and in some areas, maltreatment prevention.

Developmental Psychopathology The interdisciplinary study of developmental domains emphasizing the relevance of normal development to pathology and pathological development to normality.

Ecological Model A model emphasizing the interactions of individuals, family, community, and sociocultural factors in relation to maltreatment.

Emotional Maltreatment Verbal and nonverbal parent-to-child communications that may be psychologically injurious to the child given the child's age and developmental status.

Neglect Parent or caregiver failure to provide adequate health care, supervision, home safety and cleanliness, nutrition, personal hygiene, or supervision.

Physical Abuse Any parent or caregiver act causing nonaccidental physical injury or death.

Risk Assessment A procedure for evaluating the likelihood of maltreatment repetition given initial maltreatment substantiation.

Sexual Abuse Sexual exposure or contact by a person older than a child for the purpose of sexual stimulation or exploitation regardless of the use of force or any accompanying physical injury.

Substantiation Process by which CPS confirms a case as one of maltreatment.

CHILD MALTREATMENT is a major social problem with long-term consequences for affected individuals and society. This article reviews current knowledge and thought about maltreatment's causes, consequences, reporting, treatment, prediction, and prevention.[1]

I. HISTORY

Child maltreatment has long been a problem. The Bible contains many instances of maltreatment beginning with Abraham's emotionally traumatizing, threatened murder of Isaac. Similar examples of emotionally traumatizing and physically injurious practices occur in every culture. In China girls' feet were bound to constrain growth, making walking difficult.

---

[1] It is important to recognize that this article provides the briefest of overviews of a complex area that has yet to be adequately studied. Generalities cannot be avoided in this discussion and readers should refer to the bibliography for additional information sources.

In parts of Africa it has been routine to circumcise girls in a potentially fatal and often disabling way.

Some argue that these acts are culturally normative. The Chinese found the bound foot sexually stimulating; continuing the procedure until the early twentieth century. Issues of what is and is not maltreatment continue to be debated. This topic is discussed more fully in the next section on definition.

The modern concern about maltreatment is commonly traced to the 1874 case of Mary Ellen, a physically abused and neglected 9-year-old girl. The absence of laws protecting children led to her removal and both her step-mother's imprisonment under animal cruelty laws and to the founding of the New York Society for the Prevention of Cruelty to Children.

The concern about maltreatment expanded and the first Juvenile Court was established in Illinois in 1899. By application of the *parens patriae* principle where the state can act in place of parents in order to protect a child, children were given special status under the law.

Major societal concern about maltreatment only developed following the 1962 description of the "battered child syndrome." This medical diagnosis was applied to children with such unexplainable injuries as repeated bone fractures. Awareness that children could suffer nonaccidental injuries led to laws mandating reporting of suspected abuse and the 1974 passage of the federal Child Abuse Prevention and Treatment Act (CAPTA).

In summary, the history of child maltreatment is part of a continuing development of concern for children and their welfare. Children in the United States are now offered many rights, protections, and services that were unavailable in prior eras.

II. DEFINITION

It is hard to define the various maltreatment forms. Definitions may vary along six dimensions: the effects of the behavior on the child, the number of maltreatment subtypes, how frequently the maltreatment occurred, identity of the perpetrator, intent of the perpetrator, and the age of the child.

At the most basic level, children's advocates disagree about the number and importance of different types of maltreatment. Almost all conceptualize physical abuse, sexual abuse, emotional maltreatment, and neglect as discrete phenomena. Beyond this differences abound. Is neglect, for example, one phenomenon or the 14 different subtypes that have been proposed? Some believe that there is too much overlap across subtypes to make their use fruitful.

The present discussion examines four primary types of maltreatment: physical abuse, sexual abuse, emotional maltreatment, and neglect. There can be overlap within this categorization. Some definitions hold that physical and sexual abuse and neglect all incorporate a component of emotional maltreatment due to the psychological damage they cause to the child. Readers might find it useful to remember that abuse typically represents an act of commission, where something is done to a child, while neglect is an act or omission, where requisite care or nurturance is *not* provided.

Definitions vary across and within professional groups. Across professions, judges prefer broad definitions allowing discretion in case-handling; defense attorneys prefer limited, specific criteria; physicians focus on diagnostic criteria; and social service workers concentrate on consequences to the child. These differences were examined by asking members of different professions whether each of a set of circumstances was abuse, was not abuse, or whether they were undecided. A child injured when struck too hard was seen as abuse by 75% of public social workers and 44% of emergency room physicians. Only 6% of the former group saw this as nonabusive compared to 22% of the latter. More physicians than social workers were undecided.

In summary, the definition of child maltreatment is a complex, critically important task. Definitions relate to all other aspects of this discussion. They play roles in determining maltreatment substantiation, incidence, causes, consequences, treatment, and so on. While there is agreement that such acts as infanticide, incest, and leaving a 2-year-old home alone constitute maltreatment, there is uncertainty about such acts as spanking and parental nudity in the home. The dividing line between what is and what is not maltreatment is unclear.

This entry discusses work using a variety of definitions. Aspects of definitions that are critical to understanding a specific finding are discussed where relevant.

III. INCIDENCE

The incidence of different forms of maltreatment varies by information source. The lowest rate is for substantiated cases. However, substantiation procedures vary widely across jurisdictions. At a second level, many cases known to professionals may or may not be known to CPS. Such cases have been the focus of several National Incidence Studies (NIS) and lead to still higher incidence rates. The highest incidence estimates come from general population surveys. These have been done for physical and sexual abuse but not for neglect and emotional maltreatment. In addition, incidence data are influenced by the definitions used. For example, physical abuse and neglect are related to caregiver acts while sexual abuse may be perpetrated by either relatives or by strangers.

A. Substantiated Cases

The most recent available national data are for 1994 when 1,011,628 cases (18/1000 children) were substantiated, an increase of 27% since 1990. Neglect was most common (55% of cases, 8/1000 children), followed by physical abuse (26%, 4/1000), sexual abuse (14%, 2/1000), and emotional maltreatment (5%, > 1/1000). An additional 19% (3/1000) of substantiated cases were for other forms including "abandonment" and "congenital drug addiction." Some children were victims of multiple types of abuse.

Substantiation rates decline with child age. More than a quarter (27%) of cases are for children less than 4, 20% from 4 to 6, 17% from 7 to 9, 15% from 10 to 12, and teenagers represented 21%. Rates were the same for boys and girls, although racial/ethnic differences were found. More than half of cases were white, a quarter were African-American, and a tenth were Hispanic.

B. Reported and Unreported Cases Known to Professionals

NIS results differ from the preceding conclusions about substantiated cases in several ways. First, when both substantiated cases and unreported cases known to professionals are considered, there is a higher overall maltreatment rate of 25/1000 children. Only half of the children categorized as maltreated using the NIS definitions had been reported to CPS. Professionals know of significant numbers of cases that they do not report in spite of legal reporting requirements. Again, the highest incidence was for neglect (14/1000), followed by psychological maltreatment (7/1000), physical abuse (6/1000), and sexual abuse (2.5/1000).

NIS results also indicate that girls are more often maltreated than boys (13/1000 versus 8/1000), due to greater sexual abuse (4/1000 versus 1/1000). Maltreatment incidence increases with child age and decreases with higher family income but is unrelated to race, ethnicity, and community size.

C. Cases Known to Individuals

Many surveys have asked individuals about their victimization experiences. The questions asked, groups sampled, and other procedures vary markedly making it hard to compare findings across studies. Surveys have been done for physical and sexual abuse and emotional maltreatment, but not for neglect.

A recent Gallup Poll of 1000 parents estimated that a minimum of 49 children per 1000 had been physically abused in the year prior to the survey with 74/1000 being abused at some point in their life. These data are much higher than the substantiated case numbers. Abuse was defined as hitting the child with a hard object on some body part other than the bottom and other, more severe, acts. Overall, 50/1000 parents admitted ever hitting their child in such a manner, 15/1000 hit with their fist or kicked the child, 8/1000 threw or knocked down their child, 7/1000 beat their child up, and 7/1000 choked their child. In addition, an estimated 31,000,000 children had been physically punished in the prior year even though their parents stated they did not deserve the punishment. Abuse rates were higher for children under age 13, for lower income families, and in single-parent families.

Results of surveys about the prevalence of sexual abuse vary from 3% to 62% of respondents reporting unwanted sexual contact prior to age 18. The higher rates are for women who were asked about a wide variety of sexual experiences using detailed questionnaires and the lower rates are for men evaluated with less complex questionnaires.

Perhaps the best information about sexual abuse rates comes from a national survey of 2627 adults. An estimated 270/1000 women and 160/1000 men reported childhood sexual abuse, most often at 10 years of age. The incidents typically were severe, with over half involving intercourse. About a quarter of the perpetrators were relatives. The Gallup Poll results indicate somewhat lower sexual abuse rates: 19/1000 children in the prior year and 57/1000 ever. Teenagers were at the highest risk, followed by preteens. Surprisingly, rates were similar for boys and girls. As was the case for physical abuse, sexual abuse was more common in lower income families where there was one parent. [See CHILD SEXUAL ABUSE.]

The Gallup Poll also provides data concerning parental verbal aggression. While most parents yell at their children, 33% engaged in severe verbal aggression in the prior year. Severe verbal aggression was more commonly used with older children, was slightly more common among single parents, and did not vary across income groups.

D. Summary

Millions of children are maltreated each year. Many, if not the majority of, these cases are never reported to CPS by the affected individuals or professionals who are mandated reporters. Child maltreatment is a major social problem regardless of the type of incidence data considered.

IV. THEORY

The complex nature of maltreatment has led to the development of scores of causal explanations. Theories range from a focus on perpetrator psychological characteristics and psychopathology, to sociocultural determinants including stress and poverty, to the interaction of social and biological factors, to an emphasis on the child as playing a causal role.

At present, the most broadly accepted conceptual approach, an ecological model, emphasizes developmental, social, and interactional factors that influence behavior at multiple levels. This approach incorporates knowledge about human development, the contexts influencing its course, and interactions occurring within and across contexts. Four levels of context relate to maltreatment: (1) the individual including developmental changes and biological characteristics, (2) the family including the interactions among members, family functioning, and parenting methods, (3) the community including schools, religious institutions, work settings, peer groups, and social supports, and (4) cultural values and beliefs about corporal punishment, appropriate sexual behaviors, and family privacy. Maltreatment is multiply determined and related to risk factors and compensating, protective factors at each level.

V. CAUSES OF MALTREATMENT

Research on maltreatment causes has focused on physical and sexual abuse. Few studies have examined neglect and emotional maltreatment.

A. Individual Factors

Individual factors that have been studied include adult personality, attitudes, and cognitions, the intergenerational transmission of maltreatment, the role of substance abuse, biological factors, and child characteristics.

1. Adult Personality

Research has not identified adult or child factors that typify either maltreating adults or maltreated children. While early writers proposed that abuse was caused by perpetrator psychopathology, few perpetrators have been found to have severe mental illness.

The largest amount of research has focused on developing personality profiles of male sexual abusers. One approach incorporates four individual factors that may lead a man to sexually abuse children. They are: (1) children have specific emotional meaning for perpetrators who may lack self-esteem; (2) perpetrators are sexually aroused by children, perhaps due to childhood victimization of the perpetrator or even biological predispositions; (3) perpetrators are unable to achieve emotional and sexual satisfaction through relationships with adults and turn to children; and (4) perpetrators are not inhibited about sexual contact with children due to alcohol abuse, impulsivity, or other factors. Evidence supports each of the four components although specific precipitating factors vary for each case.

Research on physically abusive parents suggests that they tend to be depressed and anxious, and to exhibit antisocial behaviors. Resulting symptoms include impulsivity, poor self-esteem, negative affect, aggression, and substance abuse, and have been related to stress, a lack of social support, and interpersonal problems. However, child age is the only factor significantly related to physical abuse severity. Younger children are more often severely injured.

Neglectful parents have been described as apathetic and experiencing a sense of futility. These behaviors are exhibited in overall immaturity and impulsivity.

2. Attitudes and Cognition

Research on physically abusive and neglectful parents suggests that they perceive their children more negatively and lack knowledge about child rearing and development. However, such research is limited with some studies reporting negative findings.

3. Intergenerational Transmission of Maltreatment

Authors have long hypothesized a strong relation between being abused as a child and becoming an abusive parent. Research provides limited support for this contention. The above-mentioned Gallup Poll found that, while parents reporting childhood physical abuse more frequently reported using severe punishment on their own children, the combined rate of moderate and severe punishment did not differ for abused and nonabused parents. Additionally, some data suggest mothers reporting childhood physical or sexual victimization have more empathetic child-rearing attitudes.

4. Substance Abuse

The presence of a relationship between substance abuse and maltreatment has intuitive appeal. Indeed, many see prenatal substance use as automatically classifiable as maltreatment. However, research on the relation between long-term parental drug use and developmental consequences has yielded contradictory findings. Problems obtaining accurate substance abuse histories and the co-occurrence of such factors as poverty and substance use make substance abuse difficult to study. [*See* SUBSTANCE ABUSE.]

5. Biological Factors

Research has yet to indicate that factors such as a biological tendency toward aggression play a role in maltreatment. Ongoing studies may provide relevant data.

6. Child Characteristics

Research does not indicate any set of child characteristics that contribute to abuse. For example, some propose that children with handicaps are more likely to be maltreated while others have found that being disabled is not a risk factor. These contradictory findings may be due to a greater maltreatment risk for some handicapping conditions than others. For example, behaviorally difficult children who have hidden disabilities and children with limited communication ability may be at higher risk while children with clearly identifiable handicaps who receive appropriate services may be at lower risk.

7. Summary

Research suggests that single, individual characteristics typically are not direct factors leading to maltreatment. It is more likely that individual factors will be found important only when considered in relation to other individual factors and ecological levels. For example, it may be important to evaluate parental personality and child-rearing attitudes in relation to their interactions with their children or the relation between substance abuse and social supports.

B. Family Factors

Research on family factors contains the same complexities that are involved in understanding studies of individual characteristics. Thus, the differences between maltreating and nonmaltreating families are ones of degree, not of kind. No single set of descriptors can be applied to a family where a given type of maltreatment has occurred. Studies have focused on family functioning, and parenting practices and physical discipline.

1. Family Functioning

Family functioning is related to abuse. Physically abusive families are often characterized by chaos, disruption, anger, conflict, and violence. Sexual abuse is more common when step-fathers are present, when mothers are not available, and where the abused child is isolated.

Neglecting families are often chaotic, having unpredictable routines. Frequent family constellation changes cause increased social isolation and additional stress. Neighbors state they avoid contact with neglecting families.

2. Parenting and Discipline

Research on the parenting and discipline practices of physically abusive and neglecting parents suggests they are more negative. They control their children with physical punishment rather than love and reasoning. Additionally, abused children often respond negatively to their parents, resulting in rapidly escalating, coercive conflicts. Their parents use more authoritarian—punitive and restricting—child-rearing practices and are less warm. However, such practices may be adaptive for children raised in violence ridden, inner cities than would be more authoritative practices. In spite of this, studies do not find differences between African American and White families in their reported use of corporal punishment.

Neglecting parents are disengaged, neither initiating interactions with nor responding to initiations from their children. Additionally, households are often disorganized and chaotic. [*See* PARENTING.]

3. Summary

Family factors have been studied in physically abusive and neglecting families but not for other maltreatment types. It is important to recognize that many maltreating parents do not display the characteristics discussed and, similarly, many nonmaltreating parents do. Additionally, there has been little research on maltreatment correlates in cultural groups characterizing American society.

C. Community Factors

Community and neighborhood factors are related to the occurrence of maltreatment. Environmental stressors and how they are buffered or balanced by compensating formal and informal social supports have been emphasized.

Poverty was one of the first community factors to be linked to physical abuse and neglect. While it occurs in all social classes, corporal punishment is more common and reporting occurs disproportionately among impoverished families. This is particularly true for neglect, which is most common among the poorest families. However, it is not known whether this finding is the result of the stress of extreme impoverishment or to the greater surveillance of such families by social agencies. [*See* POVERTY AND MENTAL HEALTH.]

Many, if not most, poor families do not maltreat their children. This finding has led to examination of neighborhood factors that increase the probability of maltreatment. High-risk neighborhoods have fewer resources and maltreating parents make less use of available resources for support. It is not certain whether a lack of neighborhood support is a cause or a consequence of maltreatment or a correlated feature of multiproblem families.

D. Culture

Culture is a factor in most aspects of abuse and neglect. For example, a major question is whether certain cultural practices represent maltreatment. In many cultures the ideal of each child sleeping in their own bedroom would constitute maltreatment, while female circumcision might be normative. The limited research on cultural factors supports their importance. Many questions remain to be answered, including the role of our acceptance of violence, the impact of the high value placed on family privacy, the effects of racism, and a lack of systematic, societal help to families raising children.

E. Summary

Maltreatment is complex and multiply determined by many factors that operate at levels ranging from the individual to cultural. While research supports the importance of examining the relationships of these variables both within and across levels, little research has been done to clarify causal relationships. A full understanding will only occur when we know much more about such interrelationships.

VI. CONSEQUENCES OF MALTREATMENT

Attention has focused on the psychological effects of maltreatment. This section summarizes a multitude of controlled studies and clinical reports concerning the specific consequences of maltreatment. Difficulty in separating cause and effect make this issue complex. Different aspects of child behavior interact with each other, with adult responses to the child, and, more broadly, to aspects of the larger social ecology. For example, a child's difficult temperament may be both a cause and a consequence of physical abuse.

A. Neglect

The limited research on the consequences of neglect suggests that they are particularly severe. It causes both cognitive and socioemotional problems and is the major cause of death among maltreated children.

Studies have found language and intellectual deficits as well as poor academic performance in neglected children. Neglect in the early years of life is associated with the presence of such problems in adolescence. No data are available on the cognitive functioning of adults neglected during childhood.

Children neglected early in life experience disturbed caregiver attachment patterns and are withdrawn. With age they have problems with peers, remaining aloof and isolated, having more behavior problems than non-neglected peers.

Neglect has been linked to adolescent delinquency and adult violent criminality. However, studies typically do not differentiate the consequences of physical abuse and neglect. Between 20% and 30% of abused or neglected children become delinquents. Some studies suggest that abuse is related to more violent offenses. [See CRIMINAL BEHAVIOR.]

B. Physical Abuse

Research findings on the consequences of physical abuse parallel those for neglect in many ways. However, physical abuse may cause permanent central nervous system damage that can have life-long effects.

Abused children exhibit attachment problems, low self-esteem, and more affective disorders, including depression. Research supports a link between physical abuse and later physically aggressive and antisocial behaviors during childhood and adolescence. As adults, abused children are more violent toward their children. As with neglect, few studies have examined other long-term consequences of abuse. The nature of these relationships is complex and not well understood at present. [See AGGRESSION; ATTACHMENT; DEPRESSION; SELF-ESTEEM.]

C. Sexual Abuse

The consequences of sexual abuse range from sexually transmitted diseases to severe emotional problems. Sexually abused children often exhibit inappropriate sexual behaviors including self-stimulation and sexually approaching other children. Emotional problems include nightmares, posttraumatic stress disorder (PTSD), and dissociation including multiple personality disorder. Recent evidence suggests that early sexual abuse may alter hormonal balances in girls. The degree to which these symptoms are due to the sexual act or to accompanying emotional and physical trauma is unknown. [See DISSOCIATIVE DISORDERS; POSTTRAUMATIC STRESS.]

Sexually abused adolescents are more likely to run away from home, although most runaways do not report sexual abuse. Clinical reports suggest a link between sexual abuse and later problems such as self-destructive acts, prostitution, and illegal drug use. Supporting empirical evidence is lacking.

PTSD and increased revictimization are the most common abuse-specific problems affecting women sexually abused in childhood. Additional problems have been found in affect (anxiety, anger, and depression), behavior (self-mutilation, sexual difficulties, substance abuse problems, and suicidal tendencies), psychiatric symptoms (dissociation, obsessive/compulsive problems, and somatic symptoms), self-concept, and interpersonal relations.

A recent controversy has involved the question of whether forgotten memories of childhood sexual abuse can be recovered in adulthood. While many adults forget such abuse, the key question is whether accurate memories can be elicited from them. Research has yet to clarify this issue.

Understanding the consequences of sexual abuse is complicated by the relation of perpetrator and victim. Unlike other forms of maltreatment, sexual abuse can involve both familial and unrelated perpetrators. Research has only begun to explore the relationship of perpetrator identity to consequences.

D. Emotional Maltreatment

Few studies have examined emotional maltreatment in isolation from other types of maltreatment. However, when the severity of the physical, sexual, or neglectful maltreatment is controlled, emotional maltreatment and symptom severity are correlated. This supports the earlier conclusion that a major reason for concern about maltreatment is its psychological consequences.

Research suggests emotional maltreatment has

cognitive, social, and affective consequences. Limited research has found associations with poor school performance and disruptive classroom behavior, social isolation and aggression, peer relationship problems, antisocial behaviors, low self-esteem, and depression.

E. Compensating Factors

Research has begun to identify mitigating protective factors. These include social support, out-of-home placement, high IQ, and event appraisal. A loving parent may reduce the trauma of maltreatment, particularly in sexual abuse where having a supportive person who accepts the child's story is related to decreased problems. While there is considerable debate about the effects of out-of-home placements, a supportive foster parent along with the removal of a child from disorganized family and neighborhood settings may be protective. Bright children appear to be less affected by maltreatment. However, the nature of this effect is poorly understood. Finally, how a person cognitively appraises an event is related to their coping. For example, a physically abused child who is self-blaming for the abuse may fare less well than a similar child who sees the abusing parent as at fault. [See INTELLIGENCE AND MENTAL HEALTH; PROTECTIVE FACTORS IN DEVELOPMENT OF PSYCHOPATHOLOGY; SOCIAL SUPPORT.]

F. Limitations in Knowledge of Consequences

Several issues complicate maltreatment research. We know little about the role of child age, maltreatment frequency and severity, and perpetrator identity in relation to consequences. Many, if not most, maltreated children have experienced more than one type of maltreatment. Researchers have yet to consider the effects of multiple and differing maltreatment types. Relatively little work has been done on the consequences of maltreatment for boys versus girls.

Most of our knowledge about consequences is based on clinical samples or retrospective studies. The subjects were either self-selected based on symptoms or were selected because of a maltreatment history. In either case the information obtained is likely to be distorted by memory, social desirability, and other factors. Few prospective studies have been done.

G. Summary

Maltreatment has many adverse affective, cognitive, social, and behavioral consequences. While this section has focused on the relationship of consequences to maltreatment type, it needs to be noted that, in general, the effects of maltreatment are similar across types. Physical abuse and emotional maltreatment may both be important in the development of sexual problems even when there is no sexual component to the maltreatment.

It is important to recognize that many if not most maltreated children grow up without experiencing the sequelae discussed in this section. For example, Mary Ellen, the abused girl mentioned at the start of this entry, was happily married and a warm, loving mother. We do not know what accounts for her resilience. Her temperament and intelligence, loving foster parents, an ability to positively appraise the events of her life, or some other factor may have been critical.

VII. TREATMENT

Treatment and intervention programs target the individual and family levels of the ecological model. Individual level interventions focus on either the perpetrator or the maltreated child. Perpetrator treatments focus on eliminating the maltreating behavior and associated individual or environmental factors. Child treatments emphasize moderation of the short- and long-term effects of maltreatment.

Many interventions have been used, including individual, group, and family therapy; self-help groups such as Parents Anonymous; individual social and emotional support by parent aides (trained laypersons); economic and material assistance; ecologically based, broad interventions tailored to family needs; and legal actions such as perpetrator removal and child out-of-home placement. All of these are based on a belief that they will reduce maltreatment recurrence and decrease or eliminate adverse child consequences. [See FAMILY THERAPY.]

Most treatments have not been rigorously evaluated and long-term follow-up is rare. Additionally, there currently are no guides for reliably targeting specific interventions to specific types or combinations of maltreatment. Despite this, some contend that clinical data provide sufficient information to intervene effectively with both perpetrators and victims.

The few large-scale evaluations of intervention programs do not allow optimism about treatment effectiveness. For example, one major study of several intervention programs concluded that about a third of families repeat the maltreatment in spite of costly, multi-component interventions. Additionally, only about half of the treated families showed a decreased propensity for maltreatment.

A. Prediction and Risk Assessment

Investigators have been working on reliable and valid ways of predicting maltreatment and risk assessment. Prediction efforts generally have proved to be impractical. Families at high risk for physical abuse can be identified moderately accurately. However, the use of screening procedures results in dramatically higher numbers of families that are classified as potentially abusive but who do not go on to abuse a child. We lack methods for differentiating between such non-abusive and actual abusing families. While it would be desirable to intervene with all such families, we lack resources to work with even a majority of substantiated cases. The expense of working with substantially larger numbers of cases that would be detected through predictive screening is prohibitive.

Risk assessment measures have been developed to allow the focusing of intervention resources on physically abusive and neglecting families where the child is in the greatest danger of maltreatment recurrence. Many problems need to be overcome before risk assessment measures can be meaningfully applied. For example, evaluation research is needed to assess instrument reliability and validity.

B. Individual and Group Treatments

Individual treatment approaches have been used with children at the time of maltreatment disclosure, victims who exhibit sequelae as adults, and perpetrators.

1. Maltreated Children

Little literature has focused on intervening with maltreated children independent of approaches working with families. In general, the therapies used are adaptations of existing approaches.

More recently there has been a theoretical emphasis on the field of developmental psychopathology. This focuses on the relationship between infant and child attachment and the development of self-regulatory behaviors in childhood. The attachment component is related to the need for therapy to provide a secure base for a traumatized child. A secure attachment is important in a child's ability to express and control positive and negative emotions and behaviors. Abuse-related trauma and the chaotic lifestyle accompanying maltreatment interfere with attachment and appropriate self-regulation throughout childhood. Many of the consequences of maltreatment detailed above are theoretically linked to difficulties in self-regulation. These include anxiety, an inability to self-sooth resulting in somatic problems, aggression, and interpersonal problems. Research demonstrates that cognitive behavior therapy effectively reduces symptoms such as anxiety.

Evidence suggests that group settings including therapeutic nursery and school programs are beneficial for physically abused children. Improvement has been noted across developmental domains. The use of multiple therapeutic strategies in such programs limits our understanding of the effectiveness of components of such therapy.

2. Adult Survivors

We have almost no empirical knowledge specific to the appropriate treatment approaches for adult survivors. Published reports focus on women sexually abused in childhood and the procedures used have rarely been evaluated. Limited evidence from a study of different forms of group therapy suggests that they are effective with more structured programs producing greater anxiety reduction, and less structured ones improved social skills.

The clinical literature builds on the attachment and developmental psychopathology frameworks. One approach, a self-trauma model, views symptoms as attempts to adapt to trauma. Carefully timed interventions help avoid excessive anxiety, encourage growth, build a differentiated sense of self and develop appropriate affect modulation. Only when these skills have been developed do therapists work directly with trauma-related material using such procedures as systematic desensitization. To date, this therapeutic model has not been evaluated.

3. Perpetrators

Perpetrator treatment focuses on the group treatment of pedophiles. Tactics used range from imprisonment to psychotherapy to "chemical castration." Imprisonment does little to change behavior unless it is accompanied by other therapeutic approaches. Most commonly, psychotherapy has involved several components, including education, behavior therapy, and cognitive behavioral efforts to prevent relapse. However, the success of such programs has not been demonstrated. Hormonal treatment approaches must still be considered experimental. [*See* BEHAVIOR THERAPY; COGNITIVE THERAPY.]

Work with maltreating parents has focused on group programs with an emphasis on self-help groups such as Parents Anonymous and Parents United. These are based on a belief that help is best provided by "someone who has been there." Evidence suggests that participation in Parents Anonymous along with social services casework reduces a parent's potential to reabuse a child by about half.

C. Family Interventions

Many professionals view maltreatment as a familial problem and support family-oriented interventions that modify parental behavior and the family's environment. While studies show a variety of interventions to be effective few have followed families for more than 12 months posttreatment and many reports are for limited samples or individual families.

Parent training is widely used. Evidence indicates that parents can develop child-management skills in clinical settings. Project 12-Ways, a successful program based on the ecological model, used detailed family assessments to determine which of a variety of targeted interventions best met a family's needs.

A still broader intervention strategy involves home-based services or family support and preservation programs. These emphasize the multiple problems of maltreating families and work on improving relationships between individuals, the family, and the family environment.

Home-based services combine casework with therapy. Evidence suggests that long-term intervention using this approach effectively modifies the chaotic interactions and environment of neglectful families. However, the high caseloads of social service agencies often do not allow meaningful intervention to occur over such extensive time periods.

More recently there has been a focus on family preservation and support programming in order to avoid the costly and potentially damaging family disruption of out-of-home placement. Family preservation and family support programs have different histories. The former was developed by public welfare agencies to prevent out-of-home child placement. The latter is a grass-roots response emphasizing parent education and self-help groups. The two program types were combined into a continuum of service by the passage of federal law in 1993.

Families involved with preservation programs are provided with an intense level of service for a relatively short period. Services are supposed to be targeted to family needs and are available 7 days a week and for 24 hours a day. While the results of formal evaluations are not available some advocates claim out-of-home placements are reduced while others condemn the programs as placing many children at undue risk of further maltreatment. Additionally, evidence suggests that preservation programs are less effective with the chronically neglectful families who need such extended programming.

Several family support programs have already been discussed in this section, including Parents Anonymous. They are generally used with families with less critical needs or as part of a multicomponent treatment program.

D. CPS Interventions

It is important to mention the role of the CPS system as a component of treatment, although a detailed discussion is beyond the scope of this entry. During the reporting process CPS must investigate, decide which cases will be provided services, and provide or secure appropriate protection and treatment.

About half of reported cases are not substantiated and services typically are not provided. Some contend that these cases should be served in that many may involve subclinical maltreatment or escalate into maltreatment. However, treatment is not guaranteed even for substantiated cases. Recent findings indicate about 40% of families where abuse was substantiated do not receive even the most minimal service or help.

Out-of-home placements are a common, major intervention. Placements involve either foster care by an unrelated caregiver or kinship care by a relative. Proponents argue that placements protect children from further maltreatment. Opponents argue that the separation from the family is even more damaging. Kinship care is being increasingly used to provide some continuity of caregivers and avoid some problems of foster placement. Some professionals argue that such factors as lower cost and difficulty in finding foster parents are partial reasons for this trend and note that children may remain at risk due to the similarity of kinship caregiving and the maltreated child's family environment.

Research on both program types suggests that placed children typically do not receive other needed services such as medical care and psychotherapy. Additionally, children in foster care usually experience multiple placements and accompanying disruptions in caregiver continuity.

VIII. PREVENTION

Prevention programs are based on a belief that children are entitled to a life free of maltreatment, a belief that it is easier to prevent a problem than to treat it once it occurs, a desire to optimize children's development, and the relative ineffectiveness of treatments. Programs range across the components of the ecological model with different ones being developed for pregnant women, children and teens, and parents.

A. Individual and Family-Based Programs

Individual and family-based interventions focus on physical abuse and neglect. They include lay or professional home visitors, parent education, programs where the two are combined, and programs for pregnant or parenting teens.

Parent education, either prenatally or during the first years of life, is the most common intervention. They emphasize eliminating negative parenting; providing information about child development; improving parent-child interactions; and improving maternal self-esteem, problem-solving, and emotional well-being. They are based on a belief in the need for intervention before problems develop, a lack of more general parenting education programs, parental dif-

ficulties in making the transition to raising a child, and the receptiveness of new parents to caregiving information.

Home visiting programs have attracted much attention. Universal nurse visitation programs have served every new mother in many European countries for years. However, few data are available concerning their effectiveness in preventing maltreatment.

Studies in the United States support the value of services provided by professional staff prenatally and during infancy. Some evaluations show decreased maltreatment reports, decreased corporal punishment, and improved parenting. However, not all studies find decreased maltreatment. This may be due to the greater surveillance for potential maltreatment and accompanying increased risk for reporting for home visited than nonintervened families. However, even the most comprehensive program may not help some families. Unfortunately, we do not know the characteristics of such families.

Effective efforts involve support before or soon after birth; a broad service array; frequent home visits promoting positive mother–child relationships and providing social support over relatively long time periods; professional visitors; a focus on impoverished, multiproblem families; and are integrated with other community services. Programs also need to be culturally appropriate and matched to each child's developmental level.

While there remain many questions about the components of effective programs and their overall impact, advocates promote the preventive potential of home visiting. They stress the need for prevention; the human, social, and economic costs of maltreatment; and the role of research in improving prevention programs.

B. Community-Focused Programs

Community programs have been developed for physical and sexual abuse. Efforts include respite or crisis child care; sex-abuse prevention and conflict resolution programs for children; training for latchkey children; and media campaigns. Most programs are school-based and concentrate on preventing sexual abuse by strangers.

These programs teach children about the privacy of their bodies; good, bad, and questionable touching;

and that they can disclose inappropriate touching to adults even though they had been sworn to secrecy. Programs are framed in the context of personal protection training because of the controversial nature of sex education in schools. There has been controversy about the age at which children should be trained, the appropriateness of a focus on potential victims rather than perpetrators, possible behavioral consequences for children, and the overall usefulness of programs.

Programs have been found to have some benefit. Children show small gains in knowledge about abuse and what to do if it occurred and are more likely to disclose prior abuse. However, children may experience problems believing that strangers are less likely to maltreat than people that they know and retaining all of the information presented. Younger children have more problems with more abstract concepts. The youngest age at which some children remember key concepts is around four years.

Community programs have not explicitly stressed the prevention of physical abuse. Rising levels of school and community violence have led to a variety of violence prevention and conflict resolution programs. Efforts include workshops and group review of videotaped role-playing situations. Limited evaluations suggest the programs can alter knowledge, attitudes, and behavior. However, the generalizability of these results across settings is not known. Additionally, more comprehensive programs operating across the family and community levels have been developed but no evaluations are available.

C. Societal Interventions

Societal interventions have examined such factors as media's role, the need to eliminate corporal punishment, and increased criminal justice system involvement.

Media play major roles in setting the social agenda. Child abuse did not become part of the agenda until the "battered child syndrome" concept was proposed in 1962. The media seized upon this sound bite concept leading to political action and society's current concern about maltreatment. Media-based prevention efforts started appearing in the 1970s. To date, however, we know little about their impact.

Campaigns often note that while a majority of parents spank their children and believe it is effective research does not support this belief. While parents view spanking as a discrete disciplinary act, many professionals see it as one risk factor for abuse. They believe that we must eliminate all corporal punishment as has been done in six European countries. Data are lacking about whether no-hitting advice is effective in influencing parental disciplinary acts and decreasing abuse.

The relative failure of the social services system in maltreatment prevention and treatment efforts has led some to advocate greater law enforcement involvement. Some believe that threatened incarceration or actual imprisonment are effective behavior controls. Others point to increased crime and rising prison populations as indicators of system failure. The real situation is more complex; some perpetrators cannot be effectively treated and should be imprisoned.

The incarceration of parents creates problems. Children may need to be placed out-of-home, the potential for family treatment is eliminated, and the family may be deprived of income leading to greater stress and potential further maltreatment.

Some authors support involvement of the criminal justice system but view imprisonment as a last resort. They see the threat of prison as influencing behavior and the authority of judges to mandate intervention as important. However, the effectiveness of forced treatment has been questioned and in many cases of intrafamilial maltreatment there is insufficient evidence to secure a criminal court conviction. Research needs to be done to determine when legal system involvement is appropriate.

D. Summary

The prevention of maltreatment is a valuable social goal. Few of the many prevention programs that have been used have been adequately evaluated. We know most about family interventions that center on improving parenting. Beyond this we know little about what other programs directly influence maltreatment rates.

IX. CONCLUSIONS

Child maltreatment is a social problem of major importance. Its causes are rooted at many levels from individual perpetrator and child characteristics, to the community, and to society as a whole. Maltreating families typically have multiple problems with poverty being a strong correlate, particularly of neglect.

Maltreatment is linked to developmental, social, and emotional difficulties in childhood and to problems in adulthood. In spite of these consequences, the typical maltreated child and his or her family receive little in the way of service. Untreated child problems are related to adult problems, including parenting difficulties. However, we know relatively little about what types of intervention are most effective.

Prevention of recurrence and future occurrence are critical to maltreatment reduction. This involves not only intensive work with already abused or neglected children but also with families and perpetrators. Both treatment and intervention need to occur at multiple levels including communities and society as a whole.

Relatively few resources have been directed toward maltreatment research, treatment, and prevention. More than a million families need treatment resources in any year. Slightly more than half of these receive any help at all. Prevention efforts are expensive and necessary.

There is optimism for the future in spite of the complexity of the issues, a relative lack of understanding, and a lack of societal support for children and families. We have knowledge that can be applied to society generally and maltreatment specifically. We know that good housing, quality schools, available health care, sufficient income, and other services are necessary. We know the components that make home visiting an effective treatment and prevention approach. We know that programs need to be integrated and to meet the many needs of families at multiple system levels. While many problems exist, the world in general has less infanticide than in biblical times and less of the sexual abuse of boys that characterized Grecian society. Progress has been slow but will continue with further action and advocacy.

BIBLIOGRAPHY

Briere, J., Berliner, L., Bulkley, J. A., Jenny, C., & Reid, T. (Eds.). (1996). *The APSAC handbook on child maltreatment.* Thousand Oaks, CA: Sage.

Cicchetti, D., and Carlson, V. (Eds.). (1989). *Child maltreatment.* New York: Cambridge.

Garbarino, J. (1995). *Raising children in a socially toxic environment.* San Francisco: Jossey-Bass.

National Center on Child Abuse and Neglect. (1992–1995). *The user manual series.* Author, Washington, DC. [A series of 15 manuals on most aspects of maltreatment available from: Clearinghouse on Child Abuse and Neglect Information, P.O. Box 1182, Washington, DC 20013-1182]

National Research Council. (1993). *Understanding child abuse and neglect.* Washington, DC: National Academy Press.

Sagatun, I. J. & Edwards, L. P. (1995). *Child abuse and the legal system.* Chicago: Nelson-Hall, Chicago.

Starr, R. H., Jr., & Wolfe, D. A. (Eds.). (1991). *The effects of child abuse and neglect.* New York: Guilford.

Child Sexual Abuse

Kathleen Coulborn Faller

University of Michigan School of Social Work

Analogue Studies Research studies, involving staged events (e.g., a visit to a stranger in a trailer) or naturally occurring events (e.g., a medical exam) in children's lives that have some characteristics in common with situations of sexual abuse. Researchers then question children in a variety of ways, some of which may involve attempts to manipulate children or to contaminate their responses, and draw parallels between their responses in these experiments and memory and suggestibility regarding allegations of sexual abuse.

Cognitive Distortions Rationalizations (in the case of sexual abuse) of sexual acts that are considered abusive; another term used for this phenomenon is "thinking errors."

Criminal Sexual Conduct Sexual acts that are crimes, with penalties of incarceration, probation, and parole. These acts either are nonconsensual or involve minors or others unable to give informed consent (developmentally disabled individuals; persons under the influence of alcohol or drugs). These acts are usually subcategorized in terms of degree, with first degree being the most serious.

Incest Sexual activity between two people related by blood.

Polygraph A lie detector test. It relies on measures of autonomic system arousal, usually heart rate, breathing rate, and galvanic skin response. Autonomic arousal is supposed to be associated with lying, but this has not been empirically demonstrated. The polygraph has high rates of false negatives and false positives and is inadmissible in most court proceedings.

Plethysmograph A means of measuring erectile response, using a strain gauge that encircles the penis. It is used in some sexual abuse treatment programs to measure changes in arousal to various sexual stimuli.

Prognosis Prospects for improvement. In the case of mental health treatment, it refers to appropriate response to therapy.

Sequelae Consequences or effects. In the case of sexual abuse, these are sexual and nonsexual behavioral and affective symptoms.

Statutory Rape Consensual sexual activity between a child who is below the age of consent (14 to 16, depending upon the state) and an adult. The activity usually involves sexual penetration.

CHILD SEXUAL ABUSE is an important mental health issue, and one characterized by significant advances in the last 20 years, with continuing developments and refinements. However, it is also a very controversial issue. In part, the controversy can be understood in light of the emotional dilemma sexual abuse creates. On the one hand, we assume that to sexually abuse a child is to engage in monstrous behavior with devastating consequences. On the other hand, we find it virtually impossible to believe that an adult would behave so reprehensibly toward a child. Thus, allegations of sexual abuse evoke the competing reactions of rage and denial. In some respects, these reactions are manifested in the quandary of whether to believe the child or believe the offender. Often this dilemma is heightened because the child is reticent in disclosure, and the offender is insistent and persuasive in denial.

The goal of this article is to enlighten this controversy and put the problem of sexual abuse in perspective, relying upon existing knowledge about sexual abuse. In fact, child sexual abuse is common, may have many manifestations—from horrendous acts to those that differ in degree from acceptable behavior, and results in a spectrum of *sequelae*—from pervasive to negligible.

In this article, sexual abuse will be defined, its prevalence and incidence addressed, its impact described, and professional interventions discussed. These interventions include child protection investigation, mental health assessment, treatment, and prevention.

I. DEFINITION OF CHILD SEXUAL ABUSE

For an event to meet the definition of child sexual abuse, there should be a victim, an offender, and a sexual act. Characteristics and subcategories of each component of the definition will be discussed in this section. In addition, the variability in definitions employed in both research and clinical practice will be noted. Finally, situations that are regarded as "gray areas" will receive attention.

A. Child Victim

Child victim status is defined primarily by age. However, there is some variability in what is considered the upper age limit. Research definitions, legal definitions, and treatment definitions of child victims may differ in their determination of when adult status or informed consent begins. Legal definitions of the upper age limit may differ by state and by statute (e.g. statutory rape, incest, criminal sexual conduct statutes). Also, some researchers have used a lower maximum age for boys than for girls. The maximum age used in research for girls is generally 16 or 18, but some researchers have used a maximum age of 12 for boys. Interesting assumptions about gender underlie this differential. This lower age seems to be based upon assumptions that boys are more capable of protecting themselves than

girls and more desirous of sexual activity than girls. Hence boys' sexual experiences during adolescence that otherwise meet the definition of sexual victimization may not be considered abusive by researchers and others.

Research findings indicate that victims are fairly evenly distributed across the age span of childhood, that is preschoolers, latency-aged children, and adolescents. Diagnosis is more difficult for preschoolers because of their less well-developed communication skills and concerns about their suggestibility. Nevertheless, because of increased awareness of sexual abuse, allegations involving younger and younger children are coming to professional attention. Thus, there are cases involving the sexual abuse of infants.

For the relationship to be considered abusive, there usually is an age differential between the victim and the offender, the victim generally being at least 5 years younger than the offender, and 10 years younger when the victim is an adolescent. However, based upon her research of 930 women, Diana Russell pointed out that acts can be abusive without the age differential; for example, a brother may be only 3 years older than his sister, but still can impose his will for sexual activity upon her. A gray area is how to handle a situation of what appears to be consensual sexual activity between a teenager and a significantly older person, for example a 14-year-old girl and a 30-year-old man, or a 13-year-old boy and a 25-year-old woman.

More girls are reported than boys as victims, boys constituting one-fifth to one-third of cases, depending upon the source of the statistics. Although girl victims remain the majority, the proportion of girl victims is higher in intrafamilial cases than in extrafamilial ones. Thus, girls may be more vulnerable to family members, such as fathers, stepfathers, uncles, and grandfathers, and boys at relatively greater risk from persons in the community, such as coaches, boy scout leaders, and adolescents whom they admire.

Professionals who work with boy victims believe there is a greater failure to disclose sexual victimization by boy victims than by girls. This differential reporting is thought to be related to more support for girls, in the process of their socialization, to talk about their problems than for boys, and the fact that boys must overcome not only the taboo of sexual activity with an adult, but usually the taboo associated with homosexual activity, when they disclose.

B. Offender

A sex offender may be a male or female, although the vast majority are males, between 85 and 99% depending upon the study. As awareness of sexual abuse grows, so does the proportion of female offenders identified. Generally, offenders are adults or adolescents. A gray area in definition is how to classify latency-aged or even younger children who are sexual predators. Although many of these children are "abuse reactive," that is, maladaptively coping with their own sexual victimization by sexually accosting sexually naive or younger children, a substantial minority of child predators have not been sexually victimized. Some researchers and clinicians characterize them as "children with sexual behavior problems" to avoid stigmatizing them as sex offenders. Nevertheless, the acts they perpetrate may be quite serious.

There is some controversy about offender motivation, for example, some individuals asserting that the offender is motivated by a desire for dominance, not sexual gratification. Sexual abuse, like any sexual act, may fulfill a variety of needs, including the assertion of power, but what differentiates it for other exercises of power is its sexual content.

For some offenders (pedophiles), their preferred sexual object is a child, while other offenders experience and act upon sexual arousal to children because of a range of circumstantial factors. These factors include the availability of a child, the absence of an adult sexual partner, and an assault on the offender's self-esteem, such as a divorce or employment loss. Nevertheless, an initial act because of circumstances appears to enhance risk for subsequent sexual abuse to children. The proportion of sexual offenders who prefer children to those who do not is not known, but it is generally assumed that pedophiles are the minority. However, on average they have a greater number of victims.

C. Abusive Acts

Sexual abuse involves the full spectrum of sexual activity. These acts are designated and illustrated in Table I.

This list of sexual acts progresses from the least intrusive and therefore possibly least traumatic to the most intrusive and possibly most traumatic. However,

Table I Sexually Abusive Activities

Activities	Examples
1. Noncontact behavior	
A. Exposure	A. A coach wore his sweatpants low in front, with his penis hanging over the top, during girls' gym practice.
B. Voyeurism	B. A stepfather drilled a hole in the bathroom wall so he could observe his daughter toileting and bathing.
C. Lewd and lascivious talk	C. A mother told her son she wanted to suck his penis.
2. Fondling/sexual contact	2. A mother's boyfriend rubbed a 7-year-old girl's genital area on top of her panties while they watched *Pocahontas*.
	2. A 15-year-old brother grabbed his little sister's hand and placed it on his penis, saying "rub it."
3. Oral–genital contact	
A. Fellatio	A. A camp counselor cornered a 10-year-old boy in the shower and put his penis in the boy's mouth.
B. Cunnilingus	B. A grandfather bit his granddaughter's vagina.
C. Analingus	C. A 6-year-old boy described how it tickled when his friend's father "licked his butt."
4. Digital penetration of the vagina or anus	4. A 6-year-old girl said her brother's friend put a finger in her peepee and it hurt.
5. Penile penetration of the vagina or anus	5. A 4-year-old boy said, "Uncle Jimmy poked me in the butt and it stinged."
6. Sexual exploitation	
A. Child prostitution and	A. Sisters, aged 4 and 5, were fondled while naked, by men who were strangers and their pictures were taken. Their mother
B. Child pornography	B. Received money from the men.

the judgment regarding trauma is from a professional perspective, not from a child's. Victims may have a different perception. Most clinicians and some researchers include noncontact behaviors—exposure, voyeurism, and lewd and lascivious remarks, in the definition of abusive acts. Activities that do not involve the adult in the sex acts directly, such as prostituting a child or using the child in pornography, are also subsumed under the definition.

II. THE EXTENT OF SEXUAL ABUSE

How widespread is the problem of child sexual abuse? We know about its extent from studies of prevalence and reported incidence. Both sources of information tell us sexual abuse is experienced by large numbers of children. How serious a problem is false allegations? Making this determination is more difficult, but there is some useful research. Prevalence, incidence, and the issue of false reports will be discussed in this section.

A. Prevalence of Child Sexual Abuse

The term, prevalence, is used to refer to the proportion of a designated population that has a particular problem or characteristic. In the case of sexual abuse, prevalence refers to the number of people who were sexually abused during childhood. Data about prevalence are gathered in retrospective studies of adults. This research may involve face to face interviews, self-administered questionnaires, or telephone surveys. Researchers may ask a single general question, such as "were you sexually abused as a child?" or multiple questions designed to approach the topic from several perspectives and gather information about a variety of relationships and experiences. Findings vary depending upon methodology, with studies using face-to-face interviews and multiple questions yielding higher rates of child sexual abuse. Taking into account the variability in findings, estimates are that, in the general population, between 1 in 3 or 4 women were sexually abused during childhood and between 1 in 6 to 10 men.

B. Incidence of Reported Sexual Abuse

Incidence refers to the number of reports of a particular phenomenon, usually occurring during a circumscribed time frame. In the United States, there are governmental and nongovernmental initiatives to gather incidence data on child sexual abuse.

Illustrative of governmental efforts is a provision in the Child Abuse Prevention and Treatment Act of 1974, which requires that the federal government collect annual statistics on reports of child maltreatment received by local Child Protection Agencies. These data include reports of child sexual abuse. Over the 20 years this information has been collected, there has been a steady increase in reports of child abuse and neglect, and a fairly steady increase in the proportion of sexual abuse cases among reports. According to the National Committee for the Prevention of Child Abuse (NCPCA), sexual abuse cases constitute about 11% of cases currently reported—in 1995 almost 350,000 cases. Currently, approximately one-third of reports are substantiated after investigation by Child Protective Services (CPS), or about 110,000 cases of child sexual abuse annually.

Although the number of cases from the CPS reports is considerable, a study of 1000 parents conducted by the Gallup Poll in 1995 yielded a projection 10 times larger, of one million children sexually abused during the previous year. Part of the reason that the Child Protective Services number is lower is that CPS only concerns itself with situations in which a caretaker is the abuser. Most extrafamilial sexual abuse cases are not handled by CPS, but by law enforcement. However, the higher number in the Gallup Poll projection likely also indicates a substantial number of cases do not come to professional attention. Moreover, even the Gallup Poll figure is probably a low estimate because parents would be unlikely to report themselves if they were sexually abusing their children, and they might even be reluctant to report relatives and friends.

C. False Allegations of Sexual Abuse

The modest substantiation rate noted in the discussion of NCPCA findings raises the question of false allegations. Why are so many more cases being reported than are being substantiated? Does this mean that two-thirds of the reports made are false? It does not. There are many reasons that a case may not be substantiated, other than that someone made a false claim of sexual abuse.

In studies conducted at the Kempe National Center on Child Abuse and Neglect, a very small proportion of unsubstantiated cases were determined to be false allegations, altogether about 5%. Another interesting finding is that adults are more likely to make false reports of sexual abuse to children than are children. The largest proportion of unsubstantiated cases involved "insufficient information." Illustrative would be situations in which the child protection caseworker could not locate the family, or the child refused to talk to the caseworker. The next largest proportion were "legitimate cause for concern, but no sexual abuse." In these cases, reporting was appropriate, but some more plausible alternative explanation for the source of concern about abuse was found. An example might be a case in which the source of the child's advanced sexual knowledge was observing adults engaging in sexual activity. This is not to say that false allegations are nonexistent. They do exist, but research to date indicates that true reports are very much more common.

III. EFFECTS OF CHILD SEXUAL ABUSE

The impact of sexual abuse depends upon many factors: the offender–victim relationship, the particular sexual act(s), the frequency and duration of the sexual abuse, the nature of inducements to participate and admonitions regarding disclosure, the response of nonabusive caretakers to disclosure, and the personality and personal history of the child. Research documents that the most important element in the child's recovery is having a caring and concerned, nonoffending parent. Thus, being believed and supported makes a great deal of difference in the long-term well-being of the victim.

Clinicians and researchers generally divide the effects of sexual abuse into sexual and nonsexual effects. These sexual and nonsexual emotional and behavioral impacts of sexual abuse also serve as indicators of its likelihood, when professionals are making a determination about whether a child has been sexually abused.

A. Sexual Sequelae

William Friedrich, a clinician and researcher at the Mayo Clinic, has played a leadership role in cataloging the sexual effects and researching differences in the rates of sexualized behaviors in children with and without a history of sexual abuse. Table II is drawn from version 3 of Friedrich's Child Sexual Behavior Inventory (CSBI).

Table II Items from the Child Sexual Behavior Inventory

1. Dresses like the opposite sex.
2. Stands too close to people.
3. Talks about wanting to be the opposite sex.
4. Touches sex (private) parts when in public places.
5. Masturbates with hand.
6. Draws sex parts when drawing pictures of people.
7. Touches or tries to touch mother's or other women's breasts.
8. Masturbates with toy or object (blanket, pillow, etc.).
9. Plays with a friend.
10. Touches another child's sex (private) parts.
11. Tries to have sexual intercourse with another child or adult.
12. Puts mouth on another child's/adult's sex parts.
13. Touches sex (private) parts when at home.
14. Touches an adult's sex (private) parts.
15. Touches animals' sex parts.
16. Makes sexual sounds (sighs, moans, heavy breathing, etc.)
17. Asks others to engage in sexual acts with him or her.
18. Rubs body against people or furniture.
19. Puts objects in vagina or rectum.
20. Tries to look at people when they are nude or undressing.
21. Pretends that dolls or stuffed animals are having sex.
22. Shows sex (private) parts to adults.
23. Tries to look at pictures of nude or partially dressed people.
24. Talks about sexual acts.
25. Kisses adults that they do not know well.
26. Gets upset when adults are kissing or hugging.
27. Overly friendly with men he/she does not know well.
28. Kisses other children he/she does not know well.
29. Talks flirtatiously.
30. Tries to undress other children against their will (opening pants, shirts, etc.).
31. Eats breakfast.
32. Wants to watch television or movies that show nudity or sex.
33. When kissing, he/she tries to put his/her tongue in other person's mouth.
34. Hugs adults that he/she does not know well.
35. Shows sex (private) parts to children.
36. Tries to undress adults against their will (opening pants, shirts, etc.).
37. Is very interested in the opposite sex.
38. Puts his/her mouth on mother's or other women's breasts.
39. Knows more about sex than other children their age.
40. Other sexual behaviors (please describe).

Sexualized behavior is the most common impact of sexual abuse, but according to Friedrich's research, it is present in only about 40% of children with a history of sexual abuse. Friedrich and his colleagues have assessed for the presence of sexualized behaviors separately for males and females and for children from ages 2 to 6 and 7 to 12 years. Preliminary data are available from research on version 3 of the CSBI. Children with a history of sexual abuse were compared to children from psychiatric and normal populations. Children with a history of sexual abuse rank higher than children in the other two groups on total score for sexualized behavior (sexually abused, 14.2; psychiatric population, 3.45; normal population, 3.5). In addition, 22 of the 40 items differentiate children with a history of sexual abuse from the other two groups, regardless of age and sex. These items are numbers 6, 8, 10–12, 17–19, 21, 23–28, 30, 32, 33, 35–37, and 39.

B. Nonsexual Symptoms of Sexual Abuse

Nonsexual symptoms are less definitively linked to sexual victimization because they are more likely than sexual symptoms to derive from other experiences and traumas. For example, while such behavioral and emotional symptoms can come from being sexually victimized, they can also be the result of physical abuse, neglect, divorce, auto accidents, or natural disasters. Nevertheless, Table III lists nonsexual symptoms and, where relevant, their possible relationship to subgroups of victims.

Table III Psychosocial Symptoms of Sexual Abuse: Nonsexual Behavioral and Emotional Indicators of Distress

1. **Sleep disturbances**
   A. Night waking
   B. Nightmares
   C. Night terrors
   D. Refusal to go to bed (in some cases, because it is the site of the sexual abuse)
   E. Refusal to sleep alone
   F. Inability to sleep
2. **Toileting disturbances**
   A. Previously toilet trained (more common in young victims)
      1. Enuresis
      2. Encopresis

Table III *Continued*

   B. Refusal to go into the bathroom (in some cases, because it is the site of the sexual abuse)
   C. Smearing feces (more common in very disturbed victims)
   D. Hiding feces (more common in very disturbed victims)
3. **Eating disturbances**
   A. Anorexia (characteristic of adolescent girl victims)
   B. Bulimia (characteristic of adolescent girl victims)
4. **Avoidant reactions**
   A. Fear of the alleged offender
   B. Fear of persons of the same sex as the alleged offender
   C. Refusal to be left alone
   D. Fear of particular places that may be associated with abuse
5. **Somatic complaints**
   A. Headaches (associated with nondisclosure)
   B. Stomach aches (associated with nondisclosure)
   C. Pelvic pain (may be related to affect or injury)
6. **Behavioral problems**
   A. Firesetting (more characteristic of boy victims)
   B. Cruelty to animals (more characteristic of boy victims)
   C. Aggression toward more vulnerable individuals (younger, smaller, more naive, retarded individuals)
   D. Delinquent behaviors (characteristic of older victims)
      1. Incorrigibility
      2. Running away (may be an adaptive response to avoid the offender)
      3. Criminal activity
   E. Substance abuse
   F. Self-destructive behaviors (characteristic of adolescent girl victims)
      1. Suicidal gestures, attempts, and successes
      2. Suicidal thoughts
      3. Self-mutilation
7. **School problems**
   A. Inattention
   B. Sudden decline in school performance
   C. School truancy
8. **General disturbances of affect**
   A. Low self esteem
   B. Anxiety
   C. Fear
   D. Anger
   E. Dissociation
   F. Posttraumatic stress disorder

Caveat: A determination of sexual abuse cannot be made based upon the presence of these factors alone; however when noted in conjunction with sexual indicators and other positive findings, they increase the likelihood of sexual abuse.

The array of possible impacts is considerable. However, not every child is seriously affected. In fact in a 1993 survey of 45 comparative studies of the impact of sexual abuse, Kendall-Tackett, Williams, and Finkelhor found that about a third of the victims of child sexual abuse were reported to be asymptomatic. In addition, about two-thirds of children showed recovery during the first year to year-and-a-half after the abuse. Although children with a history of child sexual abuse had more symptoms than both clinical and nonclinical comparison groups—fear, PTSD, behavior problems, sexualized behaviors, and low self-esteem being the most frequently noted, no single symptom characterized the majority of children.

IV. INTERVENTION IN CHILD SEXUAL ABUSE

Awareness of the extent of sexual abuse and its effects on functioning have led to positive outcomes. First, the problem of child sexual abuse is being taken seriously. The time has passed when sexual abuse was regarded as a problem of insignificant proportions and an experience that was not very harmful. Second, the fact that there are mechanisms for reporting child maltreatment is illustrative of government and social policy commitment to address the problem of child sexual abuse, and child maltreatment more generally. Third, with reporting statutes has come greater professional and public awareness of child sexual abuse. Professionals are more likely to consider sexual abuse as a possible source of children's symptoms, and children's caretakers and others are more likely to notice symptoms. Moreover, media attention to sexual victimization has made the public more cognizant of the problem and may serve to decrease victims' sense of isolation.

In addition, there have been refinements in how governmental and mental health systems address child sexual abuse. In part, because of controversies about the truth of children's assertions about their sexual abuse, there have come advances in expertise in case investigation and assessment, the development of sexual abuse specific treatment programs, and efforts to prevent sexual abuse before it happens.

Crucial to long-term child well-being is sensitive and well-orchestrated intervention. If professionals can effectively investigate, evaluate, and ameliorate in situations of sexual abuse, children can survive their victimization and lead productive lives. The advances in assessment and treatment of child sexual abuse will be described in this section.

A. The Child Protection System (CPS)

Each state has a Child Protection System, whose responsibility includes investigation and intervention in all cases of child maltreatment involving children's caretakers. These investigations take place at the local, usually county level, and are conducted by child protection caseworkers. This response is structured to be immediate, and the involvement of CPS short term. Child protection caseworkers act as case managers and are supposed to refer children and families to ongoing therapy and other services. Not all of these caseworkers have mental health or competent, on the job training; their case loads are usually high; and the availability of treatment and other services may be limited. Consequently the promise of the Child Protection System is greater than the delivery.

B. Mental Health Assessment

In addition to CPS investigations, mental health professionals in a variety of contexts have become involved in the assessment of sexual abuse allegations. The goals of these mental health assessments are several: determining the likelihood of sexual abuse, making recommendations about child safety, proposing treatment plans, predicting *prognosis* for response to treatment, and assisting in legal intervention. With regard to the final goal, because sexual abuse is not only a mental health problem, but also a crime, mental health professionals may assist in litigation to protect children, to criminally prosecute alleged offenders, and to exact civil damages in cases involving sexual abuse.

There are a number of models for mental health assessment of possible sexual abuse. For example, models can involve the child alone, the child and other family members, and the offender alone. The appropriate model depends on the goals of the assessment, the nature of the child–alleged offender relationship, and the age and functioning of the child. Sensitive and careful assessments assist the child and others affected by the allegation in seeing the assessment process as health promoting rather than traumatic.

A somewhat unique characteristic of sexual abuse assessments for mental health professionals is the importance of determining whether an event (sexual abuse) occurred. Mental health skills need to be adapted and expanded to address this requirement. Mental health professionals must usually engage in direct inquiry about sexual abuse with the child and others, using nonleading questions. A variety of child interview questioning protocols have been developed to guide evaluators. One example is shown in Table IV.

Evaluators employing this protocol are urged to use open-ended questions (found at the top of the continuum) and only to resort to more close-ended questions when open-ended ones do not assist the child in communicating his/her experience. For example, if a

child does not respond to a focused question, "Are there things you like about your grandpa?" the mental health evaluator might ask a multiple choice question, "Does he ever do special things with you, buy you things, or do any other nice things you can think of?" The more open-ended the question, the more confidence the mental health evaluator should have in the child's response and visa versa. However, both *analogue studies* and clinical research indicate most children require direct or focused questions to disclose sensitive material. If information is elicited using a close-ended question, the interviewer should follow this disclosure with a more open-ended question. Leading questions and coercion are inappropriate for use in an evaluation of a child for sexual abuse.

Other special features of sexual abuse assessments include the following: Mental health professions should gather information on past and current history of the abuse allegation and of the people involved. Collaboration with other professionals, for example, examining physicians, child protection caseworkers, police officers, and lawyers, is integral to such assessments. The mental health professional must be able to clearly articulate criteria he/she uses in determining the likelihood of sexual abuse. In a review of such decision-making strategies in 1995, Faller found 12 sufficiently elaborated to be discussed. The criteria shown in Table V are found in these decision-making strategies.

An interesting and somewhat surprising finding from Faller's review was the number of mental health professionals who endorsed medical findings as an important factor. This is interesting because, of course, medical evidence is not gathered by mental health professionals. Furthermore, most cases of sexual abuse have no medical findings. The other items endorsed by the majority of mental health professionals were criteria derived from child interviews, specifically details about the sexual abuse and details about the context of the abuse.

Table IV A Continuum of Questions for Assessment of Possible Sexual Abuse

Question type	Example
Open ended	More confidence
1. General question	1. Why did you come to see me?
2. Focused question	
A. People	A. What kind of a guy is your dad?
B. Body parts	B. Did you ever see a penis?
C. Circumstances of abuse	C. Tell me everything you remember about daycare?
D. Circumstances of prior disclosure	D. Did you tell your mom something happened?
3. Follow-up question	
A. Narrative cue	A. What happened next?
B. Repeat disclosure	B. You said he touched you?
C. Clarification	C. He touched you where?
D. Details of abuse	D. What did that touching feel like?
E. Details of context of abuse	E. Do you remember where this happened?
4. Multiple choice	4. Did it happen before or after Christmas or both?
5. Direct question	5. Did your daddy put his peepee inside?
6. Leading question	6. Your mom makes you suck her breast, doesn't she?
7. Coercion	7. You can't leave until you tell me what happened.
Close ended	Less confidence

C. Treatment

Mental health professionals assume that every sexually abused child deserves and needs treatment. And in fact, children who are victims of sexual abuse are more likely to receive treatment (from 44 to 73% of them receiving treatment, according to Finkelhor and Berliner) than are victims of other types of child maltreatment.

Table V Criteria Included in Guidelines for Decision Making about Sexual Abuse

1. **Child interview information**
   A. **Sexual abuse description from the child**
      1. Detail about the sexual abuse
      2. Child's perspective evident in the description of abuse
      3. Advanced sexual knowledge for the child's developmental stage
   B. **Offender behavior description, as described by the child**
      1. Use of inducements to participate in the sexual activity
      2. Admonitions not to tell about the sexual abuse
      3. Progression of abuse from less to more intrusive sexual acts
   C. **Information about the context of the sexual abuse**
      1. Idiosyncratic event
      2. Where the abuse occurred
      3. When the abuse occurred
   D. **Emotional reaction to the abuse by the child**
      1. Affect consistent with the abuse description
      2. Affect related to the offender
      3. Recall of affect during abuse
      4. Reluctance to disclosure
   E. **Child functioning**
      1. Competency
         a. Cognitive test results
         b. Recall of past events
         c. Ability to differentiate the truth from a lie
         d. Ability to differentiate fact from fantasy
         e. Child is not suggestible
      2. Child is motivated to tell the truth
      3. Consistency of the child's accounts
      4. Feasibility of the events the child describes
   F. Structural qualities of the child's account

2. **Information from other sources**
   A. **Child's behavior in other contexts**
      1. Statements to others about the abuse
      2. Nonsexual behavioral and emotional symptoms
      3. Sexualized behavior
      4. Evidence of advanced sexual knowledge
   B. **Offender characteristics**
      1. Overall functioning
      2. Results of *polygraph*
      3. Results of *plethysmograph*
      4. Psychological test results
      5. Evidence of other victims
      6. Confession/admission
   C. **Family**
      1. Information related to nonoffending parent

Table V   *Continued*

      2. Marital functioning and family functioning
      3. Family history of abuse
   D. **Other**
      1. Medical findings
      2. Police evidence
      3. Witnesses

Treatment of child sexual abuse may only involve the child, the child and his/her family, or the offender and sometimes the offender's family. The relationship of the victim to the offender will usually have an impact on the structure of treatment. However, in intrafamilial sexual abuse, the offender's prognosis also affects whether his treatment will prepare him/her for some level of future contact with the child. Because of space limitations, the focus in this article will be on child victim treatment.

A variety of theoretical frameworks related to treatment and rehabilitation are being used in victim treatment, including psychodynamic, play therapy, cognitive behavioral, and eclectic, drawing upon psychodynamic, behavioral, and family systems frameworks. However, one thing they have in common is that they dictate a direct focus on the abuse in the course of treatment. For example, it is not recommended that the therapist merely focus on the child's self-esteem or avoidance of men without addressing the underlying cause of these problems, the experience of sexual abuse. [*See* BEHAVIOR THERAPY; COGNITIVE THERAPY; FAMILY SYSTEMS; PSYCHOANALYSIS.]

A variety of treatment modalities are employed, the most common being individual, group, and family therapies. These may be employed concurrently or in progression, depending upon the structure of the treatment program, the functioning of the child, and the treatment issues being addressed. [*See* FAMILY THERAPY.]

Common treatment issues for victims are fears and phobias associated with the sexual abuse, the inability to trust adults, altered body image, guilt and responsibility associated with the abuse and its aftermath, anger because of the abuse, sexualized behavior, a need to understand aspects of the sexual abuse experience, and personal boundary and prevention issues. [*See* ANGER; BODY IMAGE; PHOBIAS.]

A number of treatment manuals and descriptive writings have been developed that propose the structure of the treatment and even provide specific exercises to address treatment issues. These are geared to children at different developmental stages, and some have been especially developed for boys.

Illustrative of treatment manuals is one developed by Mandell and Damon for group treatment of 7- to 12-year-old sexually abused children. It includes guidelines for group membership selection and a rationale for group treatment. It also contains 10 modules and provides topics and exercises for each module. Issues covered in the curriculum are shown in Table VI.

Outcome studies of treatment efficacy for victims of sexual abuse are just beginning to be conducted. In 1995, Berliner and Finkelhor provided a summary of 29 treatment outcome studies. All of these treatments lasted less than a year and most were treatment of a few weeks. These studies demonstrated that children who receive treatment for sexual abuse improve, but only 5 studies demonstrated that it was the therapy, itself, rather than, for example, the passage of time, that led to the children's improvement.

In providing appropriate treatment, the mental health professional must consider the nature of the abuse, the child's age and functioning, the offender–victim relationship, and the impact and symptomology. The treatment approach and modality should take into account the child within his/her context and should be of sufficient length to address the child's

Table VI Treatment Issues Developed by Mandell and Damon

---

1. Learning to trust others, beginning with other members of the group.

2. Identifying feelings (e.g., proud, special, jealous, worried, embarrassed, ashamed).

3. Telling the secret (i.e., disclosing the sexual abuse).

4. Feelings related to sexual abuse (e.g., betrayal, shame, guilt, responsibility, secrecy, protectiveness, helplessness).

5. The effect of sexual abuse on the victim, caretakers, and the family unit.

6. Recovery from sexual abuse.

7. Rebuilding and enhancing self esteem.

8. Protecting oneself in the future from sexual abuse and other harms.

9. Preparation for puberty.

---

treatment issues and symptoms. A systematic way of measuring the child's functioning before and after treatment is advisable. The child may need to return to treatment as subsequent developmental stages raise new concerns about past abuse and when new crises and traumas reactivate issues related to the sexual abuse.

V. PREVENTION OF SEXUAL ABUSE

Prevention of sexual abuse can be conceptualized as encompassing the following endeavors: (1) community and professional education; (2) prevention programs targeted at specific populations; and (3) prevention programs targeted at particular institutions.

A. Community and Professional Education

The Federal Statute that defines Child Protective Services (The Child Abuse Prevention and Treatment Act) restricts its federal grants for child abuse and neglect prevention and treatment services to states that provide education about child maltreatment (among other provisions). This provision is aimed at identifying maltreating families so that abuse can be stopped and its causes and effects ameliorated. However, because such education must define child maltreatment, it puts the community and professionals on notice about inappropriate forms of behavior toward children and, by doing this, can prevent some instances of child maltreatment, including sexual abuse. [*See* CHILD MALTREATMENT.]

Awareness of the unacceptability of child sexual abuse that derives from education also may serve as a deterrent for potential offenders. Some potential offenders may actually be ignorant about what sexual abuse is. In addition, it is fairly common for actual offenders to engage in "*cognitive distortions*" or rationalizations of their behavior. Examples might be telling themselves that because the behavior does not involve penile penetration, it is not abuse, or because the child is too young to understand, the abuse will not be harmful. It is possible, therefore, that potential offenders could be deterred and actual offenders could be led to cease sexual abuse by information that, for example "just touching" is abuse.

In addition, some potential offenders might be deterred by knowledge of the consequences of getting caught, information that could come from education. This might be professional education, community education, or information reported in the media. Although the media have provided some misinformation in their coverage of sexual abuse, they also have been the source of news stories that could have a deterrent effect, could lead to reporting of cases by victims or others, and could help victims feel less stigmatized and alone.

Another way education can be preventative is by causing earlier reporting of cases. That this is happening is suggested by changes in the types of cases that are being reported. In the 1950s and 1960s the clinical literature suggested that the modal case was one of an adolescent, who disclosed in the course of family conflict or after marital dissolution. Statistics from the most recent National Incidence Study, which gathers data on cases of child maltreatment coming to the attention of professionals, indicate that the children ages 3 through adolescence are at relatively equivalent risk for being identified as victims of sexual abuse.

B. Prevention Programs Targeted at Specific Populations

The dominant approach to prevention of child sexual abuse has been to rely on victims to avoid potentially abusive situations, to resist attempts to victimize them, and to report attempted and successful sexual abuse. This approach has been summarized as "say no, yell, and tell." Sexual abuse prevention programs have been developed for and delivered to children from preschool age through adolescence. Most are delivered in school settings. Some programs involve classroom teachers and parents. There were initial concerns by program designers about program content because of the sensitivity of the topic and anticipated parental resistance. Because of this, many programs focused on "stranger danger" and avoided addressing the possibility that the offender could be, and in fact was much more likely to be, someone known to the child. Presently, many programs are imbedded in broader "personal safety" programs that address a variety of risks children may encounter. These include safety when crossing the street and riding a bike, physical abuse, bullying, and kidnapping.

These prevention programs have been the targets of considerable criticism. First, and justifiably, they have been criticized for making the child responsible for prevention. This especially is an issue with preschoolers. There have been concerns that the victims will not be successful at saying no, resisting, and yelling help and then will blame themselves if they are unable to protect themselves. Critics have queried, "Why not target the offenders rather than the potential victims?" Better still, programs in high school aimed at potential parents and potential perpetrators might be more efficacious.

Prevention supporters counter these arguments as follows: If children receive this training as children, they will not victimize children when they become adolescents and adults. Further, supporters state that the fact children receive this kind of training may inhibit offenders from trying to abuse them. Offenders will fear children are on guard.

Second, prevention programs have been criticized because of their impact on the recipients. Specifically, there are worries that the programs may engender fear and cause trauma. Moreover, they may create a gulf between children and important adults in their lives because these programs put children on notice that adults, even those closest them, may not be trustworthy. In addition, prevention programs have been criticized as the source of some false allegations of sexual abuse. However, outcome studies indicate that only a very small minority of children experience an elevation in anxiety because of participation in prevention programs. No empirical support has been found for the assertions that prevention programs result in fears of caretakers or generate false allegations of sexual abuse.

Third, prevention programs have been challenged for their lack of effectiveness. For example, children may not understand all of the concepts they are being taught; may not be able to use the concepts to defend themselves; and may soon forget what they have learned. These criticisms have especially been leveled at preschool programs. Prevention program supporters reply that critics are expecting too much of the programs. These programs should be one of several approaches to preventing sexual abuse. Moreover, it is unrealistic to expect a program of an hour or even of several hours over time, to have a lasting or lifetime effect. Regular, periodic doses of prevention that occur at least on a yearly basis are what is needed.

Although prevention programs are far from a panacea, they can be beneficial. Finkelhor and colleagues recently conducted a national telephone survey of youth and their parents related to these programs. This study was funded by the Boy Scouts of America and intended to address some of the above noted criticisms. Using a representative sample of 2000 young people, ages 10 to 16, these researchers found that about 70% had participated in a prevention program, 36% in the past year. Younger children were more likely to have participated in the previous year. The vast majority of both the youth and their parents rated the programs positively and 26% of youth reported using some of the skills they had learned. Girls, African American children, and children from lower socioeconomic status families rated programs more positively.

C. Prevention Programs Targeting Particular Institutions

With the growing awareness of the problem of child sexual abuse has come an appreciation that certain institutions are vulnerable. That is, they may attract adults with a sexual interest in children. These persons are drawn to these institutions, sometimes because they naively find children's company preferable, without any awareness of their sexual attraction to children, but other times with the clear knowledge they are looking for prey. Both types of adults choose vocations and avocations that afford them ready access to children. These include jobs in day care centers, positions as boy scout and cub scout leaders, volunteer assignments as big brothers and big sisters, work as camp counselors, employment in recreational programs for youth, religious vocations such as the priesthood or the ministry, work in group homes for trouble youth and in residential treatment programs, and positions as foster parents.

Compared to prevention programs that target children, those in vulnerable institutions have been slow to develop. Generally they have been inspired by the surfacing of scandalous cases. As a rule, these prevention programs include five components: (1) screening for potential pedophiles; (2) prevention material that is delivered to children in these institutions; (3) educational material provided to adults in the institutions; (4) rules that reduce risk; and (5) procedures for investigating complaints.

Since these institutions either rely on volunteers or pay staff modestly, their reluctance to take on the issue of sexual abuse and develop prevention programs is understandable. Nevertheless, the importance of prevention in these contexts cannot be overstated. The majority of youth affected in these institutions are males, and boy victims are more likely than girls to respond to the trauma of sexual abuse by victimizing others. Therefore, preventive interventions in these institutions can have far-reaching impacts, because of the number of children they can save and the number of perpetrators they can stop.

VI. CONCLUSION

Although child sexual abuse is a common and serious mental health problem, it is not unmanageable nor unspeakable. Prevention programs and early identification can decrease the extent of sexual abuse and ameliorate its impact. Impressive progress has been achieved in the last 20 years. Despite present challenges to children describing sexual victimization, adults recalling abuse during childhood, and mental health professionals who attempt to assist child victims and adult survivors, the prospects for further progress in preventing and treating child sexual abuse are good.

BIBLIOGRAPHY

Executive summary of the third National Incidence Study (NIS-3). Washington, DC: USDHHS, National Center on Child Abuse and Neglect.

Faller, K. C. (1996). Evaluating children suspected of having been sexually abused: APSAC Study Guide. Newbury Park, CA: Sage Publications.

Finkelhor, D., & Berliner, L. (1994). Research on the treatment of sexually abused children. Journal of Child and Adolescent Psychiatry, 34(11), 1408–1422.

Finkelhor, D., & Dziuba-Leatherman, J. (1995). Victimization prevention programs: A national survey of children's exposure and reactions. Child Abuse and Neglect: The International Journal, 19(2), 129–141.

Friedrich, W. (1993). Sexual victimization and sexual behavior in children. Child Abuse and Neglect: The International Journal, 17(1), 59–66.

Gil, E., & Johnson, T. C. (1993). Sexualized children. Rockville, MD: Launch Press.

Jones, D., & McGraw, M. (1987). Reliable and fictitious accounts of sexual abuse to children. Journal of Interpersonal Violence, 2, 27–45.

Kendall-Tackett, K., Williams, L. M., & Finkelhor, D. (1993). Impact of sexual abuse on children: A review and synthesis of recent empirical studies. *Psychological Bulletin, 113(1),* 164–180.

Mandell, J., & Damon, L. (1989). *Group treatment for sexually abused children.* New York: Guilford Press.

Saunders, B., & Williams, L. (Eds.). (1996). Special section: Treatment outcome research. *Child Maltreatment 1(4),* 293–352.

Wurtele, S., & Miller-Perrin, C. (1992). *Preventing child sexual abuse: Sharing the responsibility.* Lincoln, NE: University of Nebraska Press.

Chronic Illness

Robin Leake and Ronald Friend

State University of New York, Stony Brook

Behavioral Control   The belief that the aversiveness of a situation can be personally influenced.

Body Image   The part of self-construct relating to physical representation of the body or physical self.

Cognitive Control   A strategy for thinking about a situation in order to reduce its stressful impact.

Denial   Failure to acknowledge or accept the full implications of a situation.

Family Stress Theories   Theories designed to explain the relationship between physiological and psychosocial variables in adjustment to chronic illness.

Nonadherence   Failure of patients to follow the preventative or therapeutic orders of a health care practitioner.

Quality of Life   The presence of personal and social positive well-being.

Relationship-Focused Coping The balance achieved in a dyadic relationship by meeting the needs of the partner while keeping individual stress levels to a minimum.

CHRONIC ILLNESS has replaced acute illness as the most common health threat in our society. As well as billions of dollars in medical costs, other costs of chronic illness include quality of life, burden to friends and family members, and, often, the patient's life. The last century has seen improved living conditions, less infectious disease, and better medical care, which has reduced the number of deaths and increased life expectancies, especially in Western countries. In 1992, the average life expectancy for men and women was estimated to be 75.8 years, which is higher than it has ever been. By the year 2005, life expectancies are expected to increase to 81 years for women, and 74.1 years for men. People who are 85 years and older are the fastest growing segment of the population. In 1980, only 4% of the population was 65 or over, but by 1990, this statistic had increased to 11%. By the year 2050, the elderly are expected to make up 20% of the population. This elderly cohort is also the group with the greatest risk for chronic illness. Advances in medical technology now make it possible to survive, but not fully recover from illnesses and diseases that were once fatal. Furthermore, because fewer people are dying of illnesses such as cardiovascular disease (still the leading cause of death in the United States, although steadily declining), they are vulnerable to other chronic illnesses later in life. The result of new technology is an increasingly larger segment of the population having limited functional status, often referred to as the "medicated survivors." According to the 1994 National Health Interview Survey, 10.6% (about 30 million people) have some limitation of activity and function due to chronic illness, compared with 9.4% in 1988. As many as one third of these chronically ill patients are not able to work, attend school, or perform daily living activities because of functional disability. Chronic illness is an irreversible impairment that affects the total environment, including the afflicted individual, the family, and the community. Therefore, scientific research must include a comprehensive examination of psychosocial factors that impact chronic illness, such as quality of life, the family system, and adjustment factors such as adherence to treatment regimens and denial.

I. TYPOLOGY OF CHRONIC ILLNESS

This entry focuses on broad psychosocial issues that apply generally to most medical chronic illnesses rather than on specific conditions. Although people suffering from different illnesses face similar issues, there is also a large degree of diversity inherent in diseases that affect psychosocial adjustment. Often findings from studies of a particular illness are wrongly assumed to generalize to all illnesses. On the other hand, if results cannot be generalized, studies within illnesses become too narrow and lose their practicality. Similarities and differences among chronic illnesses have been organized across several dimensions by John Rolland, and are discussed throughout this entry. Rolland's organization was designed to be used in conjunction with family systems theories, but it is useful in conceptualizing the impact of other individual psychosocial processes as well.

The first distinction drawn by Rolland is whether onset of the illness is acute or gradual. The onset of symptoms is the focus, rather than the biological development of the condition. Acute illness onset requires rapid mobilization of crisis management and adjustment skills by the individual and the family. With acute illnesses such as strokes or myocardial infarctions, families must quickly attend to threats of death and deterioration while also using active coping and problem-solving skills to make decisions. The amount of stress and coping might be the same for illnesses with a more gradual onset, such as AIDS or rheumatoid arthritis, but the family often has more time to adjust. Waiting for a diagnosis of a gradual condition, however, may provoke higher levels of anxiety. [*See* COPING WITH STRESS.]

Whether the course of the illnesses is progressive, constant, or relapsing has important implications for adjustment. Progressive illnesses, such as Parkinson's disease or lung cancer, are continuously symptomatic and worsen in severity with few periods of relief from illness-related demands. Continuous adaptation is necessary, and the strain on even the most resourceful and flexible family caregivers often causes exhaustion. For more slowly progressive illnesses, such as emphysema, stamina rather than continual adaptation is required of the entire family. Illnesses with a more constant course, such as stroke or asthma, stabilize after the initial event. The individual is usually left with some permanent disability or loss of function that does not necessarily worsen over time and is fairly predictable. Although constant adaptation and flexibility are not required, depression and exhaustion of family caregivers is a threat. Finally, relapsing or episodic illnesses are characterized by periods with no evident symptoms interrupted by flare-ups or worsening of symptoms. Examples of relapsing illness include asthma and multiple sclerosis. Although periods of normal functioning and routine activity are possible, the constant threat of relapse can be detrimental to adjustment, requiring vigilance and constant readiness for crisis behaviors.

The outcome of an illness, whether it is death, shortened life-span, or permanent disability greatly impacts appraisal, coping, and adjustment to the illness. There is some evidence that the initial expectation of the outcome is an extremely important predictor of adjustment. For illness diagnoses that portend eventual death (shortening of the natural life-span), such as AIDS and Huntington's chorea, expectations of loss of control and separation can be overwhelming. Reactions of family and friends can range from desire for closeness to pulling away from the ill member in anticipatory grief. This "letting go" can lead to isolation of the ill member and feelings of alienation that are associated with poorer adjustment and medical outcome.

The degree of incapacitation caused by an illness, including cognitive, motor, sensation, energy impairment, or disfigurement, is another important distinction to make in chronic illness. Research has found that expectations that the ill member can function independently with little impairment is associated with better long-term adjustment and rehabilitation. The more actual incapacitation caused by the illness, the lower these expectations are likely to be, and the lower the subsequent adjustment by the ill member. Obviously, different impairments carry different adjustment demands and these also significantly interact with onset, course, and outcome, as well as with the roles that the individual held before the onset of the illness.

Finally, the evolving "time phases" of an illness must be considered, as each phase has different adjustment requirements. Three major time points in a chronic illness identified by Rolland are the crisis, chronic, and terminal phases. The crisis phase is used to describe the time preceding the diagnosis when symptoms become present and suggestive of a serious problem. It also includes the period of readjustment immediately after diagnosis. The chronic phase describes the period after the initial readjustment and before the terminal phase, and can vary greatly in duration depending on the illness. Problems with daily living are confronted and resolved during this phase. Finally, the terminal phase describes the end of the illness when death is inevitable and apparent. The individual and the family adjust to the impending death of the ill member during this phase by coping with grief, separation, loss, and other crisis issues. This model can be used to explain disparate research findings between previous studies examining a particular illness or population. It is also useful for designing studies that will yield more consistent and interpretable results. Finally, it is a practical model for the clinician when treating patients with chronic illness and their families.

II. QUALITY OF LIFE

Quality of life, at one time thought to by synonymous with *quantity* of life and symptomatology, had little bearing on how people thought about chronic illness until quite recently. Important changes in the way quality of life was conceptualized corresponded with the World Health Organization's recognition that quality of life is not simply the absence of disease, but the presence of positive personal and social well being. Although the basic elements of quality of life may be agreed on, these vary widely across individuals and illnesses, making quality of life an extremely subjective concept. For example, early studies using physicians' ratings of quality of life found that these assessments were not associated with patient and family ratings of quality of life. Research also suggests that quality of life, however subjective it might be, is an important

psychosocial concept related to illness outcome and functional status. Studies examining how chronic illness affects quality of life focus on the changes in personal, social, and employment activities as well as on how the illness interferes with daily living. These findings are important for designing interventions to improve compromised quality of life. Using the typology described earlier, it is evident that different illnesses will affect quality of life in different ways. For instance, patients with end-stage renal disease might experience problems with time-consuming treatments, whereas reduction of functional ability will be more common for patients suffering from Parkinson's disease. Another important consideration is whether the treatment of an illness has more severe consequences than the illness itself. For instance, whether chemotherapy in response to cancer is more harmful than the cancer itself in terms of survival rate and deleterious side effects can be assessed by quality of life information.

What is quality of life? Quality of life is usually assessed across several dimensions, including objective variables that are usually physical in nature and can be determined by other people, and psychological measures assessed by subjective self-reports. Objective measures of quality of life may include employment status, functional ability, health status, co-morbidity, and income, whereas subjective measures examine family functioning, social well-being, life satisfaction, affect, and depression. Usually, quality of life is assessed by self-report questionnaires and a composite score is assigned. One reliable measure frequently used to assess quality of life is the Sickness Impact Profile (SIP), a behaviorally based instrument that measures physical, psychosocial and other functioning. Other commonly used instruments based on activities associated with daily living are the Karnofsky Index of Physical Function and the Activities of Daily Living scale (ADL). In addition, other measures have been developed for assessment of specific illnesses.

A common assumption often made is that people suffering from chronic illness will have lower quality of life than their healthy counterparts. In a society that cherishes individualism, the ideology of individual control and responsibility for one's life is a strong cultural and psychological force. Many chronic illnesses are characterized by a loss of autonomy and dependence on life-sustaining treatments. Therefore, it is not surprising that healthy individuals view chronic illness and the corresponding loss of control as threatening. Yet research has shown that these bleak views may be a projection of fear and uncertainty rather than the reality that chronically ill individuals face. For example, studies with renal dialysis patients show that the only indicators of quality of life that the renal patients fall short on by a sizable margin when compared with healthy people are the objective quality of life indicators. However, their evaluations of their subjective quality of life are remarkably similar to what healthy individuals report. Other studies with patients suffering from diabetes, cancer, arthritis, and skin disorders yield similar results. This indicates that peoples' psychological interpretation of their experience of chronic illness is much more resilient than many realize.

Helping patients adapt to their illness may lead to improved quality of life. Although there is scant research on improving quality of life in chronically ill patients, one study found that an intervention to help patients keep their jobs greatly improved their subjective as well as objective quality of life. Many researchers believe that patients need to be taught what they should realistically expect so that they can make correct attributions for changes that occur as a result of their illness or medical treatment. Without corresponding psychological treatment, changes from physical interventions may be attenuated, misperceived, or misinterpreted. How physical changes are subjectively experienced, how they translate psychologically, and the interpretations patients make may be crucial to maintenance of quality of life and efficacy of physical interventions.

III. ADJUSTMENT TO CHRONIC ILLNESS

If quality of life is partly a function of how well patients adjust to their illness, then it is important to identify specific psychosocial factors that influence adjustment. Chronic illness can affect every aspect of a patient's life, requiring drastic lifestyle changes, such as dealing with symptoms and incapacitation, coping with treatment regimens, and maintaining emotional balance in the face of crisis. Many factors determine how well patients meet these challenges and cope with their illness. Because these factors are too numerous to discuss in detail here, several key variables that

have been shown to influence how well patients adjust will be examined, namely, denial, control, and body image.

A. Denial

Denial is an important psychological construct that affects adjustment. It is also perhaps the most controversial construct. It is thought to be adaptive in some cases, but dysfunctional in others. Research has found that denial is a commonly used, if primitive and often pathological defense mechanism in response to chronic illness. Denial has not been sufficiently operationalized, however, and studies measuring denial rarely, if ever, clarify what is actually being denied. The term is used generally to describe when the implications of an illness are either not recognized or are avoided. Studies looking at denial have yielded conflicting results. Some studies have found that patients who exercise denial have less medical complications, report fewer symptoms, and adhere better to their treatment regimens. Other studies, however, find that denial is associated with anxiety and depression and leads to poorer adjustment. One reason for these discrepant findings may be that denial may impact adjustment differently throughout the course of an illness. For instance, denial of symptoms indicative of illness, such as a cancer victim ignoring a suspicious lump in her breast, might prevent someone from seeking timely treatment. On the other hand, denial may be beneficial directly after a crisis such as a myocardial infarction, when it may serve the protective function of staving off panic or extreme distress. Denial may be harmful again, however, later in the course of the illness when the patient must learn to live with the illness, if it results in disregarding treatment demands. In fact, patients who deny the implications of their illness 1 year after a myocardial infarction show poorer adherence, higher relapse rates, and poorer quality of life.

B. Control

Whether or not a person feels able to control important life events has a large impact on adjustment. One of the frequently unavoidable consequences of chronic illness is loss of control, the extent to which is determined by the type of illness. Illnesses with acute onset often lead to greater feelings of loss of control because the patient is faced with sudden and frightening changes in functioning. Usually, an acute onset of disease necessitates hospitalization, which can magnify these feelings. In addition to relinquishing control to an unknown and often impersonal medical staff, patients are seldom given much information about what is happening to them, causing great anxiety and confusion. Even after the crisis period is over, patients are still unable to control the changes in their bodies and often the behavioral responses required of them for treatment. In fact, studies have found that patients who feel able to control their illness are better adjusted than those who do not. Therefore, restoring control to chronically ill patients can reduce distress, contribute to effective coping, and increase overall adjustment to the illness.

There are two major types of control that people can have over their lives. The first is behavioral control, or a belief in the ability that one can influence a negative event, whether by terminating the stimuli, mitigating its aversiveness, or shortening its duration. Behavioral control does not require actual coping behaviors, merely the belief that the outcome of an event is controllable. Studies that induce behavioral control find that patients have less anxiety and report their illness experience as less stressful than patients without behavioral control. Cognitive control refers to changes in thinking about a situation in such a way as to reduce its stressful impact. Strategies to attain cognitive control might involve gathering information, engaging in distracting activities, or reevaluating the level of threat that the illness poses. For example, a cancer patient might think about the positive consequence of illness, such as having a new appreciation of their life or having a second chance at living.

These beliefs about control, either behavioral or cognitive, do not have to be accurate to positively influence adjustment. "Perceived" control has been mentioned previously, because the idea that one can influence the effect of an illness may be just as important as the actual ability to do so. Some types of cognitive control, such as having a positive attitude about an illness or the philosophy of "taking things one day at a time," may help reduce stress and improve adjustment without affecting medical outcome. On the other hand, perceptions of control might induce a patient to make adaptive behavior changes which could reduce the likelihood of illness-related complications, or relapse.

C. Body Image

Body image refers to self-evaluation and perception of one's functional ability as well as physical appearance. Chronic illness often results in physical changes that can threaten self-esteem and self-image. For instance, breast cancer victims who must undergo mastectomies often feel a loss of femininity, and stroke victims who suffer motor and speech impairments may also experience feelings of inadequacy. Similarly, illnesses that require dependence on life-sustaining machines such as pacemakers or dialysis equipment often threaten patients' independence and feelings of "wholeness." Patients who suffer from illnesses with a progressive course must frequently cope with deteriorating changes in appearance and loss of physical function. As self-worth is already very closely tied to body image for adolescents because of the developmental changes that occur normally, for adolescents with chronic illness negative body image has an even more deleterious effect. Sexual dysfunction, characteristic of many illnesses such as renal failure, myocardial infarction, diabetes, stroke, and arthritis also threaten body image as well as overall self-esteem. How much body image is threatened depends not only on the nature of the threat, but also on personal factors such as body image before illness onset and self-image as it relates to the specific loss. For example, weight loss that accompanies diabetes might impact a patient who is a professional wrestler, and who depends on body mass, more severely than it would an accountant with a desk job.

Physical appearance is extremely important, both in the way people view themselves and in the way they imagine others see them. Several studies have found that internal appraisals of appearance influence adjustment and self-esteem much more strongly than external evaluations. Illnesses in which physical impairment or changes in appearance are not immediately evident or visible to others are often just as stressful. Often patients feel as if they are "passing" or masquerading as a healthy person and that they face the constant threat that someone will find out about the illness inadvertently. For example, a diabetic patient might be afraid of having a hypoglycemic reaction at work, and a renal patient might fear that others will notice the needle marks on their arm or the peritoneal dialysis bag they wear on their abdomen. Illnesses that are not visible can also be traumatic because others may not acknowledge the presence and legitimacy of disease without physical signs. For example, patients suffering from rheumatoid arthritis experience extreme pain, but the lack of visibility of their illness may fail to elicit understanding or help from others. Although the importance of body image is now recognized, very little is known about how to improve patients' perceptions of their physical self. Some studies suggest that getting patients to focus on more positive aspects of their appearance or functioning can be beneficial, as can increases in physical exercise and activity. Clearly, more research needs to be done on improving body image compromised by chronic illness. Denial, control, and body image are just a few of the many emotional and personal variables that may influence adjustment to chronic illness. Interventions designed to improve overall adjustment, as well as quality of life or adherence, must recognize the importance of these factors and target these areas for behavior change. [See BODY IMAGE.]

IV. CHRONIC ILLNESS AND THE FAMILY

A growing body of research has been addressing the realization that the family plays a key role in the development, course, and outcome of chronic illness. Attitudes about illness and coping originate within the family system, and these attitudes influence a wide range of health-relevant behaviors. Research on family and chronic illness is diverse and includes many perspectives, such as the family's influence on the cognitions, behaviors, and adjustment of the individual, as well as the impact of chronic illness on the family itself. Research on the influence of marriage on health has found that married patients have better outcomes for several chronic illnesses. For example, married patients who suffer myocardial infarction have higher survival rates, and those with rheumatoid arthritis have less functional disability.

Although family support has been found to improve coping, adjustment, and outcome of chronic illness, the family can also hinder outcome and actually increase depression and disability. Several models have been proposed and examined in order to understand the relationship between chronic illness and family functioning. One of the earliest models to recognize the social pressures that are exerted on the ill individual is the sick-role model. Development of the sick role is influenced by the expectations of the family, spouse, physician, and society in general. Four major expectations are identified: (a) the individual must see the ill state as undesirable and try to get well, (b) competent help must be sought by the individual, (c) the ill individual is not responsible for the illness, and (d) the ill individual is exempt from normal social-role obligations. Development of the sick role from a well state includes coping with the negative consequences of acute illness. The sick role may lead to the return of the well state, or may develop into a chronic state of illness. The sick role will be bestowed and socially reinforced as long as the ill individual meets the preceding expectations. Whether or not an individual retains the sick role is best predicted by social support, further demonstrating the important role that significant others play in the course of illness. Although highly influential in promoting research on social factors that influence illness, there are criticisms of the sick-role model, namely, that it is not really relevant for chronic illnesses. Although the identity of a chronically ill person may become salient to the self-concept of a person suffering from an illness, the social expectations that accompany the "sick role" as traditionally defined can never be met, because there is no recovery from chronic illness. Therefore, research differentiating the social factors (including family interactions) that influence chronic illness rather than acute illness was necessary for better understanding and treatment of chronic illness.

Many family-systems models were later proposed which focus on how transitions within the family influence the development and course of health problems. A common hypothesis of most of these models is that dysfunction in one part of the family system leads to dysfunction in other parts. The goal of family behavior is to maintain a homeostatic balance between family members. These models helped operationalize and more reliably measure important concepts such as family adaptation to the development of chronic disability in a family member. [See FAMILY SYSTEMS.]

Family stress theories were designed to explain the relationship between physiological and psychosocial variables in the adjustment to chronic illness. According to the family adjustment and adaptation response (FAAR) model proposed by Patterson, the amount of stress experienced by the family is determined by the interaction of stressful events and the family's available resources. Resources to cope with these stressors can be psychological, social, or physical. This relationship is also moderated by the family's appraisal of the stressor and subsequent coping responses. This model is used to predict how families will cope with the stress of chronic illness once their personal resources are taxed and homeostasis is not maintainable.

Research based on these models has provided support for the notions that chronic illness in one family member influences every other aspect of family life and that the family has enormous impact on the onset, course, and outcome of the illness, as well as on the way the illness is perceived and experienced. Studies specifically focused on marital coping examine many interdependent systems. When looking at coping processes, the individual coping responses of the ill family member must be examined within the context of the marriage or the family. Chronic illness can be intrusive, requiring routine hospitalization or complicated, time-consuming medical treatments that disrupt family dynamics. This often requires family members to assume new or different roles, to make physical and emotional adjustments, and to change routine activities. Furthermore, if the illness is progressive, or the functional ability of the patient fluctuates, the disruption of a structured family life causes additional stress.

Nonetheless, close family relationships can help the ill individual cope with chronic illness in a variety of ways. Individual coping strategies have been described by Lazarus and Folkman as either problem-focused, where the goal of coping behavior is to eliminate the stress, or emotion-focused, which helps manage negative appraisals of stress. In recent research, this paradigm has been applied to coping within dyadic relationships. Social support has been hypothesized to aid in coping with chronic illness by providing information, reinforcement, and feedback to help coping efforts.

Taking this a step further, relationship-focused coping has been described as the balance couples must reach in meeting each other's needs while managing individual levels of stress and not unduly burdening the other partner. One strategy of relationship-focused coping is active engagement, which refers to instrumental coping behaviors such as openly discussing reactions to the illness and possible solutions to illness-related problems. The second strategy is protective buffering, giving in to the partner in order to avoid conflict, and denying worries and concerns in order to avoid upset or disagreement. In a study examining

couples where the husband had suffered a recent myocardial infarction, the husbands' functional impairment level influenced levels of distress in both partners as well as the wives' coping responses. Wives' coping responses (managing their own stress as well as supporting their spouse) in turn affected their husbands' emotional responses. Protective buffering by husbands and wives was found to increase wives' distress levels, but was positively associated with husbands' self-efficacy. These results suggest that what is beneficial for one spouse might be deleterious to the other, and a balance must be reached for both partners to adjust to the illness.

The family can also be a source of stress and ultimately have a negative impact on the illness outcome. One member's reaction to the illness directly or indirectly impacts the coping responses of the spouse or the other family members. For example, behavior that the spouse intends to be supportive, such as urging the partner to comply with the prescribed medical regimen, may be perceived by the ill partner as controlling or overprotective. As previously discussed, many chronic illnesses are disabling and result in loss of control in many domains of life. Overprotective family members may unwittingly enhance these feelings by regulating an area, such as personal compliance, that the patient could have control over. Supportive behavior toward an ill spouse can also have negative health effects on the healthy spouse. For instance, caregiving spouses of Alzheimer's patients showed decreased immune functioning, and caregivers of heart disease patients experiencing psychological stress also experienced distress.

Marital dissatisfaction has been associated with increased physical illness and poorer adjustment in dialysis and cancer patients. Recovery of myocardial infarction is also hindered by poor marital relationship factors, such as intrusiveness, lack of confidence in the ill spouse, and overprotectiveness. Families can also influence the adoption of negative health behaviors that lead to the development of chronic illness, such as smoking and poor exercise and dietary patterns. The role that families play in the initiation and maintenance of these negative behaviors has been the focus of many studies. Several of these support the idea that family members share behavior patterns and risk factors such as sedentary lifestyles and obesity. Families also greatly influence individual members' conceptions of illness and behavior change. For instance, spousal support is one of the best predictors of successful smoking cessation. Conversely, if other family members share the risk behavior, they may inadvertently reinforce or undermine efforts to change the negative behavior. [*See* MARITAL HEALTH.]

V. ADHERENCE TO TREATMENT REGIMENS

Poor adherence to maintenance regimens for chronic illness has been a pervasive problem and a long-standing dilemma for clinicians and researchers. The rate of patient noncompliance has been estimated to be up to 80%, varying with the demands of different regimens. Nonadherence can be defined as the failure of patients to follow medical practitioners' preventative or therapeutic orders. The negative consequences of nonadherence may include reduced health and life expectancy, as well as emotional and economic strain for the family. Research has shown, for instance, that 39% of single and 31% of multiple admissions of insulin-dependent diabetics are due to poor adherence. In addition, 33% of elderly patients (who have the highest rate of noncompliance of any population) are admitted to the hospital because of poor compliance. Noncompliant medicated schizophrenics patients are more than twice as likely to be readmitted to the hospital than compliant patients. Improving adherence, therefore, is important for reducing unnecessary hospital costs. More tragically, thousands of patients die each year simply from failure to take prescribed medication either correctly or at all, and studies show that 30 to 50% of all prescriptions are taken incorrectly by patients. With such high levels of noncompliance for pill-taking, it is not surprising that few patients adhere to regimens that require more arduous behavior changes such as changing dietary, exercise, and smoking behaviors. Adherence rates seem to be just as low for pediatric patients, especially those with chronic illness. For example, children with asthma reportedly adhere to their regimen as little as 17% of the time. Compliance rates of children with juvenile rheumatoid arthritis and renal failure are only slightly higher at 55% and 57%, respectively.

Poor adherence is particularly common among patients with chronic illness because complex treatment regimens that require intrusive changes in lifestyle must be followed for long periods of time, or even indefinitely. For instance, patients with end-stage renal disease must not only undergo rigorous dialysis treatments on a daily or triweekly basis, but must also reduce their fluid intake and monitor their diet closely. For diabetics, treatment includes daily injections of insulin, close monitoring of blood glucose levels, and also strict control of their diet. Complicating the issue, compliance in one area of health behaviors is not always related to compliance in others. For instance, a patient with coronary heart disease may quit smoking but fail to modify his or her diet or increase exercise.

There are many reasons why patients fail to comply with treatment demands. First of all, the side effects of a given treatment may reduce quality of life to such a degree that they do not seem worthwhile. For instance, immunosuppressant medications that keep the immune system from rejecting a translated organ cause many adverse side effects such as nausea, weight gain, and susceptibility to other illnesses. Often, patients will stop taking the medication in order to avoid these effects. Once they stop taking the medication, they immediately feel better, which serves as positive reinforcement for the noncompliant behavior. The consequences of cessation of the medication, namely the rejection of the transplanted organ, may not occur for weeks or even months, depending on the degree of noncompliance. In addition, after patients have been taking the medication for a long time, they may become complacent or forgetful about maintaining the regimen without the presence of symptoms to remind them. Similarly, engaging in protective health behaviors might sustain life indirectly, providing no immediate reward or gratification. Research has shown, however, that patients are more likely to comply with treatments that are medical and monitored by health professionals, such as chemotherapy or kidney dialysis. Health care practitioners may also share the responsibility for poor patient adherence. Failure to motivate patients and to provide feedback concerning treatment responses have been associated with poor compliance, as well as lack of communication and empathy toward the demands and corresponding behaviors that patients must engage in to manage their illness. For example, physicians may sometimes interrupt their patients and fail to let them finish describing their symptoms and concerns.

One interesting way that chronically ill patients often fail to adhere to their treatment regimens has been labeled "creative nonadherence." This occurs when the patient intentionally changes or supplements a treatment prescribed by a health professional. One study of elderly patients, for instance, reported that 73% of nonadherence was intentional. There are many reasons why creative noncompliance occurs. First, as patients become more familiar with their illness and with how their body responds to treatment, they feel more comfortable trusting their own judgment concerning treatment modifications. For example, patients with asthma might vary their medication levels depending on environmental factors that they recognize might exacerbate their symptoms, such as weather conditions or the presence of allergens. Monitoring and self-treating their symptoms are means by which patients may feel they have more control over their illness. High rates of co-morbidity, or the presence of two or more illnesses at one time, often complicate treatment regimens. Patients may feel that the practitioner is failing to take into account the presence of co-morbid conditions and the complications that may arise as a result, or that they are simply not receiving adequate care. Sometimes the patients are correct in their assumptions that they know their bodies better than most people, and alternative treatment methods can have beneficial results.

However, creative nonadherence can have unfortunate consequences if mistakes are made. Often, patients modify their regimen by taking over-the-counter remedies in conjunction with their prescribed medication or by engaging in other alternative treatments that may have unpredictable or dangerous results. Patients may be familiar with their own responses to certain treatments but still lack the general knowledge and expertise of health-care professionals. Good patient–practitioner communication and feedback is necessary to avoid problems with creative nonadherence.

Measuring patient nonadherence has proven to be almost as difficult as improving it. Several different methods are used to assess compliance, but no one technique is completely successful. Behaviors such as keeping appointments or immunization records are relatively easy to measure as records are kept, but even evaluating behaviors that appear simple, such as pill-taking can be difficult. Although the amount of pills taken can be counted and compared to the amount prescribed, it is impossible to know whether they were taken in a timely manner or in the correct environment or circumstances, such as with food or without other medications, without actually asking the patient. In fact, patient self-reports are a common way to assess

adherence even though questions remain about the validity of such reports. One apparent source of invalidity is patients' desire to report "good" or correct behaviors, and, in fact, studies show that patients frequently overestimate their own compliance when compared with objective medical laboratory values. The advantage of using such physiological measures is their objectivity, but they are often expensive and can be influenced by factors other than compliance, such as when the measures are taken and individual differences. A third way to measure patient compliance is by using assessments of the medical staff treating the patient. Several studies have found that medical staff assessments of patient compliance are the most accurate of the three methods discussed, although these have been shown to account for only 50% of compliance variance. These studies further suggest that using multiple methods is helpful in attaining a more accurate and comprehensive assessment of compliance.

Efforts by both clinicians and researchers to improve patient compliance have yielded equivocal results. Because there are so many possible reasons for nonadherence—individual personality factors such as coping style and self-efficacy, patient–physician communication problems such as confusing or conflicting information or incomplete instructions—improving compliance remains a complex and continuous challenge. Currently, there are very few randomized and controlled intervention studies designed to improve adherence, and even fewer that examine long-term effects of specific interventions. Some clues to designing successful interventions can be found within existing research measuring patient adherence. For instance, several studies have noted that the best predictor of patient adherence 6 months to 2 years into a given regimen is the adherence rate at the onset of treatment. In other words, patient adherence does not vary much throughout the course of an illness. It is reasonable, therefore, to design interventions that motivate patients to adhere to their regimen from the beginning of their treatment.

Whether patient adherence is targeted at treatment inception or at another time during the course of their illness, the question still remains: What is the most effective way to reduce nonadherence? Educational interventions, especially those that include family support and that are home-based as well as hospital-based have been shown to improve medication and dietary adherence to several illness regimens. Similarly, modeling techniques, such as viewing videotaped instructions on self-administering insulin shots or dietary planning, also result in improved adherence.

The use of a variety of behavior strategies to change adherence is an important intervention. Behavior strategies most commonly used are training medical staff to provide better and more immediate feedback to patients as well as reinforcement for adherent behaviors. The importance of the immediacy of patient feedback is often overlooked. Patients with end-stage renal disease, for instance, are often able to control their fluid compliance because they know immediately how much weight they gain between treatments. On the other hand, patients often have inaccurate perceptions of their dietary compliance, overestimating their adherence behavior, because they are not given immediate feedback. Thus, patients may benefit from more externally validated feedback about their compliance. Providing cues or other reminders for patients, such as mailed cards or telephone calls, to remind them of appointments or treatment schedules is also helpful in promoting compliance behaviors, as is modifying treatment regimens so that patients can incorporate them into their existing daily lives more easily.

Social support interventions in the form of social support groups, family and community support, and support from medical staff have also been shown to be quite effective in reducing nonadherence and even prolonging life. Religious interventions, such as church support groups, have been effective in promoting adherence, particularly for African American and Latino patients. Social support, particularly from the family, can be instrumental in physically implementing treatment regimens by changing cooking habits, helping administer medication and other behavioral treatments, and providing emotional support, as discussed in the section on family influence on chronic illness. Finally, interventions aimed at improving patients' self-efficacy are particularly important for improving adherence. Patients must feel capable of carrying out treatment regimens and meeting the present and future demands of their illness. Self-efficacy at the beginning of treatment has been shown to predict adherence behaviors, especially with exercise and dietary compliance.

VI. PSYCHOSOCIAL INTERVENTIONS

As previously discussed, psychosocial factors greatly impact on the prevention, course, treatment, and out-come of chronic illness. It is reasonable to suggest, then, that interventions designed to manipulate these factors might lead to greater adjustment to chronic illness, ranging from less depression and anxiety to better quality of life and adherence to treatment regimens, and even longer survival. Various manipulations based on previous research have been tested in health-care settings, with some promising results. It is hoped that as this research continues, therapeutic interventions designed to improve adjustment to chronic illness will be routinely implemented in patient care. Three of the most common types of interventions are educational, cognitive–behavioral, and social support intervention programs.

A. Education

The primary purpose of education interventions is to alleviate feelings of helplessness that arise from uncertainty or lack of knowledge about the illness, as well as to relieve anxiety and increase coping and pain management. Educational techniques include increasing knowledge about illness and treatment effects as well as providing information about coping. These techniques have been shown to improve functioning and to increase feelings of control in patients with cancer, end-stage renal disease, cardiovascular disease, and stroke victims. Research results emphasize the necessity of good patient education, which is often neglected for several possible reasons. Health-care practitioners often overestimate the amount of knowledge that patients have about their illness or fail to realize how important it is for patients to develop realistic expectations of how they will be affected by their illness. In addition, patients often hold misconceptions or are unwilling to ask questions that will help them better understand and cope with their illness.

B. Cognitive–Behavioral Interventions

These interventions help patients accurately appraise or reconceptualize the impact of illness and to adjust positively to their illness through the development of coping skills. Cognitive–behavioral interventions usually include coping-skills training, such as relaxation techniques, problem solving, and distraction techniques, as well as communication skills training. All of these methods foster intrinsic motivation and self-efficacy so that patients will continue the positive behaviors beyond the actual intervention. Specifically, the purpose of these interventions is to reduce stress, improve overall functioning, and ameliorate symptoms by addressing the patients' perceptions about their illness rather than their objective physical limitations. Coping-skills training involves several techniques. One of the most common is progressive relaxation training, which increases feelings of control and reduces muscle arousal and physical tension. Problem-solving is important when helping patients identify and cope with illness-related stress, and distraction training helps patients cope with pain and other negative symptoms by directing attention to specific areas of the body. Finally, communication skills training can help patients adjust to their illness within the family system and to make other necessary social adaptations. Cognitive-behavioral interventions, although diverse, have been shown to be effective in improving overall adjustment across different illnesses. Several studies using interventions to help patients reduce the physical severity and negative affect associated with chemotherapy treatment in cancer patients found that progressive muscle relaxation and guided imagery techniques (where patients use their imagination to visualize their immune system battling cancer cells) significantly reduced the adverse side effects of chemotherapy. Training in cognitive coping skills has been shown to improve functional status, pain management, and psychosocial adjustment in patients with chronic back pain, sickle cell disease, arthritis, and renal disease. [*See* BEHAVIORAL THERAPY; COGNITIVE THERAPY.]

C. Social Support Interventions

Social support predicts better adjustment to illness, improved adherence to medical regimens, and positive outcome in chronically ill patients. However, patients with chronic illness often have fewer social support resources because of the stress that illness places on relationships. Family and friends who are adversely affected by the illness may be less able to provide necessary support to the ill member. Social support interventions, therefore, are often designed to promote family involvement and improve communication among family members. When family members are taught through therapy to integrate the patient's treatment regimen into their daily lives, adherence to treatment greatly improves. Peer support group interventions with patients who are coping with similar illness experiences can provide patients with emotional support, as well as practical knowledge from similar others. Recent research indicates that providing emotional and practical support is as beneficial as receiving it, suggesting that intervention strategies that pair beginning patients with a more experienced "sponsor" patient might lead to greater illness adjustment for both patients. Studies with cancer, rheumatoid arthritis, renal, and cardiovascular patients find that social support groups lead to better adherence behaviors, coping skills, and even survival. Although these interventions are promising because of their practicality and cost-effectiveness, the majority of patients who participate in support groups are well-educated, middle-class, and represent a small proportion of chronically ill patients. Therefore, these patients might already be more self-motivated and have better coping skills than those patients who are not involved in support groups. Overall, however, increasing social support, whether through family therapy, individual therapy, or peer support groups is an important way to mitigate the negative effects of chronic illness for patients and their families. [*See* SOCIAL SUPPORT.]

BIBLIOGRAPHY

Bishop, G. D. (1994). *Health psychology: Integrating mind and body*. Boston: Allyn & Bacon.

Cassileth, B. R., Lusk, E. J., Strouse, T. B., Miller, D. S., Brown, L. L., Cross, P. A., & Tenaglia, A. N. (1984). Psychosocial status in chronic illness. *New England Journal of Medicine, 311*, 506–511.

Coyne, J. C., & Smith, D. A. F. (1991). Couples coping with a myocardial infarction. A perspective on wives' distress. *Journal of Personality and Social Psychology, 61*, 404–412.

Fawzy, F. I., Fawzy, N. W., Arndt, L. A., & Pasnau, R. O. (1995). Critical care review of psychosocial interventions in cancer care. *Archives of General Psychiatry, 52*, 100–113.

Nicassio, P. M., & Smith, T. W. (1995). *Managing chronic illness: A biopsychosocial perspective*. Washington DC: American Psychological Association.

Revenson, T. A. (1994). Social support and marital coping with chronic illness. *Annals of Behavioral Medicine, 16*, 122–130.

Rolland, J. S. (1984). Toward a psychosocial typology of chronic and life-threatening illness. *Family Systems Medicine, 2*, 245–259.

Taylor, S. E. (Ed.). (1995). *Health psychology*. New York: McGraw-Hill.

Vamos, M. (1993). Body image in chronic illness—A reconceptualization. *International Journal of Psychiatry in Medicine, 23*, 163–178.

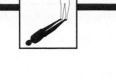

Classifying Mental Disorders:
Nontraditional Approaches

Theodore R. Sarbin

University of California, Santa Cruz

Ernest Keen

Bucknell University

Contextualism A worldview that requires taking into account the entire context in which actors' behavior takes place. For human beings, the context is largely symbolic and languaged so that one must consider the meanings that persons assign to aspects of their worlds.

Discourse Analysis Analysis of the verbal and non-verbal communication contexts within which meanings of the world and its events and objects are constructed.

Historical Act The root metaphor of contextualism, the basic concept for interpreting conduct as addressing the world in its narrative flow, thus assuming a past and anticipating a future.

Internality A characteristic of traditional diagnostic language that locates the crucial context for understanding the causes of conduct as internal to the actor, tending to neglect other contexts.

Mechanistic A worldview for understanding conduct in terms of the properties of machines, such as the transmission of energy.

Narrative The story, implicit or explicit, that contextualizes and gives meaning to human conduct; the story may be idiosyncratic but most often is borrowed from the stock of stories that comprise a culture.

Nosology A classification system of diseases assumed to be discrete entities, such as tuberculosis or measles.

Root Metaphor The basic concept, often implicit, of a particular worldview that facilitates some interpretations of the world and forecloses others. The machine and the historical act are root metaphors for, respectively, the mechanistic worldview and the contextualist worldview.

Strategic Actions Intentional acts performed by a person directed toward solving identity and existential problems.

Classifying for purposes of research or intervention is a feature of the scientific method. Traditional methods for **CLASSIFYING MENTAL DISORDERS** emerged from 19th century advances in the biological sciences basic to the science and practice of medicine. Underlying such advances was the explicit adoption of the world view of mechanism, the root metaphor of which was the transmittal of forces. In this context, physicians constructed systems for classifying organic disease. These systems provided the model for traditional psychiatric diagnostic and classification systems.

Nontraditional classification systems flow from an alternate worldview—contextualism, the root metaphor of which is the historical act in all its complexities. Instead of relying on the medically inspired concept of psychopathology, nontraditional practitioners speak of "unwanted conduct." This practice explicitly recognizes that a moral judgment is being made on the strategic actions that people employ to solve their problems in living. In the nontraditional method described in this article, classification is not of disease processes but of interactional strategies and the conditions that influence the success or failure of such strategies.

I. INTRODUCTION

As a preamble to an article on alternate ways of classifying mental disorders, we point to a built-in source of ambiguity. The use of the construction, "mental disorders," together with the phrase "mental health" in the title of the encyclopedia, reflects an implicit acceptance of a particular worldview from which the traditional approaches to classification are generated. The use of the word "mental" implies an assured and nonproblematic ontological status for the concept of mind, notwithstanding the many critiques of the concept, and by the claim that "mind" is an exemplar of the human tendency to transfigure a metaphor to a literal entity. Lost in the history of lexicography is the recognition that at one time mind was a verb, useful for talking about silent and unseen actions, such as thinking, imagining, and so on.

For the most part, the traditional approach treats "mind" as a literal entity, often as a quasi-organ parallel to the brain, or as an epiphenomenon arising from the workings of the brain. In actual practice, mental health professionals do not deal with "minds," but with persons whose actions fail to meet a particular society's standards of propriety or fail to meet self-imposed standards. It is an illusion that therapists aid in reconstructing "minds," although they may be instrumental in modifying beliefs and values, in reinforcing strategies for managing interpersonal relations, in changing habits, and in acquiring self-knowledge.

"Disorders" is also an unsettled concept. The term implies a departure or deviation from "ordered" conduct. It is important to note that the supraordinate concepts "ordered" and "disordered" (staples of mental health and mental illness doctrines) are derived

from a particular worldview, probably unrecognized by the vast majority of mental health workers. The worldview is that of the machine, the root metaphor of which is the transmission of forces. Being "in order" or "out of order" (disordered), although apt constructions for describing the condition of a clock, a motor, or a computer, are misleading when applied to the acts of human beings. As a descriptor for unacceptable conduct, "disorders" is derived from traditional practices for classifying absurd or unwanted conduct—such practices being consistent with the mechanistic worldview that the "mind" operates like other machines—as a vehicle for the transformation of forces.

Related to the mechanistic conception of order is another implicit meaning of "disorder." The concept of "social order" grew out of the belief in an orderly universe. Thus, "disorder" is applied to violations of the normative expectations for human conduct in everyday life. Shared constructions of the social order supply the context within which conduct may be classified as mentally disordered, deviant, nonconforming, abnormal, inept, or improper. Further, the shared constructions provide the background for legitimating interventions such as hospitalization, incarceration, or other systematic effort to restore order to the social group the equilibrium of which has been disrupted by the conduct of the "disorderly" or "disordered" person.

II. THE PURPOSES OF CLASSIFICATION

Behind any classification system is one purpose or more that provides the basis for distinguishing and defining categories. In Western culture, classifications of "mental disorders" have been designed to serve the purposes of the science and practice of medicine: (1) to select and guide treatment and (2) to facilitate research. In medical science, classifications are employed as a means of identifying diseases. For historically documented reasons, the classification of unwanted conduct has followed the patterns laid down by medical science for classifying organic disease. In regard to treatment, there are marked differences in the goals of treatment of measles and treatment for unwanted conduct (such as phobias). For measles, the ministrations of the doctor are in the service of providing a *cure*. For the person seeking help to control unwanted conduct, "cure" may be a less apt term than one that describes helping an individual to achieve his or her purposes in ways that are less objectionable to relevant others or more acceptable to oneself.

Medical research also explores the causes and treatments of diseases. Knowledge of treatment efficacy depends on research. However, in order to conduct research, particular instances must be located in classes in order to process data from a collection of similar cases. The literature of psychiatry and clinical psychology is replete with research reports that are indeterminate because traditional classification by "disorders," which, like diseases, are categories based on "symptoms," has not been sufficiently reliable nor valid.

If we add to treatment another purpose of classification, prevention, then examining the contexts that influence persons to engage in unacceptable conduct will influence the choice of categories for distinguishing among kinds of unwanted behavior. Such a move in the purpose of classification would require abrogating pretensions to being "objective" and value-free. The problem with the value commitments that attend the notion of "disease" is not that they are value commitments, for example, that the patient is not responsible for behavior "caused" by some internal happening. Any intervention into the life of another person engages a value commitment. The problem rather is that practices based on the notion of "disease" or "disorder" follow from the profession's commitment to a counterproductive set of values that positions the person as without agency.

III. THE TRADITIONAL APPROACH TO CLASSIFICATION

To write about nontraditional ways of classifying persons whose conduct fails to meet contemporary standards of propriety requires that we first lay out the boundaries of traditional classification systems the better to show contrasting features. We take as the prime exemplar of traditional classification systems the *Diagnostic and Statistical Manual of Mental Disorders*, Fourth Edition, published by the American Psychiatric Association, with the most recent edition (hereinafter referred to as *DSM-IV*) published in 1994. *DSM-IV* provides a detailed nosology, a critical analysis of which opens the door to an understanding of the underlying worldview that guides the practice of classifying deviant conduct. The claimed purpose of the nosology is to provide a means of establishing reliable diagnoses. [*See* DSM-IV.]

A. The Mechanistic Conception of Unwanted Conduct

The history of science makes clear that the mid-nineteenth century witnessed tremendous progress in the science of biology. This progress was directly related to the mechanization of biology. All biological phenomena were to be explained in terms of the mechanistic transmission of physical and chemical forces. Scientific explorations sought principles that were invariant. During this period medical doctors took on the task of explaining abnormal behavior by extrapolating from the findings of the rapidly developing field of neuropathology. The context for this development was the surface resemblance of symptoms of neuropathology to unwanted conduct for which no neuropathology could be found. During this period Emil Kraepelin formulated his initial classification of psychiatric diseases, a classification that assumed all abnormal behavior to be related to organic causes, even in the absence of organic signs and symptoms. "Organic" and "functional" were the terms of convenience to identify whether or not neuropathology was demonstrable. The remote influence of the ideology that influenced Kraepelin's formulations can be deduced from the explicit claim in *DSM-IV* that "nonorganic" mental disorders have a biological basis.

The mechanistic framework inherited from Kraepelin creates serious problems for professionals engaged in the therapeutic enterprise. First, *DSM-IV* continues to manifest only marginal reliability, in spite of Herculean efforts by its creators. Second, the validity of the categories all too often fails traditional scientific tests and settles for negotiation and consensus among professionals. And third, the tendency to expand both the number of diagnoses, as well as the number of criteria, yields a continuing expansion of the category "mental disorder" into what might, from a less mechanistic point of view, be seen as the necessary travails and tragedies of everyday life. (The first *Manual*, published in 1952, listed 106 categories. *DSM-IV* lists 357 diagnostic categories.)

Beginning with the question of reliability, it has

been convincingly demonstrated that the accumulation of more categories and more criteria adds only marginally to the reliability of diagnostic practice. The self-advertised theoretically neutral "descriptive" character of diagnostic language may minimize unproved explanatory hypotheses, but it can yield no more agreement among practitioners than the language it uses to describe persons or behavior. For example, the stipulation that something must have been present for "at least 6 months" offers precision in a fairly trivial way compared to the difficulties of reliably assessing whether a set of actions is "disabling" or "not disabling." No behavior exists as simply disabling or not disabling, independent of the social and psychological context, most of which is beyond the specifiable stipulations of diagnostic manuals.

Marginal reliabilities compromise research by including in samples persons whose conduct is heterogeneous but who are lumped together into diagnostic categories. More serious is the questionable validity of diagnostic categories in the course of selecting treatment programs. Traditional classification manuals fail to deal with the question of whether a "mental disorder" exists apart from a culturally specific context—whether, in other words, the label for a disorder names a part of nature that is independent of the social constructions of clinicians and the authors of diagnostic manuals. The controversy of a quarter century ago, whether homosexuality is a "disorder," is not an exception in its clear dependency on normative judgments and negotiations that occur in a historical and cultural context. Most unacceptable conduct, even if reliably identified, is "disordered" only in terms of a culturally relative standard. Cross-cultural research has shown no consistency across cultures in the use of traditional diagnostic categories, for example, "schizophrenia." It is unclear whether this lack of consistency indicates different social constructions by clinicians or different causal antecedents. Professionals are not justified in construing that the meaning of a set of behaviors in one culture is the same in another culture, in the same way that diabetes in one culture is the same in other cultures. [See MYTH OF MENTAL ILLNESS.]

Finally, in addition to the expansive and fluid character of the catalogue of disorder through its five editions, the *Manuals*' tendency to medicalize all human discomfort inspires even more questionable logic. The latest such version is the creation of "shadow syn-

dromes," which are formulated to legitimate treatment for persons whose conduct fulfills only some of the *Manual*'s criteria for a disorder. Extrapolating from the proliferation of diagnostic entities over the various editions of the *Manual,* one might predict that through the typical negotiation process of the experts, some of these syndromes will come out of the shadows and enter the next version of the *Manual* as certified "disorders."

IV. THE CONTEXTUALIST CONSTRUCTION OF DEVIANT CONDUCT

But there are practitioners and scholars who operate from a different worldview, namely, contextualism—a worldview the root metaphor of which is the historical act in all its complexity. Novelty and change are features of this alternative worldview that provides the foundation for a nontraditional approach to the classification of intentional actions. Historical acts are engaged in by people. Further, historical acts are narrated, told as accounts, anecdotes, and stories in which men and women make choices to resolve their everyday problems of living. Because contextualists construct the world in terms of historical actions, they look for *reasons* for such actions, unlike the mechanistically inclined clinician who would look for *causes*.

The contextualist worldview directs us to see human beings not only as biological specimens, but as agents, as doers, as performers and problem solvers. In so doing, we are perforce obliged to develop understandings of how human beings employ narrative structure to shape their life histories.

A. Happenings and Doings

Completely overlooked in the constructions of traditional psychiatric classification is a simple distinction, that of *happenings* and *doings*. Examples of happenings are ruptured spinal discs, toothaches, brain tumors, and carcinoma. Such happenings are attributable to causes, empirically established or hypothesized. As exemplified in *DSM-IV,* abnormal actions are caused by happenings—the transmission of forces in the brain or in the metaphorical mind. Neurotransmitters, phrenological bulges, chemical anomalies have been sought as the causes of abnormal behavior. The diagnostic drama guided by traditional classification has no room for the client as agent, as doer, as capable of intentional action.

On the other hand, doings are the agential, intentional, purposeful actions of persons attempting to participate in a drama based on their self-defining narratives. Slapping a child, seeking a mystical experience, declaring that one is host to multiple personalities, avoiding a confrontation, are examples of doings, of actions.

The distinction between happenings and doings is helpful in understanding how the traditional diagnostic system and its vocabulary of symptoms has contributed to the medicalization of distress. In the absence of a strong competitor, the language of the medical model was embraced by neighboring professions to describe unwanted conduct. To refer to an action as a "symptom" is to adopt a special linguistic system. The use of "symptom" carries the implication "symptom of something." The "something" is a happening that is the presumed *cause* of the symptom—in traditional medicine, a microbe, a tumor, a morphological anomaly, a toxin, a chemical imbalance, and so on.

The application of the mechanistic worldview with its emphasis on causal happenings has worked well in organic medicine. A perusal of *DSM-IV* makes clear that the model was adopted in its entirety by modern biological psychiatry. The *Manual* is explicit in proclaiming that the diagnosis and treatment of "mental disorders" belong to the domain of medical practice.

Classifications of any kind must follow from some articulated theory. Although the authors of *DSM-IV* claim to being atheoretical, it is apparent that the claim is a veiled cover for a weakly defined theoretical system that is reminiscent of Kraepelin's mechanistic framework, that is, that all deviant conduct is caused by anomalies in organic systems. On this framework, *DSM-IV* fails because of the large proportion of cases for which no biochemical or other organic substrate can be found.

B. Unwanted Conduct

We employ "unwanted conduct" rather than "psychopathology" to emphasize the moral judgmental component of diagnosis. Every society creates procedures and practices for marginalizing persons whose public actions fail to meet propriety norms. Beginning in the mid-nineteenth century, the responsibility for controlling such marginalized persons was assigned to physicians practicing in institutions variously named mad houses, lunatic asylums, and mental hospitals. The criteria for detention included atypical imaginings ("hallucinations"), nonconforming beliefs ("delusions"), and incomprehensible or absurd gestural or speech behavior. Behind these criteria were implicit premises about maintaining public order. Authority figures (parents, police, magistrates, and doctors) made the initial judgment whether any particular item of conduct was to be classified as unwanted. Those whose nonconforming behavior was under scrutiny were labeled as mad, insane, lunatic, crazy, and more recently, mentally ill.

In the twentieth century, the scope of psychiatric practice included diagnosing and treating men and women who were self-referred. Not regarded as mad or insane, such self-referred patients sought help from medical doctors on the belief that they were suffering from ill-defined but nonetheless genuine "nervous" ailments. Hysteria was the diagnostic label employed to denote a wide variety of such "nervous" conditions. In due course, clinicians sorted the presenting complaints into a number of classes identified by labels derived from Greek or Latin roots, such as neurasthenia, psychasthenia, anxiety, hypochondriasis, and depression. These terms sometimes reflected unwanted "feelings." Persons seeking help for dealing with unwanted "feelings" would verbalize their complaints with vague and ambiguous expressions, such as "I am anxious," "I am depressed," "I can't concentrate," "I'm sitting on a volcano." Taken together, these complaints are subsumed under the general medical term "dysphoria."

Clinicians who subscribe to the medical model regard dysphoric complaints as symptomatic of a bodily dysfunction. It has become common practice among physicians to prescribe medications to reduce the extent of the dysphoria by altering the body chemistry. A radically different approach would be taken by contextualist clinicians who are sensitive to the notion that distress follows from the failure of strategic actions to solve problems of living. The self-reports of distress that are expressed in the language of "feelings" are construed as the patient's sense-making of proprioceptive and interoceptive changes associated with failed strategies to solve existential or identity problems. Contextualist clinicians direct their attention to the *reasons* for the unresolved strains-in-knowing rather than to reports of "feelings" that are adjuncts to personal problem solving. Their focus is on understanding the antecedents of the unsatisfactory attempts at problem solving, or expanding the library of plots for interpreting distress, and on the exploration of alternative strategies for maintaining an acceptable self-narrative.

V. ASSUMPTIONS AND ALTERNATIVES

The difficulties with traditional methods of diagnosis can be specified in terms of four assumptions routinely built into diagnostic manuals (1) internality; (2) physicality; (3) individuality; and (4) the value judgments accompanying the concept of disease. For each of the assumptions undergirding traditional modes of classification, we propose an alternative assumption that is consistent with the contextualist perspective.

A. Internality

The current system envisions each abnormal psychological condition to be a malfunction generated from within the person. In a given situation, one person may behave in accordance with common sense expectations while another may not. The latter will be labeled abnormal, deviant, disordered, disturbed, and so on. The difference between the two cases does not come from the social context that traditional diagnosticians assume to be the same for both. What is taken to produce acceptable conduct from one and unwanted conduct from the other are processes internal to the person.

The most elemental of diagnostic decisions, for example, that of orientation to time, place, and person, depends on this diagnostic procedure borrowed from the standard neurological examination. Like that examination, what is being assessed is assumed to be inside the person. More elaborate diagnostic judgments, such as deciding between "depression" identified as a disease, and "mourning a death in the family," which is not so identified, depend, for example, on sadness in the absence of mourning. Such a judgment influences the traditional clinician to locate the cause of the phenomenon inside the body rather than externally, in human relationships.

It is clear that most human behavior is oriented to concrete immediate situations. Human behavior is jointly produced not only by a person and a situation, but each of these factors also responds to the other over time to create a dialectical whole, such as a relationship. When a relationship contextualizes a behavior, as is always true even in diagnosis, the meanings of any behavior must take into account the dialectical determinants. The complex of avoidant actions identified by the label "agoraphobia," for example, does not exist inside the person. The actions are ways of coping with situations that have developed over time. Nontraditional approaches that depart from the disease model begin with the individual's history of trying various ways to cope with his or her environment. Traditional diagnosis underplays the agential character of human behavior because "diseases" are ordinarily understood to be happenings that take place inside the person.

B. Physicality

The traditional diagnostic system construes a person as a complex biological machine the controlling mechanisms of which are the neurochemical patterns of the brain. Information processing is seen as the central function of the brain, a conception that extends from neural transmissions to perceptions of the environment. This information is selected for its relevance to a given stimulus situation. Such selection is not always without error. The result of acting on mistaken perceptions is conduct that may violate social norms, leading to a psychiatric diagnosis.

Observing a person confounding imaginings, rememberings, and current perceptions, a clinician would invoke the diagnostic label "hallucinating schizophrenic." Or, observing a person confounding irrelevant sad feelings with nonpresent situations, the clinician might entertain the diagnosis "depression." In these instances, information appears to be scrambled, and there is a strong presumption that the brain, as the organ of information processing, is malfunctioning and the unwanted behaviors are thus believed to be caused by chemical imbalances in the brain.

Information, however, is not merely physical. To be sure, information can be reduced to a "signal" that can be described in the vocabulary of physics, but the signal never embodies meaning. In this sense, meaning is not physical but is constructed—the achievement of human beings who have acquired linguistic and epistemic skills. To sustain the premise that abnormal behavior is the product of exclusively physical processes would be like saying that the science of acoustics can reveal to us the meanings carried by human speech. The concepts and theory of sound waves and temporal patterns can tell us about human speech in their own terms, and that is hardly trivial. But scientists who do such work make no claims that their instruments can tell us anything about the meanings of words and sentences, the logic of theory, or the motives of actors who try to communicate with one another. To extend physical science into realms of meanings and motives is to claim too much. It is to persevere in a metaphysical belief that the only reality is the reality of the physical world, a belief that ignores the arguments and demonstrations that realities are social constructions.

C. Individuality

The current system envisions abnormal psychiatric conditions as affecting encapsulated individuals. While cultural differences in the incidence of unwanted conduct are well known, and some patterns of behavior are culturally specific, as anorexia is to modern industrially advanced cultures, the goals of treatment, as well as the interpretation of the problem, rarely extend beyond the distressed individual. Although the stresses of poverty, for example, may increase the incidence of many abnormal conditions, current practice assumes that abnormal behavior happens to individuals independent of social contexts. To take more seriously conditions such as poverty, and to make them medically relevant, one can of course add a note to the diagnostic statement, codified as the marginally salient Axis IV in *DSM-IV*. An impartial examination of demographic data of persons diagnosed as psychopathological would suggest that the mental health professions should advocate as therapeutically relevant such conditions as full employment, adequate welfare safety nets, and a livable minimum wage. But this practice is marginal exactly because taking it seriously would require economic, political, and governmental intervention rather than psychiatric or psychological attention. The entry of the treatment professions into politics would undermine the value-free pretenses of the diagnostic system. Such political involvement, especially since it pretends to be scientific rather than political, runs many risks already revealed to us in the awkwardness of courts of law where psychiatric (diagnostic) testimony becomes a part of society's decision

to blame wrongdoers—or to excuse them. The risks already incurred by our diagnostic pretenses to scientific accuracy could stretch wildly the current legitimacy of the treatment professions. There is, of course, no simple solution to these problems, but it is clear they are made much worse by the notion of discrete diseases, some of which traditionally supply an excuse, others of which do not.

Empirically demonstrable is the fact that such socioeconomic variables as poverty can be relevant to diagnosis, a fact that cannot be acknowledged so long as mental illness is seen as an individualistic phenomenon. Behavior that has traditionally been labeled mental illness is hardly a private matter analogous to such patently medical conditions as diabetes or cancer where internality and physicality are demonstrable.

D. Value Judgments Accompanying the Concept of Disease

The current system envisions mental illnesses, like other illnesses, as conditions to be eliminated. Diseases, in our current understanding, rarely have value and meaning beyond that of deserving the most concerted efforts to eliminate them. The more internal, physical, and individual the diagnostic concepts and procedures, the less are abnormal actions perceived as addressing some aspect of a person's effort to position himself or herself in the world of social norms and moral expectations. An individual's complaints of depression and anxiety are not valued for their indexing a struggle with a personal decision or with a moral dilemma. They are merely "symptoms" that, when sufficiently aggregated, indicate a disease, and a disease is to be cured.

Just as the elimination of pain by analgesic drugs may mask a bodily ailment, so may the elimination of anxious or depressed behaviors mask a moral crisis. Furthermore, the individual diagnosed may, on the authority of the mechanistically oriented professional, misinterpret his or her own life narrative as internal happenings. Beyond that, the profession might address the possibilities for preventive measures. It can of course be argued that such a "public health" approach in psychiatry may have to pretend to know with some precision the societal and family conditions that engender contranormative behavior. The parameters of the ideal family or neighborhood or school have yet to be spelled out. The prevailing practice of dealing with instances of human distress as "diseases" removes from the profession any pressure to allocate research resources to filling gaps in knowledge necessary for implementing prevention programs.

VI. DIAGNOSING WITHIN A CONTEXTUALIST FRAMEWORK

A. Early Efforts to Construct a Contextualist Framework

The diagnostic procedures based on Kraepelinian doctrine have been the subject of earlier critical works. During the first four decades of the twentieth century, the Swiss-American psychiatrist, Adolf Meyer, promoted a contextualist view of unwanted conduct. He rejected the idea that the causes of deviant conduct would be discovered with advanced anatomical and histological technology. Instead, he urged his colleagues and students to attend to the whole person in his or her social and cultural milieu. His focus was not on purported biological happenings but on the person's ineptitude in adjusting to his or her life circumstances.

The history of the first half of the twentieth century credits Meyer's contextual approach with having a widespread impact on the direction of American psychiatry. A number of well-known texts promoted Meyer's contextualist views. These texts made use of formulations drawn from the social sciences and the humanities, among them discourse analysis, role-taking, socialization, learning theory, pseudocommunity, overinclusion, and so on.

Meyer's approach had a positive impact on the development of American psychiatry, but his contextualism faded into obscurity when the psychiatric profession enthusiastically adopted psychoanalysis as its quasi-official theory. The displacement of Meyer's contextualist framework by psychoanalytic doctrine may be attributed to the fact that the hydraulic model advanced by Freud was consistent with the mechanistic perspective that was already entrenched in the medical sciences. In addition, Meyer, unlike Freud, had no self-proclaimed disciples, no professional institutes to promote his contextualist formulations, and no organized corpus of writings.

More recent challenges to the validity of the Kraepelinian-inspired *DSM-IV* have been made in critical works by scholars working from contextualist behaviorism and from social psychological orientations.

B. The Narrative Framework

The contextualist model sensitizes the clinician to focus on the master question: "what is the client or patient *trying to do?*" Answers to this question will inevitably be in the form of a narrative that includes the parts played by other actors in the client's drama. The constructed narrative provides clues for a diagnosis in terms of the class of strategic actions employed. The clinician's answer to the master question satisfies the original purpose of diagnosis—namely, to guide the therapist and the client in developing a treatment plan.

Classification for purposes of scientific research should consider the narrative context within which a distressed person is trying to do something. Also relevant to scientific classification is the issue of how the client's narrative fits or fails to fit into the narratives of the client's family, social group, or subculture. Sorting cases into categories to explore differences and similarities requires attention to crucial attributes, including meanings, of the behavior itself. Science cannot ignore these narrative meanings and contexts in deciding whether cases are similar or different.

Unwanted behavior, then, is performed by agents whose purposes are crucial, even if such purposes may not be clear to relevant others or to the agents themselves. The talk, actions, and expressions of feelings that are the results of failed strategies to fulfill the requirements of an ongoing self-narrative are the raw data from which the clinician formulates a diagnosis. This alternative approach assumes that the narrative context must be understood if the puzzling behavior is to be understood. The narrative that guides a particular failed effort must be specified, as well as the fit or lack of fit, between such a narrative and the larger narratives of the social context. Usually, there is a lack of fit, which appears as a violation of norms and values held by social groups and codified in cultural traditions.

The narratives that fit these traditions may be referred to as "conventional," and those that do not, as "unconventional." Those people whose behavior issues from a life-narrative that is incomprehensible or grossly nonconforming become candidates for psychiatric diagnosis. These are not people without self-narratives; they are people with unconventional narratives, and/or an unwillingness to disclose them. For example, it is not comprehensible to most of us how someone might seriously suspect a man's unconventional narrative in which he identifies himself as Jesus Christ. In the case of such a client who is apparently convinced of the authenticity of his claims, diagnosticians have no way to understand this conviction and this narrative except to construct the inference: "the man is psychotic." The logic of that inference is consistent with *DSM-IV* criteria that qualifies the client's claim as a delusion and as sufficiently "bizarre" to assign the diagnosis of schizophrenia (if the belief had been held for 6 months or more). [*See* SCHIZOPHRENIA.]

While this diagnostic term ought scientifically be seen as a *description* of the patient's conviction, it is usually taken as an *explanation*. This elision of description to explanation is one of the outcomes of employing the disease model. It renders unnecessary any understanding of the narrative as a context for unwanted conduct, or understanding the social or moral circumstances that provided the context for the particular narrative. The illicit shift from description to explanation is in great measure responsible for the standard professional practice of ignoring the patient's life story.

However, it is important to note that not all behavior that is subject to professional diagnosis is merely an unconventional narrative. In a case of homicide, a truck driver strangled his wife in the heat of an argument in which she declared she had been unfaithful and was about to leave him for her lover. This threat not only confirmed his prior suspicions, it enraged the client. "I couldn't control myself, I was so mad. The anger inside me had to come out. I exploded." While this case is not one of clinical diagnosis for purposes of treatment, it is one of legal diagnosis for purposes of adjudication. To call him "insane" at the time of the murder would be to say that his behavior was caused by stimuli the provocative power of which controlled his behavior. He himself was helpless, the argument would go (and has gone); his being an agent of his actions would not be considered a factor.

At the same time, we recognize that the man was following a well-known and not unpopular narrative plot of "punishing an unfaithful wife." The narrative does not excuse his behavior, but it makes it intelligible. It collects those circumstantial factors together in a way that, in fact, is how we understand his behavior. It bears on why he did it, when we understand the "why" as searching for reasons, rather than causes.

This kind of contextual understanding does not resolve the question of whether or to what degree the man should be excused for his actions. It certainly avoids the possibility that the extreme behavior was caused by a diagnosable disease. And yet such contextual understanding is absolutely essential in order to understand the action, which, given the circumstances and the stock of cultural narratives about unfaithful wives and angry husbands, is quite easy to understand. This understanding addresses the question of what this man was trying to do. It opens up a psychological investigation of his strategic actions, given a particularly vivid set of circumstances.

This case, like most behaviors that come to professional attention, deals with a struggle in which both social and moral questions abound—questions about what one is to do, who one is to be. Except for behavior that is casual or genuinely accidental, human beings behave in such a way as to work toward achieving their goals, one of which is to be a certain kind of person. Was the truck driver to perceive himself as a cuckold? Was he to perceive himself as a failure in not controlling his wife? He not only wanted to punish her, but also likely wanted to persuade her, and he certainly did not want his manhood challenged.

These themes are congruent with common narratives in certain pockets of society, and they are not without influence. Grasping such meanings is what clinicians must do in order to have any intelligent grasp of clients' conduct. Such interpretive psychological work certainly does not suggest that a disease was the proximate cause of a death, as traditional diagnostic thought could imply. Finding a basis for such interpretive work is the point of the alternative model to which we now turn.

C. Strategic Actions

As an alternative construction to the implicit theory underlying *DSM-IV*—that unwanted conduct is caused by anomalous happenings in the biological machinery—the contextual construction takes its point of departure from the premise that people are agents. They are performers, actors, doers, discourse partners. This premise turns attention to a person's actions, not to postulated happenings in the brain or in the metaphorical mind. The actions of interest are in the service of resolving strain-in-knowing, particularly those actions that give rise to self-judgments or to other-declarations that such actions are unwanted. Strain-in-knowing is a response to conditions that interfere with the continuity of the person's self narrative. These are the conditions that are ordinarily subsumed under the heading of emotional life.

Strain-in-knowing occurs when there is a discrepancy between the demands of emotional life and the actor's current constructions (beliefs and values). An alternate way of formulating strain-in-knowing is the expenditure of effort to locate or position oneself in relation to the world of occurrences. Sometimes identified as anxiety, disequilibrium, threat, or unassimilated input, the center of the concept is "I have a problem."

The implicit and explicit behaviors intended to resolve strain-in-knowing may be called "strategic action." Often intelligible to the actor, strategic actions are not necessarily intelligible to others, for only the actor is the potential beneficiary. In cases we call abnormal, such strategic actions may become habitual and automatic, a condition that makes it difficult for actors to explain their conduct in ways that are intelligible to others. Strategic actions to resolve strain-in-knowing may appear to others as obscure or meaningless, or as potentially dangerous or embarrassing.

It is important to add a disclaimer that strain-in-knowing is not a passive phenomenon taking place in the metaphorical mind. The multifarious behaviors that are traditionally regarded as abnormal or incomprehensible may be parsimoniously classified as phases in the construction of a self-narrative. Whether successful or not, strategic actions in the service of resolving strain-in-knowing become a part of the lived narrative.

We present herewith a brief sketch of a model that derives from various contextualist frameworks. The model returns personal agency to the matrix of constructions that are employed to understand human action. The central feature of the model is a list of "strategic actions" that can serve as the scaffolding for a contextualist classification system. Strategic actions may be classified as follows:

- instrumental acts (including rituals);
- tranquilizing and tension-releasing acts;
- attention deployment acts;
- acts to change beliefs and values;
- nonaction.

These classes of strategic actions are connected to antecedent events and subsequent effects, the latter having a feedback function. Strategic actions are employed to neutralize strain-in-knowing. Any particular strategic act has two potential effects: the first, if successful in satisfying the intentions of the actor, would eliminate or modify the perceived source of strain, the second would provide a relevant audience with opportunities to give warrants of social validation or invalidation for the particular strategic action. In this model, the persons and institutions that enforce values are part of the external world of occurrences. The moral judgments of others are inputs that must be instantiated, matched against the beliefs and values that make up the person's self-narrative.

The antecedent events to strain-in-knowing require no detailed analysis—the cognitive psychology of the 1960s and 1970s has given us a template. The world of occurrences may be sorted into discrete domains or ecologies: the self-maintenance domain, the time–space domain, the social domain, the moral domain, and the transcendental domain. Sensory inputs are also generated within the body, the proximal world of occurrences. Human beings (and other sentient organisms) try to match sensory inputs with their systems of knowledge. In problematic situations, the actor directs his or her efforts to the world of occurrences to gain confirming or disconfirming inputs. During the interval when no match is made, the condition of strain-in-knowing prevails. In short, the actor strives to match the inputs against a construction—a self-narrative—derived from his or her prior experience. Of special interest is the observation that efforts to find a match are not always successful.

The prototype for sense-making is the ethological concept of vigilance. When an animal, human or other, registers inputs through vision, hearing, olfaction, and so on, it tries to match the sensory inputs against its available constructions. In the primeval world, the construction might be represented by the question: Is the stimulus event to be instantiated as benign or hostile? The choice of subsequent actions follows from the type of instantiation.

The problems in living that are the starting places for both traditional and nontraditional professionals are in the social, moral, and transcendental domains.

Positioning oneself in these domains or ecologies involves mapping input against existing constructions, that is, against the beliefs and values that have become part of the actors' ongoing self-narratives. Any particular self-narrative is built up from answers to the social identity question: Who am I? to the moral identity question: What am I in relation to moral standards? and to the transcendental identity question: What am I in relation to such abstractions as God, the universe, departed ancestors, and so on. When inputs from the social, moral, or transcendental domains produce incompatible or conflicting answers to the identity question, the person experiences strain-in-knowing, a condition that involves *effort* to match inputs with existing constructions and/or to seek confirming or disconfirming inputs for putative matches. This is a proactive process. Effort involves physiological participation that produces interoceptive and proprioceptive inputs. These inputs feed back into the proximal world of occurrences, thus, the actor's task includes attending to the additional sensory inputs generated in efforts at sense-making.

The use of strategic actions is not exclusive to people in distress who are the clients and patients of mental health professionals. We are all strategists in order to deal with our everyday strains-in-knowing, in our need to make sense of the welter of inputs from the various domains. It is only when the strategies fail to resolve the strain and/or are not given warrants of validation by significant figures—parents, spouses, teachers, employers, doctors—that the person becomes a candidate for diagnosis and treatment.

Each class of actions has a target: *instrumental acts* are directed to the external world, to change the relations between the person and some aspect of the world of occurrences. Inputs from the social domain, for example, that cannot be matched to one's self-narrative lead to an unvoiced interpretation: my identity is at risk. The person may choose between the traditional fight-or-flight instrumentalities in their many attenuated forms. A particular instrumental act may reduce strain-in-knowing and simultaneously be validated (or invalidated) by persons who have the power to pass moral judgment. The alleged Oklahoma City bombers are said to have constructed a belief that "the government" was evil. They equated a federal building with "the government" and destroyed it. Other citizens engage in less extreme forms of instrumental action: they write letters to their senators or change

the relation to the distal domains by withdrawing from social relations, or becoming a hermit. *Ritual behavior* is included in the strategy of instrumental acts because it is mediated by the belief that, like direct action, rituals and ceremonials can influence the world of occurrences.

The *tranquilizing and releasing* strategy is directed toward changing bodily sensations that may be indirect effects of sense making efforts. Alcohol, drugs, sex, hot baths, cold showers, vigorous exercise, and the excitement of gambling are examples of the choices of actions that modify inputs from the internal ecology. The use of the strategy by itself does not certify that one is a candidate for a clinic or a sanitarium. The moral judgment of relevant others on the particular tranquilizing or releasing strategy is the act that identifies the strategy as acceptable or as not acceptable.

Examples of the strategy of *attention deployment* are the acts that are subsumed under such traditional labels as hypochondriasis, conversion reactions, and participation in imaginary worlds. The person's attentional resources focus on inputs other than those from the social and moral domains that are the usual antecedents to strain-in-knowing among humans. A common deployment is to attend to bodily sensations, thus avoiding critical inputs from the social world. A variant of the strategy of attention deployment is involved participation in an invented set of self-narratives, as in classic multiple personality.

Changing one's beliefs and values is a strategy directed to influencing the structure of knowledge. It is the strategy of choice for clinicians who work in the tradition of cognitive psychology. For example, a suicidal client holds the belief that suicide (an instrumental act) will solve his or her problems. The clinician takes on the task of modifying that belief. For example, a sample of women who held suicidal beliefs repudiated such belief following individual and group therapy, skills training, and other interventions. As with other strategies, change in beliefs may neutralize strain. When the person acts on the beliefs, or makes them public, the possibility exists for others to declare the beliefs good or bad. Persons who claim to have been abducted by extraterrestrial aliens, for example, are likely not to receive warrants of validation from most professionals.

The fifth category is labeled *nonaction*. The person may have tried the available strategies and they have not worked, either in the direct reduction of strain or in gaining social validation. Under these conditions, strain-in-knowing increases. Not succeeding in neutralizing strain, the person may strive to reduce involvement in the world, lest any actions may lead to inputs that would increase the strain. Traditional diagnosticians would scan the *DSM* categories for one of the 10 mood disorders, a procedure that would locate the individual's suffering as a happening.

In this connection, an alternative approach to "depressive disorders" should be mentioned. The nonaction of the so-called depressed person is interpretable as a subtle form of strategic action, the goal of which is to convince others that one is a helpless, hopeless, or worthless figure in a self-narrative. Specific kinds of "depressed" actions influence others to respond in specific ways. The "helpless" person, for example, calls out responses from others that are qualitatively different from the responses called out by persons who claim to be "hopeless."

This briefly sketched model is radically different from the medical model in that moral judgment is an acknowledged component. The appellation "unwanted conduct" and similar terms are moral judgments rendered either by relevant others or by self. This component is ordinarily omitted from psychiatric discourses that focus on hypothesized internal mechanisms only after the initial moral judgment has been rendered by relevant others or by self.

VII. CODA

The dominance of *DSM-IV* has clouded the fact that a variety of alternative approaches have been, from time to time, put forth for diagnosing psychological problems. These approaches have been eclipsed by the attempt to standardize procedures—an effort driven more by bureaucratic and insurance pressures than by scientific goals. In a historical and critical analysis of *DSM* some of these motivations have been laid bare. At century's end, the economic goals of the therapeutic professions continue to favor quick categorization of patients. A convincing argument has been made that the *DSMs* have evolved into instruments that serve bureaucratic and financial functions more fully than they do scientific ones. When critically examined the *DSM*'s claim to theoretical neutrality cannot be sustained. In fact, the *DSM* authors take pains not to conceal a strong biological bias. Critics have argued that the current dominance of *DSM* prematurely closes off scientific analysis. More specifically, the authors of *DSM* have failed to examine their underlying assumptions, particularly those embedded in their unarticulated theoretical structure and in their choice of root metaphors. Given the state of knowledge, it is premature to posit a theoretical structure that would support the notion of clearly delineated diseaselike entities. The root metaphor of mechanistic causal forces defines not only the clinical reality but human behavior in general, and it does so in a way that transforms historical actions of persons in identifiable sociocultural contexts into physicalistic happenings like infections and mechanical breakdowns that occur independent of human intentionality.

The narrowness of this perspective is obvious. It not only neglects most of the considerable advances made in social psychology and social anthropology in recent decades, it negates common sense views like those of Adolf Meyer half a century ago to be examined to construct systems for organizing the actions of people.

"Problems in living" are neither "mental" in any simple distinction from somatic, nor are they "disorders" in any obvious contrast to an order we can identify as natural. The intellectual resources available to the task of classifying people's problems in living are rich, varied, and often very much more precise and elaborate than the *DSMs*, but they have been neglected for reasons other than their scientific relevance to the task.

DSMs of the traditional kind are bound to become increasingly unworkable as the number of diagnoses approaches 500 and as the number of criteria approaches 2000. This development, together with the promulgation of critical inquiries that continue to illuminate the flaws in *DSM* systems, will direct professionals to entertain nontraditional theoretical premises. It is our belief that *DSM* systems will be replaced with systems based on the premise that human beings are agents that engage in intentional strategic actions to maintain their self-narratives. It is likely that scientists of the next century will look back at traditional *DSMs* with somewhat the same puzzlement that is now expressed about the claims of phrenology in the nineteenth century and the claims of lobotomists in the twentieth century.

ACKNOWLEDGMENT

We acknowledge with thanks critical readings of an earlier draft by Ralph M. Carney, James C. Mancuso, and Karl E. Scheibe.

BIBLIOGRAPHY

Berger, P. L., & Luckman, T. (1967). *The social construction of reality: A treatise on the sociology of knowledge.* Garden City, NY: Doubleday.

Borges, E. (1995). A social critique of biological psychiatry. In C. Ross & A. Pam, *Psychology, 64,* 1117–1119.

Follette, W. C., & Houts, A. C. (1996). Models of scientific progress and the role of theory in taxonomy development: A case study of the DSM. *Journal of Consulting and Clinical Psychology, 64,* 1120–1132.

Goffman, E. (1959). *The presentation of self in everyday life.* Garden City, NY: Doubleday.

Kirk, S. A., & Kutchins, H. (1992). *The selling of DSM: The rhetoric of science in psychiatry.* Hawthorne, NY: Walter deGruyter.

Kleinman, A. (1988). *Rethinking psychiatry: From cultural categories to personal experience.* New York: Free Press.

Lief, A. (Ed.). (1948). *The commonsense psychiatry of Adolf Meyer.* New York: McGraw-Hill.

Mirowski, J., & Ross, C. E. (1989). *The social causes of psychological distress.* New York: Aldine de Gruyter.

Sarbin, T. R. (1997). On the futility of psychiatric diagnostic manuals (DSMs) and the return of personal agency. *Applied and Preventive Psychology, 6,* 568–570.

Sarbin, T. R. (1977). Contextualism: A world view for modern psychology. In Landfield, A. (Ed.), *1976 Nebraska symposium on motivation.* Lincoln, NE: University of Nebraska Press.

Sarbin, T. R., & Keen, E. (1997). Sanity and Madness: Conventional and Unconventional Narratives of Emotional Life. In W. Flack & J. Laird (Eds.), *Emotions and psychopathology: Theory and research,* pp. 130–142. New York: Oxford University Press.

Wiener, M. (1989). Psychosocial transactional analysis of psychopathology: Depression as an exemplar. *Clinical Psychology Review, 9,* 295–321.

Clinical Assessment

Eileen Gambrill

University of California, Berkeley

Antecedents Events that immediately precede behavior and influence its frequency.

Behavior Any measurable or observable act or response. Behavior is defined broadly in some perspectives to include cognitions, feelings, and physiological reactions which, although they are not directly observable, are defined so that they can be measured.

Behavioral Approaches to understanding behavior in which learning histories and current environmental contingencies of reinforcement are emphasized. Behavioral approaches differ in the relative degree of attention devoted to thoughts and images.

Clinical Inference Assumptions about the causes of a problem.

Cognition Internal events such as thoughts (beliefs, self-statements, attributions) and images.

Consequences Events that follow behavior and influence its frequency.

Contingency The relationship between a behavior and the events that follow (consequences) and precede (antecedents) the behavior.

Diagnosis A label given to a client with particular characteristics that is assumed to reflect etiology and to have intervention implications.

DSM-IV Official classification system of mental disorders published by the American Psychiatric Association.

Psychodynamic Approaches to understanding behavior, in which unconscious mental and emotional processes (e.g., motives and conflicts) stemming from early childhood experiences are emphasized. Approaches differ in attention given to interpersonal processes, biological factors, and the cultural context.

Validity The extent to which a measure measures what it was designed to assess. There are many different kinds of validity (e.g., predictive, content, concurrent, construct).

CLINICAL ASSESSMENT involves the clarification of presenting problems and related factors including identification of outcomes that will be focused on. It should offer guidelines for selection of intervention methods.

Goals of assessment include describing clients, their problems and desired outcomes as well as their life situations, understanding why problems occur (inferring causes), deciding on what methods are most likely to achieve desired outcomes, and obtaining a base from which to evaluate progress. Assessment requires the search for and integration of data that are useful in deciding how to remove complaints. It involves (1) detecting client characteristics and environmental factors related to problems; (2) integrating and interpreting data collected; and (3) selecting outcomes to focus on. It should indicate what situational, biological, or psychological factors influence options, create demands, or cause discomfort. Decisions must be made about *what* data to collect, *how* to gather this, and *how* to organize it. Assessment should indicate the specific outcomes related to complaints, what would have to be done to achieve these outcomes, how these could most effectively be pursued, and the potential of attaining them.

The assessment methods that are used differ because of differences in theoretical perspectives which influence the kind of data collected as well as the uses and functions of these data. Clinical inferences vary in how closely they are tied to concrete evidence. Carrying out an assessment is like unraveling a puzzle or locating the pieces of the puzzle. Certain pieces of the puzzle are sought rather than others depending on the clinician's theoretical orientation and knowledge, and puzzle completion may be declared at diverse points. Issues of practicality also arise. The aim of all methods is to yield data that are useful, reliable, and valid. Specialized knowledge may be required and critical thinking skills are needed to weigh the value of evidence and examine the soundness of assumptions. Although decisions must typically be made on the basis of incomplete data, without a sound assessment framework, opportunities to gather useful data may be lost and ineffective or harmful plans may be suggested. Data should be gathered that are of value in helping clients. Collecting irrelevant data wastes time and money and increases the likelihood of incorrect decisions. Assessment should offer clients more helpful views of problems and a more helpful vocabulary for describing problems and options.

There is general agreement that an individualized assessment should be conducted which considers cultural differences. This does not mean that this is indeed done and practice perspectives differ in what is focused on. Individualized assessment avoids the patient uniformity myth in which clients (or families, or groups) are mistakenly assumed to be similar. Behavior consists of different response systems, which may or may not be related depending on the unique history of each individual: (1) overt behavior (for example, avoidance of crowds) and verbal reports (verbal descriptions of anxiety); (2) cognitions (thoughts about crowds); (3) physiological reactions (for example, increased heart rate when in crowds). Each person may have a different pattern of responses in a situation. Only through an individualized assessment can these unique patterns and related situations be discovered. Suicidal potential should be assessed as relevant. Recognizing the signs of pathology is important anytime this would be helpful in understanding what can be accomplished and how it can be accomplished. A clear agreement between clinicians and clients about the focus of helping efforts increases the likelihood that intervention will focus on outcomes that are of concern to clients.

I. THE GUIDING ROLE OF PRACTICE THEORIES

How problems are structured is a key part of clinical decision-making. Assessment frameworks differ in what is focused on, the kinds of assessment methods used, and how closely assessment is tied to selection of intervention methods. Preferred practice theories influence what clinicians look for and what they notice as well as how they process and organize data collected. Practice theories favored influence beliefs about what can be and is known about behavior and how knowledge can be developed. Dimensions along which theories differ include the following:

- Unit of concern (individual, family, community)
- Goals pursued (e.g., explanation and interpretation alone or understanding based on prediction and influence)
- Clarity of goals pursued
- Criteria used to evaluate the accuracy of explanations (e.g., consensus, authority, scientific)
- Range of problems addressed with success
- Causal importance attributed to feelings, thoughts, and/or environmental factors
- Range of environmental characteristics considered (family, community, society)
- Causal importance attributed to biochemical causes
- Attention devoted to past experiences
- Degree of optimism about how much change is possible
- Degree to which a perspective lends itself to and encourages empirical inquiry (finding out whether it is accurate)
- Degree of empirical support (evidence for and against a theory)
- Attention given to documenting degree of progress
- Ease with which practice guidelines can be developed
- Degree of parsimony

Practice frameworks differ in the value given to observation of interactions in real-life settings, in whether significant others are involved in assessment, and how directive clinicians are. They differ in degree of attention paid to cognitions (thoughts), feelings, environmental characteristics (such as reactions of significant others), genetic causes, and/or physiological causes. Different frameworks are based on different beliefs about the causes of behavior. Beliefs about behavior, thoughts, and feelings, and how they are maintained and can be changed influence what data are gathered and how data are weighted and organized. History shows that beliefs can be misleading. For example, trying to assess people by examining the bumps on their head was not very fruitful. However, for decades many people believed that this method was useful.

Problems can be viewed from a perspective of psychological deficiencies or from a broad view in which both personal and environmental factors are attended to. For example, a key point of feminist counseling is helping clients to understand the effects of the political on the personal, both past and present. Frameworks that focus on psychological characteristics are based on the view that behavior is controlled mainly by characteristics of the individual. In interactional perspectives, attention is given not only to the individual but to people with whom he or she interacts. The unit of analysis is the relationship between environmental events and psychological factors. It is assumed that both personal and environmental factors influence behavior. Interactional views differ in how reciprocal the relationship between the individual and the environment is believed to be and in the range of environmental events considered. In contextual, ecological perspectives, individual, family, community, and societal characteristics are considered as they may relate to problems and possible resolutions. A contextual framework decreases the likelihood of focusing on individual pathology (blaming the victim), and neglecting environmental causes and resources. Practice perspectives that focus on individual causes of personal problems may result in "psychologizing" rather than helping clients. Assessment frameworks differ in the extent to which they take advantage of what is known about behavior, factors related to certain kinds of problems, and the accuracy of different sources of data.

Forming a new conceptualization of presenting problems, one that is shared by both the clinician and the client that will be helpful in resolving problems is an integral aspect of assessment. The kind of conceptualization suggested will depend on the theoretical orientation of the clinician. It is important to arrive at a common view of the problem, as well as agreement as to what will be done to change it. This common view is a motivating factor in that, if clients accept it and if it makes sense to clients, there will be a greater willingness to try out procedures that flow from this account. Mutually agreed-on views are fostered in a variety of ways, including questions asked, assessment procedures used, and rationales offered. Focused summaries help to pull material together within a new framework. Identifying similar themes among seemingly disparate events can be used to suggest alternative views.

II. SIGN AND SAMPLE APPROACHES

Traditional assessment is based on a sign approach in which observed behaviors are viewed as indicators of more important underlying (and unobserved) personality dispositions (typically of a pathological nature) or traits. Traits can be defined as a general and personally determined tendency to react in consistent and stable ways. Examples are "aggression" and "extraversion." Inherent in sign approaches such as psychoanalytic approaches is the assumption that observable behavioral problems are only the outward signs of some underlying process, which must be altered to bring about any lasting change. A focus of change efforts on the behavior itself, according to this model, would not succeed, because no change has supposedly been brought about in underlying causative factors. A clinician may conclude that a child who has difficulty concentrating on his school work and sitting in his seat is hyperactive. The observed behaviors are viewed as a sign of an underlying disorder. The underlying hypothetical constructs are viewed as of major importance in understanding and predicting behavior. Dispositional attributions shift attention away from observing what people *do* in specific situations to speculating about what they *have*. Inconsistencies in behavior across situations are not unexpected within this approach because it is assumed that underlying motives, conflicts, wishes may be behaviorally manifested in many different ways.

The interactions between wishes, the threats anticipated if wishes are expressed, and the processes used to cope with or defend against conflictual situations are of interest in psychodynamic frameworks. Important elements in such processes are believed to be beyond conscious recognition of the individual experiencing them even when they may be recognized or inferred by others. The concepts of "positions" (developmental stages) and "mechanisms" (psychological processes such as defense mechanisms) are central concepts. Defensive aims, processes, and outcomes are of interest. Defense mechanisms include suppression, undoing, repression, role reversal, projection, and regression. The defenses are believed to be heightened under conditions of high emotion, stress, and conflict. Motives include the wish to avoid unpleasant, overwhelming, or out-of-control states. Some unconscious processes anticipate such outcomes. Classification of phenomena is in terms of deflections from volitional consciousness and rationally intended actions: as intrusions and omissions. For example, recurrent dysfunctional alterations in self-esteem and interpersonal behavior (such as those seen in the personality disorders) are viewed as involving both intrusive, inappropriate schemas and omissions of realistic learning of new schemas. It is assumed that the "dynamic unconscious" constantly undergoes symbolic changes which in turn affect feelings and behavior. Other aspects of psychoanalytic approaches include an emphasis on verbal reports concerning early histories and efforts to alter inner processes by verbal means. Compared to behavioral assessment, less attention is devoted to environmental variables that may influence behavior because of the assumed core relevance and stability of underlying dispositions. [*See* DEFENSE MECHANISMS.]

There are many different kinds of psychodynamic assessment frameworks. For example, there are variants of object relations theory, each of which may have a somewhat different approach to assessment. The nature of a client's past interactions with their parents is viewed as central. However, there are differences in what is focused on by clinicians of different psychodynamic persuasions. In object relations theory, the concepts of mirroring and self objects are key ones. Attention is given to internal mental representations of the self and significant others. It is assumed that how we feel about ourselves and act toward others is a reflection of internal relationships based on experience. The term "object relations" refers to the interplay between the images of self and others. This interplay results in wishes, impulses, thoughts, and feelings of power

(or its lack). Ego psychology emphasizes identification and support of strengths and working within the "defenses" rather than breaking them down. Proponents consider resistance to change natural and work with and support adaptive strengths. Defense mechanisms, such as rationalization of actions and projection of feelings onto others are identified but not necessarily discussed.

Behavioral assessment involves a sample approach. In a sample approach, direct observation of behavior in real life settings (or, if this is not possible, in situations that resemble these) is valued. A behavioral approach is based on an interactional view in which it is assumed that behavior is a function of both organismic variables (genetic history and physiological states) and the environment. Labels are used as summarizing categories rather than as terms indicating some underlying characteristic (usually a disorder). Unlike in sign approaches where the cause of behavior is assumed to be underlying dispositions, the cause of behavior is assumed to lie largely in environmental differences. Behavioral frameworks differ in the relative amount of attention devoted to thoughts and environmental contingencies. Differences in focus are so marked that they have resulted to the formation of different journals and societies. Differences in emphasis are related to the role attributed to thoughts in influencing behavior. This role varies from a causal to a mediating role. In the former, reflected in cognitive–behavioral frameworks, thoughts are presumed to cause changes in feelings and behavior. In the latter, reflected in applied behavior analysis, thoughts are assumed to influence feelings and behavior in a mediating (not causal) manner. It is assumed that one must look to past and present environmental contingencies to account for both thoughts and feelings.

In cognitive–behavioral methods, attention is devoted to thoughts as well as behaviors. Thoughts of interest include attributions for behavior, feelings, and outcomes, negative and positive self-statements, expectations, and cognitive distortions. Attention is devoted to identifying the particular kinds of thoughts that occur in problem related situations. Cognitive–behavioral approaches differ in their assumptions about the kinds of thoughts that underlie behavior. However, all share certain assumptions such as the belief that individuals respond to cognitive representations of environmental events rather than to the events per se. It is assumed that learning is cognitively mediated and that cognition mediates emotional and behavioral dysfunction. [*See* BEHAVIOR THERAPY; COGNITIVE THERAPY.]

In applied behavior analysis, environmental contingencies are focused on. A contingency analysis requires identification of the environmental events that occasion and maintain behavior. There is an interest in describing the relationships between behavior and what happens right before and after as well as "meta-contingencies"—the relationships between cultural practices and the outcomes of these practices. There is an emphasis on *current* contingencies. Attention is directed toward the change of "deviant" environments rather than the change of "deviant" client behaviors. There is an interest in identifying functional relationships. A behavioral analysis includes a description of behaviors of concern as well as evidence that specific antecedents and consequences influence these behaviors; it requires a functional as well as a descriptive analysis.

Although there are differences, all behavioral approaches share many characteristics that distinguish them from sign approaches. Assessment is an ongoing process in behavioral assessment. This contrasts with some traditional assessment approaches in which assessment is used to "diagnose" a client in order to decide on treatment methods. What a person *does* is of interest in behavioral approaches rather than what she *has*. Behavior is of great interest, especially the behaviors of individuals in real-life contexts. Identifying variables that influence the frequency of behaviors of interest is a key assessment goal. Behavior is assumed to vary in different contexts because of different learning histories and different current contingencies as well as different levels of deprivation and fatigue. There is an emphasis on clear description of assessment methods as well as clear description of problems and outcomes. It is assumed that only if complaints are clearly described can they be translated into specific changes that would result in their removal. The emphasis on behavior and the influence of environmental contingencies call for the translation of problems into observable behaviors and the discovery of ways in which the environment can be rearranged. Clients are encouraged to recognize and alter the role they play in maintaining problems. For example, teachers and parents often reinforce behaviors they complain about. Assess-

ment is individualized; each person, group, family, organization or community is viewed as unique. Data about group differences do not offer precise information about what an individual does in specific situations and what cues and consequences influence their behavior.

The focus on behavior has a number of implications for assessment. One is the importance of observing people in real-life contexts whenever feasible, ethical, and necessary to acquire helpful data. A range of assessment methods is used including observation in real-life settings as well as role plays. Multiple assessment methods are also called for because of the lack of synchrony in overt behavior, physiological reactions, cognitions (thoughts), and feelings. Assessment and treatment are closely related in a behavioral model. It is assumed that assessment should have treatment utility. There is an emphasis on the use of validated assessment methods. The principles of behavior are relied on to guide assessment and intervention. There is a preference for limited inference and a focus on constructing repertoires (on helping clients to acquire additional knowledge and skills that will increase opportunities for reinforcement). Clients are viewed in terms of their assets rather than their deficiencies. The preference for enhancement of knowledge and skills requires a focus on behaviors that are effective in real-life contexts. In a task analysis, the specific behaviors that are required to achieve an outcome are identified. For each step, performance is clearly described as well as the conditions in which it is expected to occur.

A. Some Important Distinctions

The form of a behavior (its topography) does not necessarily indicate its function (why the behavior occurs). Identical forms of behavior may be maintained by very different contingencies. Just as the same behavior may have different functions, different behaviors may have identical functions. The distinction between motivational and behavioral deficits is also important. If a desired behavior does not occur, this may indicate either that the behavior exists but is not reinforced on an effective schedule or is punished (a motivational deficit) or that the behavior is not present in the client's repertoire (a behavior deficit). Motivational deficits are often mistaken for behavioral deficits. Motivational and behavioral deficits can be distinguished by arranging conditions for performance of a behavior. For example, clients could be requested to role play behaviors and asked whether similar or identical behaviors occur in other situations. Behavior surfeits are often related to behavior deficits. For example, aggression on the part of a child may be related to a lack of friendship skills. It is also important to distinguish response inhibitions from behavior deficits. Emotional reactions such as anxiety may interfere with desired behavior.

B. Past History

Although the past is viewed as important in influencing current behavior in just about all perspectives, assessment frameworks differ in how much attention is devoted to the past and what is focused on. Past experiences are a major focus in psychodynamic assessment frameworks. Knowledge about past circumstances may be of value when it is difficult to identify current maintaining factors and may be helpful in preventing future problems. Information about a person's past may provide valuable information about unusual social histories related to problems. An understanding of how problems began can be useful in clarifying the origins of what seem to be puzzling reactions. New ways of viewing past events may be helpful to clients. Information about the past can be useful in encouraging clients to alter present behaviors and may help clients understand the source of current reactions. Demographic indicators about a client's past behavior in certain contexts may be better predictors of future behavior than personality tests or clinical judgments.

Information about the past offers a view of current events in a more comprehensive context. Major areas include medical history, educational and work history, significant relationships, family history and developmental history. Helpful coping skills may be discovered by finding out what clients have tried in the past to resolve problems. Research concerning autobiographical memory suggests that memories change over time, making it difficult to know whether reports are accurate. From a psychodynamic perspective, accuracy would not be an issue. Rather, the client's memories of events, whether accurate or not, are the substance of import. It is assumed in fact that memories may be distorted by unconscious motives/conflicts and so on. Excessive attention to past troubles may create pessimism about the future and encourage rational-

izations and excuses that interfere with change, especially if this is not fruitful in selecting effective plans.

C. What about Psychiatric Labels?

Labels are used in assessment in two main ways. One is as a shorthand term to refer to specific behaviors. The term hyperactive may refer to the fact that a student often gets out of his seat and talks out of turn in class. A counselor may use "hyperactive" as a summary term to refer to these behaviors. Labels are also used as a diagnostic category which is supposed to offer guidelines for knowing what to do about a problem. Here, a label connotes more than a cluster of behaviors. It involves additional assumptions about the person labeled which should be of "diagnostic" value. The *Diagnostic and Statistical Manual of Mental Disorders* (*DSM-IV*) of the American Psychiatric Association describes hundreds of terms used to describe various disorders. [*See* DSM-IV.]

Methodological and conceptual problems connected with the use of diagnostic categories include lack of agreement about what label to assign clients and lack of association between a diagnosis and indications of what intervention will be effective. Psychiatric labels have been criticized for being imprecise (saying too little about positive attributes, potential for change, and change that does occur, and too much about presumed negative characteristics and limits to change). Both traits and diagnostic labels offer little detail about what people do in specific situations and what specific circumstances influence behavior. There is no evidence that traits have dispositional properties. Little cross-situational consistency has been found in relation to "personality traits." Some behaviors may appear "trait-like" in that they are similar over time and situations because of similar contingencies of reinforcement. Degree of consistency should be empirically explored for particular classes of clients and behavior rather than assumed. Acceptance of a label may prematurely close off consideration of promising options. The tendency to use a binary classification system (people are labeled as either having or not having something, for example, as being an alcoholic or not), may obscure the varied individual patterns that may be referred to by a term. Critics of the *DSM* highlight the consensual nature of what is included (reliance on agreement rather than empirical criteria) and the role of economic considerations in its creation. Some argue that psychiatric classification systems encourage blaming victims for their plights rather than altering the social circumstances responsible for problems.

Labels that are instrumental (they point to effective interventions) are helpful. For example, the understanding of anxiety disorders has advanced requiring the differential diagnosis among different categories (simple phobia, generalized anxiety, panic attacks and agoraphobia). Failure to use labels that are indeed informative may prevent clients from receiving appropriate intervention. Labels can normalize client concerns. Parents who have been struggling to understand why their child is developmentally slow may view themselves as failures. Recognition that their child has a specific kind of developmental disability that accounts for this can be a relief.

III. SOURCES OF INFLUENCE

Influences on behavior include other people's actions, the physical environment, tasks and materials, physiological changes, thoughts, genetic differences, and developmental factors. Material and community resources and related political, economic, and social conditions influence options. It is important to obtain an overview of the client's current life as this may relate to problems, including relationships with significant others, employment, physical health, recreational activities, and community and material resources available. Antecedents of behavior, like consequences, have a variety of sources. In addition to proximal antecedents (those that occur right before a behavior), distal antecedents may influence current behavior. Past or future events may be made current by thinking about these. These thoughts may then influence what we do, feel, and think. *Setting events* are antecedents that are closely associated with a behavior but are not in the situation in which behaviors of concern occur. For example, an unpleasant exchange with a teacher may influence how a child responds to his parents at home. The earlier event alters the likelihood of given reactions in subsequent situations. Preferred practice theories influence the attention given to various sources. Problems vary in the complexity of related factors. Problems may be complex because significant others lack needed skills, have interfering beliefs, or are threatened

by proposed changes. Distinguishing between problems and efforts to resolve these will avoid confusion between the results of attempted solutions and effects of the original concern. Expected role behavior in a certain culture may limit change. Ongoing discrimination against a group may limit opportunities. Clients may lack needed information or skills. A *behavior deficit* may exist (the client may not know how to perform a given behavior).

A. Other People/The Nature of the Client's Social Relationship

With any presenting problem, the possible influence of significant others in the maintenance of a problem should be explored. Behavior occurs in a context. How significant others respond makes up an important part of our environment. Significant others are those who interact with clients and influence their behavior. Examples include family members and staff in residential settings. Significant others are often involved in assessment. For example, in family therapy, family members participate in assessment. Understanding relationships among family members is a key part of assessment in family therapy. Interactions between couples is closely examined in relationship counseling. Clients may lack social support such as opportunities for intimacy, companionship, and validation or the opportunity to provide support to others. Social interactions may be a source of stress rather than a source of pleasure and joy. It is important to assess the nature and quality of the client's social network and social support system. [*See* SOCIAL NETWORKS; SOCIAL SUPPORT.]

B. The Physical Environment

The influence of the physical environment should be examined. Physical arrangements in residential and day care settings influence behavior. Unwanted behaviors may be encouraged by available materials. For example, toys that are visible to children may distract them from educational tasks. Temperature changes affect behavior as do degree of crowding and noise level. Characteristics of the community in which clients live that may influence complaints and possible intervention options should be assessed. Neighborhood quality influences well-being. For example, children who live in lower quality environments (e.g., there is little play space, housing is in industrial neighborhoods, upkeep of streets is poor) are less satisfied with their lives, experience more negative emotions, and have more restricted and less positive friendship patterns. There is a relationship between number of nonaccidental injuries to children and the physical conditions of the home which is related to socioeconomic status.

C. Tasks and Activities

The kind of task confronting an individual may influence the rate of problem behavior. Particular tasks or activities may be high-risk situations for unwanted behavior. Many studies have found a relationship between the kind of task and deviant behavior such as self-injury. Problems may occur because a task is too tedious or difficult or because an individual is uncomfortable or bored, or is told to do something in an unpleasant manner. In these instances, altering antecedents may correct the problem.

D. Biophysiological Factors

Presenting problems may be related to neurological or biochemical factors. Such factors may place boundaries on how much change is possible. Malnutrition, hypoglycemia, and allergic reactions have been associated with hyperactivity, learning disabilities, and mental retardation. Biochemical abnormalities are found in some children with serious behavior disturbances such as those labeled autistic. However, this only establishes that abnormalities in biochemistry are present, not that they cause a certain disorder (e.g., cause certain behaviors). Biochemical changes may be a result of stress related to social conditions such as limited opportunities due to discrimination. Drugs, whether prescribed or not, may influence how clients appear and behave. Certain kinds of illness are associated with particular kinds of psychological changes.

Drugs, alcohol, environmental pollutants, and nutritional deficiencies may influence health and behavior. Accidents may result in neurological changes which result in concomitant psychological changes. Even when brain damage can be shown to exist, this does not show that it causes any particular behavior. Premature acceptance of biophysical explanations will interfere with discovering alternative explanations that yield intervention knowledge. Behavior changes may be due to brain tumors. Hormonal changes associated with menopause may result in mood changes which may be misattributed to psychological causes. On the other hand psychological changes may be misattributed to hormonal changes. There are gender differences in return of diffuse physiological arousal (DPA) to baseline levels; men take longer to return to baseline levels. These gender differences have implications for understanding and altering aggression among family members. Whenever physiological factors may be related to a problem as, for example, with seizures, depression, fatigue, or headaches, a physical examination should be required. Overlooking physical causes including nutritional deficiencies and coffee, alcohol, or drug intake may result in incorrect inferences.

E. Cognitive–Intellectual Characteristics

People differ in their intellectual abilities which may influence problems and outcomes. Genetic differences have been found in intelligence as well as in shyness, temperament, and conditioning susceptibility. The importance of assessing what people say to themselves in relevant situations is emphasized in many assessment frameworks. For example, in cognitive–behavioral approaches, clients' internal dialogues (what they say to themselves) and the way this relates to complaints and desired outcomes is explored and altered as necessary. Certain thoughts may occur too much, too seldom, or at the wrong time. A depressed client may have a high frequency of negative self-statements and a low frequency of positive self-statements. In a radical behavioral perspective, thoughts are viewed as covert behaviors to be explained, not as explanations for other behaviors, although it is assumed they can serve a mediating function and influence both feelings and behaviors. The thoughts and feelings in a situation are assumed to be a function of the contingencies experienced in this situation or in situations that are similar or associated in some way. A causal role may be misattributed to thoughts because the histories related to the development of thoughts is overlooked. The role of thoughts can be examined by varying certain ones and determining the effects on behavior.

F. Feelings

When feelings are presented as a problem or are related to a problem, associated personal and environmental factors must be identified. Assessment frameworks differ in the role attributed to feelings and in factors sought to account for feelings. Some emphasize the role of thoughts in creating feelings. Others emphasize the role of unconscious conflicts and motives related to early childhood experiences. Other frameworks focus on the role of environmental contingencies in influencing emotional reactions. For example, in a radical behavioral approach, feelings are viewed as by-products of the relationships between behavior and environmental events. Feelings can be used as clues to contingencies (relationships between behavior and environmental events). Changing feelings will not make up for a lack of required skills, or rearrange contingencies required to attain desired outcomes.

G. Cultural Differences

Cultural differences may affect both the problems that clients experience as well as the communication styles and assessment and intervention methods that will be successful. An individualized assessment requires attention to cultural differences that may be related to problems and potential resolutions. Culturally sensitive practice requires knowledge of the values of different groups and their historical experience in the United States, and how these differences may influence the client's behavior, motivation and view of the helping process.

Different groups may prefer different problem-solving styles and have different beliefs about the causes of problems. The norms for behavior vary in different groups. It is important to be knowledgeable about cultural differences that may be mistakenly viewed as pathology. The degree of acculturation (the process of adaptation to a new or different culture) is important to assess. This influences drop-out rate, level of stress, attitude toward clinicians, and the process and goals that are appropriate. Knowledge of problems faced and preferred communication styles of people in different generations will be useful. Bicultural individuals are members of two or more ethnic or racial groups.

H. Developmental Considerations

Assessment requires knowledge about developmental tasks, norms, and challenges. Information about required behaviors at different ages and life transitions can be helpful in assessment. Knowledge of what is typical behavior at different times (developmental norms) can be useful in "normalizing" behavior—helping clients to realize that reactions they view as unusual or "abnormal" are in fact common. Knowledge about typical changes in different phases of the life cycle (e.g., adolescence, parenthood, retirement) allows preventative planning. The following kinds of information will be helpful: (1) norms for behavior in specific contexts; (2) tasks associated with certain life-situations such as parenthood and retirement; (3) the hierarchical nature of some developmental tasks (some behaviors must be learned before others can be acquired). Different kinds of norms may be used in the selection of outcomes. Criterion referenced norms rely on what has been found to be required to attain a certain outcome through empirical analysis. Another kind of norm is what is usual in a situation. However, what is usual may not be what is desirable. For example, although it may be typical for teachers to offer low rates of positive feedback to students in their classroom, it is not optimal. The similarities of contingencies for many people at a given age in a society may lead one to assume incorrectly that biological development is responsible. The role of similar contingencies may be overlooked. Acceptance of a stage theory of development may get in the way of identifying environmental factors that can be rearranged.

I. Reviewing Resources and Obstacles

Assessment involves identification of personal assets and environmental resources that can be used to help clients attain desired outcomes, as well as personal and environmental obstacles. Personal resources and/or obstacles include cognitive–intellectual abilities and deficiencies, physical abilities and handicaps, social skills and social-skill deficits, vocational and recreational skills, financial assets, and social support systems. Clients differ in their "reinforcer profile" and in degree of motivation to alter problematic circumstances. Environments differ in opportunities for certain kinds of experiences (see discussion of physical environment). Resources such as money, housing, vocational training programs, medical care, or recreational facilities may be unavailable. Limited community resources (such as day care programs, vocational training programs, recreational centers, high-quality educational programs, parent training programs) and limited influence over environmental circumstances may pose an obstacle. Child maltreatment is related to poverty. Unemployment is related to substance abuse and spouse violence. Agency policies and practices influence options. Lack of coordination of services may limit access to resources. Clients may receive fragmentary, overlapping, or incompatible services.

IV. SOURCES OF INFORMATION

Sources of data include interviews, responses to written or pictorial measures, data gathered by clients and significant others (self-monitoring), observation in the interview as well as in role play or in real-life settings, and physiological indicators. A variety of electromechanical aids are available for collecting data such as wrist counters, timers, biofeedback devices, and audio- and videotape recorders. Familiarity with and knowledge about different methods, as well as personal and theoretical preferences and questions of feasibility influence selection. Preferred practice theories strongly influence selection of assessment methods. For example, in individually focused psychodynamic approaches, self-report and transference effects within the interview may be the main source of data used.

In behavioral approaches, self-report is supplemented whenever possible by other sources of data such as observation in real-life settings, role play, and/or self-monitoring. (Clients keep track of some behaviors, thoughts, or feelings and surrounding circumstances in real-life). Some sources, such as self-report in the interview, are easy to use and are flexible in the range of content provided. However, accuracy varies considerably. The question is: what methods will offer a fairly accurate description of reactions or conditions of concern and related events? Individual differences will influence a client's willingness to participate in a given manner. Accuracy of decisions can be improved by using multiple methods, drawing especially on those most likely to offer accurate relevant data.

Self-report is the most widely used source of information. There are many different types of self-report including verbal reports during interviews and answers on written inventories. Interviews also provide an opportunity to observe clients. Advantages of self-report include ease of collecting material and flexibility in the range of material that may be gathered. Structured in-

terviews have been developed for both children and adults in a number of areas. These may be completed by the clinician, the client, or significant others. The accuracy of self-reports depends on a number of factors including the situation in which data are collected and the kinds and sequence of questions asked. Helpful questions in assessing the accuracy of self-reports include the following: (1) Does the situation encourage an honest answer? (2) Does the client have access to the information? (3) Can the client comprehend the question? (4) Does the client have the verbal skills required to answer questions? Special knowledge and skills may be required when interviewing children. Play materials and storytelling may be used to gather data about children's feelings and experiences.

Measures that have uniform procedures for administration and scoring and that are accompanied by certain kinds of information are referred to as *standardized measures*. Thousands of standardized questionnaires have been developed related to hundreds of different personal and/or environmental characteristics. Standardized measures are used for a variety of purposes including: (1) describing populations or clients, (2) screening clients (for example, making a decision about the need for further assessment or finding out if a client is eligible for or likely to require a service), (3) assessing clients (a more detailed review resulting in decisions about diagnosis or assignment to intervention methods), (4) monitoring (evaluating progress), and (5) making predictions about the likely futures of clients (for example in relation to use of a particular intervention method). As always, a key concern is validity. Does a measure assess what it is presumed to assess? Reliability must also be considered. How stable are responses on a measure given a lack of real change? Unstable measures are not likely to be valid. How sensitive will a measure be to change?

Personality tests may be used to collect assessment data. *Objective tests* include specific questions, statements, or concepts. Clients respond with direct answers, choices, or ratings. *Projective tests* such as the Thematic Apperception Test, incomplete sentences test, and the Rorschach Inkblot Test are purposefully vague and ambiguous. It is assumed that each person will impose on this unstructured stimulus presentation unique meanings that reflect his or her perceptions of the world and responses to it. Psychoanalytic concepts underlie use of most projective tests. These tests focus on assessing general personality characteristics and uncovering unconscious processes. Tests are used not as samples of the content domain (as in behavioral approaches), but as signs of important underlying constructs. Whereas content validity is of great concern in a behavioral perspective, this is not so within a traditional approach. In fact, items may be made deliberately obscure and vague.

Valuable information can be obtained from data clients collect (self-monitoring). As with any other source of data, not all clients will be able or willing to participate. Observation of relevant interactions in real-life settings offers a valuable source of information. This is routinely used in applied behavior analysis. If observation in real-life settings is not possible, observation in role plays may provide a useful alternative. Physiological measures have been used with a broad array of presenting problems including illness such as diabetes and dermatitis and problems such as smoking, anxiety, sexual dysfunction, and rape. Measures include heart rate, blood pressure, respiration rate, skin conductance, muscle tension, and urine analysis. Physiological measures are useful when verbal reports may be inaccurate. Certain kinds of desynchronies between verbal reports of fear and physiological measures may provide useful assessment data. Whenever presenting problems may be related to physical causes, a physical examination should be obtained. Failure to do so may result in overlooking physical causes.

V. ASSESSING THE VALUE OF DATA

Assessment methods differ in their accuracy. For example, self-report of clients or significant others may not accurately reflect what occurs in real life. Observers may be biased and offer inaccurate data. Measurement inevitably involves error. One cause of systematic error is social desirability; people present themselves in a good light. Criteria that are important to consider in judging the value of assessment data include: (1) reliability, (2) validity, (3) sensitivity, (4) utility, (5) feasibility, and (6) relevance. *Reliability* refers to the consistency of results (in the absence of real change) provided by the same person at different times (time-based reliability), by two different raters of the same events (individual-based reliability) as in inter-rater reliability, or by parallel forms of split-halfs of a measure

(item-bound reliability). Reliability places an upward boundary on validity. For example, if responses on a questionnaire vary from time to time (in the absence of real change), it will not be possible to use results of a measure to predict what a person will do in the future.

Validity concerns the question: Does the measure reflect the characteristic it is supposed to measure? For example, does behavior in a role play correspond to what a client does in similar real-life situations? Assessment is more likely to be informative if valid methods are used—methods that have been found to offer accurate information. *Direct* (e.g., observing teacher–student interaction) in contrast to *indirect* measures (e.g., asking a student to complete a questionnaire assumed to offer information about classroom behavior) are typically more valid. Validity (accuracy) is a concern in all assessment frameworks; however, the nature of the concern is different in sign and sample approaches. In a sign approach, behavior is used as a sign of some entity (such as a personality trait) that is at a different level. The concern is with *vertical* validity. Is the sign an accurate indicator of the underlying trait? *Horizontal* validity is of concern in a sample approach. Different levels (e.g., behavior and personality dispositions) are not involved. Examples include: (1) Does self-report provide an accurate account of behavior and related circumstances? (2) Does behavior in role play reflect what occurs in real life? Different responses (overt, cognitive, and physiological) may or may not be related to an event. For example, clients may report anxiety but show no physiological signs of anxiety. This does not mean that their reports are not accurate. For those individuals, the experience of anxiety may be cognitive rather than physical.

The *sensitivity* of measures is important to consider; will a measure reflect changes that occur? The *utility* of a measure is determined by its cost (time, effort, expense) balanced against information provided. *Feasibility* is related to utility. Some measures will not be feasible to gather. Utility may be compromised by the absence of empirically derived norms for a measure. *Norms* offer information about the typical (or average) performance of a group of individuals and allow comparison of data obtained from a client with similar clients. The more representative the sample is to the client, the greater the utility of a measure in relation to a client. *Relevance* should also be considered. Is a measure relevant to presenting problems and related outcomes? Do clients and significant others perceive it as relevant?

VI. THE SOCIAL CONTEXT OF ASSESSMENT

Assessment takes place in the context of a helper–client relationship. The nature of this relationship is considered important in all practice frameworks. Influence of the clinician on the client has been found even in very nondirective approaches. The role of the relationship is viewed differently in different practice perspectives. Great attention is given to the diagnostic value of transference and countertransference effects in psychodynamic therapies and the relationship itself is viewed as the primary vehicle of change. Traditionally, transference has been viewed as a reenactment between the client and the counselor of the client's relationship with significant others in the past, especially parents. Countertransference effects refer to feelings on the part of helpers toward their clients. Transferences are distinguished from therapeutic or working alliances within psychodynamic perspectives. Understanding and analyzing how the client relates to the clinician are of major importance. The way the client relates to the clinician is considered to be indicative of the client's past relationships with significant figures in the past and is thus viewed as a key source of information about the client. Within other perspectives such as cognitive–behavioral approaches, the relationship is viewed as the context within which helping occurs. The interpersonal skills of the clinician are viewed as essential for facilitating a collaborative working relationship, validating and supporting the client, and encouraging clients to acquire valued behaviors.

There is a continuing need throughout assessment to explain the roles and requirements of the client and the counselor, the process that will occur, and the rationale for this. Introductory explanations include an overview of mutual responsibilities and of the framework that will be employed. Because different client behaviors may be required during different phases of assessment and intervention, this "socialization" of the client is an ongoing task. Behavioral clinicians tend to be more directive than psychoanalytically oriented clinicians. They more frequently give instructions, provide information, influence the conversation, and talk more. Clinicians may err by being too directive or too nondirective. Overly directive clinicians may not recognize the need to help clients to explore and to understand their behavior. In contrast, nondirective counselors may err by assuming that self-understanding is sufficient to achieve desired outcomes (when it is not).

VII. COMMON ASSESSMENT ERRORS AND THEIR SOURCES

Errors may occur in any of the three steps involved in assessment: (1) detection of characteristics of the client and his or her life situation that are related to problems and desired outcomes; (2) integration and interpretation of data gathered; and (3) selection of outcomes to pursue in order to remove complaints. Errors made in the first two steps will result in errors in the third step. Examples of common errors are noted below. They result in incomplete or misleading assessment. Some errors involve or result in inappropriate speculation—assuming that what is, can be discovered simply by thinking about the topic.

- Hasty assumptions about causes (failure to search for alternative accounts)
- Speculating when data collection is called for
- Confusing the form and function of behavior
- Using misleading and/or uninformative labels
- Confusing motivational and behavior deficits
- Focusing on pathology and overlooking assets
- Collecting irrelevant material
- Relying on inaccurate sources (e.g., anecdotal experience)
- Being unduly influenced by first impressions
- Being misled by superficial resemblances of a client to other clients in the past or to a stereotype

Errors in detection include inadequate selection of modalities (e.g., confining attention to thoughts), inadequate selection of data collection methods (e.g., reliance on the interview alone), and errors in the data collection method itself (e.g., observer bias). Inaccurate or incomplete accounts of problems and related factors may occur because attention is too narrowly focused on one source (for example on thoughts or feelings). The fundamental attribution error is made when behavior is attributed to internal dispositions of the individual, overlooking the role of environmental causes. Sources of error in integrating and interpreting data include focusing on consistency rather than informativeness of data, hasty generalization based on limited samples, and inadequate conceptualization of problems due to theoretical biases (e.g., focus only on environmental factors) or superficial knowledge of practice frameworks. Another source of error at this stage is use of vague language that is not informative (e.g., psychological jargon). Errors in selection of outcomes to focus on may occur due to error in the first two phases.

Studies on clinical decision-making indicate that decisions are made on the basis of quite limited data. Even though a great deal of data are gathered, only a small subset is used. Clinicians tend to gather more data than are needed and, as the amount of data gathered increases, so does confidence in its usefulness, even though accuracy may not increase. Clinicians have a tendency to confuse consistency of data with informative value. Irrelevant as well as relevant data may be influential. Clinicians, like other individuals, are affected by limited information-processing capacities and motivational factors. As a consequence, they do not see all there is to see. Because of preconceptions and biases, things that are not actually present may be reported and events that do occur may be overlooked. There is a behavior confirmation tendency. Data are sought that are consistent with preferred theories and preconceptions, and contradictory data tend to be disregarded.

It is easy to recall bizarre behavior and pay excessive attention to this, ignoring less vivid appropriate behavior. The frequency of data that are available is overestimated. Many factors that are not correlated with the true frequency of an event influence estimates of its frequency and how important it seems (such as how visible it is, how vivid it is, and how easily it can be imagined—that is, how available it is). Chance availability may affect clinical decisions—that is, certain events may just happen to be available when thinking about a problem, and these have an impact on what is attended to. Clinicians in given settings are exposed to particular kinds of clients, which may predispose them to make certain assumptions. For example, a psychologist who sees many severely depressed individuals may be primed to attend to signs of depression. Base rate data that are abstract tend to be ignored, which increases the probability of inaccurate inferences. A lack of concern for sample size and sample bias can lead to incorrect judgments. General predictions about a person that are based on tiny samples of behavior in one context are not likely to be accurate, especially when behaviors of interest

occur in quite different situations. Not distinguishing between description and inference may result in incorrect assumptions. Use of multiple methods in a contextual practice framework provides the greatest opportunity for sound assessment.

VIII. ETHICAL ISSUES AND FUTURE DIRECTIONS

Lack of assessment competencies may result in the selection of ineffective and/or harmful intervention methods. It is thus incumbent on clinicians to use valid methods that are useful in selecting effective intervention plans. This may require training. There are great stakes in how problems are framed and considerable resources are devoted to influencing how people think about problems. Many problems once viewed as sins were then seen as crimes and more recently are considered to be mental disorders. Explanations influence how people are viewed. In past years, pathology was often attributed to housewives who wanted to work. Incorrect explanations of problems often harm clients. Knowledge about social, political, and economic factors that influence the very definition of personal and social problems will help clinicians to consider problems in their social context and decrease the likelihood of pathologizing clients.

A discussion of clinical assessment would not be complete without noting the increased attention given to evolutionary influences. It is easy to lose sight of the fact that humans are the result of a long evolutionary process and that we carry anatomical, physiological, and psychological characteristics related to this history. An evolutionary perspective adds a valuable dimension to understanding aggression and caregiving in society, whether directed toward family members or strangers, as well as defeat states such as depression and the experiences that may be responsible. Computers will play an increasing role in helping clinicians to handle the many different kinds of data that must often be integrated. There has been considerable interest in the integration of different approaches to clinical practice. Some have explored the possible integration of behavioral and psychoanalytic approaches. Others have investigated the relationship between classical psychodynamics and object relations perspectives. Discussions here concern the nature of inferred conflict and how mental phenomena of interest are formed. Accurate descriptions of assessment perspectives will increase the likelihood that points of convergence and differences are correctly identified. Continuing research efforts are needed to identify valid assessment methods and indicate assessment frameworks that are most likely to help clients. Increased interest in clinical reasoning bodes well for enhancement of assessment competencies.

This article has been reprinted from the *Encyclopedia of Human Behavior, Volume 1.*

BIBLIOGRAPHY

Bellack, A. S., & Hersen, M. (Eds.) (1988). "Behavioral Assessment," 3rd ed. Pergamon, New York.

Bergen, J. R., & Kratchowill, T. R. (1990). "Behavioral Consultation and Therapy." Plenum, New York.

Ciminero, A. R., Calhoun, K. S., & Adams, H. E. (1986). "Handbook of Behavioral Assessment," 2nd ed. Wiley, New York.

Gambrill, E. (1990). "Critical Thinking in Clinical Practice." Jossey-Bass, San Francisco, CA.

Gilbert, P. (1989). "Human Nature and Suffering." Erlbaum, Hillsdale, NJ.

Goldstein, M., & Hersen, M. (Eds.) (1990). "Handbook of Psychological Assessment." Pergamon, New York.

Horowitz, M. J. (1987). "States of Mind: Configurational Analysis of Individual Psychology," 2nd ed. Plenum, New York.

Kirk, S., & Kutchins, H. (1992). "The Selling of DSM: The Rhetoric of Science in Psychiatry." Aldine de Gruyter, Hawthorne, NY.

Nay, W. R. (1979). "Multimethod Clinical Assessment." Gardner, New York.

Wetzler, S., & Katz, M. M. (1989). "Contemporary Approaches to Psychological Assessment." Brunner/Mazel, New York.

Cognitive Development

Rochel Gelman

University of California, Los Angeles

Accommodate   To change one's concept on the basis of new knowledge.

Assimilate   To take in a new information and incorporate it into an existing concept.

Concept   An abstract or generic mental representation generalized from particular instances.

Habituation   Decrease in responsiveness upon repeated exposure to a stimulus.

Stage Theory Assumption   Development occurs through qualitatively different stages in a given order.

The study of **COGNITIVE DEVELOPMENT** is concerned with how our young come to share with us knowledge about the world of objects, people, and ideas. Answering these questions requires suitable methods of observation and experimentation, on the one hand, and good ideas about what to look for, on the other hand. Often what one looks for is tied to one's theories about cognitive development, in general, and the nature of concepts, in particular. This essay begins by asking "what is a concept" and embeds in the answer a review of theories of cognitive development and relevant findings. Evidence for the conclusion that there are some universal (core) kinds of concepts is presented.

I. ABOUT CONCEPTS

Our concepts do not stand alone, each separate from the other. For example, our concept of a dog is related to our knowledge of other animals, and our concept of a bicycle is related to what we know about other wheeled artifacts. Concepts are organized into coherent groupings or structures; at the same time, what we know about one concept in a grouping is interrelated with what we know about others in the same organization. This fact about mental organizations is extremely important. It underlies our ability to generalize what we know to novel instances in the same conceptual structure, to make inferences about the meaning of names for new objects, and so on. When we are told that a picture of an unfamiliar animal depicts a species living in a far-away place, we can infer that it is the kind of thing that breathes, eats, reproduces, probably makes communicative noises, has sensory receptors, interacts at least some times with others of its kind, and is capable of moving itself from place to place. Such inferences are possible even if we will never see the animal and despite the fact that, in a picture, it resembles a cactus. When told the creature is an echidna, we will assume that all items that look like it are also echnidas and will be able to answer questions that refer to it, for example, "Does an echidna bear young?" versus "Does one wear an echidna in cold weather?" Our understanding of the world is not a collection of random facts joined together by pairs of associations. Therefore, when we are told that an unknown animal is an echidna, we do not have to start from scratch and build an understanding of the animal as described above, one piece at a time.

The challenge for students of cognitive development is to characterize how our young accomplish the task of acquiring concepts and the related abilities to apply them to novel cases. Any answer to this question must account for the fact that children do not merely develop concepts. We need to explain how they develop concepts that they share with others and therefore can communicate about. Psychologists' realization that knowledge about concepts is organized goes hand in hand with a new theoretical concern in cognitive development—the nature of domain-specific knowledge structures and how they develop.

II. AN OVERVIEW OF COGNITIVE DEVELOPMENT THEORIES

There are at least five different kinds of accounts of cognitive development. Learning theory account is based on the assumptions of associationism: All knowledge is due to sensory and motoric experiences and the capacity to form associations. Information processing theorists focus on the role of information processing and problem solving capacities for explaining how children learn to understand the world. With time, experience, and practice, children acquire organized memories and develop ways to circumvent processing limits on attention, short-term memory, and perception. Learning theory and information processing accounts of cognitive development share the assumption that cognitive development is a linear function of experience. The sociocultural account of cognitive development places emphasis on the assumption that concept acquisition is facilitated by infants' inclinations to pay attention to the social agents who serve as transmitters and presenters of key information. Still, it shares the assumption that the acquisition of concepts is a protracted process, taking as much as two years before a child reaches the point where he or she has the ability to represent the world in terms of concepts and to communicate with others.

Some sociocultural theorists like Vygotsky incorporate a stage theory assumption, showing development as a passage through qualitatively different stages in a given order. At each stage, the child actively engages the environment with existing structures of mind

so much that it is possible for the child to "misinterpret" inputs about concepts. For example, in Piagetian theory, cognitive development proceeds through four stages: from the sensorimotor (0 to 2 years of age), to preoperational (2 to 5 or 6 years), to concrete operational (6 to 10 or 11 years), and finally, the formal operational (12+ years) stage. The Piagetian child who is still at the preoperational stage will fail to conserve quantity across transformations because she still has to acquire the structures that will support quantitative reasoning, a hallmark of Piaget's concrete operational stage. At the preoperational stage, children also fail perspective-taking tasks as a result of focusing on their own views.

The fact that all four theories named above differ in notable ways becomes more apparent in studies of post-infancy cognitive development. For example, since scholars working in the information processing tradition emphasize the general limits on processing, they do studies that show how success varies as a function of real-time processing demands. Those who emphasize the social aspects of cognitive development might focus on the acquisition of shared conversational rules. Despite the fundamental differences, all four classes of theories converge on a common view about infant cognition. This view is that infants come to the world without any mental structures that relate to the kind of conceptual, linguistic, and social world they will live in. The general idea for association, information processing, and stage theories is that infants first learn about sensory and action experiences. These lay the foundation for developing perceptions which in turn form the basis upon which concept acquisition can proceed. The cultural account also shares the sensation to perception to cognitions view of development; but it adds the assumption that acquisition is facilitated by infants' inclinations to pay attention to the social agents who serve as transmitters and presenters of key information.

Thus, all four of the above theoretical accounts embody the view that the start of concept acquisition takes as much as 2 years to get off the ground, to reach the point where the child has the ability to represent the world in terms of concepts. On first blush, this seems reasonable. After all, newborn infants are extremely helpless and human infants take a fairly long time to get beyond the many limits on their motoric, sensory, and communicative abilities. The delayed onset of language use until around 2 years of age is consistent with the ideas that neonates' conceptual knowledge is nonexistent and that of older infants is extremely shallow. Indeed, one might ask, how could anyone think otherwise? Those who answer to the contrary do so because of the accumulating body of evidence that infants, toddlers, and preschoolers have some remarkable conceptual competencies. Such evidence, some of which is presented below, has contributed to the emergence of a fifth theoretical account of cognitive development that can be dubbed a rational-constructivist theory of cognitive development. The rationalist side of the theory captures the assumption that our young bring a skeletal outline of domain-specific knowledge to their task of learning the initial concepts they will share with others. The constructivist side of the theory captures the assumption that, from the start, our young actively join in their own cognitive development. Even as beginning learners, skeletal principles motivate them to seek out and assimilate inputs that nurture the development of these structures.

Like stage theorists, rational-constructivist proponents hold that there are universal structures of mind. These theories differ, however, on whether there is some innate conceptual knowledge at the start. Piaget held that the processes of assimilation and accommodation are innate, but he denied the presence of any innate structures of mind. In contrast, the rational-constructivist position joins two assumptions: innate inclinations to actively process (assimilate and accommodate) the environment, along with an assumption of innate skeletal structures of knowledge. The rational constructivist position also differs from stage theories in its commitment to the view that there are domain-specific, as opposed to domain-general, structures of mind. For example, whereas Piaget's theory grants the mind general structures such as concrete operations, rational constructivist theories hold that different knowledge domains, for example, number and space are represented by domain-specific structures. Universally shared domains, also called core domains, benefit from innate, skeletal, domain-specific structures. The common underlying set of skeletal, domain-specific structures are learning-enabling engines of mind. Given that infants actively apply whatever structures of mind they might have—skeletal or otherwise—data (i.e., inputs from the environment) that have the capacity to nurture these structures are privileged as targets of attention and then assimilation

to the structures. As a result, these data nurture rapid learning about many of the objects and events they encounter. As skeletal as these structures might be, they nevertheless facilitate selective attention and assimilation of structure-relevant data and therefore serve much like engines of learning about their domains.

We turn to evidence, starting with the fact that infants learn quickly about core domains of knowledge. Thereafter, the text turns to a review and assessment of some of the classical experiments, the traditional interpretations of these, and then examines ways to reconcile the seeming differences between the new and old findings. To end, we discuss the fact that, although people all over the world develop core concept domains, with or without formal instruction or intentional practice, acquisition of noncore domains is much more idiosyncratic. The development of conceptual mastery in noncore domains requires organized lessons, study, and years of learning.

III. EVIDENCE

A. Recent Findings about the Capacities of Infants

In their 1973 pioneering study, Kalnins and Bruner showed that infants use their well-developed sucking responses to explore and learn about the world of objects and even representations of them. Not only will infants suck on a nipple (specially constructed with a transducer linked to a recording machine) to get access to an interesting picture, they learn to adjust the rate at which they suck in order to bring the picture into focus. Young infants also adjust their sucking rate, signaling when they are bored with a particular picture. They habituate; that is, they slow their sucking in the presence of a given picture and thereby let it go out of focus. Given a new picture, infants once again resume sucking at a high rate. This conjugate reinforcement method is also used to show that 1-month-old infants are capable of making categorical distinctions between different phonemes, for example, ba and pa, la and ra.

The discovery that infants have potent tendencies to attend actively and learn about novel inputs quickly turned into a major research tool for investigations of infants' perceptual and conceptual abilities. Across a range of studies, infants have attended to and learned about a wide range of structurally complex data. Six-to 8-month-olds can match the number of items they see with the number of drumbeats they hear. Young infants also know that objects continue to exist even when they cannot see them. Other studies expand on these conclusions, as described below.

Baillargeon and her colleagues provide evidence that infants interpret motion paths for inanimate objects in ways that are consistent with an external-agent causal principle. That is, inanimate objects require a source other than themselves to move. Baillargeon, Spelke and Wasserman's demonstration of object permanence in 6- to 8-month-old infants is one example of this. In their 1985 experiment, infants saw the same motion path at two different times. First, during the habituation phase, infants saw a screen rotate towards and away from them, through a 180° arc. Nothing was behind the screen. When their interest in the moving screen declined, that is when the infants habituated, the experimenters set the stage for creating the viewing conditions of the same 180° rotating screen for a second time. This time, the experimenter showed infants an object placed to the left side of the rotating screen. While infants watched, the experimenter moved the object behind the screen while it was upright. Then the post-habituation phase of the experiment began. Once again, the screen rotated toward and away from the infant. On alternating trials it either traversed a novel 120° arc or the familiar 180° arc. Given that there was an object in the path of the rotating screen, the screen should have stopped at about the 120° position of its rotation. When it continued through a 180° arc (thanks to the use of trick mirrors and invisible doors), it contributed to the adult perception of an impossible event, an unseen block being repeatedly crushed and uncrushed as the screen circumscribed its 180° arc. The event is impossible for adults because for them—save in the world of spirits and ghosts—one solid object cannot move through another one. If infants are restricted to perceptual analyses of motion paths, they should see no difference between 180° arc rotation that was shown in both the habituation and post-habituation phases. They should therefore continue to be uninterested in this event and prefer to look at the 120° event, the one that generates a novel perception. If, however, infants interpret the motion paths in terms of causally relevant variables, they should treat the second showing of the 180° event as different from the first showing

of the 180° event. In fact, they attended more to the 180° event, from which we conclude that infants interpreted the perceptual information about the motion path in ways that we know are causally relevant.

Studies by Spelke and colleagues demonstrate that 7-month-olds know that, whereas two inanimate objects have to contact each other if a causal event that involves them is to occur, the same is not true for two people. To show this, the authors constructed infants' reactions to two pairs of videotaped displays. The inanimate pairs of stimuli were two 5- and 6-ft. tall objects that had distinctive novel shapes and contrasting bright colors and patterns. The animate pairs were two people. In the inanimate test condition, infants watched two events: (a) the objects moved toward each other, touched each other, and changed direction; (b) the objects moved toward each other, stopped before reaching the point of contact for a brief time, and changed direction. In the people condition, the structure of the two events was identical to that of the inanimate events. For example, the parallel event for the person-contact condition showed a person holding her arms up and close to her body as she brushed up alongside another person. During test conditions, infants looked reliably longer at the no-contact inanimate event; they showed no such preference in the animate event trials. Spelke's findings are buttressed by other findings that 9-month-old children organize their exploration of toys so as to keep examples of animals and vehicles in separate categories.

These demonstrations are especially surprising given the longstanding assumption that infants enter the world with a mind that is a blank slate and only the abilities to sense bits of light, sound, and so on. Piaget's idea that these perceptions are brought together as bits of schemata and the associationist view that infants gradually contribute to the building of associations about these punctate sensory experiences are consistent with the widespread belief that infants start out in a "blooming, buzzing, confusing" world. It is therefore no surprise that researchers have challenged the idea that studies like those presented above demonstrate early conceptual competence and instead try to find "simpler" explanations. Nevertheless, the continued demonstrations of early competence provide a series of converging lines of evidence. This makes it harder and harder to reject the viability of some variant of the rational-constructivist theory. The challenge remains to reconcile the traditional findings with the new findings, not to try and explain away the new. That is, it is important to take a hard look at the studies showing infants do have concepts and can learn rapidly about numbers, causes, categorical differences between animate and inanimate objects, and people, and then ask what distinguishes these studies from those that do not.

B. Some Traditional Findings

Some of the best evidence in favor of stage theories comes from the various classification tasks that Bruner, Piaget, and Vygotsky used. Across a set of different tasks, preschool-aged children will fail to apply a classification structure. That is, they do not use consistent criteria to sort a pile of objects, be these different colors and shapes; and they do not solve problems that require reasoning about the hierarchical relationships between superordinate and subordinate categories. For example, when children who were 7-years-old or younger were asked whether a bouquet of flowers made up of six roses and four tulips contains more roses or flowers, children invariably answered, "More roses."

Other results add weight to the idea that young children cannot classify consistently. Specifically, children will not pick out all and only those exemplars that are examples of the concept. In a study in Bruner's lab, subjects ranging in age from 6 to 19, heard a series of concrete nouns and had to answer how each new item was both similar to and different from a pair of items presented. For example, a child first heard "banana," "peach," and then "potato." Then she was asked, "How is potato different from a banana and peach and how is it similar?" The youngest children answered on the basis of perceptual attributes like color and size, not categorical membership or even functional similarity. In a second task, participants were shown a large number of photographs and then asked to pick out groups that were alike. Again, responses of the young children were based predominantly on shared perceptual attributes as opposed to shared conceptual criteria.

Vygotsky described a similar pattern of findings, with younger children focusing on common perceptual or thematic criteria. Given the robustness of the developmental classification data, it is easy to see why

so many people believed that preschool-aged children have pseudoconcepts, pre-concepts, or idiosyncratic concepts that lead them to put together items older children and adults would never put together. From such results, it is an easy step to infer a stage theory that says older children and adults have mental structures that support hierarchically organized concepts, but young children, toddlers, and infants do not. This is especially so when we consider the many cases where younger children seem indeed to be perception-bound, as Piaget's conservation tasks suggested.

Preschool children's persistent failure on Piagetian conservation tasks is used as a salient example of their reliance on surface perceptual attributes of the displays. When shown two identical glasses with equal amounts of water that obviously reach the same level, all children aged 4 to 8 years of age agree that two amounts are equal. However, when one glass is poured into a tall, thin beaker, the 4- and 5-year-olds deny that equivalence is maintained, either because one column of water is taller or one is shorter. Piaget's work on early causal reasoning adds weight to the idea that preschoolers reason on the basis of the superficial appearance of things. For example, young children seem to think that the sun and the moon move when (and because) they themselves are moving.

Turning to infants, there are the traditional Piagetian tests of object concept and the famous "A-not-B error" that is characteristic of 8- to 12-month-old infants. At this range, infants will reach out for an object (say, a toy), watch as it is covered, and even remove the cover to get the hidden object. However, if, while the baby is watching, the object is put under a second cover, the infant no longer uncovers the desired toy. Instead she continues to look under the first cover where they toy no longer is. An amazing performance! It is as if the infant believes the existence of the object is related to his or her own earlier successful action and not that an object is a permanent entity that continues to be somewhere "out there." That is what Piaget concluded and what many take to be true.

C. Contradictory Findings?

The main question one has to ask about seemingly contradictory findings is this: Is there a coherent interpretation of performance variability within and across conditions? Is it possible that there are systematic variables contributing to failure across tasks that are meant to tap the target competence in question? If so, it may be possible to validate interpretations of competence with either new evidence or manipulations of the hypothesized interfering variable.

Infants are immature planners and information processors. Piaget's tests of the infant's understanding of the object concept all require the deployment of a competent plan of action. However, if the planning system needed to generate a competent plan of action is limited or not even developed, then the risk is high that a child will fail no matter how much she knows about the content domain at hand. There are reasons to presume that infants' abilities to generate coordinated actions go through a protracted developmental course. Therefore, perhaps Piaget's conclusions about the development of object permanence are better thought of as gains in infants' abilities to assemble suitable plans and related action sequences.

To start, we know that the information processing demands of a task vary as a function of development. In a 1991 study Diamond reported clear effects from varying the time before an experimenter allows the infant to reach for the hidden object. If the delay between the end of the hiding phase and the beginning of the retrieval phase is less than 2 seconds, 7½- to 8-month-old infants do not make the A-not-B errors instead they look for the object in its second hiding place. If the interval exceeds 2 seconds, they make the standard error of seeking the object in the original hiding position. By 9 months of age, infants can succeed after delays of up to 5 seconds, and by 12 months can do well on delays of up to 10 seconds. Other studies show that infants who erred had a clear tendency to choose an item that was near the first hiding place, thereby adding another dimension to what we know about information processing demands in the A-not-B task.

Limits on memory are not the only factor hindering the immature infant's ability to reach for the item in the correct location. Diamond details a number of variables that limit 5- to 7-month-old infants' ability to assemble and produce a competent plan of action. For example, younger infants have trouble inhibiting reflexes that are elicited if they accidentally touch an object that happens to be near the one they have to get. Baillargeon, Kotovsky, and Needham make it clear that the requirements of the task (i.e., ones that are not tied to knowledge about object permanence), can

mask the infant's knowledge of objects. In a 1995 study, they showed that 5-month-old infants know the difference between actions that can and cannot support the retrieval of an object that is hidden behind a screen. In one experiment, infants watched an object being retrieved under a possible and impossible action condition. To set the stage for the relevant part of the experiment, infants first watched one of two hiding events. One involved showing the hand of an experimenter placing a teddy bear on a table; a screen was then moved in front the display, and infants saw a hand reaching behind the screen and pulling out the teddy bear—a perfectly possible event. In the other hiding event, a teddy bear was placed on a table with a transparent cup over it and then a screen was moved to occlude the display. Then, while the screen was in place, the infant again watched as the experimenter's hand reached behind the screen and pulled out the teddy bear—an impossible outcome. Infants responded differently to these two different events by showing surprise and looking longer at the impossible event condition. Thus at least some of the differences in results from studies using reaching tasks rather than looking habituation paradigms to evaluate object permanence in infants has to be attributed to general limits on their ability to produce suitable action sequences. There is much to learn about the development of action planning, and therefore procedural competence, during the first few years of life.

Infants in habituation and visual preference studies have been tested under a wide range of stimulus conditions, including ones where balls fall to the floor, trains go down tracks, blocks and toys are hidden, and objects are felt but not seen. The studies that show infants are able to discriminate between relevant and irrelevant retrieval acts and succeed on Piagetian tasks, if they are tested under the right conditions, help corroborate the conclusions that were based on habituation methods. Additionally, they give further reason to argue that part of what develops is an ability to relate conceptual competence to procedural competence.

Thus, there is a sense in which Piaget was right to focus on the role of action in thought. However, for Piaget thought and action are almost one and the same. An alternative view assumes that infants start life with immature and limited abilities to perform, let alone put acts together into a competent plan that can demonstrate underlying conceptual competence.

It is wise therefore, to use assessment techniques that minimize demands on the procedural side if the question of interest concerns conceptual competencies that infants might have. A better approach is to find and use more than one such method, or at least vary the test materials across experiments. As these variations increase, so does one's confidence in the attribution of conceptual competence. Because there are many different studies of very young infants' ability to treat objects as permanent, we are now able to show that there are systematic sources of variability of performance in Piaget's tasks that are not due to the kinds of conceptual limits Piaget would want us to place on infants.

Conversational rules can confound assessments. The experimental setting often violates the rules of everyday conversations, especially the rule that one should not repeat what already is known by the listener. A question about available information presents an especially flagrant violation of that rule. Yet this typically occurs in experiments with young children. Imagine the quandary of a child who knows not to say the obvious when shown five items and is asked by an adult, "How many?" She knows the experimenter knows the answer, so she may do one of the following: violate a rule of conversation and state what she takes to be obvious, find something else to talk about, or decide to remain quiet. Even if a child realizes that she is supposed to tell what anyone could know, there is a further hurdle. In many studies of cognitive development the same question is asked more than once, and the repetition often follows right on the heels of the question's first presentation. There is nothing malicious about this. Researchers often want to know how children respond to irrelevant transformations of the stimulus arrays. Still, from the child's perspective, she must answer once again even though everyone in the conversation knows the answer. It therefore should be of little surprise when the child changes her answer or brings up another subject to talk about.

Because we are not supposed to repeat what is known, the child who shares knowledge of verbal counting principles with an interviewer might assume that it is sufficient to provide the cardinal value or count when answering the question, "How many?" When a speaker counts aloud, there is no need to repeat the last count to signal its status as the cardinal value of the set; the auditor can hear the last count word. It would be a violation of conversation rules to

signal something so obvious to an adult listener. Conversely, a statement of cardinal numerosity may be taken to imply that there was a count. These suggestions are more than speculations; they are supported by a study in which undergraduates were asked the "How many?" question about 18 blocks. All of them counted aloud but only one bothered to repeat the last count word. Repeats of the question elicited puzzlement, some recounting, and so on; the responses suggest we violated the conversational rule, "Don't ask about what has been communicated"—in this case the numerosity implied by the count. The implication is clear: Repeating the "How many?" question risks confounding assessments of interpretative and conceptual competence.

Because the experimental setting is hardly an everyday experience for any major culture or ethnic group of preschool children, we might expect the rules that apply here to be relatively late to develop—even for those who are encouraged to initiate talk about what they know. A particularly interesting illustration of this comes from a finding that 4- and 5-year-old children who "fail" the two-question conservation task probably do so because they are motivated to please the experimenter. Researchers had children watch puppets who either passed or failed conservation tests. The children were to indicate whether the puppets' answers served to "tell what they knew" or "please the experimenter." The children said that the nonconserving puppets were trying to please the experimenter and that the conserving puppets were telling what they knew. These findings are relevant to any situation where children must answer the same question again and again, as for example, in a therapeutic interview or court setting.

Toddlers and preschoolers are novices in noncore domains. It is hard to underestimate the effect that knowledge about a domain has on anyone's ability to engage in sensible problem solving, produce coherent classifications, and reach inferences. A given set of principles, the rules of their application, and the entities to which they apply together constitute a domain. Different domains are defined by different sets of principles. Therefore, we can say that a body of knowledge constitutes a domain of knowledge if we can show that a set of interrelated principles organizes its rules of operation and entities. For example, the mental operations of addition and subtraction in combination with the cardinal (count) numbers constitute one domain. The intuitive understanding of principles of mechanics, as applied to objects and their motion and existence conditions, make up another domain. Note that from this perspective, discrimination learning tasks or general processes like problem solving do not constitute a domain.

Some of the many domains that people can acquire have an innate basis but not all domains are core domains. Core, or innate, domains are universally shared; they develop from a common set of existing skeletal structures. Given their presence, learners already have the wherewithal to find and assimilate relevant data. If the data are present in the surrounding environments, learning can proceed without the explicit help of others. In this sense, learning can take place "on the fly," as the learner encounters domain-relevant inputs to assimilate to an existing structure. Learning in a noncore, novel domain, however, must proceed without the benefit of even a skeletal structure, so the acquisition of knowledge in the domain will be more difficult.

Extensive work on the differences between adults who are novices and experts underscores this point. In one study, novices and experts were asked to sort physics textbook problems in any way they wished. Novices did so on the basis of the perceptual aspects of the diagrams or the apparatus; for example, inclined plane and pulley problems were grouped separately. Experts classified the problems on the basis of underlying physics principles needed to solve the problem, for example, Newton's Second Law. They were able to apply the organizing principles of their acquired (noncore) domain of knowledge to the different problems. Because the novices did not share this principled knowledge, they did not categorize the problems based on the laws of physics. Therefore, they could either use a default strategy based on perceptual cues to classify problems, or map the input to whatever existing mental structures they had available. Both kinds of strategies were used: the former are classified as examples of perceptual solutions, the latter as examples of misconceptions. Neither are examples of conceptual understanding on the part of the novices. Yet it is unlikely that a reader would conclude that the adults in this study were at a stage of cognitive development that is best characterized as perception-bound. Instead, one might argue that in order to gain an understanding of Newtonian physics, one needs extensive time to build up new conceptual structures. These new ones differ from those that serve our every-day cognitions about objects in the world, which are more qualitative than quantitative in form. Further, one might ask whether the conceptual structures for children and adults are all that different when the focus is a core, as opposed to a noncore, domain of knowledge. The animate–inanimate distinction is an example.

Young children, as a group, know a great deal about the different kinds of causes for movement. Massey and Gelman showed this in their 1988 study of whether 3- and 4-year-old children are able to indicate whether novel objects depicted in photographs could move themselves both up and down a hill. The pictures showed objects drawn from five categories: mammals, nonmammals, statues that share animal parts, wheeled devices, and rigid complex objects. The young children were extremely good at the task. They did not rely on surface perceptual similarity rule. For example, they denied that statues could move by themselves even if they had arms and legs. When probed further, children left no ambiguity in their replies, saying, for example, "does not have real legs," or "just a furniture-animal." Gelman also found that young children can give sensible answers to questions about the insides of objects, a result that complements their knowledge that animates and inanimates use internal rather than external sources of causal energy.

The literatures on early numerical and spatial concepts add weight for a theory that assumes very young children are inclined to learn about some domains with facility. The case for an early principled understanding of addition and subtraction in combination with counting principles that render cardinal representations of collections is supported by a variety of converging lines of evidence. Preschoolers can detect principled counting errors, invent counting strategies to solve addition and subtraction problems, and deal with novel counting problems. They can also disambiguate ambiguous instructions and settings. Cross-cultural work shows commonalities in how young children learn the first nine digits in count lists and in error patterns in addition and subtraction.

IV. FROM CORE TO NONCORE DOMAINS OF KNOWLEDGE

The young child's competence with natural numbers does not guarantee clear sailing when it comes to learning numerical concepts that are not represented by a core domain. This is a problem for all theories of cognitive development. Movement to formal operations, whether one is a school-aged child or college-educated adult, does not assure parallel passage to understandings of probability, rational numbers, mechanics, evolution, and chemistry. This is a startling fact given the Piagetian school's emphasis on these in the discussions of formal operations. People all over the world have a persistent problem with the concept of rational numbers, even with years of instruction, which constitutes a serious challenge to associationist theories of concept learning. Despite a great deal of exposure to examples meant to foster associative strength for new concepts, there is little advance toward learning these with understanding.

In the end, new understanding in a domain will proceed rapidly when the structure of the target domain is consistent with that of the existing mental structure. However, if the structure of the target domain is different from existing knowledge structures, new learnings will be difficult to acquire. In order for learning with understanding to occur in a noncore domain, the mind has to acquire both the structure and the domain-relevant database of the novel domain. Learning in noncore domains can be handicapped for a straightforward reason: there is no domain-relevant structure, not even a skeletal one, to start the ball rolling. This means that the mental structures have to be acquired de novo for noncore domains like chess, sushi making, computer programming, literary criticism, and so on. In these cases, learners have the twofold task of acquiring both domain-relevant structures and a coherent base of domain-relevant knowledge about the content of that domain. It is far from easy to assemble truly new conceptual structures and it takes a very long time. Some training such as formal instruction is usually required, and still this is not effective unless there is extended practice and effort on the part of the learner. Efforts to provide domain-relevant instruction in noncore domains must recognize and overcome a crucial challenge: Learners may assimilate inputs to existing conceptual structures even when those inputs are intended to force progress in the mental structures and conceptual change. That is, learners may fail to interpret novel inputs as intended and instead treat it as further examples of the understanding they currently have. The risk for this happening is especially high in mathematics classes, to give one example. Harnett and Gelman illustrate this contrast between learning in core and noncore domains. They contrasted elementary school children's rapid acquisition of understanding that every natural number has a successor with their painfully slow progress in understanding rational numbers. The difference is so pronounced that high school and college students around the world cannot be counted on to interpret rational numbers correctly.

V. SUMMARY

The evidence favors a theory that posits skeletal structures and grants the mind an ability to use them and engage actively in its own cognitive development. Domain-specific and stage theories are consistent with this conclusion and present challenges for domain-general theories of conceptual change. A domain-specific theory is consistent with the idea that development involves qualitative shifts in understanding, especially regarding advanced understanding of mathematics, science, and the acquisition of other noncore expertise that characterizes master chefs, chess players, professors of psychology, and so on. Success in these latter domains requires the construction of new conceptual structures, something that is extremely hard to do. Building these structures requires mastery of the specialized language and tools of the domain. As an example, second language learning for adults is never easy. Ponder then, the problem of mastery when there is no understanding of the concepts to which the specialized language maps onto, and we see then that cognitive development is a lifespan endeavor.

BIBLIOGRAPHY

Baillargeon, R., Spelke, E. S., & Wasserman, S. (1985). Object permanence in five-month-old infants. *Cognition, 20,* 191–208.

Baillargeon, R., Kotovsky, L., & Needham, A. (1995). The acquisition of physical knowledge in infancy. In D. Sperber, D. Premack, & A. J. Premack (Eds.), *Causal cognition: A multidisciplinary approach* (pp. 79–116). Oxford, England: Oxford/Clarendon Press.

Brown, A. L. (1990). Domain-specific principles affect learning and transfer in children. *Cognitive Science, 14,* 107–133.

Carey, S. (1985). Are children fundamentally different kinds of thinkers and learners than adults? In S. Chipman, J. Segal, & R. Glaser (Eds.), *Thinking and learning skills: Research and open questions.* Hillsdale, NJ: Lawrence Erlbaum Associates.

Diamond, A. (1991). Neuropsychological insights into the meaning of object concept development. In S. Carey & R. Gelman (Eds.), *The epigenesis of mind: Essays on biology and cognition* (pp. 67–110). Hillsdale, NJ: Lawrence Erlbaum Associates.

Gelman, R. (1993). A Rational-constructivist account of early learning about numbers and objects. In D. Medin (Ed.), *Learning and motivation* (Vol. 30). New York: Academic Press.

Gelman, R. (in press). In Craik, F. (Ed.), Domain specificity and cognitive development: Universals and non-universals. *International perspectives on psychological science. Vol. 2.* Hove, UK: Lawrence Erlbaum. (Based on a State of the Art Address, International Congress in Psychology, International Union of Psychological Science, Montreal, 1996).

Harris, P. L. (1983). Infant cognition. In M. M. Haith & J. J. Campos (Eds.), *Handbook of child psychology: Vol. 2. Infancy and developmental psychobiology* (4th ed.). New York: Wiley.

Harnett, P. M., & Gelman, R. (In press). Early understandings of number: Paths or barriers to the construction of new understandings? *The Journal of the European Association for Learning and Instruction, 4.*

Kalnins, I. V., & Bruner, J. S. (1973). The coordination of visual observation and instrumental behavior in early infancy. *Perception, 2,* 307–314.

Massey, C., & Gelman, R. (1988). Preschoolers decide whether pictured unfamiliar objects can move themselves. *Developmental Psychology, 24,* 307–317.

Siegler, R. S. (1991). *Children's thinking* (2nd ed.). Englewood Cliffs, NJ: Prentice Hall.

Spelke, E. S., Phillips, A., & Woodward, A. L. (1995). Infants' knowledge of object motion and human action. In D. Sperber, D. P. Premack, & A. J. Premack (Eds.), *Causal cognition: A multidisciplinary debate* (pp. 44–78). Oxford, England: Clarendon Press/Oxford University Press.

Cognitive Therapy

Marjorie E. Weishaar

Brown University School of Medicine

Automatic Thoughts Thoughts that are involuntary and difficult to inhibit.
Cognitions Thoughts and images.
Cognitive Distortions Habitual errors in logic.
Cognitive Organization A model of cognitions arranged hierarchically which reflects the accessibility and stability of various types of thoughts, beliefs, and assumptions.
Cognitive Shift The change from flexible thinking, which allows reappraisal and reevaluation, to more rigid thinking characteristic of psychological distress.
Cognitive Specificity Thoughts and images that are specific to diagnostic categories. For example, the cognitive themes of anxiety are danger and threat.
Continuity Hypothesis Hypothesis that psychological syndromes are exaggerated and persistent forms of normal emotional responses.
Schemas Cognitive structures that hold core beliefs and, when triggered, generate affect-laden thoughts and images.

COGNITIVE THERAPY is a form of psychotherapy that posits that how an individual perceives and interprets events strongly influences how that person responds emotionally and behaviorally. It combines cognitive and behavioral techniques to teach patients to challenge biased perceptions and the underlying assumptions that may cause them to distort current situations. It is best known as an effective treatment for unipolar depression. Since its establishment 30 years ago, it has been applied to a wide range of psychological problems and clinical populations. Outcome studies have demonstrated its usefulness in the treatment of depression and have suggested that cognitive therapy has some preventive effects against future depressive episodes. Current research is investigating whether cognitive therapy can prevent a first episode of depression among those at risk. In addition, cognitive therapy techniques are being used in schools to promote cooperation and self-esteem. Thus, this form of therapy can be used to promote mental health at the individual and community levels.

I. COGNITIVE THERAPY AND MENTAL HEALTH

Cognitive therapy is a system of psychotherapy that emphasizes the role of information processing in human behavior and psychological distress. It posits that how people perceive, interpret, and assign meanings to events strongly influences their emotional and behavioral reactions. It also maintains that significant life experiences shape core beliefs about the self and the world. These core beliefs, in turn, affect how new information is incorporated. Cognitive therapy is thus concerned with both the idiosyncratic meanings of events for people and the ways in which these meanings are generated and maintained. Although the content of cognitions (i.e., thoughts and images) may be highly personal, the mechanisms of cognitive processing are believed to be universal.

Cognitive therapy was developed in the 1960s by psychiatrist Aaron T. Beck. It is derived from empirical findings from studies of depressed patients. Beck found that depressed patients' thinking is saturated with themes of deprivation, defeat, and loss. Moreover, their judgments are absolute and rigid. Usually, information processing proceeds in a fairly flexible manner, so that initial impressions or primary appraisals may be checked and verified or adjusted. Beck observed that during depression this flexibility is lost, making it extremely difficult for depressed persons to generate alternative interpretations of events, solutions to problems, or new ways of behaving. Cognitive deficits, such as impaired perception, recall, and long-term memory, interfere with reasoning. Errors in logic, or *cognitive distortions,* become more apparent and create a negative bias to thinking.

Cognitive distortions are present in the thinking of nondepressed persons as well, for no one has perfect understanding. However, in the case of depression, anxiety, or other syndromes, these distortions are rigidly applied and initial impressions are not reevaluated. Self-correction is limited. In addition, in psychological distress, errors in thinking are combined with maladaptive assumptions, leading the patient in a negative spiral. Cognitive distortions include overgeneralization, dichotomous thinking, arbitrary inference, selective abstraction, personalization, and maximization and minimization. The goals of cognitive therapy are to return the person to more flexible thinking and to modify maladaptive beliefs and assumptions which may be risks for further depression. Cognitive therapy teaches people to identify and correct the distortions in their thinking to regain flexibility. It also teaches them to assess the utility of their beliefs and assumptions and to modify them if necessary. Beliefs are modified by examining them logically and considering alternative interpretations and through behavioral experiments designed to challenge specific assumptions.

The cognitive model of depression has found support for descriptive aspects of its theory and for its treatment efficacy. Cognitive therapy has also been applied to a number of other psychological disorders, including anxiety, personality disorders, substance abuse, eating disorders, stress, and marital conflict. More recently, it has been applied to nonclinical problems, such as management problems in business and conflict resolution in schools.

An important finding of treatment outcome studies in depression has been the apparent benefit of cognitive therapy in relapse prevention. This finding has generated studies of depression prevention with populations at risk. Thus, cognitive therapy may be helpful in preventing depression, not just in treating people once they have become depressed. Additionally, school intervention programs that teach cognitive skills such as problem solving, disputing negative self-talk, and improving self-esteem promote positive adjustment at a community level. In this sense, cognitive interventions may contribute to public health.

In theory and in practice, cognitive therapy addresses a spectrum of mental health, from treating psychiatric diagnoses to enhancing the functioning of those at risk for depression or poor social adjustment. This article reviews the cognitive model of psychopathology, describes characteristics of healthy cognitive functioning and presents information on how cognitive therapy may be used to promote mental health.

II. PRINCIPLES OF COGNITIVE THEORY

A. Cognitive Organization

Cognitive therapy envisions a cognitive organization that is hierarchically structured and cognitive mechanisms that selectively take in or screen out relevant information. The most accessible cognitions in this hierarchy are voluntary thoughts which appear in stream-of-consciousness reports. Less accessible, but more stable, are automatic thoughts, which arise without awareness and are difficult to inhibit, especially at times of emotional arousal. At the next level are beliefs and assumptions, including values. At the deepest level, out of the person's awareness, are core beliefs embedded in cognitive structures called *schemas.* The cognitive model proposes that these schemas are latent until triggered by a personally relevant life event. In depression, for example, a life event might trigger a schema of loss, deprivation, or defeat. This would be the mechanism that sets in motion the negative cognitive shift. As a consequence of the cognitive shift, much positive information is filtered out by cognitive distortions, and negative self-relevant information is accepted. The person is thus flooded by negative automatic thoughts.

Automatic thoughts are important in cognitive therapy because they are accessible and reflect core beliefs. They are also full of cognitive distortions. Cognitive therapy works directly on correcting biased thinking by challenging the validity of automatic thoughts. It also works at a structural level to modify maladaptive beliefs and assumptions contained in schemas. It is presumed that these schema-level beliefs are a cognitive vulnerability to various psychological disorders and, if not addressed, pose a risk of recurrence for that disorder.

B. Cognitive Specificity

Although individuals have idiosyncratic thoughts, themes appear within diagnostic categories. Studies comparing the cognitive content of depression and anxiety have found that the cognitions of depressed patients reflect themes of loss, defeat, worthlessness, and deprivation, and anxious patients express themes of danger and threat.

C. Continuity Hypothesis

The cognitive model of psychopathology emphasizes well-being on a continuum. Various psychopathological syndromes are viewed as exaggerated and persistent forms of normal emotional responses. Thus, there is "continuity" between the content of normal reactions and the excessive responses seen in psychological disorders. This hypothesis fits an evolutionary perspective, for it suggests that disorders are extreme manifestations of adaptive strategies. In addition, the notion of continuity makes psychological syndromes more understandable, because people in general can identify with the less severe forms of the behaviors. Indeed, extrapolating from observations of psychopathology gives information about the more subtle biases common in everyday reactions. For example, the intense fear of negative evaluation in social phobia is an exaggeration of the normal social vulnerability and self-consciousness felt in many social interactions.

Positive bias and positive illusion, noted in many non-depressed individuals, have an extreme expression in the expansiveness and self-aggrandisement of mania. [*See* PHOBIAS.]

Cognitive therapy research has identified cognitive risk factors for various disorders. As a psychotherapy, it is biased in its attention to deficits and limited in its generalizability from clinical samples. Thus, conceptualizations of mental health must be tempered with evidence from social, developmental, and cognitive psychology, which investigate normal populations but are often biased in the direction of generalizing from contrived, laboratory situations. Cognitive models of several disorders are presented here to elucidate cognitive risk factors to mental health. These risk factors are considered in the design of interventions to treat and prevent psychological distress. In addition, contributions from other branches of psychology are presented to consider how healthy cognitive functioning can be promoted.

III. COGNITIVE MODEL OF DEPRESSION

The cognitive model posits that in nonendogenous, unipolar depression, life events activate highly charged negative schemas which override more adaptive schemas and set negatively biased cognitive processing in motion. The activation of schemas is the mechanism by which depression occurs, not its cause. Depression may be caused by any combination of genetic, biological, stress, or personality factors. Regardless of its cause, the same cognitive changes occur in depression. Cognitive distortions bias perceptions and interpretations, judgments and problem-solving skills become limited, and thinking reflects the cognitive triad: a negative view of the self as a failure, a negative view of one's personal world as harsh and unyielding, and a negative view of the future as hopeless. As a consequence of pessimism, hopelessness, or apathy, the depressed person becomes less active, avoids social contact, and takes fewer risks. Reduced performance is then taken as a sign of failure or worthlessness, reinforcing the negative view of the self.

Although the cognitive model is not explicitly causal, it does propose that schemas containing negative beliefs about the self and the world are a cognitive vulnerability to depression. Examples of depressogenic schemas are, "I am unlovable" and "I can never get what I want." Schemas are believed to be established by early learning experiences which are reinforced over time. As they are used to explain further events, schemas become anchored and are both self-perpetuating and difficult to change.

Cognitive therapy also considers the interaction of personality and stressful life events in the onset of depression. Two broad personality types have been identified among depressed patients: autonomous and sociotropic. Autonomous individuals are most likely to become depressed when thwarted from achieving their goals or when confronted with failure. Sociotropic types are most sensitive to personal rejection or to loss of a relationship. Although these are pure types at opposite ends of a continuum of personality styles, they allow investigation of the relationship between life events and various cognitive vulnerabilities. Current research supports the association between sociotropy and depressive symptoms.

Beck's original formulation of depression describes nonendogenous, unipolar depression. He later refined his theory to include six separable but overlapping models: cross-sectional, structural, stressor–vulnerability, reciprocal interaction, psychobiological, and evolutionary. This reformulation was made to describe comprehensively the onset and maintenance of various types of depression. It was articulated in response to such developments in psychology as the growing interest in Bowlby's attachment theory, the emergence of evolutionary psychology, and findings on marital interaction and depression. For example, the original cognitive model exemplifies the stressor–vulnerability model. The maintenance of depression seen in marital discord demonstrates the reciprocal interaction model.

A further clarification of the cognitive theory of depression addressed the misconception that cognitive therapy states that only the thinking of depressed persons is inaccurate or distorted. Research from the field of social cognition demonstrates that the thinking of nondepressed persons tends to be distorted or biased in an optimistic way, rather than being entirely realistic or rational. It also appears that the thinking of mildly depressed persons is more accurate in some specific ways than is the thinking of euthymic individuals. Beck conceives of bias as operating in either a positive or negative direction. According to his formulation, the nondepressed cognitive organization has a positive bias, as it shifts toward depression, the posi-

tive cognitive bias is neutralized, and as depression develops, a negative bias occurs. In bipolar cases, there is a pronounced swing into an exaggerated bias as the manic phase develops.

A negative bias in thinking is most likely to occur when data are not immediately present, are not concrete, are ambiguous, and are relevant to self-evaluation. An important feature of the cognitive bias in depression seems to be a perception that current negative circumstances cannot improve. Thus, a depressed person may perceive a situation accurately, but lack the persistence and creativity necessary to solve the problem. [*See* DEPRESSION.]

IV. COGNITIVE RISK FACTORS IN SUICIDE

Research on suicide risk was a natural outgrowth of Beck's depression research, and his prospective studies have contributed to the understanding of psychological processes in suicide, particularly the role of hopelessness in predicting suicide. Hopelessness is conceived of as a relatively stable schema, incorporating negative expectations of the future.

Other researchers have identified additional cognitive risk factors for suicide that emerge even with the level of depression and degree of pathology controlled. They are low self-concept, dysfunctional assumptions, the absence of positive beliefs or reasons for living, cognitive rigidity, and poor problem-solving skills. The last two risk factors, cognitive rigidity and poor problem-solving skills, have received attention recently because of their pervasiveness in psychological disorders. Two examples of cognitive rigidity are dichotomous thinking and perfectionism. Evidence for the relationship between all-or-nothing thinking and suicidal behavior is long-standing. In addition, dichotomous thinking is found in a range of psychological disorders, including personality disorders. It is also characteristic of the thinking of normal adolescents.

Recent research also indicates a relationship between perfectionism and suicide risk. Among inpatients, for example, a perfectionistic attitude toward the self and sensitivity to social criticism have been found to be associated with suicide ideation independent of depression and hopelessness. Other research has found that a certain type of perfectionism—perceived expectations for the individual by society—is related to suicide ideation. The belief that the world holds unrealistic and unbending expectations for an individual represents a component of the cognitive triad, the negative view of the world.

Perfectionism may generally inhibit healthy functioning. Analysis of the data from the Treatment of Depression Collaborative Study, which compared the efficacies of pharmacotherapy, cognitive therapy, and interpersonal therapy, found that subjects who had perfectionistic attitudes had a significantly negative relationship to therapeutic outcome, regardless of the type of treatment modality they received. In contrast, subjects with relatively low levels of perfectionism were responsive to all forms of intervention. Perfectionism may be thought of as a risk factor for depression and suicide, and as a challenge to psychotherapy in general.

Problem-solving deficits are of interest not only because of their demonstrated relationships to depression and suicide, but also because social problem-solving is an important skill in general adjustment. Problem solving is being taught in schools as a way to reduce conflict and promote mental health.

Problem-solving deficits have been found in suicidal children, adolescents, and adults, and these deficits become compounded as problems become interpersonal in nature. Suicidal persons have difficulty accepting problems as a normal part of life and are not inclined to engage in problem solving. Once they engage in problem solving, their solutions show more avoidance, more negative affect, less relevance, less versatility, and less reference to the future than do the solutions of nonsuicidal persons.

An important aspect of problem solving among suicide ideators appears to be a tendency to focus on the potential negative consequences of implementing any solution. This feature reflects how pessimism affects motivation in depression and is congruent with the theory of helplessness depression.

A number of researchers have constructed and tested models of how various suicide risk factors might interact. It appears that hopelessness, problem-solving skills, and self-concept are independent risk factors. Beck's observations of patients hospitalized for suicidal ideation shed some light on how self-concept, problem-solving skills, and hopelessness may appear statelike for some patients and traitlike for others. One group studied was composed of depressed persons. Their hopelessness, suicidal ideation, self-concept, and problem-solving abilities improved when their depression remitted. The second group was composed of patients with alcoholism, personality disorders, and antisocial behavior problems. Their negative views of themselves were reinforced by society. This group was characterized by cognitive rigidity, impulsivity, and poor problem-solving skills, which persisted between suicidal crises. Indeed, these characteristics may have predisposed these patients to future suicidal episodes. Thus, for some, poor problem-solving is temporary; for others, it is more chronic. It appears that once suicide becomes an alternative, restricted problem-solving ability can establish it as a stereotyped response in a very limited behavioral repertoire. [See IMPULSE CONTROL; SUICIDE.]

V. COGNITIVE MODEL OF ANXIETY DISORDERS

Whereas the cognitive themes in depression are deprivation, defeat, and loss, the cognitive theme in anxiety disorders is danger. Following the continuity hypothesis, anxiety reactions are on a continuum with normal physiologic responses, but are exaggerated reactions to perceived threat. Cognitive therapy views anxiety from an evolutionary perspective, as originating in the flight, freeze, or fight responses apparent in animal behavior. These innate responses to physical danger became less adaptive in humans over the millenia as danger became less physical and more psychosocial in nature.

The cognitive model of anxiety emphasizes the roles of beliefs and interpretations of events in maintaining and escalating anxiety. Anxious cognitions reflect unrealistic perceptions of danger, catastrophic interpretations about loss of control, or perceived negative changes in a relationship. As in depression, there are underlying beliefs, such as, "the world is a dangerous place," which make one vulnerable to anxiety. Cognitive distortions support those underlying beliefs and contribute to the overestimation of the probability of a feared event, the overestimation of the severity of the event were it to happen, the underestimation of one's ability to cope with the feared event, and the underestimation of "rescue factors" such as the presence of people or environmental factors that could help or reduce risk.

The contribution of cognitions to anxiety is exemplified in the cognitive model of recurrent panic. In this case, the person's catastrophic misinterpretation of his or her own physiology escalates anxiety to the point of panic. The sequence is as follows: a variety of factors (e.g., mild anxiety, caffeine, exercise, excitement) create mild sensations that are interpreted as signs of internal disaster. Consequently, there is a marked increase in anxiety which leads to a further heightening of bodily sensations. This creates a vicious cycle, which culminates in a panic attack. Stress-induced hyperventilation may be part of this cycle if somatic sensations are interpreted as a sign of imminent danger. In the case of panic, the feared stimulus is one's own physiology. Once a person has had a panic attack, he or she becomes hypervigilant to any signs of physiological arousal. One's own physiology becomes the feared stimulus. Treatment, therefore, includes exposure to physical sensations.

Cognitive therapy, which uses cognitive techniques alone or in combination with behavioral techniques, can almost eliminate panic attacks after 12 to 16 weeks of treatment. [See ANXIETY; PANIC ATTACKS.]

VI. COGNITIVE MODEL OF PERSONALITY DISORDERS

Cognitive therapy conceptualizes personality disorders as legacies of hominid evolution. They are seen as exaggerated expressions of primitive "strategies," which at one time influenced survival and reproductive success. For example, the adaptive strategy of attachment becomes exaggerated as "I am helpless" in the dependent personality.

In addition, the repetitive nature of maladaptive behaviors seen in personality disorders indicates the frequency with which maladaptive schemas are triggered. Beck and his associates have found that the maladaptive schemas in personality disorders are triggered in many if not most situations, have a compulsive quality, and are extremely difficult to modify or control. Compared with other people, the dysfunctional attitudes found in persons with personality disorders are rigid, overgeneralized, absolute, and resistant to change.

The dysfunctional beliefs in personality disorders are thought to be a result of the interaction between the person's genetic predisposition and exposure to specific undesirable or traumatic events. Maladaptive behavior patterns may result from reinforcement of such behaviors over a person's lifetime. Such maladaptive behaviors may arise from avoidance or from compensation or overcompensation for dysfunctional beliefs. For example, a person who fears abandonment might avoid relationships altogether, cling to partners and drive them away, or end relationships before they can be left by the other parties. Any of these behaviors can reinforce the dysfunctional belief that the person will inevitably be abandoned. [See PERSONALITY.]

VII. WHAT DOES HEALTHY COGNITIVE FUNCTIONING LOOK LIKE?

Cognitive therapy is derived from research on clinical populations, particularly depressed patients. Characteristics of the diagnostic groups studied are assumed to be extreme manifestations of qualities that are also found in normal people. Among depressed patients, for example, thinking is characterized by cognitive distortions or errors in logic, by cognitive rigidity, and by maladaptive core beliefs. Does this mean that the thinking of nondepressed people is free of distortions or an accurate reflection of reality? It does not.

Considerable evidence from cognitive and social psychology testifies to the presence of illusion or a general, enduring pattern of error, bias, or both in the information processing of normal people. However, the bias in thinking is positively skewed. Experimental studies, typically done with college student volunteers, show that nondepressed thinking is characterized by unrealistically positive views of the self, exaggerated perceptions of control, and unrealistic optimism.

This is apparent in attributional or explanatory style. The explanatory style of depressed persons is to attribute causality of negative, uncontrollable events to internal, stable, and global causes. One fails a test because one is stupid, not because that particular test was especially difficult. Nondepressed people, who have positive illusions concerning control and self-perception, are better able to externalize failure and thus not damage their general sense of self-esteem.

It appears from several lines of evidence that mildly depressed people, those with low self-esteem, or both have more balanced self-perceptions, more evenhanded assessments of their future circumstances, and a more accurate sense of personal control than do nondepressed persons. In contrast, both clinically depressed and euthymic people have biased thinking.

It is not surprising that many of the same cognitive mechanisms operate in different mood states, but they operate to different ends. Studies in social cognition support many of the clinical observations on which cognitive therapy is based. In 1989, Janoff-Bulman wrote about the benefits of illusion for mental health. She describes how preverbal interactions with responsive caregivers establish supraordinate schemas that are positively biased and largely reflect reality at the time they are established. One need only substitute the experience of a child with unresponsive, neglectful, or depriving caregivers to arrive at maladaptive schemas. The early interactions among people receiving good care teach them that the world is benevolent and controllable, and that they are worthy of care. Although later experience may somewhat contradict or qualify these assumptions, they will remain fundamentally intact. Evidence that does not confirm positive assumptions can be ignored, dismissed, or reinterpreted to fit previously held beliefs. This process is the same as that in depression: cognitive distortions screen out positive information or distort neutral information to maintain negative schemas. Only traumatic negative events pose a serious challenge to the equilibrium of positive illusions.

Parallels between the cognitive processes in depression and those in well-being also appear in Taylor and Brown's theory of cognitive adaptation. They present a model of normal cognitive processing in which social and cognitive filters make information largely positive as opposed to the disproportionately negative bias that results from the mental filters operating in depression. These authors conclude that the mentally healthy person appears to have the capacity to distort reality in a direction that enhances self-esteem, maintains a sense of personal efficacy, and promotes an optimistic view of the future. This positive triad is in striking contrast to the cognitive triad in depression.

For both depressed and nondepressed people, biased thinking is most apparent in situations that are ambiguous and that are relevant to self-evaluation. For both negative and overly positive thinking, ambiguous information tends to be interpreted to fit with prior beliefs or schemas.

Just as the cognitive model of psychopathology

might overemphasize the negative aspects of biased cognitive processing and thus appear to endorse rationality, models from cognitive and social psychology might overemphasize the benefits of positive illusion for mental health. Some researchers have addressed various types of illusions and the circumstances under which they appear helpful and not so helpful.

Taylor's research on cognitive adaptation to threatening events such as rape and cancer found that illusions of meaning, mastery, and self-esteem fostered positive adjustment. Individuals who made causal attributions that maintained a sense of personal control and who could construct some personal benefit from the negative experience fared better psychologically than those unable to use illusion. Taylor concludes that illusion is essential for normal cognitive functioning. She also argues that having an accurate self-perception should not be a criterion of mental health, as has been customarily believed. [*See* CANCER; RAPE.]

It also appears from the work of others that illusions are only adaptive if they do not stray too far from the truth. Illusions that are too inflated may lead to self-defeating behavior. A small positive distortion of the truth, rather than unbridled optimism, seems optimal.

Janoff-Bulman proposes that positive illusions are most beneficial at the level of core beliefs or schemas. She sees conceptual (or cognitive) systems as hierarchically organized. Higher-order postulates represent one's most abstract, global, and generalized theories about oneself and the world. Lower-order postulates are narrow generalizations that relate to specific domains of life, such as one's abilities. These hierarchical distinctions are compatible with Beck's notions of core schemas and more accessible assumptions, respectively. Janoff-Bulman argues that higher-order postulates, which are least subject of all cognitions to empirical validation or invalidation, may contain positive inaccuracies without being problematic. However, inaccuracies and positive illusions at the level of lower-order postulates are maladaptive. In other words, it is not harmful to have a generally positive view of oneself as a competent person as long as one is aware of one's limitations in specific areas.

According to Janoff-Bulman's theory, the advantage of positive higher-order assumptions (or schemas) is that they enable a person to attempt to tackle new situations. Thus, positive illusion at this level benefits affect and motivation. One can see how such optimism might allow someone to engage in creative problem solving when faced with a novel situation. [*See* OPTIMISM, MOTIVATION, AND MENTAL HEALTH.]

Another benefit of generalized positive illusions about the self relates to efficacy in problem solving. People with high self-esteem appear better able to discriminate soluble from insoluble problems than are people with low self-esteem. They are more able than people with low self-esteem to know when to quit and to feel comfortable quitting. They may also choose to work only on problems that can be solved, thereby reinforcing their sense of self-efficacy. [*See* SELF-ESTEEM.]

In contrast to Taylor, Janoff-Bulman believes the healthiest people probably have a good sense of their strengths and weaknesses, their possibilities and limitations. The key appears to be maintaining positive illusions at the level of fundamental beliefs while aiming for and accepting accuracy at the level of everyday, specific interactions with the world. Healthy people can thus respond to environmental feedback and learn.

Healthy cognitive functioning is creative and flexible enough to reexamine strategies that no longer work. No doubt, healthy beliefs contain inaccuracies, but they are adaptive in that they allow one to maintain a sense of self-worth while trying to learn from one's experiences. Healthy functioning also recognizes emotions as important sources of information about the self and the environment. Cognitive therapy allows patients to reappraise and empirically test their lower-order postulates within the context of a caring and collaborative therapeutic relationship. Although schema change at the level of higher-order postulates is more difficult to achieve, longer term cognitive therapy may allow for these fundamental changes.

VIII. SOME DEVELOPMENTAL CONSIDERATIONS

Research in cognitive development, social cognition, and child psychology lends further insight into what healthy cognitive functioning looks like. The unrealistic optimism and self-confidence apparent in well-adjusted adults has also been found in healthy children. Studies have compared "helpless" and "mastery-oriented" children in their responses to failure. Mastery-oriented children are those who have a sense

of control over an experimental task; helpless children have no such sense of control. Mastery-oriented children were less discouraged by failure than were helpless children. In fact, they did not seem to recognize that they had failed. Instead, they focused on how to overcome defeat. In addition, they expected success in the future and attributed success to their own ability. They exemplified the nondepressed explanatory style articulated by the learned helplessness model of depression. In contrast, the helpless children demonstrated an explanatory style that may be a cognitive vulnerability to depression.

The adaptive explanatory style may not be exclusive to confident children, but may be the rule for all very young children. Some developmental psychologists report that learned helplessness is relatively rare in very young children. They review studies that demonstrate that children around 3 years of age typically overestimate their skills on a wide variety of tasks and have unrealistically positive expectations for success. This may be highly adaptive for the same reason it is adaptive in adults: self-efficacy motivates further action. Unrealistic optimism gives young children the opportunity to try new skills and to practice them. Researchers hypothesize that ignorance of their limitations allows children to try more diverse and complex behaviors that exceed their grasp at the present time. This allows them to practice skills and may foster long-term cognitive benefits.

Kendall's research in cognitive–behavior therapy with children has identified two types of thinking errors in children, cognitive deficiencies and cognitive distortions. Cognitive deficiencies refer to an absence of thinking. Youngsters with such deficiencies lack careful information processing and often act without thinking. Impulsivity is a result of cognitive deficiencies. Cognitive distortions occur among those who engage in information processing, but who do so in a biased or dysfunctional way. Depressed and anxious children demonstrate cognitive distortions in their misperceptions of social and environmental situations and in their self-perceptions. Children with aggressive behavior demonstrate both cognitive deficiencies and cognitive distortions, because they overinterpret signs of hostility and react without careful thought. Targeting cognitive deficiencies in therapy requires stopping nonthoughtful activity and channeling activity into problem solving. Targeting cognitive distortions calls for the identification of faulty thinking and the correction of misperceptions, misattributions, and misinterpretations.

Both developmental theory and clinical studies support the notion that particular types of cognitive distortions are to be expected at certain stages of normal development. For example, dichotomous thinking and overgeneralization emerge in the preoperational stage of cognitive development. Dichotomous thinking is also viewed as characteristic of normal adolescent thinking. However, these natural proclivities may interact with maladaptive schemas and persist into adulthood.

IX. HOW DOES COGNITIVE THERAPY WORK?

Cognitive therapy combines behavioral and cognitive techniques in a collaborative effort with the patient to examine and test the validity and utility of the patient's maladaptive beliefs. The patient's beliefs and assumptions are viewed as hypotheses to be tested. In the course of therapy, alternative perspectives, interpretations of events, and solutions to problems are considered. Through logical examination of beliefs and behavioral experiments to test specific assumptions, the patient learns more adaptive ways of thinking.

Despite the demonstrated efficacy of cognitive therapy, the mechanisms by which it works have not yet been determined. Beck and others believe that cognitive therapy relies on empirical hypothesis testing to produce changes in beliefs. An explicit goal of the therapy is to teach patients this strategy so that they may apply it in the future, thereby preventing relapse. Some developmental psychologists explain change in cognitive therapy with Piagetian theory. In cognitive therapy, the presentation of contradictory evidence creates a cognitive imbalance or disequilibrium which can lead to a new and improved balance of knowledge.

There has been some debate as to whether cognitive therapy works by teaching compensatory skills to manage triggered schemas or whether schema change itself can be achieved. It may be that schema change is only possible with longer treatment, whereas compensatory skills operate early in therapy.

One cognitive feature that seems to change with cognitive therapy is explanatory style. Research has found that explanatory style and severity of depression improved together over a course of cognitive therapy and remained stable at follow-up. It has therefore been hypothesized that explanatory style is a mechanism of change for depressed patients receiving cognitive therapy. Undoing a pessimistic explanatory style may be an active ingredient in the therapy. If it is possible to reduce a pessimistic style, it may be possible to reduce the risk of future depressive episodes. Evidence for change in explanatory style among euthymic groups demonstrates that such training is feasible, so perhaps cognitive therapy can be used to prevent an initial depressive episode. For use with euthymic groups, such as business managers or students, cognitive therapy is modified slightly. There is less emphasis on behavioral activation strategies, which occur early in the treatment of depression, and greater emphasis on cognitive strategies to challenge maladaptive thoughts and change explanatory style.

X. THE PREVENTION OF DEPRESSION

A number of outcome studies that examined the efficacy of cognitive therapy for depression found differential relapse rates among those treated with cognitive therapy, with or without medication, and those treated with medication alone. Specifically, it appears that cognitive therapy for depression prevents relapse. Currently, there is no evidence of a preventive effect after termination of antidepressant medication or any other psychotherapy. Interpersonal psychotherapy, another efficacious treatment for depression, appears to reduce risk only as long as it is continued.

As a result of these findings, there is interest in discerning whether cognitive therapy can truly prevent relapse and whether it can prevent a first episode of depression among populations at risk.

The Penn Prevention Program used a school-based, cognitive–behavioral intervention to prevent a first episode of depression in 10- to 13-year-old children. The children were identified as being at-risk for depression on the basis of depressive symptoms and their reports of parental conflict. The cognitive–behavioral techniques were designed to teach children coping strategies to use when confronted with negative life events, thereby increasing their sense of mastery and competence. In addition to preventing depressive symptoms, the intervention attempted to address problems associated with depression, such as academic difficulties, poor peer relations, low self-esteem, and behavior problems. [*See* COPING WITH STRESS.]

The program consisted of a cognitive component, a social problem-solving component, and a coping skills component. The cognitive component taught flexible thinking and how to evaluate the accuracy of beliefs. It also included explanatory style training to foster more accurate, less pessimistic attributions. For situations in which an accurate interpretation of events was negative, children were taught to focus on solutions or on ways to cope with emotions. Coping techniques included decatastrophizing about potential outcomes of the problem, distraction, steps to distance oneself from stressful situations, relaxation training, and ways to seek social support. In this way, investigators tried to address both cognitive distortions and cognitive deficiencies. The cognitive interventions addressed dysfunctional thinking, and the problem-solving and coping skills components prevented impulsive actions.

Those children who received the intervention showed significant reductions in depressive symptoms and improved classroom behavior compared with controls. These differences persisted at 6-month follow-up. The decrease in depressive symptoms was greatest in the children most at risk for depression.

A controlled prevention trial was conducted by Munoz among adults at risk who comprised a multiethnic, low-income sample. This cognitive–behavioral intervention also resulted in a significantly lower incidence of depressive symptoms among those receiving treatment than those in the control group. In addition, there was a lower incidence rate of major depressive episodes in the treatment group, but the cases were too few to be statistically significant.

Prevention of actual depressive episodes was an outcome criterion in a study by Clarke and associates of adolescents at risk by virtue of their subclinical, depressive symptomotology. This 15-session, cognitive–behavioral intervention taught adolescents to identify and challenge negative or dysfunctional thoughts. Participants had a total incidence of unipolar depression of about half of that of the control group, and this persisted through a 12-month follow-up.

Other controlled trials of cognitive therapy and other modalities for the prevention of depression are underway. In the meantime, cognitive therapy skills are being used to promote general social adjustment in school settings. School-based programs nationwide are applying cognitive–behavioral techniques as part of interpersonal skills training and conflict resolution. Cognitive skills such as disputing negative self-talk and problem solving are part of programs that typically include emotional awareness, communication skills, and behavioral self-control strategies. These programs are an example of health promotion, because they are applied at the community level and decrease the likelihood of occurrence of a range of psychological problems. Although cognitive therapy was designed as a treatment for psychological disorders, it may be beneficial in the prevention of psychological distress and in the promotion of well-being.

BIBLIOGRAPHY

Beck, A. T. (1987). Cognitive models of depression. *Journal of Cognitive Psychotherapy: An International Quarterly, 1*(1), 5–37.

Beck, A. T. (1991). Cognitive therapy: A 30-year retrospective. *American Psychologist, 46*(4), 368–375.

Beck, A. T., Emery, G., & Greenberg, R. (1985). *Anxiety disorders and phobias: A cognitive perspective.* New York: Basic Books.

Beck, A. T., Freeman, A., & Associates (1990). *Cognitive therapy of personality disorders.* New York: Guilford Press.

Beck, A. T., Rush, A. J., Shaw, B. F., & Emery, G. (1979). *Cognitive therapy of depression.* New York: Guilford Press.

Clark, D. M., & Beck, A. T. (1988). Cognitive approaches. In C. G. Last & M. Hersen (Eds.), *Handbook of anxiety disorders.* New York: Pergamon.

Janoff-Bulman, R. (1989). The benefits of illusion, the threat of disillusionment, and the limitations of inaccuracy. *Journal of Social and Clinical Psychology, 8*(2), 159–175.

Salkovskis, P. M. (Ed.). (1996). *Frontiers of cognitive therapy.* New York: Guilford Press.

Seligman, M. E. P. (1991). *Learned optimism.* New York: Knopf.

Weishaar, M. E. (1993). *Aaron T. Beck.* London: Sage.

Community Mental Health

Edward Seidman and Sabine Elizabeth French

New York University

Deinstitutionalization The movement to reduce the number of patients kept in mental institutions by releasing them to the care of the community. The original intention of this movement was to maintain former patients in the community with a wide array of comprehensive and supportive services.

Inoculation Programs Programs that are designed to build and strengthen skills in groups of individuals in order to protect them from, and prepare them for, future difficulties.

Primary Prevention Programs that intervene with a population or setting to reduce the incidence, number of new cases, of one or more emotional disorders.

Promotion of Well-Being Programs that foster the development of healthy environments that encourage positive mental health; in turn, these programs reduce the incidence of one or more psychiatric disorders in the population or setting.

Restructuring The alteration of the unwritten rules of a setting in order to facilitate the development of new rules and an environment that facilitates positive mental health; indirectly, such a change reduces the incidence of disorder in the setting.

Risk and Protective Factors Circumstances in an individual's life, a population, or setting that either increase or decrease the chances of suffering from or manifesting problems-in-living. Stressful life events, for example, death of a parent or divorce, and daily hassles are common risk factors, while positive social support is a common protective factor.

Secondary Prevention Programs that identify early signs of a disorder and intervene quickly or at the point of a crisis to short-circuit the problem from developing into a full-blown mental health problem.

Tertiary Prevention Programs that intervene directly with patients to reduce the duration of their career as a patient, that is, to rehabilitate or treat them; thereby reducing the prevalence of psychiatric disorder in the community.

The confluence of two salient events in the early 1960s—efforts to deinstitutionalize the chronically mentally ill and legislation to create **COMMUNITY MENTAL HEALTH** centers across the nation—launched the community mental health movement. With the aide of a prevention framework adapted from the field of public health, this movement has continued to evolve and grow. Initial emphases on tertiary prevention, often in the form of alternative community-based methods of treatment for the severely mentally ill, were followed by efforts aimed at early detection and intervention (secondary prevention), for example, suicide prevention telephone "hotlines." In both tertiary and secondary forms of prevention, emotional and behavioral problems, or early antecedents thereof, continued to be identified at the level of the individual. Interventions were implemented within institutions in contrast to within communities. However, to reduce the incidence of disorder in the population, primary prevention programs aimed at communities, population groups, or settings were developed and implemented. The positive concept of promoting well-being was a further evolution from the notion of preventing disorder. This article describes, explains, and illustrates with exemplary programs the evolution from tertiary prevention to the promotion of well-being that has characterized the community mental health movement during the second half of the twentieth century.

I. ORIGINS OF THE COMMUNITY MENTAL HEALTH MOVEMENT IN TWENTIETH-CENTURY AMERICA

Widespread implementation of conceptions of community mental health did not begin in America until the early 1960s, even though these ideas and practices had numerous roots that originated both in previous centuries and in other nations. In fact, several scholars date the origins of interest in prevention as an alternative to treatment back to the twelfth-century Spanish philosopher Maimonides who spoke of "preventing poverty."

Returning to more recent history, in 1961, in response to a Congressional mandate the final report of the Joint Commission on Mental Illness and Health entitled *Action for Mental Health* was released. Among other things, it called for improved and expanded mental health services including: (a) improved care in small psychiatric hospitals of chronically mentally ill patients; (b) improved and expanded aftercare services, both partial hospitalization and rehabilitation in the community; (c) intensive care for acutely disturbed mental patients in mental health clinics in the community, general hospital psychiatric units, or in small intensive psychiatric centers; and (d) increased efforts at public education about both psychological disorders and the citizenry's inclination to reject the mentally ill.

President John F. Kennedy was extremely receptive to the *Action for Mental Health* report. In a message delivered in 1963, he stated:

we must seek out the causes of mental illness . . . and eradicate them . . . For prevention is far more desirable . . . more economical and it is far more likely to be successful. Prevention will require both specific programs directed especially at known causes, and the general strengthening of our fundamental community, social welfare, and educational programs which can do much to eliminate or correct the harsh environmental conditions which are often associated with mental retardation and illness (p. 2).

Comprehensive care available to all people in their local communities was central to his clarion call for a "bold new approach." These concepts were enacted into legislation as part of the Community Mental Health Centers Act of 1963.

As a result of this legislation, some 1500 catchment areas (currently referred to as mental health service areas) with populations ranging from 75,000 to 200,000 people were created in the United States; each catchment area was eligible for federal construction and staffing funds for a community mental health center. These centers were mandated initially to offer inpatient care, outpatient care, emergency services, partial hospitalization, and consultation and education, and ultimately to include diagnostic services, rehabilitation services, precare and aftercare services, training, and research and evaluation.

Both implicitly and explicitly, the goals of the Joint Commission on Mental Illness and Health, the Kennedy Administration, and the Community Mental Health Centers Act were to provide more humane and effective rehabilitation to those who were severely mentally ill. Patients needed to be integrated into their local communities and smaller treatment settings in contrast to huge, anonymous state hospitals in remote physical locations. Most importantly, they needed continuity of care, as indicated by the array of services to be offered by the local community mental health center.

Several other factors converged with this more humane and progressive approach to the treatment of the chronically mentally ill that were critical to the implementation of this movement toward deinstitutionalization. The use of phenothiazines made it more feasible to return patients to their communities as they were less likely to engage in the extremes of deviant behavior. At the same time, deinstitutionalization was seen as a dramatic cost-saving device by fiscally conservative legislators. As we describe below, ultimately, these fiscal motives undermined the continuity of care and services in the community envisioned by its originators. [*See* MENTAL HOSPITALS AND DEINSTITUTIONALIZATION.]

Other salient factors that drove the community mental health movement included well-publicized, analytic reports that indicated that the mental health needs of the population far outstripped the resources of trained personnel. Moreover, those that needed services the most, for example, urban and rural poor, children, adolescents, and the elderly, received them least often and, generally paid more for these services when they did receive them. If prevention was to fulfill its promise, hard-to-reach, unserved, and underserved populations needed to be reached.

The principles of comprehensive community-based treatment, prevention and the promotion of well-being inherent to the ideology of the community mental health movement have continued to hold sway among practitioners and scholars to the present time. However, presidential support, implementation mechanisms, and financial resources at the national level were seriously undermined during the Nixon and Reagan Administrations.

II. PRINCIPLES OF PREVENTION

As we have seen, the preceding policy initiatives in the area of community mental health were inextricably intertwined with the idea of prevention. In 1964, Gerald Caplan published his classic book entitled *The Principles of Preventive Psychiatry*. Using public health concepts, he described three types of prevention—tertiary, secondary, and primary—as they related to mental health and illness.

The overriding goal of prevention is to reduce the prevalence or number of cases of mental disorder(s) at a specified moment in time in the population or community. Prevalence is, however, a function of both the incidence (the number of new cases diagnosed during a specified time period) and duration (the time between the initial diagnoses and recovery) of a disorder. Reducing duration, incidence, or both, reduces prevalence. Tertiary prevention reduces prevalence by decreasing the duration of a disorder. Secondary prevention can reduce prevalence either by short-circuiting the duration of a disorder or by intervening in the developmental course of a disorder before it has become fully manifested (and so labeled) to decrease in-

cidence. Primary prevention reduces prevalence solely by decreasing the incidence of disorder.

In tertiary prevention, the goal is to reduce the duration of an individual's career as a patient. Here, the patient has already been identified with a problem(s) in living. Thus, tertiary prevention is more appropriately referred to as rehabilitation. In secondary prevention, the goal is to identify early signs or antecedents of psychopathology in an individual so that intervention can be implemented promptly to alter the developmental course, duration, and/or severity of psychopathology. Here, short-circuiting a disorder's duration is the primary means of diminishing prevalence. Early treatment or crisis intervention represent the most common forms of secondary prevention or intervention.

In both tertiary and secondary prevention, problem identification and change take place at the level of an individual person. This distinguishes them from primary prevention. In primary prevention, the prevalence, and more specifically the incidence of a disorder, in a population or setting is reduced. Thus, primary prevention is mass in contrast to individually oriented. It also differs from tertiary and secondary prevention by occurring "before-the-fact." With regard to the nature/target of intervention, the distinction between tertiary/secondary and primary prevention is less clear. While most often the target of intervention in tertiary and secondary prevention is an individual, as we will see below, occasionally the target is the creation or alteration of a setting that a group of problem-identified individuals inhabit. However, based on the sharp differences in problem identification and the locus of change, some authors have suggested that referring to tertiary and secondary prevention as prevention makes the concept of prevention meaningless.

As early as 1964, Caplan offered a compelling definition of primary prevention:

> Primary prevention is a community concept. It involves lowering the rate of new cases of mental disorder in a population over a certain period by counteracting harmful circumstances before they have had a chance to produce illness. It does not seek to prevent a specific person from becoming sick. Instead, it seeks to reduce the risk for a whole population, so that, although some may become ill, their number will be reduced. It thus contrasts with individual patient-oriented psychiatry, which focuses on a single person and deals with general influences only insofar as they are combined in his unique experience (p. 26).

In primary prevention (or "true" prevention), the level of assessment or target of intervention is not an individual, but instead the reduction of the prevalence of disorder in an entire population or setting before it occurs. A vaccine can inoculate an entire population from contracting an illness before anyone has been affected, as exemplified by the polio vaccine or fluoride in water. Similarly, effective social policies can reduce the incidence and prevalence of unwanted problems in a society, as in the case of an effective gun control policy that reduces the homicide rate or a policy of availability and accessibility of condoms for sexually active adolescents that reduces unwanted pregnancies. An example specific to mental health is pellagra that is accompanied by psychotic-like symptoms. Pellagra is a disease that stems, in part, from a deficiency of niacin in the diet. Today, the disease is prevented with a dietary intake that includes a sufficient amount of niacin.

In an effort to reduce the prevalence of a disease, the progression from tertiary to primary prevention points the way toward the promotion of well-being. To the degree that interventions or policies can successfully promote well-being in the population, we will have succeeded in reducing the incidence and prevalence of a wide array of disorders and undesirable outcomes.

In the subsequent sections of this article, we will utilize the preceding principles and articulate more specific ones. These principles will be underscored with the use of exemplary programs in each area: tertiary, secondary, and primary prevention, and the promotion of well-being.

III. TERTIARY PREVENTION

Long-term hospitalization of the mentally ill seemed to do little more than guarantee a chronic pattern of institutionalization. Thus, with the ideology and resources behind the community mental health movement in the 1960s, we began to see the development of a variety of innovative, experimental alternatives to institutional treatment. The goals were to remove patients from state psychiatric or Veteran's hospitals and reintegrate them into local communities with the provision of a comprehensive and critical array of supportive services ranging from housing and employment to cooking, personal grooming, and treatment. These innovative community-based alternatives were not viewed

as magical cures, but instead as the best means to provide patients with some semblance of "normal" lives, and at a minimum, a way to halt the well known iatrogenic effects of institutional treatment.

As a result of the Community Mental Health Movement, the number of state hospital beds were dramatically reduced over the years. Unfortunately, many of the patients who were deinstitutionalized did not receive the continuity of community-based services called for by the architects of this movement. Many patients would quickly return to the hospital for services. They would stay for a short period of time and, then again, be released to the community. This pattern would repeat itself; it came to be known as the "revolving door" phenomena.

Closing state hospitals and reducing the number of beds available did save money, but over time, fewer and fewer of these revenues were returned to local communities to provide for the continuum of services that were essential to community-based treatment. To date, this paradoxical pattern has not abated. Thus, an increasing number of people with serious problems in living are found roaming the streets; they lack access to a comprehensive array of essential residential and rehabilitative services.

While many in politics and the media have judged deinstitutionalization to have been a failure, this verdict is misleading. As envisioned by its architects, the policy of deinstitutionalization was never genuinely implemented since a continuum of comprehensive services tailored to the needs of individual patients was never put into place. However, though isolated, exciting and promising innovative experiments were implemented. Unfortunately, the results of these demonstration programs were ignored as fiscally minded politicians seized upon the opportunity to cut mental health budgets on the basis of the savings realized from the reduction in the number of hospital beds.

One such example of a successful demonstration program in the 1960s was developed by Fairweather and his colleagues; they created an innovative setting as an alternative to institutionalization, known as the community lodge program. Here, 8 to 10 long-term mental patients worked and lived in an autonomous unit outside the hospital. The "lodge" was often located on the border between a middle class and a poor neighborhood. In this way, the residents were able to create a small business and, at the same time, they were less likely to be rejected by their neighbors. The lodge residents shared household management and tasks ranging from cooking and cleaning to budgeting. They established a joint business, for example, a janitorial service, that enabled them to earn income and develop a sense of accomplishment. They ran their own "show" with leadership emerging from their ranks. Professional services, ranging from psychotherapy and medications to accounting, were available to them, but on an as needed basis, and after a time, only when the residents requested these services. Thus, unlike institutional treatment and many group homes that appear similar on the surface, patients no longer found themselves in the characteristic "one-down" relationship with the "doctor who knows best." Results demonstrated that they were able to remain in the community for a longer period than were patients who were assigned to traditional outpatient care upon their release from the hospital.

To prevent the negative effects of institutionalization a number of exemplary innovations were implemented at the point of psychiatric admission. For example, in the 1970s, the Stein, Test, and Marx group in Madison, Wisconsin, developed, implemented, and evaluated an intriguing program that occurred within 1 week of hospitalization. Patients with extensive histories of psychiatric hospitalization who were deemed "unreleasable" by hospital personnel were placed into independent living situations based on their individual resources and needs. The goal was for these patients to make it in the natural environment. In that vein, staff took on the roles of advocate, resource finder, and teacher. Initially available on a 24-hour basis, staff gradually phased themselves out. Staff endeavored to keep patients independent of the usual mental health system and to help them obtain the resources needed for daily living by prodding and supporting job finding, grooming and cooking skills, recreational and social activity, and so forth. Staff also encouraged others to view patients as responsible citizens, even if it meant allowing the patient to spend a day or two in jail for breaking the law. In research evaluating this program, as in the community lodge program, the experimental group of patients was far more successful at maintaining themselves in independent living arrangements than the control group, yet few differences in psychiatric symptomatology were demonstrated between the two groups of patients.

A dramatically different alternative to psychiatric hospitalization became more ascendant in the 1980s—

self-help groups and mutual support organizations. Although self or mutual help groups often are viewed as adjuncts to traditional treatment, as illustrated in the next paragraph, mutual help organizations have greater potential as a true alternative, in that, beyond the weekly group meetings, there are many other ways that members engage themselves in each others' lives as prodders and supporters. Moreover, some of these organizations view themselves as an international community health movement.

GROW, a mutual help organization, came to the United States in the late 1970s. The organization was created in Australia in the late 1950s by a group of former mental patients seeking more appropriate ways to deal with their problems in living than what they were receiving within the state institutions. In part, they modeled their mutual help group meetings along the lines of Alcoholics Anonymous meetings, which some of them had attended. Over time they developed a far more elaborate structure and set of principles, both for the group meetings, per se, and for the larger and more encompassing "sharing and caring community" that they established for their members. The organization's most fundamental principle is not to do "to" or "for" people, but "with" people. Roles and niches are created, at whatever level of functioning people are at, where individuals can attain a sense of accomplishment and pride. In this way, their members can feel empowered and begin to grow. Members create friendship networks that provide support and assistance beyond the weekly group meetings. Local groups are organized into a regional network and they create other social functions; the regional network often establishes a small residential setting where they can tend to members at crisis times. Mutual help organizations clearly provide people with serious problems in living a social and psychological community in which to grow in contrast to institutional treatment and living.

Grassroots mutual help organizations such as GROW have a complete philosophy of treatment, offer a continuum of services, and operate relatively inexpensively. Because they are less dependent on outlays of financial resources from the government and, at the same time, are free of many bureaucratic constraints, they are more likely to be sustained and disseminated in contrast to many innovative demonstration programs that, most often, erode and disappear after the initial funds have been exhausted, no matter how effective they had been. The "catch 22" is that while mutual help organizations offer considerable therapeutic promise, their ascendance runs the risk of allowing governmental bodies to continue to rationalize their decreasing financial commitment to a continuum of mental health services.

As we have seen, several innovative treatment methods have been developed as alternatives to institutional treatment. They reduce the duration, and thus, the prevalence of serious problems in living. These alternatives are community-based and provide a continuum of supportive and residential services that keep people out of hospitals. Most often, these programs are characterized by a philosophy that dictates that they work *with* individual patients, in contrast to doing things to or for them. In essence, the traditional pattern of "one-up, one-down" role relationships between patients and service providers is restructured in these innovative and successful tertiary prevention programs. Nevertheless, these innovative methods provide rehabilitation to individuals constituting forms of tertiary prevention. They do not short-circuit problems, nor do they prevent groups/populations from developing mental health problems in the first place.

IV. SECONDARY PREVENTION

In secondary prevention, problem identification and intervention occur much earlier in the process than in tertiary prevention. The duration or magnitude of a mental health problem can be short-circuited by identifying and intervening early in the problem's developmental course, thus, reducing its prevalence. On the other hand, if a problem is identified early enough in its course that it is not even considered a mental health problem, its incidence and, in turn, its prevalence can be reduced. Here, the potential problem can be thought of as being "cut off at the pass." In both forms of secondary prevention, intervention occurs at the level of the individual; intervention is not mass-oriented as it is in primary prevention. However, in the latter form of secondary prevention, problem identification can occur at the level of a population or setting.

Once individuals enter the mental health system, they seem to become entrapped within it. From a secondary prevention perspective, we might want to examine gateways to the mental health system—how individuals enter the system. In some communities this gateway is the State's Attorney's Office, who must file a petition in order to legally involuntarily commit someone who appears disturbed. The State's Attorney is often asked to file petitions for involuntary commitment on persons who would profit more from other services, for example, short-term housing, a friendship network, help in finding employment, or intensive outpatient counseling regarding a recent family crisis. Unfortunately, given limited resources and options, involuntary commitment is too often the easiest and most expedient action for the legal system.

In the Midwest during the 1970s, Delaney, Seidman, and Willis developed and evaluated an innovative and successful crisis intervention program for individuals in jeopardy of being involuntarily committed to a psychiatric hospital. They negotiated an arrangement in which they would immediately be notified by the State's Attorney that they were considering filing a petition for involuntary commitment. Within 24 hours, the crisis intervention team would see the person in their natural environment, fully assess the problem, and develop a comprehensive plan of intervention, and set the plan into motion. State hospitalization was often deemed inappropriate or was used only as a last resort for a seriously disturbed individual. This program reduced the number of state hospitalizations in the area, provided persons with more appropriate services, thereby reducing many of the iatrogenic effects of hospitalization. (Were the focus of the program tertiary prevention, researchers would have aided the patients only *after* they had been involuntarily committed.)

Many secondary programs intervene with children since it is believed that the seeds of many problems are sown in childhood. Early detection and intervention is viewed as optimal. Since most children go to school, early identification programs often take place within schools, where populations of individuals can be screened.

One of the earliest exemplars of early detection and intervention programs was known as the Primary Mental Health Project developed by Cowen and his associates. Mass screening allowed early identification of children thought likely to manifest future adjustment problems. (This differs from a tertiary prevention program, which would focus on children that have already been identified as exhibiting problem behaviors.) The identified children were then assigned to minimally paid volunteer child aides (housewives or college students) to work one-on-one with them after school. These aides were trained and closely supervised by university personnel. By using paraprofessionals, the program extended the limited numbers and reach of mental health professionals.

Secondary prevention reduces incidence and prevalence by short-circuiting problems before they are fully realized. In this way it is clearly preferable to the rehabilitation strategies of tertiary prevention. However, intervention remains at the level of the individual and, thus, still runs the danger of stigmatizing and "blaming the victim."

V. PRIMARY PREVENTION

Primary prevention programs endeavor to reduce the incidence of disorder, or unwanted outcomes, in a population or setting, such as the school, the workplace, or the community. Problem identification occurs at the level of a population or setting, not at the level of an individual. In contrast to tertiary and secondary prevention, the population or setting's constituents have *not* been screened to determine if they have symptoms or problems.

Primary preventive interventions are mass-oriented; some programs are aimed at entire populations or communities, while others are aimed at population groups at high risk for negative outcomes. For example, poverty places some demographic groups at greater risk for maladaptive mental health outcomes. A variant of the high-risk approach is that a setting or transition can be considered "risky," where residing in a particular setting or making the particular transition is associated with a higher likelihood or negative outcomes. For example, the work environment of air traffic controllers is considered a risky setting because of the high rates of physical and psychological stress reactions controllers experience. Similarly, the movement from elementary to junior high school is often deemed a risky transition because of the concomitant and precipitous drops in self-esteem and academic performance. In these examples, the social and environmental organization and structure of these risky settings and transitions need to become the focus of primary preventive interventions.

Regardless of the scope of the preventive intervention, malleable risk and protective factors take on increased importance. Stressful life events, for example, the death of a parent or divorce, and daily hassles are common risk factors, while positive social support is a common protective factor. The immediate goal of many recent primary prevention programs has become the reduction of risk factors and/or the enhancement of existing protective factors with regard to a specific risk–disorder linkage. However, the relationship between a particular risk and disorder, by no means, manifests a one-to-one correspondence. The same risk may be linked to several outcomes. For example, the risk of parental discord is related to both conduct disorder and depression. Consequently, the reduction of a single risk (or enhancement of a specific protective) factor may lead to reductions in the prevalence of several disorders. Thus, primary preventive interventions may be most powerful when they target a broad range of disorders with a set of salient risk and protective factors. [*See* PROTECTIVE FACTORS IN DEVELOPMENT OF PSYCHOPATHOLOGY; STRESS.]

When the focus of intervention is a population or subpopulation, "inoculation" methods are the most common type of preventive intervention. Such programs endeavor to provide individuals *directly* with the skills, resources, and know-how to cope with future stresses, strains, and interpersonal encounters that might lead to problems—that is, inoculate them beforehand. Such a repertoire is intended to make the individual stronger and better prepared to deal with whatever may occur in the future. Inoculation programs are often administered to entire classrooms as part of the educational curriculum. In this type of primary prevention program, individuals remain the agents of change, although they are less likely to feel "blamed" than in tertiary and secondary prevention programs since they have not been singled out; everyone is receiving the inoculation.

When the focus of an intervention is a setting, inoculation methods are not employed. Instead, the prevention strategy is more often to restructure the social regularities of the setting. The goal is to modify the setting to become more facilitative of positive mental health outcomes. Thus, strategies to restructure settings characterize efforts more aptly depicted as the promotion of well-being than primary prevention. *Indirectly* these strategies reduce the incidence of an array of disorders for members of the setting. A more detailed example is presented in the next section.

When one thinks of primary prevention, one generally envisions programs for children. However, there are many adult problems that cry out for preventive interventions. For example, unemployed workers often suffer from depression and diminished self-efficacy after a futile search for new employment. In true cyclic form, depression and diminished self-efficacy can make finding a job more difficult and thus lead to greater depression. [See DEPRESSION.]

At the University of Michigan, the Jobs Project was designed by Price, Caplan, and Vinokur to inoculate a high-risk population of recently unemployed individuals from the sequelae of depression and to evaluate the program's success. Participants were recruited from the lines of the recently unemployed at the Michigan Employment Security Commission and randomly assigned to either an experimental or control group. The experimental group received an eight-session curriculum, while the control group received a brief booklet in the mail with general information about job seeking. The curriculum included topics such as dealing with obstacles to reemployment, handling emotions related to unemployment and job seeking, thinking like an employer, identifying sources of job leads, contacting potential employers, completing job applications, preparing a resume, conducting the information interview, rehearsing interviews, and evaluating a job offer. A second part of the intervention was participation in discussion and analysis of the unemployment situation; the researchers felt that when individuals felt empowered to solve their problems they would experience greater self-efficacy and be more committed to follow through and implement the strategies for seeking reemployment.

Participants in the program were assessed at 1 month and 4 months after the intervention program. At both times, program participants had a higher reemployment rate and reported a better quality of working life than the control group. Among those who were re-employed, program participants were more likely to report finding jobs in their main occupation and reported higher earnings. Participants who remained unemployed reported higher levels of job-search self-efficacy than the unemployed control group members. Even more importantly, long-term effects for the intervention were found in a follow-up approximately 3 years later. Program participants continued to report higher earnings and more stable employment than the control group. In addition, a cost-benefit analysis confirmed the utility of this program. Finally, central to our primary prevention focus, among participants deemed

high risk for a depressive episode (based on their initial scores on depression, financial strain, and low social assertiveness), this intervention reduced both the incidence and prevalence of depressive symptoms. Had the researchers taken a secondary prevention perspective, they would have selected only individuals who manifested early signs of depression.

A different approach to primary prevention begins at the earliest point in human life—the unborn fetus. When carried by a poor, teenage mother, a baby is more likely to be delivered preterm and/or low in birth weight. As a result, these infants and children are at greater risk for physical and mental health problems. These poor, teenage mothers often do not get the necessary prenatal care to ensure a healthy and safe delivery. For many of these mothers, the lack of resources and social support often result in their dropping out of school and/or having difficulty maintaining stable employment; in turn, these negative outcomes further compound the negative effects and risk of disorder for their children. [See PRENATAL STRESS AND LIFE SPAN DEVELOPMENT.]

To address these issues, David Olds and his colleagues developed the Prenatal/Early Infancy Project. It was designed as a population-level prevention program in which nurses went into the homes of teenagers in the early stages of their first pregnancy as well as during the first 2 years of the infant's life. Initially, the nurses educated the mothers about fetal and infant development and helped the women improve their diet and try to eliminate the use of cigarettes, alcohol and drugs, they identified signs of pregnancy complications, they encouraged rest and exercise, they prepared parents for labor and delivery and early care of the newborn, and they encouraged use of the health care system and future family planning. Once the infant was born, the nurses would visit the families weekly for the first 6 weeks, gradually reducing the frequency of their visits from every other week to every 6 weeks until the infant was 2 years of age. During these visits the nurses would improve parents' understanding of infant temperament, and they would promote socioemotional and cognitive development and the physical health of the child.

The Prenatal/Early Infancy Project focused on reducing the risk factors associated with being a teenage mother and provided the mothers-to-be with positive social support, a well-documented protective factor.

The program promoted the involvement of family members in and around the mother's home in the development of the infant. The nurses also provided connections to other formal health and human services. Moreover, the nurses paid special attention to the culture and the norms of the family, and they were respectful if they differed from that of the nurse and the program. Once again, this program illustrates an inoculation design because it prevents maladaptive outcomes by preparing and educating the mothers.

Research on this intervention revealed that participants in the home visit program manifested many positive outcomes when compared with a control group who only received free transportation for regular prenatal and well-child visits. During pregnancy, program mothers made better use of formal services, reported greater informal social support, improved their diets, and reduced smoking more than the control group. As a result, among the very young teenagers in the program, the birth weight of their babies was higher, and they were less likely to have preterm deliveries. Among the program mothers at higher risk—poor, unmarried adolescents—their children were less likely to have verified cases of child abuse and neglect and they had fewer emergency room visits. In a 15-year follow-up, program families had fewer subsequent pregnancies, approximately half the number of child abuse cases, and spent approximately half as long on welfare as the control group. Clearly, this primary prevention program was beneficial to the teenage mothers and their offspring. In a secondary prevention program, mothers would not have been targeted until after they had delivered a low birth-weight baby or had been accused of neglect.

In sum, primary prevention programs are generally targeted to populations or subpopulations before problems or even signs of problems are manifested. Individuals, per se, are not identified, but instead a population or group placed at increased risk for one or more disorders or unwanted outcomes, often on the basis of a developmental transition that members of the group experience. Inoculation programs are administered to these populations in order to reduce the incidence of one or more disorders. By providing skills and resources, individuals are able to cope more effectively with future stressful and problematic situations that they may encounter. On the other hand, because individuals are not singled out at the stage of problem identification, individuals are much less likely to be (or feel) blamed.

VI. PROMOTION OF WELL-BEING

There has been a recent movement to go beyond a prevention mindset to focus on promotion of well-being. Focusing on promotion of well-being leads us away from simply thinking in terms of defining problems, their negative outcomes, and ways to prevent them; instead we focus on methods for improving the lives of individuals, and making them healthier and more positive. Promotion of well-being interventions generally move beyond the population level and focus on the setting level, although they may target both or solely a population. To the degree that well-being is promoted, problems are inevitably, although indirectly, prevented.

In New Haven, Weissberg and his associates from Yale University joined together with the superintendent of schools, the Board of Education, parents, community leaders and school staff to develop an organized approach to the promotion of socio-emotional development in the public school system. A Department of Social Development was created with the central element being a comprehensive inoculation program. For every public school in the city, the Social Development Program was incorporated from kindergarten through twelfth grade. This program had from 25 to 50 hours of classroom instruction at each grade level, which focused on problem solving, self-monitoring, conflict resolution, communication skills, respect, responsibility, health, substance abuse, culture, and citizenship. Realizing that there was a need to provide children with activities and outlets outside of the school, and in order to reinforce lessons taught in the classroom, the program moved beyond mere classroom curricula and developed school and community activities. Students participated in mentoring, afterschool clubs, an outdoor adventure class, peer mediation, and leadership groups. Finally, the new department took advantage of previously existing mental health teams in the schools (made up of mental health workers, school staff, and parents). These teams effectively restructured the nature and quality of communication patterns and relationships among the three groups in order to focus on the climate of the schools, needs of the community and the issues that pertained to the growth and development of the students. They ensured that additions to the program were implemented and supported by the school and community.

The majority of school personnel supported the comprehensive and integrative strategy. Lessons taught to the students about problem solving were not only implemented by the students, but actively used by teachers and other school staff. Rather than detaining children for fighting, children received peer mediation or discussed the issues in a life skills class. School hallways were filled with the Traffic Light diagrams illustrating the six problem-solving steps taught in the life skills component. This was not your typical primary prevention program because it did not focus on one problem or even a few problems; rather, it focused on promoting positive social and emotional development and it embraced the entire school day and system.

This comprehensive strategy had many positive outcomes, including reduced problem behaviors. Evaluation research with sixth graders indicated that the curriculum improved students' problem-solving skills, social relations with peers, and behavioral adjustment. Follow-up evaluations illustrated that students who received 2 versus 1 or no years of training had more durable improvements in problem-solving skills.

Often, enduring effects are also hindered by the unwritten social and organizational rules and procedures, or social regularities, that govern a setting. The best exemplars of programs that promote well-being challenge the social regularities of a setting and alter them so that they foster positive development and mental health. An excellent example of a promotion of well-being program is one that altered the social regularities involved in the transition from junior to senior high school.

Normative school transitions may be disruptive and negatively impact adolescents' self-esteem and academic achievement. Often, adolescents make a transition into a more chaotic, more impersonal, less nurturing, and larger school where they have to contend with new routines and demands, numerous different teachers for short periods of time, and a completely different set of peers in each class. In these situations, the social regularities of the new school setting are critical to student well-being.

In the School Transitional Environment Program (STEP), Felner and his colleagues sought to reduce the chaos and flux upon entry into an inner-city high school. STEP students from each homeroom class took all their primary subjects together as a group. The homeroom teachers also taught the students one of their primary classes so they saw their homeroom students at least twice a day. In addition, the five STEP classrooms were in close proximity to each other in order to reduce the distance students traveled, and to keep them close to each other and in less contact with older, perhaps more intimidating students. STEP students experienced a very different environment than their peers, despite being in the same school.

The program was designed to provide adolescents with greater social support from school staff. Homeroom teachers served as the primary liaisons between the students and their parents and the school. Students received a counseling session with their homeroom teachers once every 4 to 5 weeks to discuss any school or personal problems. The homeroom teachers contacted parents of students during the summer before the transition to explain the purpose of the program and that they wanted to be accessible to the parents. Whenever a student was absent, the homeroom teacher would contact the family and follow-up on excuses. The teachers had regular meetings to discuss the students and the program. If a particular student was having a problem, all the STEP teachers were aware of it and tried to work together to help the student.

Research findings revealed that by the end of the first marking period, a comparison group of students declined in academic achievement and increased in absenteeism, whereas STEP students remained stable. By the end of the first year, 19% of comparison students dropped out compared to 4% of STEP students. In terms of academic achievement and absenteeism, the STEP students had significantly higher grades and lower absenteeism than the comparison group in both the first and second years of high school. Moreover, STEP students perceived the school environment to be more stable, well-organized, and supportive than the comparison group.

Although the STEP program was only in place for the incoming freshmen, the researchers felt that this program should have a long-term effect on the students because the transitional year is often the most vulnerable year for students. The researchers followed up their study of the original cohort by examining their school records after they should have graduated from high school. The most impressive finding was the difference in drop-out rates between the STEP students and the comparison students. The drop-out rate was 43% for the comparison group, which was similar to the drop-out rate of other students from the school in previous years. However, the drop-out rate was only 21% for the STEP students. The STEP program has been replicated in many sites, both at the senior high school level and the junior high (and middle) school level. The results are generally consistent across sites. This program illustrates an ideal promotion of well-being program that targets the school environment and makes it less chaotic, rather than a prevention program, which would most likely try to prevent school drop-out by targeting all students and providing them with extra help or supportive services to deal with the school transition.

VII. CONCLUSIONS

The evolution of the Community Mental Health Movement from tertiary prevention to the promotion of well-being demonstrates the field's growth, development and increased knowledge of mental health and the factors necessary to promote positive mental health. Although tertiary (rehabilitative) and second-ary (early intervention) programs are still necessary and very much in practice today, it is clear that to incorporate prevention in their names is a misnomer. True prevention can only be through primary prevention and promotion of well-being programs. These types of programs, especially promotion of well-being are the present and future of the development and maintenance of positive mental health. Healthy, positive behavior in the individual cannot be maintained in a negative or chaotic environment. We must move away from solely targeting individuals to targeting the environments in which people live, work and learn.

BIBLIOGRAPHY

Albee, G. W., & Gullotta, T. P. (Eds.). (1996). *Primary prevention works*. Thousand Oaks, CA: Sage.

Bloom, B. L. (1984). *Community mental health: A general introduction*. (2nd ed.). Monterey, CA: Brooks/Cole.

Caplan, G. (1964). *Principles of preventive psychiatry*. New York: Basic Books.

Price, R. H., Cowen, E. L., Lorion, R. P., & Ramos-McKay, J. (1988). *14 ounces of prevention: A casebook for practitioners*. Washington, DC: American Psychological Association.

Salem, D. A., Seidman, E., & Rappaport, J. (1988). Community treatment of the mentally ill: The promise of mutual help organizations. *Social Work, 33*, 403–408.

Commuting and Mental Health

Meni Koslowsky

Bar-Ilan University

I. Background
II. Objective Stressors
III. Moderators
IV. Subjective Stress
V. Coping Techniques
VI. Summary

Commuting Impedance Obstacles or behavioral constraints on movement or goal attainment. As applied to commuting, impedance consists of stimuli that frustrate the commuter from achieving a goal such as arrival at work or home.

Commuting Stress The stimuli or independent variables, usually a characteristic of the ride to work or of the commuting environment, are considered as the causes of various negative affective and physical consequences.

Coping Techniques A method for reducing or, in some cases, preventing the onset of negative consequences. In the present context, two techniques for coping with the negative consequences of commuting are suggested: individual and governmental/organizational.

Flextime In organizations that implement flextime, employees are allowed to vary (or control) their work arrival and departure times.

Moderator Variable A variable that is said to interact with the independent variable to produce a consequence beyond that predicted by the variables independently; in the present context, a moderating effect is said to exist if the relationship between commuting stress and some consequence differs by subgroup of the moderator.

Telecommuting Working away from the office. Although the concept is often used for people who work at home and are "electronically" attached to their office, it is also relevant for others who are on the road and check in periodically with headquarters.

The relationship of **COMMUTING** with various affective and physical consequences has become an important topic for social and mental heath investigators. A model that describes the process includes three main antecedent variables: objective (commute-related and environmental) stressors, moderators, and subjective (perceived difficulty of the trip) stressors. Recent research has provided better definitions for the stressor stimuli and suggested moderators that may influence the relationship between stressors and consequences. In addition, methods for coping so as to reduce or eliminate the effects of the stressors are suggested.

I. BACKGROUND

Every day tens of millions of men and women from every social strata commute between home and work in the United States and most other industrialized countries. This morning and evening ritual involves billions of person-hours every year, and it has wide-ranging implications for the way urban environments and societies function, for how business is conducted, and, perhaps, most important, for the way that individuals feel and behave. Perhaps a few statistics describing the magnitude of the problem will put the commuting situation in proper perspective. Between the years 1970 and 1989, the number of cars on the road increased by 90%, whereas urban road capacity increased by less than 4%. The 10-mile commute in Los Angeles, which took 20 minutes to complete in 1990, took 30 to 35 minutes in 1992—an increase of about 50% in just two years.

Besides the loss in productivity experienced by profit making as well as nonprofit organizations, the direct and indirect costs to the individual and society cannot be measured solely in financial terms. On a general level, deleterious effects on the environment, employer, and the family have been reported. For the individual commuter, research findings support the notion that the commuting experience is related to emotional and physical consequences. Although studies have used different indicators for the independent and dependent variables and the statistics are usually correlational—not experimental—there seems to be a trend in the literature linking commuting stressors to mental health-related outcomes, mood level, job and life satisfaction, and physiological behavioral effects. Moreover, investigators have argued that commuting stress seems to be an interdomain phenomenon and manifests itself in many settings. Thus, the worker who experiences commuting stressors on the way to work may not be at his/her peak level at work and, as a result or, in addition, may be tired or frustrated at home or during leisure activities. For this reason, investigators have collected both residential and work data from subjects, and inferences relate to both work and nonwork settings.

Findings in the field are not always significant or consistent, yet there is a strong trend that supports the notion of a commuting effect on mental and physical health. Investigators have reported that employees who live far from work are more tense and nervous than their counterparts who live closer. Similarly, increased levels of anxiety, aggravation, tension, and health symptoms have been attributed to the commuting experience. In addition, certain subgroups (moderators, in the terminology, used below) showed a commuting stress effect. For example, data collected from car drivers, as compared to users of mass transportation, showed a higher correlation between commuting time and a measure of affective symptoms. In another study, women reported less satisfaction with their commutes and considerably greater negative affect than men. Other moderators that may have an impact on the relationships between independent and dependent variables will be discussed below.

Besides emotional reactions, physiological and physical changes have also been observed after certain types of commutes. Increases in blood pressure, epinephrine or norepinephrine secretions, and cold/flu symptoms were shown to be associated with the time or travel distance between home and work. Lower back pain, one of the more ubiquitous problems in Western society, may also be a consequence of commuting. In particular, elevated risk for acute herniated lumbar intervertebral disk was associated with driving on the job (e.g., truck driver) and to driving in general (work or leisure).

Another domain that has direct implications for the organization are work-related behavioral measures, which often serve as indicators of effectiveness and productivity. Investigators have found that absence, lateness, and turnover may all be affected by the commuting experience. According to this notion, workers who live far from their jobs were absent, late, and left their jobs for other places of employment at much higher rates than those who lived close. Another related indicator that seems particularly influenced by the commute is performance. For example, one study found that subjects whose average speed was low had lower scores on a proofreading task administered immediately after arriving at work than subjects whose average driving speed was higher. Similar trends have been shown on discrimination tasks and on performance on a critical thinking test.

In order to better understand the commuting experience and its effects, the present article considers the variables as linked in a process that has several distinctive stages. As such the following discussion is divided into several sections: (a) a description of the objective stressor (or stressors) in the commuting experience; (b) moderator variables that interact with these stressors; (c) subjective or perceived stress that is the psychological outcome of the interaction and the direct influence of the first two groups of variables; and (e) methods of coping with the negative effects of commuting. A graphical description of the linkages between variables is presented in Figure 1. In stage 1, two types of variables are identified: stressors and moderators, stage 2 contains perceived stress, and stage 3 various outcome measures. Between stages 2 and 3, coping techniques are identified. These techniques can prevent negative outcomes or mitigate

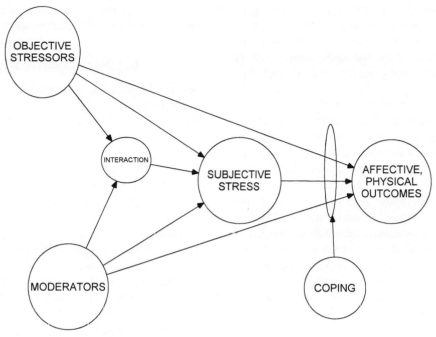

Figure I   A model of the effects of commuting stress.

their effects. Finally, arrows in the figure represent direct effects of one variable on another. Thus, the effect of objective stress on outcome measures is direct and also indirect through perceived stress.

II. OBJECTIVE STRESSORS

According to the usage adopted here, stressor refers to the stimulus or independent variable that is posited as a potential cause of strain response. Strain is the response part of the equation and refers here to the emotional and physical outcomes of the commute. In the present context, objective stressors refer to the features of the commute itself (e.g., time, distance) or the environment (e.g., noise, crowding). Table I contains the commute-related stressors and the environmental stressors that are relevant in the model presented in the article. [*See* STRESS.]

A. Commute-Related Stressors

Over the years, several attempts have been made to define the precise stressor in the commuting experience. Initially, the commuting experience for both car

drivers or users of mass transportation was defined in terms of distance or time traveled. In 1988, Schaeffer and colleagues argued that average speed, a combination of distance and time, should be the best measure with low values more likely to be associated with negative outcomes. However, extraneous variables (e.g., type of commute) may very well play a role in determining average speed and they may distort any relationship. Thus, a commuter who uses local streets and travels at a speed of 30 miles per hour may feel quite good and indeed considerably better than an-

Table I   Objective Stressors in the Commuting Process

A. Commute-related stressors
   1. Time
   2. Distance
   3. Average speed
   4. Impedance

B. Environmental stressors
   1. Noise
   2. Crowding
   3. Thermal conditions
   4. Pollution
   5. Illumination

---

other commuter who can maintain an average speed of 40 miles per hour but is traveling on a highway with a speed limit of 55 miles per hour. As compared to the former, the latter may encounter many more negative stimuli and obstacles and perceive them as such during the commute.

Based on a series of studies in the early 1990s, Novaco and colleagues developed a measure that they felt would better describe the commute. By combining time and distance and creating three "impedance" categories (high on time and high on distance; middle, middle; and low, low), they argued that this measure should predict negative outcomes quite well. Commuting impedance was seen as an indicator of behavioral constraint on movement or goal attainment. The authors were able to find support for several of their hypotheses linking stressors with strain responses.

Although they did not systematically measure objective indicators outside of commuting time or distance, it is possible to extend their definition of impedance to include any potential obstacle that frustrates the goal to arrive at a particular destination—for example, traffic congestion or road construction. For commuters who use public transportation, impedance would include such potential "obstacles" as the number of stages or transfers from one train to another, the crowded conditions of the commute, which may prevent one from even getting onto the train, and the time interval between train arrivals in a station. This last "obstacle" is one of the reasons often cited by drivers for preferring their automobile to public transportation. An employee who drives to work decides when to go to work and when to leave whereas workers who use public transportation are at the mercy of the train schedule.

As with all of the stressors discussed here, there are both objective and subjective components that influence the individual's reaction. Novaco and colleagues refer to the obstacles mentioned above as subjective impedance (see discussion below of subjective stress). Nevertheless, it is possible and quite useful in understanding the process to also try to obtain some objective measure of the stressor. This may require the experimenter to drive to work under the same conditions as the subject and to note the value or degree of stress exposure. In such cases, an interesting comparison could very well include examining the relationship between objective stress, as measured by some

source outside the commuter, and subjective stress as obtained from a self-report measure.

B. Environmental Stressors

Besides the purely quantitative indicators of the commuting experience, it is possible to identify certain features or qualities of the commute that have been associated with emotional and physical reactions in other contexts. These variables come from the domains of social and environmental psychology and have been shown both in the laboratory and the field to be meaningful stressors.

I. Noise

Typical of most commuting experiences is some sort of noise factor. Whereas car drivers may experience this stimulus less than other commuters, noise is, at the very least, in the background in all modes of travel. The manner in which noise affects people has been investigated in several other settings including worksites and airports. According to one theoretical approach, noise stimulates a form of arousal that forces individuals to attend to specific features of the environment and not to others. Performance that requires a wide range of cues may be affected as noise often limits the individual's ability to focus attention and perform accurately or quickly. Researchers also argue that the decrement in performance in a noisy environment is not only a function of the magnitude of the stimulus but also of its meaning, appropriateness, and degree of control. Thus, a driver who has made a decision to actively choose the music that is being played in the car may indeed perform better and be more alert regardless of the noise volume. In situations where the noise is not under the individual's control and has no particular meaning, as occurs when a subway enters a station or a commuter passes near a construction site, the stimulus may be perceived as noxious and a negative reaction is likely.

Several findings from other contexts, particularly the laboratory, are relevant here. Driving tasks such as vigilance and monitoring the environment may be adversely affected by environmental noise. In the same vein, the cessation of the noise itself does not indicate that its effects are over. Thus, after exiting a bus or train, a commuter's subsequent behavior at work or at home may continue to be affected from the previous exposure. Thus, eliminating the noxious stimulus may be efficacious and not only for the period of time the commuter spends on the bus or train. Finally, studies have shown that noise that has been present for a considerable period of time and is no longer attended to loses its potential to be a noxious stimulus. For the commuter, this finding is quite salient as it says that it is possible to "tune" out noxious stimuli and attend only to relevant ones.

2. Density and Crowding

Epstein, one of the main researchers in the field of density (number of people per unit space) and crowding, suggests a model for understanding the problems identified with these variables. Although technically the first term is the objective measure and the second the subjective measure, the terms will be used interchangeably here, as is often the case in the social/ environmental psychology literature. Epstein's formulation is particularly relevant to the commuting experience. When other people enter into someone's proximity, activities, level of interpersonal reaction, and spatial location are all affected. If there is enough space for all and interference is not a problem, then the effect is minimal. However, if the number of people in a particular location begins to increase, competition for the available space becomes more pronounced and tasks such as reading, concentrating, even talking to a fellow passenger are, at least, partially thwarted. This is especially apparent in a situation where others in the environment are competing for similar goals. A crowded train, bus, or subway may make it impossible to read a paper or to just sit and relax. In some cases, a densely populated platform may not permit people to board.

For many commuters, crowding, pushing, and shoving are an integral part of their daily routine. Researchers argue that such chronic, repeated, and unwanted experiences are particularly stressful. Several irritants can be identified here; all of which make the commute uncomfortable. The violation of spatial norms that in another type of social situation would be considered unacceptable is taken for granted in the train or subway experience. Finally, crowding is a group phenomenon with inherent competition. Commuters, generally, do not cooperate with each other. Each one wants to get on the train, available seats are fought over, and reading a paper may encroach on someone else's space. Although in other contexts it has been shown that cooperation or planning together is the best method for allocating available resources, in commuting environments, this is not really practical. In trying to increase the use of mass transportation in Western societies, it will be necessary to control for the negative effects of crowding. [See Co-OPERATION, COMPETITION, AND INDIVIDUALISM.]

3. Other Environmental Variables

Of the variables typically considered as environmental, noise and crowding are the most salient for the commuting experience. Nevertheless, a few other environmental stimuli that have been investigated in other contexts and which may contribute to the quality of the trip between home and work will be discussed briefly. For example, thermal stress (heat and cold), pollution, and illumination have been found to have a wide range of effects on humans and, in situations, where the individual has little control, these effects may be magnified.

With each of these stressors, physical functioning of the individual may be particularly vulnerable. Thus, a passenger train that is not cooled in the summer may cause a commuter to feel extremely uncomfortable during the commute and, probably, begin the work day tired and exhausted. Pollutants in the air are well-known potential health hazards that appear to be particularly prominent during rush hour driving. Toxic fumes that are spewed into the commuter's immediate environment are potential causes for such ailments as headaches, nausea, vertigo, and over the long run, may be responsible, at least partially, for many chronic diseases. Research, as it relates to the effects of commuting, is scarce and some of the principles discussed in relationship to noise and crowding may be relevant here.

III. MODERATORS

Moderators are so called third variables (in addition to the independent and dependent variable) that interact with an independent variable to influence an outcome that would not be predicted by examining the sum of effects of each one of the variables. Discovery of a significant moderator in an analysis will, generally, result in new inferences and conclusions. This section reviews some moderators that have been discussed previously in other stress contexts and suggests how they can be applied to commuter stress research.

A. Control

Inferences concerning the impact of control in work stress and its role as a moderator are derived from laboratory work where subjects are given a chance to exercise control over a specific situation. When demand is high and control (actual or perceived) is low, strain reactions are expected. In the present context, a car driver *expects* control during the drive to work and when traffic congestion prevents it from occurring, negative consequences may ensue; this contrasts with a bus or train passenger who has voluntarily relinquished control when boarding and a traffic problem does not have as much of an effect. There are several types of control, actual or perceived, that may be relevant for commuting.

I. Sense of Motion

A particularly relevant aspect of control is the sense of motion experienced by the commuter during the journey to work or home. If the trip to work or home is accompanied by movement, the driver does not feel a loss of control and the destination is perceived as within reach even if arrival may be delayed. In contrast, a lack of motion may be quite frustrating. In the latter situation, uncertainty and a perception of lack of control is introduced as the driver is not sure when the end of the journey will be reached.

Perhaps the best practical illustration of this concept occurs in large amusement parks such as Disneyland where visitors are usually moving while waiting to enter an attraction. It is likely that visitors while moving, even if only sideways, will experience less anxiety than an equivalent group that must stand still for a long period of time. Similarly, a car driver may choose to get off a highway and increase total mileage but, nevertheless, feel that the goal is getting closer all the time.

2. Predictability

In situations where circumstances do not permit control of the environment, people may be satisfied with being able to predict it. The implications for the commuter are quite apparent. The time to get to work is often unpredictable and variable. One day the trip is relatively quick and the next it is dragged out. Differences of an hour or more between a good and bad day are not uncommon and such variability prevents an individual from planning his (her) arrival time at work or at home. Similar to what was described before when a car is stuck in traffic and does not move, the unpredictability does not let the commuter relax during the trip. Several ways of operationalizing unpredictability in a commuting context can be devised. Alternatively, the variance of commuting times for a month or a year can be determined. In either case, it would be expected that the greater the difference or variability, the greater the negative consequences. Finally, a subjective measure of commuting predictability can be obtained by asking the commuter if he (she) feels the drive to work takes about the same time each day or not. Again, a negative response would be expected to predict strain.

B. Personal Moderators

I. Gender

One of the variables that appears to act as a moderator in commuting is gender. Investigators have found that commuting distance and lateness are positively correlated for women but not for men. Similarly, an interaction between gender and objective stress measures was found with women showing greater discontent at home after a long journey back from work. Nevertheless, it is likely that gender, similar to other biographical indicators, acts as a surrogate for other constructs such as "activities in route." It is possible that women are possibly doing more on their trip to work (shopping, picking up the children, etc.) than men. Further investigations of the underlying construct in the gender phenomenon are needed.

2. Time Urgency

Although industrial/organizational psychologists have traditionally not had much luck in finding correlates of work behavior among personality traits, recent findings show some promise in changing this impression. The aspect of personality that seems to be particularly relevant to a wide group of areas including commuting is time urgency. An individual who has an exaggerated concern about time may be vulnerable to strain reactions that are time related. If this is coupled with time delays on the roads, the reaction may be quite negative.

Time urgency also has a cognitive component associated with it. During the commute, this manifests itself in the commuter who is acutely aware of the passage of time. Such an individual may look at his (her) watch all the time, may ask others if the time on the dashboard or overhead clock is really correct, or may turn to the news station each hour or half-hour. For a commuter who is time urgent, the whole experience may be quite negative and strain responses may occur even before the commute actually begins. Deadlines, train schedules, and making connections are all time contingent and exaggerated awareness of these critical points may be sufficient to bring about strain reactions.

IV. SUBJECTIVE STRESS

As with other areas of stress, perceptions, as well as the objective dimension, must be considered in understanding the effects of the process. In operationalizing the concept of subjective impedance, researchers have identified four components: evening commute congestion (e.g., self-report of times brakes were deemed necessary, etc.), aversiveness of travel (e.g., ratings of the commute in terms of slow-fast, stop-and-go, etc.), morning commute congestion (e.g., necessity to apply brakes on the way to work, etc.), and surface street constraints (subjects reactions as to whether travel speed was reduced by stop signs, etc.). For Koslowsky and colleagues the perceived stress stimuli, purportedly a function of the objective stressors, were viewed as both significant determinants of outcomes and as mediating variables, that is, constructs that explain (fully or partially) the relationship between the independent and dependent variable.

Data on the subjective stressor is obtained through self-report. Potential bias in such instruments is not particularly important here as we are actually interested in the subject's perception. Thus, the researcher or practitioner is not concerned with the actual number of traffic lights encountered by the commuter but rather how many he thought were there, or, stated somewhat differently, his or her reaction to the question: are there many traffic lights during your commute? As illustrated in Figure 1, perceived stress or the subjective stressor is a function of the objective stressor and a series of moderators. According to this formulation, subjective stress is the link between an-

tecedents in stage 1 and outcome in stage 3. In a study by Novaco and colleagues on the impact of subjective impedance on strain reactions, the authors found that subjective impedance did indeed mediate between objective stressors and personal home affect (e.g., mood, conflicts in family, general spirits).

V. COPING TECHNIQUES

It is apparent that an individual's reaction to stress is a function of the variables or potential causes that were discussed above and the way he or she deals with mitigating or eliminating these influences. In the case of commuting, it is possible to identify two sources for coping strategies: the individual and the organization (including governmental agencies and private corporations). In the following few pages, some of the techniques as well as their rationale are discussed. A more detailed presentation is given in Koslowsky *et al.*

A. Individual Coping Strategies

One method of understanding individual coping strategies is to divide them into two categories: instrumental or problem-focused approaches and palliative tactics that focus on regulating emotional distress. As discussed by Koslowsky *et al.*, instrumental coping includes time management, organization problem solving, information gathering, and communication skills training. Essentially these procedures are employed to change the environment or remove oneself from it. Palliative tactics focus on reducing emotional distress through the application of techniques such as cognitive relabeling or reframing, relaxation, diverting attention, search for meaning, and positive thinking. This second method is concerned with teaching the commuter strategies for applying coping skills to fit the situation. Such procedures would include relaxation and learning how to control physical stress responses.

1. Mental Preparation and Time Management

When facing the morning rush hour with its potentially noxious stimuli, an aware commuter can prepare for the trip to work (or home) by taking special precautions. Rather than trying to cope with all potential impediments or obstacles that may be encountered, he (she) can try to cope with the commute as a whole by conceptualizing it as a part of the time that must be allotted so as to come prepared for work. Such commuters reduce time pressures by organizing their lives, taking care of physiological needs by getting enough sleep, maintaining proper diet and following recommendations for proper nutrition, and creating opportunities for dialogue with spouses and children. The less rushed one is in the morning, the less the influence of the commuting stimuli.

One way of preparing for the trip to work is through exercise. Studies have shown that exercise increases cardiovascular fitness, releases muscle tension, lowers blood pressure, and helps improve self-image and appearance. The exercise may be done before work, after work, and in many places, even during the workday. Some, who bike to work or walk to work, are actually integrating the exercise routine into their commute. In addition, they are avoiding many of the negative stimuli experienced by most commuters. A related technique for coping with commuting stress is meditation. Although this is not the place to describe them in detail, many variations of this technique are available with nearly all of them geared toward reducing strain reaction and inducing relaxation. [*See* Exercise and Mental Health; Meditation and the Relaxation Response.]

Much of the field of cognitive psychology is based upon the idea that between every stimulus and response there is a thought process that takes place. During the commuting experience, there is generally a time pressure involved and a high level of motivation to get to work on time. When the realization sets in that the commute will be longer than usual, one may choose to react by becoming angry or irritable or, alternatively, by taking a more rational and positive view of the situation and accepting the reality and focusing one's thoughts in other directions. This may be the time to plan the day's activities or to review a speech that will be delivered at the office. As the cognitive literature supports the notion that processing or attending to stimuli involves a degree of individual choice, it may be possible to focus on non-negative issues and, therefore, reduce negative reactions to the commute. By developing positive thinking skills a commuter can turn a difficult situation into a much more tolerable one.

Besides some of the cognitive approaches for coping with commuting stressors, several behavioral suggestions may be quite appropriate also. If the commuter can take advantage of the commute, the stressors that do exist may take on less importance. CD tapes or audio tapes are available for learning various skills or for self-improvement. Communicating and handling business affairs is now possible during the commute. For example, a cellular phone could be used by the commuter to begin the workday earlier. The concept of a moving office is already here and, for many commuters, this may make the commute a positive, beneficial experience rather than a negative, costly one.

B. Government and Organizational Coping Methods

In addition to individual coping techniques, the government and the organization can help the commuter in solving some of the basic problems of getting to work and returning home. This intervention does not have to wait for commuting problems to manifest themselves. It can begin with proper government planning, including road construction, public transportation, and other methods so as to create a better commuting infrastructure. Thus, before approval of a new factory or office, factors such as traffic patterns, parking spaces, access to roads, and many other features must be taken into consideration. Below is a list of areas where the government and the organization can make a difference in reducing the negative effects of commuting.

1. Carpooling

As studies have shown that carpooling is likely to be less stressful than solo driving, it would be useful for governments and organizations to encourage such modes of travel to work. Unfortunately, carpooling, long viewed by governmental agencies as a possible remedy for worsening traffic, has simply failed to catch on in metropolitan areas around the United States. Despite a decade-long effort to persuade people to double, triple, and even quadruple up in the interest of reducing traffic congestion and pollution, the campaigns are not heeded by the public and little behavior change is observed. Some commuters drive alone because they want to be able to leave work early or stay late and not be bothered by someone else's schedule. Others want their own cars on hand so that they can run errands at lunch, or depart immediately in case of family emergencies.

Does psychology have anything to say in persuading people to change their choice of travel mode? Based on the work in learning and social theory, it may be possible for governments and organizations to apply some of the lessons gleaned from these areas to the commuting situation. Government policy that uses positive reinforcement including charging less for parking spaces taken by carpoolers, reducing tolls for them, and providing special lanes in addition to organizational guidelines that set realistic goals and delineate the means for achieving them through publicity, financial incentive, and other rewards are legitimate means for encouraging behavioral change. At the worker–manager level, "power" or influence tactics discussed in the social psychology literature including expertise, information, and reference can be used to show the workers the potential psychological, economic (to the company, in higher efficiency and to the individual, as savings in commuting expenses), and social benefits of carpooling versus automobile usage.

2. Specific Company Coping Strategies

One of the first steps that an organization can take in order to help employees cope with work stress is to recognize that a commuting-related problem may exist. As we have pointed out previously, negative emotional and physical effects are a possible outcome of the trip to work. An organization can do internal studies to confirm that such a problem actually exists and must be dealt with. Surveys, meetings with employees, some simple statistical analyses of commuting distance, time, or impedance data correlated with outcomes such as sick days, blood pressure readings, lateness, and absences may be quite informative. Assessment of the stressors is the essential first step before any action can be recommended. At the organizational level, even a small association between stressor and outcome may have meaningful implications, as its effects are multiplied many times over. Once a commuting-related problem is identified, several possible solutions may be explored by the organization:

a. Telecommuting This concept has developed in the last few years and describes the situation where workers do not have to arrive at a specific office or factory but can do their work at home or on the road. With the advances made in technology, including laptops, fax machines, and cellular phones such communication with a supervisor or colleague is quite common and efficient. The obvious advantage of telecommuting is that the drive to work on a regular basis is eliminated or vastly reduced. Several other organizational benefits of telecommuting can be identified, including the possibility of drawing workers from a much larger pool. With the level of communications in the international community as it is today, employees of a particular firm can be scattered around the world. An excellent example of this is the software industry where it is possible to find programmers in various countries all working for one multinational company. Many of these employees never even leave their homes but are, nevertheless, in constant contact with headquarters.

b. Flextime The concept of flextime refers to the organization allowing employees to decide which eight hours during the day they prefer to work. The worker who wants to avoid rush hour traffic may want to start earlier (or later). Within limits, the worker is given control over the beginning and end of the workday. Data shows that by the early 1990s about 40% of organizations had instituted some type of flextime schedule. The motivation for these changes was the hope that flexibility at work can lead to many positive consequences for the worker and organization in addition to reducing commuting-related and environmental stressors.

VI. SUMMARY

The field of commuting stress is a rather new one in applied social psychology. By borrowing ideas from both the laboratory and other related fields, it is possible to study the positive and negative effects of this phenomenon in a more efficient fashion. As the links in the model become more clearly defined and identified, researchers will be able to recommend the best coping methods both for the individual and the organization.

BIBLIOGRAPHY

Epstein, Y. (1982). Crowding stress and human behavior. In G. W. Evans (Ed.), *Environmental stress* (pp. 133–148). London: Cambridge University Press.

Koslowsky, M., Kluger, A. N., & Reich, M. (1995). *Commuting stress: Causes, effects, and methods of coping.* New York: Plenum.

Novaco, R. W., Kliewer, W., & Broquet, A. (1991). Home environmental consequences of commute travel impedance. *Am. J. Comm. Psych. 19,* 881–909.

Novaco, R. W., Stokols, D., Campbell, J., & Stokols, J. (1979). Transportation, stress, and community psychology. *Am. J. Comm. Psych. 7,* 361–380.

Novaco, R. W., Stokols, D., & Milanesi, L. (1990). Objective and subjective dimensions of travel impedance as determinants of commuting stress. *Am. J. Comm. Psych. 18,* 231–257.

Schaeffer, M. H., Street, S. W., Singer, J. E., & Baum, A. (1988). Effects of control on the stress reactions of commuters. *J. Appl. Soc. Psych. 18,* 944–957.

Conduct Disorder

Alan E. Kazdin

Yale University

Antisocial Personality Disorder A set of symptoms recognized as a psychiatric disorder among adults that includes a pervasive pattern of disregard and violation of the rights of others. The main characteristics include criminal behavior, impulsivity, aggressive acts, consistent irresponsibility, and lack of remorse. This disorder reflects a continuation of conduct disorder into adulthood.

Attention Deficit-Hyperactivity Disorder A set of symptoms recognized as a psychiatric disorder among children that includes as its central characteristics impulsivity, inattentiveness, and overactivity. The disorder is usually first evident in childhood.

Externalizing Symptoms Symptoms that are directed toward the environment and considered to reflect undercontrolled behaviors. Examples include aggressive, delinquent, and hyperactive behavior.

Internalizing Symptoms Symptoms that are directed inward and considered to reflect overcontrolled behaviors. Examples include withdrawal, anxiety, and depression.

Oppositional Defiant Disorder A set of symptoms recognized as a psychiatric disorder among children that includes as its central characteristics stubbornness, temper tantrums, and noncompliance. For some children, this is an early stage that leads to conduct disorder.

Prevalence The rate or proportion of cases of a particular characteristic or problem (such as conduct disorder) within the population at a given point in time.

Prevention Systematic efforts to avert the onset of a problem and to decrease further problems among those who already show the problem.

Protective Factor Among individuals who are at risk for an outcome (e.g., conduct disorder), many will not develop that outcome. Characteristics, events, or processes that attenuate the impact of risk factors on the outcome are referred to as protective factors. These factors appear to increase resilience in the face of influences that ordinarily increase risk.

Risk Factor Characteristics, events, or processes that increase the likelihood (risk) for the onset of a problem or disorder (e.g., conduct disorder). Risk factors are not necessarily causes of the problem, but rather are correlated features that can be identified in advance of the onset.

CONDUCT DISORDER refers to antisocial behaviors in children and adolescents. These behaviors encompass a variety of acts that reflect social rule violations and actions against others. Such behaviors as fighting, lying, and stealing are common examples of behaviors evident among youth referred for conduct disorder. It is important to note that many of these behaviors are seen in most children over the course of development. Conduct disorder refers to antisocial behavior that is clinically significant and clearly beyond the realm if "normal" functioning.[1] Whether antisocial behaviors are sufficiently severe to constitute conduct disorder depends on several characteristics of the behaviors, including their frequency, intensity, and chronicity, and whether they are isolated acts or part of a larger "package" or syndrome with other deviant behaviors. Typically, conduct disorder is reserved for instances in which antisocial behaviors lead to impairment in everyday functioning, as reflected in unmanageability at home and at school or dangerous acts that affect others (peers, siblings).

Conduct disorder is identified in childhood as a pattern of clinical dysfunction, usually during elementary school years. Yet, for many individuals, conduct disorder is a pattern of functioning over the life span. This article discusses characteristics of conduct disorder, continuities and discontinuities over the course of development, issues and challenge for research, and implications of selected findings for social policy.

I. CONDUCT DISORDER IN CHILDHOOD AND ADOLESCENCE

A. Diagnosis and Prevalence

Extremes of conduct problems are delineated in contemporary diagnosis, as represented by the *Diagnostic and Statistical Manual of Mental Disorders*. Conduct Disorder (CD) is the diagnostic category for coding antisocial behavior among children and adolescents. The essential feature is a pattern of behavior in which the child ignores the rights of others or violates age-appropriate norms and roles. Table I lists the main symptoms that conduct youths exhibit. In contemporary psychiatric diagnosis, a diagnosis of CD is pro-

---

[1] Two issues related to terminology and meaning warrant comment here. First, the term conduct disorder here is used generically to delineate clinically severe levels of dysfunction. The proper noun, Conduct Disorder, will be used to refer specifically to the formal psychiatric diagnosis with its associated criteria. Second, the terms "normal" and "normal development" will be used to refer to youths functioning in the community and who are not referred for mental health services. These terms do not necessarily refer to youths without clinical dysfunction. The reason is that a significant proportion of youths (e.g., 17 to 22% under age 18) functioning in everyday life and who are not clinically referred show clinical symptoms and impairment.

Table I Symptoms Included in the Diagnosis of Conduct Disorder

1. Bullying or threatening others.
2. Fighting.
3. Using a weapon that can cause serious physical harm to others.
4. Being physically cruel to people.
5. Being physically cruel to animals.
6. Stealing and confronting a victim (e.g., mugging, purse snatching, extortion, armed robbery).
7. Forcing someone into sexual activity.
8. Firesetting.
9. Destroying property of others.
10. Breaking into someone else's house, building, or car.
11. Frequent lying or "conning" others.
12. Stealing without confronting a victim.
13. Staying out late at night despite parental prohibitions.
14. Running away from home.
15. Being truant from school.

vided if: (1) the individual shows at least 3 symptoms of those listed in Table I; (2) the symptoms were evident within the past 12 months; and (3) at least one of the symptoms was evident in the last 6 months.

Using diagnostic criteria such as those in Table I or prior versions of the *DSM*, the prevalence of the disorder among community samples of school-age youth is approximately 2 to 6%. One of the most frequent findings is that boys show approximately 3 to 4 times higher rates of CD than girls. The sex differences may be explained by differences in predispositions toward responding in aggressive ways and in socialization through parent–child interactions in relation to aggression, expression of anger, experience of empathy and guilt. Differential responding on the part of parents may contribute to greater sensitivity of girls to the emotions of others, to their higher levels of empathy, and their reduced outward expression of aggression, compared to boys.

Differences in the base rates of boys and girls for a number of behaviors such as engaging in rough and tumble play, bullying others, not complying with requests, and fighting have implications for the greater prevalence of conduct disorder. The symptoms that are listed in the diagnostic criteria emphasize confrontive and violent acts that are more likely in boys than girls. Because of low rates of these behaviors in girls, even a few instances, albeit below the threshold of existing diagnostic criteria, may be clinically important.

These base-rate differences have raised the possibility of a sex bias in the diagnostic criteria which would also explain, or at least contribute to, the greater prevalence of CD in boys than in girls. In general, research on normative development has revealed qualitative and quantitative differences between boys and girls in behaviors related to aggression and antisocial acts, but the information has not yet influenced diagnostic practices. [*See* GENDER DIFFERENCES IN MENTAL HEALTH.]

Age variations reveal interesting patterns in prevalence rates. Rates of conduct disorder tend to be higher for adolescents (approximately 7% for youths ages 12 to 16) than for children (approximately 4% for children age 4 to 11 years). The increase seems to be due to increases in onset among adolescent girls and among youths who engage in nonaggressive forms of antisocial behavior (e.g., truancy, running away). Sex differences are apparent in the age of onset of dysfunction. The median age of onset of dysfunction is 8 to 10 years of age. Most boys have an onset before age 10 (median = 7 years old). For girls, onset of antisocial behavior is concentrated in the 14-to-16 year age range (median = 13 years old). Characteristic symptom patterns are different as well. Theft and aggression are more likely to serve as a basis of referral among antisocial boys. For girls, antisocial behavior is much more likely to include sexual misbehavior.

B. Age of Onset and Subtypes of Conduct Disorder

Conduct disorder includes a heterogeneous set of problem behaviors. Research has identified subtypes in an effort to find meaningful ways of grouping various sets of symptoms and to understand processes leading to onset and course of conduct disorder. Many different ways of delineating subtypes and patterns have emerged. Recent attention has focused on age of onset as a way of accounting for prevalence differences over the course of development and sex differences in symptom patterns.

Child-onset conduct disorder consists of youths whose dysfunction is evident early in childhood, beginning with stubbornness, noncompliance (e.g., Oppositional Defiant Disorder [ODD]) and hyperactivity (e.g., Attention-Deficit/Hyperactivity Disorder

[ADHD]). The symptoms may progress to those of CD, even though many of the youths retain the symptoms from these other diagnoses. Youths with child onset are more likely than those with adolescent onset to engage in aggressive and criminal behavior and are more likely to continue their dysfunction into adulthood. Thus, child-onset conduct disorder is the more severe form. [*See* ATTENTION DEFICIT HYPERACTIVITY DISORDER (ADHD).]

Adolescent-onset conduct disorder is more common than child onset. During adolescence, many youths engage in criminal behavior. For many of these youths, the acts are isolated; for others, the pattern meets criteria for CD. Both child- and adolescent-onset conduct disorder youths engage in illegal behavior during adolescence. However, those with child onset are more likely also to engage in aggressive acts and to be represented primarily by boys. Those with adolescent onset are more equally distributed between girls and boys. Peer group influences are considered to play a central role in emergence and onset of adolescent conduct disorder.

Child onset has been particularly well studied in relation to parent–child interaction. Evidence suggests that parent child-rearing practices contribute to child onset by inadvertently promoting aversive behavior in the child. Reinforcement of deviant behavior, inattention to positive, prosocial behavior, and coercive interactions between parent and child lead to escalation of aggressive child behavior. This, in turn, leads to stable patterns of child aggression that has other consequences (e.g., poor peer relations, association with deviant peers, school failure). [*See* PARENTING.]

Child and adolescent onset subtypes, at this point in the research, do not yet offer an explanation of the different patterns. Even so, age of onset may be a useful point of departure for connecting subtypes of conduct disorder to specific developmental processes. Perhaps influences studied in developmental research (e.g., regulation and dysregulation of emotions, bonding to parents, peers relations) and transitions over the course of development (e.g., school entry) can be readily integrated with these different patterns. Also, developmental work on understanding peer socialization may provide clues regarding early patterns and how they lead to different trajectories. In this regard, work on child popularity and rejection may be important because peer reactions predict later dysfunction.

C. Correlates and Associated Features

1. Child Characteristics

Children who meet diagnostic criteria for CD are likely to show a number of other problem behaviors than those included in the diagnosis. They are likely to argue with adults, lose their temper, actively defy and refuse to comply with requests, deliberately annoy others, and they are angry and resentful. These behaviors, as a group, are occasionally referred to as oppositional behavior and comprise their own diagnostic category (Oppositional Defiant Disorder), alluded to previously. Developmentally, oppositional behaviors are precursors to conduct disorder for many youths. Most children who evince conduct disorder probably have this early history of oppositional problems; but most children with oppositional problems are not likely to progress to conduct problems. Longitudinal research is critical in delineating the conditions leading to the continuation and escalation of behavioral problems.

In addition to oppositional behavior, many youths with severe conduct problems are considered by their teachers and parents to be "hyperactive." There is a reasonable basis for this. A large percentage of children (e.g., 40–70%) diagnosed with CD also meet criteria for Attention-Deficit/Hyperactivity Disorder. The core symptoms of ADHD include inattention, impulsiveness, and hyperactivity. The general point to underscore here is that children and adolescents with the diagnosis of CD are likely to have many other symptoms.

There are other characteristics that affect diverse facets of functioning as well. Children with conduct disorder are also likely to show academic deficiencies. They are more likely to repeat a grade, to show lower achievement levels, and to end their schooling sooner than their peers matched in age, socioeconomic status, and other demographic variables. Such children are often seen by their teachers as uninterested in school, unenthusiastic toward academic pursuits, and careless in their work.

Poor interpersonal relations also are associated with conduct disorder. Youths with conduct disorder often are socially ineffective in their interactions with adults (e.g., parents, teachers, community members) and engage in behaviors that promote deleterious interpersonal consequences such as peer rejection. Conduct disorder youths are often deficient in attributional processes and cognitive problem-solving skills that underlie social behavior. For example, such youths are more likely than their peers to interpret gestures of others as hostile and are less able to identify solutions to interpersonal problem situations and to take the perspective of others.

2. Parent and Family Characteristics

Several characteristics of the parents and families of conduct disorder children are relevant to conceptualization of the dysfunction. Among the salient characteristics are parent psychopathology and maladjustment, criminal behavior, and alcoholism. Parent disciplinary practices and attitudes also are associated with conduct disorder. Parents are likely to show especially harsh, lax, erratic, and inconsistent discipline practices. Dysfunctional relations are also evident, as reflected in less acceptance of their children, and in less warmth, affection, and emotional support, compared to parents of nonreferred youths. At the level of family relations, less supportive and more defensive communications among family members, less participation in activities as a family, and more clear dominance of one family member are also evident. In addition, unhappy marital relations, interpersonal conflict, and aggression characterize the parental relations of antisocial children. These characteristics are correlated with, and often antecedent to, conduct problems, but do not, of course, necessarily cause or inevitably lead to those problems.

3. Contextual Conditions

Conduct disorder youths are likely to live in conditions of overcrowding, poor housing, and high crime neighborhoods, and to attend schools that are in disadvantaged neighborhoods. Many of the untoward conditions in which families live place stress on the parent or diminish the threshold for coping with everyday stressors. The net effect can be evident in adverse parent–child interaction in which parents inadvertently engage in patterns that sustain or accelerate antisocial and aggressive interactions. Also, contextual factors (e.g., poor living conditions) are associated with other influences (e.g., deviant and aggressive peer group, poor supervision of the child) that can further affect the child. [See SOCIOECONOMIC STATUS; STRESS.]

D. Factors that Influence Onset of Conduct Disorder

1. Risk Factors

Risk factors refer to characteristics, events, or processes that increase the likelihood (risk) for the onset of a problem or dysfunction (e.g., conduct disorder). Risk factors, as antecedents to the dysfunction, may provide clues as to development and progression of conduct problems, possible mechanisms and processes through which the dysfunction comes about, and periods during development that might be used to identify cases at risk and to intervene. The factors that predispose children and adolescents to conduct disorder have been studied extensively in the context of clinical referrals and adjudicated delinquents. Numerous factors have been implicated. Table II highlights several risk factors that have been studied along with a general statement of the relation that has been found.

Merely enumerating risk factors is misleading without conveying some of the complexities in how they operate. These complexities have direct implications for interpreting the findings, for understanding the disorder, and for identifying at-risk children for preventive interventions. First, risk factors tend to come in

Table II Factors that Place Youths at Risk for the Onset of Conduct Disorder

Child factors

Child Temperament. A more difficult child temperament (on a dimension of "easy-to-difficult"), as characterized by more negative mood, lower levels of approach toward new stimuli, and less adaptability to change.

Neuropsychological Deficits and Difficulties. Deficits in diverse functions related to language (e.g., verbal learning, verbal fluency, verbal IQ), memory, motor coordination, integration of auditory and visual cues, and "executive" functions of the brain (e.g., abstract reasoning, concept formation, planning, control of attention).

Subclinical Levels of Conduct Disorder. Early signs (e.g., elementary school) of mild ("subclinical") levels of unmanageability and aggression, especially with early age of onset, multiple types of antisocial behaviors, and multiple situations in which they are evident (e.g., at home, school, the community).

Academic and Intellectual Performance. Academic deficiencies and lower levels of intellectual functioning.

Parent and family factors

Prenatal and Perinatal Complications. Pregnancy and birth-related complications including maternal infection, prematurity and low birth weight, impaired respiration at birth, and minor birth injury.

Psychopathology and Criminal Behavior in the Family. Criminal behavior, antisocial personality disorder, and alcoholism of the parent.

Parent–Child Punishment. Harsh (e.g., severe corporal punishment) and inconsistent punishment increase risk.

Monitoring of the Child. Poor supervision, lack of monitoring of whereabouts, and few rules about where youths can go and when they can return.

Quality of the Family Relationships. Less parental acceptance of their children, less warmth, affection, and emotional support, and less attachment.

Marital Discord. Unhappy marital relationships, interpersonal conflict, and aggression of the parents.

Family Size. Larger family size, i.e., more children in the family.

Sibling With Antisocial Behavior. Presence of a sibling, especially an older brother, with antisocial behavior.

Socioeconomic Disadvantage. Poverty, overcrowding, unemployment, receipt of social assistance ("welfare"), and poor housing.

School-related factors

Characteristics of the Setting. Attending schools where there is little emphasis on academic work, little teacher time spent on lessons, infrequent teacher use of praise and appreciation for school work, little emphasis on individual responsibility of the students, poor working conditions for pupils (e.g., furniture in poor repair), unavailability of the teacher to deal with children's problems, and low teacher expectancies.

Note. The list of risk factors highlights major influences. The number of factors and the relations of specific factors to risk are more complex than the summary statements noted here.

"packages." Thus, at a given point in time several factors may be present such as low income, large family size, overcrowding, poor housing, poor parental supervision, parent criminality, and marital discord, to mention a few. Second, over time, several risk factors become interrelated, because the presence of one factor can augment the accumulation of other risk factors. For example, early academic dysfunction can lead to truancy and dropping out of school that further increases the risk for conduct disorder. Third, risk factors may interact with (i.e., be moderated or influenced by) each other and with other variables. As one example, large family size has been repeatedly shown to be a risk factor for conduct disorder. However, the importance of family size as a predictor is influenced by income. If family income and living accommodations are adequate, family size is less likely to be a risk factor. As another example, risk factors often interact with age of the child (e.g., infancy, early or middle childhood). For example, marital discord or separation appear to serve as risk factors primarily when they occur early in the child's life (e.g., within the first 4 or 5 years). How risk factors exert impact in childhood and why some periods of development are sensitive to particular influences underscore the importance of understanding "normal" developmental processes.

2. Protective Factors

Research on risk factors leads naturally to the study of positive outcomes. The reason is that even under very adverse conditions with multiple risk factors present, many individuals will adapt and will not experience adverse outcomes. A conceptually interesting and potentially critical set of influences that may affect onset are referred to as protective factors. These are characteristics, events, or processes that decrease the impact of a risk factor and likelihood of an adverse outcome. Although protective factors have been less well studied than have risk factors, significant progress has been made.

Researchers have identified protective factors by studying individuals known to be at risk (i.e., show several risk factors) and by delineating subgroups of those who do, versus those who do not, later show conduct disorder. Youths can be identified who are at risk for delinquency based on a number of factors. Yet, not all at-risk youths become delinquent. Those who do not evince delinquency by adolescence are more likely to be first born, to be perceived by their mothers as affectionate, to show higher self-esteem and locus of control, and to have alternative caretakers in the family (than the parents) and a supportive same-sex model who played an important role in their development. Other factors that reduce or attenuate risk include above average intelligence, competence in various skill areas, getting along with peers, and having friends. In many cases, these protective factors seem to be the absence or inverse of a risk factor. For example, easy temperament, academic success, and good relations with parents reduce risk, as does a good relationship with an emotionally responsive, caregiving adult, whether a parent or nonparent figure.

Among the many protective factors, three general categories help to organize current findings. The first is personal attributes of the child. Beginning in infancy and unfolding throughout development, these include such factors as easy temperament, sociability, and competencies at school. The second category is family factors and includes such characteristics as caretaking style, education of the parents, and parent social competence. The third category consists of external supports and includes friendships, peer relations, and support from another significant adult. The categories are useful ways to describe protective factors, but it is important to bear in mind that they tend to be interdependent and reciprocal. For example, child attachment to the parent is important as a protective factor and probably reflects personal attributes of the child in combination with characteristics of the parent. In general, it is useful to conceptualize many of the protective factors as part of transactions between the child and the environment. [See PROTECTIVE FACTORS IN DEVELOPMENT OF PSYCHOPATHOLOGY.]

3. General Comments

Risk and protective factors refer to variables that influence the probability of onset of an outcome in a population. Although many risk and protective factors have been identified, we do not understand how most of the factors operate. In some cases, there are clues as to the processes and mechanisms that have direct influences on the outcome. For example, harsh punishment practices serve as a risk factor for conduct problems. Punishment is part of a broader set of inept child-rearing practices that have been shown to escalate coercive and aggressive behavior directly. How the parent responds (e.g., coercively or passively) in response to the demands of the child has been shown to increase systematically the level of aggressive child behavior. Moreover, intervening with special training programs that alter how the parents respond to their children decreases child aggression and antisocial behavior. Research on parent discipline practices has made significant gains in moving from identification of a descriptor (risk factor) to the process (means of operation). Understanding the processes leading to dysfunction provides an excellent basis for preventive interventions. Also, understanding discipline practices and their relation to conduct problems draws attention to broader developmental issues. For example, inept discipline practices do not invariably lead to behavior problems. Understanding influences that may attenuate the role of these practices in development could be important. Thus, the study of conduct problems draws attention to discipline practices more generally in development, as well as to the search for protective factors among youths who are subjected to those practices that promote antisocial behavior.

II. CONDUCT DISORDER OVER THE COURSE OF DEVELOPMENT

The manifestations of conduct disorder are likely to change over the course of development. Even so, there may be a continuity in the inferred trait or characteristic that underlies these manifestations. For example, young children (3 to 4 years of age) with conduct problems may be mildly stubborn, break other children's toys, and "borrow" (take) things that belong to their friends. These behaviors may not predict these same behaviors 10 years later. Yet, these early behaviors may predict other behaviors, such as stealing from stores and confronting strangers with a weapon, that are conceptually related or that belong to the same general class of behaviors. A life-span perspective emphasizes continuities and discontinuities over time and paths and progressions. Behavioral and other manifestations may be discontinuous but still reflect continuity at a broader level of conceptualization. Charting the course over the life span begins with descriptive characterization of conduct problems at different points in development. The period of school-age years through early adolescence has been especially well studied. The present discussion of conduct

disorder focuses on early development and adult outcomes, to fill out the life course of the problems.

A. Early Development: Infancy and Preschool Years

Risk-factor research suggests that a number of signs may be evident in the child, parent, and family context beginning in infancy. Child characteristics (e.g., difficult temperament, neuropsychological deficits, high activity), parent characteristics (e.g., prenatal and perinatal birth complications, parental punishment of the child), contextual characteristics (e.g., stress, marital conflict), and other factors, noted earlier, are likely to be present. In addition, diverse psychological processes and experiences (e.g., development of affect, attachment, and cognition) are likely to be implicated. It is likely that a set of general factors may emerge in early development that increase vulnerability to dysfunction and some set of more specific factors that move the child more specifically to conduct disorder.

Charting the influence of any single factor is difficult because characteristics of child, parent, and contexts are dynamic rather than static. The dynamic feature emphasizes complex interrelations such as the reciprocal and mutual influence of the child on the parent and the parent on the child. As the child interacts with others (e.g., peers), reciprocal and dynamic influences continue and have their own consequences (e.g., early aggression may lead to peer rejection).

In addition to dynamic influences at a given point, there is a developmental progression over time. The influences can place children on a trajectory or path that refers to a course leading to a particular outcome such as conduct disorder and criminality. The trajectory or path is not necessarily a fixed or determined course, but rather a matter of increased likelihood (probability) that specific behaviors will unfold in the short run and lead to other outcomes in the long run. Some outcomes become more probable (e.g., being arrested, bonding with delinquent peers), and other outcomes become less probable (e.g., graduating high school, sustaining employment). A variety of influences can converge to alter the probabilities. [*See* CRIMINAL BEHAVIOR.]

The progression of characteristics in early development toward conduct disorder has been examined in longitudinal studies from birth through adolescence and young adulthood. In such research, the same individuals are studied at multiple points in time (e.g., every few years) and then early predictors of later behavior can be identified. Through longitudinal studies, one can chart the course over short and long periods and identify transitions from one time to another and the relations among proximal and distal manifestations. Recent research has characterized progressions and different paths and how conduct disorder symptoms and their associated features emerge. Among the salient findings is a progression of severity of conduct problems over time. Trivial antisocial acts precede more severe acts in the child's repertoire. Youths who show the more serious behaviors (e.g., assault, firesetting) are likely to have progressed through the less severe behaviors (e.g., temper tantrums, noncompliance) but, of course, not all youths who engage in less severe antisocial behaviors progress to more severe antisocial behaviors.

B. Adult Outcomes

1. Antisocial Personality Disorder and Psychopathy

Longitudinal studies show that conduct disorder in childhood predicts conduct disorder up to 10, 20, and 30 years later. Antisocial behavior when continued into adulthood falls into another diagnostic category, namely, Antisocial Personality Disorder (APD). The essential features include a pervasive pattern of disregard of others, violation of the rights of others. The main symptoms of APD include repeatedly engaging in unlawful behavior, deceitfulness (e.g., repeated lying, conning others), impulsivity, irritability, aggressiveness (repeated fighting), disregard for the safety of others, consistent irresponsibility (e.g., repeated failure to retain a job), and lack of remorse.[2] The presence of CD in one's youth is a prerequisite for the diagnosis of APD. The criteria include many concrete behavioral acts of CD but also encompass more pervasive personality patterns, as reflected in deceit, manipulation, impulsivity, and irresponsibility.

Large-scale epidemiological research has revealed

---

[2] The symptoms noted here are based on the *DSM-IV*, referred to previously. The diagnosis of Antisocial Personality Disorder requires evidence of a pervasive pattern of disregard for and violation of the rights of others occurring since age 15 years, as indicated by 3 or more of the symptoms noted here. In addition, the individual must be at least 18 years of age and with evidence of a history of Conduct Disorder before the age of 15.

a life-time prevalence rate of APD of 2.1 to 3.3%. Males are approximately 4 to 8 times more likely to be diagnosed with the disorder. The greater prevalence of APD among males compared to females is in keeping with the sex-difference pattern evident in childhood. Follow-up of child conduct disorder has elaborated this sex difference. Boys are much more likely to continue conduct disorder into adulthood and show APD. In contrast, girls are likely to shift into more internalizing types of disorders (e.g., depression, anxiety) in adulthood. This pattern is especially interesting in light of research showing different reactions of boys and girls who are exposed to factors that might increase risk for conduct disorder. For example, exposure to family violence in childhood (ages 6 to 11) is associated with externalizing and internalizing symptoms in boys but primarily internalizing symptoms among girls. The process leading to symptom pattern differences have yet to be elaborated. [*See* ANXIETY; DEPRESSION.]

The symptoms required for a diagnosis of APD, noted previously, emphasize overt behavioral signs. Over the history of the study of antisocial behavior in adulthood, emphasis has also been accorded internal experience such as lack of guilt or remorse, lack of empathy, and egocentricity. A distinction has been drawn between APD, which emphasizes the behavioral components, and psychopathy, which focuses more on the motivational and interpersonal processes. APD has as its characteristics adverse family background (e.g., low socioeconomic status) and lower IQ. Psychopathy is correlated negatively with anxiety and positively with narcissism. Interestingly, individuals with both APD and psychopathy are those who exhibit the most severe and enduring patterns of antisocial behavior in adulthood. The distinction in the adult literature between behavioral and motivational/interpersonal components is important from a developmental perspective because it identifies different end points of earlier developmental trajectories. Unfortunately, to date there have been few efforts to connect the different outcomes of adulthood with characteristics of early development.

2. Other Outcomes

Among youths who are severely antisocial during childhood, slightly less than 50% continue their conduct disorder into adulthood. What happens to the remainder of youths? If all diagnoses are considered,

Table III Long-Term Prognosis of Youths Identified as Conduct Disorder: Overview of Major Characteristics Likely to Be Evident in Adulthood

Characteristics in adulthood
Psychiatric Status. Greater psychiatric impairment including anatisocial personality, alcohol and drug abuse, and isolated symptoms (e.g., anxiety, somatic complaints); also, greater history of psychiatric hospitalization.
Criminal Behavior. Higher rates of driving while intoxicated, criminal behavior, arrest records, and conviction, and period of time spent in jail.
Occupational Adjustment. Less likely to be employed; shorter history of employment, lower status jobs, more frequent change of jobs, lower wages, and depend more frequently on financial assistance (welfare). Served less frequently and performed less well in the armed services.
Educational Attainment. Higher rates of dropping out of school, lower attainment among those who remain in school.
Marital Status. Higher rates of divorce, remarriage and separation.
Social Participation. Less contact with relatives, friends, and neighbors; little participation in organizations such as church.
Physical Health. Higher mortality rate; higher rate of hospitalization for physical (as well as psychiatric) problems.

Note. These characteristics are based on comparisons of clinically referred children identified for conduct disorder relative to control clinical referrals or normal controls or from comparisons of delinquent and nondelinquent youths.

rather than continuation of conduct disorder alone, 84% of the full sample received a diagnosis of psychiatric disorder as adults. Moreover, diagnosis of dysfunction does not adequately characterize the scope of adjustment difficulties in adulthood. There are many other outcomes identified by following conduct disorder children. As adults, multiple domains may show continued dysfunction, as reflected in psychiatric symptoms, criminal behavior, physical health, and social maladjustment. The characteristics that conduct disorder youths are likely to show when they become adults are presented in Table III. As the table indicates, individuals with a history of conduct disorder evince a broad range of untoward outcomes.

C. General Comments

From a developmental standpoint, it is important to understand the continuities and discontinuities of conduct disorder over the life span. Longitudinal studies have identified intriguing patterns, yet to be explained. For example, the continuity of conduct disorder among boys (ages 7 to 12) is influenced by APD of a parent or child intelligence. With either an APD parent and lower level of intelligence, boys are likely to continue conduct disorder symptoms. How these characteristics operate and combine and the other variables with which each is associated has yet to be studied. The continuity of conduct disorder over the life span warrants mention in another light. The continuity extends beyond the life of the individual,

because conduct disorder extends across generations. For example, children are more likely to show antisocial behaviors if their grandparents have a history of these behaviors. Similarly, one of the best predictors of how aggressive a boy will be in childhood is how aggressive his father was when he was about the same age. Thus, the life-span perspective requires consideration of how the dysfunction is extended to one's offspring and whether there are different modes of transmission.

III. ISSUES AND CHALLENGES OF DEVELOPMENTAL PERSPECTIVES

A. Continua of Dysfunction and Risk

Research often focuses on youths who meet diagnostic criteria for CD. In principle, it is quite useful to specify criteria in this fashion so that diagnoses can be made reliably and that research on these samples can be replicated. Yet, the criteria themselves are difficult to defend. Where one draws the cutoff point to decide dysfunction (e.g., 3 symptoms rather than 4 or 8; duration of 12 months rather than 18, 24, or more) is likely to lead to different findings with regard to risk and protective factors, developmental trajectories, responsiveness to treatment, and prognosis.

Clearly, youths who meet the criteria are likely to be significantly impaired. Yet to understand the nature of conduct disorder more generally, it would be important to extend research to the full spectrum of severity of impairment and dysfunction. For example, youths who show symptoms of CD but who are below, at, and above threshold (e.g., fewer than 2 symptoms, 3 symptoms, or more than 4 symptoms, respectively, as only one way to operationalize threshold) for meeting the diagnosis would be important to study. This type of analysis would permit evaluation of factors that predict functioning across the spectrum of severity and frequency, as well as those that are only predictive of more severe levels or types of dysfunction. In general, conduct disorder is a "fuzzy" insofar as some individuals are at each extreme (clearly conduct disorder, and clearly not) with many shades in the middle. Presumably, there are points on the continuum at which there is a particularly poor prognosis, failure to respond to treatment, and so on. The full spectrum warrants much more attention to understand where the points are warranted to be delineated for intervention and for policy decisions as well.

In a similar vein, many of the factors that contribute to conduct disorder can be conceived along continua. In much of the research that focus on risk factors, groups are selected and compared based on their exposure to and experience of an event. For example, the effects of abusive child-rearing practices on children and adolescents are often studied in this way. Typically in research, one selects abused and nonabused children and then identifies the other characteristics they might show at some later point in time (e.g., symptoms of psychopathology, poor school performance, dysfunctional peer relations). Identification of extreme groups is an excellent point of departure, but we wish to understand the continuum of the risk characteristic. Evaluation of the continua of discipline practices is required to understand the impact of various levels and types of punishment and the point at which these practices become risk factors for various outcomes.

Studying multiple levels of a proposed risk factor is important to reveal the function (or relation) in a more fine-grained fashion than the study of two groups or the presence or absence of a particular characteristic. Many influences are likely to bear curvilinear relations to an outcome of interest, and assessment of different levels of the risk characteristic can reveal this. For example, parental efforts to control their adolescents is related to externalizing symptoms and drug use. However, the relation between degree of parental control and symptoms is not linear. Extremely high or low parental control, but not intermediate control, is associated with adolescent dysfunction. Similarly, adolescent substance abuse is correlated with current dysfunction and predicts lack of academic pursuits, job instability, and disorganized thought processes years later. Yet, the relation of substance use and untoward consequences is not linear. Heavy alcohol or drug use predicts later problems; no alcohol or drug use or consumption whatsoever is associated with undesirable personal and social characteristics as well. Use of a small amount of alcohol or drugs (primarily marijuana) is associated with positive outcomes such as decreased loneliness, reduced self-derogation, improved relationships with family, and increased social support. [*See* SUBSTANCE ABUSE.]

The point of these examples is to convey the need to study multiple levels of factors presumed (or indeed known) to increase risk for dysfunction. There may be points at which a given factor has one effect (risk), another at which it has no effect, and another level at which it has an opposite (protective) effect for an outcome of interest. Developmental research examines continuities and discontinuities over time for individuals and groups. Research is needed that examines continuities and discontinuities over dimensions of behavior (e.g., conduct disorder), risk factors (e.g., child-rearing practices), and contextual influences (e.g., socioeconomic status). How the dimensions influence development and the points at which risk and impairment are especially likely are not well known.

B. Packages of Influences and Outcomes

A significant challenge for research is the finding that many influences and outcomes come in "packages." It is difficult to identify simple profile of risk factors that are associated with and are unique to conduct disorder. The reason is that many influences and outcomes come in "packages," that is, sets of factors that go together and have multiple deleterious outcomes. For example, socioeconomic disadvantage, adverse child-rearing practices, parental neglect, and low parental interest in the child's academic accomplishments are interrelated. The presence of one or two of these risk factors increases the likelihood of a child accumulating more of them. Thus, early child aggression or academic retardation is often associated with peer rejection, association with deviant peers, and placement in a class designed for socially and emotionally disturbed youths. These qualities in turn can lead to a "snowballing" of additional risk factors.

"Packages" are also evident in the outcomes (e.g., problem behaviors, disorders). Although we are interested in understanding the development and course of specific emotional and behavioral patterns, many of these are embedded in, or are part of, larger packages. For example, antisocial acts often are part of a larger cluster involving multiple problem behaviors (e.g., substance abuse, early sexual activity, and academic dysfunction). A challenge is to explain how these behaviors come together developmentally. A prominent view, referred to as problem behavior theory, suggests that problem behaviors serve similar functions in relation to development. Autonomy from parents and bonding with peers are two of the functions that may be served by such behaviors. Another view is that there is a trait or pervasive tendency to engage in deviant, delinquent, and criminal behavior. The tendency, referred to as low self-control, reflects a propensity to seek pleasures of the moment and short-term solutions to problems.

What has been well established is that multiple deviant behaviors co-occur. Evidence points to complex interrelations among behaviors and patterns that are idiosyncratic and that vary reliably across individuals, situations, and contexts. Understanding the organization of affect, cognition, and behavior and how they emerge and evolve developmentally are central to understanding problem behavioral patterns. No doubt specific factors (e.g., risk and protective) relate to specific outcomes (e.g., conduct disorder), and these are obviously important to identify. Yet from what we know so far, two general conclusions can be reached: (1) multiple paths (e.g., different packages of risk factors) can lead to a specific outcome (e.g., conduct disorder); and (2) a single path (e.g., single or seemingly identical packages of risk factors) can lead to multiple outcomes (e.g., diverse types of dysfunctions or other outcomes). Elaborating specific lines of development and exploring the bases for variation are rich in opportunities for both theory and research.

C. Variations in Patterns of Influence and Outcome

A challenge for research stems from the prospect that some influences and relations may vary systematically as a function of other variables. For example, the relation between characteristics of early development and outcome in relation to conduct problems varies as a function of child sex. It is not merely the case that boys and girls differ on a particular characteristic (e.g., degree of aggressiveness), but rather how the relations among other variables differ as a function of sex. We know, for example, that early signs of aggression in the school is a risk factor for conduct disorder, delinquency, and crime in adulthood for boys but not for girls. The issue in relation to the present discussion is not merely the fact that there are sex differences, but rather the relation between antecedents and outcomes and how and why they are influenced by sex.

Race and ethnicity are also likely to influence relations among factors related to conduct disorder. Differences are known to exist among European American, African American, Asian American, and Hispanic American children in relation to prevalence, age of onset, and course of dysfunction. For example, among youths with substance abuse, one of many behaviors associated with conduct problems, ethnic variation exists in the specific substances used, degree of family monitoring, and amount of exposure to substance use. In addition, whether a particular influence emerges as a risk factor varies as a function of ethnicity. That is, a relation between a particular antecedent and outcome is moderated by ethnicity. [See ETHNICITY AND MENTAL HEALTH.]

Sex and ethnic differences are not the only factors that influence the relations among other variables. Yet, these two are important and serve as a basis for articulating the challenge for research. Investigators are often interested in developing theories of dysfunction with implied widespread generality of explaining conduct disorder. It is likely that key variables such as sex and ethnicity, but no doubt others as well, influence onset and course of conduct disorder and the suitability of various interventions.

IV. INTERVENTIONS TO PROMOTE PROSOCIAL AND TO DECREASE ANTISOCIAL BEHAVIOR

Conduct disorder represents a serious clinical problem for individuals and their families, as well as a major mental health problem for society at large. From a social perspective, conduct disorder is considered to be the most costly mental disorder, at least in the United States. The costs stem from the fact that for many youths conduct disorder is a life-long problem. Over the course of childhood and adolescence, youths are likely to enter into many systems and programs, including special education classes, mental health services (inpatient or outpatient treatment), and the juvenile justice system. As adults, entry into mental health services and the criminal justice system may continue. Thus, the costs that accrue to care for conduct problem individuals is exorbitant. These costs extend beyond the individual's lifetime, insofar as conduct disorder tends to be transmitted from one generation to the next. With these considerations in mind, identifying interventions to combat the problem is obviously important. Three broad levels of intervention can be delineated, namely, treatment, prevention, and social policy. An overview of each is presented next.

A. Treatment

Treatment refers to a broad range of interventions that are applied to youths who have been identified as showing conduct disorder symptoms and who experience impairment in their everyday lives. Conduct problem symptoms constitute the most frequent basis for which children and adolescents are referred for treatment. Consequently, there is a need for effective interventions. Many different treatments have been applied to youths with conduct disorder, including psychotherapy, pharmacotherapy (medications), psychosurgery, home, school, and community-based programs, residential and hospital treatment, and assorted social services. Few treatments have been carefully evaluated in controlled studies and shown to reduce conduct disorder problems and to improve functioning of the child in everyday life (at home and at school). A few treatment approaches have been studied and show considerable promise in treating children and adolescents who are referred for treatment. Three of the more well studied treatments are highlighted here.

Parent management training refers to a treatment in which parents are trained to interact with the child in ways that promote prosocial behavior. The treatment is based on learning research from psychology and focuses on the use of reinforcement (e.g., use of contingent consequences), mild punishment (e.g., very brief

time out, response cost), and a variety of related techniques (prompting, shaping) to develop child behavior. Extensive research has shown that many parent–child interaction patterns in the home unwittingly foster and escalate child aggressive behavior. Parent management training teaches skills to the parent, develops interactions between parents and the child that promote positive parent and child behavior, and in the process decreases aggressive and antisocial behavior. Several controlled studies have shown that parent management training reduces oppositional, aggressive, and antisocial behavior at home, at school, and in the community. The effects have been maintained in many studies up to 1 to 2 years. Few studies have evaluated the longer term impact of treatment, but evidence has been favorable for these studies.

Another technique is *cognitive problem-solving skills training*. This technique is based on research showing that conduct problem youths often show distortions in various cognitive processes. Cognitive processes reflect how individuals perceive, code, and experience the world, as reflected in beliefs, attributions, and expectations. A variety of cognitive processes pertain to interactions with others, including the ability to generate solutions to interpersonal problems, to identify the means to obtain particular ends (e.g., making friends) or consequences of action (e.g., what would happen after a particular behavior), and to make attributions to others of the motivation of their actions. Distortions and deficits in these and related cognitive processes relate to conduct problems at home and at school. Problem-solving skills therapy develops skills in approaching interpersonal situations. Youths learn a series of steps or self-instruction statements that help identify prosocial or adaptive solutions and alternative consequences of actions. Children practice using the approach in treatment sessions and at home with their parents. Within the sessions, several techniques are used, including modeling by the therapist, practice, role playing, and reinforcement to shape appropriate behavior of the child. Several controlled studies have shown that problem-solving skills training can reduce aggressive and antisocial behavior in children and adolescents. The effects have been maintained up to one year after treatment.

Multisystemic therapy is a family systems approach to antisocial behavior. The treatment focuses on the child behavior within the context of various systems (e.g., the family, peer group, schools) which may contribute to the child's problem behavior or could be used to help alter that behavior. Many different techniques are applied within the context of treatment to modify specific behaviors of the child and others whose behaviors may be affected by the child. Parent management training and problem-solving skills training, mentioned previously, often are incorporated into treatment. A focus on the family as a system is designed to build better communication, to reduce negative interactions, and to improve the ability of the parents to function. Factors that can affect these interactions and the child's problems, such as stress that the parent experiences, marital conflict, association of the child with a deviant peer group, are focused on as well. Several controlled studies have shown that multisystemic therapy reduces delinquency and antisocial behavior. The effects of treatment surpass the effects achieved with other types of treatment routinely provided to antisocial youths (e.g., counseling, probation) and have been maintained up to 5 years after treatment.

There are other promising treatments for conduct disorder, but only a small number of techniques have been carefully evaluated. Although the promising treatments have evidence from controlled studies in their behalf, they still leave many questions unanswered. For example, we do not yet know the long-term effects of even the best available treatments, whether they influence adaptation into adulthood, and for whom they are likely to be most effective. Considerable attention in the field focuses on these questions with the goal of improving treatment.

B. Prevention

Ideally we would like to prevent the onset of conduct disorder so there would be no need for treatment. Actually, prevention includes a number of goals. *Primary, secondary,* and *tertiary* prevention have been delineated to note whether the intervention is designed to prevent the onset of dysfunction (incidence), to reduce the severity, duration, or manifestations among cases with early signs (prevalence), and to delimit the disability or dysfunction and its complications among persons who have early signs or the dysfunction itself, respectively. A more recent classification distinguishes types of interventions and includes: *universal* interventions, which are designed

for the general population, are low cost, and deemed beneficial for persons in general; *selective* interventions, which are targeted to subgroups that have elevated risk for the disorder; and *indicated* interventions, which are targeted to high-risk individuals who already show detectable signs or symptoms of developing the problem.

Research on risk factors has been very helpful in guiding preventive efforts. Because many risk factors for conduct disorder are known, we can identify youths who are at high risk and provide preventive interventions. In addition, the risk factors may suggest processes through which antisocial behavior may emerge. For example, we know that harsh punishment practices can contribute to antisocial behavior and that altering these practices reduces antisocial behavior. Parenting is one of the foci of many early intervention programs.

Prevention programs come in many different forms. Early intervention programs with the family have been effective in altering conduct problems. High-risk families are identified, usually by such factors as low socioeconomic status, low educational attainment, and high-stress living conditions. Intervention programs sometimes begin before the child is born to provide counseling regarding maternal care, to provide support in the home to reduce stress, and to prepare the parents for child-rearing demands. After the infant is born, the program may continue for a few years to help support parents, to develop cognitive skills of the child, and to enroll the child in a preschool program. Programs of this type can have broad impact beyond reducing the incidence of conduct problems. Adolescents who have received such programs when they were young, compared to those who did not, show lower arrest rates, higher educational attainment, less substance use and abuse.

Prevention programs are often conducted in the schools because there are opportunities to provide programs to youths in larger numbers, in the context of peers, and on a regular basis for protracted periods. Programs often focus on developing positive skills and success experiences at home and at school. The reason for this focus is that bonding to deviant peers and poor connections with the family are risk factors for such behaviors as delinquency and substance abuse. Developing such success experiences in the schools among elementary school children has increased bonding to families and decreased rates of antisocial behavior and substance abuse.

Prevention is an obviously critical focus. To date, the evidence shows that preventive interventions can have impact on child functioning and onset of conduct problem behaviors. At the same time, the very best and most effective programs show that the incidence of conduct problems can be reduced, but by no means eliminated. The long-term effects of prevention are not well studied. However, the value of preventive efforts is that many outcomes may be improved by early intervention.

C. Social Policy and Action

Social policy refers to governmental and legislative efforts to implement changes to benefit society or a particular segment of society and, in this sense, is a social intervention. In principle, the interventions rely on practices that have emanated from research on the nature of the problem (e.g., risk and protective factors) and intervention practices that are or appear to be promising. Thus, policy interventions are not necessarily different from those discussed in the context of treatment or prevention. As an example, Head Start has been implemented as an early preschool program to have broad impact on child development and families. Many of the practices are designed to improve educational and social goals of the children and to improve conditions that in the long term will have impact on children.

Efforts to influence policy are reflected in recommendations to alter or modify practices with the goal of decreasing aggression, violence, and other conduct problems on a large scale. As a recent example, a Commission on Violence and Youth of the American Psychological Association (1993) completed a 2-year study and concluded that, "society can intervene effectively in the lives of children and youth to reduce or prevent their involvement in violence" (p. 5). Several specific suggestions were elaborated to convey how this can be accomplished. Table IV summarizes the categories of actions that can be taken. Each of these was developed in detail to convey their connection to what is known from current research on risk factors, onset of dysfunction, and interventions.

There are multiple opportunities within society to reduce influences that can contribute to conduct problems and aggression more generally. For example, the use of corporal punishment in child-rearing and school discipline, violence in the media, especially television and films, and social practices that permit, facilitate, or tacitly condone violence and aggression (e.g., availability of weapons), to mention salient issues, are some of the practices that are relevant to the issue of aggression and antisocial behavior in society. We take as giv-

Table IV   Overview of Recommendations to Curb Violence

- Early childhood interventions directed toward parents, child-care providers, and health-care providers to help build the critical foundation of attitudes, knowledge, and behavior related to aggression.
- School-based interventions to help schools provide a safe environment and effective programs to prevent violence.
- Heightened awareness of cultural diversity and involvement of members of the community in planning, implementing, and evaluating intervention efforts.
- Development of the mass media's potential to be part of the solution to violence, not just a contributor to the problem.
- Limiting access to firearms by children and youth and teaching them how to prevent firearm violence.
- Reduction of youth involvement with alcohol and other drugs, known to be contributing factors to violence by youth and to family violence directed at youth.
- Psychological health services for young perpetrators, victims, and witnesses of violence to avert the trajectory toward later involvement in more serious violence.
- Education programs to reduce prejudice and hostility, which are factors that lead to hate crimes and violence against social groups.
- Efforts to strengthen the ability of police and community leaders to prevent mob violence by early and appropriate intervention.
- Efforts by psychologists acting as individuals and through professional organizations to reduce violence among youth.

From the Executive Summary of the Report of the American Psychological Association Commission on Violence and Youth (1993). *Violence and youth: Psychology's response* (Vol. 1). Washington, DC: American Psychological Association.

ens a backdrop of factors and practices that contribute in significant ways to aggression and antisocial behavior in society. The factors need to be scrutinized in relation to policy regarding child management and care.

As an illustration, the use of corporal punishment (e.g., physical aggression against children) is already implicated as a contributor to child aggression. The extensive use of corporal punishment is one of the givens in our society—a right that accompanies parenting and often teaching—that might be challenged if there is broad interest in delimiting aggression and antisocial behavior. Corporal punishment in child discipline at home and at school has been banned in a number of countries (e.g., Austria, Denmark, Finland, Norway, and Sweden). Large-scale efforts to reduce risk factors in this fashion are critically important in addition to the more common prevention and treatment efforts.

It might be useful to conceptualize the full range of influences in terms of a risk-factor model in which there are multiple influences that contribute to the outcome. Yet, in a risk-factor model, multiple influences add and combine to increase the likelihood of the outcome (e.g., aggression). Small influences can combine (additively and synergistically) and have significant impact, even if their individual contribution would be nugatory. We want to reduce risk factors not because individually they are the cause or because they will eliminate the problem, but because they are likely to have a palpable impact.

Limiting violence in the media can be seen as one influence likely to affect the level of violence and aggression in society. Efforts to quell gross displays of violence in the media are countered with arguments noting the benefits of television (e.g., education) and the responsibilities of others (e.g., parents) in policing what children watch. Yet, the significant impact of the media on antisocial and at-risk behaviors already has been well documented. Reducing aggression in the media is likely to have impact, even though media violence is not "the cause" of violence in society.

A commitment at the policy level and at the level that can mobilize social forces that influence, express, or model aggression could have significant impact on the problem. Social influences involving the matrix of societal displays, encouragement, and implicit endorsement of aggression including the media at all levels ought to be mobilized more systematically for a broad effort to ameliorate aggression and antisocial behavior. Again, this is not the solution nor a reflection on the cause of aggression in society, but rather a way to have impact in one more incremental way.

V. CONCLUSIONS

Conduct disorder represents a special challenge given the multiple domains of functioning that are affected. For many individuals, severe antisocial behavior and associated dysfunction in multiple spheres represents a lifelong pattern. Advances have been made in understanding the characteristics and patterns evident in school-age children and adolescents. Also, efforts have been made to chart the life course longitudinally, different paths leading to conduct disorder in childhood and adulthood, and the role that specific influences play (e.g., parent child-rearing practices, peers) at different points in development. Research has identified characteristics of the child, parent, family, and contexts that contribute to the emergence and maintenance of conduct disorder.

The lifelong pattern of conduct disorder and the transmission of the problems within families from one generation to the next underscore the importance of a developmental and life-span perspective. It will be important to identify the course and various paths and to examine developmentally opportune points of intervention. Over the course of development, influences vary in their contribution to conduct disorder. For example, during adolescence, the influence of peers on the appearance of conduct problem behavior is marked. Peer influences have been implicated in the onset, maintenance, and therapeutic change of antisocial behaviors. Identifying how such influences operate and precursors to such influences has obviously important implications for intervening.

Although many fundamental questions remain about conduct disorder over the course of development, sufficient information is available to advance policy recommendations, a few of which were noted previously. A broad range of social interventions are required to have impact on such conduct problems. Specific programs and interventions developed by mental health professionals play a major role, but these programs do not exhaust the options. Broader social practices warrant scrutiny in ways that balance individual freedoms and responsibilities. Recommendations from research on ways of reducing conduct problems require addressing these broader issues.

ACKNOWLEDGMENTS

Completion of this article was supported in part by a Research Scientist Award (MH00353) and a grant (MH35408) from the National Institute of Mental Health.

BIBLIOGRAPHY

American Psychiatric Association (1994). *Diagnostic and statistical manual of mental disorders.* (4th ed.). Washington, DC: Author.

American Psychological Association, Commission on Violence and Youth (1993). *Violence and youth: Psychology's response* (Vol. 1). Washington, DC: American Psychological Association.

Kazdin, A. E. (1995). *Conduct disorder in childhood and adolescence* (2nd ed.). Thousand Oaks, CA: Sage.

Ketterlinus, R. D., & Lamb, M. E. (Eds.) (1994). *Adolescent problem behaviors: Issues and research.* Hillsdale, NJ: Erlbaum.

McCord, J., & Tremblay, R. E. (Eds.) (1992). *Preventing antisocial behavior.* New York: Guilford.

Mrazek, P. J., & Haggerty, R. J. (Eds.) (1994). *Reducing risks for mental disorders: Frontiers of preventive intervention research.* Washington, DC: National Academy Press.

Patterson, G. R., Reid, J. B., & Dishion, T. J. (1992). *Antisocial boys.* Eugene, OR: Castalia.

Pepler, D. J., & Rubin, K. H. (Eds.) (1991). *The development and treatment of childhood aggression.* Hillsdale, NJ: Erlbaum.

Peters, R. D., McMahon, R. J., & Qinsey, V. L. (Eds.) (1992). *Aggression and violence throughout the life span.* Newbury Park, CA: Sage.

Robins, L. N. (1991). Conduct disorder. *Journal of Child Psychology and Psychiatry, 32,* 193–212.

Robins, L., & Rutter, M. (Eds.) (1990). *Straight and devious pathways from childhood to adulthood.* Cambridge: Cambridge University Press.

Constructivist Psychotherapies

Robert A. Neimeyer and Alan E. Stewart

University of Memphis

Constructivism An epistemological position that emphasizes the personal and collective processes of meaning-making and their implications for psychotherapy. Human beings are viewed as active creators of constructions that vary in the extent to which they help a person adjust to life's challenges.

Narrative Therapeutic Approaches A way of thinking about psychotherapy that views the client's life as a story or text. The life-as-narrative metaphor suggests that problems in living result from gaps, incongruities, or problematic passages in one's life story. Narrative therapeutic approaches seek to restore the client as an active narrator of his/her life by helping the person re-author aspects of experience to give events greater meaning or the plot structure of life new direction.

Postmodernism A philosophical position, deriving in part from constructivism, that acknowledges the multiplicity of constructions that can be developed for people, things, ideas, or institutions. Postmodernism assumes that no definition, characteristic, or attribute of something is fixed and invariant across either time or context. Adherents of postmodernism recognize that efforts to understand the "truth" or "essence" of an experience ultimately lead instead to constructions about those experiences.

Social Constructionism An epistemological approach that emphasizes the socially shared meanings developed between people about phenomena experienced by a culture or society. In contrast to constructivism this approach emphasizes the ambient meanings that exist prior to any individual and that serve as the basis for people's identity and forms of relating.

Systemic Approaches A general psychotherapeutic approach common to family therapy that emphasizes the ways in which one's embeddedness in a network of interpersonal relationships (which can encompass family, community, and organization) affects the experiences and behavior of persons in the system as well as the functioning of the system as a whole.

CONSTRUCTIVISM, a philosophical position that emphasizes the human penchant for meaning making in understanding both psychological distress and therapeutic intervention, has influenced several current traditions of psychotherapy. Following a review of the historical contributions to this approach, we consider two critical issues: the relationship between language and reality and the construction of the self, as viewed from both constructivist and related social constructionist perspectives. We then trace the implications of constructivism for the practicing therapist, reviewing four traditions that are characterized by a central concern with the person as interpreter of experience: personal construct therapy, developmental cognitive therapies, narrative approaches, and sys-

Encyclopedia of Mental Health
Volume 1

547

temic orientations. We conclude that constructivism is making a robust contribution to the further development of psychotherapy, both in terms of research and practice.

I. INTRODUCTION

In both popular and professional writing, many schools of therapy are distinguished by their concrete clinical procedures, the fund of therapeutic techniques most closely associated with particular traditions. Thus, psychoanalysis is characterized by its historical preference for free association and dream reporting on the part of the client, and the interpretation of transference and defense by the therapist. For its own part, cognitive therapy is linked with various methods for evaluating, monitoring and disputing dysfunctional thoughts or beliefs both in and between therapy sessions (e.g., homework assignments). Likewise, behavior therapy is associated with counterconditioning procedures (such as systematic desensitization), and contingency management (through the manipulation of reinforcement to increase or decrease desired or undesired behavior). Even family therapy is associated with a distinctive set of procedures, ranging from the use of paradoxical interventions to the challenging of dysfunctional coalitions or boundaries among family members. In each case, these approaches to therapy are linked in the popular and professional imagination with a preferred set of techniques, which govern the pattern of therapeutic interaction in a way that sets them apart from others. [*See* BEHAVIOR THERAPY; COGNITIVE THERAPY.]

In contrast, constructivist psychotherapy is characterized by the distinctive *mind-set* that guides it, more than by any particular set of procedures that distinguish it from other clinical traditions. Of course, the unique philosophical position that informs constructivist practice does subtly encourage some ways of working with clients, while constraining others, as we shall see below. But to understand the evolution of this form of practice, it is helpful to view it against the backdrop of what constructivist therapists *believe,* in order to gain a deeper appreciation of what they *do.* This will then allow us to consider variations in the constructivist tradition, which has begun to permeate traditional schools of therapy, ranging from the psychodynamic and behavioral to the humanistic and

systemic. As the "family" of constructivist therapies has grown, so too has the repertory of clinical strategies associated with them, and the body of qualitative and quantitative research emanating from them. While a thorough review of the theoretical, empirical, and applied literature associated with this perspective is clearly beyond the scope of this article, the present article provides an initial point of entry into this burgeoning contemporary therapeutic tradition, and offers some leads for the reader interested in pursuing its implications for clinical scholarship, research, and practice in greater detail.

We begin with an examination of the philosophical heritage of constructivism and discuss the emergence of psychological theory from constructivist epistemology, the study of knowledge. We then consider two current issues pertaining to constructivist theory and therapy: first, the relationship between language and reality, and second, the construction of the self. Next, we compare and contrast four traditions of constructivist psychotherapy, including personal construct theory, narrative approaches, family systemic orientations, and developmental perspectives. Finally, we conclude by considering the implications of constructivism for psychotherapy research, and offer a critical evaluation of the current status of constructivist practice.

II. PHILOSOPHICAL HERITAGE OF CONSTRUCTIVIST ASSUMPTIONS

A. Constructivist Epistemology

Although most constructivist scholars and practitioners acknowledge that a real, ontologically substantial world exists, they are much more interested in understanding the nuances of the person's construction of the world than in evaluating the extent to which it accurately "represents" some external "reality." Constructivists emphasize the development of a viable or workable construction of people, things, and events over the attainment of a singularly "true" rendering of one's surrounds. This suggests that multiple meanings can be developed for the events in one's life, and that each may have some utility in helping the person understand his or her experience and respond creatively and adaptively to it.

The idea that people actively and continuously engage in meaning-making processes, that is, construction, dates at least to the ancient Greek philosopher Epictetus who maintained people were more perturbed by their views of reality than by reality itself. But it was the Italian rhetorician Vico (1668–1744) who systematized the rudiments of a truly constructivist philosophy, tracing the origins of human mentation to the gradual acquisition of the power to transcend immediate experience. Vico argued that the origins of human thought lay in the attempt to understand the mysteries of the external world by projecting upon it the structures of human motives and actions in the form of myths and fables. This tendency to order experience through the application of such "imaginative universals" was eventually displaced, he thought, by the development of linguistic abstractions that permitted categorization of events and objects on the basis of single characteristics.

The work of Kant (1724–1804) also contributed significantly to a conception of the human mind as an active, form-giving structure. Specifically, Kant believed that experience and sensation were not passively written into the person, but that the mind transforms and coordinates the multiplicity of sense data into integrated thought. Because human beings can come to "know" only those phenomena that conform to the structures of the human mind, with its penchant for organizing the world in three-dimensional terms and imputing causality to events, humans are forever barred from contacting the "thing in itself," a "noumenal" reality uncontaminated by human knowing.

At the threshold of the twentieth century, the German analytic philosopher, Vaihinger (1852–1933), embraced constructivist epistemology in asserting that people develop impressions of the real world and create *workable fictions* that help them to adjust and to meaningfully respond to people and events. Conceptual "artifices" (e.g., of mathematical infinity or of a "reasonable man"), while having no exemplars in reality, performed a heuristic function in helping the person organize and integrate disparate pieces of knowledge or sensory data. Vaihinger categorized his *Philosophy of 'As If'* as a kind of "idealistic positivism," to acknowledge the dual reliance upon hard data and impressions received by the sensory system along with a purposive, form-giving activity of the mind to create useful constructions.

Avenarius (1843–1896) and Mach (1838–1916) espoused a unique form of impressionistic positivism, known as empiriocriticism, that also contributed to

the history of constructivist epistemology. Contemporaries of Vaihinger, Avenarius and Mach placed heavier emphasis on raw sensory data as the beginning point for human knowing processes. While maintaining that people constructed an understanding of the world based upon sensory data, their principles of economy and parsimony maintained that sense data were minimally embellished by activities of the mind. Despite this more empirical emphasis, these two authors, working separately, both recognized an active, organizing role of mental processes in rendering sense data more holistically.

Within this century, the work of Vaihinger, Mach, Avenarius, and others influenced Korzybski's development of general semantics. Korzybski (1879–1950), a Polish intellectual working independently of established academic circles, essentially criticized the use of the verb "to be" and its conjugations because it tended to identify people or things, in an Aristotelian sense, with qualities or characteristics that often were meant only to describe them (e.g., "Terry is lazy"). Such identity, Korzybski maintained, de-emphasized the multiplicity of meanings and modes of existence that characterize most phenomena, living or inanimate, and obscured the role of the speaker in attributing meaning to events. Korzybski's negation of the use of "to be" makes it possible for people or things to be construed in different ways and provides a linguistic basis for a constructivist epistemology. Korzybski developed an approach to language usage, known as E′ (E-prime), that recommended persons use conjugations of "to be" sparingly or not at all in written or spoken language. The idea behind E-prime is that the map (in this case, language) is not the territory (other persons or things in the world).

B. Constructivist Psychologies

Constructivist epistemology provided a conceptual basis for three distinct psychologies in this century. First, the British researcher, Bartlett (1886–1979), applied constructivist concepts in his investigations of human memory processes. In his classic work on remembering, Bartlett maintained that memories were reconstructed out of bits and pieces of recollected information. That is, memories did not consist of stored, complete representations of past events that were recalled *in toto*. Bartlett viewed memories as past information unified by *schemas,* the threads of constructive processes that exist at the time information is remembered.

The Swiss genetic epistemologist Piaget (1896–1980) was the second psychologist to establish a coherent theory founded on a constructivist basis. As a developmental psychologist with interests in children's forms of knowing, Piaget chronicled how children's meaning-making capacities changed as a function of both physical growth and active adaptation upon exposure to a succession of conceptually challenging experiences. Piaget contended that rather than representing a smooth "learning curve" over time, cognitive development was punctuated at critical points by qualitative transformations in the very style and form of thinking, permitting the eventual emergence of abstract, formal thought having a level of plasticity unavailable earlier in childhood. Subsequent developmentalists in the Piagetian tradition have extended this model into adult life, when still more subtle dialectical forms of thinking emerge to permit more adequate accommodation to the complexities of social life.

Finally, the American clinical psychologist, Kelly (1905–1967), became the first to develop a personality theory and psychotherapeutic interventions based upon a constructivist epistemology. Influenced by both Korzybski and the psychodramatist, Moreno, Kelly's psychotherapeutic system exemplified constructivist thinking in that he viewed people as incipient scientists, striving to both anticipate and to control events they experienced through developing an integrated hierarchy of personal constructs. As will be discussed in a later section, Kelly viewed psychological intervention as a collaborative effort of the therapist and client to help the latter revise or replace personal constructions that were no longer viable. By making the reconstruction of personal belief systems the focus of psychotherapy, Kelly anticipated the work of later cognitive theorists and therapists. More generally, Kelly's position that multiple, viable constructions can be developed for a given phenomenon and that no single version of reality is prepotent over others heralded the arrival of postmodern critiques of the humanities and social sciences.

Although overshadowed by psychology's embrace of information processing perspectives on human mentation in the 1960s and 1970s, constructivist approaches experienced a strong resurgence of interest in the 1980s with the founding of *The International Journal of Personal Construct Psychology* in 1988. This forum was renamed *Journal of Constructivist Psychology* in 1994 to accommodate the growing diversity of constructivist scholarship beyond Kelly's personal construct psychology. Increasing interest in constructivist theory, research, and practice in both individual and family therapy has enriched the field, spawning the diversity of constructivist perspectives outlined below.

A common thread among various constructivist scholars is that human psychological processes are proactive and form generating. Thus, rather than viewing people's behavior as a mere reaction to the "stimuli" of the "real world," constructivists view humans as actively imposing their own order on experience and shaping their behavior to conform to their expectations. Thus, a fundamental concern of constructivist psychotherapists becomes the study of the personal and communal *meanings* by which people order their experience, meanings that must be transformed if clients are to envision new (inter)personal realities in which to live. While most members of the broad family of constructivist approaches would endorse this basic position, they differ significantly in the emphasis they place on the individuality or communality of meaning making, and their corresponding emphasis on private interpretations of experience as opposed to broad linguistic and cultural processes that shape human action. For this reason, it is useful to examine two central issues in constructivist epistemology from the standpoints of both (personal) constructivist and social constructionist positions, to lay a groundwork for understanding the different foci and methods of the various "schools" of constructivist therapy that follow.

III. CURRENT ISSUES IN CONSTRUCTIVIST THEORY

Two areas in which there has been continuing elaboration of constructivist ideas involve first, the relationship between language and reality, and second, the construction of the self. The former issue bears directly on constructivist epistemology and the central role of language in ordering experience. The latter issue relates to the structural aspects of meaning systems and how they function together in creating temporally or situationally coherent identities. Each of these issues also carries direct implications for psychotherapy, although with different nuances in the case of constructivist versus social constructionist accounts.

A. Language and Reality

1. Constructivist Perspective

Perhaps the pivotal concept in a constructivist account of human nature concerns the relationship between human knowledge and reality. Specifically, constructivists reject or at least suspend the implicit epistemology of the modern social sciences, which assumes that one's understanding of the world, especially the world of complex and dynamic interpersonal systems, can be considered "true" or justified to the extent that it corresponds to a reality external to the person's knowing system. Instead, they posit that human knowers have no direct confirmatory access to a world beyond their grasp, no firm contact with a bedrock of reality that would provide a secure foundation for their constructions.

This posture of epistemological humility, for most constructivists, stops short of an "anything goes" relativism, insofar as the development of personal knowledge is constrained by the need for varying degrees of internal coherence, on the one hand, and the quest for consensual validation of our private constructions on the other. While the resulting meaning systems cannot be strictly "validated" in the sense of matching some objective criterion independent of the observer, they can nonetheless be judged more or less viable as guides to organizing our anticipations regarding our activities in and our accounts of our experiential world.

Language, in this constructivist view, represents a medium for articulating private discriminations, enabling us both to manipulate them symbolically and to inject them into the medium of public discourse. Using language as a straightforward instrument of "communication" is viewed as problematic insofar as commonality of construing becomes more of an aspiration than an assumption. This view of meaning as resident primarily in individual construction systems, which are bonded together by the thin substantiality of language, is most evident in "cognitive constructivist" accounts like Kelly's that consider persons as agents capable of making choices and creating original, personal constructions with minimal interference by larger social systems or structures.

2. Social Constructionist Perspective

Social constructionists largely agree with cognitive constructivists in rejecting objectivist epistemologies that a real world exists and can be discovered by establishing a correspondence between the knower and the phenomenon to be known. Social constructionists, however, differ with constructivists regarding the centrality accorded to individually constructed experiences. That is, constructions of people, things, or events in the world arise from negotiations between persons rather than within them. The implication of this sociocentric view is that individuals' constructions both derive from and contribute to the social and cultural contexts with which they are associated.

Given their attention to collective, rather than individual experience, language and linguistic processes occupy an even more central role for social constructionists than for constructivists. This increased emphasis is also reflected in social constructionists' broader definitions of language to include all manner of semantic, semiotic, and symbolic methods of negotiating and disseminating meaning, rather than restricting it to the spoken or written word alone.

As a form of collective meaning making and coordinated social action, language can be used to create cultural tales that become repositories of socially constructed meanings from the past or from other societies or cultures. The availability of ready-made meanings that embody the local "truths" of one's place and time implies that cultural narratives may "author" people, rather than vice versa, in the sense that they constitute prefabricated and socially validated patterns to which individual identities are expected to conform. Thus, in this constructionist view, language and culture predate the experience of any particular individual, and provide the ineluctable scaffolding for constructing one's identity in relation to others.

B. The Construction of the Self

1. Constructivist Perspective

The personal quest for coherent and socially warranted knowledge carries with it clear implications for an image of the *self*. Like the "world," the "self" is relativized and problematized in constructivist accounts, stripped of stable traits or enduring features that define its essence. Instead, selves are constructed as a by-product of our immersion in language and practical activity, as one strives for personally significant ways of thematizing, organizing, and narrating experiences. Stated differently, *people are their constructs,* so that at least in a distributed sense, selfhood consists of an entire repertory of shifting and provisional patterns for understanding, engaging, and "storying" the world and other people. Because the majority of these patterns are tacit, only rarely articulated in symbolic or explicit ways for either for the person or for others, clear limits are imposed upon self-knowledge. At best, efforts to "know oneself" represent an attempt to impose an explicit order on the relatively abstract and durable themes that punctuate one's lived engagement in the world.

Viewing self-development as oscillating between an extension of our forms of concrete activity in the world and the effort after an abstract reflexivity toward the self poses major challenges to modernist goals associated with an essentialized image of human nature. In particular, the loss of a fixed and "real" self erodes the value of "genuineness" or "congruence" in one's relationships to others. That is, the multiplicity of selves that exists for each of us across time and contexts precludes the discovery of a primary or essentialized self, just as it undermines the quest to discover who a person "really is." Thus, this postmodern conception emphasizes narrative elaboration over authenticity, and self-explanation over self-actualization.

2. Social Constructionist Perspective

Social constructionists and constructivists agree in rejecting the concept of a single, essentialized self. The social constructionist critique, however, runs deeper to challenge the very category of "self" as an individually based construct, viewing it instead as an historically circumscribed concept arising only fairly recently in Western culture, with its pervasive emphasis on individuality, autonomy, and personal responsibility. In contrast to this cultural trend, social constructionists view discussions of the "self" as merely one possible form of *discourse,* one that may be insufficiently attentive to the numerous ways in which our sense of identity is penetrated by relationships to significant others and even impersonal media, especially in the electronic age. In making this critique, social constructionists emphasize the fragmentation and in-

coherence of self in divergent social contexts rather than embracing the idea of an integrated agent whose coherence transcends such divergent social realities. In this view, therefore, characteristics of the self such as responsibility, purpose, agency, and so forth are seen as fictions derived from society's construction of the individual, rather than as universal "facts" or ideals that generalize across different times and settings.

As might be expected in view of these differences, constructivism and social constructionism also differ in their endorsement of self-knowledge as a goal of life in general, or psychotherapy in particular. Whereas constructivists encourage the conscious elaboration of a multifaceted "self" and reflexive recognition of this process, social constructionists focus more upon the implicit ways in which practical engagement in specific contexts shapes one's mode of self-presentation, with or without one's conscious awareness or "choice." This divergence contributes to a differential use of self-reflective versus social-conversational methods in various traditions of constructivist therapy, a topic to which we shall now turn.

IV. CONSTRUCTIVIST PSYCHOTHERAPIES

A. General Orientation

Just as constructivists are suspicious of a psychological science that pursues a universal set of factual observations concerning human nature, they also distrust "scientific" forms of psychotherapy that establish highly standardized and manualized procedures for modifying human behavior. In addition, the growing family of constructivist interventions eschews methods that simply supply clients with supposedly more "functional" or "adaptive" ways of existing, thinking, or feeling rather than helping persons or families find their own unique way to adaptive meaning making. This suggests that at the level of clinical practice, constructivists accord both therapist and client an "expert" role in understanding what changes are necessary in the assumptive foundation of the client's life.

Consistent with this emphasis, constructivists reject pathologizing diagnostic systems that focus on client deficits and deviations from supposedly "normal" patterns of behavior. Accordingly, they resist the common practice of applying universal categories of disorders that fail to capture the richness and subtlety of any given individual's way of interpreting the social world and constructing relationships with others. For instance, a diagnostic category such as "major depression" merely describes a presumably maladaptive "mood disorder," without conveying any information about the way the person's meaning-making processes have ceased to be viable for construing life's experiences. In contrast, constructivists prefer assessment techniques and working conceptualizations that are idiographic or tailored to each use, which examine both the positive and negative implications (from the client's, family's, or society's standpoint) of clients' ways of construing their lives and problems.

Because both therapist and client lack access to a straightforward "truth" beyond their constructions, neither can define hard and fast criteria for distinguishing "healthy" or "rational" beliefs or actions from those that are "disordered" or "irrational." Given this "level playing field," the therapist is left with the somewhat daunting task of building an empathic bridge into the lived experience of the client by attempting to construe his or her process of meaning making. Establishing this connection will help the therapist to understand the entailments of the client's constructions of events and help negotiate their possible deconstruction and elaboration. The personalism of this encounter requires that the therapist have a sensitive attunement to the unspoken nuances in the client's conversation, and skill in using evocative and metaphorically rich language to help sculpt their mutual meaning making toward fresh possibilities. To be successful, such "structural coupling" between client and therapist systems must ultimately move beyond bland generalizations about the nature of the "working alliance" and banal prescriptions for "effective interventions," and instead foster a unique "shared epistemology" irreducible to the individual systems of either partner in the therapeutic relationship.

What "outcomes" might be valued in this constructivist approach to the counseling process? While the specific aims of psychotherapy are necessarily defined by the participants, at an abstract level, the goals of constructivist therapies include adopting a "language of hypothesis" by recognizing that one's constructions are at best working fictions rather than established facts. As such, they are amenable to therapeutic deconstruction (e.g., through subjecting the same events to alternative "readings") and reconstruction (e.g.,

through acting upon alternative interpretations to realize their effects).

Although enhanced reflexivity toward the "self" may be a legitimate aim of this work, it is ultimately subordinated in importance to the aim of constructing a self with sufficient narrative coherence to be recognizable, but sufficient fluidity to permit continued tailoring to the varied social ecologies the client inhabits. Because new and tentative reconstructions of the self require social support, therapy typically also fosters a deepened engagement with selected others who can function as "validating agents" for the growing edges of the client's provisional attempts at meaning making.

B. Distinctive Traditions

The last 10 to 20 years have witnessed a growing diversity of psychotherapeutic approaches that have embraced a constructivist epistemology. There is no single or unique constructivist psychotherapy, no single "approved" set of techniques that define constructivist interventions. Instead, a constructivist mind-set has percolated into most major traditions of therapy, from the psychoanalytic to the cognitive-behavioral, producing novel ways of conceptualizing therapeutic practice as well as a broad variety of associated change strategies or techniques. Our goal in this section will be to survey some of these developments, concentrating on four discernible therapeutic traditions within constructivism that make somewhat different assumptions about human change processes, and carry distinct implications for the role of the therapist.

1. Personal Construct Theory

The first tradition we will consider is Kelly's personal construct psychology, which despite its status as the first consistent expression of clinical constructivism, continues to attract fresh adherents and generate new therapeutic strategies. Kelly's psychotherapeutic approach derived from his unique conception of personality. Kelly employed the metaphor of the "person-as-scientist" to characterize the ways in which people attempt to formulate personal theories to both anticipate regularities in their environments and to channel their behavior in relation to them. Central to Kelly's theory is the idea that people create constructs, or basic dimensions of contrast, that help them to discover relevant similarities and differences arising from the people, situations, and events with which they interact.

More than other forms of constructivist intervention, personal construct therapy emphasizes the hierarchical nature of the person's construct system. That is, some constructs are more central to the person's meaning-making processes than other, more peripheral and subordinate constructs. For example, one person may evaluate all others primarily in terms of whether they are likely to form accepting, close relationships with him or her, or are likely to reject and abandon the person without warning. Moreover, the construing of another on either the "accepting" or "abandoning" pole of this construct is likely to carry sweeping implications for the person, resulting in a global appraisal of the other as an individual and the prospect of constructing a meaningful relationship with him or her. Another person may employ this construct in a much less central way, perhaps to understand the behavior of potential dating partners, and may see it as carrying fewer implications for the other's personality or the relationship as a whole. Key to Kelly's theory is that such constructs ultimately say more about the individual who formulates them, than about the person to whom they are applied.

Systems of personal constructs operating as an organized whole affect what phenomena a person can construe as well as how these phenomena will be interpreted. Continuing with the example above, the person who views others in "close versus rejecting" terms may not be able to understand the behavior of a person who wishes to form a friendly, but casual relationship. An implication of this, again echoing the sentiments of Epictetus, is that people are not victims of problems in reality as much as they suffer from the constraints and limitations of their construct systems.

Personal construct therapists believe that psychological problems stem from anomalies in the structure or operation of the person's construct system. More specifically, a disorder consists of any personal construction that is used continually despite its repeated invalidation. Given this general conception of problems in living, various kinds of problematic experiences can be predicted.

Threat, for instance, results when the individual feels on the brink of an imminent, comprehensive change in core identity constructs, as when marital discord reaches a crisis point, and the threatened spouse recoils from the awful recognition that divorce will mean a wholesale reworking of his or her view of the self and world. *Anxiety* arises with the awareness that

critical events are outside of the range of the person's current constructs, that one confronts experiences that cannot be meaningfully construed or anticipated. Another problematic experience, *hostility,* results when the person continues to garner or even force support for one or more constructs after they have repeatedly led to unsuccessful predictions. For example, a husband who maintains that his wife should assume a subservient, domestic role and not seek employment, and who uses verbal or physical threats or abuse to keep her in the role he has constructed for her would be manifesting hostility in Kelly's sense. Finally, personal construct therapists view the experience of *guilt* as stemming from the client's awareness that he or she has been dislodged from central value commitments, as defined idiosyncratically within his or her construct system.

At a general level personal construct therapy helps the client examine his or her repertory of constructs and to find more meaningful constructions with which to face life challenges. In particular, the therapist first may help the client articulate constructs of significant others through use of the repertory grid or laddering techniques. In the former exercise the client may be asked to consider two or more persons he or she knows and then describe how the people differ. In this way the client's basic dimensions of meaning are articulated as successively different groups of people are considered. The laddering technique helps the person examine the implications of systems of constructs as they are applied to some real life problem.

The therapist may then help the client expand the construct system so that a wider or more diverse range of people or events may be construed without the person experiencing fear or anxiety. The therapist may also help the client to create new constructions that revise or replace previous constructs. Therapy may also help to "tighten" a construct by requiring the client to examine its concrete, specific implications for the people and events encountered in life. Alternatively, it may be therapeutic for the client to "loosen" certain constructs so they become more flexible and are applied provisionally to a wider range of experiences. In the case of the person who perceived all relationships in terms of acceptance or rejection, therapy may help the person to apply this construct more selectively and discriminately than before. In summary, from this general perspective the therapist helps the client identify interesting problems that derive from his or her view of life, gather evidence in daily life about their viability or utility, and experiment with new or revised constructs. Thus, the role of the personal construct therapist is analogous to that of a *co-investigator,* with the important questions to be researched being defined by the unique affordances and limitations of the client's personal meaning system, rather than the therapist's.

A specific technique pioneered by Kelly and modified by subsequent personal construct therapists is the fixed role technique. This technique was based upon Kelly's observation that the dramatic license to portray a role sometimes led to the actor retaining some of the mannerisms and modes of thinking associated with the role after he or she stepped out of it. That is, temporarily assuming the role helped the person to develop or elaborate his or her construct system in useful and enduring ways.

The technique begins with the client writing a self-characterization sketch that the therapist then uses in drafting a new role for the client to enact. The new role may help the person to construe a wider range of people or events, to revise old constructs, or to help create new constructs. To be useful, the exercise must allow the client to enact a rather different—although not simply opposite—way of approaching life for a fixed period of time. As the therapist and client practice relating to an increasingly intimate set of figures from the client's life in therapeutic role plays, and then experiment with generalizing the new role to real-life situations, the client may come to realize that "personality" is itself a construction, one that can (with effort) be reconstructed as one evolves. Thus, at the end of a time-limited period (typically only a few weeks), the client explicitly relinquishes the new role and considers its implications for his or her ongoing engagement with social life.

Despite its appearance more than 40 years ago, personal construct theory and therapy continue to attract the interests of new generations of researchers and clinicians. Repertory grid methodology has been used to review clients' life histories, their vocational interests and preferences, and their construal of group members' behavior, among other uses. Recent work on personal construct therapy has focused upon death and loss issues, agoraphobia, marriage and family interventions, and life-span development. This level of continued interest by researchers and clinicians underscores the enduring heuristic value of Kelly's original vision, while permitting accommodation of the theory as it comes into contact with more recent additions to the constructivist family of approaches described below.

2. Developmental Perspectives

A second tradition in constructivist therapy includes a "fuzzy set" of approaches that share a focal concern with psychological development, and especially the development of self. Like personal construct theory, they view the evolution of personal meaning systems as the individual's progressive attempts to create "working models" of self and significant others, but they place greater stress than does personal construct theory on the origin of these models in childhood attachment relationships. In keeping with constructivist epistemology, determining the authenticity of reported childhood events (e.g., whether the client as a child was or was not incestuously abused by a stepfather) is less critical than the conclusions the client has drawn about herself and others (e.g., that she must always accede to others' needs, or that others cannot be trusted). In this sense, therapy consists of a sensitive search for the *narrative truth* of the client's life, rather than detective work to "uncover" the literal events that supposedly shaped the client's personality. By focusing attention on the domain of meanings, the therapist also is sensitized to the considerable range of personal reactions to any given "objective" event, as when childhood sexual involvement with a parent is viewed by one client as a shameful secret to be maintained, and by another as indisputable evidence for the contemptability of the opposite sex. Still a third client may view such involvement as an emotionally complicated but essential haven from the still more painful abuses of the other parent. In developmental perspective, these highly individualized themes are viewed as core ordering principles that shape much of the person's subsequent experience of reality, identity, emotionality, and control.

In developmental therapies of this type, the therapist functions as a kind of *psychohistorian,* prompting the client to link current distress to problematic experiences from the recent or more distant past, and explore them more deeply. Theoretically, this involves helping the client subtly shift between two aspects of him- or herself, the experiencing "I," which engages life in all of its emotional immediacy, and the explaining "me," which attempts to give a coherent account of these experiences in rational terms. Because the tacit experience of events tends to precede the ability to articulate and evaluate them, the therapist frequently must assist the client to focus closely on problematic events, reliving them in "slow motion" in all of their emotional intensity in the session, to provide the "raw material" for interpreting the experiences in more useful ways. For example, a confused and self-critical client might trace her recent seemingly inexplicable loss of initiative to her sense of discomfort following an interaction with a male employer. The therapist might then encourage her to "unpack" the interaction in all of its sensory detail, discovering that the client experienced heightened anxiety at the point that her employer rolled his eyes during her presentation, in a way that was reminiscent of her father's silent dismissal of her as a child. This might lead to further exploration of more remote scenarios, and to the thematization of her sense of insufficiency, especially in relation to men.

Among the specialized techniques that are compatible with this developmental perspective is the life-review procedure, which involves attempting to piece together a more continuous sense of one's biography by organizing one's own memories by year, noting significant events, feelings, and developments in one's self understanding on a chronological series of index cards that are added to over the course of therapy. Other forms of reflective writing (e.g., exploring one's changed sense of self after a major early loss) are also frequently used by developmental therapists, either as an adjunct to formal therapy or a means of ongoing self-exploration. More than any specific outcome, the goal of such work is to develop the ability to transition between delicate attention to the nuances of one's engagement in life, and the attempt to interpret them in a way that promotes ongoing reconstruction of one's sense of self.

3. Narrative Approaches

The third tradition, the narrative approach, views life as organized by personal, familial, and cultural themes, and regards therapy as an intimate form of collaboration in editing the client's life story. Narrative perspectives have burgeoned over the last 15 years as clinicians have found the generative and integrative characteristics of stories to be apt metaphors for individuals' meaning-making processes. Most narrative therapeutic perspectives share the common view of

the person as both author and hero of a life story that invariably includes an unexpected (and often unchosen) cast of characters, events, and twists on the temporal and situational plots of one's life. In this way narratives lend coherence and integrity to one's past as well as contribute to the way one anticipates the outcomes of a life story in the future.

Clinicians working in the narrative vein view emotional distress as resulting from or marked by a break, failure, or gap in one's ongoing autobiography. Such narrative suspension leaves the person with a diminished capacity to emplot experienced events or subjected to unanticipated subplots that are markedly discrepant with what the person expected from life. For instance, the traumatic loss of a spouse later in one's life removes a highly valued figure from the partner's life story and necessitates the tragically painful revision of the partner's storied role as companion, friend, caretaker, and lover, among others.

Most narrative therapeutic approaches share the goal of weaving painful, negative, or other unexpected events into the client's dominant life narrative. That is, the client and therapist collaborate to help the person both live and author an active, integrated story. Here, the therapist functions as an *editor or co-author* in attempting revisions of the client's life narrative. For instance, treatment for the bereaved spouse might focus on grieving the loss of the partner by examining how the person dealt with previous losses and the way these were integrated or interpreted in the larger framework of meaning that informs the person's life. Emphasis also may be placed upon developing further roles with children, other family, and friends as a way to emplot a new life "chapter" without the deceased spouse.

Given the goals of narrative repair and reconstruction, therapists working from this perspective may employ a variety of literary techniques. Developing metaphors to help clients more clearly define problems, tease out the meanings of significant struggles and emotional experiences, and find solutions may provide benefits at all phases of therapy. Structured reminiscence may help the client identify salient events, people, and plots in their own stories over the course of their lives. Reminiscence for the grieving spouse may reveal how emotions of sadness, anger, or betrayal from previous losses were incorporated into the life narrative. Writing assignments, such as a letter to the deceased partner, journals, and dialogues may help to both bring problems into greater relief and to help transform them so they may be integrated with existing life stories. Other written documents exchanged between the client and therapist such as certificates of "readiness for change" or "completion of therapy" may help to document and certify real changes in the client's life story.

In summary, narrative approaches to therapy include a rich and growing collection of constructivist methods for acknowledging and creating change in clients' lives. As exemplified by the recent growth in both the number and types of books and scholarly articles on narrative themes, this field of endeavor appears to be among the most rapidly growing areas of constructivism.

4. Systemic Approaches

The fourth set of approaches includes variants of systemic family therapy, which generally reflect a social constructionist concern with "languaging" and its role in shaping the family's definition of the problem. From this perspective, "psychological disorders" are not viewed as syndromes or symptoms that attach themselves to persons, but instead are defined in language through the interaction of those persons—including the identified "client"—engaged in the problem. For example, whether a woman's depressive withdrawal after the death of her stillborn child is considered "normal" or "pathological" is very much a matter for social negotiation, especially within the family context. Problems arise and are sustained in language when they are conferred a "reality" by individuals, family members, and the broader society, and particularly when they are attributed to deficiencies, deficits, or diseases in one individual. Therapy, in this perspective, consists of creatively helping participants in a problem system "language away" the difficulty by reframing it in a way that it is either viewed as no longer problematic (e.g., the mother's continuing sadness is reconstrued as an attempt to maintain her connection to her deceased child) or becomes amenable to solution (e.g., her sense of loss might be validated by a shared family ritual acknowledging the place of the child in their collective lives).

In this approach to therapy, the therapist assumes the role of *conversation manager,* artfully eliciting divergent views of the problem within the family system and exploring their implications for each member. Because family members are often engaged in interlocking patterns of recursive validation (e.g., when the be-

reaved father's confused withdrawal from his wife is viewed by her as emotional abandonment, and her resulting tearfulness is construed by him as further evidence for her "falling apart"), the therapist must often find ways of exposing the hidden premises of each family member's view, and prompting them to view their interaction, at least temporarily, in novel terms. Among the many techniques for accomplishing this are the use of circular questions, which inquire about perceptions among family members (e.g., "Who is most convinced that mom is suffering from major depression? Who is least convinced that this is what is going on?") and their relationships to one another (e.g., "Who in the family is next most depressed? Next? Least?").

Systemic therapists who operate from a constructivist standpoint also make use of novel therapy formats, such as the reflecting team, in which a group of clinicians observes a family therapy session, and then joins the therapist and family to share divergent, but provocative interpretations of the family's difficulty. The aim of such interventions is not to determine the single "correct" interpretation of the complaint, but to dislodge both therapist and clients from habitual ways of thinking about the problem in a way that contributes to its maintenance. As the systemic therapies have continued to evolve, they have become increasingly open to "importing" concepts from more individual constructivist approaches (e.g., personal construct and narrative models) that help reveal the "selves" within the system, and that provide a means of tacking back and forth between individual and family level work across the course of a given therapy.

V. IMPLICATIONS OF CONSTRUCTIVISM FOR PSYCHOTHERAPY RESEARCH

Constructivism and the epistemological approach that undergirds it possess profound implications for guiding inquiry in science in general and for the social and psychological sciences in particular. Work in all science is essentially a human enterprise because people formulate hypotheses, devise working models, conduct experiments, interpret data, and prepare scientific papers and reports. To the extent that the constructivist image of human nature questions our degree of contact with either a knowable world or a knowable self, it shakes the foundations of modern psychological science conceived as the cataloging of factual observations and their systematization into unified theories in the natural, physical, or social sciences.

Constructivists view science instead as continuous with other forms of knowing, yielding inherently partial and positional perspectives reliant on the models and metaphors of a particular place and time, even when it formulates general "laws" of human functioning. This implies that the theories and "laws" that have been developed in all of the sciences represent complex and organized constructions that have been elaborated to varying degrees. Each field also may enjoy different amounts of coherence among theoretical constructions.

Conceptualizing science in this manner may raise fundamental and provocative questions for some about whether observing the same results about a thing, event, or a person with different methods or at different times reveals successively more "accurate" or "real" characteristics or just reflects a coherent system of constructions that function somewhat equivalently. The former position seems to assume a realist or objectivist position that reality can be known and that science incrementally advances by developing more accurate or realistic knowledge through successive approximations of theories and their research paradigms. The latter position of constructivism deemphasizes "knowing reality" by focusing instead on coherent, viable, and workable constructions of relevant phenomena. A question that follows from the constructivist perspective concerns the methods and criteria for determining how construction systems are viable and workable. When and under what conditions is a construction system viable and when does it appear to lose its ability for meaning making?

Within psychology, tensions exist between realist/objectivist positions and those that assume a more constructivist stance. These tensions can, in part, be traced to the long-standing dialectical relationship between nomothetic and idiographic perspectives on psychological inquiry. Typically the experimental psychologies (social, cognitive, biological, and so forth) have attempted to catalog observations about human nature that are invariant over time and place, that is, to use a nomothetic approach. In focusing more on the life phenomena of individuals, the clinical sciences have developed a more idiographic approach to their field of inquiry. While nomothetic and even quantifiable generalizations about human behavior may be attempted at the level of abstract theory, constructivists ultimately contend that the lived particulars of the person's knowing systems can be best understood through adopting an idiographic and qualitative approach to the study of concrete individuals in their unique social ecologies.

The differing foci of constructivist and realist/objectivist approaches in psychology presents a dilemma for how these methods of inquiry may interface with each other and how the fruits of each paradigm may be incorporated by the other. How can generalizations about the "average anorexic" from the nomothetic perspective be of use to the therapist engaging this *particular* client and the way she constructs her role in life? Similarly, what is the utility of individual constructions, no matter how rich and clinically informative, when trying to discover and articulate fundamental principles of human behavior? At a more general level, what would psychological science look like if all research were conducted at the idiographic and qualitative level associated with constructivist inquiry?

Such questions face those who study psychotherapy outcome. In trying to document the "real world" effects of therapeutic interventions, researchers may use instrumentation and assessment techniques that fail to capture the subtle nuances of human change. Yet, persons may report greater happiness, adjustment, or ability to proceed with life despite producing unremarkable profiles on standard instruments. How does the realist/objectivist outcome researcher account for this phenomenon? Constructivists would propose using idiographic and ipsative measures that are uniquely tailored to the work that is being undertaken in psychotherapy. Methods such as goal-attainment scaling, content analysis procedures, and repertory grids may both help trace the client's level of achieved change and permit the outcome researcher to compare the extent to which clients as a group received benefits.

Beyond these issues in the assessment of therapeutic outcome, lie the questions of what constructivism has contributed to psychotherapy research, and what psychotherapy research has revealed about the nature of constructivist psychotherapy. As implied above, constructivists have actively pursued the development of both qualitative and quantitative procedures for tracking human change processes, particularly at the level of meanings that reflect one's evolving appraisal of the self, life problems, and significant relationships over the course of therapy. While such procedures add refinement to nomothetic measures of personal change, they essentially operate within the traditional paradigm for the study of psychotherapy.

A bolder contribution being made by some constructivists is the development of new paradigms for research on psychotherapy process, which attempt to identify "markers" of significant in-session change episodes (e.g., points of sensed internal conflict or confusion) and then pinpoint the processes that facilitate their positive resolution (e.g., therapist initiated confrontation of the inner "split," or use of metaphor to place experiences in a new perspective). At a more general level, constructivists have also pioneered the development of models of research that actively involve clients as co-investigators and interpreters of a study's results, and that foster deep-going reflection on the part of investigators about shifts in their methodological and conceptual commitments across the course of their research programs.

What has research taught us in turn about the distinctive processes or outcomes of constructivist therapies? In a sense, a definitive answer awaits further study. As fairly recent contenders in the psychotherapy arena, the approaches described in this article have yet to receive the empirical attention given to more "mature" therapeutic traditions. In addition, the abstract and philosophic nature of constructivist theory has discouraged more traditionally trained investigators, who are understandably drawn to simpler models that work with a limited range of concepts and techniques. However, the preliminary research that has been conducted on these novel forms of practice suggests that they are often more acceptable to clients than more regimented, prescriptive alternatives, that they can be effective for even quite discrete problems such as speech disfluencies, phobias, and social anxieties, and that they are adaptable to a range of formats including individual, group, and family therapy. With recent and ongoing efforts to examine their efficacy in the treatment of eating disorders, sexual abuse, and other serious clinical problems, we are optimistic that they will continue to contribute to the refinement of both psychotherapy research and practice.

BIBLIOGRAPHY

Mahoney, M. J. (1991). *Human change processes*. New York: Basic Books.

McNamee, S. & Gergen, K. J. (Eds.). (1992). *Therapy as social construction*. Newbury Park, CA: Sage.

Neimeyer, R. A., & Mahoney, M. J. (Eds.). (1995). *Constructivism in psychotherapy*. Washington, DC: American Psychological Association.

Rosen, H., & Kuehlwein, K. T. (Eds.). (1996). *Constructing reality: Meaning-making perspectives for psychotherapists*. San Francisco, CA: Jossey-Bass.

Journal of Constructivist Psychology, published quarterly. Philadelphia, PA: Taylor and Francis.

Control

Beth A. Morling* and Susan T. Fiske

University of Massachusetts, Amherst

Control The ability intentionally to influence environmental, psychological, or behavioral events.
Mental Control Control over one's own thoughts and feelings.
Outcome Control Control of external events motivationally relevant to the self.

CONTROL, the ability intentionally to influence environmental, psychological, or behavioral events, appears to be fundamental to people's well-being. People who feel they have control also perceive that they are competent, that they can influence events, and that they can predict what happens to them. People who temporarily feel out of control may be upset that they cannot alter events, and may engage in compensatory behaviors to restore a feeling of control. People who consistently feel out of control may give up, feel helpless, and cope less well with adversity. Psychological research in Western industrialized cultures indicates that people who feel in control live longer, suffer from fewer serious illnesses, and have better psychological health than people who do not feel in control. And regardless of culture, people everywhere strive to influence, learn about, and gain competence in cultur-

ally relevant areas of experience. Robert White's concept, "competence motivation" or "effectance," perhaps best captures this universal goal of control. From infancy, all animals exhibit a fundamental motivation to explore, act upon, and master their environment. People's motivation for effectance is reflected in their desire to control events and have an impact on the world.

I. INTRODUCTION TO CONTROL RESEARCH

Because of its fundamental importance to people, control plays an important role in theories of human behavior. Many psychologists view control as a motivation for human action; others cite it as an important individual difference. Psychologists study control from two perspectives: (a) individual differences in control, especially as it relates to the self-concept and psychological health, and (b) environmental effects on control, including contexts that make people feel out of control and people's reactions to control deprivation.

Control can be directed internally or externally (toward the self or toward others) in order to influence different environmental or psychological events (outcomes or mental processes). Most psychological research deals with perceived outcome control, that is, people's perceived control over external, self-relevant events (for example, a student's feeling that studying will produce a passing grade, or a patient's feeling that a change in diet will affect the course of a disease). Outcome control is the focus of the first two parts of this article. Other psychological research studies mental control, people's perceived control over their own internal thoughts and feelings (for example, a dieter's

*Beth A Morling is presently at Union College, Schenectady, New York.

attempts to avoid thinking about food, or an anxious person's intrusive worries about physical danger). Mental control is covered in the third and last section of this article. Thus, the entire article covers attempts by individuals to control their *own* outcomes and mental processes. People can also control another person's thoughts, feelings, and behavior, which psychologists call social influence, or they can control another person's outcomes, which psychologists call social power.

In this article, we first describe personality psychological approaches to own-outcome control: individual differences and correlates of feelings of outcome control. There we describe how feelings of outcome control are related to a stable self-concept and to general coping ability. We also list some of the many theories that treat an individual's sense of outcome control as an important mediating or moderating variable. Second, we describe the social psychological approach to outcome control: ways that feelings of control can be manipulated, and what people do when they feel deprived of control. There we explain that people's strategies for control involve either acting on the environment or thinking about a situation differently. In addition, we explain that when people feel control-deprived, they search for information to regain control, or they may give up trying. In the last section of the article, we describe theory related to mental control, the control over one's own thoughts and feelings. In that section, we focus on the degree of control people have over their own cognition and affect.

II. PERSONALITY APPROACHES: INDIVIDUAL DIFFERENCES IN PERCEIVED OUTCOME CONTROL

Personality approaches to control have traditionally focused on differences between people who believe they can control their own outcomes and people who believe they cannot. One of the most well-known attempts to measure these differences is Rotter's Internal–External Locus of Control construct, based in learning theory. We will explore this construct and its limitations in some depth, because many of the same assumptions, predictions, and criticisms can apply to constructs to be described later.

A. Locus of Control Theory

According to Rotter, people with an internal locus of control (LOC) perceive contingencies between their behavior and subsequent events (such as reinforcements), whereas people with an external locus of control do not. Implied in the construct is that people's behavior will, to some extent, be determined by their control expectancies. Rotter's Internal–External Locus of Control scale contains 23 forced-choice items measuring the extent to which people believe that the things that happen to them are caused by their own actions or are caused by external forces such as chance, luck, or powerful others. People who score low on the scale have an internal locus of control, meaning they believe their outcomes result from their own efforts. People who score high on the scale have an external locus of control, meaning they believe their outcomes result from environmental forces. Importantly, the scale, and the construct itself, concerns people's *beliefs* about outcome contingencies; it does not concern the *actual* correlation between people's actions and subsequent events.

Much research has explored social correlates of the LOC construct, and the studies suggest that people who have an internal LOC are more likely to resist persuasion, to try to act on their environments, and to place a high value on achievement. Studies show that people with an internal LOC conform less to external standards, have higher self-esteem, are more creative, are more optimistic, and persevere longer at difficult tasks. Internal LOC is related to political activism among students, to knowledge of prison regulations among inmates, and to knowledge of one's physical condition among hospital patients. Most researchers have concluded from these studies that an internal LOC is more psychologically healthy and adaptive than an external LOC.

Rotter's locus of control construct has been extremely widely used in personality, social, and health psychology, but it has also been criticized. Behavioral correlates (such as activism and achievement) of LOC often fail to replicate in different studies. And many writers have debated the construct, addressing its implication that an internal LOC is always preferable and an external LOC is always devalued. Furthermore, many studies show that lower social classes tend to score in the external direction, and thus are more prone to an external LOC's achievement "deficits."

One common critique separates locus of control beliefs into two separate constructs. One, perceived personal control, addresses individuals' beliefs about control in their own lives. The other, control ideology, is an individual's philosophy about how rewards are distributed in the larger world. Critics hold that the two kinds of control are independent. Therefore, for example, someone from a lower socio-economic status might hold an internal control ideology that individuals, in general, should be rewarded for their actions, but may also have an external sense of personal control reflecting that, in the past, his or her own actions have gone unrewarded.

Others have criticized the explicit bias toward an internal locus of control on the grounds that an accurate assessment of reward contingencies is more important than whether a person's LOC is internal or external. For some people, particularly those in lower social classes, an external locus of control may be an accurate picture of their worlds. Furthermore, an internal locus of control can be used by middle- or upper-class people to justify their position in life; thus, advantaged people hold a philosophy that one deserves one's superior position. The LOC construct (and also the related constructs of self-efficacy and learned helplessness, discussed below) may ignore or oversimplify the social contexts that surround individuals and influence their feelings of control. Control theories may be biased by an individualistic context, common to Western cultures, in which individuals are expected to stand out and make their own way instead of working together and fitting in with others.

B. Related Control Theories

Several personality constructs are related to the locus of control construct (Table 1). To the extent that they are similar to locus of control, they are also subject to the same criticisms for being biased toward internality. Two of these theories (self-efficacy and learned helplessness) treat individual differences in outcome control as a central variable, much like locus of control theory.

I. Self-Efficacy Theory

First, Bandura's self-efficacy theory addresses people's feelings of competence regarding an activity. Like locus of control theory, self-efficacy theory studies how

Table I Summary of Major Personality Approaches to Individual Differences in Outcome Control

Major theorist	Construct	Variables affecting and affected by feelings of control
Rotter	Locus of control	Perceived contingency between one's actions and subsequent events leads to feelings of internal control
Seligman	Learned helplessness	Perceived lack of contingency between one's efforts and subsequent aversive events leads to feelings of no control
Bandura	Self-Efficacy	Perceived ability to enact a behavioral outcome enhances feelings of personal control

people perceive their own abilities to act successfully in the world. If people feel they will be successful at an activity, they express agency, initiative, and achievement; i.e., they put more active, persistent, effort into that activity and are more likely to succeed. Self-efficacy is related to setting high goals for oneself, being optimistic about achieving those goals, and being motivated to try again if progress toward the goal is frustrated. Bandura explicitly relates self-efficacy to the ability to control and predict one's outcomes. Bandura extends the self-efficacy construct to groups, with a parallel theory of collective efficacy, which refers to groups acting together to achieve some outcome, for example, social change. Like self-efficacy, collective efficacy involves agency, initiative, and achievement, and describes how groups can influence outcomes that are related to the welfare of the group or the larger world. [*See* Self-Efficacy.]

2. Learned Helplessness Theory

Learned helplessness, first studied in dogs who became passive in an experiment in which they received uncontrollable shocks, is also used to describe people who perceive their own outcomes to be uncontrollable. Because learned-helpless people do not feel they have control over outside events, they act passive and persist less in activities. Learned-helpless people resemble those with an external locus of control; they do not perceive a contingency between their efforts and their outcomes. The learned helplessness construct has been used as a model for depression.

3. Control as Moderator or Mediator

Scores of psychological theories include an individual's feelings of outcome control as a variable that moderates people's behavior (i.e., people who feel in control act one way and people who do not feel in control act another way) or mediates people's behavior (i.e., one variable influences people's feelings of control, which then influence a third variable). Still other theories view people's strivings for control as motivation for their behavior or beliefs about the world. There are simply too many theories that use control to catalog them all here; briefly mentioning the scope of the theories will suffice. For instance, research on stressful life events has studied how feelings of control can sometimes, but not always, help people cope. Other theories that focus on everyday life have used control to predict what people will do, such as when they will act on their attitudes, attend to their environments, feel good about things they have done, or try hard at an academic task. Still other theories have used the desire for prediction and control to explain why people tend to act in certain ways, such as why they choose particular romantic partners. The wide range of theories that have found control to be a useful predictive and explanatory variable attests to how important it is to people to influence environmental, psychological, and behavioral events.

III. SOCIAL PSYCHOLOGICAL APPROACHES: SITUATIONAL DETERMINANTS OF PERCEIVED OUTCOME CONTROL

Whereas personality theories of control describe how people differ in their relatively stable, dispositional feelings of outcome control, social psychological theories of outcome control focus on more temporary, changeable feelings of control. In particular, they focus on the techniques people use to feel in control, the effects of control feelings in stressful situations, and the effects of control deprivation on people's behavior.

A. Ways of Feeling in Control: Techniques for Mastering the Situation

This section first addresses six major avenues to feeling in control, first identified by Suzanne Thompson. Each of these has been related to how people cope

in stressful situations. Although there are six main control behaviors, they can all be summed up in two general techniques: acting to influence an aversive situation or thinking about the situation differently (Table II).

First, in *behavior control* people take steps to end an event, make it less likely, or change its timing or intensity. An example of behavioral control is people having the opportunity to press a button to control the intensity of an impending shock or loud noise, or a cancer patient having control over when to administer his or her own pain medication. Behavior control can still be effective even if it is illusory (that is, even if a person never uses the response and does not know whether it would actually reduce the loudness of a noise). Perceptions of behavior control reduce people's distress before and after an aversive stimulus. People with behavioral control can also tolerate higher levels of the aversive stimulus. However, it is less clear whether people feel less distress during the event as a result of behavioral control.

In *cognitive control,* people think differently about an impending or ongoing noxious event through (a) avoidant strategies, for example, directing attention away from the stressful aspects of the event; or (b) nonavoidant strategies, for example, coping with the event by focusing on benefits of the event, conjuring images inconsistent with the stressful event, or talking calmly to the self. For example, a beginning graduate student might focus on the benefits, instead of the trials, of years of graduate training, or a person might mentally withdraw from a fight with a romantic partner. In general, cognitive control appears to help people cope with stressful events before, during, and after the event. However, specific kinds of cognitive control appear to help in particular ways: Mental withdrawal appears more effective in reducing pre-event distress, whereas reinterpretation (focusing on benefits) reduces postevent distress more effectively.

Decision control refers to the ability to make decisions about the type of aversive event, its onset, or its timing. For example, a patient might be given a choice between two kinds of surgery, or a student may be given a choice of several courses to take in fulfilling a requirement. In some cases, decision control can be illusory, when the choices are presented in such a way that people almost always choose one particular option. Decision control appears effective if the choice leads to positive outcomes (e.g., the surgery is success-

Table II   Summary of Types of Control and Their Effects on Adjustment to Stress

Type of control	Definition	Example	Effects
Behavior control	Acting in a concrete way to reduce aversiveness of a negative event	Pressing a button to reduce the intensity of a loud noise	Reduces pre-event anxiety, increases tolerance for the aversive event, reduces post-event distress
Cognitive control	Thinking about an aversive event differently or focusing on non-noxious features of event	Focusing on benefits of a noxious medical procedure while it is occurring	Appears to improve coping with all phases of an aversive event
Decision control	Ability to make decisions regarding timing, onset, or type of aversive event	Choosing between two types of surgery	Is beneficial if the outcome of the event is favorable, but may not help if outcome is unfavorable
Information control	Obtaining or seeking information about details of an aversive event (e.g., sensations, duration, timing)	Learning the side effects of surgery	Sensation information and procedure information reduce the stress of an aversive event
Retrospective control	Beliefs that one can control an event that already occurred	Believing that one could have prevented an accident	Effects are yet unknown, may improve adjustment to some noxious events but not others
Control achieved through mastering the self. Techniques: predictive control, vicarious control, illusory control, and interpretive control	Bringing thoughts and behaviors in line with environmental forces	Carefully learning what might happen, aligning oneself with a powerful group, accepting what fate brings, or viewing events in beneficial terms	May help adjustment to events when situation mastery is not possible; may be a culturally proscribed control expectancy

Source: Fiske, S. T., and Taylor, S. E. (1991). "Social Cognition," 2nd ed. McGraw-Hill, New York.

ful) or to outcomes that can be reinterpreted with dissonance-reduction strategies (e.g., the chosen class is not really as boring as the other students say). But it is unclear whether decision control helps people cope when the outcome of the choice is decidedly unfavorable (e.g., when the surgery is unsuccessful).

When people gather information about an aversive event, they practice *information control*. The information can include details about how the event will feel, how long it will last, or what will cause it. Having a general understanding of what will happen, and why, appears to help people adjust to and cope with noxious events. Information control may be an easy way to implement control when more direct forms of control are less possible. In this particular way, it is related to predictive control, a form of mastering the self (described below).

In *retrospective control,* people construct control-related beliefs about an event that has already occurred. For example, a rape victim might blame herself for not locking her windows or for walking alone at night. Retrospective control beliefs might help vic-

tims feel more control over the event and over future recurrences of the event, perhaps restoring a positive sense of self. Another kind of retrospective control concerns beliefs about how replicable, rather than how controllable, a past event is. For example, cancer patients might not feel they had control over the onset of their disease, but may feel they can prevent a recurrence by changing their diet. Retrospective control is still relatively unstudied in social psychology.

B. Ways of Feeling in Control: Techniques for Mastering the Self

Control attempts in which individuals attempt to master the self (traditionally called secondary control) differ from the previous five types of control. These five, behavior control, decision control, retrospective control, and, to a lesser extent, information control and cognitive control, are all examples of attempting control through mastering the situation (also called primary control). When people master the situation, they take action to bring the environment in line with their wishes. But when people attempt control by mastering the self, they do not attempt to influence the environment; instead, they attempt to bring themselves in line with it. Whereas the targets of mastering the situation are other people, objects, or environmental conditions, the targets of mastering the self are the *self's* expectations, goals, perceptions, or interpretations. Some theorists suggest that people from Western cultures are more likely to attempt situation mastery and that people from Eastern cultures are more likely to attempt self mastery; however, both kinds of control are prevalent in both cultures.

Mastering the self can take many forms. In *predictive control,* people attempt to avoid uncertainty by accurately predicting a future event. For example, they may learn their status in an impending social situation and the relevant rules of etiquette to avoid feeling unprepared or uncomfortable. (Note that predictive control is similar to information control, described earlier). In *vicarious control,* people align themselves closely with people or groups who have power, in order to participate indirectly in their control. For example, people may derive feelings of self-esteem by their close alignment with a successful work group. In *illusory control,* people align themselves with chance and accept their fate. People practice illusory control when they accept streaks of good and bad luck as they come. Finally, in *interpretive control,* people perceive events as purposeful and meaningful. An example of interpretive control is viewing a failure as an opportunity for growth, or interpreting a chronic anxiety problem in more positive terms (e.g., it makes one more vigilant and alert).

Theory on self-mastery control techniques is an important complement to the situation mastery research. It suggests that people can feel in control even when opportunities to alter the environment are unavailable. Control-theories focusing on self-mastery grew out of cross-cultural research in much the same way that critiques of the personality approaches to control (see Section II) reacted to findings of external control expectancies in lower social classes. In particular, some cultures appear to encourage self-mastery control expectancies by emphasizing a close relationship with one's social group. In such cultures, people may be encouraged to fit in and go along rather than stand out and make their own way without the group. Similarly, systems in society may reduce opportunities for situation mastery for people from lower social classes.

Self-mastery implies that even when people's actual opportunities to alter the environment are low (as may be the case for lower social classes or in cultures where social behaviors are more strictly proscribed), people can still feel in control by altering the self or identifying with a group. It therefore brings a broader and more universal perspective to control theory.

Although much of the social psychological work on control has focused on how feelings of control can help buffer stress, some research indicates that control is not always adaptive. In some situations, having control can actually cause higher distress. One such situation occurs when people have high levels of control but low levels of perceived self-efficacy. A person who is placed into a powerful position may have high control, but may feel incapable of fulfilling the responsibilities of the position, creating significant distress. Another situation occurs when people have too much control, so that the amount of control becomes overwhelming (for example, a medical procedure in which a patient is given too much information about the experience *and* given choices about treatment). Attempts at control can also be stressful when they require much more effort than not attempting control. Control is also aversive when efforts at control are unsuccessful. Some people may be able to identify situations when attempts at control are likely to be effective and situations when they are not, an ability that is part of a more general theory of coping called constructive thinking. Finally, some people prefer to cope with negative situations by repressing them. For these people, control options are aversive.

C. Effects of Control Deprivation

The previous discussion has focused on the effects of perceived control on people's coping with aversive life events. In social psychology, perceived control has also been tied to other psychological responses: increased information search, psychological reactance, and helplessness. These three responses are people's typical reactions to control deprivation. People can feel control-deprived when they experience a lack of contingency between their efforts and their outcomes or when they perceive a restriction of behavioral choice. Each of these three reactions and the specific type of control deprivation that typically causes them follows next.

One typical response to control deprivation is to

look for more information. This *information search* likely responds to the kind of control deprivation caused by noncontingent or unpredictable outcomes. At times, control-deprived people become desperate for information, making them more susceptible to social influence and less able to process the information carefully. An indiscriminate information search can lead people to make inappropriate decisions or inaccurate predictions about their outcomes. But other times the search is more careful (and more adaptive), as when people vigilantly scan the environment.

Information search is significantly related to control motivation in impression formation. Heider, Kelley, and Jones, all original attribution theorists, unanimously proposed that people make attributions (i.e., casual judgments) about others to render the world more predictable and controllable. It follows that attributions should be especially important when control is threatened. Pittman and Heller proposed three kinds of situations in which people's feelings of control deprivation lead to more careful, information-driven impressions of others. The first occurs when people feel momentarily control-deprived, such as when they experience noncontingent feedback. Second, some interpersonal situations take control away from an individual. For example, people who are dependent on another person for an outcome (such as a reward) lose sole control over their own outcomes. Third, a situation that contains negative or surprising information threatens people's model of a predictable and benevolent world, so it also leads to increased information search. In these three situations, people respond to the lack of outcome control by paying more attention to interpersonal information and processing it more thoroughly and carefully.

Information search, then, is one typical reaction to control deprivation. Another common response is *reactance*. Reactance is most likely to occur when people's control is arbitrarily withdrawn or when people's previous freedoms are taken away. Reactance leads to anger and hostility, efforts to restore the lost freedoms, and a higher evaluation of the restricted option. For example, if a class originally had a choice between two paper topics and were then arbitrarily told to write on a particular one, the students might feel angry, might protest the action, and might also evaluate the unassigned topic as the better one. Reactance often causes physiological responses that can persist a long time and exacerbate health problems.

Another typical response to control deprivation is helplessness. In this response, people typically give in to the situation and act passively. People often act helpless when they feel that events are completely beyond their control: for example, an extremely stressful or shocking event (such as the death of a spouse) or alternatively, attempts at control that have been unsuccessful (such as repeated, vain attempts to escape an aversive situation). In addition to promoting passive behavior, helpless reactions are related to anxiety, depression, and depleted physiological reserves. Helplessness is directly related to learned helplessness theory. It also resembles the lack of persistence and low desire for achievement hypothesized in people with an external locus of control or low feelings of self-efficacy. In addition, it ties in with the theory of mindfulness, in that people who act mindlessly give up control over their environment by resorting to default levels of processing. A helpless reaction to control deprivation is therefore similar to people's more dispositional differences in low feelings of outcome control.

To summarize, social psychological approaches to outcome control have covered two domains. First, people can use a variety of strategies to feel in control, and often people's control attempts help them cope with stressful events. Second, people react to control deprivation by seeking information, reacting to restore lost freedoms, or by withdrawing effort when they perceive that they will have little impact.

Thus, the social psychological perspective on outcome control in many ways parallels the personality psychology approaches. Just as dispositional differences in control beliefs are related to perseverance, optimism, information-seeking, self-esteem, creativity, and other positive variables, social environments can create similar effects on a situationally specific (though not necessarily less potent) scale. Environments that provide choices for behavior and in which a person feels competent lead to greater personal interest, less tension, more trust, more creativity, improved mood, higher self-esteem, greater persistence, and better health. In large doses, such environments may well change people's dispositional differences in control beliefs.

Control beliefs in social environments also play a role in current theories of social cognition, the study of how people think about other people. Recently, social cognitive theorists viewed social perceivers as "cognitive misers," doing only as much mental work as they had to to get by. But currently, social perceivers are being viewed as "motivated tacticians." The current view emphasizes that people's social thinking is pragmatic: purposeful and affected by people's plans and goals. Therefore, sometimes it is in the interest of people's goals to make a careful, thoughtful impression, whereas other times, people may find a simple, "good-enough" impression suitable. Both the variations in the amount of control a situation affords and people's changing motivations for control can influence people's impression goals. In addition, social perceivers can use different degrees of controlled mental processing (discussed next) when they allocate their attention according to relevant goals.

IV. APPROACHES TO MENTAL CONTROL

People's ability to control their thoughts and feelings varies tremendously. Some types of thinking are highly deliberate and controlled, whereas other types of thinking do not require as much effort or allow as much conscious intervention, so they qualify as less controlled processing. This section briefly describes the differences between controlled and uncontrolled (typically called automatic) mental processes. Psychological approaches to mental control appear to have little in common with the psychological approaches to outcome control mentioned in Sections I and II. Indeed, the domains of research do not overlap much, and very little research has explored the links, if any, between people's relative control over their thoughts and feelings and their control over their outcomes.

A continuum from automatic to controlled mental processes, outlined by John Bargh and James Uleman, provides a framework for a discussion of mental control. Starting at the most automatic end of the continuum, automatic processes include: preconscious automaticity, postconscious automaticity, and goal-directed automaticity. Moving toward the more controlled end of the continuum, controlled processes include: spontaneous thought, ruminations, and intentional thought. We discuss automatic and controlled thinking in separate sections; however, they are theoretically arranged on a single continuum. Criteria and forms of both automatic and controlled mental processes are presented in Table III.

Table III Automatic and Controlled Mental Processes

Type of process	Criteria	Forms (corresponding to the criteria for each process)
Automatic	Process must be unintentional, involuntary, effortless, and outside awareness	Preconscious automaticity (most automatic) Postconscious automaticity Goal-dependent automaticity
Controlled	Process must be able to be started, monitored, and terminated at will	Spontaneous thought Ruminative thought Intentional thought (most controlled)

Source: Fiske, S. T., and Taylor, S. E. (1991). "Social Cognition," 2nd ed. McGraw-Hill.

A. Types of Automatic Processing

Automatic (uncontrolled) processes are so called because they are unintentional and occur without a person's awareness. They do not require cognitive capacity or mental effort to operate. Different types of automatic processes adhere to a greater or lesser extent of these criteria. *Preconscious* automaticity is a name for the most automatic kind of mental processing, conforming to all of the criteria. When people process information preconsciously, they react immediately and spontaneously. People are not aware of a preconscious mental process. An example is subliminal encoding, where stimuli are presented at a rate too fast for conscious processing, but they are still processed and can still affect people's subsequent judgments.

A less pure form of automaticity on the continuum is called *postconscious* automaticity. This form occurs when people are aware of a stimulus in the environment, but are not aware of its effects on their mental processes. For example, people are often aware of their moods, but may not be aware that their moods affect the way they make judgments about stimuli. Similarly, sometimes activated schemas spur immediate, category-based affective responses. Such "schema-triggered affect" is postconscious in that people are aware of the stimulus, but not necessarily of their retrieval of the schema and its accompanying affective response.

An even less pure form of automaticity is *goal-dependent* automaticity. In this kind of processing, people need to initiate the processing, but once it is started, it does not require conscious effort to continue. For example, people may have a conscious goal of forming an accurate impression of another person, but their increased attention and individuating processes occur without intentional monitoring.

B. Types of Controlled Processing

Controlled processes are characterized by people's ability deliberately to stop and start them, and by people's ability consciously to monitor their progress. As with automatic processes, controlled processes adhere more or less to these criteria. The first form of controlled mental processes, which is the least controlled of the three, is *spontaneous* thought. Spontaneous thought begins without intent or awareness, but takes up cognitive capacity and can be terminated or inhibited at will. It overlaps to some extent with the least automatic of automatic mental processes, goal dependent automaticity; indeed, the two are next to each other on the continuum from controlled to automatic processes. An example of spontaneous thought is people's rapid judgment of other people in terms of dispositional traits. People categorize others into traits relatively easily and with little cognitive effort; however, the trait judgments can be altered if people's goals or the situation changes. Therefore, spontaneous processes occur rapidly and unintentionally, but they can also be controlled.

A more controlled kind of thought is *ruminative* thought. Ruminations are controlled in that people are aware of the thoughts, but they are uncontrolled in that people are unable to end them at will. Ruminations are common when people's goals are interrupted. Ruminative thought can focus on searching for alternative means to achieve an interrupted goal, or, if alternative means are unavailable, ruminations focus on the feelings associated with the goal. It appears that as long as a goal remains unmet, ruminations continue unless people find a way to overcome the obstacle or abandon the goal altogether.

Related to rumination is a more general inability for people to prevent an unwanted thought from coming into consciousness. People have a difficult time purposefully suppressing thoughts (for example, it is difficult for a dieter to suppress thoughts of tempting foods). Furthermore, after a period of attempting to suppress a thought, people often experience a rebound, in which they think the unwanted thought more than people who had not been deliberately suppressing it. Focusing on an alternative thought during the suppression period can help prevent this rebound effect.

Thought suppression and ruminations appear prevalent in depression and coping with traumatic events. Depressed people ruminate about failures more and have more trouble suppressing negative thoughts than nondepressed people do. And people who experience negative life events often ruminate about them until they have worked them through. For these people, ruminations can be helped by intentionally focusing on the very thoughts they are trying to suppress. Talking or writing about the negative event appears to lower victims' distress, helps prevent ruminations from recurring, and attenuates medical complaints for weeks after the talking or writing. [*See* DEPRESSION.]

At the most controlled end of the continuum are *intentional* processes. When people perceive that they have choices or different interpretations of a situation, whatever choice they make can be said to be an intentional one. People's intent is especially obvious when they make a more difficult choice (one requiring more mental effort). People enact their mental intents by paying attention to the chosen alternative. For example, if a person intends to view a group of people in less stereotypical terms, he or she would consciously attend to stereotype-inconsistent information, instead of relying on the easier process of attending only to stereotype-consistent information.

V. SUMMARY

In their efforts to feel in control of their worlds, people can attempt to control their outcomes or their own mental processes. People differ in the extent to which they feel their actions can alter their outcomes, a difference that personality psychologists have sometimes labeled locus of control, self-efficacy, or learned helplessness. Social psychologists have shown that people can feel in control by actually influencing an event or by changing the way they think about it. These attempts at control can help people adapt to stress and lead to improved physical health and longer life expectancy. When people's outcome control is threatened, they may seek information, protest to restore lost freedoms, or give up trying. And when people process information, they sometimes have considerable control over their thoughts and feelings, and other times they operate more automatically. People's desire for mastery and competence, reflected in their need to control events, is a primary motivating force. When this motivation is challenged, people react strongly: they fight or they give up. When it is promoted in culturally appropriate ways, people try, persist, learn, cope, and thrive.

This article has been reprinted from the *Encyclopedia of Human Behavior, Volume 1.*

BIBLIOGRAPHY

Averill, J. R. (1973). Personal control over aversive stimuli and its relationship to stress. *Psychol. Bull.* **80,** 286–303.

Bandura, A. (1989). Human agency in social cognitive theory. *Am. Psychol.* **44,** 1175–1184.

Bargh, J. A. (1989). Conditional automaticity: Varieties of automatic influence on social perception and cognition. In "Unintended Thought." (J. S. Uleman and J. A. Bargh, Eds.), Guilford, New York.

Dépret, E., & Fiske, S. T. (1993). Social cognition and power: Some cognitive consequences of social structure as a source of control deprivation. In "Control Motivation and Social Cognition," G. Weary, F. Gleicher and K. Marsh, Eds.), Springer-Verlag, New York.

Fiske, S. T., & Taylor, S. E. (1984). "Social Cognition," Chapt. 5. Addison-Wesley, Reading, Ma.

Fiske, S. T., & Taylor, S. E. (1991). "Social Cognition," 2nd ed., Chapt. 6. McGraw-Hill, N.Y.

Lefcourt, H. M. (1973). The function of the illusions of control and freedom. *Am. Psychol.* **28,** 417–425.

Pittman, T. S., & Heller, J. F. (1987). Social motivation. *Annu. Rev. Psychol.* **38,** 461–489.

Rotter, J. B. (1966). Generalized expectancies for internal versus external control of reinforcement. *Psychol. Monogr.* **80** (1), 609.

Strickland, B. R. (1989). Internal-external control expectancies: From contingency to creativity. *Am. Psychol.* **44,** 1–12.

Thompson, S. C. (1981). Will it hurt less if I can control it? A complex answer to a simple question. *Psychol. Bull.* **90,** 89–101.

Uleman, J. S. (1989). A framework for thinking intentionally about unintended thoughts. In "Unintended Thought," J. S. Uleman and J. A. Bargh, Eds.), pp. 425–449, Guilford, New York.

Wegner, D. M., & Pennebaker, J. W. (Eds.) (1992). "Handbook of Mental Control." Prentice-Hall, Englewood Cliffs, N.J.

Weisz, J. R., Rothbaum, F. M., & Blackburn, T. C. (1984). Standing out and standing in: The psychology of control in America and Japan. *Am. Psychol.* **39,** 955–969.

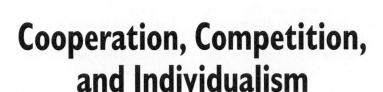

Cooperation, Competition, and Individualism

George P. Knight
Arizona State University

Gustavo Carlo
University of Nebraska, Lincoln

Scott C. Roesch
University of California, Los Angeles

Altruism Resource distributions that maximize the resources of another.

Competitive Preference A tendency to choose either a superiority or rivalry resource distribution.

Cooperative Preference A tendency to choose either an equality, group-enhancement, or altruism resource distribution.

Equality Resource distributions that minimize the difference between one's own and others' resources.

Group-Enhancement Resource distributions that maximize the resources of two or more individuals as a group irrespective of the specific distribution of resources to oneself or to another.

Individualistic Preference A preference for a resource distribution that maximizes one's own resources.

Resource Distribution Preference A tendency to divide valuable commodities between oneself and one or more others in a specific manner.

Rivalry Resource distributions that minimize the resources of another.

Superiority Resource distributions that maximize one's relative resources compared to another.

Here we examine existing major theories and research relevant to **COOPERATIVE, COMPETITIVE,** and **INDIVIDUALISTIC BEHAVIORS.** Although a number of theoretical perspectives on these behaviors exist, we focus on social psychological and developmental theories of cooperative, competitive, and individualistic behaviors. In addition to the review of major theories and empirical findings, methodological issues in research on cooperative, competitive, and individualistic behaviors are also covered.

I. DEFINITIONS

Defining cooperative, competitive, and individualistic behaviors is necessary for understanding the antecedents of these behaviors. To date, there are at least two types of definitions in the literature regarding these social behaviors. Many researchers have begun to refer to these behavior patterns as either a preferred interaction style or as a resource distribution preference.

A. Social Behaviors as Preferred Interaction Styles

Among researchers who refer to "preferred interaction styles," cooperation is defined as a preference for working together with another person in a coordinated fashion. In contrast, a preference for working against another person is referred to as competition, and individualism is defined as a preference for working alone. Investigators who view these behaviors as preferred interaction styles often point out that these styles have different consequences across different social contexts. For example, cooperation may be the behavior pattern most preferred in a context where resources are not limited and when coordinated efforts are most useful to attain some goal. On the other hand, competition may be preferred to obtain some desired goal in a context where resources are finite. Individualism is often preferred when acquiring resources depends on consistent individual performance and when other individuals are merely social distractions.

B. Social Behaviors as Resource Distribution Preferences

A second approach to investigating cooperative, competitive, and individualistic behaviors is to view these behaviors as resource distribution preferences. This refers to allocation preferences and how they reflect underlying social values. In this approach, cooperative, competitive, and individualistic behaviors are specific forms of outcomes or consequences which are based on the individual's value system. There are at least six resource distribution preferences that are likely to occur in any given real-world context. Three of these preferred resource distributions are considered cooperative: equality, group-enhancement, and altruism. Equality is a preference for resource distributions that minimize the difference between one's own and others' resources. Group enhancement is a preference for resource distributions that maximize the resources of two or more individuals as a group. This occurs irrespective of the specific distribution of resources to oneself or to another. Altruism is a preference for resource distributions that maximize the resources of another. There are also two competitive resource distribution preferences: superiority and rivalry. Superiority is a preference for resource distributions that maximize one's relative resources compared with those of another. Rivalry is a preference for resource distributions that minimizes the resources of another. Finally, there is one individualistic resource distribution preference—individualism. Individualism is a preference for resource distributions that maximize one's own resources without regard for the impact on others.

Although a number of theorists have suggested these resource distributions as the most likely preference behaviors, the measurement of these behaviors has proven to be somewhat difficult. Part of the difficulty stems from the forced interdependency among the various resource distributions within any given circumstance. For example, there are contexts in which behaving in a manner that maximizes one's own resources simultaneously maximizes a peer's resources, creates parity in the resources for oneself and a peer, and maximizes the resources of the group. In contrast, there are also real-world contexts in which maximizing one's own resources simultaneously leads to minimizing the resources of a peer and maximizing relative resources compared with those of a peer. In some real-world contexts it is difficult to determine whether a person is distributing resources in a way that is individualistic or cooperative; in other contexts it is difficult to determine whether a person is distributing resources in an individualistic or competitive manner.

One solution to the problem of inferring the individual's preferred resource distribution pattern has been to look at the individual's resource distributions across a variety of contexts and to infer the preferred resource distribution from the overall pattern of distributions. For example, if a person chooses a resource distribution that reflects individualism, altruism, equality, and group enhancement in one situation but chooses a resource distribution that provides individualism, rivalry, and superiority in another situation, it is reasonable to infer that the person has been attempting to express an individualistic preference, that is, attempting to maximize his or her own resources across situations. Indeed, there has been considerable research of this nature, and based on this research there are more recent views regarding the actual occurrence of different preferred resource distributions. In particular, individualistic, equality, group enhancement, and superiority resource distributions are relatively common, but altruism and rivalry resource distributions occur relatively infrequently.

C. Conclusions

Most researchers have defined cooperation and competition as preferred interaction styles, and cooperative, competitive, and individualistic behaviors as social resource distribution preferences. Although many researchers have defined these behaviors in one of these two ways, there has been relatively little consideration of the relations between the two different characterizations of these behaviors. That is, there has been little attention to how these different social interaction frameworks facilitate or mitigate specific resource distributions in different situations. Further examination of the relations between these two types of conceptual frameworks is needed. Given that there have been few investigations of the relations between these two types of social behaviors and that there is a substantially larger knowledge base regarding resource distribution preferences, we will focus on the research on cooperative, competitive, and individualistic resource distribution preferences.

II. SOCIAL PSYCHOLOGICAL PERSPECTIVES AND RESEARCH

A. Measurement Issues

By far the majority of research on cooperative, competitive, and individualistic behavior has been conducted from the social psychological perspective. In this research, investigators place individuals in a social dilemma that provides some resources or payoffs for themselves and another person. Thus the situation is one of mutual interdependence.

A commonly used social dilemma is the "Prisoner's Dilemma," in which each of the two participants receives some payoff depending on their decision to cooperate or defect (see Figure 1). In the Prisoner's Dilemma, the payoffs are defined such that "T" > "R" > "P" > "S" and "R" > ("S" + "T")/2. In effect, R is the reward both individuals receive for mutual cooperation, P is the punishment both individuals receive for mutual competition, T is the temptation to defect or compete if one believes the other person will cooperate, and S is the sucker's payoff the cooperator receives if the other person competes. The "Prisoner's Dilemma" label refers to a much discussed hypothetical situation that exemplifies these contingencies. Anatol Rapaport and Albert Chammah described this anecdotal situation as follows:

> Two suspects are questioned separately by the district attorney. They are guilty of the crime of which they are suspected, but the D.A. does not have sufficient evidence to convict either. The state has, however, sufficient evidence to convict both of a lesser offense. The alternatives open to the sus-

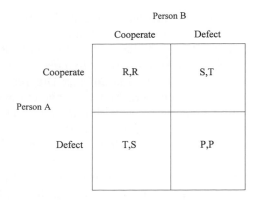

Figure 1 The payoff matrix for the Prisoner's Dilemma is defined by the inequalities "T" > "R" > "P" > "S" and "R" > ("S" + "T")/2. The left number in each cell represents the payoff for Person A and the right number in each cell represents the payoff for Person B. For an example Prisoner's Dilemma matrix substitute the following payoffs: "T" = 18, "R" = 12, "P" = 6, and "S" = 0.

pects, "A" and "B", are to confess or not to confess to the serious crime. They are separated and cannot communicate. The outcomes are as follows. If both confess [defect], both get severe sentences ["P"], which are, however, somewhat reduced because of the confession. If one confesses (turns state's evidence), the other gets the book thrown at him ["S"], and the informer goes scot free ["T"]. If neither confesses, they cannot be convicted of the serious crime, but will surely be tried and convicted for the lesser offense ["R"].

The dilemma is whether or not each individual should attempt to obtain their best outcome. Each individual's best outcome results from defecting (confessing), but only if the other does not defect. However, if both reason that defecting is the only way to obtain the best possible outcome (no jail time), then both will defect and each will receive more jail time than had they trusted each other. The situation for Prisoner A is as follows: If Prisoner B fails to implicate him or her, then he or she should implicate Prisoner B in order to get T instead of R; and if Prisoner B implicates him or her, then he or she should implicate Prisoner B in order to get P instead of S. Of course, the situation for Prisoner B is precisely the same as that of Prisoner A.

Although most social psychologists have assessed cooperative and competitive behavior with individual's choices in the Prisoner's Dilemma, a wide variety of dilemmas have been used. These dilemmas differ in the contingencies associated with cooperative and competitive decisions. For example, Charles McClintock has conducted extensive research on behavior in the Maximizing Difference Dilemma. The defining inequalities for the Maximizing Difference Dilemma is "R" > "T" > "P" = "S" and "R" > ("S" + "T")/2 (see Figure 1). In effect, the contingency structure of the Maximizing Difference Dilemma makes the cooperative alternative the mathematically logical choice for both individuals. Harold Kelley, John Thibaut, and Morton Deutsch have provided analyses of the various forms of interdependence that can be created through subtle manipulations of the contingencies (i.e., the defining inequalities) in the preceding types of social dilemmas. In addition, Robyn Dawes has described the logic associated with a variety of other social dilemmas in which the individual's resources are maximized by competing (defecting). However, if all individuals involved in these dilemmas defect, then those individuals will receive fewer resources than if they had all cooperated.

In recent years, social psychological researchers have relied on decomposed dilemmas to measure cooperative and competitive preferences. Dean Pruitt was among the first to use a decomposed dilemma when he used a decomposed form of the Prisoner's Dilemma. In a decomposed dilemma the individual is presented with a choice of two or more alternatives that completely define some resource distribution for themselves and one or more other individuals (see Figure 2). This is in contrast to the standard form of this type of social dilemma in which the distribution of resources depends on the choices of two or more individuals. Thus, in the decomposed dilemmas there is a more direct connection between the individual's

choice and the distribution of resources, thereby reducing the need for strategic behaviors aimed at influencing other participants. Although the decomposed dilemmas are structured differently from the more standard form of social dilemma, these decomposed dilemmas can be constructed such that they conceptually present the same dilemmas as the standard dilemmas. For example, the numerical resource distributions are such that two individuals making choices in the decomposed Prisoner's Dilemma jointly could receive a better outcome if both selected the cooperative distribution, jointly receive a poorer outcome if both selected the competitive distribution, individually receive the best possible outcome if one selected the competitive distribution while the other selected the cooperative distribution, or they could individually receive the worst possible outcome if one selected the cooperative alternative while the other selected the competitive alternative.

Furthermore, some researchers have assessed cooperative, competitive, and individualistic social values by having individuals rate the desirability of different resource distributions. These researchers present a resource distribution, such as one row of a decomposed dilemma, and then ask the individual to rate that resource distribution on, for example, a seven-point scale ranging from very desirable to very undesirable. The systematic analysis of these desirability ratings allows more accurate inferences of the social values underlying the individual's resource distribution preferences.

All of the measures mentioned have been used to investigate the personal and social factors that may influence the frequency of cooperative and competitive behaviors. These factors can be classified into one of three types of influences: those due to characteristics of the target individual whose cooperative, competitive, and individualistic behavior is being assessed; those due to the characteristics of the individual or individuals who will receive some resources based on the target individual's behavior, and those due to the characteristics of the situation in which the individuals find themselves.

	Self	Other
Choices:		
Cooperative	**W**	**X**
Competitive	**Y**	**Z**

Figure 2 The payoff matrix for a decomposed dilemma. This would represent a decomposed Prisoner's Dilemma if "y" > "w," "x" > "z," and "w" + "x" > "y" + "z." This decomposed dilemma would be analogous to the Prisoner's Dilemma matrix noted in Figure 1 if "w" = 6, "x" = 6, "y" = 12, and "z" = 6. (Note that "T" = "x" + "y," "R" = "w" + "x," "P" = "y" + "z," and "S" = "w" + "z.")

B. Individual and Group Differences in Social Values

Most researchers interested in individual differences in cooperative, competitive, and individualistic behaviors have focused on the characteristics of the individual and their expectations of others. Two major conclusions have been drawn from this research: (1) there are relatively stable individual differences in values that lead to relatively consistent resource distribution preferences, and (2) there are individual differences in expectations of others' behaviors.

Several lines of evidence support the notion of individual differences in social values. Wim Liebrand has shown that individuals with different social values (i.e., altruists, cooperators, individualists, and competitors) make different choices in a variety of social dilemmas. Michael Kuhlman and colleagues have demonstrated that individuals with these different social values respond to cooperative and competitive overtures in quite different ways. Cooperators cooperated unless the partner was extremely competitive, competitors were competitive regardless of the behavior of the partner, and individualists were competitive unless the partner mimicked their behavior and mutual cooperation occurred. Kuhlman et al. have also shown that cooperators expect that others will be cooperative and competitors expect that others will be competitive. These findings, in conjunction with evidence that peers can reasonably accurately predict which classmates will make cooperative, competitive, or individualistic resource distributions, clearly demonstrate individual differences in social values. Further support of these stable individual differences is evident in cross-cultural, cross-ethnic, cross-race, and cross-class research that demonstrates group differences in social values.

C. Research on the Influence of the Recipient

Of particular interest to other investigators is the influence of the characteristics of the partner on the cooperative, competitive, and individualistic behavior of the subject. This research has led to the conclusion that conditionally cooperative behavior on behalf of the partner leads to mutually cooperative interactions. That is, if the partner responds to an individual's cooperative resource distribution preference with a cooperative resource distribution preference, the individual will display more cooperative preferences toward the partner. For example, copying the previous trial behavior of a partner leads to the highest rates of mutual cooperation in the Prisoner's Dilemma.

D. Research on Situational Influences

Investigators of the influence of situational factors on cooperative, competitive, and individualistic behaviors have studied factors such as the motivational structure of the situation, the individual's involvement in the situation, the communication opportunities in the situation, the public versus private nature of behavior in the situation, and the group size. Researchers have concluded that certain motivational structures, high involvement in the situation, more communication, public behavior, and small group size lead to more cooperative and less competitive preferences.

As mentioned previously, there are real-world situations where dual motives are not uncommon. The motivational structures created by dual motivational confounds may have a substantial influence on cooperative and competitive preferences. In some real-world settings and in some social dilemmas, individualistic and cooperative outcomes may coexist or individualistic and competitive outcomes may coexist. Specifically, it is possible for individuals to maximize their own resources through cooperative responses in some situations or for individuals to maximize their own resources through competitive responses in other situations. Thus individualistic values may lead to quite different behaviors depending on the motivational structure of the situation. A number of studies have demonstrated more frequent cooperative behavior when such behavior also results in an individualistic resource distribution. In this case, however, some individuals may be engaging in cooperative behavior in order to satisfy equality or group-enhancement values, and other individuals may be engaging in cooperative behavior to satisfy an individualism value. It is often difficult to discern the underlying value associated with resource distribution preferences.

Evidence of the influence of involvement in the situation comes primarily from studies of the effect of the value of the resources available. Although there are some mixed findings, when the assessment procedure involves resources of substantial value (usually substantial amounts of money), there is often an increase in the frequency of cooperative behavior observed. Possibly the mixed findings are a function of the motivational structure of the situation. Some researchers have found that as the value of the resources to be distributed increases, then individuals who value individualism tend to modulate their behavior in accord with the situation. Those individuals tend to behave cooperatively if that is what will maximize their own resources or they may behave competitively if that is what they expect will maximize their own resources.

Other researchers have examined how communication among participants influences cooperative, competitive, and individualistic behaviors. Overall, this research has yielded relatively consistent evidence that increases in the opportunity and occurrence of communication among participants result in increases of cooperative behavior. Some researchers have provided evidence that suggests that group discussion increases cooperative preferences because it arouses group-regarding motives. That is, the communication between individuals in the situation creates motivation to want other group members to do well in the situation.

Finally, there is consistent evidence that there is likely to be more cooperative preferences and less competitive preferences when there is public disclosure of one's behavior and when the behavior occurs in a small group setting. This greater frequency of cooperative behavior may be the result of social norms and sanctions. Clearly, in these latter contexts, cooperative preferences are the socially desirable behavior.

III. DEVELOPMENTAL PSYCHOLOGY PERSPECTIVES AND RESEARCH

A substantial body of recent research has addressed the issue of the development of cooperative, competitive, and individualistic behavioral styles. Most of this research has assessed the age differences in cooperative, competitive, and individualistic preferences across the 3- to 12-year-old age range. Although there are some inconsistencies in the research findings, probably due to measurement difficulties, recent research has clarified the developmental patterns. It appears that the most accurate description of the age differences is that there is a developmental shift from individualistic to cooperative or competitive preferences across the 3- to 8-year-old age range and a shift toward increasing cooperative preferences after 8 years of age. From 3 to 8 years of age, there is a shift from individualistic to equality or superiority preferences, and after 8 years of age there are increasing equality and group-enhancement preferences. Furthermore, some

researchers have attempted to explain these developmental patterns as a function of cognitive development and learning processes.

A. Measurement Issues

Research on the development of cooperative, competitive, and individualistic social values and behaviors has often used experimental game measures, choice card measures, decomposed dilemmas, or individualized regression techniques. Experimental game measures usually put two or more children in a situation where they must complete a task in order to receive some desirable resource such as a toy. Millard Madsen's Cooperation Board is a representative example of this assessment method. The Cooperation Board consists of a flat posterboard with a circle drawn on each side and an eyelet at each corner, a ring which holds a marker in an upright position, with four strings attached to the ring and each passing through one eyelet. A child stands at each side of the board holding on to one string. By coordinating the tension on each of their strings the four children can move the marker around the board. The children are told (at least in some conditions) that they will receive a toy every time the marker passes through the circle in front of them within a limited time frame. Note that this is clearly an interaction style measure of cooperation and competition, as are nearly all of the experimental measures. Cooperation is defined as the coordinating of actions during the task. Unfortunately, inference of social values and resource distribution preferences from the behavior is difficult in this measure, as it is for most of the experimental measures, because of the inherent motivational confounds and the group nature of this measure. That is, individuals can only maximize their own resources (i.e., express an individualism value) by cooperating. In addition, the presence of only one uncooperative child results in all children in the task scoring low on cooperation because it takes all four children to coordinate the movement of the marker.

The choice card measures are similar to the decomposed dilemma measures described earlier (see the section on social psychological perspectives). They are different, however, in that they are usually designed to assess specific resource distribution preferences and may provide the child with more than two alternatives to choose from. Figure 3 shows a choice card that is

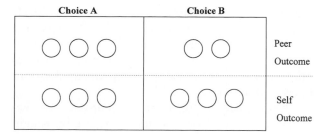

Figure 3 A choice card. The circles within each box represent valuable resources, usually money or tokens, that can be used to trade for desirable toys.

a representative example of choice card measures. In this case, a child is given a choice between two different resource distributions that represent the theoretically prescribed social values. Choice card measures, and the decomposed dilemmas described earlier, are more useful for identifying resource distribution preferences and inferring social values. However, there are other inherent difficulties even with the relatively good measures. For example, the choice on the right (choice B) in the choice card in Figure 3 offers superiority, but it also offers rivalry. The choice on the left (choice A) offers equality, group enhancement, and altruism. Furthermore, neither alternative offers more of an individualistic outcome than the other. Therefore, there are certain motivational confounds within these two resource distribution alternatives. Other choice pairs like those in Figure 3 may produce differing motivational confounds. Most importantly, individualism is sometimes confounded with the cooperative alternative in some resource distribution choices and, in the competitive alternative, in other resource distribution choices. Because of the motivational confounds within these constrained sets of alternatives, developmental researchers have moved toward inferring social values from resource distribution preferences across a variety of choice cards or decomposed dilemmas to clarify the preferred underlying social value.

A more recent approach to examining developmental issues in cooperative, competitive, and individualistic preferences involves a relatively sophisticated analytical approach. George Knight and colleagues have used an individualized regression analytic approach to disentangle the motivational confounds. Similar to the choice card procedure, individuals are presented with a number of choice cards sequentially (see Figure 3)

and asked which resource distribution on each choice card they prefer. Using a statistical technique that assigns a weight to their choices according to the number of times they chose a specific distribution over the other distributions, the researchers are able to determine the strength of each individual's references for each of the six theoretically described resource distribution preferences (i.e., equality, group-enhancement, altruism, superiority, rivalry, and individualism). Then, the researcher can use this individualized score to predict other behaviors and to examine the relations to other factors (e.g., age, gender). There is much promise in the use of this procedure to assess cooperative, competitive, and individualistic behaviors.

B. Research on the Influence of Cognitive Development

Emmy Pepitone has suggested that the age differences in these social behaviors are a function of developmental decreases in egocentrism and centration. Egocentrism refers to the tendency of young children to see the world from their own viewpoint with no awareness of the existence of other viewpoints. Centration of thought refers to the tendency of the young child to be able to attend to only one dimension of an object or situation at a time. As thought becomes less egocentric and more decentered, and as the child becomes more capable of perspective taking (i.e., understanding others' thoughts, feelings, and situations), the child becomes more capable of other-oriented, cooperative behavior. Unfortunately, there is little direct empirical evidence addressing this causal mechanism. Although several studies have examined the relation between perspective taking and cooperative/competitive behaviors, this research has generally produced inconsistent findings.

Linda Keil and Charles McClintock have suggested that age differences in cooperative, competitive, and individualistic social behaviors are a function of cognitive–numerical development. The numerical operations necessary for the expression of fairness rules such as equality and equity, as well as superiority rules, are related to the abilities to make quantitative judgments of more than, less than, and equal. Thus as the child's understanding of the mathematical concepts of more than, less than, and equal develop, the child may be more likely to engage in social behaviors such as equality and superiority. Knight and colleagues have also suggested that some of the age differences in cooperative, competitive, and individualistic preferences are a function of the development of the mathematical operations required by each preference. Other authors such as Jay Hook and Thomas Cook have also suggested a strong link between mathematical abilities and these kinds of social behaviors.

Indeed, there is evidence quite supportive of the cognitive–numerical development explanation. Hook and Cook found that from 6 to 14 years of age resource allocations went from equality to ordinal equity to proportional equity. In this study, children were allowed to distribute resources to two hypothetical children who had contributed in varying degrees to the product for which the children were to be rewarded. The youngest children generally divided the resource equally between the two hypothetical children. The middle-aged children generally divided the resources such that the child who contributed the most to the product received the most resource (ordinal equity). Finally, the older children divided the resources such that each of the two children received a number of resources proportional to their contribution to the product (proportional equity). Furthermore, these age differences occurred at the same age as the development of the logical mathematical concept of proportionality. Another series of studies demonstrated that children's numerical ability to estimate elapsed time is related to their equal sharing of a desirable object. Furthermore, when young children are provided with a means of performing a numerical operation of estimating elapsed time, these young children engage in equality distributions if the motivational properties of the situation encourage sharing.

A number of authors have suggested that the age differences in cooperative, competitive, and individualistic preferences may be a function of the development of the executive control functions that guide the use of mathematical abilities. For example, Knight et al. have suggested that the expression of individualistic preferences requires the same mathematical operations as the expression of equality or superiority preferences. That is, the identification of the individualistic resource distribution requires making the same kind of more than, less than, and equal judgments that are required in identifying the equality or superiority resource distributions. However, identification of the equality and superiority resource distributions

requires using these mathematical abilities repetitively in a systematic and functional order. Thus, young children may make individualistic decisions because of the need to appropriately sequence mathematical operations to make equality or superiority decisions taxes their abilities.

The evidence supporting this executive control explanation is based on a series of studies by Knight et al. that indicate that it takes longer, and is more difficult, to identify accurately equality and superiority resource distributions than individualism distributions, that those children who spontaneously make individualism decisions have greater difficulty identifying equality and superiority distributions than those children who spontaneously make equality or superiority decisions, and that reducing or eliminating the relatively greater executive control demands of the equality and superiority decisions reduces or eliminates the age differences in these preferences.

Further support for the role of limited cognitive processing capabilities comes from two studies conducted by Willard Hartup, Judith Brady, and Andrew Newcomb. In these studies, children completed a cooperation/competition task in either a cooperative or competitive incentive condition and with either a cooperative or competitive partner. In the first study, the frequency of cooperative behavior among young children was influenced by the partner's behavior but not by the incentive manipulation. In contrast, the behavior of the older children was influenced by both the partner's behavior and the incentive manipulation. In the second study, the frequency of cooperative behavior among young children was influenced by both the partner's behavior and the incentive manipulation when the children were instructed to use specific information processing strategies. Thus, it appears that the young children were capable of understanding and using the contextual features of the situation unless the cognitive demands of the situation exceeded their cognitive processing capabilities. [*See* COGNITIVE DEVELOPMENT.]

C. Research on the Influence of Socialization Experiences

There have also been attempts to link the age differences in cooperative, competitive, and individualistic social values and behaviors to socialization experiences. One of the most significant functions of socialization is the transmission of cultural, societal, and familial values. Socialization is a broad range of experiences that control the process through which prescriptions and prohibitions are transmitted to members of a social group. Thus, family and society create opportunities for the child to learn values and to use those values in day-to-day behaviors. Cooperative, competitive, and individualistic values are among the many societal-based values children internalize through socialization.

The socialization mechanisms that have been linked to social behaviors similar to cooperative, competitive, and individualistic behaviors can be grouped into those of direct instruction, modeling, regulation practices, and/or affective relationships. Instruction is the use of verbal prompts or commands to induce specific behaviors. Exhortations are similar verbal attempts to influence future behaviors by communicating what the child ought to do and why the child ought to behave in that manner. Modeling involves exposure to the behaviors of others and provides an opportunity for the child to acquire information about specific behaviors. Specifically, the observation of others may increase the salience of specific behavioral alternatives and social norms and provide information about the appropriateness of behavioral alternatives.

Regulation practices include a variety of processes involving the reward or reinforcement of desired behaviors, the assignment of responsibilities that foster desired behaviors, and the discipline of undesired behaviors. The reward or reinforcement of specific behavioral alternatives provides the child with guidance regarding the expected mode of behavior. The assignment of responsibilities that foster specific behaviors provides the child with specific opportunities to engage in the desired behaviors. The discipline of specific behavioral alternatives provides the child with guidance regarding which behavioral alternatives are prohibited. Relationships with a socialization agent include affective qualities such as acceptance, affection, and nurturance. A positive affective relationship with the key socialization agents is essential for emotional security, which enhances the occurrence of prosocial behaviors by lessening the child's preoccupation with their own needs.

Thus the child will likely come to value cooperative behaviors if the parents and other socialization agents instruct the child in how, when, and why the child should behave cooperatively, model cooperative behaviors before the child, reward cooperative behaviors, assign roles and responsibilities that require cooperative behaviors, discipline behaviors that are incompatible with cooperative behaviors, and have a positive affective relationship with the child. Furthermore, the specific combination of practices may be particularly important because these mechanisms function interactively or jointly in the socialization of the child. For example, in addition to the intended effects of discipline, the form that the discipline takes may affect behavior. Thus, victim-centered or psychological discipline may help put the feelings and thoughts of the other into the child's consciousness and thus help guide the child's behavior in a prosocial direction. Particularly when this discipline style suggests concrete acts of reparation, the socialization agent is not only focusing attention on the other but is also providing the child a prosocial model and instruction on how to be prosocial. In contrast, when the agent uses physical punishment, the agent is focusing the child's attention on themselves and at the same time providing an antisocial model. Thus, disciplinary practices may also influence the child through one or more of the other socialization mechanisms. Similarly, as Martin Hoffman has suggested, acceptance, affection, and nurturance may foster identification with and imitation of the socialization agent while also providing a prosocial model. If the values that are communicated by the socialization practices are culture-specific, as may be the case in cooperative, competitive, and individualistic preferences, then these values may become part of the child's ethnic or cultural identity.

The most direct support for the influence of socialization on cooperative, competitive, and individualistic behaviors comes from a recent study by Marya Cota, George Knight, and Martha Bernal. In this study with Mexican American children and their mothers, the researchers showed that mothers' ethnic knowledge and preferences and teaching about ethnic culture predicted the child's ethnic identity, and this in turn predicted the child's cooperative, competitive, and individualistic behaviors. The greater the level of ethnic identity, the greater the level of cooperation and the lower the level of competitive behaviors. Unfortunately, to date, there is little other direct evidence for the socialization model, particularly on the acquisition of cooperative, competitive, and individualistic resource distribution preferences.

There is, however, indirect evidence that attests to

the importance of socialization in the transmission of social values. The differences in cooperative, competitive, and individualistic behaviors across ethnic groups, racial groups, socioeconomic status groups, genders, and birth orders could well be the result of differential socialization experiences associated with group membership. Furthermore, there is substantial research literature describing investigations of the socialization of other prosocial and antisocial values and behaviors. However, our current view of the socialization of cooperative, competitive, and individualistic social values and behaviors must be considered speculative because of the limited empirical base.

D. Integration of Cognitive Development and Socialization

The cognitive development and socialization explanations of the age differences and individual differences in cooperative, competitive, and individualistic social values and behaviors are not necessarily incompatible. The age differences in cooperative, competitive, and individualistic social values and behaviors are consistent with the possibility that the complexity of the child's resource distribution preferences is largely determined by the child's cognitive abilities and the cognitive demands of the context, whereas the prosocial/antisocial quality of those preferences may be largely determined by the child's socialization history. That is, perhaps the young child's behavior in many contexts is individualistic because the cognitive demands of equality or superiority taxes their cognitive abilities. In contrast, the older child's behavior may be more flexible because the child's cognitive abilities may facilitate equality, superiority, or individualistic behaviors. Once the child has sufficient cognitive abilities, the child's specific behavioral preferences may be based on the social values the child has acquired through socialization. The child may encounter socialization experiences that direct him or her toward valuing cooperative behaviors, and this socialization pressure may lead to internalized cooperative values once the child has the necessary cognitive abilities. Perhaps perspective taking, decentered thought, and increases in reasoning about moral situations are among the requisite skills for acquiring these values. Moreover, once these cooperative values are acquired, they may be selectively applied to vari-

ous contexts depending on the cognitive demands of the context. At this point, cognitive–numerical or executive control skills may become necessary skills for enacting these internalized values.

Although this model emphasizes largely different roles for cognitive development and socialization, this is not to imply that these are independent processes. Indeed, as described, cognitive development likely impacts socialization. Furthermore, it is likely that socialization impacts on cognitive development. For example, parents who consistently use combinations of socialization practices designed to enhance the child's understanding will most likely have children who acquire social values at an early age. Parents who consistently reward equal sharing of resources and at the same time verbally describe the appropriateness of equally sharing will have children who understand and adopt a sharing value at an earlier age than parents who use only reward contingencies. In the former case, the verbal information may help the child to abstract the appropriate rule correctly rather than require the child to make inferences about the reasons for rewards and punishments.

Although socialization probably affects cognitive development, it is not likely that the socialization of specific cooperative or competitive values is the mechanism by which the requisite cognitive abilities are acquired. That is, although we assume that socialization does influence cognitive development, and vice versa, we do not believe that exposure to pressure to value cooperative or competitive behaviors in and of itself causes the child to acquire the specific cognitive skills we have discussed. The more likely case is that the development of those types of cognitive skills is the result of interaction with the environment in the broadest sense. There is a vast array of socialization experiences that create momentum for cognitive development to proceed. The socialization pressure to value either cooperative or competitive behaviors is but a small part of this vast array of pressures, and the presence or absence of any small set of specific socialization pressures is likely to be inconsequential for cognitive development to proceed.

The integration of cognitive developmental and socialization explanations hold much promise for further understanding cooperative, competitive, and individualistic behaviors, as well as other forms of prosocial and antisocial behaviors. However, studies to examine these ideas are needed. In a recent unpublished study, Scott Roesch and colleagues found that age differences in cooperative, competitive, and individualistic behaviors were moderated by the nationality, the cognitive demands of the situation, and the gender of the child. Thus there was some evidence that cognitive development and culturally related factors interact to predict this set of behaviors. These findings suggest that examination of integrative models such as the one described here may be a fruitful endeavor for future investigators.

IV. GENERAL CONCLUSIONS AND FUTURE DIRECTIONS

As can be surmised from the review, much has been done to further our understanding of the origins and correlates of cooperative, competitive, and individualistic behaviors. Social psychologists and developmentalists have provided the underlying theoretical basis that has spurred a number of investigators into examining these behaviors. There have been some dramatic advances in clarifying definitional and measurement issues for future researchers. Thus far, the brunt of the research on cooperative, competitive, and individualistic behaviors has focused on individual and group differences, the influence of cognitive development, the social context, the recipient, and on socialization experiences.

Although cooperative, competitive, and individualistic behaviors may be relevant to mental health issues, comparatively little research has been devoted to examining the links between these factors. From a socialization perspective, the development of cooperative, competitive, and individualistic behaviors enhances the successful adaptation of the individual to its social environment. Some social environments may reinforce specific resource distributions and punish other specific resource distributions. An individual deficient in applying the appropriate resource distribution in the appropriate social context may be subject to rejection, scorn, or ridicule from others and may be perceived as socially unskilled. In turn, these social reactions may have long-term mental health consequences for the individual. For example, striving for cooperative resource distributions in a business environment in which competition is necessary for success

may lead to punishment (e.g., demotion, pay cut, layoff) and, over time, lead to negative mental health outcomes (e.g., depression, anxiety). Unfortunately, as mentioned previously, there is a lack of research that examines these links.

A second need for future research is to investigate the role of emotions and affect on cooperative, competitive, and individualistic behaviors. There is a rapidly developing literature that shows the importance of sympathy and other affective responses to other prosocial behaviors and to social cognitions (e.g., perspective-taking and prosocial moral reasoning). Ultimately, the understanding of the development of cooperative, competitive, and individualistic values and behaviors may require research efforts that address the role of affect in these types of social behaviors.

Finally, there is reason for concern over the relatively exclusive reliance on cross-sectional methods and on select nonrepresentative samples. Differences between age groups could result from development or from any nonequivalence in the representation of the two samples. Thus it is necessary to verify the nature of the developmental findings with longitudinal methods and with a variety of samples in which the developmental changes in cooperative, competitive, and individualistic social values and behaviors are observed within individuals as they develop.

BIBLIOGRAPHY

Dawes, R. M. (1980). Social dilemmas. *Annual Review of Psychology, 31,* 169–193.

Derlega, V. J., & Grzelak, J. (Eds.). (1982). *Cooperation and helping behavior: Theories and research.* New York: Academic Press.

Kagan, S. (1977). Social motives and behaviors of Mexican American and Anglo American children. In J. L. Martinez (Ed.), *Chicano psychology* (pp. 45–86). New York: Academic Press.

Keil, L. J., & McClintock, C. G. (1983). A developmental perspective on distributive justice. In D. M. Messick & K. S. Cook (Eds.), *Equity theory: Psychological and sociological perspectives* (pp. 13–46). New York: Praeger.

Knight, G. P., Bernal, M. B., & Carlo, G. (1995). Socialization and the development of cooperative, competitive, and individualistic behaviors among Mexican American children. In E. E. Garcia & B. M. McLaughlin (Eds.), *Yearbook in early childhood education: Vol. 6. Meeting the challenge of linguistic and cultural diversity in early childhood* (pp. 85–102). New York: Teachers College Press.

Knight, G. P., & Chao, C.-C. (1991). Cooperative, competitive, and individualistic social values among 8- to 12-year-old siblings, friends, and acquaintances. *Personality and Social Psychology Bulletin, 17,* 201–211.

Knight, G. P., Dubro, A. F., & Chao, C.-C. (1985). Information processing and the development of cooperative, competitive, and individualistic social values. *Developmental Psychology, 21,* 37–45.

Rapoport, A., & Chammah, A. M. (1965). *Prisoner's dilemma.* Ann Arbor: The University of Michigan Press.

Staub, E. (1978). *Positive social behavior and morality: Social and personal influences* (Vol. 1). New York: Academic Press.

Wilke, H. A., Messick, D. M., & Rutte, C. (Eds.). (1986). *Experimental social dilemmas.* New York: Verlag.

Coping with Stress

Anita DeLongis and Sarah Newth

University of British Columbia

Coping   Cognitive and behavioral efforts to manage stress.
Emotion-Focused Coping   Coping responses that are geared toward managing one's emotions during stressful episodes.
Problem-Focused Coping   Coping responses that are geared toward directly changing some aspect of the stressful situation.
Relationship-Focused Coping   Coping responses that are geared toward managing and maintaining one's social relationships during stressful episodes.
Stress   Situations that the person cognitively appraises as taxing or exceeding his or her resources.

COPING refers to a person's cognitive and behavioral responses to a stressful situation. This article reviews literature on coping with stressful experiences. It discusses the antecedents and consequences of various strategies for coping with stress, including the role of coping in health and well-being. It describes three functions of coping: problem-focused, emotion-focused, and relationship-focused.

I. CONCEPT OF COPING

In common parlance, "coping" is often used to suggest that individuals are handling stress well or that they have the situation under control. However, most health psychologists who study stress and coping would define coping broadly to include all thoughts and behaviors that occur in response to a stressful experience, whether the person is handling the situation well or poorly. Coping includes what we do and think in response to a stressor, even if we are unaware of why or what we are doing. This broad definition is important for two reasons. First, if we limit the definition of coping to thoughts and behaviors that the individual purposefully and intentionally engages in as a way of handling the stressful situation, we may exclude a wide array of responses that typically remain outside of awareness. These can include, for example, believing in unrealistically positive illusions, escaping through the use of alcohol and other drugs, or fleeing from stress in one area of life (e.g., family) by immersing oneself in some unrelated activity (e.g., work). Second, this definition of coping does not assume a priori that some forms of coping are bad and others are good. *All* of the person's responses to the stressor are considered coping, whether or not they help to resolve the situation. This is important, as in recent years researchers have found that many forms of coping that have traditionally been considered bad coping, such as escape-avoidance, may actually have beneficial effects when coping with certain types of stressors under specific circumstances.

A. Why Is Coping Important for Mental Health?

Many disorders of mental health are either directly caused by stress or their expression is triggered by stress. In cases where a person is already experiencing poor health, stress can exacerbate and maintain the problems. However, there are wide individual differences in the effects of stress, and these are thought to be largely due to individual differences in coping with stress. Therefore, many health psychologists have turned their attention in recent years to trying to understand the antecedents and consequences of various ways of coping with stress.

B. Historical Overview

In early models, certain forms of coping (and people who used them) were viewed as immature, dysfunctional, or maladaptive. Many emotion-focused strategies were not even considered forms of coping, but merely defenses. These models lost favor as evidence accumulated that many forms of coping previously assumed to be maladaptive could sometimes have positive effects, at least in certain circumstances. Researchers such as Lazarus conceptualized coping as a process in constant flux, responsive to changes in situational demands. The focus on situational factors as primary determinants of coping responses was welcomed as a correction of previous tendencies to treat coping in trait terms. Claims made by Mischel in 1968 that personality traits are poor predictors of behavior were also influential. Furthermore, the findings of a number of studies suggest that in general, situational factors play a larger role in determining responses to stress than do personality traits. Thus, earlier notions of rigid "styles" of coping have been replaced by an understanding that coping is best conceived in process terms. Given this new understanding of coping that emerged during the 1970s and 1980s, the role of personality in coping was given scant attention during those years. Recently, it has been acknowledged that although personality may not be the single most important determinant of coping responses to stress, its role is nonetheless quite important. In the past few years, health psychologists have again turned their attention to examining personality factors that might determine how people cope with stress. Currently, most researchers in the field would agree that how a person copes with stress will shift over time depending on an array of factors that can be broken down into two broad categories: person and situation. [*See* PERSONALITY.]

II. DETERMINANTS OF COPING RESPONSES

A. Personality Characteristics as Determinants of Coping

Clinicians and researchers alike have examined the role of personality in coping in an attempt to predict and explain which individuals are at risk for experiencing psychological maladjustment. The underlying assumption is that personality can influence how one copes with stress, and coping determines whether stress will have deleterious effects on health and well-being. A consistent set of personality traits have emerged as significant predictors of the ways in which people cope and the impact coping has on their health. The following is a brief summary of the various personality traits that have been empirically related to coping.

The last 50 years have seen a growing interest in the role of personality as measured by the big five personality traits of neuroticism, extraversion, openness to experience, agreeableness, and conscientiousness. These five factors are believed by many personality researchers to be the five basic underlying dimensions of personality. Researchers have tended to find that neuroticism (the tendency to experience negative affect) is related to maladaptive coping efforts and poor psychological well-being. In comparison, researchers have tended to find that extraversion (the tendency to be gregarious and to experience positive affect) is related to adaptive coping and better psychological well-being. Individuals high on openness (the tendency to be creative and open to feelings and experiences) remain strong in the face of adversity and are more able to engage in coping that is sensitive to the needs of others. Given that two defining features of openness to experience are originality and creativity, future research may show individuals high on openness to be particularly effective and flexible copers. Those individuals high on agreeableness (the tendency to be good-natured) also appear to cope in an adaptive manner that is sensitive to the needs of others. Individuals high on agreeableness tend to engage in less negative interpersonal coping strategies (e.g., confronting others), more positive interpersonal coping (e.g., seeking social support), and lower levels of maladaptive emotion-focused coping (e.g., escape avoidance). Individuals high on agreeableness may seek to avoid additional conflict and distress when coping. Finally, those individuals high on conscientiousness (the tendency to be careful and reliable) have been found to engage in lower levels of maladaptive emotion-focused coping (e.g., escape avoidance) and higher use of problem-focused coping. Individuals high in conscientiousness may seek to engage in the most responsible and constructive forms of coping.

The way in which one anticipates future events has also been established to have an impact on well-being. The tendency to anticipate positive outcomes for the future is referred to as optimism. Carver, Scheier, and others have reported this trait to be associated with both adaptive coping and good mental health. High levels of optimism may lead to higher levels of constructive coping, which in turn reduce distress, making positive expectations highly adaptive. In contrast, pessimistic individuals (those who do not generally anticipate positive future outcomes) tend to use more maladaptive coping strategies, which in turn are related to higher levels of both anxiety and depression. [See ANXIETY; DEPRESSION; OPTIMISM, MOTIVATION, AND MENTAL HEALTH.]

An internal locus of control (i.e., feeling a sense of personal control) over the events and experiences in one's life is often positively related to psychological well-being, whereas an external sense of control (i.e., lacking a sense of personal control and feeling that control over events is external to oneself) is often negatively related to mental health criteria. Research examining locus of control as a stable personality trait has identified several ways in which this trait influences both coping and psychological adjustment. For example, studies have found that an internal locus of control is related to greater use of problem-focused coping. It appears that a belief in one's ability to impact or change events is related to constructive attempts to alter or change aspects of the environment or oneself under times of duress. Given that such problem-focused coping efforts are generally associated with better psychological outcomes, at least when used with stressors that are controllable, an internal locus of control can have beneficial effects upon mental health.

B. Situational Specificity in Coping

Currently, there is much interest among researchers in studying the factors within a given situation that de-

termine how an individual will cope, how the chosen coping strategies influence mental health, and how this process varies from situation to situation. In 1984, Lazarus and Folkman identified a number of dimensions of stressful situations that are important determinants of the stress and coping process. Novelty (has the individual coped with this type of stressor in the past?), predictability (are there signs that will alert an individual to the onset of the stressful event/situation?), event uncertainty (how likely is it that the situation will occur?), imminence (is the event likely to occur in the near future?), duration (how long will the experience last?), and temporal uncertainty (is it possible to identify whether the event will occur?) all impact affective, cognitive, and behavioral reactions to stress. That is, these situational factors play a role in determining the extent to which a person experiences a situation as stressful, and in turn, how he or she copes with the stressful situation.

Several researchers have conducted studies that explore a variety of situational determinants of coping. Consistent with the hypothesis that situational factors do influence the coping process, researchers have tended to find that different situations elicit different forms of coping, and similar situations elicit similar modes of coping. In addition, similar coping strategies have been found to have different effects across different situations, in that the effectiveness of any one coping strategy and its impact on well-being varies from situation to situation. This points to the importance of a match between a chosen coping strategy and the situationally specific demands of a stressor to maximize emotional adjustment and minimize ongoing struggles. Thus, the particular characteristics of a stressful situation determine both coping choice and coping effectiveness. For example, positive reappraisal is generally an effective coping strategy related to psychological well-being. However, in 1991, Wethington and Kessler noted that when the stressful situation calls for some form of action to be taken, the use of positive reappraisal alone is related to psychological maladjustment. Likewise, in 1994, Aldwin pointed out that emotion-focused coping is more effective when coping with a situation that is perceived as involving loss, whereas problem-focused coping is more effective when coping with a situation that is appraised as a threat or challenge. Therefore, one must be cautious in making generalizations about the relation of specific coping strategies to mental health, as this relation will vary according to the situational demands.

Empirical evidence supports the hypothesis that individuals will vary their coping efforts and choices systematically to fit a given stressor. General coping styles aggregated over time tend to be poorly correlated with the ways in which one copes in a specific situation. That is, researchers or clinicians cannot accurately predict how an individual will cope with any one specific stressor by relying on the average way in which the same individual copes across a variety of situations over time. To illustrate, an individual may engage in moderately high levels of a particular coping strategy over time but not use this particular strategy at all when coping with a certain type of stressor. Averaging coping responses across multiple situations, therefore, obscures important information about how coping is related to well-being under specific and well-defined circumstances.

Researchers such as Wethington and Kessler have identified several ways in which coping varies from situation to situation. First, the ways in which individuals cope with an acute but short-term stressor often differs from the ways in which they cope with an ongoing chronic stressor. Second, the ways in which individuals cope can also be influenced by the coping responses of others around them. Third, individuals tend to use different strategies depending on the role domain in which stress occurs. Fourth, situations are defined by a multitude of demands and therefore any one stressor may demand multiple coping strategies in order to be resolved effectively. Those with the highest psychological well-being may well be those individuals who can successfully engage in a variety of coping strategies. Rigid adherence to a small set of coping strategies geared toward direct resolution of the stressor, at the expense of those that might help to reduce stress-related negative emotions, could be maladaptive in many circumstances.

Researchers have begun to examine the ways in which situational factors interact with person factors in determining how people cope with stress. Existing evidence suggests that coping varies as a function of both the situation and the person. For example, in 1986, Parkes found that individuals low in neuroticism varied their use of direct action according to the level of work demands. In comparison, those individuals high in neuroticism did not vary their use of direct action in response to changing levels of work demands. Furthermore, although situational factors play a larger role overall in determining coping responses, the more ambiguous a stressful situation is, the greater the influence of person factors on the coping process.

III. WAYS OF COPING

Historically, coping has been seen as serving two basic functions: problem-focused (active attempts to alter and resolve the stressful situation) and emotion-focused (efforts to regulate one's emotions). Recently, a third function that concerns relationship-focused coping (efforts to manage and maintain social relationships during stressful periods) has been studied as well.

A. Problem-Focused Coping

Problem-focused coping includes those forms of coping that are geared directly toward solving the problem or changing the stressful situation. Most of the research examining problem-focused coping has been on planful problem-solving. Coping strategies based on planful problem-solving involve conscious attempts to determine and execute the most appropriate course of action needed to directly prevent, eliminate, or significantly improve a stressful situation. Making a plan of action and following it is an example of the sort of cool deliberate strategy that typifies this form of coping. Although the primary effect of problem-focused modes of coping is to change or eliminate the stressful environment, it is not unusual for such coping to result inadvertently in a reduction in negative affect and/or an increase in positive affect (e.g., devising and carrying out a plan to finish a task that one has felt pressured to complete). The increase in positive affect following the use of planful problem-solving may be the result of an improvement both in the way one perceives the stressful situation and in the direct changes in the stressful situation itself. In general, planful problem-solving tends to be associated with less negative emotion, more positive emotion, positive reappraisals of the stressful situation, and satisfactory outcomes.

Important moderators of this strategy and its influence on psychological well-being have been documented. First, it appears that individuals engage in a higher use of planful problem-solving when they perceive a situation or encounter as one in which something can be changed for the better. Furthermore, the use of this strategy in uncontrollable or unchangeable situations seems to have a negative impact on psychological health. It appears that pursuing a futile course of action can interfere with the adaptive function of accepting those things that cannot be changed or altered. Second, when a loved one has something to lose in a stressful situation, individuals tend to use lower amounts of planful problem-solving than when a loved one does not have something to lose. Individuals seem to experience difficulty formulating a plan of action when coping with the added emotional distress invoked by concern for a loved one's well-being. Third, when the stress occurs at work, individuals tend to use higher levels of planful problem-solving. In this context, many forms of emotion-focused coping strategies may be viewed as ineffective and socially inappropriate.

In summary, in situations that require a course of action to minimize or reduce stress, the individual may be better off engaging in planful problem-solving efforts rather than in emotion-focused strategies such as denial. Such efforts will more likely improve the interactions between an individual and their environment, and have a positive impact on well-being.

B. Emotion-Focused Coping

Emotion-focused modes of coping include those forms of coping that are geared toward managing one's emotions during stressful periods. A larger number of studies have examined emotion-focused modes of coping than either problem- or relationship-focused modes of coping. All of the many forms of emotion-focused coping that have been described in the literature cannot possibly be discussed here. Instead, we focus on those forms that have received the most attention in the scholarly literature.

I. Emotional Expression

Emotional expression is the active expression of one's thoughts and feelings about an experience or event, and is a common way to cope with stress. The expression can take place through a variety of interpersonal, verbal, and artistic means, including talking or corresponding with someone, keeping a diary, and drawing or painting.

Pennebaker reviews the historical relation of emotional expression to mental health, as reflected in Maslow's notion of self-expression and Freud's concept of emotional catharsis. However, modern researchers studying this phenomenon have construed emotional expression as more than simply the venting of emotions. Pennebaker and his colleagues suggest that it is the active expression of both thoughts and feelings surrounding experiences that makes emotional expression a beneficial form of coping with stress. Pennebaker suggests that this expression can aid in deriving a sense of meaning, insight, and resolution by initiating a process in which facts, feelings, thoughts, and options can be organized effectively.

Pennebaker and colleagues have found across several studies that emotional expression is positively related to both psychological and physical well-being. These studies used a variety of modes of emotional expression, such as writing essays about one's experiences, talking out loud into a tape recorder, or talking to another individual. In comparison, active inhibition (i.e., the deliberate and conscious nonexpression of one's thoughts and feelings) has been found to be negatively related to psychological well-being. In addition, emotional expression that is inappropriately disclosing (e.g., telling a nonreceptive stranger), overly self-absorbed (i.e., disengaging and isolating the listener), overly intellectualized (i.e., lacking acknowledgment and expression of one's feelings), or done in the presence of an unsupportive and critical person, is less likely to have beneficial effects.

There are individual differences in people's ability and desire to engage in emotional expression. For example, some people tend to engage in high levels of emotional expression, whereas others do not. This area of research suggests that the degree of emotional expression may reflect a general personality trait. Gender differences in emotional expression have also been found as women tend to report higher levels of emotional expression than men.

There are a variety of contexts in which individuals coping with stress may engage in emotional expression. As Pennebaker points out, support groups, self-help programs (e.g., Alcoholics Anonymous), telephone crisis lines, psychotherapy, pastoral counseling, and even internet discussions all provide a context in which emotional expression is supported, if not actively encouraged. Evidence suggests that emotional expression has a disease-preventative effect.

2. Seeking Social Support

Another common way of coping with stress is to seek some form of social support. The social support sought may be informational support (e.g., an individual recently diagnosed with HIV contacting a support group to find out more about the virus), tangible support (e.g., a grieving widow asking a friend to help baby-sit her children for an afternoon), or emotional support (e.g., a recently laid-off worker accepting sympathy and understanding from a friend). In general, higher levels of social support are associated with better psychological and physical well-being. However, the quality of available social support is more important to well-being than the absolute amount of available social support. To illustrate, an individual who has a few constructively supportive friends and family members may receive better social support and experience greater health benefits than an individual who has many friends and family members but who do not provide constructive social support. In this context, constructive social support consists of support provision that meets the needs of the individual seeking such support.

In 1988, Fisher and colleagues differentiated between solicited versus unsolicited social support. There are times when members of one's social support network provide unsolicited social support. Unsolicited support tends to occur when the stressor is highly visible and there exist social norms as to how members of the social network should behave (e.g., a death in the family, loss of a child, dissolution of a marriage). However, individuals often have to cope with stressors that are not readily apparent to those around them. During such times, an individual must actively seek social support in order to receive it. Furthermore, a variety of factors seem to play a role in the extent to which individuals will seek social support as part of their coping with such stressors. For example, if individuals blame themselves for the occurrence of a stigmatizing stressor (e.g., contracting HIV after having unprotected sex), they may be less likely to seek social support because of the potential for embarrassment, stigmatization, judgment, and further blame. Given that nondisclosure of stressful experiences has been associated with threats to psychological well-being, not seeking social support may result in an increase risk for disorders of health and well-being.

Individuals may also resist seeking social support when the support available has the potential to add stress to an already stressful situation. Social support would be feared when the support provider delivers social support in an excessive or inappropriate manner. To illustrate, an individual suffering from a chronic, debilitating illness such as rheumatoid arthritis (RA) may avoid seeking social support if doing so threatens their independence (e.g., a support provider insists on doing everything for the individual with RA rather than simply facilitating the sufferer's own coping efforts).

In addition, individual differences have been found in both the extent to which individuals will seek social support and the degree to which they perceive seeking social support to be an effective coping strategy. For example, Thoits, in 1991, found that women engage in higher levels of support seeking than men and perceive seeking social support as a more effective coping strategy than do men. Personality differences also influence the extent to which seeking social support is an effective coping strategy. Recent research has indicated that certain personality traits may explain some of the individual differences in the seeking and receiving of social support. To illustrate, individuals high in neuroticism may tend to elicit negative reactions from others when they seek social support, whereas individuals low in neuroticism may tend to elicit positive reactions. Therefore, different individuals may seek social support to varying degrees and invoke different reactions from others depending on their particular personality and interpersonal style. This suggests that the very individuals most likely to experience threats to their psychological well-being (e.g., those high in neuroticism) and therefore most in need of social support may be those individuals least likely to seek and receive social support in a way that is beneficial to their mental health. [See SOCIAL SUPPORT.]

3. Escape-Avoidance

There are times when individuals fail to cope actively with a stressful situation and instead engage in efforts to avoid confronting the stressor. Attempts at escape and avoidance can take a variety of cognitive or behavioral forms, such as wishful thinking, distancing, denial, or engaging in distracting activities. For example, an individual may attempt to repress thoughts of a recently deceased spouse as a cognitive means of escape-avoidance. Likewise, one could immerse oneself in cleaning the house as a way of avoiding a stressful task such as paying bills. As Aldwin noted, certain ways of coping can serve as avoidant coping strategies on one occasion despite serving as approach coping strategies on another. As an example, Aldwin suggests that cognitive reappraisal may function as a constructive approach strategy when used to view a stressful situation more positively and when acting as a catalyst for further action. Conversely, cognitive reappraisal may serve as an avoidant coping strategy when used to rationalize a lack of action or justify engaging in actions that lead to further avoidance (e.g., drinking to make oneself feel better).

Avoidant coping strategies are often a response to the negative affect that results from a stressful situation. For example, some individuals may initially deny that a stressful situation has occurred in an effort to minimize their distress (e.g., not accepting the possibility that a lump in one's breast may be cancer). Researchers such as Lazarus have suggested that in the early stages of a stressor, such avoidant type strategies may be adaptive in that minimizing distress levels allows one time to adapt and to gather one's resources. By decreasing levels of distress, short-term escape-avoidance may increase one's ability to engage in active problem-focused coping. Similarly, the use of escape-avoidance may minimize negative affect while one is waiting for a potentially short-term stressor to pass (e.g., reading a magazine to relieve anxiety while waiting to hear the results of an important medical test).

Despite the positive short-term effectiveness of escape-avoidance in reducing psychological distress, the long-term use of escape-avoidance is generally associated with lowered psychological well-being. For example, although distraction is useful when coping with short-term stressors (e.g., medical and dental procedures), long-term use of distraction with an ongoing stressor (e.g., coping with unemployment) is associated with maladjustment. The negative association between the use of escape-avoidance strategies and well-being may result from the lack of constructive action that the continued use of escape-avoidance can entail. That is, when avoiding thoughts or behaviors that are directed at a stressor, one also tends to avoid engaging in constructive efforts that could potentially reduce both the source and degree of one's distress. In extreme situations, the use of prolonged escape-avoidance can backfire by amplifying a stressful situation and creating added emotional distress (e.g., avoiding obtaining medical attention until it is too late to receive basic treatment).

4. Positive Illusion

Historically, it has been assumed that reality-based perceptions are essential to the maintenance of mental health and psychological well-being. However, in 1988, Taylor and Brown suggested that "positive illusions" (i.e., unrealistically positive perceptions) are related to several common criteria of mental health, such as feelings of contentment and the ability to care for others. They argue that a positive misconstrual of experiences over time is beneficial to the psychological adjustment of the individual engaging in such perceptions. Research suggests that more positive views of the self are associated with lower levels of distress, and Taylor and Brown have argued that a relatively unbiased and balanced perception of the self tends to be related to higher levels of distress. Given that distress tends to be related to less constructive forms of coping, a positive view of the self may have beneficial effects through an increase in constructive coping efforts, even if the positive self-view is illusory. For example, individuals fighting life-threatening illnesses such as diabetes may perceive themselves to be higher in personal strength than others, which in turn may lead to more persistent and effective attempts to cope with their disease.

In a similar vein, Taylor reviews research that establishes a positive relation between illusory perceptions of control and mental health. For example, depressed individuals have been found to have perceptions of control closer to reality than nondepressed individuals. Research assessing control has also demonstrated that when coping with a stressful experience, those individuals who feel a greater sense of control will tend to experience better psychological well-being, even when the sense of control is overestimated. For example, a patient dying of AIDS may experience better psychological well-being by choosing to use alternative medicine, thus obtaining some sense of personal control over the treatment of a disease that remains incurable.

Various mechanisms may explain the relation between positive illusions and mental health when individuals are faced with coping with stress in their lives.

For example, Taylor hypothesizes that positive illusions are related to positive mood, which in turn is related to social bonding, which in turn is related to higher levels of well-being. Given the adaptive role that constructive social support plays in the coping process, the potential ability of positive illusions to increase social bonding could be highly beneficial. Taylor also suggests that illusions may enhance creative functioning, motivation, persistence, and performance. Higher levels of all of these factors may lead to more effective coping and better well-being (e.g., higher levels of motivation and creativity could increase one's ability to develop an unusual but highly effective coping strategy).

Recently it has been suggested that conclusions regarding the relation between positive illusions and mental health are an artifact of methodological problems inherent to this area of study. Specifically, Colvin, Block, and Funder, in 1991, argued that previous research has not used valid criteria for establishing objective reality. Without such criteria, it is difficult to verify which individuals are truly engaging in positive illusions. Therefore, conclusions regarding the relation between positive illusions and psychological adjustment may have been premature. These researchers found empirical evidence suggesting that positive illusions can have negative influences on both short-term and long-term mental health. [*See* POSITIVE ILLUSIONS.]

5. Social Comparison

In 1954, Festinger suggested that individuals are driven to compare themselves to others as a means of obtaining information about oneself and the world during times of threat or ambiguity (i.e., stress). Although the patterns of findings are diverse and sometimes complex, most research in this field suggests that social comparison processes have important implications for psychological well-being. In fact, several researchers have proposed that social comparisons play a central role in the way in which people cope with stressful experiences. For example, social comparisons can help individuals evaluate their resources and provide information relevant to managing emotional reactions to stress. However, the underlying motivation and purpose that each individual has for engaging in this type of coping and the resultant psychological outcomes can be diverse.

In 1989, Wood described three classes of motivational factors that drive a person to engage in social comparisons: self-evaluation, self-improvement, and self-enhancement. All three purposes can be relevant to coping with stress and may aid the individual in striving toward an adaptive outcome. Self-evaluation motivations to engage in social comparison stem from an individual's desire to obtain information regarding his or her standing on a particular skill or attribute. Self-improvement motivations to engage in social comparison suggest that individuals are interested in deriving information regarding another's standing on a particular skill or attribute in order to improve their own standing on the same dimension. Self-enhancement motivations to engage in social comparison stem from a need to see oneself in a more positive manner; that is, the results of the social comparison are used to make one feel better about one's own standing on a particular skill or attribute relative to others.

When an individual seeks a social comparison target as a means of coping with an ambiguous or threatening situation, several options are available. One can select an individual who has a higher or more positive standing than oneself on the dimension in question (i.e., an "upward social comparison"). Alternatively, one can select an individual who has a lower or more negative standing than oneself on the relevant dimension (i.e., a "downward social comparison"). Presumably, comparisons against others who differ from oneself produce distinctive and discriminating information that has immediate and practical implications for the individual when engaging in coping efforts.

In general, research suggests that when people engage in downward comparisons, they feel more positive and less negative about themselves than when they engage in upward comparisons. Individuals engaging in downward social comparisons because of self-enhancement motivations tend to experience reduced levels of negative affect and feel better about themselves in both field and experimental studies. For example, in their 1985 study of women coping with breast cancer, Wood and her colleagues found that downward comparisons appeared to help women feel better about how they were dealing with their illness by yielding positive evaluations relative to women who were not coping as effectively. However, research has also demonstrated that when individuals are motivated by self-improvement or self-evaluation needs, there is a clear preference for upward comparison information. Under these circumstances, comparisons may help determine what kinds of interventions or efforts are both possible and necessary to cope more effectively with a particular stressor.

Collins proposed in 1996 that the outcomes of social comparisons are not predetermined by the direction in which one makes a comparison. Instead, evidence supports the notion that both upward and downward comparisons can have both positive and negative impacts on psychological well-being. First, upward comparisons can generate negative psychological outcomes through a contrast effect (i.e., one feels inferior to the comparison target). Second, upward comparisons may also yield positive effects through the inspiration and hope they generate. These types of comparisons may be especially helpful for problem-solving activities, as they can provide constructive information that suggests specific coping strategies. Third, downward comparisons can lead to positive outcomes presumably because they allow one to focus on ways in which one is doing well relative to others. Such comparisons may be especially helpful in regulating negative emotions. Finally, downward comparisons can lead to negative outcomes from the fear that one will "sink" to the lower level of the comparison target at some future point in time. Such comparisons may have special significance for individuals coping with illness, where it is feasible that their disease will progress negatively. Given that both downward and upward comparisons contain both positive and negative information relevant to the self, the particular aspect the individual focuses on while coping will determine the valence of the outcome.

A growing number of moderating variables are being identified as important factors in determining the impact social comparison will have as a coping strategy during times of stress, threat, or ambiguity. For example, it appears that individuals with high self-esteem have a greater tendency to derive positive outcomes from either upward or downward social comparisons than individuals with low self-esteem. Other researchers have also noted the important role played by perceived control. Individuals with high degrees of perceived control over the dimension in question may be less likely to experience negative reactions to social comparisons in contrast to those with low levels of control. Individual differences in familiarity with a stressor may also moderate the process of social comparison. For example, an individual who has just discovered they have HIV (unfamiliar dimension) may

select different comparison targets for coping than an individual who has been living with the illness for some time (familiar dimension). Presumably, the type of information one needs in order to adapt to threats will vary according to how long one has been dealing with the threat. In addition to individual differences, it appears that the situational context in which the social comparison process takes place is an important determinant of the impact of the comparison itself. For example, different contexts vary in terms of the potential social comparison targets they provide.

At times, individuals will actively self-select when to engage in social comparison and with whom they wish to compare themselves. However, as Collins noted, social comparisons can sometimes be forced on the individual. For example, researchers have found that someone who needs health care services for a serious condition may have no choice but to sit in a waiting room with other individuals who also have the same condition, making social comparisons unavoidable. Such comparisons most likely make it difficult for an individual to avoid the possibility that his or her own illness and condition could get worse. In addition, researchers have suggested that the impact of forced comparisons can be particularly aversive when the comparison target is someone with whom the individual is interdependent (e.g., close friend, co-worker). This suggests that individuals may sometimes have to cope with the stressful nature of the social comparison itself.

Regardless of whether or not one chooses to engage in social comparison, once the social comparison process is underway (i.e., target is compared against), there are some active strategies that individuals can use to maximize the probability of obtaining a positive outcome. First, peripheral dimensions can be used to moderate comparison outcomes. If a comparison produces an unfavorable outcome (e.g., an upward comparison that leaves one feeling inferior), one can always attribute the lower standing to differences between oneself and the target on other related variables (e.g., sex, ethnicity, duration of stressor). Alternatively, as previously discussed, individuals can actively distort information to maintain a more positive perception of reality.

In summary, social comparison processes provide valuable information that individuals can use for a variety of purposes when coping with stress, threat, or ambiguity. The target selected, the situation or context in which the comparison is made, and the unique traits of both the individual and the comparison target have an impact on the outcome of the comparison process. As a result, social comparison may have a positive impact on well-being for particular individuals in certain situations, and a negative impact on well-being for other individuals in different situations. Research has demonstrated the relevance of social comparison to coping with a variety of stressors such as illness and marital problems.

C. Relationship-Focused Coping

Relationship-focused coping refers to the various attempts made by the individual to manage, regulate, or preserve relationships when coping with stress. Recently, there has been growing interest in the interpersonal dimensions of coping as distinct from the intrapersonal dimensions of emotion- and problem-focused coping.

1. Empathic Responding

Empathic coping is one such form of relationship-focused coping. The use of empathy has been related to positive social behaviors such as providing social support and caring for others. Recently, O'Brien and DeLongis have suggested that empathic coping includes the following elements: (a) attempts to see the situation from another's point of view, (b) efforts to experience personally the emotions felt by the other person, (c) attempts to read between the lines in order to decipher the meaning underlying the other person's verbal and nonverbal behavior to reach a better understanding of the other person's experience, (d) attempts to respond in a way that conveys sensitivity and understanding, and (e) efforts to validate and accept the person and their experience while avoiding passing judgment. One may engage in empathic coping either verbally (e.g., telling a spouse that you understand what they are feeling) or nonverbally (e.g., tenderly holding someone's hand as they talk).

Empathic coping can play a significant role in coping with stress, particularly stress caused by interpersonal problems. Research suggests that empathic coping is related to a decrease in distress caused by interpersonal tension and an increase in relationship satisfaction. The increased understanding gained from

empathic coping may result in more appropriate and well-considered coping choices that will maximize the benefits for all involved. Empathic coping may also lead to further benefits for psychological adjustment because of its impact on concurrent or subsequent use of problem- and emotion-focused coping. For example, in 1993, Kramer found that caregivers who engaged in empathic coping strategies were more likely to engage in planful problem-solving than caregivers who did not engage in empathic coping. The greater use of these strategies was related to greater caregiver satisfaction with the caregiving role. In the same study, lower use of empathic coping was related to more maladaptive emotion-focused coping efforts, which were in turn related to depression.

Individuals vary in how often and how effectively they use empathic coping. For example, O'Brien and DeLongis have found that when a close other is involved in a stressful situation, those high in neuroticism are less able to use empathic coping than are those low in neuroticism.

2. Active Engagement and Protective Buffering

In addition to empathic coping, other forms of relationship-focused coping are also receiving attention. In 1991, Coyne and Smith identified active engagement (e.g., discussing the situation with involved others) and protective buffering (e.g., attempting to hide worries and concerns from involved others) as two forms of relationship-focused coping. They found that higher degrees of protective, relationship-focused coping (e.g., not conveying fears to one's spouse) among wives of myocardial infarction patients was related to higher degrees of distress among the wives. Note that this is consistent with research suggesting that suppression of emotional expression is related to lowered psychological well-being. However, wives' use of protective buffering was positively related to self-efficacy among their husbands. It appears that the wives were coping with the stress of their spouse's illness in a way that maximized the benefits for their sick husbands (i.e., interpersonally adaptive) yet threatened their own well-being (i.e., intrapersonally maladaptive). Such results point to the need to include interpersonal dimensions of coping in addition to the traditional intrapsychic dimensions of coping in order to understand the relation of coping and health outcomes.

IV. FINAL COMMENTS

In conclusion, there is no one "good" way to cope with stress. Stress takes on many forms, and likewise, so must coping. The most adaptive way to cope with any given stressor depends on both the personality of the stressed individual and the characteristics of the stressful situation. Dimensions of the stressful situation that must be considered in determining the best way to cope with a given stressor include (a) whether others are involved in the situation, how they are coping, and the relationship of these people to the stressed individual; (b) the timing of the stressor and the degree to which it is anticipated or controllable; (c) the types of specific demands inherent to the stressful situation, the duration of such demands, and one's prior experience with similar stressors; and (d) what is at stake in the stressful situation. Perhaps the key to good coping is flexibility. That is, the ability to vary one's coping depending on the demands of the situation. What is clear is that no one form of coping will be effective in dealing with all stressors. There are times when attempts at problem-focused coping will be a waste of time and energy that could be better spent engaged in emotion- and relationship-focused coping. At other times, when something can be done directly to prevent or alter the stressful demands, energy may be better spent doing something concrete to solve the problem rather than concentrating on emotion management. Perhaps it is the wisdom to know the difference, and then to act on that knowledge, that is essential to successful coping. [*See* STRESS.]

BIBLIOGRAPHY

Aldwin, C. (1994). *Stress, coping, and development: An integrative perspective.* New York: Guilford Press.

Collins, R. (1996). For better or for worse: The impact of upward social comparison on self-evaluations. *Psychological Bulletin, 119,* 51–69.

Eckenrode, J. (Ed.). (1991). *The social context of coping.* New York: Plenum Press.

Gottlieb, B. (Ed.). (1997). *Coping with chronic stress.* New York: Plenum Press.

Lazarus, R. S., & Folkman, S. (1984). *Stress, appraisal, and coping.* New York: Springer.

Goldberger, L., & Breznitz, S. (Eds.). (1993). *Handbook of stress: Theoretical and clinical aspects.* New York: Free Press.

O'Brien, T. B., & DeLongis, A. (1996). The interactional context of problem-, emotion-, and relationship-focused coping: The role of the Big Five personality factors. *Journal of Personality, 64,* 775–813.

Pennebaker, J. W. (1990). *Opening up: The healing power of confiding in others.* New York: William Morrow.

Taylor, S. E. (1989). *Positive illusions: Creative self-deception and the healthy mind.* New York: Basic Books.

Zeidner, M., & Endler, N. S. (Eds.). (1996). *Handbook of coping: Theory, research, applications.* New York: John Wiley & Sons.

Couples Therapy

Kieran T. Sullivan

Santa Clara University

Andrew Christensen

University of California, Los Angeles

Differentiation   The degree to which a person (or a couple) is able to differentiate between his or her *emotional system* (i.e., instinctual reactions) and his or her *intellectual system* (i.e., the ability to use reason and to communicate complex ideas).

Emotional Joining around the Problem   Focusing partners on the pain each is experiencing rather than on the blame each deserves.

Negative Attributions   Distressed partners' tendencies to attribute each other's negative behavior to unchangeable characteristic of the partner rather than to temporary, external circumstances.

Problem–Solution Loop   Attempted solutions that partners use to control or alleviate the problem that actually make the problem persist.

Projective Identification   One partner projects onto the other his or her repressed objects or aspects of the self.

Securing the Frame   The therapist outlines the parameters for therapy, including setting the fee and scheduling the sessions, which creates a safe and stable environment for partners.

Selective Inattention   Distressed partners' tendencies to remember negative relationship events with great clarity, but to have little recall of positive events.

This article presents five major approaches to **COUPLES THERAPY** and discusses their relative effectiveness in treating relationship distress. Each of these approaches is based on a theory of the development of relationship distress and uses specific therapeutic techniques to help alleviate this distress. In addition, two recent integrative approaches are presented that combine elements of the previous approaches in an attempt to increase the effectiveness of the intervention. Interventions for couples with psychiatric disorders and alternative interventions, such as group couples therapy and prevention, are also discussed.

I. INTRODUCTION

Joe and Diane have both been feeling very unhappy lately with their marriage. Diane feels that Joe spends too much time at work and has been neglecting his responsibilities at home, particularly child care with their daughter. She is lonely and angry at him. Joe thinks that Diane is too demanding and feels overwhelmed when he comes home to her criticism and nagging. They seem to be fighting more and more, and their sex life has diminished considerably. Unable to work these problems out on their own, they seek the help of a couples therapist.

When faced with a distressed couple like Diane and Joe, there are many different ways to conceptualize and treat their problems. Some therapists might focus on the couple's negative interactions, for example, when Diane becomes very angry at Joe and Joe withdraws from Diane. Others might emphasize the problems in the family system, exploring Diane's relatively stronger alliance with their daughter compared with Joe. Still others might explore Diane's and Joe's relationships with their own families of origin and try to discover how those relationships have affected their marriage.

Over the last two decades, many models have emerged to explain and treat relationship distress. This article begins with a history of the development of couple's therapy and then presents five empirically validated therapeutic approaches to treating couples in distress, using the preceding example to illustrate each type of intervention. It is important to note that these approaches may not correspond with approaches typically practiced in the community. They are theoretically based models of couples therapy, most of which have been subject to controlled clinical trials in order to evaluate their effectiveness. The results of these outcome trials are presented after the description of each approach.

In an attempt to provide optimal treatment for couples, couples researchers have begun to develop interventions that integrate effective aspects of different theories into one general approach. Two of these integrative models are briefly described after the five core models. The term *marital therapy* is avoided in favor of *couples therapy* (except in historical contexts) to reflect the recent shift away from a marriage bias to include all types of couples who seek treatment.

II. HISTORY OF COUPLES THERAPY

The identification of couples and families as a system for which psychological intervention is appropriate and even advantageous is a relatively recent phenomenon. In this section, we highlight important movements, historical developments, and influential contributors to the development of couples therapy from the post-World War I era to the present.

In the period after World War I, professionals from various disciplines began to promote human sexuality as a legitimate area of scientific study and to call for public education regarding sexual and reproductive issues. Spearheaded by Hirschfeld in Germany, Ellis in Great Britain, and Kautsky in Austria, public centers were founded throughout Europe to promote

awareness and knowledge of these issues. In these centers, advice was given on contraception, eugenics, and psychological and relational issues. Concurrent with the rise of Nazi Germany, however, the focus of the centers became increasing eugenic. As noted by Kopp in 1938, "In the United States of America marriage counselling to date has in the main been concerned with the solution of the problems related to the psychology and physiology of sex, reproduction, family and social relationships. In Europe, on the other hand, the main objectives are the betterment of the biological stock" (p. 154).

Although the idealistic vision of sexual reformers was impeded in Europe, the development of couples and family therapy continued in the United States. Social workers emphasized the need to expand interventions to include the family. Educators implemented home economics courses in high schools nationwide. Workshops addressing family and marital issues were offered through churches and universities. Finally, new psychoanalytic theories (such as object relations theory) opened the door for psychological interventions beyond just one individual.

Emerging from such varied fields, the marriage counseling movement was both eclectic and pragmatic. Early couples counseling was mainly conducted as a secondary profession by college professors, physicians, and gynecologists. In the early 1930s, the first institutes were opened whose primary function was to provide couples therapy. These institutes included the American Institute of Family Relations in Los Angeles, an ecumenical marriage center in New York and the Marriage Council of Philadelphia.

The American Association of Marriage Counselors (AAMC) was established in 1945 for establishing standards, exchanging information, and helping in the development of interest in marriage counseling. Of the professionals who initially formed the AAMC, "no less than fifty percent came primarily from the medical specialties, while the rest represented such fields as social work, psychology, and sociology" (p. 433). During the 1950s and early 1960s, centers for marriage counseling were opened across the country, marriage counseling textbooks were produced for a general professional audience, standards were proposed for marriage counselors, and training centers were accredited. Despite this progress, however, the new profession of marital counseling had yet to establish a clear sense of professional identity. Marriage counseling continued to be a secondary profession for most practitioners, leaving the status of marriage counseling as a profession marginal.

In the late 1960s and early 1970s, the profession matured. Perhaps the most important development during this period was the establishment of a common journal, the *Journal of Marital and Family Counseling* (now the *Journal of Marriage and Family Therapy*). It was also during this period that varying approaches to conjoint therapy were developed and proposed by marital therapists and researchers. In 1970, the AAMC changed its name to the American Association for Marriage and Family Counselors (AAMFC) to reflect the convergence of marriage and family counseling during this period.

In the last two decades, many marital and family therapists have worked for the recognition of their profession as autonomous and distinct. In 1992, regulations in the Federal Register officially declared marriage and family therapy to be the fifth core mental health profession (along with psychiatry, psychology, social work, and psychiatric nursing). By 1993, 31 states had implemented licensing procedures for marital and family therapists. The struggle for an autonomous profession is not without controversy, however. Proponents of marital and family therapy remaining within an established profession (e.g., psychology, psychiatry, etc.) have specific advantages, such as ease in obtaining funding and reimbursement for research and clinical work. Today, marital and family therapy "is partially established as a major profession, but its status in the broader society remains frustratingly marginal" (Shields et al., 1994). [*See* FAMILY THERAPY.]

III. THEORETICAL APPROACHES IN CONDUCTING COUPLES THERAPY

A. Behavioral Couples Therapy

1. Theory of Distress

Behavioral couples therapy (BCT) emphasizes the behaviors that partners exchange and the antecedents and consequences of those behaviors. Although behaviorists acknowledge the role of affect and cognition in the development and maintenance of distress, they target the external determinants of behavior as the point of intervention for distressed couples. Ther-

apists help couples to define their problems in behaviorally specific terms and to gain control over them by manipulating the conditions that precede the problematic behavior and those that are consequent to it. By teaching couples various communication and problem-solving skills, therapists help couples minimize distressing exchanges and maximize rewarding exchanges. [*See* BEHAVIOR THERAPY.]

2. Development of Dissatisfactions

According to behavior theory, people select mates based on the actual and anticipated reinforcers received in the relationship (e.g., sexual pleasure, emotional intimacy, wealth, etc.). Couples who are initially satisfied with these reinforcers may become less satisfied over time because reinforcements become habitual and routine or because greater contact and/or life changes may expose important incompatibilities that were not apparent to the couple during the courtship phase of their relationship. When faced with important incompatibilities, partners may cease previously rewarding behaviors and engage in coercive techniques in an effort to get their own way. When one partner gives in to such aversive techniques, his or her partner is reinforced for using these techniques and will therefore be more likely to use them in the future. For example, Diane may nag Joe to complete his share of the housework. When Joe finally gives in to her nagging, her nagging is reinforced. The partner who gives in is also reinforced by the removal of the aversive stimulus. Thus, Joe is more likely to give in to the nagging in the future, because it is reinforcing for him to have the nagging stop. As partners become habituated to these aversive stimuli, the coercing partner must use them in greater amounts. Also, the coerced partner may engage in coercion to achieve his or her own goals. Thus, an initially satisfied couple may develop negative interaction patterns that cause them both distress, but which they are unable to stop.

3. Intervention

The emphasis in BCT is on behavioral change, specifically, behaviors that contribute to a partner's satisfaction and distress. The techniques most frequently used to promote these changes are behavior exchange and communication/problem-solving strategies. In behavior exchange, the therapist helps the couple to identify behaviors that are reinforcing and through various strategies directs them to increase these reinforcing behaviors. This exchange of behaviors provides some immediate relief of distress and paves the way for more difficult negotiations which require communication and problem-solving strategies. The therapist then teaches the couples noncoercive ways of discussing and resolving conflicts and practices these skills with the couple using conflicts that the couple is currently experiencing. The final goal is for the couple to learn to apply these skills on their own whenever a new conflict arises.

4. Specific Therapeutic Techniques

In behavior exchange, therapists guide partners in the selection of reinforcing behaviors, direct them to increase the frequency of these behaviors, and debrief their experiences with these change efforts. Ideally, couples select behaviors that are maximally reinforcing to the receiver and of minimal cost to the giver. Typically, low-cost behaviors are behaviors that are not a current source of conflict, do not require the learning of new skills, and are positive. Therapists may directly assign partners to increase the overall frequencies of the selected behaviors or direct each partner to increase the target behavior within a certain time frame, as in "love days" or "caring days." Finally, therapists debrief these behavior change experiences. In these sessions, receivers are encouraged to acknowledge and positively reinforce the increase in positive behavior by the giver.

In communication/problem solving training, couples are taught to approach problem solving in two distinct steps, problem definition and problem solution. The distinction between these two steps is made to avoid premature problem solving. During the problem definition phase, partners are encouraged to begin by acknowledging some positive part of the problem. They are then encouraged to state their problems in specific behavioral terms, to express their feelings, to acknowledge their own role in the problem, and to devise a brief summary statement of the problem. For Joe and Diane, one problem might be that Joe frequently comes home late from work and is criticized for his lateness when he comes home. Diane would be encouraged to acknowledge that her criticism may be part of the reason why Joe comes home late and to discuss how she feels when he is late. Joe would be encouraged to acknowledge his lateness and to discuss his feelings in response to Diane's criticism. During

the problem–solution phase, the couple begins by brainstorming all possible solutions, without further elaborating on the problem. Then, the couple evaluates these solutions based on a cost–benefit analysis. Finally, a specific agreement is reached, which is often set in writing. Throughout the discussion, couples are instructed to address only one problem at a time, to focus on their own views without presupposing what their partner's views are, and to paraphrase what their partner just said to ensure listening and to avoid interruptions.

5. Efficacy of Treatment Approach

More controlled, clinical trials have been conducted on BCT than on any other modality. The results have been mixed. Although about two thirds of couples who receive BCT show an increase in satisfaction at the end of therapy, long-term follow-up data suggest that about 30% of couples who were successfully treated relapse after 2 years. Thus about one half of couples treated with BCT experience lasting improvement in their relationships.

B. Cognitive Behavioral Couples Therapy

Cognitive behavioral couples therapy (CBCT) emerged in response to a number of studies that revealed the importance of cognitions in the development and maintenance of couples' distress. It uses the same basic structure and therapeutic strategies as BCT, but it also includes assessment of and intervention in partners' maladaptive cognitions. The following description focuses solely on the cognitive components of CBCT, as the behavioral components have been described previously.

1. Theory of Distress

Researchers have identified five areas of cognition that are related to distress. *Selective inattention* refers to distressed partners' tendencies to remember negative relationship events with great clarity, but to have little recall of positive events. *Negative attributions* occur when distressed partners attribute each other's negative behavior to unchangeable characteristic of the partner rather than to temporary, external circumstances. Partners may also have unrealistic *expectancies* about the future and *assumptions* about how relationships operate that contribute to their distress.

Finally, partners' *standards* about what a relationship should be like often interfere with their ability to be satisfied with their current relationship.

2. Development of Distress

The conceptualization of the development of distress in CBCT is similar to the conceptualization used in BCT. One difference is that maladaptive cognitions are seen as contributing to the behaviors that lead to distress as well as to the distress itself.

3. Intervention

The structure of the sessions in CBCT is flexible to allow for varying focus on behavior, cognition, and emotion. Therapists address maladaptive cognitions when they emerge as the main problem or when they are clearly interfering with behavioral skills training. The therapist's role is active and directive. When assessing or evaluating cognitions, the focus is on the content of the cognitions rather than on the process that is occurring between the partners. This is done to get a clear understanding of problematic cognitions. Couples are taught about cognitions and how they can influence behavior and emotions. Over the course of therapy, couples learn how to become more aware of cognitions, how to evaluate them, and how to challenge them when necessary.

4. Specific Therapeutic Techniques

One technique that CBCT therapists frequently use to help partners become more aware of selective inattention, unrealistic expectancies, assumptions, and standards, and maladaptive attributions is the use of daily logs. Couples write down their automatic thoughts as they occur and this material is used for later evaluation. For example, when Joe does not come home in time to say good night to their daughter, Diane might think "He doesn't love her," or "He is a very selfish person." During actual sessions, therapists use open-ended questions, coaching, and direct questions to uncover relationship standards and beliefs that are difficult to access. To modify cognitions, partners learn to challenge their own cognitions as they make them, evaluating whether their inferences make sense logically. They are also trained to identify alternative, relationship-enhancing attributions. Diane would be encouraged to rethink her automatic attribution that Joe is late because he does not love her daughter and

instead attribute Joe's lateness to his temporary and stressful project at work. Finally, therapists teach couples about specific types of distortions (e.g., personalization, overgeneralization) so that they can be aware of them when they occur. Therapists also help to uncover deeply held relationship standards and assumptions and to evaluate the advantages and disadvantages of maintaining these standards.

5. Efficacy of Treatment Approach

A series of clinically controlled outcome studies have consistently shown that CBCT is equally effective in treating marital distress when compared to other treatment strategies, including BCT. In addition, CBCT has been shown to affect partners' actual cognitions. Baucom, Epstein, and Rankin (1995) have identified several reasons why CBCT has not been shown to be more effective than BCT alone. First, couples were randomly assigned to either BCT or CBCT. Because the need for cognition restructuring varies in couples, matching couples to treatment is necessary to determine whether CBCT will be more effective in helping those couples with distorted and maladaptive cognitions. Second, the interventions (skills training and cognitive restructuring) were separated in time rather than integrated. This is inconsistent with a naturalistic intervention, which would use cognitive restructuring when needed by the couple, not when dictated by the protocol. Finally, the cognitive restructuring phase was often very brief (about 3 weeks), which is probably insufficient. For these reasons, it remains unclear whether adding cognitive components to BCT increases the effectiveness of BCT.

C. Systemic Couples Therapy: Bowen Family Systems Therapy

Several distinct approaches for couples therapy have been developed based on systems theory. One of the most prominent and widely practiced is Bowen Family Systems Therapy (BFST). This section begins with a general overview of systems theory followed by a more in-depth description of BFST. The systems approach emphasizes the organization of the family as a whole and the patterns of interaction that the family engages in. The family, or in this case the couple, is seen as made up of elements that are organized by the consistent nature of the relationship between them.

Systems theory states that all systems work to maintain balance and stabilization. Each part of the system plays an important role in maintaining that balance. For families and couples, mechanisms can be identified whose primary purpose is the maintenance of an acceptable behavioral balance within the family. Families tend to establish a behavioral balance and to resist any change from that predetermined level of stability. [*See* FAMILY SYSTEMS.]

1. Theory of Distress

In BFST, a key concept in understanding couples distress is *differentiation,* which refers both to individuals and to couples. Differentiation is the degree to which a person (or a couple) is able to differentiate between his or her emotional system (i.e., instinctual reactions) and his or her intellectual system (i.e., the ability to use reason and to communicate complex ideas). Persons or couples who are unable to make this differentiation consistently respond to their environment using the emotional system, which makes them vulnerable to distress. In contrast, persons and couples who are able to regulate their behavior using their intellectual system are less likely to develop symptoms of couples' distress. Symptoms of distress appear when a couple encounters anxiety; these symptoms include emotional distancing, conflict, development of dysfunction in one partner, and, in the case of families, projection of the problem onto a child.

2. Development of Dissatisfaction

The BFST approach relies on an intergenerational theory that suggests that degrees of differentiation do not change much from generation to generation. This is based on two assumptions. The first is that parental differentiation affects how well children are able to separate emotionally from their parents. Adult children of undifferentiated parents will experience unresolved emotional attachment to parents that will prevent them from becoming differentiated themselves. Second, people pick marital partners who have similar levels of differentiation. When undifferentiated partners marry, they tend to be overly dependent on one another and are very vulnerable to the development of distress when anxiety is encountered. Differentiated adults, in contrast, tend to have a strong sense of self within their own marriages, and their functioning is

less dependent on the behavior of their partner. They are able to tolerate the anxiety that is generated when inevitable differences appear.

3. Intervention

The overall goal of BFST is not to relieve the immediate symptoms, but to increase the level of differentiation of the members and of the unit. Symptom relief without increased differentiation leaves the couple vulnerable to developing new symptoms when additional anxiety is encountered. In BFST, the therapist functions as a coach who creates a climate in which each individual can reach their highest potential level of differentiation and in which the relationship can assist the individuals to develop further than they might have alone. The couple or family system is viewed as the patient, and the therapist attempts to interact with the system to enhance its own natural restorative processes. This is accomplished by focusing not on the content presented during therapy, but on the emotional processes of the couple over time. In particular, the therapist wants to prevent the couple from engaging in an *emotional chain reaction* of instinctive, emotionally laden reactions to one another. To accomplish this, it is critical for the clinician to understand and control his or her own emotional reactivity to provide a safe environment in which the couple can discuss emotionally charged issues. The therapist must remain emotionally neutral, unembroiled in the family system, and maintain his or her own differentiation.

4. Specific Therapeutic Techniques

The BFST therapist begins with a thorough history of the immediate and extended family to formulate a picture of the family emotional system. The survey should give the therapist a working knowledge of the current symptoms as well as the mechanisms that the couple uses to manage anxiety and to keep the relationship stable. Bowen (1978) identified four main functions of the clinician. First, the clinician defines and clarifies the emotional processes between partners. Because partners are preferentially sensitive to one another, each behavior is perceived, interpreted, and reacted to by the other. These reactions are often based in the emotional system in distressed couples, guided more by feeling than by thinking, with each reaction generating its own counterreaction. The therapist's goal is to get couples to become more aware of and to think about this process (i.e., use their intellectual system) rather than simply to enact it. Thus, when Joe feels nagged by Diane to do housework, he becomes aware that he is having this feeling and is more able to discuss this with Diane, rather than to react by withdrawing and neglecting the housework. Second, it is critical for the clinician to remain detriangulated from the emotional process. "Conflict between two people will resolve automatically if both remain in emotional contact with a third person who can relate actively to both without taking sides with either." (Bowen 1978, p. 224). Third, the therapist teaches the couple about the emotional system. Fourth, the therapist models differentiation of self for the couple. To do so, the therapist must be aware of his or her own viewpoint and values, and how he or she typically responds to a variety of situations. The usual format is for the therapist to talk with one person while the other listens, using low-key questions aimed at clarifying the emotional reactivity of the person and the chain reaction between partners. Overall, the questions are used to elicit thinking and to tone down emotional responses.

5. Efficacy of Treatment Approach

To date, there are no controlled outcome studies examining the efficacy of the Bowenian approach with couples or with families. There have been studies examining other family systems approaches; a review of the few *controlled* outcome studies found that family therapy, compared with no treatment and alternative treatments, did have positive effects. Because the studies varied in the type of family therapy and in the type of alternative therapy, it remains unclear how effective a systems approach is in treating couples' distress.

D. Psychoanalytic Couples Therapy

1. Theory of Distress

Psychoanalytic theories of marriage emphasize the interplay of unconscious wishes, fears, and fantasies between spouses. According to object relations theory, all adult individuals have "lost" parts of themselves which were "split off" and repressed into the unconscious during infancy. This happened as a result of the inevitable gap between the infant feeling a need and the satisfaction of that need. This gap leads to feelings of frustration in the infant and to the perception of

the mother (the object) as rejecting. Because the infant is unable to tolerate the ambiguity of a giving mother who is sometimes rejecting, it splits off the image of the rejecting mother from the image of the ideal mother and represses it into the unconscious (as the rejecting object), along with the part of the self that related to the rejecting mother. When individuals choose a mate, they do so at both a conscious and an unconscious level. Unconsciously, they are attracted to mates whose unconscious objects and selves are complementary to their own. Ideally, this complementarity helps partners to regain lost parts of themselves in relation to their partner. When the unconscious interplay between partners causes partners to repress further rather than reintegrate lost parts of the selves, distress can occur.

2. Development of Dissatisfaction

Partners' unconscious communication takes place through a process called *projective identification*. In projective identification, one partner (e.g., the wife) projects onto her husband her repressed objects or aspects of the self. Ideally, her husband is able to identify temporarily with and embody these projections. Through this process, the projection is modified and "detoxified" for the wife, who can then consciously assimilate this new view of herself. As a result, she is better able to distinguish herself from her husband and to love him for who he is and not for what she projects onto him. This process takes place simultaneously for both partners. Thus, through the complementarity of unconscious objects, partners facilitate growth and reintegration in one another. When partners' projective identification is not mutually gratifying and objects are more firmly repressed rather than modified, distress occurs.

3. Intervention

The main focus in intervention is the unconscious projections that each person is making and the partners' responses to these projections. The overall goal of therapy is to increase partners' abilities to contain, modify, and reintegrate aspects of the self that they project onto one another. Through this reintegration, the partners become more able to give and receive genuine love. This is accomplished through careful observation of partners' defenses and anxieties and through creating an environment in which these anxieties can be worked through. Psychoanalytic couples therapy is ideally a long-term, in-depth enterprise, which typically requires a period of 1 to 2 years.

4. Specific Therapeutic Techniques

The techniques used in psychoanalytic couples therapy are more attitudinal than behavioral. The therapist typically engages in careful, undirected listening and, later, in interpretations. The therapist begins with a period of assessment that allows the couple to understand the nature of the undertaking so that they may freely choose to enter into psychoanalytic couples therapy. In this assessment process, called *securing the frame*, the therapist outlines the parameters for therapy, including setting the fee and scheduling the sessions, which creates a safe and stable environment for the partners. It is also the first opportunity for partners to attempt to gratify unconscious wishes by encroaching on the frame, which provides insight into the unconscious difficulties affecting the marriage. For example, Joe might object to the therapist's policy that he must attend therapy every week and that he must pay the therapist her usual fee if he misses an appointment. He may feel infantalized and "nagged" to attend therapy regularly. This feeling gives the therapist some insight into Joe's unconscious processes and the current difficulties in the marriage. As mentioned previously, the therapist attempts to listen primarily to the unconscious and to make use of countertransference (the therapist's feelings regarding the couple) for clues into the unconscious. The therapist maintains a neutral position and uses his or her own self as a "holding place" where the couple can recognize and modify their own dysfunctional unconscious patterns. The therapist is able to create this holding place based on the intimate knowledge of his or her own unconscious attained through rigorous training, supervision, and personal psychotherapy. As the therapist begins to understand the unconscious dynamics between the partners, he or she begins to offer interpretations to help the couple gain insight into their process of projective identification. Termination is initiated once the couple is able to "internalize" the therapist and create their own holding space within which to work through anxieties and defenses. Ideally, the couple will also have recognized, modified, and taken back much of their projective identifications, although usually this process must continue even after therapy has ended.

5. Efficacy of Treatment Approach

In the first controlled outcome study comparing a variant of psychoanalytic couples therapy (Insight-Oriented Marital Therapy, IOMT) with BCT, Snyder and colleagues found IOMT and BCT equally effective at termination and at a 6-month follow-up. Four years after treatment, however, a significantly larger percentage of couples had divorced when treated with BCT (38%) than when treated with IOMT (3%). These findings have been disputed, with critics questioning whether therapists using the BCT intervention used state-of-the-art behavioral interventions. Nevertheless, Snyder et al. have provided at least preliminary evidence that psychoanalytic couples therapy may have more long-term effectiveness than behavioral approaches. [*See* PSYCHOANALYSIS.]

E. Brief Problem-Focused Couples Therapy

Short-term, problem-focused couples therapy was developed in response to the difficulties that arise in treating two individuals who may have different agendas and intentions for entering into therapy as well as for the current difficulties in receiving reimbursement for couples treatment from insurance companies. Two major models of brief couples therapy have been developed and evaluated in the last three decades. Brief problem-focused therapy was developed at the Mental Research Institute (MRI) in the late 1960s and early 1970s. The model was further developed at the Brief Family Therapy Center in Milwaukee, Wisconsin (the Milwaukee model), as brief solution-focused therapy beginning in the late 1970s.

1. Theory of Distress

Brief couples therapy was developed to be as efficient and parsimonious as possible. The goal of brief couples therapy is to address and provide relief for the presenting complaint. Therapists do not probe for underlying emotional or unconscious issues, they do not seek to promote personal growth in their clients, nor do they spend time teaching communication or problem-solving skills. Consistent with these goals, brief couples therapy offers no developed theory regarding couples distress or its development. Instead, it takes couples' complaints at face value and works for the relief of those complaints through lessening the behaviors related to the presenting problem (the MRI model) or through finding alternative solutions for the presenting problem (the Milwaukee model).

2. Development of Distress

Although brief couples therapy offers no theory about the development of distress, it does focus on the perception of distress. A couple has a problem when they perceive a problem, and the problem is alleviated when the couple perceives such alleviation. Brief couples therapy makes no attempt to objectively define dysfunction or normality in marriage. Furthermore, brief couples therapy does not seek to understand the origin of the particular presenting problem, but rather to identify and alter the behaviors of both partners that serve to maintain the current problem.

3. Intervention

In brief problem-focused couples therapy, the clinician works with the couple to identify the presenting problem and the interactional patterns that are perpetuating the problem. Usually, the attempted solutions that partners use to control or alleviate the problem are the very behaviors that make the problem persist (this phenomena is called the problem–solution loop). For example, Diane's solution to Joe's lateness is to nag him to come home on time. However, it is her nagging that causes him to dread coming home and to want to work longer. Likewise, it is his hiding at work that motivates Diane to nag him. Once problem-maintaining behaviors are identified, the therapist encourages the couple to lessen those behaviors. For Diane and Joe, this would mean less nagging from Diane and less lateness from Joe. Because the continuance of the problem is contingent on the problem-maintaining attempted solutions, once these are eliminated the problem itself should be alleviated. In brief solution-focused therapy, the emphasis in intervention is on identifying exceptions to the problem and encouraging the couple to increase those behaviors that are effective solutions to the problem. Here, the therapist would ask Diane and Joe to remember times when Joe did come home from work early and they shared a pleasant evening together. This approach is more cognitive than the MRI approach, assuming that behaviors will change once the couple perceives the problem differently. Clinicians attempt to reframe the problem as not so overwhelming and the solution as something the couple already has in their behavioral repertoire. The clinician's main goal

is to increase the couple's sense of mastery over the presenting complaint.

4. Specific Therapeutic Techniques

Therapy in the MRI approach begins with a thorough behavioral understanding of the presenting complaint and the related behaviors that contribute to its perseverance. Through this formulation, the therapist identifies specific problem-maintaining behaviors that should be lessened in specific situations. The therapist then communicates this to the client using three important principles. First, the change is prescribed in a way that is consistent with the client's own goals and views of the relationship. Second, the therapist works with the customer by targeting the person most concerned about the problem. In fact, therapists will often work individually with a concerned person whose partner is resistant to therapy. Theoretically, intervention with even one partner's maladaptive solutions should have an impact on the problem–solution loop. Third, the therapist maintains maneuverability by avoiding premature commitments to therapeutic strategies. Overall, the therapist consistently reminds couples that change takes time and encourages them to make small changes at a slow rate. In contrast, therapists using the Milwaukee approach bypass examination of the problem relatively quickly and instead ask questions designed to influence the client's view of the problem in a manner that leads to solutions. An example is miracle questions. Clients are asked what their relationship would look like if a miracle occurred and the problem disappeared overnight. The therapist also asks about times in the past when the problem has not occurred or when they have dealt with it successfully. The therapist may also probe the degree of distress and commitment to change (scaling questions), how well the couple is managing given their difficulties (coping questions), and what changes have they already made before therapy began (questions about presession change). These questions are designed to challenge feelings of hopelessness by highlighting the small, positive changes that couples have managed on their own. Therapists also use tasks to help couples recognize possible solutions that they are already using. For example, couples are asked at the end of their first session to observe things about their relationship that they would like to have *continue*. Throughout therapy, the therapist provides ample praise for positive changes and continually inquires about and highlights use of constructive solutions whenever they occur.

5. Efficacy of Treatment Approach

Both centers have conducted follow-ups on many of their cases to find out whether a complaint has been resolved. The MRI team has called clients 3 and 12 months posttreatment and evaluates "success" based on whether the treatment goal was attained, whether the complaint has been resolved, other areas of improvement in the relationship, and the emergence of new problems. For the first 97 cases, 40% were deemed successful, 32% significantly improved, and 28% failures. Two recent studies by Shoham and colleagues reported outcome rates of 44%, 24%, and 32%, respectively, and a success rate of 86% at an 18-month follow-up, with an average of 4.6 sessions. However, there are several reasons to interpret these numbers with caution. These include the lack of detail in describing follow-up procedures, which prevents analysis of reliability or validity of the results, and the fact that the same clinical team was used to conduct therapy and to conduct follow-up interviews. To date, no controlled clinical outcome trials have been conducted on either approach.

IV. INTEGRATIVE APPROACHES TO COUPLES THERAPY

A. Integrative Behavior Couples Therapy

Integrative Behavior Couples Therapy (IBCT) was developed by Andrew Christensen and Neil Jacobson to increase the power and effectiveness of Behavior Couples Therapy. It is strongly rooted in behavior theory and uses many of the same treatment strategies as BCT. It does not, however, focus on promoting behavioral change exclusively, but gives equal emphasis to *acceptance* of partners' behavior the way it is. This shift in focus has both theoretical and practical implications for therapy. First, IBCT targets major controlling variables for change, rather than derivative variables. In BCT, because of the exclusive emphasis on discrete, currently observable behavior, functional analysis often focuses on variables only indirectly related to partners' dissatisfaction, for example, Diane's complaint that Joe comes home late from work. The IBCT therapist would attempt to uncover the underlying controlling variable, that is, the wife's desire for more closeness with her husband. The IBCT therapist

looks for affect (especially "softer" feelings such as sadness or fear) and themes in couples' interactions to help uncover the crucial variables for the couple.

Once the crucial variables are identified, IBCT therapists work simultaneously for change and emotional acceptance. Emotional acceptance is a shift in the way a partner reacts to the problematic behavior. Behaviors that were once seen as intolerable and blameworthy are now seen as tolerable or even desirable. For example, Joe may begin to perceive Diane's "nagging" as a desire to be more closely involved with him, and Diane might see Joe's intense work involvement as his desire to provide material comforts for the family. Change and acceptance are mutually facilitative, with greater change leading to greater levels of acceptance, and greater levels of acceptance leading to more spontaneous and long-lasting change.

The IBCT therapists use several strategies to promote acceptance. They facilitate an emotional joining around the problem, focusing partners on the pain each is experiencing rather than on the blame each deserves. Therapists promote this by reformulating recurring problems as differences between partners to which each person has an understandable emotional reaction. Therapists also encourage partners to talk about their own feelings and emphasize "soft" disclosures which make each partner appear more vulnerable and thus more acceptable and less blameworthy. They encourage partners to see the problem as a common external enemy to facilitate emotional acceptance through unified detachment of the problem. In emotional acceptance through tolerance building, therapists use a number of techniques designed to increase partners' tolerance for negative interactions, such as role playing, faked incidences of negative behavior, and emphasizing the positive features of negative behavior. Finally, therapists encourage emotional acceptance through greater self-care by helping partners to identify alternative methods of getting their needs met and additional options when faced with a partner's negative behavior.

Preliminary data from a clinical trial that compared IBCT to BCT has provided some promising support for IBCT and suggests its superiority over BCT.

B. Emotionally Focused Couples Therapy

In Emotionally Focused Couples Therapy (EFT), Susan Johnson and Leslie Greenberg integrate psychoanalytic theory, specifically attachment theory, with recent research on negative behavioral interactions to formulate an intervention for distressed relationships. According to EFT, couples' adjustment involves both the intrapsychic emotional experiences of each partner and the couples' interpersonal interaction patterns. These processes are mutually determined and both are targeted for intervention in BFT.

Intrapsychic emotional experiences are rooted in partners' internal models of attachment, learned from past attachment experiences, particularly the infant's attachment to the mother. These working models affect how partners respond emotionally to negative interpersonal experiences and are in turn affected by these experiences as well. Distressed relationships are insecure bonds in which the attachment needs of one or both partners are not met because of rigid interaction patterns that block emotional engagement. The core problem in these relationships is partners' inaccessibility and inability to respond to or engage the partner. Therapists target both the underlying emotions and the rigid, negative interaction patterns in order to restore accessibility and form a new, secure bond between partners where each can have his or her innate needs for protection, security, and connectedness met.

The core of EFT is the accessing and reprocessing of the emotions underlying negative interaction patterns and the enactment of new patterns in which partners are affiliative and engaged. Distress is alleviated, not through new skills or new insights, but through the *experience* of new aspects of the self and new interaction patterns that take place in the therapy sessions. Thus, when Diane begins to nag Joe in therapy, the therapist helps Diane to focus on the underlying sadness she feels at not being close to Joe. Joe is better able to respond to her feeling of sadness than to her nagging, and the two experience a moment of closeness and understanding. The EFT therapist uses several general techniques to create this experience for the couples. First, a strong positive alliance is established with both partners. This alliance is critical if the couple is to feel safe enough to express and process their underlying emotions. Second, the therapist focuses on the moment-by-moment experience of the clients to help them reshape interactions and emotional experiences as they occur. Third, as interactions are tracked and emotions restructured, the therapist encourages the clients to replay their interactions to create new, more positive relationship events.

Initial studies have indicated that EFT is more effective than a waiting period of no therapy and at least as effective as CBCT and BCT. In comparing EFT, CBCT, and BCT, EFT was found to be more effective than BCT on marital adjustment, intimacy, and target complaint level.

V. COUPLES THERAPY FOR SPECIFIC PSYCHIATRIC DISORDERS

Couples and family therapists have developed specialized interventions for a wide variety of psychiatric disorders, including depression, alcohol, and a variety of anxiety disorders. Outcome studies have generally found that intervening with couples and families (rather than individuals) leads to lower drop-out rates and higher treatment success rates. Behavioral and cognitive couples treatments for depression have been found to reduce depression and increase satisfaction when the depressed person is in a distressed relationship. Behavioral Couples Therapy has also been shown to reduce alcoholism and to improve couples' satisfaction. Finally, spousal involvement has been shown to increase the effectiveness of behavioral treatments for agoraphobia.

VI. ALTERNATIVE APPROACHES TO COUPLES TREATMENT

Alternative treatments for distressed couples have been developed to improve the success rates of more traditional couples treatments as well as to provide less costly interventions. Two prevalent alternative approaches are group couples therapy and prevention/enrichment programs. In group couples therapy, couples help each other as firsthand observers of couples' conflict and provide perspective on the problems each couple is experiencing. The group process provides an arena where couples can learn from one another, obtain insight, experience support, and receive feedback. Preliminary descriptive data on the outcome of group therapy indicates that most couples experience improvement at termination in areas as diverse as communication, reframing problems, appreciating each other more as individuals, and feeling more acceptance toward the partner's family of origin.

Premarital programs designed to prevent future marital distress and programs designed to enrich couples' relationships attempt to spare the couple and their children from the negative consequences of distress. Like traditional couples therapy, these programs vary theoretically and methodologically, with some programs focusing on teaching communication and problem-solving skills and others promoting awareness of underlying emotional or unconscious factors that might make a couple vulnerable to the development of distress. A review of 85 controlled outcome studies found that the average participant in one of these programs improved more than did 67% of those in corresponding control groups at termination. A recent longitudinal study of a behavior intervention program (PREP) demonstrated that couples who received the intervention had significantly higher relationship satisfaction than the control couples 18 months after the intervention and reported significantly higher sexual satisfaction, less intense marital problems, and higher relationship satisfaction than control couples at the 3-year follow-up. Because prevention spares couples (and their children) from the detrimental effects of distress that many couples experience before they seek couples therapy, prevention models may prove more efficient and effective than treatment models of already distressed couples.

VII. CONCLUSION

The need for effective treatments for couple distress has grown in the last few decades for several reasons: the United States has the highest divorce rate of any major industrialized country, there has been a sharp increase in divorce rates from 1960 to 1980, and there is unambiguous evidence that marital distress and divorce have harmful consequences for spouses and children. As a result, couples therapists and researchers have de-

veloped therapies that appear to be effective, at least in the short run. The comparative effectiveness of the different types of therapeutic approaches remains unclear, however. Further study is needed to clarify the comparative effectiveness of different approaches and to begin to understand how approaches and techniques might be matched to couples to maximize the effectiveness of the intervention for each couple that seeks treatment.

BIBLIOGRAPHY

Baucom, D. H., & Epstein, N. (1990). *Cognitive-behavioral marital therapy.* New York: Brunner-Mazel.

Bowen, M. (1978). *Family therapy in clinical practice.* Northvale, NY: Aronson.

Giblin, P., Sprenkle, D. H., & Sheehan, R. (1985). Enrichment outcome research: A meta-analysis of premarital, marital, and family interventions. *Journal of Marital and Family Therapy, 16,* 257–271.

Gurman, A. S., & Kniskern, D. P. (Eds.). *Handbook of family therapy.* New York: Brunner-Mazel.

Jacobson, N. S., & Christensen, A. (in press). *Integrative couple therapy.* New York: Norton.

Jacobson, N. S., & Gurman, A. S. (Eds.). (1995). *Clinical handbook of couple therapy.* New York: Guilford Press.

Johnson, S. M., & Greenberg, L. S. (1985b). Differential effects of experiential and problem-solving interventions in resolving marital conflict. *Journal of Consulting and Clinical Psychology, 53,* 175–184.

Lebow, J. L., & Gurman, A. S. (1995). Research assessing couple and family therapy. *Annual Review of Psychology, 46,* 27–57.

Sheilds, C. G., Wynne, L. C., McDaniel, S. H., & Gawinski, B. A. (1994). The marginalization of family therapy: A historical and continuing problem. *Journal of Marital and Family Therapy, 20,* 117–138.

Snyder, D. K., Wills, R. M., & Grady-Fletcher, A. (1991). Long-term effectiveness of behavioral versus insight-oriented marital therapy: A four-year follow-up study. *Journal of Consulting and Clinical Psychology, 59,* 138–141.

Creativity and Genius

Dean Keith Simonton

University of California, Davis

Desurgency Factor F on Cattell's Sixteen Personality Factor Questionnaire. Those scoring high on this dimension are introspective, restrained, brooding, and solemn (as opposed to surgency).

Emergenesis The inheritance of characteristics that require the co-occurrence of multiple genetic traits (i.e., multiplicative rather than additive heredity).

Historiometry The method of applying quantitative techniques to biographical and historical data in order to test nomothetic hypotheses about human behavior.

Overinclusive Thought An attention deficiency in which there occurs a failure to eliminate responses that are irrelevant or inefficient within a given behavioral situation.

Psychoticism A scale of the Eysenck Personality Questionnaire. High scorers on this dimension have tendencies toward being criminal, impulsive, hostile, aggressive, psychopathic, schizoid, unipolar depressive, affective disorder, and schizophrenic, whereas low scorers tend toward the conformist, conventional, empathetic, socialized, and altruistic.

Schizothymia Factor A on the Cattell Sixteen Personality Factor Questionnaire. High scorers are withdrawn, internally preoccupied, precise, critical, and skeptical (low scorers being labeled cyclothymic).

CREATIVITY AND GENIUS are closely related concepts. Although there can exist creativity without genius, and genius without creativity, creative genius is often considered the highest or purest manifestation of both creativity and genius. To appreciate better their connection, it is first necessary to specify what each term is usually taken to signify in the psychological sciences.

I. INTRODUCTION

Of the concepts of creativity and genius, creativity is perhaps the hardest to define in a scientifically satisfactory manner. The only secure statement on which there is some scientific consensus is that creativity concerns the production of creative ideas. An idea is called "creative" if it meets two requirements. First, the idea must be original in the sense that it represents a relatively rare response. Ideas that arise from just a single person are more original than those that emerge from numerous individuals. Many people have used a shoe to keep a beach blanket from blowing away, but only one person revolutionized physics by developing the general theory of relativity. Second, the idea must be adaptive in some significant manner. For example, it must solve some important problem or accomplish some worthwhile task. Without this second condition, one could not discriminate the strange mental meanderings of a psychotic from the breakthrough ideas of a scientific genius. Hence, creative ideas must be at once original and adaptive.

When we try to obtain a more specific definition, however, various researchers will often exhibit contrary conceptions of what creativity entails. There are three main viewpoints.

1. Creativity may be taken as a mental process, or a set of mental processes, that generates creative ideas. These cognitive operations might include insight, intuition, and imagination. This is the definition adopted by cognitive psychologists who study problem solving in laboratory experiments.

2. Creativity may be considered to represent a characteristic of concrete products, such as a painting, poem, or invention. Those products that satisfy certain standards—such as novelty, elegance, beauty, and technical virtuosity—are called creative. This is the orientation favored in theoretical and empirical aesthetics.

3. Creativity may be seen as a special personality trait, or cluster of traits, on which individuals may differ. For example, individuals who exhibit sufficient intelligence, ambition, determination, independence, and originality may be defined as creative. This is the definition preferred by personality psychologists who examine the traits that distinguish creative persons from everyday populations. [*See* PERSONALITY.]

Hence, creativity may be examined as a process, a product, or a person. Despite this conceptual divergence, the three perspectives can overlap and converge in various forms. For instance, researchers might study individual differences in cognitive styles—or preferred modes of information processing. This variation may then correlate with the production of creative ideas. Other investigators may examine individual differences in the output of creative products. Those persons who are the most prolific may then be said to be the most creative by this criterion. Thus, there exists a tremendous variety of ways that creativity may be provided an operational definition.

The term "genius" has a long history that harks back to Roman times, when genius was a "guardian angel" that looked out for a person's fate. Later the word became extended to include the unique qualities and abilities of individuals that led to distinctive achievements. When the term entered the behavioral sciences, it acquired a more objective and highly quantitative meaning. In fact, psychologists developed two rather different operational definitions, one psychometric and the other historiometric.

The psychometric definition of genius was established by such pioneers as Lewis Terman and Leta Hollingworth. According to this conception, a person can be considered a "genius" if he or she scores exceptionally high on a standard intelligence test. Often IQ scores of 140 are taken as indicative of genius, although sometimes the cutoffs will be higher or lower than this figure. For example, the Mensa Society requires its members to exhibit IQs at least two standard deviations above the mean (a figure around 130 to 132 on most intelligence tests). Of course, it is also possible to take the IQ score as simply indicating the relative magnitude of genius an individual displays, rather than attempting to identify some discrete threshold for inclusion. Nonetheless, the key problem with the psychometric definition is that there is no good evidence that performance on intelligence tests has a strong positive correlation with actual achievement. The most highly creative individuals in a discipline, for example, will not necessarily claim higher IQs than will their less successful colleagues. The strongest assertion that can be made for intelligence tests is that those who earn low IQ scores are rather unlikely to demonstrate any kind of notable creativity. It is not clear what the minimum level of intelligence may be, although the literature often mentions an IQ of 120 as demarcating the most common lower bound. [*See* INTELLIGENCE AND MENTAL HEALTH.]

The historiometric definition avoids this validity problem. According to this alternative conception, which dates back to Francis Galton, genius is directly defined in terms of actual overt impact. A genius is someone who makes contributions to a domain that are so numerous and so distinctive the domain is noticeably, if not fundamentally, transformed. The greatest geniuses literally make names for themselves, often becoming eponyms for discoveries, movements, or events. Examples include the Copernican revolution, Newtonian physics, Darwinism, Pasteurization, and Freudian slips. Moreover, like the psychometric definition, the historiometric assessment can be used to gauge degrees of genius. That is, researchers can speak of the magnitude of impact, so that Mozart exhibits more genius than Salieri, and Salieri more genius than Türk.

One special virtue of the historiometric definition of genius is that it can provide a comprehensive perspective on creativity. Although genius may appear in many forms—including political, military, religious, and entrepreneurial—it is creative genius that is most universally recognized. In fact, when the word "genius" first emerged to label those individuals who made a mark by their achievements, it was initially applied to outstanding creators. Only later was the term extended to cover exceptional leaders. Moreover, it is clear that creative genius encompasses the process, product, and person definitions of creativity. Creators of this caliber are supposed to possess a distinctive personality profile and a set of mental processes that permit them to generate the products by which they leave their mark on their chosen domain. Even if in more everyday forms of creativity the process, product, and person perspectives might be isolated, in genius-level creativity these three viewpoints become intimately connected.

This linkage will become more apparent in the next section, where we examine one of the central debates in the psychology of creativity and genius.

II. THE MAD–GENIUS CONTROVERSY

Ever since the ancient Greeks, philosophers have speculated about the possible connection between creative genius and madness. For instance, Aristotle was reputed to have said that "Those who have become eminent in philosophy, politics, poetry, and the arts have all had tendencies toward melancholia." Centuries later Seneca made the more general observation that "no great genius has ever existed without some touch of madness." Notions such as these continued right down to more modern times, as is evident in Shakespeare's remark that "The lunatic, the lover and the poet / Are of imagination all compact."

Nor was this belief confined to works of philosophy or imaginative literature. The scientific tradition that developed during the nineteenth century put considerable stress on the pathological nature of genius. Perhaps the most influential proponent of this view was the Italian criminologist Cesare Lombroso. In his classic *The Man of Genius,* which appeared in 1891, he affirmed that genius could be linked with "degenerative psychosis," especially that of the "epileptic group." Similar ideas were expressed by William James, Sigmund Freud, and other early psychologists, the only grounds for debate being the specific nature of the disorder involved. Freud, for one, viewed

creative genius as a guise of neurosis rather than psychosis, but nonetheless agreed with the rest that such outstanding creativity is not symptomatic of psychological and behavioral normality. In fact, when Freud and other psychoanalysts began publishing psychobiographies of creative geniuses, almost invariably it was "pathographies" that emerged—works dedicated to proving that some notable figure from the past had serious psychological problems.

With the advent of humanistic psychology, a dissenting view appeared. Carl Rogers, Abraham Maslow, and Rollo May, among others, saw creativity as a sign of mental health, not illness. In Maslow's study of "self-actualizers," for example, he identified several creative geniuses as indicative of the best in human intellectual and emotional functioning. His cases included such big names as Spinoza, Haydn, Goethe, Renoir, and Einstein. Moreover, not only was genius-grade creativity positively associated with psychological well-being, but more everyday forms of creativity were also taken as indicative of an adaptive, flexible, open personality. For the humanistic psychologists, creativity became a "good thing" to which all individuals should aspire as an integral part of personal growth and adjustment. Rather than pity the great creators of history, we all should emulate them as models of maximal mental, emotional, and behavioral vigor.

Of course, ultimately this debate can only be resolved by looking at scientific data on whether creative personalities, and especially creative geniuses, display more or less psychopathology.

III. THE EMPIRICAL EVIDENCE

The research literature addressing this issue falls into three broad categories. First, some investigators have applied historiometric methods to the biographies of historic personalities, most of whom are deceased. Second, other researchers have relied on psychiatric diagnoses of contemporary creators of genuine stature. Third, still other investigators have also used contemporary creative individuals, but in this case requiring that the persons be subjected to standard psychometric assessment. Despite the divergence of approach, the three methods converge on the same broad conclusions.

A. Historiometric Studies

Publications on the mad-genius relationship will often include long lists of famous creators who showed signs of mental disorder, such as schizophrenia, manic-depression, or some personality disorder. Table 1 provides just such a partial list. The individuals included are those who are most frequently mentioned in this literature. However, it must be observed that these assignments are seldom predicated on clinical diagnoses of psychometric assessments. Instead, the judgments are most often based upon a tentative reading of appropriate biographical material, which may not always lead to an unambiguous determination. In any case, the main inference that can be drawn from Table I is that at least some personalities have managed to exhibit both psychopathology and history-making achievement.

Nevertheless, it is impossible to consider such tabulations as coming anywhere close to a scientific demonstration. After all, the number of geniuses in the sum total of history is very large. As a consequence, even if the risk for psychopathology were *lower* than average for eminent creators, we would still predict the occurrence of a very large absolute count of disordered personalities. Therefore, to make any headway using this type of data we have to begin calculating incidence rates so that comparisons can be made with the general population. The first person to do so was Havelock Ellis at the turn of the century. Looking at over 1000 creators and leaders with entries in the *Dictionary of National Biography,* he found that 4.2% demonstrated some extreme psychopathology, such as insanity, another 8% exhibited melancholia, and a further 5% showed some personality disorder. He also noted that 16% had been imprisoned. Nowadays this figure may seem unrelated to the rest, but at the turn of the century its relevance would have been immediately apparent. The psychiatric literature of the time contained many claims that geniuses, the mentally dis-

Table I Eminent Creative Personalities with Supposed Mental Illnesses

---

Schizophrenic disorders (and other cognitive psychoses):

Scientists: Tycho Brahe, Cantor, Copernicus, Descartes, Faraday, W. R. Hamilton, Kepler, Lagrange, Linnaeus, Newton, Pascal, Semmelweiss, Weierstrass, Horace Wells;

Thinkers: Kant, Nietzsche, Swedenborg;

Writers: Baudelaire, Lewis Carroll, Hawthorne, Hölderlin, S. Johnson, Pound, Rimbaud, Strindberg, Swift;

Artists: Bosch, Cellini, Dürer, Goya, El Greco, Kandinsky, Leonardo da Vinci, Rembrandt, Toulouse-Lautrec;

Composers: Donizetti, MacDowell, Felix Mendelssohn, Rimsky-Korsakov, Saint-Saëns.

Affective disorders (depression, mania, or bipolar):

Scientists: Boltwood, Boltzmann, Carothers, C. Darwin, L. De Forest, J. F. W. Herschel, Julian Huxley, T. H. Huxley, Jung, Kammerer, J. R. von Mayer, V. Meyer, H. J. Muller, J. P. Müller, B. V. Schmidt, J. B. Watson;

Thinkers: W. James, J. S. Mill, Rousseau, Schopenhauer;

Writers: Balzac, Barrie, Berryman, Blake, Boswell, Byron, Chatterton, J. Clare, Coleridge, William Collins, Conrad, Cowper, H. Crane, Dickens, T. Dreiser, R. Fergusson, F. Scott Fitzgerald, Frost, Goethe, G. Greene, Hemingway, Jarrell, Kafka, Charles Lamb, Jack London, Robert Lowell, Maupassant, O'Neill, Plath, Poe, Quiroga, Roethke, D. G. Rossetti, Saroyan, Schiller, Sexton, Shelley, C. Smart, T. Tasso, V. Woolf;

Artists: Michelangelo, Modigliani, Pollock, Raphael, Rothko, R. Soyer, Van Gogh;

Composers: Berlioz, Chopin, Elgar, Gershwin, Handel, Mahler, Rachmaninoff, Rossini, R. Schumann, Scriabin, Smetana, Tchaikovsky, Wolf.

Personality disorders (including severe neuroses):

Scientists: Ampère, Cavendish, A. S. Couper, Diesel, Einstein, Frege, Freud, Galton, Heaviside, Huygens, Marconi, Mendel;

Thinkers: Beccaria, Comte, Descartes, Hegel, Hobbes, Hume, Kierkegaard, B. Russell, Spencer, Voltaire, Wittgenstein;

Writers: H. C. Andersen, E. B. Browning, R. Browning, Bunyan, Carlyle, Dickinson, Dostoevski, T. S. Eliot, Emerson, Flaubert, García Lorca, Gide, Allen Ginsberg, Gogol, Heine, G. M. Hopkins, A. Huxley, W. M. Inge, Melville, Pavese, Proust, S. Richardson, Rimbaud, Ruskin, Tennyson, Tocqueville, Tolstoy, Verlaine, Tennessee Williams, Zola;

Artists: Borromini, Bramante, Caravaggio, Cézanne, Munch, Romney;

Composers: Beethoven, Bruckner, Orlando de Lasso, Schubert, Wagner.

---

turbed, and criminals all originated in the same underlying genetic degeneracy. In any case, these statistics are complemented by another study that concentrated solely on twentieth-century personalities and focused on a single symptom of mental disorder, namely suicidal inclinations. This inquiry found that 5% displayed suicidal tendencies, either actually committing suicide (2%) or attempting to do so (3%). Indeed, many of the individuals with affective disorders given in Table 1 died suicides, including Boltzmann, Chatterton, Van Gogh, Hemingway, Plath, Tchaikovsky, and Virginia Woolf.

Unfortunately, although the foregoing figures appear impressive, they do not lend themselves to easy interpretation. One problem is that creators are combined with leaders. Yet other evidence indicates that the incidence of mental disorder among creative personalities is higher than what holds for individuals who are notable for their leadership.

Hence, of more direct relevance are those investigations that focus on creative genius. Two studies, for example, concentrated on illustrious poets. One study found that 13% were either insane or else showed symptoms of hallucinations and delusions. The other inquiry obtained even more impressive figures: Almost half had pathological symptoms of some kind, and 15% became outright psychotic. Yet another historiometric inquiry focused on 100 eminent scientists, including such figures as Pascal, Newton, Lavoisier, Dalton, Avogadro, Faraday, and J. J. Thomson. The investigation was conducted by R. B. Cattell, who adapted his Sixteen Personality Factor Questionnaire (16 PF) for use with biographical data. He found that these scientific geniuses had distinctly abnormal profiles. In particular, they scored especially high on schizothymia and desurgency. Hence, they tended to be withdrawn, internally preoccupied, brooding, solemn, and introspective—often to a decidedly maladaptive degree.

The most comprehensive historiometric inquiry is also the most recent: Arnold Ludwig's 1995 *The Price of Greatness*. He examined more than 1000 eminent personalities, including both creators and leaders. Although the empirical results are too complex to summarize completely here, four key results must be mentioned:

1. The incidence rate of various disorders among these individuals was clearly higher than what is normally seen in the general population. The disorders included depression, mania, psychosis, pathological anxiety, suicide, alcoholism, and drug abuse, with incidence rates sometimes ranging between 70% and 80%.

2. There was actually a positive relationship between the presence of psychopathology and the magnitude of a person's accomplishments. To establish this relationship, Ludwig had devised a reliable and valid measure of lifetime creative achievement.

3. There were tremendous contrasts across different domains of achievement in terms of the incidence rates. Not only were the rates lower in leaders than in creators, but the artistic creators exhibited much more psychopathology than did the scientific creators.

4. The specific type of disorder varied greatly across the various forms of creative achievement. That is, the relative representation of schizophrenics, affective psychotics, neurotics, and other syndromes depends very much on the area in which creative genius is displayed. For example, within the creative arts the architects exhibited relatively few syndromes, whereas the poets were susceptible to almost every major type of mental disturbance. Moreover, whereas poets and fiction writers often suffered from drug abuse, the nonfiction authors did not experience this difficulty.

The overall conclusion to be drawn from these diverse studies is that the historical record does seem to support the inference of some association between psychopathology and creative genius.

B. Psychiatric Studies

A totally different approach is to determine whether eminent contemporaries exhibit clinical-level symptomatology. The usual criterion is whether a creative person had to receive clinical treatment, whether therapy, medication, or hospitalization. Two investigations using this approach have received the most attention.

First, Nancy Andreasen conducted some interesting studies of writers of sufficient acclaim that they had been invited to attend the prestigious Writers Workshop at the University of Iowa. These creative personalities were compared to controls who were matched for age, education, and gender. The incidence of affective disorders, alcoholism, and suicide were 3 to 5 times higher in the creators than in the controls. Indeed, about 80% of these writers were plagued by mood disorders, especially bipolar manic-depressive symptoms. During the course of her study, she even lost 7% of her sample to suicide. [*See* MOOD DISORDERS.]

Second, Kay Jamison surveyed notable artists and writers of Great Britain. Almost two-fifths had sought treatment for affective disorder, the incidence rates being especially high for writers. And among the writers, the poets were the highest of all. In fact, fully half of the distinguished poets reported the need to receive medical treatment for depression, and around a fifth had to be treated for mania. This higher pathology in the poets parallels what Ludwig observed in his historiometric sample. Finally, all groups reported a high incidence of mood swings, with the exception of those writers who specialized in biography.

These two studies have been the subject of some methodological criticisms. By themselves, they probably would not offer strong evidence for a connection between creativity and mental illness. Even so, these results are consistent with what has been found in historiometric work, and are compatible with the outcome of the psychometric findings to be described later. Moreover, there exist other psychiatric investigations that do not suffer from the same problems and yet which arrive at comparable conclusions. Of special interest is an extensive study that examined around 19,000 persons drawn from German-speaking nations, including 294 highly gifted creators. Not only were the rates of psychopathology in creative artists and scientists found to be much higher than in the general population, but, in addition, those individuals who could claim only intermediate levels of creative achievement had incidence rates that fell between those of the truly successful and those of the population at large. Hence, just as Ludwig's investigation suggested, increased psychopathology may be associated with increased creativity.

This same study arrived at another critical fact: The relatives of creative individuals also displayed higher than normal rates of psychopathology. In particular, the parents, siblings, children, and grandchildren of the highly gifted creators often had incidence rates that were 2 to 7 times greater. This provocative finding has been replicated in another epidemiological investigation conducted in Iceland. Taking advantage of the records of the Reykjavik mental hospital, it was found that the relatives of schizophrenics and manic-

depressive patients were 2 to 6 times more likely to become an artist or scientist of sufficient importance to earn a listing in *Who is Who in Iceland*. Furthermore, by exploiting three comprehensive genealogies, the investigator could show that eminent Icelanders tended to originate in family lineages with unusually high risk for psychopathology. In particular, mental illness was found in the pedigrees of between 25% and 40% of the illustrious novelists, poets, painters, mathematicians, and philosophers.

Because we know that many forms of mental illness have a genetic component, these findings are most important. These data suggest that creativity may itself have an inheritable component, and that a portion of this component may entail the endowment of a certain proclivity toward mental disturbance. This conclusion fits in nicely with the historiometric findings that Francis Galton reported in his 1869 *Hereditary Genius*. There he showed that eminent creators and leaders tend to form family pedigrees. Although his own explanation of these lineages involved the inheritance of intellectual ability, we cannot dismiss the possibility that the endowment of talent may actually involve psychopathological tendencies.

In sum, the psychiatric investigations appear to add further support to the generalizations abstracted from the historical record. Not only may creativity be associated with some inclination toward mental disorder, but at least some of this association may be the repercussion of genetic endowment. [*See* GENETIC CONTRIBUTORS TO MENTAL HEALTH.]

C. Psychometric Studies

Although the logistics of the research is often difficult and expensive, it is sometimes possible to administer personality inventories to a sample of willing creative contemporaries. For instance, R. B. Cattell has conducted studies in which creative artists, writers, and scientists have taken his Sixteen Personality Factor Questionnaire. In general, he received results complementary to his historiometric inquiry mentioned earlier. It is clear that these eminent creators do not usually exhibit trait profiles typical of normal personalities, and that some of these differences may be considered indicative of some psychopathology. One particularly interesting finding was that the artistic creators, in comparison to the scientific creators, displayed much more emotional instability. This is consistent with the historiometric studies that suggest that psychopathology is much more strongly associated with artistic creativity than with scientific creativity.

Even more convincing are the results of a series of investigations carried out at the Institute for Personality Assessment and Research (IPAR) at the University of California, Berkeley. The IPAR group, which included Donald MacKinnon and Frank Barron, invited many illustrious personalities to undergo rather extensive psychological assessment. These subjects included world-famous architects as well as notable American writers. The personality profiles of these creative individuals departed significantly from what was observed in more normal samples. In addition, the observed departures were in the direction of psychopathology. For example, the creative architects received high scores on the psychopathic-deviate and schizophrenia scales of the Minnesota Multiphasic Personality Inventory (MMPI). The results for the creative writers were even more dramatic, since they showed elevated scores on all of the clinical scales of the MMPI (viz., depression, hypomania, schizophrenia, paranoia, psychopathic deviation, hysteria, hypochondriasis, and psychaesthenia). This is not to say that these creative authors suffered from severely diminished mental health. Quite the contrary, in two crucial ways the creative writers differed from those individuals who cannot adapt well to the demands of everyday life. First, the creators tended to exhibit considerable ego-strength, an asset that allowed these individuals to channel their psychological eccentricities into more healthy and productive directions. Individuals who succumb to their pathological tendencies, in contrast, do not have the ability to prevent an inherently incoherent personality from falling apart. Second, the creators tended to score at subclinical levels—somewhere between the normal and the abnormal ranges. This seems consistent with Dryden's often-quoted claim that "Great Wits are sure to Madness near ally'd, / And thin Partitions do their Bounds divide."

Finally, we must acknowledge the implications of those psychometric inquiries that have applied the Eysenck Personality Questionnaire (EPQ) to creative and noncreative populations. This research indicates that creative people score higher on the psychoticism scale of the EPQ, and that the greater the amount of creativity the higher the scores tend to be. Yet just as was found for the MMPI, creative individuals do not score high enough to lead to a prognosis of outright mental breakdown. There are four reasons why an association between psychoticism and creativity would make theoretical sense.

1. Individuals who score high on psychoticism are less prone to conform to social norms. As a consequence, they will thereby exhibit the kind of nonconformity that is essential for bold innovation. Many people who have some creative potential fail to realize it owing to an unwillingness to appear odd or different.

2. Closely related to the preceding is the fact that those who score high on psychoticism are often more disposed toward the solitary, energetic, and single-minded commitment to certain ideas. This quality is highly desirable in a creative individual who must often be monomanical in the pursuit of an original vision.

3. High scorers on this dimension tend to exhibit a distinctive style of cognitive functioning that may more likely lead to original ideas. For instance, they often display overinclusive thinking as well as certain peculiarities in latent inhibition and negative priming. Although these thought patterns are frequently associated with mental disorder, in the creative individual they permit the intrusion of "irrelevant" associations that often lead to critical insights.

4. There is evidence that psychoticism has a sizable heritability coefficient, and therefore this may define one of the traits that underlie the genetic basis for creative genius. In fact, in his 1995 book on *Genius,* Eysenck proposed a comprehensive theory of creative genius in which the trait of Psychoticism plays a critical explanatory and predictive role.

When this psychometric literature is combined with the findings of the psychiatric and historiometric inquiries, there can be little doubt that some relationship exists between creative genius and psychopathology. Moreover, there is also good reason for believing that the same conclusion holds for more mundane forms of creativity, albeit the connection would be less pronounced. For example, Ruth Richards and her colleagues have shown that patients with psychiatric symptoms tend to score higher on an index of everyday creativity, such as participation in arts and crafts. Furthermore, the first-degree relatives of these psychiatric patients also exhibited higher creativity by this more relaxed criterion. The most important question, accordingly, is not whether a relationship exists, but what this relationship means from the standpoint of theory and practice.

IV. INTERPRETATIVE ISSUES

What exactly are the implications of the findings just reviewed? That question does not allow an easy answer. Like so often happens in the behavioral sciences, each empirical datum may have more than one interpretation. Even worse, an explanation that might be adequate for interpreting one finding may prove incapable of explicating another finding. The only thing that we know for sure is that a great many questions must be resolved before it will be possible to offer an integrated account of the facts. The following six issues are especially urgent.

A. Magnitude of Creativity

Does psychopathology bear the same relationship with everyday creativity as it does for genius-level creativity? Note that the answer to this question would help resolve the controversy between those who believe that creativity is a sign of mental health and those who think that creativity is indicative of mental illness. It could be, for example, that psychopathology is negatively correlated with everyday creativity, as the humanistic psychologists argue, while still being positively correlated with genius-caliber achievement, such as stated in the received tradition. Unfortunately for this compromise solution, what little evidence we have seems to support the conclusion that the relationship is positive no matter what the degree of creativity may be. Mildly creative individuals will exhibit more symptoms of mental illness than noncreative but normal individuals, and highly creative individuals will simply display an even more pronounced symptomatology. After all, many researchers in this area will point out that creativity is not a discrete trait, but rather it forms a dimension on which people may vary, from the normal person on the street to the supernormal genius. Even more importantly, many of the traits that correlate positively with everyday creativity, such as the capacity for divergent thinking, also correlate positively with such diagnostic dimensions as psychoticism.

B. Degree of Pathology

Is mental illness sine qua non of creativity, or is it merely one of many predictors? One conclusion is quote obvious from the historiometric, psychiatric, and psychometric study of creative personalities. A large percentage of even the most acclaimed creative geniuses seem to display no signs whatsoever of mental illness. Indeed, in line with the humanistic psychologists' assertions, such individuals may even be sublimely happy and well adjusted. How can such a fact be accommodated if we think that genius and madness are intimately connected?

One solution would be to simply reject the evidence. Perhaps the healthy souls are only putatively so. Maybe these are individuals with such substantial ego-strength that they can easily hide their moments of deep depression or manic elation. This conjecture, unfortunately, runs away from the question rather than really answering it. Nonetheless, it is worth a close look in future research.

Another response is to say that mental illness is just one of dozens if not hundreds of factors that contribute to a person's ability to conceive innovative ideas. As a consequence, so long as an individual is sufficiently high on the other predictive variables, that person can be relatively low on the proclivity toward mental illness. Perhaps if a talent is extremely bright, extraordinarily ambitious and persistent, and completely independent of conformity pressures in a completely healthy, self-possessed manner, there is not as much need for the crazy thinking and asocial commitments that figure so prominently in the daily routine of creative genius. This explanation, of course, can only be established after a considerable amount of effort devoted to constructing an inventory of variables that predict creative achievement, especially variables that are orthogonal to any tendency toward mental illness.

C. Types of Psychopathology

Which psychopathology is most strongly associated with creativity? The historiometric, psychiatric, and psychometric studies do not always concur on what syndromes or symptoms are the most frequently found among creative individuals. For example, the psychiatric investigations seem to identify the affective disorders as the most prominent, especially the depressive and bipolar syndromes. The historiometric inquiries, in contrast, have often isolated a significant proportion of schizophrenic disorders. And, finally, the psychometric studies sometimes find that the psychopathology spans several syndromes that are normally distinct. [See DEPRESSION; SCHIZOPHRENIA.]

Maybe these discrepancies should not surprise us, given the divergent nature of the data sources, measurements, and symptom criteria. Even modern diagnoses by trained clinicians will often differ greatly from each other and from the implications derived from psychometric assessments. In addition, it is very possible that the resolution of this irksome issue is closely tied to that of the next question.

D. Domain of Creative Achievement

How does the type and intensity of psychopathology vary across the domain of creative activity? One conclusion on which the historiometric, psychiatric, and psychometric studies uniformly agree is that different creative domains tend to feature characteristic types of mental illness, or at least manifest the various symptoms in differing degrees. For example, it is clear that creative personalities have a higher risk for psychopathology than equally eminent individuals who attained distinction in other fields, such as political leadership. Moreover, scientists seem to exhibit more mental health than do artists, and when an eminent scientist does suffer some difficulties, they may be more of a neurotic than of a psychotic kind. Even among artistic creators, the symptom profiles may vary dramatically from one domain to another. Where creative architects often display a pattern closest to the scientists, creative writers, and especially poets, frequently appear to totter on the outer fringe of mental and emotional stability.

E. Nature versus Nurture

What is the relative influence of genetic endowment versus environmental conditions in producing both the creativity and the psychopathology? The classic nature–nurture issue that plagues the psychological sciences is no less irksome here. And as has been the case in other substantive domains of psychology, it seems that both factors seem to have an important role to play.

On the one hand, we have already cited evidence from psychiatric and historiometric studies that suggest not only that creativity and psychopathology may each run in family lines, but also that those pedigrees may significantly overlap. Lineages that produce a disproportionate number of creative personalities may also generate a high percentage of mentally disturbed individuals. However, because we cannot identify a gene or set of genes that underlying these patterns of intergenerational inheritance, it is not easy to rule out other, nongenetic interpretations of the data. More critically, modern behavioral genetics has introduced the concept of "emergenesis," a phenomenon where genetic traits combine in a multiplicative rather than additive fashion. One peculiar implication of emergenetic traits is that they may not necessarily run in families, a possibility that greatly complicates the picture. This is especially true given that some recent studies have suggested that to some extent creative genius may entail emergenetic inheritance.

On the other hand, there is ample reason for believing that environmental factors have an important role in the determination of creativity and mental illness. Furthermore, these factors can sometimes overlap. For example, the experience of a traumatic childhood, such as parental loss, can contribute to the development of a creative personality, but the same circumstances can contribute to the emergence of sociopathic and depressive personalities as well. It is possible that environmental influences such as this interacts with genetic endowment in the determination of whether the ultimate consequences are constructive or destructive for the individual. In addition, we must acknowledge the possibility that the environmental factors may operate at various points during the course of development, including even prenatal stages. It is intriguing to note, for instance, that there exists a tendency for eminent creators to be born in the first few months of the year, a tendency that corresponds quite closely with a calendrical bias in the births of schizophrenics. Although we are a long way from understanding the etiology of these patterns, the congruence may not be coincidental. The prenatal environment may be affected by the special conditions that attend the winter months, yielding circumstances that favor both creativity and psychopathology.

F. Causal Relationships

What is the precise causal relation between creativity and psychopathology? This question is clearly the most important of all. If this issue were resolved, the answers to the preceding five queries would probably become almost straightforward. The number of possible causal models is very large, but three deserve special attention.

1. Psychopathology may contribute to creativity, at least so long as the disturbances are kept within bounds. This is the position taken by many researchers in the field, such as Hans Eysenck. Creative genius may require a capacity for anticonforming behavior, manic preoccupation, and unconstrained imagination—qualities that demand that the individual's intellectual and emotional functioning lean at least part way toward psychopathology. This explanation is consistent with the positive correlation between the magnitude of psychopathology and the degree of creative achievement exhibited.

2. Creativity may contribute to psychopathology. A considerable body of research shows that mental illness can be triggered by extreme environmental stress, and the life of a creative genius can be considered among the most stressful. It may require a constant struggle to win acceptance, and even after some success has been obtained, the creator is not isolated from future failures and disappointments. The very circumstance of attaining fame may prove extremely stressful as well. The famous creator may suddenly become idolized by the wrong people, who take away the last vestiges of that solitude that is so essential to the creative process. Even worse, the external pressure on the creator to outdo what has already been accomplished may put excessive strain on an already fragile personality. It is interesting, for example, that many illustrious creators become alcoholics and drug abusers *after* they made it big, not before. Alcoholism and drug abuse may become a self-handicapping strategy used so that they have an excuse for not living up to the unrealistic expectations of their fans.

3. Creativity and psychopathology may simply share some underlying causal antecedents, making any observed association between them causally spurious. For example, it may be that creativity depends to a certain extent on the early acquisition of unconventional attitudes and nonconformist behaviors, and

that this development is encouraged by an upbringing that does not adhere to normal socialization practices. The frequent and intense experience of trauma early in childhood and adolescence is one way to disrupt conventional development, and yet this same condition may encourage the growth of psychopathological symptoms. These symptoms not only may have nothing whatsoever of value to contribute to adulthood creativity, but they might even interfere with creative activity to some noticeable degree.

Or, to offer an even more curious possibility, it could be that the sole reason that creativity is associated with psychopathology is that creativity represents one of the few occupational activities that does not always have to select against individuals with some amount of mental disturbance. Persons with bizarre thoughts and eccentric behaviors are not going to make it far in the business world, nor in any other domain where the emphasis is on reliability, stability, rational decision making, and impression management. Yet a poet or an artist can engage in their creative activities while dwelling at the margin of society—holding odd jobs and drifting from place to place with absolute professional impunity. Indeed, this selection process would account for why the incidence of psychopathology varies according to the domain. Architects and scientists, unlike artistic creators, must often work for organizations (whether firms or universities) that may not tolerate the expression of anything extremely unconventional.

These alternative causal models are not of merely theoretical interest. Determining the correct interpretation has great practical importance besides. After all, the most appropriate therapeutic intervention depends on the answer. If psychopathology contributes directly to the creative process, then creative persons suffering from mental illness would have to evaluate carefully whether they should seek or accept therapy. To be sure, if an individual is so depressive that suicide becomes a very real possibility, then a creative life may be at risk—making intervention mandatory. Even so, there may exist a delicate line between a treatment that prevents such a catastrophe from happening and a treatment that stifles the creative expression that constitutes an essential part of the person's identity. In contrast, if psychopathology bears only a spurious or coincidental connection to creative behavior, then therapeutic inventions may be able to extend an individual's productive life, besides making that life a more pleasant one to live.

V. CONCLUSION

It will take considerably more historiometric, psychiatric, and psychometric research before we can make practical recommendations. We need more assessments of the correct mix of traits, both abnormal and normal, that nourish creative activity. For instance, how much ego-strength is required to compensate for a certain observed level of affective or schizophrenic disorder? It may be particularly crucial for future investigations to conduct longitudinal analyses that can detect how creative output and psychopathology symptoms vary across time. Does an increase in productivity raise or lower the level of mental disturbance? At this point the only conclusion that we can draw with absolute confidence is that creativity and genius are positively associated with various symptoms of mental and emotional disorder.

BIBLIOGRAPHY

Eysenck, H. J. (1995). *Genius*. Cambridge: Cambridge University Press.

Jamison, K. R. (1993). *Touched with fire*. New York: Free Press.

Kessel, N. (1989). Genius and mental disorder: A history of ideas concerning their conjunction. In P. Murray (Ed.), *Genius* (pp. 196–212). Oxford: Blackwell.

Ludwig, A. M. (1995). *The price of greatness*. New York: Guilford Press.

Prentky, R. A. (1989). Creativity and psychopathology: Gamboling at the seat of madness. In J. A. Glover, R. R. Ronning, and C. R. Reynolds (Eds.), *Handbook of Creativity* (pp. 243–269). New York: Plenum Press.

Rothenberg, A. (1990). *Creativity and madness*. Baltimore: Johns Hopkins University Press.

Simonton, D. K. (1994). *Greatness*. New York: Guilford Press.

Creativity, Everyday

Ruth Richards

Saybrook Institute
University of California, San Francisco
McLean Hospital and Harvard Medical School

Acquired Immunity A biological model, for which psychological parallels have been suggested. Early exposure to disorders such as measles or whooping cough can provide a milder experience than in later years, as well as an ongoing immunity. Certain types of psychological exposures have been proposed to have similar, if perhaps more complex, effects.

Bipolar Disorders A family of mood disorders defined by multiple criteria in the American Psychiatric Association's *Diagnostic and Statistical Manual of Mental Disorders* (*DSM-IV*), but characterized particularly by their mood elevations and depressions; these may frequently alternate with significant periods of normalcy. Common disorders by current criteria are: *bipolar I disorder, bipolar II disorder*, and *cyclothymia*. Among other criteria, bipolar I disorder is characterized by major mood elevations as well as depressions. Bipolar II disorder also involves severe depressions, but relatively mild mood elevation. Cyclothymia involves milder elevations and depressions, but is characterized by a more rapid alternation of mood states. A familial liability to bipolar disorders may result in a wide *spectrum* of manifestations, including not only bipolar disorders but, even more frequently, a range of unipolar manifestations ranging from periods of major depression to milder forms of depression or dysthymia.

Compensatory Advantage Another biological model for which a psychological parallel is suggested. In biology, there are inherited familial liabilities that may not only increase vulnerability to illness, but are linked with positive characteristics that run in the same families. An example is the disabling disease of sickle cell anemia compared to the much milder carrier state. The compensatory advantage is resistance to malaria. A similar phenomenon in families has been proposed for certain psychiatric disorders with *creativity* the compensatory advantage.

Eminent Creativity Regarding creators or creative outcomes in situations where recognition has been given by society or by relevant organizations in forms including awards, prizes, honors, publication, or other recognition. These individuals and their accomplishments are widely thought in their culture to have exceptional qualities (although a different generation or culture would not necessarily agree). The term may also pertain to the creative process that generated this outcome.

Everyday Creativity Regarding creators or creative outcomes (products, ideas, or behaviors) that pertain to day-to-day activities at work or leisure and characterized both by *originality* (involving new and unusual aspects) and *meaningfulness* (it is not random or idiosyncratic, but communicates to others). The term may also pertain to the creative process that is involved.

Inverted-U Effect A curvilinear effect, relating two variables, where too little or too much of the first one is associated with low levels of the second variable, but where an intermediate level is optimal and predicts for the highest values of the criterion. This was the prediction for certain manifestations of bipolar disorder in relation to creativity.

EVERYDAY CREATIVITY refers to products, ideas, or behaviors produced or occurring in day-to-day activities. Acts of everyday creativity are characterized by originality and their meaningfulness to others.

I. EVERYDAY CREATIVITY: UNDERRECOGNIZED AND UNDERVALUED

How often do you hear someone say "I'm not very creative, I can't paint." Or they say "I can't sing," or "I can't write." This may be creativity to them: expertise in the arts, or in the sciences. Leadership, too, may be among the more "traditionally creative areas." Furthermore, to be "creative," some people feel they must perform up to a lofty standard—perhaps a gallery-level painting, or a short story that could win some award; for them, social recognition is a part of the picture. All these qualities fit much more with what might be called exceptional level or *eminent creativity*. Yet, with such a limited and dichotomous picture of creativity (either you've got it or you haven't got it), quite a few people may end up saying, "I'm not very creative."

Some people may thereby disenfranchise themselves from creativity.

A. Everyday Creativity

Everyday creativity, by contrast, may be seen as so essential to life, and to our flexible adjustment to it, that we will all inevitably need it, every one of us, in order to cope and to stay alive. It may be viewed as a fundamental survival capacity—and here is "health" with a vengeance. Everyday creativity involves the wide range of

original (and *meaningful*—see glossary) acts that help us adjust to changing circumstances, and to alter these circumstances when necessary, either at work or at leisure.

Examples include not only doing one's own private writing, sketching, designing, or experimenting, but resolving a dispute at work, finding one's way out of the woods when lost, dealing with a difficult child, fixing a broken automobile, creating a meal out of minimal ingredients. It can also include singing in an amateur group, or putting together an inviting yard sale—indeed a great many activities at work and leisure require flexibility, improvisation, new perspectives, and thinking for oneself. Included, in fact, are also activities that may end up receiving eminent recognition. In this sense, eminent creativity may be seen as one special case of everyday creativity—one that this time serves a wider social purpose.

In general, the everyday creative *product* may be a concrete outcome, idea, or behavior (e.g., an innovative newsletter column, a way of resolving a conflict, a dance step). In the language of creativity, there are three other "P's" besides *product*. We can talk as well about the creative *person*, the *process* of creation, and the environmental *press* that can help or hinder its progress.

B. Brief Historical Notes

Everyday creativity is not a new concept, and dates back at least to Sir Francis Galton, who moved away from the notion of unique genius with his proposal that "natural abilities" are normally distributed in the population. Although initial applications involved assessment of "general intelligence" or IQ, a "boom" of interest in creative ability began in the 1950s, starting with J. P. Guilford's presidential address to the American Psychological Association on the measurement of creative thinking, or divergent thinking, abilities. Other interest in a day-to-day creativity was found in Freud's conflict-oriented psychoanalytic viewpoint—where unconscious conflict could emerge transformed either as neurosis or as creative material. By contrast, humanistic psychologists such as Abraham Maslow and Carl Rogers saw creativity as an ultimate expression of health, fueling ongoing curiosity, growth, and development, and representing at best the fullest expression of human potential.

With the human potential movement of the 1960s and 1970s, creativity became all the more an everyday concern, with focus on process, or creative ways of being, as much as product. There were educational innovations as well, and a push for creativity in the schools—in one sense going back to Thomas Dewey, but greatly stimulated by a post-Sputnik Cold War concern from the late 1950s—focused on American youth's ability to compete in science. E. P. Torrance and associates did much influential educational writing and developed the most widely used creativity measures, *The Torrance Tests of Creative Thinking*. In business, J. J. Osborn's "brainstorming" became popular, along with W. Gordon's Synectics, and other idea-generating techniques.

C. Underrecognized and Undervalued

Yet for all of this past concern, we find everyday creativity is often not a priority today, even when it is touted as such. Findings on teacher attitudes, beginning with Getzels and Jackson's influential work in the 1960s, are still being replicated today, showing that teachers often prefer the less to more creative students. Teachers may even say and believe that they prefer the more creative kids while behaving otherwise, as Mark Runco and others have shown. Indeed, here are the more dutiful, neat, and orderly students who do what they are supposed to do—not the creative nonconformists who are rather less predictable and may delight in challenging the status quo. Is this phenomenon, perhaps, part of a relegation of the recognized creative work to an elite few, while the rest of us more often strive in school to learn what they have done?

After all, it can be harder for a parent to raise a more creative child than a less creative one, as writings by E. P. Torrance and others suggest. And it often is harder to *be* a more creative child than a less creative one—or at least as far as dealing with social response is concerned. Thus the great importance of environments that actively recognize and reward everyday creativity. Regarding the healthy and rewarding benefits of more creative attitudes we shall have more to say.

II. PATHOLOGY AND CREATIVITY: EVERYDAY VS. EMINENT CREATORS

One quickly sees that it is critical to distinguish everyday creativity from eminent creativity when talking about illness and health. The pictures are not neces-

sarily the same. And once again, the eminent creators have been more in the news.

A. Eminent Creativity and Bipolar Mood Disorders

One can take mood disorders as a key example, and as an important topic in its own right. People have probably heard about the very high rates of mood disorders among *eminent* creative artists and writers in the recent work of people like Nancy Andreasen, Kay Redfield Jamison, or Arnold Ludwig. Indeed Andreasen found that 80% of her creative writers had experienced at least one depression. One has perhaps also heard famous quotations such as John Dryden's: "Great wits are sure to madness near allied; And thin partitions do their bounds divide."

There is now good support for a link between artistic creativity and mood disorders (and to a lesser degree with linked problems such as substance abuse). The picture may be quite a bit healthier outside of the arts, as Arnold Ludwig's work in particular suggests. Findings of psychopathology are crucial, as is the frequent appearance among mood disorders of a bipolar disorder—either in the actual artist or in the immediate family. Among Andreasen's mood disordered writers, over half had a bipolar disorder, either bipolar type I (with major manic mood elevations as well as severe depressions) or bipolar type II (with milder hypomanic mood swings and severe depressions).

It should be underscored that, with any sort of mood disorder, long periods of normalcy may also be an important part of the picture. It is critical for the reader to note, as in Goodwin and Jamison's authoritative textbook, *Manic-Depressive Illness*, how treatable these disorders can be. People can suffer terribly, and it is important not to romanticize or to minimize these problems. Furthermore—and this is a crucial point—having a mood disorder is no guarantee of being a creatively productive individual. [*See* MOOD DISORDERS.]

B. Everyday Creativity and Bipolar Mood Disorders

When the question is turned around, and we start with the everyday person, it is truly a different question. If many eminent creative writers have mood disorders, this does not, in any way, as Ruth Richards pointed out, mean that most mood-disordered people will be creative, never mind be creative *writers*. Taking a more ludicrous example, if all poets had curly hair, one would not expect every curly haired person to be a *poet*.

Among the many people with mood disorders, some have had enough advantages—perhaps early mentors, supportive figures, exposures to creative methods, educational and financial resources, to pursue their interests—and the necessary motivation and opportunity, to become productively creative. Such advantages, as outlined by researchers including Robert Albert and Arnold Ludwig, can also raise the odds of creativity for all of us. In situations of bias or disadvantage, familial and societal advantages become more important yet, as Ravenna Helson has shown in the case of women.

Indeed, for each such creatively advantaged person, many more potential creators may have fallen by the wayside. Even if there are advantages related to mood swings that raise creative *potential* for everyone with these swings (and we don't know this), it doesn't mean this potential will be realized. Indeed, the disadvantages of mood disorders can be severe.

Beyond this, the process of becoming socially recognized in the first place, or eminent for one's creative achievements, may involve a whole other realm of motivations and skills—including ones not necessarily linked to creativity—along with the coincidence of factors in the environment, as mentioned. Therefore, rather than focus on this very tiny, although important, handful of eminent humanity, we will now turn to the many millions of other people living in this country alone, and inquire about their everyday creativity.

III. TYPOLOGY OF RELATIONS BETWEEN CREATIVITY AND PATHOLOGY

Indeed, there is no one single road to creativity. People differ in a great many ways from each other. In a 1981 monograph, Richards gave five types of direct and indirect association between creativity and psychopathology (see Table I). With the first two types, aspects of psychopathology can either directly or indirectly *raise the odds* of creative accomplishment. With the next two types, creative accomplishment in turn either directly or indirectly raises the odds of psychopathology. In the last type, a third factor independently raises the odds of both psychopathology and creativity. Here, the focus is more on creative *process* and *person* than creative *product*, although all of these are implicated, and the environment for creativity, or *press*, remains a critical background factor. These general causes are not mutually exclusive and, for a particular creative person, they may be multiple and overlapping.

Examples of each typology level follow.

1. **Direct effects of pathology on creativity:** Psychological problems may become transformed into creative *content*, as in drama drawing on Freud's Oedipus Complex, or may yield a more creative *process*, as in the availability of looser associations with clinical mood elevation.

2. **Indirect effects of pathology on creativity:** Feeling "different" and somehow handicapped over the years may stimulate qualities in some people including greater independence, risk-taking, and a desire to overcome—a style facilitating creative activity; addition-

Table I   Relations between Aspects of Creativity and Pathology or of Creativity and Health

Symbols for pathology and creativity *	Type of relationship *	Applied to health and creativity
$P > C$	1. Pathology contributes to creativity directly	$H \to C$
$P > T > C$	2. Pathology contributes to creativity through a third factor	$H \to T \to C$
$C > P$	3. Creativity contributes to pathology directly	$C \to H$
$C > T > P$	4. Creativity contributes to pathology through a third factor	$C \to T \to H$
$C < T > P$	5. A third factor contributes to both independently	$C \leftarrow T \to H$

*It is understood that some *aspect* of pathology influences some *aspect* of creativity, and so forth. Note that the symbol *T* stands for a separate third factor (or for multiple factors) that mediate an indirect relationship. Adapted from: R. Richards (1990), *Creativity Research Journal*, 3, p. 320.

ally, he or she may undergo "occupational drift," finally leading to a work setting (for instance, in the arts) more accepting of deviancy, bizarre thoughts and behavior, erratic performance, or inattention to time and other constraints.

3. **Direct effects of creativity on pathology:** Unearthing of conflicts in creative activity may lead to intolerable anxiety in some people, and direct decompensation, or stress related psychosomatic illness.

4. **Indirect effects of creativity on pathology:** Conflict from creative work may gradually draw certain people into pathological escape or attempts to limit anxiety, for instance through substance abuse. As an additional example, the creative nonconformist may provoke profound societal disapproval that, in turn, could lead to stress and decompensation.

5. **Third factor which affects both creativity and pathology:** Examples here include, first, *biological* factors (for instance, a genetic liability that runs strongly in families for the bipolar spectrum of presentations); such factors could enhance cognition, affect, and motivation for creative activity on the one hand (see later), yet also lead to great suffering. Then there are *environmental* factors, including the all too prevalent early childhood abuse; abuse may spark forms of creative expression for some people, but may readily lead to posttraumatic stress disorder, and to clinical depressions with which trauma has a very high comorbidity.

In the next two sections, this article will deal with certain of these situations. The same five-part typology will then be used to look at associations between creativity and *health*. Do note that Arnold Ludwig adapted this same five-part typology to clarify patterns of, and reasons for, alcohol abuse among eminent creative people who had indulged. The reasons can be multiple and complex. Although many other authors have also noted elevated alcohol or substance abuse among eminent artists, such use is not the rule, and is surely not prerequisite. Ludwig's and most other authors' conclusion is that substance abuse is more apt to harm creativity than to help it.

In general, it is important to note the significant concurrence or *comorbidity* of mood disorders and substance abuse. At times, this perhaps represents a misguided attempt at self-medication and symptom relief. Ludwig has also discussed high rates of early abuse and posttraumatic stress, along with elevated rates of depression, notably among eminent female creative writers. Faced with all this pathology, it is important

once again to recognize that eminent and everyday creators represent two different types of populations that should not be equated automatically with each other.

In sections below, the discussion turns sequentially to issues of creativity and (a) mood disorders in everyday life (where as much as 5% of the population may be affected); (b) overcoming personal adversity; and (c) furthering personal development and enhancing societal health.

IV. MOOD DISORDERS AND CREATIVITY

Do our moods affect our creativity? Absolutely. We can end up learning much about this from the study of mood disorders. This may even tell us something about why these disorders are so prevalent in the first place, and have persisted down through evolution.

A. Several Typology Levels at Once

Here one is dealing with, at minimum, the first, second, and last levels of the typology of creativity and psychopathology (Table I), in a situation of potential overlap. First, do mood swings directly affect the extent to which we creatively process information? Second, do they indirectly influence "something else" that ends up in turn facilitating creativity?

Thirdly, does the risk—and this is very important—including those genetic and/or familial environmental factors of vulnerability that make mood disorders more likely (for indeed they do run quite strongly in families), do these factors also sometimes lead independently to creativity by a separate path? The discussion below starts with this third possibility, focusing on everyday creativity and *bipolar mood disorders*.

B. Creativity as a Compensatory Advantage

A key term here is *compensatory advantage*. For it appears there may sometimes be another side—in individuals or in families—to the picture of pain and uncertainty involved in having abnormally high or low mood swings. One classic example of familial compensatory advantage in biology is found in sickle cell anemia. The homozygote, the person who inherits from both parents, has a terrible anemia, severe suffering, often early death. The heterozygote, however, who inherits from one parent only, may have a mild and even insignificant anemia. Plus, there is the compensatory advantage: resistance to malaria.

A genetic or genetic-environmental model for bipolar disorders would likely be more complex. Yet it is important to consider the compensatory advantage possibility—one that may even redefine some of what we consider "deviant" or "pathological." This may suggest new treatment approaches for those in pain, and even help us to understand the evolutionary significance of mood disorders. After all, if creativity is (or is associated with) a "reproductive advantage," one affecting selection and evolutionary fitness, it cannot depend entirely upon a tiny handful of eminent creators, however remarkable they may be. It must operate at the grass roots level—at the level of everyday creativity.

C. Avoiding Design Traps and False Conclusions

It is worth looking closely at one key study to highlight both the results and some design safeguards that, when unheeded, have limited other studies. (Other research which supports these findings is mentioned later.) This was the first formal study of connections between mood disorders and real-life everyday creativity—here defined very broadly in terms of all manner of life's activities. The work was done by Ruth Richards, Dennis Kinney, and associates, in conjunction with Seymour Kety's Danish study of mood disorders; this connection gave the advantage of extensive and rigorous clinical and interview data on subjects and many family members, gathered by an international team of investigators, without prejudice to creativity. The issue: If you start with patients and relatives, and look at whatever creativity may come up, however it may be expressed, compared to other people, will there be a creative advantage?

In fact, a creative advantage *was* found, and not necessarily for the most ill. This fit with an hypothesized *inverted-U* model—a little is good, but a lot isn't necessarily as helpful— regarding aspects of psychopathology. Who was studied? Manic-depressive, cyclothymes, their "psychiatrically normal" relatives, and control subjects who were either "normal," or carried a diagnosis, but who had no mood disorder them-

selves or in their families. (It takes sensitive study of many relatives to make this statement.) What was found? First, overall, people at risk for bipolar disorders *were* found to have higher creativity, on the average, compared to others lacking this risk.

Yet, breaking this down, the highest creativity was not found in the manic-depressives (although certain individuals did excel, and we cannot say there wasn't an unrealized potential, in general). The main advantage was in those with milder mood swings, the cyclothymes (including some people today who would be called bipolar II). There was also one more group that emerged as a surprise.

D. More Than Normal

The surprise was that a similar creativity was also suggested in the *psychiatrically normal* relatives of bipolars. It was not normalcy that made the difference, because the effect did not show up in the normal control subjects. Perhaps it was a subclinical *hypomania* or another clinical complex, or perhaps it was something else altogether!

This is important indeed: If mood disorders are relevant to creativity, it is not necessarily the pain and suffering that are making the difference—that are facilitating the creative results. On the contrary, it may be something much more subtle, more subclinical—or maybe not *clinical* at all. We are often so busy sniffing out abnormality, that we fail to look at what is going *right* with people who come in for help. Never mind what may be exceptional, and hold that promise of unusual talent, never mind contribution to society.

We shall return to this around issues of *state vs. trait* effects, and ways in which such findings may be important for all of us, mood disordered or not.

It is significant here that *"peak"* lifetime creativity was assessed, and that it was sought across area of endeavor. Assessments were made using *The Lifetime Creativity Scales,* which were developed and validated for this research, and were based on the originality of everyday real-life accomplishments at work and at leisure. The underlying rationale involved a creative *style* or *disposition toward originality,* thought to run in certain mood-disordered families. This disposition might come out in a variety of ways, depending upon the needs and interests of the person; it is surely a more adaptive capability to have—and to have running in families—than one that, let us say, pertains only to visual creation. The *sine qua non* of adaptation involves coping with the unknown.

Indeed, when Frank Barron and others studied eminent creative persons across fields in well-known studies at the Institute of Personality Assessment and Research at the University of California, Berkeley, they concluded that originality was habitual with highly creative persons—reflecting basically "what they were like" in general. This is not to deny the importance to creativity of special abilities, for instance the spatial ability of Rembrandt or the musical ability of Bach. Yet such special abilities can be directed toward less creative ends, as well as more creative ends. One artist might experiment, explore, take risks, and break rules, while another simply reproduces styles and themes, and works firmly within a school. It is one thing to copy a Rembrandt, and another thing entirely to *be* a Rembrandt.

In casting a wide net for creativity—and especially if not to miss any unusual or erratic creativity—the "peak" approach to measurement can be important. We all have our good years and bad years, our times of rich or limited opportunity, breaks, resources, or inspiration. Such is all the more true, perhaps, for some mood-disordered persons. Here, the goal was to pinpoint the maximum realization of creative potential in a major lifetime enterprise, and avoid missing remarkable achievements through use of some misleading average. The "peak" measure highlighted the very best each person had done, and discounted the rest.

It's also critical that subjects were chosen only by personal and family clinical history—and without any attention to what they had or had not been doing creatively. One is dealing then with a cross-section of creative possibility—with all of us and what we may choose to do. The picture isn't artificially narrowed to artists, writers, and so on. Yet, given this, we need somehow to capture the creativity of that cross-section, all at once, and without losing any pieces of the picture. Here is a creative homemaker, auto mechanic, parent, entrepreneur, and landscaper—wherever the creativity may emerge, we must be waiting.

It is also important that all assessments were made by people completely "blind" to, or unaware of, irrelevant or potentially biasing information. People making diagnoses knew nothing of subjects' creativity, and vice versa. If one were interviewing a bipolar person, might

one look more carefully for creativity, even despite one's best intentions? It is best to avoid such unintentional bias before it can even arise.

E. Related Findings and Broad Potential Applicability

Other research supports and extends such findings of compensatory advantage. Interestingly, this includes Hans Eysenck's work, linking creativity with his so-called psychoticism dimension (this pertains to unusual, but not necessarily psychotic, thinking). Psychoticism is linked in a curvilinear way, and its optimum level is intermediate (again this does not mean one is psychotic). Studies by David Schuldberg and others have associated creativity with hypomanic-like states of mild mood elevation in general college populations. Findings of Hagop Akiskal and others with patients are consistent with higher creativity in bipolar II than I disorders (involving mild mood elevations vs. full manic-depressive pictures, respectively), consistent too with results on eminent creators, and raising even further questions about mood *states* most conducive to creativity. Interestingly, normal relatives of bipolars have even shown greater achievement generally than relatives of controls, and there is also some support which Kay Jamison reviews for an above average socioeconomic status in families with a history of bipolar disorders.

It is important how common such mood-linked phenomena might be. A compensatory advantage involving creativity could affect a rather large segment of society. At one pole, Akiskal and colleagues estimate that as much as 4 to 5% of the population may have a history of a mood disorder related to an underlying genetic liability for bipolar disorders. (One should note here that manifestations of a bipolar family history go beyond the bipolar "spectrum" marked by what we have termed bipolar I and II disorders, or cyclothymia. It includes persons with major or minor depressions and no obvious mood elevations at all and, furthermore, these "pure" depressive cases are even more numerous than the bipolar ones. It is important that one preliminary study found higher creativity in "pure" depressives with, rather than without, a positive family history of bipolar disorder.)

Finally, let us not forget the psychiatrically normal relatives. Should each mood disordered person have only one normal relative carrying a bipolar liability or risk, we might be talking about even 8 to 10% of the population—a remarkable number of people who might have a heretofore unrecognized creative compensatory advantage. This is an advantage that could perhaps be built upon more, both in early development and later intervention, to benefit both: (a) the development of creativity—to explicitly realize creative potential and/or (b) mechanisms to protect one against or help cope with psychiatric disorders. Much more work is needed on these important questions.

We now look further at traits and states.

V. DOES IT MATTER IF YOU'RE IN A GOOD MOOD? STATE VS. TRAIT ISSUES

What in fact do such mood disordered people *say*? What about their states makes them *feel* more creative? We asked this of bipolars regarding everyday creativity, and the most common response was: a mildly high mood. (There nonetheless was a minority who preferred to create when depressed or in another state—people do indeed differ).

Regarding mood elevation, people's reasons fell into three general areas identified as: *positive feelings* (including confidence and enthusiasm), *spontaneous exuberance* (including expansiveness and euphoria), and a *cognitive facility* (including rapid thinking and fluent associations). Even persons with extreme mood swings didn't believe the extremes were the key states. Findings are consistent with Jamison's research with both everyday and eminent creators, and is with Andreasen's and others' anecdotal reports of eminent creators. Such findings can be considered from the viewpoint of the "psychopathology leads directly to creativity" category in Table I.

A. Indirect and Long-Term Effects: "Affective Integration"

One should keep in mind that other processes may readily coexist. For bipolar individuals, for instance, consider a mediated example, proposed by Richards. Here, an ongoing expectation that mood state will *change* could have lasting effects on cognitive style, with two classes of effect. First are effects on *creative cognition,* in which a richer mood-linked coding and cross-linking of material in memory storage could occur, along with a dilution of state-dependent learning (or learning that is linked only to a particular affective state). Hence, a richer creative repository could be created, along with more varied means of accessing it. Second are effects on *motivation for creativity,* where an active hypomanic "flight from depression" could be transformed into a creative coping strategy. If one expects that mood will change anyway, why not actively help this to occur? There could be a weakening of common human tendencies toward positive mood maintainance ("what a nice day . . . the sun feels good . . . the meeting should go well . . ."), and negative mood repair ("that's awful . . . I can't stand it . . . I'm not going to think about that."), in favor of a more conscious and accurate reading of one's emotional state, and perhaps also an intention actively to transform one's negative moods whenever possible. The distorting functions of positive mood maintainance and negative mood repair we all use could seem greatly less useful in a lifetime of moodswings where, at times, highs and lows follow each other like waves on the ocean.

Whatever the general pattern or explanation (see Table I), one should keep in mind that potential mechanisms may occur together as well as separately. They may also differ between people, and even differ within a person from one time to another. Creativity can be as individual as the experience of each one of us.

B. Trait and State Effects: Overinclusion Works in All of Us

One needs first to distinguish *trait and state* effects. Here one is distinguishing transitory *state* of mind, and not an ongoing, stable *trait* or a fluctuating condition to which as a whole we could apply an identifier, such as the name "bipolar disorder." (Indeed, it may also be misleading to apply a static label to a spectrum of states such as the word "depression" encompasses. These may differ dramatically from one person to the next, or from one year to another). We begin here with flndings that apply to all of us, mood disordered or not. Notably, Alice Isen and associates found that even a slight mood elevation—from watching a brief comedy film, for example—can directly increase creative problem solving in a general sample of research subjects, as well as increase stylistic modes of information processing such as associative originality or overinclusion.

Interestingly, overinclusive categorization has been

related to creative thinking by other investigators too. This involves the tendency (as part of one's *cognitive style,* or habitual mode of information processing reflecting underlying personality trends) to make errors of commission rather than omission in classifying information. In classifying objects as "square," for instance, the more overinclusive person might go beyond equal-sided books, mats, or napkins, and other clear geometrical figures, to put in a postage stamp that wasn't quite square, a cube despite its three dimensions, or even an awkward "out of it" person who is known as a "square." Classification rules can include ones that are more vague, distant, or developmentally primitive.

Interestingly, there are some well-known tests of divergent or creative thinking, including J. P. Guilford's original groundbreaking tests of divergent production, and the widely used *Torrance Tests of Creative Thinking,* which are in effect scored for overinclusion. Common verbal divergent production scores for a question such as "Name as many round things as you can," include *fluency, flexibility,* and *originality*—three properties related to the number of responses, the number of types of responses, and their relative rarity.

In the spirit of the "square things" example above, imagine the task is to list a great many "round things." If one sticks to the likes of "wheel, tire, ring, saucer, ball," one won't get as many points for fluency as the person who goes on to append several less likely responses such as: "the impression a bouncing ball makes in sand, a cross-section of a finger, a smoke ring, a lasso's whirling motion," and so on. Such people are indeed throwing their mental lassos more broadly. (That statement counts too.) Overinclusive responses may also, as one may imagine, raise test scores for flexibility and originality.

C. Overinclusion and Mood Pathology

Perhaps not surprisingly, overinclusion has also been associated with psychopathology, and particularly with mania and bipolar mood elevation, as Nancy Andreasen, for one, has shown. Overinclusion is also related to the loose associations found in a manic condition; similar processes have been modeled in a neural net model of mania. Richards discusses such findings in terms of the potential for sudden creative insight in an edge-of-chaos model of emergent mental structures. Interestingly, overinclusion has also been featured centrally by Hans Eysenck in connection with his "psychoticism" dimension of personality. Psychoticism, in Eysenck's work, appears to bear a curvilinear relationship to creativity (i.e., it is helpful if one has neither too much psychoticism, nor not too little). It bears reemphasizing that psychoticism regards unusual thought which, at one extreme, might become psychotic; it is not a measure of psychotic thought per se.

It is revealing to look at clinical thought disorder as measured by the multivariate Thought Disorder Index of Johnston and Holzman. Using factor analysis, this group showed that manic thought disorder takes specific forms that can be distinguished, for instance, from patterns for schizophrenics. Here is an example of looseness, for instance, in response to a Rorschach inkblot used in the assessment: "Dark, darkness, lovemaking." Such statements might not work in a business meeting, but what about in a poem? One sees it is not necessarily what is said, but *why* it is said—when, where, and under what degree of conscious control—that may make the difference between a response that is disordered, and one that is creative.

D. Overinclusion Is Only One Factor

One must indeed beware; as Nancy Andreasen points out, an overinclusive creative person and an overinclusive manic person may show similarities, but differ in a great many ways. Required in addition are the abstract and cohesive forms of thought needed to control and shape the material toward creative ends—such strengths were found in Andreasen's writers much more (at that moment at least) than in the manics. This complex mix of mental functions may relate to what Kris originally called "regression in the service of the ego." One can tap into looser, perhaps more bizarre, more primitive, and more "preconscious," thought, but can one ultimately do this in a more deliberate and consciously controlled way?

This process relates as well to the high "ego strength" measured by MacKinnon, Barron and others at U.C. Berkeley in their "live-in assessment" studies of highly creative people across varied fields. This finding created a remarkable contrast with deviant scores found on other measures, which in themselves would have raised concerns of pathology. Creative writers, in fact, scored in the *top 15%* on virtually all scales of the Minnesota Multiphasic Personality Inventory, a well-known measure of psychopathology.

The notable exception was the high score for the healthy quality of ego strength. High ego strength scores are rarely found with such pathological profiles. One must keep in mind the high rates of mood disorders among writers, found with other samples by Andreasen and others. Perhaps some psychopathology is present. On the other hand, we should weigh in Barron's remark that these eminent individuals appeared both healthier and sicker than the population at large. On the positive side of the picture, this so-called deviancy of thought could reflect the openness, complexity, and lack of defensiveness found in the richest, and perhaps even the healthiest, creativity.

E. Expanding Our Views of Normality

One may recall the normal relatives of bipolar individuals who, in the work of Richards and associates, themselves showed an advantage for creativity. As it occured, Holzman and associates looked at thought disorder, not only in manics and other patients, but in their relatives as well. The key finding: There was qualitatively similar thought disorder—albeit more muted—in the first degree relatives of patients, including relatives who are not themselves clinically ill.

Surely this is not only fascinating, but vitally important. There is great need for further research. Yet it may still be underlined that *deviant ideas do not necessarily imply pathology*. Deviancy in itself may be good; it may be full of creative potential. Here is the nonconformist who will see where we cannot. Robert Albert and others have spoken to the evolutionary significance of creativity. Consider the importance of valuing the diversity we can all co-create, and the vast potential this may offer to us individually and together for adapting to changing environments and a changing world. Indeed, to coping in an endangered world. Rather than trying to normalize everyone toward some hypothetical ideal, we need to celebrate diversity, resist pathologizing, and expand the acceptable limits of normality.

VI. PERSONAL ADVERSITY AND CREATIVITY

What does it mean that so many exceptionally creative people, as in extensive studies by Victor and Mildred Goertzel of the most written about twentieth-century individuals, or Arnold Ludwig's historiographic work on eminent men and women, came from some sort of troubled beginnings? Here, the reference is not only to mood disorders, as above, or to other psychiatric problems, but to a diverse range of adversities including early loss of important figures, unhappy or conflicted childhoods, personal disability or illness, early trauma and abuse, poverty, and parental misfortunes including physical and psychiatric disorders. Were such troubled circumstances a spur, and if so, a necessary spur, for the creative risks and tenacity needed to alter the status quo at the highest level of influence?

Even if so—and more controlled studies are needed to clarify the relevance of troubled circumstances—how might this apply to the creativity of everyday life, which is typically much quieter and potentially more personal?

A. Freudian vs. Humanistic Views

As noted earlier, in a traditional Freudian view, creativity serves primarily to resolve inner conflict and to return the person to a less troubled state. The function is compensatory. In more humanistic views, views for instance of Abraham Maslow and Carl Rogers, the goal is a positive ongoing one, involving self-development, growth, and ultimately the transcendent potential of self-actualization.

This latter viewpoint predicts for the natural pursuit of creativity in the lives of most people. And it speaks once again to an essential—if not yet fully understood—role in our evolution, an evolution both of biological organisms and of the information and culture we generate.

But let us return to early adversity as pertains to everyday creativity. First, we know that not every traumatized child becomes creative; indeed the majority may be vastly more hurt than helped by their suffering. They may be much more likely to be vanquished without such countervailing advantages as role models, mentors, helpful and protecting figures, rich resources and advantages in the home and community, and educational and professional opportunities. Without advantages, many young people might never become aware of their strengths, their potential empowerment as an innovator, or specific ways in which they might transform their problems to personal and creative advantage.

B. Beware False Conclusions or Expecting Too Much

The point is worth an additional caution. The thought that "unhappy childhoods" might reveal some universal formula for creativity is not only a dangerous and potentially devastating error, but is structurally similar to the earlier error which can lead to painful misunderstandings of mood disorders and their thoughtless romanticization. Romanticization of adversity was of such concern to the Goerztels, that they explicitly warned parents not to take their results on eminent twentieth-century persons to suggest erroneously "mistreatment of children as a way of stimulating creativity." (See Richards' monograph in the bibliography).

Similarly, authors have been concerned that one not automatically expect high creative accomplishment from anyone who has a mood disorder. Again, if many creative writers have mood disorders, this does not mean that mood disorders automatically make one more creatively accomplished, either in writing, or in anything else. Well-meaning individuals and clinicians can create yet further unrealistic expectations and struggles for people who may already be overwhelmed by their lives. (On the other hand, it is conceivable that there may be some general advantages for creative *potential*, as in an *increased sensitivity* which Kay Jamison and others have linked with depression; such possibilities need further study.)

One sees here a curious flip-flop on the harmful stigmatizing of people with mental illness or difficulties. This time it is a too-ready attribution of something considered positive that may never arrive—creativity—where, with a little more clarity and understanding by researchers and clinicians, a real *potential* advantage might be unearthed and usefully encouraged to develop.

To comprehend this literature, it is clear one must be a critical reader. High creativity appears to be a result of the interaction of many personal, familial, and social factors—and these may also differ from creator to creator. Having some particular one of them may not even be necessary, and certainly not sufficient. If this strikes someone as bad news, the good news might be a confirmation of our uniquely variable life paths—indeed the birthplaces of creativity—where our innovations may emerge unexpectedly amidst varied conditions. This is testimony perhaps to the ubiquity of creativity. Indeed, as we shall soon see, among the many varied roads to creativity are ones that do appear healthy indeed.

VII. TYPOLOGY OF RELATIONS BETWEEN CREATIVITY AND HEALTH

This discussion, once again, begins with the creative confrontation of personal adversity. But this time we follow things further, past initial resolution into positive ongoing contributions to physical health and psychological openness. These, we assert, can also eventually lead to one's greater creative expression and efficacy, and finally to awareness of universal aspects of one's conflict joined to the ability to help others along with oneself.

A. The Typology

It is worth looking again at Table I, but this time at the typology of relationships between creativity and mental or physical *well-being*, framed in terms of health. Specific findings and writers are mentioned by way of example only and are by no means exhaustive. Yet with the references appended here, they may provide directions for further reading. A few examples also draw on situations already discussed.

1. Direct Effects of Health on Creativity

Psychological openness, lack of defensiveness, access to material at the threshold of consciousness, all can facilitate creative mental activity. This is supported by writings from many individuals, including Silvano Arieti, Karen Horney, C. G. Jung, Ernst Kris, Lawrence Kubie, Abraham Maslow, Rollo May, Anthony Storr, and others.

2. Indirect Effects of Health on Creativity

Greater openness and awareness may lead, longer term, to greater affective integration of contents in memory storage, as Richards has suggested, with a richer and more interconnected intellectual–emotional mix to draw on when creating, along with less mood-congruent storage and bounded–defended access, based on "positive mood-maintenance" or "negative mood repair." This fits with writings of Alice Isen on mood and schemas in memory, and by other writers in various contexts, including Kay Jamison, Arnold Ludwig, and David Schuldberg on bipolar disorders, and Mardi Horowitz, John Kihlstrohm, and Jerome Singer on mental organization and schemas generally.

Happily, one also sees hope for lowering risk of psychosomatic and physical symptomatology when energy isn't tied up in defensive activity, as supported for instance by the work of Jerome Singer on repression, David Spiegel on trauma or group support in cancer treatment, Ian Wickramesekera on mind-body disconnection and its somatic consequences, and James Pennebaker as discussed further below. One might question whether this will inevitably facilitate creativity. (For instance, mightn't this be more the case for everyday than eminent creativity, and depend as well on one's reasons for creative expression in the first place?) Yet in situations where this *is* the case, note that emergent creativity might be more greatly energized, advance again the healing process, and create a happy loop of positive feedback.

3. Direct Effects of Creativity on Health

Dramatic effects of creative confrontation of conflict have been shown to affect biological measures of health as well as decrease number of doctors visits in James Pennebaker's work on writing and self-disclosure, below. Think too about modalities such as creative visualization in healing, as used by Jeanne Achterberg, the embodied approaches of Ilene Serlin, or the creative reframing of Joan Borysenko along with the practice of mindfulness and relaxation training.

In a somewhat different vein, consider Stephanie Dudek's work with children, in which fewer aggressive impulses appeared in the presence of higher creativity. Sandra Russ' research linked children's creativity and play with greater openness to affect-laden themes, and involved both more primitive primary process thinking, and nonprimary process thinking. Creative women, in Ravenna Helson's work, were found to show a greater flexibility and evolution of self, rather than a rigidity of personality.

In addition, creative older persons were shown to have more flexible and open attitudes toward life transitions and factors of aging in the research of Gudmund Smith and Gunilla van der Meer. There are additional benefits for health and even longevity linked to flexible conceptual capacity, as in the "mindfulness" work of Ellen Langer. Finally, despite hard-to-talk-about carts and horses, and which come first in this correlational research—never mind philosophically!—the initial associations found by Mark Runco and colleagues between creativity and self-actualization are of interest, and deserve further study. [*See* AGGRESSION; PLAY.]

4. Indirect Effects of Creativity on Health

The integrated mental openness in (2), above, brings potential for resilience, for approaching a problem rather than avoiding it, for envisioning multiple transformations of the situation, and developing an empowerment born of past successes. Rollo May has written eloquently on this in *The Courage to Create;* Mardi Horowitz, James Pennebaker and others have done related studies on adults, and Anthony, Garmezy, and Rutter on children, although not necessarily framed in the context of creativity. This also fits with Jung's writings on the need to face one's unconscious "shadow" side for ongoing personality development and growth. In addition, by analogy with biological processes, Ruth Richards has proposed an acquired immunity model as another type of prototype; here, success in coping with more manageable situations in one's past leads to increased efficacy in the present, with features including increased confidence and resilience—this is a form of risk-taking learned small that now looms large and powerful (see also below). Frederick Flach, John Gedo, Kay Jamison, Arnold Ludwig, Albert Rothenberg, Tobi Zausner, and others have addressed historical or current cases of this.

5. Third Factor That Affects both Health and Creativity

Take, for instance, optimism, which may encourage creative achievement and has been linked with health by people including Martin Seligman and Christopher Peterson. People vary in optimism in general, but this may also be a special instance where people at risk for bipolar mood disorders (including normal relatives) may cycle through positive mood states that facilitate optimism, health, and creative risk taking. [*See* OPTIMISM, MOTIVATION, AND MENTAL HEALTH.]

One should note, in general, how compelling this is; not only can health facilitate creativity, but under the right conditions, pathology may facilitate creativity as well. When defined in broad everyday terms, creativity may be as natural as breathing. Unless one's creativity is blocked through personal trauma or extreme social suppression, it may find at least some way to emerge, like a flowering plant pushing through a break in the pavement. Furthermore, one's creating is apt to leave psychological openness in its wake, with a sounder personal health, and the ability to respond to yet further challenges.

VIII. PERSONAL WELL-BEING AND BROADER PATTERNS AND PURPOSE

Should one have any doubt about the effects of creative confrontation, consider one of James Pennebaker's studies, this one with Janice Kiecolt-Glaser, and Ronald Glaser. Students were asked to write about one of their most severe problems, in fact one they had never or rarely discussed with anyone. Meanwhile a control group wrote about something much more neutral such as the appearance of their shoes. This went on for only 20 minutes at a time—and after only four sessions, some remarkable results appeared. First of all, differences were found between the first group and controls on two measures of T-cell function; there was a difference in immune systems between the two groups. In addition, over the subsequent 6 weeks, the first group made fewer visits to the student health center, showed a lower systolic blood pressure, and lower subjective distress. Other studies are consistent with various of these findings. [*See* PSYCHONEUROIMMUNOLOGY.]

A. Creative Confrontation—And a Resultant Acquired Immunity?

What exactly is going on here? Take the Pennebaker study, for instance. For one thing, these subjects who never told anyone much about their problems might not have been entirely honest or direct within themselves either. Suddenly, in their writing, the situation is revealed before them for more rational and conscious analysis—happily coming forth in a creative context where the difficulty may be described, managed, and tranformed, at least at a symbolic level. Mental walls and barriers may thereby be able to yield in one's mind, with psychic energy freed for better purpose. Perhaps there can occur as well a subtle sense of social support, based on the fact that subjects "shared," at least, with a piece of paper. Now, certainly, someone else *could* read about the situation. It is of interest what one person later reported about a traumatic childhood situation: "Now I don't feel like

I even have to think about it because I got it off my chest."

How might this experience carry forth into the future? Certainly the resulting mental openness can persist, as may a greater awareness that creative confrontation can work. Here are innovative solutions to one's pain, and an appealing route that can even carry the pleasures and rewards of creative insight and transformation. Furthermore, here are specific loci of resistance that have yielded, and strategies that have worked, for instance, in situations of abuse, or conflict, or confusion, or illness, and might be modified and used again in the future.

One can here find the analogy to biological immunization (as for instance in developing acquired immunity to whooping cough or measles), where a measured exposure to a pathogen allows antibodies to build and protects against future assaults. In psychological terms, such acquired immunity might be even more powerful than this—consider the general human potential for generalization and transfer of learning, and the important overall capacities of resilience and confidence that may result from creative confrontation, successfully carried through. Creative confrontation may have multiple effects on both creative *ability* and creative *motivation*. This too deserves much more study.

B. Sharing One's Discoveries—And One's Humanity

Now think about creators and writers who have already addressed their problems, but continue to write! Here for instance is Kay Jamison, who chronicled her own manic-depressive illness and her difficulty coping as a professional, not only for her own sake (she could have used a private journal) but to help others as well. How brave indeed was her writing of *An Unquiet Mind*; here she was, a psychologist of international renown, confessing that she had at times been completely overwhelmed by a terrible illness. Or what about William Styron, writing in *Darkness Visible* about his own depression and despair. Why after all does this work appeal, and fascinate? Surely not only because of each author's renown, but because the work also potentially touches every one of us. We too have our terrible secrets (whatever they may be) and at times may feel a similar hopelessness. There is a universal theme here, a human core, that the creator has tapped into. When we resonate with this message, we can all become part of the picture.

Here is where the momentum of problem solving can motivate the helping of others, and with even further satisfactions and rewards. Celeste Rhodes has proposed a potential movement of creative purpose from deficiency needs to self-actualization, based on Maslow's needs hierarchy (this moves stepwise upward from physiological needs, including food and warmth, through safety, love, and esteem needs, through self-actualization; some satisfaction of the lower needs are prerequisite to ongoing movement and growth). Conceivably growth will proceed organically and naturally when certain "blocks" are removed. In this model, the meeting of deficiency needs (including love, acceptance, and self-acceptance) through creative work can also bring—and can begin to instruct one in—contributions at higher levels of abstraction and creative contribution, as more universal themes are tapped. This can benefit others beyond the immediate creator. There may be higher levels of intrinsic motivation, with movement toward self-actualization, and more transcendent experience as well. This is an extremely important point, and the preliminary work above on self-actualization remains one important beginning.

C. Are Problems Needed to Stimulate Creativity?

What if no problems are to be solved? What happens then to creativity? Does it still flourish and grow when all is well? Freud might have had some questions about this. Yet we are talking about the creativity of everyday life (and one should recall, things may be different for eminent creativity, in the arts in particular). In a humanistic view, creativity serves our ongoing needs for growth, development, and an expanding capacity and personal contribution. It can bring great pleasure in the results, never mind an enterprise that can logically continue and build on itself. Why indeed would it stop?

Consider additional personality traits related to highly creative people, including preference for complexity, tolerance of ambiguity, openness to experience, flexibility, unconventional thinking, independence of judgment, intuitiveness, and a preference for challenge and risk taking. Such a profile predicts for the ongoing pursuit of creativity for its own sake, and perhaps for much of the time.

Similarly, in an evolutionary view, if creativity is seen as essential to survival—individually and culturally—this also speaks to the pursuit, and enjoyment, of creativity across a great many of life's situations, as a matter of routine, and without a prerequisite problem to be solved. Again we are not talking about painting a masterpiece—that is, about exceptional achievement. Here the concern may be more with getting to work, keeping one's job, raising one's children, maturing in one's marriage, enjoying one's friends, thriving in one's hobbies. These are the things we all do—at least when we're not watching TV or pursuing other mindless activities.

D. Chaos, Complexity, and a New Order

Finally, from a systems point of view, or the perspective of chaos theory, our roles in generating novelty in our own neighborhoods may all be part of a larger evolving social picture, a dynamic of emergent structures. At key times and places, things may change very rapidly—and perhaps creatively—across a broad field of influence in response to very small inputs. We are not isolates walking along a linear yardstick, but cohorts dancing within a complex and ever-changing field. Within this dynamic may lie perspectives on some serious global problems, as well as on the health of a more broadly conceived whole.

In this regard, Ilya Prigogine has noted how, "our vision of nature is undergoing a radical change toward the multiple, the temporal, and the complex . . . to the emergence of new conceptual structures that now appear essential to our understanding of the physical world—the world that includes us." Complex dynamic systems have been proposed and modeled in a great many areas in the physical, biological, psychological, and social sciences. Creativity researchers are being drawn increasingly to this, and have addressed issues including creative insight, and the effects of life's turning points, based on metaphor and reasoning drawn from chaos theory.

E. Considerable Social Benefit

A creative style as a way of life can push us outward to join with each other in the moment, in shared meaning and communication. At best, it can unite us in universals that have more to do with our humanity than with the constraints of our identifications, be they with nationality, ethnicity, gender, politics, or socioeconomic status. We can work to become more whole within ourselves. We can move to heal the false dichotomies of intellect and emotion, science and art, within ourselves and our culture—and maybe even learn where we are going in an overly mechanized and intellectualized age. Imagine if we could learn to thrive on process, on ambiguity, multiple possibilities, flexibility and surprise. Isn't this just what we need in a rapidly changing world, and an exponentially shrinking one?

Yet there is often a price for challenging the "certainties" in one's inner world, and in the often resistant world without. How upsetting the discoveries can be at times; how readily one may be labeled deviant, different, strange—or disruptive, foolish, and uncooperative. If this discussion is about health, we should not stop with the person, but look at the greater context, and its norms. We need to value our diverse possibilities, as well as encourage those courageous people who challenge us and let us grow in our own ways, be they parents, teachers, mentors, supervisors, employers, or poets and playwrights. Everyday creativity often goes underrecognized and underrewarded. Yet the more we encourage the creator and lower the external resistance, the more flexible, open, adaptive, and creative our society can become—and the more healthy.

BIBLIOGRAPHY

Special Issues on Creativity and Health. (1990). *Creativity Research Journal,* 3(Nos. 3 & 4).

Goleman, D., & Gurin, J. (Eds.). (1993). *Mind-body medicine: How to use your mind for better health.* Yonkers, NY: Consumer Reports Books.

Goodwin, F. K., & Jamison, K. R. (1990). *Manic-depressive illness.* New York: Oxford University Press.

Gruber, H., & Wallace, D. (Guest Eds.). (1993). Special Issue: Creativity in the Moral Domain. *Creativity Research Journal,* 6 (Nos. 1 & 2).

Montuori, A., & Purser, R. (1997, and in press). *Social creativity: An exploration of the social, historical and political factors in creativity and innovation* (Vols. 1–3). Creskill, NJ: Hampton Press.

Pennebaker, J. W. (Ed.). (1995). *Emotion, disclosure, and health.* Washington, DC: American Psychological Association.

Richards, R. (1981). Relationships between creativity and psychopathology: An evaluation and interpretation of the evidence. *Genetic Psychology Monographs, 103,* 261–324.

Runco, M. (Ed.) (1996). Special Issue Creativity from Childhood through Adulthood: The Developmental Issues. *New Directions for Child Development, 72.* San Francisco: Jossey-Bass.

Runco, M., & Richards, R. (1998). *Eminent creativity, everyday creativity, and health.* Greenwich, CT: Ablex Publishing Corp.

Shaw, M., & Runco, M. A. (Eds.). (1994). *Creativity and affect.* Norwood, NJ: Ablex.

Sternberg, R. J. (Ed.). (1988). *The nature of creativity: Contemporary psychological perspectives.* New York: Cambridge University Press.

Criminal Behavior

Joan McCord

Temple University

Index Crimes Crimes that are listed as Part I serious offenses by the Federal Bureau of Investigation.

Mala in se An act that is wrong in itself, without regard to whether the law has stipulated illegality. These are presumed to be wrong in every culture.

Mala prohibita An act or omission that is wrong only because it is prohibited or directed by the law.

Mens rea Having a guilty mind, the intent to harm that is required for most crimes.

Response Rates The proportion of those in a sample who actually respond to questions or participate in interviews.

Victimization Being the victim of a crime.

CRIMINAL BEHAVIOR includes theft and murder, trespassing and begging, destroying property belonging to someone else, and public drinking when under the age permitted. Criminal behavior includes buying and selling sex or illegal drugs, charging usurious rates for loans, and writing checks without sufficient funds. It includes political corruption and police abuse of power. In short, criminality includes a broad range of behavior.

I. WHAT IS CRIMINAL BEHAVIOR?

Just about everyone has broken some law at some time. Yet most people do not regularly break the law, nor do most people act in ways that are generally considered to be criminal.

Typically, investigators of criminal behavior select subsets of criminals, those who break laws frequently or in ways that are considered to be especially serious. Criminal behavior has been classified in a variety of ways. Some of these focus on the nature of crimes and others focus on the criminals.

One classification is based on whether or not a crime has involved only consenting participants. According to this classification, crimes such as drug use, public drunkenness, and sexual crimes between consenting adults (e.g., homosexual acts and prostitution) fall into one category and are considered "victimless" crimes. Although a drug addict may be a victim of family and social conditions that explain the addiction, a choice to use drugs does not typically involve coercion. Although families of public drunkards may suffer greatly, drunkards are not typically drinking *in order* to injure them.

Judgments that behavior among consenting parties may be criminal reflect moral judgments not shared by all members of society. Victimless crimes tend to gain public attention when the legality of behavior accepted as a right by some has been condemned by others. Despite the fact that there may be injuries involved, abortion, euthanasia, and the sale of intoxi-

Encyclopedia of Mental Health
Volume 1

635

cating liquors have been considered crimes without victims

Critics argue that victimless crimes ought not be crimes at all. Such critics note that defining behavior without victims as criminal amounts to a misguided attempt to legislate morality. Perhaps the most eloquent of the critics is John Stuart Mill who, in his treatise *On Liberty,* published in 1859, cautioned against the use of government power to restrict freedom for any reason other than preventing harm to others. Mill specifically mentioned that neither physical nor moral harm to oneself legitimizes restrictions. Proponents of legislation to regulate behavior that does not clearly injure others argue that, because the state has an interest in preserving the health and well-being of its citizens, it should legally condemn behavior that is harmful even when the only victim is the perpetrator.

Another category system that has been widely used separates white collar crimes from other offenses. In 1939, Edwin Sutherland introduced the concept of "white collar crime" to refer to illegal practices of large corporations, practices that included fraud, violations of trust, false advertising, infringement, unfair competition, and coercive labor practices. Sutherland identified such behavior as criminal even though it was not normally punished by imprisonment or brought to the attention of the public. Sutherland used illegality and potential punishment as criteria, considering crime to be "behavior which is prohibited by the State as an injury to the State and against which the State may react, at least as a last resort, by punishment" (p. 46). His work on white collar crime brought into question theories that attributed crime to poverty and located criminal behavior almost exclusively among the lower classes. In addition, Sutherland believed that white collar criminals falsified claims that crimes were caused by family dysfunction or mental disorder.

White collar crimes have subsequently been defined as crimes typically committed by the politically powerful or economically advantaged. White collar crimes are linked to occupational roles and usually involve a violation of trust. Laws proscribing behavior defined as white collar crime are typically *mala prohibita,* in contrast with index crimes, many of which are considered *mala in se.* Examples of white collar crime include tax evasion, consumer fraud, restraint of trade, and embezzlement. Those accused of white collar crime may be tried in special courts or through administrative hearings that focus on remedial action rather than punishment. White collar crimes need not require *mens rea.*

A related category identifies organized crimes or illegal enterprises. Whereas studies of white collar crimes have typically focused on crimes committed by large organizations and respected individuals, studies of organized crime and illegal enterprises focus on criminal activities such as money laundering, bootlegging, extortion, and gambling that are carried out by the relatively poor who participate in small-scale, often informal, enterprises. Illegal enterprises seem to develop in response to demands for illicit goods or services. Historically, studies of organized crime have assumed that the underworld was composed of hierarchically structured crime families, but recent careful examinations of illegal enterprises suggest that they are more likely to consist of partnerships and syndicates.

Within formal criminal justice agencies, crimes are typically divided into felonies and misdemeanors. Felonies are more serious than misdemeanors.

The Federal Bureau of Investigation provides information about crimes known to the police through two indices, known as Part I and Part II offenses. Part I offenses (index crimes) are divided into violent and property crimes. Part I violent crimes include murder and nonnegligent manslaughter, forcible rape, robbery, and aggravated assault. Part I property crimes include burglary, larceny-theft, motor vehicle theft, and arson (which was added in 1978). Males are more likely than females to commit Part I crimes.

Part II offenses are less carefully monitored than Part I offenses. Part II offenses include simple assaults and attempted assaults without weapons or those causing little injury; forgery and counterfeiting; fraud; embezzlement; buying, receiving, or possessing stolen property; vandalism; carrying or possessing weapons; prostitution and commercialized vice; sex offenses other than forcible rape, prostitution, or commercialized vice; drug abuse violations including unlawful possession, use, growing, sale, and manufacture; offenses against family and children, including nonsupport, neglect, desertion, and abuse; driving under the influence of alcohol or narcotics; violations of state liquor laws other than drunkenness and driving under the influence; drunkenness (excluding driving under the influence); disorderly conduct; vagrancy, including vagabondage, begging, and loitering; and violations of state or local laws not mentioned elsewhere—with the exception of traffic offenses. Attempts to commit many of the above crimes are also included. In addition, suspicion (no specific offense), violations of curfew and loitering laws aimed at juveniles, and running away from home as a minor are tabulated as Part II offenses.

The typologies of crime illuminate crime patterns and provide a basis for comparisons. Perhaps surprisingly, however, attempts to show the development of specialization in offending have been only moderately successful. Most studies show that people who break laws with any degree of regularity break laws of several types. Such specialization as has been found seems to come from offenders restricting their repertoires as they age.

The pattern of offending—with criminality most prevalent among the young, and most criminals committing more than one type of crime—has led to theories that criminality represents delayed maturation, acceptance of values ("definitions of situations") that are generally antisocial, a lack of attachment to families and schools, absence of social control, and lack of self-control. Studies show that criminals tend to have had rejecting or neglecting parents, they tend to have friends who also are criminals, they typically do poorly in school, and their work histories tend to be irregular. In addition, they often come from families in which there are other criminals and in which alcoholism is prevalent.

When classifications are based on characteristics of criminals, typologies refer to whether the criminal committed crimes alone or with others, whether or not the offender has a history of crime, and the age of the offender at the time of the first offense. Juvenile delinquents who commit at least some of their crimes with others tend to be more violent than those who commit all of their crimes alone. Recidivist criminals tend to be at greater risk for re-offending than first-time offenders.

Offenders whose crimes began when they were under the age of 10 have been found to be particularly prone to committing many crimes. There is disagreement about the reason for this relationship between an early age of first offense and a persistent record of offending. T. E. Moffitt has suggested that the early offenders are at particularly high biological risk for becoming criminals. Alternative interpretations include the possibility that young offenders come from particularly difficult families or that their early behavior re-

sults in a labelling process that helps to create associations with peers who reinforce antisocial values and behavior. These younger delinquents are those most likely to be diagnosed as having conduct disorder.

II. TYPES OF EVIDENCE

At least since the nineteenth century, when Adolphe Quételet pioneered the use of crime rates as a social indicator of the health of society, measures of crime have been subjected to important debates. These debates center on what to count as crimes and whose perspective to use for recording. Not only do laws change, thus shifting the nature of crimes themselves, but also public tolerance for various types of conduct shifts, creating elastic borders for the identification of particular crimes. Intentionally depriving another of life has been considered a crime (*mala in se*) at least since the Ten Commandments. Yet at various periods in American history, widespread killing of sheepherders, Mexicans, native American Indians, Blacks, Mormons, and Chinese—among others—were not counted as criminal acts. During the mid-nineteenth century, infanticide and drunken violence punctuated urban life. Yet only a small proportion of these offenses were brought to the attention of authorities. Responding apparently to the civilizing effects of industrialization and urbanization, rates of violence declined during the late nineteenth and early twentieth centuries.

Crime rates can provide a crude index of the social health of a society. Measurement of criminality across cultures is particularly difficult, however, because nations count different types of behavior as criminal and few are systematic in collecting information. For example, Sri Lanka considers accidental deaths from firearms and motor vehicle crashes, as well as intentional murder, as criminal homicide. Some countries record a crime if police receive a report that one has been committed, others only if additional investigations indicate that a crime has occurred, others only if a perpetrator has been found, and still others only after a conviction.

Information about crime rates clearly has political import. The difficulty of standardizing measurement and the sensitive nature of the information has resulted in problems for those who would evaluate the impact of population shifts, wars, industrialization, or democratization on mental health as reflected in crime.

Dane Archer and Rosemary Gartner have attempted to overcome these problems by developing the Comparative Crime Data File (CCDF). The CCDF includes data from 110 nations and 44 cities around the world. The data use definitions provided by the countries themselves and cover different crimes and a variety of time periods, leaving to researchers the issues of comparability and validity.

Several surveys have been designed to measure violence cross-nationally. These show that the United States tends to be particularly prone to violence. For example, the Third United Nations Survey, carried out in 1986, gathered data for crimes reported to the police. Robbery, a personal violent offense, appeared to have been counted similarly among 23 of the reporting nations. Rates per 100,000 ranged from 1 in Cyprus to 223 in the United States.

Because official records are subject to political control, they are suspect when the focus is on discovering differences among nations. Furthermore, official records reflect reporting practices that, in turn, are functions of standards for conduct, faith in police, and proximity to a means for notifying officials that a crime has been committed.

Victim reports reflecting descriptions of specific acts can overcome some of the problems attached to official records. Under the auspices of the United Nations Interregional Crime and Justice Research Institute, researchers gathered information about victimization from 20 nations in 1989 or 1992 (with 8 nations participating in both surveys). The surveys used standardized questions and most countries used similar sampling techniques. Recommended sample sizes were small (1500 to 2000 interviews), and response rates were low (an average of 41% for 1989 and 61% for 1992). Nevertheless, the effort marked a beginning of cross-national cooperation in understanding crime.

Four main sources have been used to gather information about criminal behavior in the United States. These include official records gathered from police and sheriffs by the Federal Bureau of Investigation, information about victimization gathered through surveys conducted by the Bureau of Justice Statistics, self-reports of crimes committed, and third-party reports about children.

A. Official Records from Police and Sheriffs

During the nineteenth and early twentieth centuries, measures of crime depended largely on prosecution and prison records. Arrests, convictions, and punishments, however, reflect public attitudes toward characteristics of crimes committed and toward the accused, police efficiency, and practical politics. Therefore, a less elastic measure of crime was thought to be desirable.

The International Association of Chiefs of Police, in 1927, proposed a solution that involved collecting data from local police departments. In 1930, the Federal Bureau of Investigation (FBI) assumed the role of clearinghouse for police records collected in the United States. Since then, the FBI has collected monthly records regarding 29 categories of offenses from participating police departments. In 1931, the Wickersham Commission published its *Report on Criminal Statistics* recommending offenses known to police as the best evidence regarding actual crimes committed. Since 1933, the Federal Bureau of Investigation has published annual summaries, known as Uniform Crime Reports (UCR). Despite endorsement of the Wickersham Commission and efforts of the United States Department of Justice to obtain full cooperation, reports have been erratic. Thorsten Sellin noted that between 1933 and 1945, only 16 states and the District of Columbia reported regularly. Even after World War II, reporting continued to be problematic. In 1988, for example, no data were available from Florida and Kentucky; in 1991, no data were available from Iowa; in 1993, complete data were not available for Illinois and Kansas.

The Uniform Crime Reports capture only part of the crime picture, one that reflects politics as well as popular beliefs about police efficacy and proper behavior. Politicians seeking increasing funds to fight crime or wanting to show success in campaigns against crime may influence how police departments record and transmit information. Citizens who believe the police will do nothing about their complaints have few incentives to report crimes, and people who believe that they deserve the injuries they receive (for example, in cases of domestic violence) will not seek police interference. These sources of unreliability plus known difficulties in ascertaining the population to use as a denominator in computing crime rates have led to a second national effort to collect data about crimes committed.

B. Reports from Victims of Crimes

In 1965 and 1966, The National Opinion Research Center undertook a study of households to determine the feasibility of gathering data on crimes from victims and other members of their households. Using definitions provided by the Uniform Crime Reports, interviewers asked 10,000 randomly selected adult informants whether they or any other member of the household had been victims of a variety of crimes. The resulting victimization reports uncovered approximately twice as much crime, including forcible rape, robbery, and aggravated assault, as had been reported to police.

Since 1973, the Bureau of Justice Statistics has published results of the National Crime Victimization Survey (NCVS). This survey is based on a stratified, multistage cluster sample of households throughout the United States. An attempt is made to interview each competent member of a selected household who is at least 12 years old. Households remain in the sample for 3 years, with interviews every 6 months.

Either in person or by telephone, respondents are asked to report being victims of rape, robbery, assault, and larceny. In addition, they are asked whether their households have been victimized by burglary, larceny, or motor vehicle theft.

Trends in crime rates recorded through the NCVS differ from those found through the UCR. Both property crimes and crimes of violence known to the police increased between 1973 and 1990. (See Fig. 1, adapted from data reported in Bureau of Justice Statistics, 1994 and by Maguire and Pastore, 1995.)

According to victim reports, however, crimes against property declined and there was almost no change in rates of violence.

The contrast between trends in crimes known to the police and those reported to interviewers could be due to a number of factors. The discrepancy should not, however, be attributed to the fact that homicides are recorded by the UCR and not by the NCVS. Even if homicide rates had risen, the fact that these were not included in victim surveys could not account for the discrepancy in rates of violence because homicide

rates are a negligible part of violent crime. Furthermore, according to the UCR, rates of murder and nonnegligent manslaughter were not rising over this period.

Some of the discrepancy might be due to changing attitudes toward police. Crime rates known to police would rise without accompanying increases in crime were there to be more confidence that reporting could be helpful (or at least not damaging). Respondents in the NCVS surveys were asked whether they had reported their incidents of victimization. Throughout the period, victims said that they reported to the police fewer than half the crimes of violence described to the interviewers. Over this period of time, the reporting rate for violent crimes exhibited no trend, ranging from a low of 44.2% in 1978 to a high of 48.8% two years before. Thus, changes in reporting rates fail to account for the difference. More likely, the difference is due to two conditions: first, changing attitudes of police toward recording as offenses those acts of violence over which they have discretion; second, memory "telescoping" that would tend to reduce changes in rates of crime reported retrospectively. Changed police practices toward recording violence, especially domestic violence, would tend to produce an increase in violent crimes reported to police coincident with rising consciousness of the rights of minorities, women, and children. Telescoping, or remembering things long past as having happened more recently than they did, would tend to reduce the amount of detectable change in criminality represented by victim surveys.

In contrast to rates of violence, changing rates of property crimes known to police (UCR) appear to be due to an increase in reporting rates. Reporting rates for personal thefts ranged from a low of 22.1% in 1973 to 28.7 in 1989. Reporting rates for household crimes ranged from 36.4% (in 1978 and 1979) to 41.3% (in 1990).

C. Self-Report of Crimes Committed

Collecting accurate information about crime clearly poses some insurmountable problems. Official statistics reflect public attitudes as well as practices of enforcement agencies. Some evidence suggests that both racial and sexual biases affect reporting. Victim surveys are affected by retrospective biases that reflect current circumstances and memory distortions. They

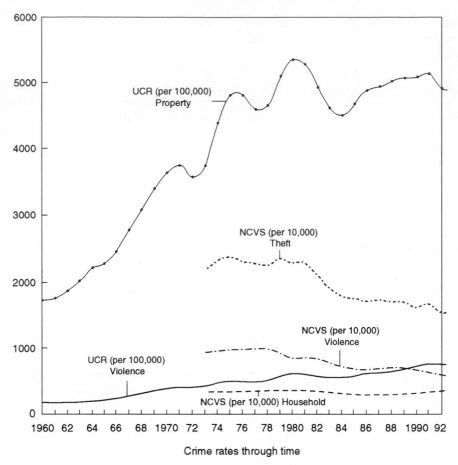

Figure I   Crime rates through time.

also reflect attitudes toward participation in government-sponsored research as well as varying discomfort with revealing information to strangers.

To overcome some of the problems involved in using official records, researchers have turned to reports by those whose behavior is being studied. Although self-reports can offer information about undetected crimes, they are subject to both underreporting and overreporting.

Self-reports must rely on voluntary cooperation, and people most heavily involved with crime are least likely to participate in the studies. In addition to the problem of winning cooperation from possibly reluctant or elusive respondents, self-report studies also face problems of memory and honesty. Some reporting errors seem to be due to the respondent's desire to appear respectable. A first arrest increases a delin-

quent's veracity about his crimes, for which one explanation is that prior to arrest, a delinquent tries to maintain the appearance of respectability.

The best known national study that uses self-reports of criminal activities is the longitudinal National Youth Survey (NYS). This survey first gathered information on families, behavior, and attitudes from a probability sample of boys and girls between the ages of 11 and 17 in 1976. After initial attrition of more than a quarter of the selected sample, response rates remained high (87%) over the next 7 years of reported data collection efforts. As with other self-reporting studies using general populations, the degree to which reported delinquent activities represent behavior serious enough to result in arrest had the activities been known by the police remains a question.

The NYS identified mental health problems as well

as delinquency and drug use through self-reports. Youths answered questions that were designed to identify lonely, isolated adolescents (for a Social Isolation/ Loneliness scale) and questions aimed at detecting youths who were labelled as having emotional problems by their peers and family (for an Emotional Problems scale). Elliott, Huizinga, and Menard report that mental health problems declined with age. Among those who reported committing serious crimes and also having mental health problems, slightly over half reported the crimes prior to the mental health problems. Mental health problems, however, tended to precede reports of marijuana or polydrug use.

D. Third-Party Reports

Studies of young children typically rely on reports by parents or teachers to identify youngsters who steal or aggressively injure others. Parents and teachers typically identify different children as particularly prone to aggression or theft. Children showing these types of problems both at home and in school tend to have the worst prognoses in terms of school achievement and criminality.

Although most researchers treat the adult reports as veridical, they may represent ongoing interactional processes. If reports of misbehavior reflect adult rejection of the child, the prognostic power of parent/ teacher descriptions may be partially due to the rejection these descriptions represent.

III. CRIMINAL BEHAVIOR AS MENTAL ILLNESS

Criminal behavior is typically distinguished from behavior produced as a consequence of mental illness on the grounds that crimes require *mens rea*. Although having a guilty mind is unnecessary for the commission of some crimes (e.g., parking on a snow route), these are generally misdemeanors. A middle ground between the actual having of a guilty mind and an assumption that one is responsible for an action has been created by the concept of "a rational man."

The crime of public drunkenness, for example, presumes knowledge on the grounds that a rational man would have known that drunkenness can result from heavy drinking. Negligent manslaughter is based on the assumption that a rational man would have con-

sidered his action from a perspective that could have prevented death.

Although in theory, those who are mentally ill ought to be distinguishable from those who merely misbehave, both in practice and conceptually, the distinction has been blurred. On the practical side, the decision whether to place a perpetrator of a crime in prison or in a mental hospital depends in large part on the nature of the crime committed, the jurisdiction, and who makes the decision—rather than on any recognizable set of symptoms that might identify the mentally ill. On the conceptual side, by providing diagnostic criteria for Conduct Disorder and Antisocial Personality, the American Psychiatric Association has erased the distinction between intentional acts and symptoms of mental illness.

The *Diagnostic and Statistical Manual of Mental Disorders,* Fourth Edition (*DSM-IV*), incorporates behavioral descriptions of theft, arson, truancy, burglary, rape, and assault as symptoms for the diagnosis of Conduct Disorder. Describing Conduct Disorder, the manual explains: "The essential feature of Conduct Disorder is a repetitive and persistent pattern of behavior in which the basic rights of others or major age-appropriate societal norms or rules are violated." It should be noted that *DSM-IV* (as did its predecessor, *DSM-IIIR*) defines the most dangerous delinquents as mentally ill. [*See* CONDUCT DISORDER.]

Crimes tend to be associated with the commission of other types of antisocial acts. Adults, according to *DSM-IV*, can have Antisocial Personality Disorder after age 18 if they evidence having symptoms of Conduct Disorder prior to reaching age 15. Antisocial Personality Disorder may manifest itself through "acts that are grounds for arrest." Thus for adults as well as for children, the signs of serious criminality are taken to be evidence of mental illness.

IV. ISSUES RELATED TO CONSIDERING CRIMINAL BEHAVIOR AS MENTAL ILLNESS

By using performance of criminal acts as evidence for mental illness, reporting biases have been imported into the system of diagnoses. Persistent criminal behavior is abnormal and distasteful to conventional society. Whether persistent criminals ought to be considered mentally ill on the grounds of their criminal behavior alone should be considered in the light of what this might do to health insurance as well as to the criminal justice system.

With the exception of a handful of prevention programs that work with families to improve management practices and with children to improve their problem solving skills, treatments to reduce criminality have not been shown to be effective. The diagnosis of Conduct Disorder usually does not occur until children are older than those effectively treated by prevention programs. It seems fair to say, therefore, that if Conduct Disorder is a genuine disease, it is one for which there is no known cure.

The criminal justice system assumes that, at least after the age of majority, people are responsible for their actions. They deserve praise for good works and condemnation for bad acts. If those who commit crimes most frequently are mentally ill, it is not reasonable to hold them responsible. Only the least offensive criminals would belong in criminal courts.

V. CONCLUSIONS

Criminal behavior includes a wide variety of actions carried out by both powerful and powerless people. The crimes that attract most attention, index crimes, provide an incomplete picture of lawless behavior.

Crime rates vary in relation to the methods for gathering data. No system seems to provide complete and accurate information, though even in rough form crime rates may be a reasonable indicator of societal mental health.

Defining mental illness in such a way as to include people because they commit crimes eliminates the possibility of learning that such people suffer from (other) specific mental health problems that might independently show causes for their behavior. In addition, the definitions of Conduct Disorder and Antisocial Personality Disorder create "mental illnesses" for behavior that may merely reflect social rejection.

BIBLIOGRAPHY

Bureau of Justice Statistics. (1994). *Criminal victimization in the United States: 1973–92 Trends.* Washington, DC: U.S. Department of Justice.

Elliott, D. S., Huizinga, D., & Menard, S. (1989). *Multiple problem youth: Delinquency, substance use and mental health problems.* New York: Springer Verlag.

Farrington, D. P. (1988). Social, psychological and biological influences on juvenile delinquency and adult crime. In W. Buikhuisen & S. A. Mednick (Eds.), *Explaining criminal behaviour: Interdisciplinary approaches* (pp. 68–89). New York: E. J. Brill.

Gurr, T. R. (1989). The history of violent crime in America: An overview. In T. R. Gurr (Ed.), *Violence in America, Volume 1: The history of crime* (11–20). Newbury Park, CA: Sage Publications, Inc.

Kelly, R. J., Chin, K-L., & Schatzberg, R. (Eds.). (1994). *Handbook of organized crime in the United States.* Westport, CT: Greenwood Press.

Maguire, K., & Pastore, A. L. (Eds.). (1994). *Sourcebook of criminal justice statistics–1993.* U.S. Department of Justice, Bureau of Justice Statistics. Washington, DC: USGPO.

Moffitt, T. E. (1993). "Life-course-persistent" and "adolescence-limited" antisocial behavior: A developmental taxonomy. *Psychological Review, 100,* 674–701.

Richters, J. E., & Cicchetti, D. (Eds.). (1993). *Development and psychopathology, special issue: Toward a developmental perspective on conduct disorder.* Cambridge: Cambridge University Press.

Sutherland, E. H. (1949/1983). *White collar crime.* New Haven: Yale University Press.

Crowding: Effects on Health and Behavior

Stephen J. Lepore

Carnegie Mellon University

Community Density   Number of people in a community area or proportion of people per available dwellings or space in a community.

Crowding   A negative psychological state that results from perceiving that there are too many people present in the available space.

Density   Number of people in a specified amount of space or proportion of people per available space.

Household Density   Number of people in a residential dwelling or proportion of people per available rooms or space in a residential dwelling.

CROWDING is a complex of undesirable or negative psychological reactions to highly populated, or high-density, settings. The experience of crowding is almost always aversive. It is the feeling of being cramped, perceiving that others are too close for comfort, or feeling that there is not enough elbow room and breathing space. People who feel crowded for prolonged periods of time can become psychologically demoralized, depressed, and anxious. People who experience crowding often exhibit a pattern of somatic and social reactions in addition to their psychological reactions. The body often responds to the experience of crowding with increased arousal, as indicated by elevated blood pressure and a faster heart rate. Social responses to crowding can include physically withdrawing from interactions with other people. Thus, crowding appears to have adverse effects on interpersonal relations, as well as undesirable effects on psychological and bodily functioning. Crowding, therefore, can be conceived of as a syndrome of psychological, somatic, and social reactions to the stress associated with high density.

I. DISTINCTION BETWEEN DENSITY AND CROWDING

It is important to distinguish between the subjective, psychological experience of crowding and the objective, environmental source of the crowding experience: high population density. Density is a property of the physical environment whereas crowding is primarily a psychological experience. The negative effects of high density on human health and behavior are strongest and most prevalent when individuals are uncomfortable or stressed by the high density. That is, high density might only affect health and behavior when individuals appraise the high-density setting as being crowded. Density is an important antecedent to the experience of crowding but is often not sufficient to explain everyone's feeling of crowding or a particular individual's experience of crowding in different settings or at different times.

Density is typically measured by calculating a ratio score of the number of people to a given amount of space. There are two broad types of density studied by social scientists, *household density* and *community*

Table I   Different Environmental Sources of Crowding

Types of household density
     Number of people per household area[a]
     Number of rooms per household
     Square footage per household
     Number of persons per room in a household

Types of community density
     Number of residents per community area[b]
     Number of households per community area
     Number of commercial buildings per residential community area
     Number of multi-unit housing structures per community area
     Proportion of households with more than one person per room
       in a community area
     Proportion of households with five or more persons in a com-
       munity area
     Number of persons per 10,000 square feet of residential space in
       a community area
     Number of persons living on a street per 1000 feet

---

[a]Household areas can be measured in square footage or meters.
[b]Community areas can be measured in acres, square miles, or by census tract.

density (see Table I). Household density can be determined in many ways. For example, one could calculate the number of people per rooms or square footage within a household. According to the U.S. census, households with more than 1.0 persons per room are overpopulated. Absolute number of people in a household in a residence also can be used as indicators of objective levels of household crowding. Community density measures reflect the amount of space for a given population over a wider space than an individual's residence. Community density can be determined by calculating the number of people per acre, people per square mile, or people per census tract. Occasionally community density will be defined as the ratio of dwellings or buildings to a given area or the total number of dwellings in a community area.

Public, health officials, city planners, housing developers, and policy analysts in charge of setting housing standards are particularly interested in understanding the effects of household and community density levels on human health and behavior. In general, ratio measures of density are better predictors of health, especially mental health, than are absolute measures, such as number of persons or number of rooms. In addition, measures of density in a dwelling, such as persons per room, are better predictors of in-

dividual health and behavior problems than are community measures of density, such as dwellings per square mile or persons per acre. These latter two findings may be explained by the fact that individuals will tend to have greater difficulty escaping from or avoiding unwanted interactions with other people when they are inside a highly populated dwelling with little available space than when they are in the outside world or in a highly populated dwelling with lots of space. The different behavioral and health effects of density in a dwelling versus density outside of a dwelling are discussed in more detail below.

II. ROLE OF SOCIAL AND PERSONAL CHARACTERISTICS

The correspondence between density and the psychological experience of crowding often depends upon the individual and the social situation. For example, people can be exposed to high levels of density in a bustling city street, a cramped apartment, a sporting event, a concert, a supermarket, or a political rally. Some of these crowded situations are exciting and inviting and some are threatening and foreboding. While many people would concede that the throngs of people cheering at a football stadium contribute to the excitement of the sport, few would agree that the clanging and banging of shopping carts and waiting in long lines to make a purchase in a crowded supermarket are enjoyable experiences.

Why do different situations evoke different experiences of and feelings toward high density? There are, of course, important differences between high density in different settings, like stadiums or supermarkets. For example, in a stadium the cheers and enthusiasm of a crowd can be stimulating and help a spectator to have a good time. In the supermarket, the presence of many people can interfere with or constrain a shopper's movement through the supermarket and his or her ability to finish shopping. When high density thwarts goal-directed behaviors it is more likely to be experienced as stressful and crowded than when it does not block goal-directed behaviors. Interference with goal-directed behaviors can diminish individuals' actual and perceived control over their environment. Lack of control over the environment can cause some people to feel psychologically distressed. The role of control in explaining the negative effects of crowding is discussed in more detail below.

There are also wide differences in peoples' reactions to high density. For example, men and women appear to experience high density quite differently. When men and women are required to interact in small groups, men are more uncomfortable and less social than are women. Thus, men appear to prefer a larger amount of personal space or physical distance between themselves and other people than do women. Different cultural groups also seem to experience density differently. For example, American college students appear to be less tolerant of household crowding than are adult males in India. Many Chinese and Japanese families appear to be relatively unaffected by living in very high-density homes. Among different American ethnic groups, household density tends to have a stronger negative effect on the mental health and social relations of black Americans than white Americans, and only a weak effect on Americans of Hispanic descent.

Why do individuals have unique reactions to similar levels of density? One explanation of the cultural differences is that people who have had long-term exposure to high-density conditions develop methods of coping with the crowding. For example, in crowded Chinese households, it is not uncommon for family members to eat at different times to reduce the amount of crowding during meals. Japanese homes often have movable walls and partitions than can be used to get the maximal function from the limited space and rooms in the homes. In addition, customs regarding appropriate social interaction distances might be developed in particular cultures to make the social environment more predictable and controllable. Gender differences in reaction to high density might be explained by adaptation to different levels of closeness in interpersonal interactions. In comparison with males, females might be socialized to expect and to engage in contact with others in closer physical proximity. As they mature, males might become more accustomed than females to having large interpersonal distances between themselves and others. Thus, experience with high-density settings can diminish the negative psychological experience of crowding because individuals can learn how to cope with the undesirable aspects of high density or they become accustomed to close physical contact with others.

III. EFFECTS OF CROWDING ON HEALTH AND BEHAVIOR

There has been a long history of interest in the effects of crowding on human health and behavior. The spread of various diseases and social pathologies is often attributed to the vast numbers of people living in urban areas. High population density is often cited as a reason for the very high rates of mental and physical health problems and various deviant social behaviors found in cities. It is not entirely clear, however, what aspects of high density might cause various social and health problems.

Observations of the negative effects of overpopulation in non-human animal species have fueled some of the concern over the effects of high density and crowding in human populations. Much of what has been learned about density and disease processes has been through experimentation with animals because of ethical limitations in experimenting with humans. However, even in animal populations it is difficult to ascertain the exact causes for the negative effects of density on health and behavior. Take, for example, the observation that high density is associated with higher rates of mortality in many animal species. Many animal species exhibit cycles of population escalation followed by a sudden and tremendous mortality, or a "population crash." Different pathways have been identified that may link density to mortality. For example, food shortages or the rapid spread of disease, as in plagues and other epidemics, could explain population crashes in high-density settings. However, starvation and contagious disease do not fully explain the effects of high population density on mortality. One group of scientists observed that deer living on an island multiplied quite rapidly until their population reached about one deer per acre, then their mortality rate skyrocketed. The deer population crashed, even though the deer had plenty of food and water and showed no signs of contagious disease spread. Examinations of the deer's internal organs, however, revealed signs of stress-related disease processes, which suggested another explanation of why high density can increase mortality: social stress.

Social stress can be caused by uncontrollable, threatening, unwanted, or otherwise negative social contacts and interactions with other organisms in an environment. High density can increase social stress, which can induce fighting between animals, interfere with reproductive behaviors, and cause unhealthy metabolic disturbances. Under high-density conditions, rodents' reproduction rates drop, cannibalism and deviant sexual behavior increase, and other social and biological pathologies all increase. In some animal studies, higher mortality among animals in high-density pens appears to be caused by overactive adrenal glandular systems. Many of the biological pathologies manifest in crowded rodents are similar to those observed in many species of animals after they have been exposed to noxious environmental stimuli, or stressors. Thus, it appears that the stress-related disease processes that might be caused by high population density could contribute to death and illness in different animal species. [*See* STRESS.]

It is tempting to draw analogies between overpopulated animal populations and overpopulation that occurs in human settlements. For example, birth and mortality rates of high-density human communities could be compared to similar outcomes in high-density rat colonies. However, many outcomes, such as criminal behavior in humans versus aggression in rats, are not so directly comparable. In addition, it is more difficult to prove that density is the cause of deviant behaviors in humans than it is to do so in animals. In animal research, scientists can control the effects of external factors other than high density that could influence the behaviors of crowded animals. Researchers studying human crowding can seldom control other factors, such as poverty and noise, that tend to accompany high density and influence humans' health and behaviors independently of density. In social science terms, the uncontrollable factors could cause a "spurious," or illusory, relation between density and human health and behaviors. Some researchers use statistical techniques to attempt to examine the effects of density independent of other social factors. The problem with making such statistical judgments is that researchers never know for certain whether they have identified all possible factors that could influence both density and the outcome of interest. These points should be kept in mind when reading the next section on the evidence relating high density to human health and behaviors.

A. Chronic versus Acute Crowding

The effects of high population density on humans do not appear to be as dramatic as in animals. This is partly due to the sophisticated and complex ways in which humans experience and adapt to noxious environmental stimuli like high density. For example, humans can hoard food supplies or increase food production to avoid starvation under high population conditions. Humans also can modify their environments, perhaps through scheduling or architectural interventions, to minimize social stress in high-density settings. Nevertheless, social research has revealed some relations between density and various health and social problems in humans.

In discussing the effects of crowding on humans, it is important to distinguish between *chronic crowding* and *acute crowding*. Chronic crowding takes place in settings where people tend to spend much of their time, like work places, residential settings, or institutional settings such as dormitories, prisons, and military barracks. Acute crowding takes place in settings where people tend to spend very little time, like stores, elevators, sidewalks, restaurants, theaters, stadiums, and other public places. The effects of acute crowding also have been examined by researchers in laboratory settings modified to represent different levels of density.

I. Effects of Chronic Community Crowding on Social Pathology

Social pathology can be defined as those phenomena that contribute to the demise of a society, typically by reducing its population, but also by disrupting its institutions and social relations. Thus, high rates of crime, mortality, accidents, disease, and divorce are indicators of social pathology. In the minds of many, social pathologies are linked to large cities, where they seem to proliferate and concentrate. Because large cities are both highly populated and full of social pathology, scientists have attempted to determine whether community crowding is at the root of the pathology evident in cities.

Interest in the relation between community density and pathology has been apparent since at least the end of the 19th century. Along with the industrial revolution came a rapid growth in cities throughout the western world. Some social theologists thought that the diversity of people, the personal anonymity, and high levels of individual autonomy existing between people in large cities would lead to psychological distress and anomie. In contrast, people from small towns and agrarian societies were expected to have richer social lives and greater morale because of familiarity and close interaction with similar others. Other social theorists argued that the high density of cities would expose people to overwhelming amounts of stimulation. In response to the stimulus overload, city-people would socially withdraw. Social withdrawal could be a strategy for reducing stimulus overload. By reducing concern for others and by interacting at a superficial level, there would be fewer stimulus inputs to cope with in day-to-day life. However, there would naturally be social costs if everyone acted this way, including apathy, frustration, conflict, and competition.

Contemporary social scientists pursue many of the same questions regarding community crowding and pathology as did their counterparts from a hundred years ago. Typically, crowding researchers investigate whether areas with high levels of community density also have high concentrations of social, psychological, and biological pathologies or problems. Community population density has been studied in relation to rates of death, infant mortality, perinatal mortality, accidental death, suicide, tuberculosis, venereal disease, mental hospitalization, birth, illegitimate birth, juvenile delinquency, imprisonment, crimes, public welfare, admissions to general hospitals, and divorce. The current evidence suggests that there is little or no relation between population density and major indicators of social pathology, such as mortality, crime, and juvenile delinquency. One research group observed that a higher ratio of persons per acre was associated with slightly elevated rates of mortality, fertility, juvenile delinquency, admissions to mental hospitals, and public assistance. However, the researchers also noted that certain ethnic and economic groups were overrepresented in the high-density areas. Thus, factors such as poverty, rather than density, could have caused the higher rates of pathology observed among individuals living in high-density areas. Indeed, when the researchers controlled for the effects of social class and ethnic background on the pathological outcomes, the relations between density and the outcomes disappeared.

On the other hand, it is possible that some community-crowding studies have underestimated the effects of high density on human pathology. Aggregate measures of density, such as persons per square mile, and aggregate measures of pathology, such as number of hospital admissions, do not precisely reveal the exposure to high density or its effects on individuals. For example, a person living in a high-density community might spend most of his or her waking hours at a job in a community that has a low-level of density. Or, a person from a low-density suburb might work all day in a high-density city. The actual exposure of these respective individuals to high density is different than what one would expect based on the density of their communities. In one instance, the negative effects of living in a high-density community could be underestimated. In the other instance, the benefits of living in a low-density community could be overestimated. If there are many of these peculiar cases in a study population, then an aggregate measure of community density will not be a good estimate of exposure to crowding. Nor would such a measure be useful for examining the effects of crowding on human health and behavior. There are also problems with aggregate measures of pathology. The principle problem is that data on social pathology originate from official public records, which can be incomplete and inaccurate.

To make matters more complicated, when analyzing aggregate data researchers can never know whether the relations between density and pathology are overestimated or underestimated. That is, the data errors caused by using aggregate measures could make the effects of density on pathology look stronger or weaker than they are in reality. One way around the problems associated with aggregate data is to study the effects of high density on individuals rather than on whole communities. That is, one could carefully measure individuals' exposure to density and their health and behaviors. This is usually done by surveying individuals about the levels of density in their households and about their health, behavior, and psychological well-being. Findings from this type of research are discussed in the next section.

2. Effects of Chronic Household Crowding on Health and Behavior

Household crowding stems from high density in the residential environment. Residential environments include individuals' homes and apartments, as well as institutional settings such as prisons, dormitories, and military bases. Household density appears to have a wide-range of effects on human health, behavior, and general well-being.

Prisoners in high-density cells, for instance, report more negative moods, discomfort, and illness symptoms than those in single-person cells or relatively low-density cells. Disciplinary problems, psychiatric commitment rates, suicide rates, and death rates also appear to increase in prison populations that grow in size without increases in prison facilities' size. Crowding also is a frequent problem in student populations. This often occurs because of a shortage of desirable housing near colleges or because students often double-up in apartments to save money on rent. In comparison with students in low-density dormitories or off-campus apartments, students in high-density residences feel more crowded, have more unwanted social contact and interactions, have more frequent negative moods, are less happy, and try to avoid interactions by socially withdrawing. In comparison with their uncrowded counterparts, crowded students are less sensitive to others' needs, less willing to help others, and less aware that others are available to provide emotional support or help to them when they need it.

People living in high-density residences can become insensitive to social cues even when they are not in the high-density setting. That is, the social insensitivity cultivated in high-density environments can carry over into low-density settings. College students who are withdrawn and insensitive to social cues in their high-density residences also act this way in low-density laboratory settings. Crowded students exhibit their withdrawn behaviors by sitting far away from others, not initiating conversation, making little eye contact with others, and not being helpful to others in need.

High household density in noninstitutional settings also results in antisocial behaviors and complaints of excessive social interaction. High household density is also related to increased negative mood and symptoms of depression and anxiety among adults. People from high-density households tend to have fewer friends and greater difficulty getting along with their neighbors than do people from relatively low-density homes. Parents tend to interact less with their young when they live in high-density homes than when they live in relatively low-density homes.

Children appear to be more negatively affected by high density than are adults, partly because they have less control over their environment than do adults. In comparison with children from low-density homes, those from high-density homes tend to have more behavioral problems in school, more anxiety, greater distractibility, more conflicts, lower achievement motivation, and poorer verbal abilities. However, cau-

tion must be applied when interpreting these results. As discussed above, density often accompanies other environmental conditions that could influence children's behaviors. Noise, for example, is likely to be greater in high-density households than in low-density households; and noise can interfere with children's attention, hearing, and learning abilities. Uncoupling the effects of density from those of noise is nearly impossible in naturalistic settings.

Earlier in this article, it was noted that social factors could influence whether an individual would perceive a particular setting as crowded. The social environment also can have a strong influence on the relation between crowding and psychological distress symptoms. As Figure 1 shows, students living in high-density households who have frequent hassles from roommates are more likely to be psychologically distressed than are students living in high-density households with relatively few hassles. Students living in low-density homes do not appear to be adversely affected by social hassles. People living in high-density households may be particularly distressed by roommate hassles because it is more difficult to avoid or escape from the hassles in a high-density home than in a low-density home. In contrast to the effects of social hassles, positive social relations can counteract the negative psychological effects of high-density living situations. As Figure 2 shows, college students living in high-density households who have supportive roommates are less likely to be distressed than are students

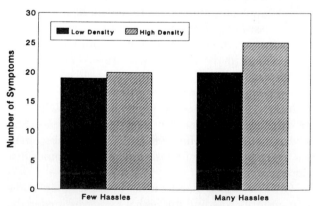

Figure 1   Psychological distress symptoms as a function of household density and levels of social hassles from roommates. [Reprinted, with permission, from S. J. Lepore, G. W. Evans, and M. L. Schneider (1992). *Environ. Behav.* **24**, 795–811. Copyright © Sage Publications.]

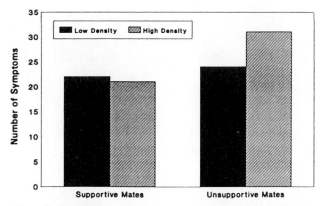

Figure 2 Psychological distress symptoms as a function of household density and levels of social support from roommates. [Reprinted, with permission, from S. J. Lepore, G. W. Evans, and M. L. Schneider (1991). *J. Pers. Soc. Psychol.* **61,** 899–909. Copyright © 1991 by the American Psychological Association.]

living in high-density households with relatively unsupportive roommates or students living in low-density households. However, as mentioned earlier, chronic household crowding can undermine socially supportive relations because people become withdrawn and insensitive to social cues. Thus, although positive social relations may be beneficial to crowded individuals, such relations may be rare in households that are chronically overpopulated.

3. Effects of Acute Crowding on Physiology and Behavior

Acute crowding has been studied in scientific laboratories and in natural settings, like trains and elevators. In the animal studies discussed above, it was noted that many animals living in high-density populations showed biological signs of stress, such as enlarged adrenal glands. Elevated and sustained physiological arousal is another sign of stress that is commonly observed in organisms under stress. In high-density laboratory settings, arousal has been exhibited in human subjects using many different measures. People exposed to acute crowding in laboratories exhibit increased perspiration, skin conductance, and blood pressure. Passengers in crowded commuter trains exhibit increases in blood levels of adrenaline. Interestingly, passengers who board a train when it is already near capacity are more negatively affected by the crowded conditions than passengers who board early, when the train is nearly empty. Even though the latter

passengers ride the train longer, they had more choice, or control, over where they could sit on the train than passengers who board the train when it is already loaded with other passengers.

It should be noted that although acute exposure to high-density settings usually increases physiological arousal, it is not clear whether there are negative health consequences of the increased arousal. It is possible that elevated and prolonged arousal can wear down the body's defenses against illness and generate illness itself, such as hypertension or ulcers. However, there is not enough evidence at this point to state unequivocally whether the arousing effects of high-density have health implications. [*See* PSYCHONEURO-IMMUNOLOGY.]

Impaired task performance is another common side-effect of acute exposure to high density. Mostly, this research has been conducted in laboratory settings that manipulate individuals' exposure to high or low density and then measure performance on problem-solving tasks or assess one's ability to concentrate or persist on a task. Although high density does not seem to interfere with performance on simple tasks, it does diminish complex task performance. It also appears that individuals are more easily distracted and are less persistent at completing challenging tasks under high- versus low-density conditions.

Short-term exposure to high density produces many of the same withdrawal behaviors observed in people chronically exposed to high density. It is not uncommon, for example, for people on crowded subways to read newspapers and books as a way of avoiding interaction with others. In laboratory settings, crowded people are more likely to leave the settings, increase social distance, withdraw from social interactions, increase defensive posturing, and reduce eye contact than uncrowded people. Another way to maintain space from others is to be aggressive and threatening. Several studies have shown increased competition and aggression between individuals in high-density settings. Interestingly, crowding is more likely to evoke aggression in men than in women and when resources in the environment are scarce rather than plentiful. The adaptive value of withdrawal and aggression in high-density settings is not completely understood, but it does appear that these social behaviors may help people to cope with crowding. For example, social withdrawal might be a way of minimizing physiological arousal by avoiding unwanted social interactions and the excessive social stimulation that is common in high-density settings.

IV. EXPLAINING THE NEGATIVE EFFECTS OF CROWDING

Several theoretical explanations of the effects of crowding on human health and behavior have been alluded to throughout this article. Below we discuss three of the more prominent of these theories: behavioral constraint, control, and overload/arousal theories.

A. Behavioral Constraint

According to this theory, high density interferes with individuals' goal obtainment by restricting or inhibiting their movements and behaviors. The diminished freedom makes the high density noxious and undesirable. When people are in high-density settings that do not thwart their goal-directed behaviors, they tend to be less negatively affected by the high density than when their goals are thwarted. Imagine, for instance, two groups of individuals performing a task in a crowded room, but one group has to complete the task while sitting still and the other group has to complete the task while moving around the room. It is more likely that crowding will interfere with the task performance of the moving group than of the still group because the crowded group will be coping with the task and the constraints on their movements caused by the crowding.

Behavioral constraints do not refer only to restrictions in bodily movement. Sometimes high density can create resource shortages, such as food shortages, which constrain behavioral choices. That is, density can restrict access to valued resources. In the case of food shortages, behaviors such as eating might be inhibited. In addition, people in such situations might act aggressively to get valued resources. Finally, it should be noted, that high density often can have negative effects on mood and performance because people perceive that there are behavioral constraints in high-density environments. That is, simply believing that high density can limit one's behaviors or access to valued resources is sufficient to diminish task performance or increase discomfort in high-density settings.

B. Control

Limits to behavioral freedom also can be construed as limits in personal control over the self and the environment. Control models of crowding hypothesize that high density is undesirable and harmful because it renders the environment more unpredictable and exposes individuals to situations over which they have little or no control. A lack of control in high-density settings has been shown to exacerbate the negative effects of density on humans, whereas the availability of control has been shown to reduce the negative effects of density.

One group of researchers tested the control hypothesis by examining the effects of control on people's moods in crowded elevators. Control in the elevator was manipulated by giving some people access to the elevator control panel and other people no access. Those who had panel access, or more control, in the crowded elevators felt less crowded and had more positive moods than those without control. As with behavioral constraint, sometimes it is enough to simply perceive, or believe, that control is available to reduce the negative effects of high density on performance or mood. However, if one's expectations for control in a high-density situation do not match the actual availability of control, then the high density can be more disturbing than if one expected little control in the situation. Thus, it appears that control or beliefs and expectations about control in high-density environments influences how strongly humans are affected by crowding. [See CONTROL.]

C. Overload/Arousal

A final theory posits that high density increases pathology because of sensory overload from excessive stimulation. Humans have a limited capacity to process information; in high-density settings the information available in the environment exceeds that capacity. This process is similar to information-overload in a computer system, which can cause a computer to make errors or shut-down operations. In humans, overarousal is often unpleasant, can diminish complex task performance, and could contribute to health problems.

Evidence for the overload/arousal model of crowding is found in studies such as those discussed above that have shown increased sympathetic arousal under high-density situations. Some scholars have suggested that heightened social withdrawal in high-density settings is a method of reducing arousal. At present, however, there is no strong evidence that social withdrawal can actually lower sympathetic arousal in crowded people. In addition, there is no evidence that the levels or duration of arousal people experience in high-density settings is significant enough to compromise health or contribute to disease processes.

V. CONCLUSIONS

Crowding in humans is a syndrome of stress associated with exposure to high-density households, community, or laboratory settings. A distinction exists between the subjective experience of crowding and the objective source of that feeling: high population density. Overpopulation in non-human animals leads to deviant social behaviors and health problems. However, exposure to high density and overpopulation in humans seldom results in extreme social pathologies. Unlike lower animals, humans appear to be able to adapt to and cope with high-density situations with a good deal of tolerance. Humans can adapt by limiting their exposure to high density through many means, including architectural interventions, careful scheduling and planning of space usage, and by engaging in distracting or withdrawal behaviors. Unfortunately, some adaptations to density, such as social withdrawal, can have unintended consequences, such as loneliness or deterioration of interpersonal relations.

The research evidence to date suggests that people do have undesirable psychological, social, and bio-

logical responses to crowding. However, it is also clear that crowding is more or less aversive and detrimental to people depending on their personal experiences with and preferences for particular levels of density. In addition, social conditions, such as the presence of supportive others or undesirable social hassles from others, can influence the strength of the relation between density and various outcomes, such as psychological well-being. Thus, density does not necessarily increase social pathology in humans. Indeed, low levels of density can be undesirable at some occasions, such as parties, sporting events, or concerts. It appears that density is most detrimental to human behavior and health when individuals feel a lack of control over their own behaviors or the environment, or when they experience excessive stimulation and arousal from the density.

This article has been reprinted from the *Encyclopedia of Human Behavior, Volume 2.*

BIBLIOGRAPHY

Baum, A., & Paulus, P. B. (1987). Crowding. In "Handbook of Environmental Psychology" (D. Stokols and I. Altman, Eds.). Wiley, New York.

Evans, G. W., & Lepore, S. J. (1992). Conceptual and analytic issues in crowding research. *J. Environ. Psychol.* **12**, 163–173.

Gove, W. M., & Hughes, M. (1983). "Overcrowding in the Household." Academic Press, New York.

Paulus, P. B., & Nagar, D. (1989). Environmental influences on groups. In "Psychology of Group Influence" (P. B. Paulus, Ed.), 2nd ed. Erlbaum, Hillsdale, NJ.

Taylor, R. B. (1988). "Human Territorial Functioning." Cambridge University Press, Cambridge.

Custody (Child)

Robert E. Emery

University of Virginia

Child Custody The rights and responsibilities held by adults responsible for the primary caretaking of children. Specific rights and responsibilities evolve over time but generally include rights to care for and make decisions for children and responsibilities to provide for children's basic safety and needs and to control children according to societal standards.

Child's Best Interest Standard The legal rule governing many issues related to child custody and other legal decisions concerning children. The standard suggests that decisions should be made according to children's future best interests, a benevolent but vague directive.

Divorce Mediator An impartial third party who helps separated or divorced partners to negotiate a legal divorce settlement.

Joint Custody The sharing of parental rights and responsibilities between parents even following separation, divorce, or extramarital childbirth. Either legal or physical custody, or both, may be shared.

Legal Custody The assignment of parental rights and responsibilities, particularly following divorce.

Open Adoption Adoption in which biological parents maintain contact with biological children.

Permanency Planning A requirement that foster care agencies form plans about the permanent placement of children in foster care—either with their biological families or in other living arrangements.

Physical Custody Where children live according to what schedule of residential arrangements. Commonly applied following separation or divorce.

Procedural Law The processes involved in legal decision making and the rules governing these procedures such as the rules for disclosing and presenting evidence in a trial.

Substantive Law The content of the law, that is, the specifics of legal rules such as which parent should get custody following a divorce.

Termination of Parental Rights The legal term for the complete and irrevocable loss of all custody rights and responsibilities. Parental rights can be terminated voluntarily as in adoption or involuntarily as (rarely) occurs in cases of severe abuse or neglect.

The topic of **CHILD CUSTODY** is controversial and often confusing. The potential loss of custody of a child is a tremendous threat to parents, whether a parent fears losing custody to the child's other parent (who may or may not be a former spouse), to some other relative (such as a grandparent), or to a social service agency acting as an agent of the state. Further controversy and confusion can be added because the different major professions involved in child custody controversies—attorneys, psychologists or psychiatrists, and social workers—often view the topic of child custody differently and bring different professional philosophies to bear on the issue. Even more controversy and confusion stem from the different circumstances in which disputes about custody may arise. Custody disputes can result from questions of paternity establishment, adoption, foster care placement, abuse or neglect, or marital separation and divorce. Most of the present discussion focuses on child custody following separation and divorce, consistent with the major emphasis of both legal proceedings and social science research. Nevertheless, it is critical at the outset to define, as precisely as possible, the diverse meanings and contexts of the issue of child custody.

I. DEFINING CHILD CUSTODY AND THE CONTEXTS OF CUSTODY DISPUTES

The term, child custody, has different meanings in different legal contexts, however, it is useful to attempt a general definition. Child custody includes a variety of rights and responsibilities possessed by the adult(s) responsible for the primary caretaking of a child or children. Custodial rights involve the authority to raise and care for a child and to make decisions about that child's upbringing. Custodians can freely make relatively mundane decisions about such topics as discipline, and they also can make broader decisions for children such as choices between alternative forms of education (e.g., public or private schooling), different religious training, and elective medical care. Custodial responsibilities include the duty to provide for and protect a child's health, physical safety, and emotional well-being, to offer children sufficient economic support to meet their basic needs, to ensure children's adequate education, and to control children so they do not violate the rights of others.

One reason why child custody cannot be defined with absolute precision is that the legal (and social) expectations concerning parental rights and responsibilities have evolved in the past and continue to evolve today. In the not-so-distant past, parents had limited legal responsibility and almost complete authority over their children who were viewed as parental "property" in early American law (and in English common law from which most American legal traditions derive). However, societal concerns for children's welfare increased in the latter part of the nineteenth and throughout the twentieth century, and the

state assumed increasing "parental" authority under its *parens patriae* (state as parent) powers to protect children. Thus, for example, child labor laws limited parents' rights to make decisions concerning children's employment, and mandatory education laws gave parents the responsibility to ensure children's school attendance. In fact, the parental rights and responsibilities that define child custody continue to evolve today, as we debate and sometimes enact legislation or support judicial rulings about such issues as allowing parents to commit minors to mental hospitals against an adolescent's wishes or holding parents criminally responsible for their children's misbehavior.

A. Biological and Social Parents

The terms "parent" and "custodian" were used interchangeably in the preceding paragraphs, and biological parents have traditionally assumed child custody in American law. In fact, custody still rests with a child's biological parents in the absence of the voluntary relinquishment of parental rights (as in adoption), the biological parents' failure to meet certain basic custodial responsibilities (as in cases of child abuse or neglect), or when disputes about custody arise for various reasons between actual or potential caregivers.

Nevertheless, the automatic preference for biological parents has been challenged in various legal cases (and in some psychological theories). Thus, some case law and some psychological recommendations favor "social parents" over biological parents. Social parents, sometimes called "psychological parents," are adults who have offered or are able to offer children extensive emotional and practical caretaking. Social parents may be relatives such as grandparents, stepparents, adoptive parents, or simply caring adults who are unrelated to a child by blood, marriage, or law.

The theory behind the concept of a social parent is that parenting is defined by the parenting role, not by biological lineage. That is, children's healthy psychological development is viewed as a product of the quantity and quality of children's relationships with their caregivers whether or not the caregivers are the children's biological parents. In fact, there is extensive psychological evidence that social parents, including members of the extended family, stepparents, and foster or adoptive parents, often can and do raise children as effectively or more effectively than biological parents.

B. The Child's Best Interests Standard

The reason why social parents may be judged to be preferred custodians over biological parents is that the overriding legal principle guiding child custody is the child's best interests standard. According to this legal rule, when disputes about child custody arise, custody determinations are to be made based on what will be in a child's future best interests. Thus, under contemporary law it is possible that a social parent might win custody over a biological parent. For example, it is theoretically possible for a judge to rule that a child is better placed in the custody of maternal grandparents rather than with a biological father following the death of the biological mother. More commonly, courts often rule that children should be removed from their biological parents in an abusive or neglectful home and temporarily placed in the custody of foster parents. [*See* CHILD MALTREATMENT.]

The best interests standard has both strengths and weaknesses. The positive and the negative aspects both flow from the fact that the best interests standard is a vague directive that gives judges and their agents great discretion in determining any given child's future best interests. The standard allows judges to make determinations based on the unique aspects of any given child's circumstances, a positive feature since the circumstances surrounding questions of custody can differ greatly and because different children can have very different childrearing needs. On the other hand, the vague nature of the best interests standard also allows the values of any given judge, or even of a broader segment of society, to intrude into family life. For example, one judge may be biased toward mothers as custodians, while a second judge may prefer fathers. Or middle class social workers may impose standards of neglect that are inappropriate and insensitive to the struggles of parents living in poverty.

A more general problem is that there often is no clear answer to the question of what will be "best" for a child—both in general and in the individual case. Is it better for children to be removed from their neglectful parents (and from their communities) and to be reared by foster or adoptive parents who have more resources? Is it better for a child to live in the custody of a divorced, biological mother who will offer the child much love but limited demands for achievement, or would it be better for the same child to live in the custody of a divorced, biological father who will instill achievement values but provide less nurturance? Aside from our present inability to make such predictions either normatively or individually, the best interest standard faces the inherent problem that questions of what is best (or better or less detrimental) for children typically include tradeoffs between better or worse outcomes in different domains of life functioning. In short, the question of what is best for children often is laden with value judgments.

The impossibility of resolving inherent value judgments is one reason why a strong preference for biological parents remains in theory and in practice both in the law and in social science. Case law documents instances where social parents have been awarded child custody over biological parents. However, our courts continue to prefer biological parents as custodians given the uncertainty about what is best for children, and also given our society's desire to protect biological parents' rights as well as to protect children's interests. Even in cases of abuse and neglect, children are likely to be removed from their biological parents only temporarily and family reunification is the eventual goal. That is, the involuntary termination of parental rights, the legal term for the complete and irrevocable loss of all custody rights and responsibilities, occurs very rarely even in cases of serious abuse and/or neglect.

C. Legal and Physical Custody

A particularly vexing problem arises when the custody dispute is between a child's two biological parents, and, in fact, the most common form of custody dispute is one that follows separation and divorce. Changes in social practices of childrearing following separation and divorce, and eventually in the legal system, have given us one of the more important ways in which the definition of child custody has evolved in the last two decades.

Following a separation or divorce, it is now common to distinguish between physical custody and legal custody. Physical custody concerns where a child will live and includes any schedule that may be devised for the child to spend time with the second parent or with other relatives. *Legal custody* includes the parents' rights and responsibilities in caring for children and in making decisions concerning their welfare. One parent may assume primary physical custody of a child, for example, so that the child lives primarily with that parent and perhaps sees the other parent every other weekend. The same two parents may jointly share legal custody, however, and divorce agreements often spell out in great detail how parents will share or separate decision making concerning their children's well-being.

D. Joint Custody

This last example leads to consideration of a second innovation stemming from divorce law, namely, the relatively new concept of joint custody, where custody is shared by a child's parents following separation or divorce. Joint legal custody involves a sharing of parental rights and responsibilities, but the shared parental authority typically is limited only to major issues such as schooling and religious upbringing. Sometimes joint legal custody also involves a commitment between the two parents to attempt to communicate about the children and to work together in devising similar rules for discipline across their two households. Joint physical custody is typically defined as an agreement that approaches an equal division of a child's residence between each of the parents. The precise definitions of joint legal and physical custody often differ in the statutes of different states, however, and parents, as well as professionals, also frequently differ in their view of joint custody. For example, some divorced parents view the only joint physical arrangement as one in which the child spends exactly the same amount of time with each parent (e.g., every other week in each parent's household). Other divorced parents view an arrangement that includes frequent or extensive contact with both parents as joint physical custody, for example, when a child spends weekends with one parent and weekdays with the other, or when a child resides with one parent during the school year and the other parent during the summer.

Thus, child custody following divorce may be held by one parent or shared jointly between two parents. Sole or joint custody includes not only residential arrangements but also a set of parental rights and responsibilities, although the parental rights and responsibilities may differ across families and surely evolve over time. Finally, we should be clear that even when sole custody is the outcome following divorce, the rights of the noncustodial parent have not been terminated. The noncustodial parent still retains various parental rights and responsibilities, including the right to spend time with the children (called visitation or access) and to have information on the children's well-being (e.g., access to school records).

II. THE PSYCHOLOGICAL HEALTH OF CHILDREN FOLLOWING SEPARATION AND DIVORCE

Do custody arrangements make a difference in terms of children's psychological health following separation and divorce? As we have noted, questions about children's best interests invariably involve questions of values. Nevertheless, empirical research on children's psychological outcomes can help practitioners and policymakers in confronting the difficult, sometimes impossible, questions that are raised about child custody following divorce. A large number of studies have been conducted on the psychological health of children from divorced families. In fact, far more research has been conducted on this topic than on other circumstances in which child custody is at issue (e.g., foster care, adoption). Thus, we focus on divorce both because it is the most common arena for child custody disputes and because it has been fertile ground for research. [*See* DIVORCE.]

In considering child custody and divorce, it is essential to call attention at the outset to the difference between substantive and procedural law. The substantive law includes laws pertaining to the content or preferred alternative outcomes of custody disputes. Historically, substantive law originally favored fathers as custodians under "chattel" or property rules. Beginning in the nineteenth century and continuing through much of the twentieth century, mothers became preferred custodians in substantive law under the so-called "tender years presumption," a view that mothers were naturally better parents than fathers. (The age range defining "tender years" originally was limited to very young children but eventually came to include children of any age.) Since the 1970s, however, substantive law has given mothers and fathers equal opportunity to be awarded custody in legal theory under the child's best interests standard. Most recently, some state laws have indicated a substantive preference for joint legal and/or physical custody following divorce.

Procedural law involves the methods used to resolve disputes. The basic, formal procedure for resolving disputes in the United States is the "adversary system." Disputants are viewed as adversaries or opponents, and our legal system offers a variety of procedural rules to ensure that both sides in a dispute have the opportunity to present their case in a fair and open forum. However, a number of commentators have raised questions about the suitability of adversary procedures for resolving child custody disputes following separation and divorce. Essentially, adversary procedures have been criticized as further undermining the relationship between former partners who remain parents, a circumstance that often is contrary to children's best interests. Thus, courts and private practitioners have developed a number of nonadversarial methods of dispute resolution that may help parents to renegotiate their coparenting relationship more successfully. The most notable alternative methods are attorney negotiation, a well-established tradition in the law, and divorce mediation, a far more recent innovation. A divorce mediator is an impartial third party (who may be a lawyer, a mental health professional, a social worker, or a lay person) who helps former partners to negotiate directly themselves.

Most divorcing parents negotiate a settlement out of court either on their own or with the aid of attorneys and/or with a divorce mediator. Nevertheless, high divorce rates make child custody disputes common either before, during, or sometimes long after a divorce settlement. In the following discussion, we focus first on substantive issues related to custody and later address procedural matters.

A. The Context of Child Custody Disputes in Divorce

Divorce rates escalated dramatically beginning in the late 1960s, and they remain at a stable but high level in the 1990s. Thus, about half of all children born to married parents in the 1990s will experience their parents' divorce. According to United States census data, of all children from divorced families, nearly 90% live in the residential custody of their mothers, and somewhat more than 10% live in the residential custody of their fathers. The census does not track joint custody, and other studies of national samples are limited in their estimate of the number of children living in joint legal and/or physical custody arrangements. Based on various state surveys, however, we can conclude that a sizable and increasing number of parents maintain joint legal custody of their children after divorce, but only a small minority—less than 10%—of children live in joint physical custody arrangements.

B. Consequences of Divorce for Children

Evidence on the consequences of postdivorce family relationships, including various child custody and visitation arrangements, is informative both in relation to divorce custody disputes and to other circumstances in which child custody may become an issue. The starting point in examining this research is to consider evidence on the consequences of divorce for children.

A large number of studies have been conducted on the consequences of divorce for children. One clear conclusion from this body of research is that divorce is not an event but a process of change that unfolds over a prolonged period of time—beginning in the two-parent family and often continuing long after the legal divorce. The actual separation or divorce can be a relief for some children but for most the process of transition is emotionally wrenching. Among the sources of distress are conflict in the family prior to a separation and following a divorce; the physical separation from and dramatically reduced contact with one parent; less adequate parenting on the part of both parents; each parent's preoccupation with their own emotional turmoil; and the financial worries and many practical adjustments that accompany the shift from one household to two, including possible changes in residence, schooling, and peer relationships.

Evidence indicates that divorce is a risk factor associated with a number of undesirable psychological outcomes for children, including increased behavioral problems, difficulties in school, more frequent use of mental health services, and more problems in relationships (including an increased likelihood of divorce during adult life). In addition, various case studies have concluded that children of divorce have many, often unseen or unanticipated, emotional problems. However, the psychological functioning of most children (and parents) improves as time passes. Despite the increased risks, moreover, most reviews of the empirical literature conclude that the differences in the psychological well-being of children from divorced and married families are modest in magnitude. Divorce may double or triple the risk for a number of problems (the increased risk for one's own divorce is notably smaller than this), but many of the psychological problems found after divorce have been demonstrated to be present *before* the divorce. Furthermore, *most* children from divorced families do not suffer from psychological, behavioral, or educational problems.

The apparently contradictory findings about risk, as well as between clinical and empirical research, can be reconciled by noting that, on average, children are resilient in coping with divorce—but there are costs associated with coping. More specifically, the resilience perspective indicates that (a) children confront many emotional, relationship, and economic stressors before and after divorce; (b) divorce is a risk factor for psychological problems but the majority of children remain psychologically healthy following divorce; and (c) even successful coping can leave children with painful memories, strained relationships, and persistent regrets about their parents' divorce. [*See* COPING WITH STRESS.]

This last point requires some further elaboration. Many of psychologists' empirical measures of children's psychological health are not especially sensitive to the subtleties of emotional experience. These measures often assess a global, concrete outcome, such as a parent's ratings of a child's behavior problems or the number of years in school a child completes. Clearly, parent-rated behavior problems and level of educational attainment are important indices of children's well-being. In fact, the positive functioning of most children from divorced families on these outcomes supports the resilience perspective. At the same time, the measures used in empirical research commonly assess children from the outside in, that is, from the perspective of adults. These objective measures may miss many of the concerns that are of emotional importance to children themselves, even among children who cope well on the outside despite their inner concerns.

In fact, recent research indicates that even very well-functioning school-aged and young-adult children from divorced families report numerous painful feelings related to divorce such as social embarrassment, uncertainty about their parents' (usually the father's) love, and feeling that their childhood was more difficult than most. Together with the many practical stressors involved in divorce, such painful feelings constitute some of the costs of coping with the break-up of one's parents' marriage. Such findings not only are important in their own right, but they also may help to explain the apparent contradiction between the findings of empirical research and clinical case studies. Empirical researchers focus on important, observable outcomes for groups of children, and these investigators invariably note children's success in completing their developmental tasks despite the stress of a parental divorce. Clinical case investigators focus on the detail of the individual's struggle in coping with divorce. In so doing, case studies accurately detect much of the pain experienced by children from divorced families that is missed in many empirical studies. At the same time, case studies can miss the forest for the trees. Case studies can overlook the successful coping of children of divorce as a group—and it is the more successful children who are less likely to be the subjects of case studies. To put the matter simply, children are resilient but not invulnerable in coping with their parents divorce.

I. Predictors of More or Less Successful Coping

Many aspects of children's psychological health are linked with how families manage the process of divorce. Conflict between parents is one central concern, as a large body of research clearly indicates that high levels of conflict between parents in marriage and following divorce are associated with more psychological difficulties among children. In particular, interparental conflict is more damaging when it is prolonged, openly angry or violent, focuses on or involves the child, and remains unresolved.

Less adequate parenting is another risk factor associated with increased psychological problems among children from divorced families. In comparison to married parents, divorced parents, on average, offer their children less affection, have more problems in communication, are worse at family problem solving, monitor children less closely, and are more inconsistent. Like parental conflict, parenting problems often begin prior to a marital separation, commonly escalate in the year or two following separation, and generally improve again as more time passes. The relationship between children and the parent with primary physical custody is most important to children's psychological health. If this parent maintains an authoritative relationship, children can thrive following divorce even if they have little contact with their other parent. [*See* PARENTING.]

Finally, divorce inevitably creates financial strain, because it is cheaper to live in one than in two households. In fact, evidence demonstrates that children living with single mothers experience the brunt of this economic hardship. Economic disadvantage is important, but less so than parenting quality or interparental conflict, to children's psychological well-being following divorce. However, the economic consequences of divorce for children are important outcomes in their own right. For example, a significant proportion of children, especially those who live in the custody of their mothers, move into poverty as a result of divorce.

III. CHILD ADJUSTMENT AND DIVORCE CUSTODY ARRANGEMENTS

A relatively small number of studies have been conducted on children's adjustment in alternative post-divorce legal and physical custody arrangements. Applied research in this area has focused on children's psychological health in relation to: mother versus father custody, contact with nonresidential parents, joint physical custody, and joint legal custody.

A. Mother versus Father Custody

The question of whether children should be placed in the custody of their mother or father is often intensely debated in individual custody battles. In fact, several studies have compared the adjustment of children living in the physical custody of their mothers versus their fathers following divorce, and researchers typically find no differences in children's well-being that are attributable to custody type. Much more controversial, however, is that several investigators have found children to be better adjusted when they live in the custody of their same-sex parent. That is, in these studies, girls appear to fare better in the custody of

their mothers while boys do better in the custody of their fathers.

If we can conclude that the custody arrangement *causes* these differences in the adjustment of boys and girls, these findings would hold numerous implications both for legal decision making and for psychological theories. However, there are important reasons to question the causal conclusion. For one, selection factors must be carefully considered in interpreting the results of research. Divorced fathers may be more likely to be awarded physical custody of their sons when they are exceptionally good parents, but fathers may be more likely to get physical custody of their daughters when the mother is particularly troubled. That is, children's (and parents') emotional well-being may be the cause of the alternative custody arrangements rather than result of them. In addition, the samples in most studies to date have been small and quite select, and one of the few investigations of a large national sample failed to find the expected interaction between gender of child and gender of custodial parent for any one of 35 different outcome measures. Finally, there is a strong bias in the law to keep sibling groups together, and at least some research indicates that sibling support is important to children's adjustment to divorce. Gender-based custody arrangements obviously would lead to splitting siblings in many families. In short, the evidence is weak at best for a preference for placing children with their same-gender parent.

B. Contact with Nonresidential Parents

Several studies, particularly those that have used survey data from large national samples, have found no relation, or only a weak one, between the frequency of contact with the nonresidential parent (typically the father) and children's adjustment following divorce. On the other hand, some studies of select samples report that children are better adjusted when they have more frequent contact with their nonresidential fathers, provided that a number of conditions hold. Moderating factors include the mental health of the nonresidential parent, whether the nonresidential parent–child relationship is positive, and the degree of conflict between parents. Other evidence indicates that positive benefits are evident only when contact is consistent, especially when contact is frequent, and one provocative study reported that frequency of nonresidential mother–child contact, but not nonresidential father–child contact, was related to more positive child adjustment.

Inconsistencies across studies are likely due in part to the number of variables that moderate the effects of contact between children and their nonresidential parents. Under differing circumstances more frequent contact may have positive, negative, or neutral effects on children's well-being. The number of moderating factors makes it difficult to draw firm conclusions from available evidence, but one inference is clear: Increased contact per se is not strongly related to measures of children's adjustment.

Two important caveats apply to this conclusion. First, we again raise a caution about measurement. Evidence indicates that children value their relationships with their nonresidential fathers even when contact is infrequent. Commonly used measures may be inadequate in assessing more subtle emotions that children feel toward their absent fathers, such as feelings of anger or rejection, yearning or love. It also is possible that the consequences of infrequent contact may only surface during certain developmental periods. For example, children may be particularly likely to feel the loss of contact during their late adolescence when identity concerns cause them to reflect on the meaning of their troubled family relationships for their developing sense of self.

A second caveat is that father contact is quite infrequent on average in studies of national samples. In terms of children's well-being, it is possible that the positive effects of father contact may not be evident when contact is so infrequent. Still, it is clear that more frequent contact with the nonresidential parent is a relatively *less* important predictor of children's psychological health than the quality of the residential parent–child relationship, the degree of interparental conflict, or economic stability.

More generally, however, the low level of contact between noncustodial fathers and their children is distressing in its own right. Based on data from a recent survey of a national sample, for example, among fathers separated for 2 years or less, 12.8% had seen their children only once a year or less, while 42.7% saw them once a week or more. Contact declines rapidly over time, particularly following the remarriage or relocation of one or both parents. Thus, among fa-

thers separated for 11 years or more, 50.4% had seen their children only once a year or less, while only 12.0% saw them once a week or more. [*See* FATHERS.]

C. Joint Physical Custody

Overall, evidence indicates that joint physical custody is associated with more frequent contact between children and their fathers, increased parental cooperation, and somewhat better functioning among children. Differences between joint and sole custody families typically are small in magnitude, however, and selection factors suggest an important caution in interpreting existing research: Parents who chose joint physical custody likely differ from other parents in many ways. These differences, not the joint physical custody arrangement, may account for the positive outcomes associated with joint custody. In addition, there are circumstances when joint physical custody is associated with worse outcomes for children, especially when there are high levels of ongoing conflict between the parents. Thus, there are some benefits linked with joint physical custody, but the benefits are linked to the parents' ability to coparent following divorce.

D. Joint Legal Custody, Father Contact, and the Payment of Child Support

The meaning of joint legal custody can be vague, but the symbolism of joint legal custody can be important to parents who do not have physical custody of their children. Apparently, symbolism matters, as fathers with joint legal custody maintain more contact with their children over time. Joint legal custody does not affect the size of child support awards, but it is related to compliance with paying child support awards. Importantly, one study found that background characteristics, including measures of the quality of the partners' relationship during marriage, did *not* explain the positive effects of joint legal custody on postdivorce parenting. Although we cannot conclude that joint legal custody causes these positive, if modest, benefits, few concerns have been raised about negative effects of joint legal custody. Thus, joint legal custody appears to be a positive alternative for postdivorce family arrangements.

E. Divorce Mediation and Children's Well-Being

Numerous efforts have attempted to replace adversary procedures with more cooperative ones in resolving child custody disputes in separation and divorce. Divorce mediation is the most prominent of these, as mediation has rapidly replaced or altered adversary practices in relation to child custody throughout the United States. Mediation is based on the assumption that cooperative negotiation can produce added benefits or so-called win-win outcomes. Divorced parents are not expected to be friends, but they are encouraged to develop a degree of cooperation in coparenting. Philosophically, mediation assumes that divorced parents should be the experts who decide what is in their own children's future best interests.

Evidence indicates that mediation greatly reduces the need for custody hearings, somewhat reduces relitigation, increases compliance with court orders, and increases parents' satisfaction with the legal system. However, research generally has not found that, as opposed to litigation, mediation leads to better outcomes for children's or parent's mental health. However, some evidence indicates that fathers who mediate maintain more contact with their children, pay more child support, and work more closely with their children's mother. These outcomes would seem to be important to children's well-being even they have not been directly linked with improved functioning on various psychological measures.

IV. CHILD CUSTODY IN FOSTER CARE AND ADOPTION

Current practices regarding foster care and adoption are outgrowths of the historical fact that a substantial number of children were orphaned and required substitute care due to the short, expected life span of adults prior to the twentieth century. Today, however, most children are placed into foster care as a result of abuse and neglect, and adoption most commonly results when living parents' voluntarily give up their parental rights.

Prior to the nineteenth century, care for orphaned or destitute children was provided mainly through indentured servitude, as children were legally bound to another adult as an apprentice or other worker. Later in the 1800s, almshouses were used to house orphaned children, together with adults who were destitute, physically ill, or mentally ill, but conditions in almshouses were deplorable and many children died in these facilities. Comprehensive adoption laws were not enacted in the United States until the middle of the nineteenth century, and the idea of foster care, involving a temporary rather than a permanent placement out of the home, was not widely embraced until early in the twentieth century. The Social Security Act of 1935 established a variety of programs for dependent children, but little federal financing was made available for foster care until 1961, when foster care funds were provide to some children who qualified for the federal Aid to Families with Dependent Children (AFDC).

A. Foster Care Placement Procedures

The 1980 Adoption Assistance and Child Welfare Act (AACWA) brought about two important and continuing influences on current foster care: Mandating services to families to avoid removal of children into foster care and implementing permanency planning, a requirement to form specific plans for children in foster care either to return them to their birth homes or to provide them with adoptive placements. The law had an important influence on the length of time children stayed in foster care, reducing the median length of stay from 2.4 years to 1.4 years.

Based on the requirements of the AACWA, children can be removed from their home and placed in foster care if a social welfare agency deems continued residence unsafe, although removal decisions must be reviewed by a judge. Once the child is in placement, the child welfare agency must develop a plan that includes reasonable efforts to rehabilitate the family so that the child can return home. A decision about permanent placement must be made by 18 months after removal. If the conditions that led to the removal of the child do not improve, the child welfare agency can pursue termination parental rights at this time, although legal proceedings and appeals can cause the process to drag on for as long as 5 years. Because of the irreversible nature of the termination of parental rights, many judges are reluctant to grant terminations, and as a result, many children remain in foster care because their parents are unable to care for them and because they cannot be adopted.

B. Procedures for Adoption and Involuntary Termination of Parental Rights

Parental rights can be terminated either voluntarily or involuntarily. The adoption of infants often follows a voluntary termination of birth parents' rights in which the parent(s) relinquish all parental rights and responsibilities including the right to see the child. (Another possibility is an open adoption, in which the birth parent can maintain some ongoing contact with the child.) Voluntary terminations must be given freely, and some states allow parents to reverse their decision to terminate their parental rights for a period of time even after the child has lived with the adoptive parents (e.g., 6 months). Birth fathers, including unmarried fathers, have rights similar to those of birth mothers. Whether an unmarried father can veto a mother's adoption and claim custody of a child is controversial, but the custody claims of fathers generally take precedence over those of strangers. Efforts must be made to locate a father who is not aware of the birth of his child and efforts also must be made to identify the father if the mother is unwilling or unable to identify him. However, a father who knows of the existence of his child but who does not participate in the life of his child may be considered to have abandoned or neglected the child, thus permitting termination of his rights.

Biological parents have a fundamental right to custody of their children, thus involuntary termination of parental rights typically involves situations in which a child has been abandoned or removed from his or her home by a social service agency. Involuntary terminations require court proceedings during which the rights and needs of the birth parents, children, and the state are weighed. The birth parents must be found to be unfit before their rights can be terminated. In this circumstance, the child's best interests are not the overriding concern, because such a circumstance would allow tremendous state intervention in families.

C. Children's Adjustment to Adoption and Foster Care

Determining children's adjustment to foster-care placement or adoption is difficult, because children in these circumstances are different from other children in many ways in addition to their placement, most notably, in terms of the family experiences that resulted in foster placement or adoption. Foster children often come from low-income homes, have had little stability in school and peer relationships, and may be vulnerable to many emotional disorders because of their prenatal and postnatal environments and/or genetic influences. Infants or children placed through adoption also may be at risk because of a number of background characteristics, including genetic factors, poor prenatal care, and maternal age. Moreover, many parents, especially parents with limited resources, find it more difficult to raise a child who has an emotional or physical handicap. Thus, children may be placed in foster care or put for adoption because of their special needs.

Case studies and uncontrolled research typically conclude that most children fare well in foster care. Similarly, no differences in adjustment usually are found in studies comparing the adjustment of children in foster care with that of children who have been investigated but not removed from their homes. Most optimistically, some evidence indicates that children's functioning *improves* when they are placed in foster care. For example, there may be a reduction in behavior problems and some gain in academic achievement. The benefits are modest, however, the weight of evidence indicates that foster care does not cause children psychological harm, and it does protect their physical safety.

In contrast to this positive outlook, the limited evidence available generally indicates that children who have been adopted have *more* psychological problems than would be expected based on the prevalence of difficulties in the general population. These findings may well be the result of select effects, however. As noted earlier, adopted children may be at risk for a variety of reasons other than their adoption.

V. CONCLUDING COMMENT

Few circumstances in life are as potentially disruptive to children or to parents as the issues discussed in the chapter. There is no doubt that the majority of children are resilient, even in the face of major changes in their life and challenges in their families. Still, there also is no doubt that the preferred living arrangement for children is to be reared in the custody of their two, loving and happy parents.

Many children are lucky enough to be reared in this ideal circumstance; however, far more children than we might like to believe grow up in the custody of only one parent, a relative, or an adoptive or foster parent. As a society, we need to come to grips with this reality, and attempt to reach greater consensus about how to balance the sometimes competing interests of children, parents, and the state. We need to do so for the sake of clarity and also for the sake of children, because the uncertainty inherent in our ambiguous stand, and the conflict that can result from it, only harm children further. When the state intervenes to protect children, it should do so with clarity and assertion. Weak and inconsistent efforts are likely to both waste resources and do more harm then good.

In considering the mental health of children, we note again that children who live in nontraditional family circumstances are resilient but not invulner-able. We need to be sensitive to their struggles in coping with upheavals in their lives, but we also need to recognize children's strength even in the face of some of the most profound stressors they could ever be expected to face.

BIBLIOGRAPHY

Emery, R. E. (1994). *Renegotiating family relationships: Divorce, child custody, and mediation.* New York: Guilford Press.
Emery, R. E. (1998). *Marriage, divorce, and children's adjustment* (2nd Ed.). Thousand Oaks, CA: Sage Publications.
Goodman, G. S., Emery, R. E., & Haugaard, J. J. (1998). Developmental psychology and law: The cases of divorce, child maltreatment, foster care, and adoption. In W. Damon, I. E. Sigel & K. A. Renninger (Eds.), *Handbook of child psychology (5th Ed. Vol. 4): Child psychology in action.* New York: Wiley.
Melton, G. B., Petrila, J., Poythress, N. G., & Slobogin, C. (1987). *Psychological evaluations for the courts.* New York: Guilford.
Mnookin, R. (1978). *Child, family, and state.* Boston: Little, Brown & Co.

Day Care

Virginia D. Allhusen and Alison Clarke-Stewart

University of California, Irvine

Attachment   A close, enduring relationship formed between child and adult that serves to bring the child close to the adult in times of need.

Avoidance   Tendency of some children to avoid proximity to and contact with the attachment figure, even when the child is stressed.

Cognitive Development   Development of increasingly sophisticated mental processes through which the child comes to know and make sense of his or her surroundings.

Day Care   Daily care of a child by someone other than the child's parents. May take place in day-care centers, preschools, family day-care homes, or in the caregiver's or child's own home, with or without other children present. Often referred to as "child care."

Nonparental Caregiver   Person other than the parents who regularly cares for the child in the care setting. May be related to the child (grandparent, aunt, cousin) or unrelated (teacher, nanny, family day-care provider).

Social Competence   Skills acquired by the child to facilitate acceptance in social groups and situations. Includes awareness of others, cooperation, empathy, compliance, negotiation of conflict with peaceful resolution, and assertiveness.

Strange Situation   Standard laboratory method for assessing the quality of 12- to 18-month-old children's attachment relationships with their mothers or other attachment figures, which presents a series of separations from the mother and approach by an adult female stranger. The child's reaction to these mild stressors and use of the mother as a source of comfort are used to classify the attachment relationship as secure or anxious.

In this article, research on the effects of **DAY CARE** on children's development is reviewed. The discussion is organized around two central questions. The first question is, "Is day care harmful for children's development, particularly in the first year or two of life?" To answer this question, research on the relation between day-care attendance and the quality of children's relationships with their mothers and with their peers is summarized. The second question is "Can it be beneficial for children to spend time in day care?" To answer this question, research on children's relationships with day-care providers, cognitive and language development, and social competence with peers is presented. The article concludes with a summary of what is known and what is yet to be learned about the effects of early day-care experience on children's development, and recommendations are made for further research to help illuminate our understanding of this complex issue.

I. WHAT IS DAY CARE?

Table I shows the distribution of the major types of child-care arrangements currently being used by working mothers of preschool children in the United States.

Table I Primary Child-Care Arrangements Used by Employed Mothers for Their Children Under 5 Years[a]

Type of care	Percent using the arrangement	
	for infants and toddlers	for preschool children
Parents themselves	25%	23%
Another relative	27%	21%
Nonrelated in-home provider	7%	5%
Day-care home	26%	18%
Day-care center	16%	33%

[a]Statistics based on the most recent available data from the U.S. Department of Labor.

All these types of care except that provided by the mother, herself, or more broadly, by both parents, are referred to as day care. Only about one-quarter of the families in which mothers work manage to cover child care by juggling the parents' schedules or by taking the child along to work. All the other families use one or more of these day-care arrangements. One-quarter use a relative—aunt, grandmother, older sibling—as a care provider. Care by relatives is especially common for infants, for poor children, and for children whose mothers work part time. A smaller number of families use a nonrelated caregiver who comes to or lives in their home—a neighbor, a friend, a paid or unpaid babysitter, a nanny, a housekeeper, a maid, a live-in student, or an au pair. The use of nonrelated babysitters in the child's own home has dropped sharply over the past decade. Only about 6% of families today use this kind of care. Again, this form of day care is relatively more common for infants. About one-quarter of the children whose mothers work are cared for by a nonrelated provider who looks after a number of children, perhaps including her own, in her home. This "family day care" arrangement is the most common type of care for 1- and 2-year-olds whose mothers work full time. The number of regulated, licensed day-care homes in the United States has increased by one-third over the past 15 years. [*See* CHILD CARE PROVIDERS.]

Day-care centers are used relatively rarely for infants and toddlers; only 16% of the infants of working mothers are in centers. But for 3- and 4-year-olds whose mothers work full time, centers are the day-care arrangement of choice. About one-third of the 3- and 4-year-olds whose mothers work are in centers. In addition, many children whose mothers are not employed attend day-care centers or nursery schools; currently about half of all 3- and 4-year-olds in the United States attend some kind of center program. It is in the use of day-care centers that we see the greatest change over the past two decades. Over the past decade both the capacity of day-care centers and the proportion of working mothers placing their infants in day-care centers have doubled. Over the past 15 years, the capacity of day-care centers has tripled.

II. IS DAY CARE HARMFUL TO CHILDREN'S DEVELOPMENT?

American society has long held a belief in the primacy of the mother–child relationship and the sanctity of the traditional nuclear family in which children are nurtured in the folds of their mothers' skirts while fathers toil in workplaces outside the home to provide for their families. Perhaps owing to this belief, the preponderance of research on day care has been focused on the question of whether day-care attendance (and therefore time spent outside this idealized nuclear family environment) is harmful to young children's development. Many of the earlier studies of the effects of nonmaternal day-care experience on children's development (done in the 1960s and 1970s) used a rather simplistic design of comparing behavioral development in groups of day-care and non-day-care children. Not surprisingly, these studies produced mixed results, with some finding no differences in the two groups and others finding significant differences in favor of one group or the other. These first studies were followed by research focused on the effects of day-care experiences varying in type and quality. More recently, studies have been designed to take account of the fact that day-care and non-day-care "groups" are each heterogeneous, with wide within-group variation in child, mother, and family characteristics. In this most recent conceptualization, day care, per se, is seen as only one factor contributing to the trajectory of a child's development, with other forces such as the child's sex and temperament, the family's affluence and attitudes, and the day-care environment's quality and features simultaneously considered.

Throughout this evolution of research on the harmful effects of day care, two child outcomes have received particular attention: (1) the quality of children's relationships with their mothers, and (2) the nature of children's interactions with their peers.

A. Children's Relationship with Mother

Perhaps more than any other issue in the day-care area, the question of whether day-care attendance disrupts the mother–child relationship has been the most hotly debated. Societal values about the primacy of the mother–child relationship provided the sociocultural backdrop for the emotionality of this debate, and the work of British psychiatrist John Bowlby provided its theoretical framework. In his observations of institutionalized infants in the 1950s, Bowlby documented a pattern of despair and detachment, in which infants who had been permanently separated from their mothers progressed through a sequence of what he termed "despair," characterized by negative affect and low activity level, to a state of "detachment," in which infants seemed to recover but were observed to be emotionally distant and incapable of forming close, trusting relationships with caregiving adults. The infants' "attachments" to their mothers had been broken, and they were emotionally crippled as a result. Based on this work, child development researchers began to wonder if the same types of negative effects might be found in children who experienced long daily separations from their mothers while in day care.

Early research findings all converged on the fact that day-care attendance in the preschool years (ages 3–4 years) did not have a deleterious effect on the quality of children's attachment relationships with their mothers. There was also some suggestion in early studies of younger children that even day care initiated in the first 2 years of life was not inherently harmful to the mother–child relationship. These studies soon came under criticism, however, for their lack of representativeness: most studies at that time were being conducted in high-quality, university-based day-care centers. Critics quite rightly argued that not only were most day-care infants not cared for in centers, but the quality of day care available to most parents in the United States was of lower quality than that found in the university-based research settings. Critics also suggested that the ways in which the mother–child relationship had been assessed in these studies were not sufficiently probing to discern emotional problems and it was premature to give day care a clean bill of health. A new set of studies was launched, taking care to include day-care centers varying in quality and, later, different types of day-care arrangements beyond day-care centers (e.g., family day care, in-home nonparental care, care by relatives, etc.), and assessing the mother–infant relationship with the best available measure of attachment the "Strange Situation." These studies produced somewhat different results, and thus was born the Great Infant Day Care Debate.

Dozens of studies were conducted between 1980 and 1995 to help shed light on the question of whether day-care attendance in and of itself threatens the development of a healthy child–mother attachment relationship. Although the variability across studies in terms of research design and subject population made it difficult to combine results into one coherent conclusion, there appeared in the studies to be a trend toward somewhat higher rates of insecure attachments among children who entered day care in their first year of life and who experienced 20 or more hours of care per week. Meta-analyses suggested there was about an 8% increase in the incidence of insecure attachments among children with extensive, early day-care experience compared to children with less, later, or no day-care experience. This difference was statistically significant.

There was also evidence, in these studies, that family factors play a critical role in determining whether day care will exert a negative effect on the development of attachment relationships. Day-care children were found to be more likely to develop insecure attachment relationships with their mothers in the context of low family social support, high stress, poor marital quality, and poor maternal psychological functioning.

Because of findings such as these, researchers began

to reconceptualize the design of studies aimed at examining the effects of day care on children's attachments. The latest studies carefully measure not just child and day-care variables, but also family variables that may account for differences among children in the quality of the relationships they develop with their mothers. In one of the most comprehensive such studies, the National Institute of Child Health and Human Development (NICHD) Study of Early Child Care, researchers found that day care alone was not a predictor of the security of children's attachment relationships with their mothers at 15 months of age. No difference in attachment security in the Strange Situation was observed to be related to the type of day care (with grandmother, in-home sitter, day-care home or center), the numbers of hours of care, the age at which care began, or the quality of caregiving received. Only when day-care experience was combined with "risk" factors in the family were children more likely to develop insecure attachments. Most notably, when day-care quality was poor *and* the mother was less sensitive and responsive, children were more likely to develop insecure attachments to their mothers. These results are particularly noteworthy given the scope and magnitude of the study—over 1000 subjects in 10 different areas around the country—and the care taken to eliminate problematic research design issues present in previous research.

Nevertheless, this may not be the last word on the subject. One issue remaining is the ecological validity of the measure used to assess attachment security. The "Strange Situation" is a lab procedure in which the child's reaction to brief (3-minute) separations from the mother and greeting behavior upon her return are assessed. In recent years, the validity of this measure for day-care children, who routinely experience separations from their mothers, has been called into question. Might it be that day-care children are less stressed by the separations presented in the Strange Situation (because they resemble their typical daily separations from the mother), and therefore they are less likely to greet mother in search of comfort when she returns and more likely to go on playing? In the NICHD study, no difference was found in the distress levels of day-care and non-day-care children when they were separated from their mothers. Nevertheless, some other research using a new measure of attachment (one that does not rely on maternal separations to elicit attachment behaviors) showed that day-care children (but not non-

day-care children) were more likely to be rated as secure in this situation than in the Strange Situation. Longitudinal research is needed to determine the later sequelae of reunion behavior in the Strange Situation for children experiencing extensive day care in their first year. The NICHD study, which is following children through the end of the first grade, will provide these data. [*See* ATTACHMENT.]

B. Children's Interactions with Peers

A second issue motivating research on day care has been concern about the development of children's social interactions in group care settings and, more specifically, whether children with extensive day-care experience exhibit maladaptive social behavior with their peers.

Beginning once again with the most simplistic models for examining the effects of day care on children's development, a number of researchers looked at differences in social competence for day-care versus non-day-care children. In general, the results of these studies showed that although day-care children are in some respects more socially skilled than their stay-at-home counterparts, they may also behave more aggressively in social encounters.

Children in day care, researchers have found, are, on average, less polite, less agreeable, less compliant with their mother's or caregiver's demands and requests, less respectful of others' rights, more irritable and more rebellious, more likely to use profane language, louder and more boisterous, more competitive and aggressive with their peers than children who are not or who have not been in day care. In three large, recent studies of preschool and kindergarten children, researchers found that children who attended day care in the earlier years were more aggressive toward their peers and more disobedient with adults than those who did not attend day care. These differences in aggressive and noncompliant behavior, although not inevitable, appear in tests and in natural observations, in classroom settings and on the playground, with adults and with other children, with strangers and with parents, for children from model and mediocre day-care programs. They are more marked for boys and for children from lower income families, but they also appear for girls and middle-class children.

This finding of heightened aggression among day-care children has been given a great deal of attention in the day-care literature. Some researchers have claimed that the aggression and noncompliance observed in day-care children reflects psychological maladjustment. They have suggested that day care places children at risk for developing emotional problems. There are several reasons to question this interpretation, however. First, although day-care children are more aggressive on the playground, they are not generally considered by their teachers to be unlikable or difficult to manage. Second, when characteristics of the child and of the family are taken into account, the apparent differences in children's aggression decrease dramatically. Third, when a curriculum that focuses on teaching children social skills is implemented in the day-care center, the heightened aggression of day-care children is reduced. Fourth, although day-care children are more aggressive from preschool through first or second grade, they are not more aggressive in the later school years. And fifth, even in studies in which statistically significant differences in aggression between day-care and non-day-care groups are found, the more aggressive children are still within the normal limits of behavior: in other words, this heightened aggression, when found, is not clinically significant. [*See* AGGRESSION.]

III. CAN DAY CARE BE BENEFICIAL TO CHILDREN?

Up to this point we have reviewed research on the question of whether day care has *negative* effects on children's development. An alternative approach is to ask whether day care *enhances* children's behavior and development. As Urie Bronfenbrenner proposed in his ecological model of human development nearly 20 years ago, children can benefit from a variety of experiences outside the home. It is reasonable to ask, then, whether *if the quality of nonmaternal day care experienced by the child is good,* experiences and opportunities in the day-care environment might augment the stimulation of the home environment and promote children's development. Experience in day care might also help young children master adjustments to other types of new environments that they will inevitably experience later in life (e.g., transition to formal school, overnight or more extended visits in the households of relatives and friends, etc.). There are three outcomes that have received researchers' at-

tention in the effort to study the potentially positive effects of day-care attendance on children's development: attachments to nonparental caregivers, cognitive development, and social competence with peers.

A. Attachments to Nonparental Child-Care Providers

Research on the quality of children's relationships with their day-care providers has arisen from the framework of attachment theory, which suggests that children form attachment relationships with those who care for them and can benefit from secure attachments with these caregiving figures. The earliest question to be asked was: Do infants develop attachment relationships with their nonparental care providers? In its earliest form, this question seemed to be motivated by a concern that the day-care provider might supplant the mother as the primary attachment figure in the young child's life. Studies were thus undertaken to compare children's attachment behaviors with their mothers and their day-care providers in settings where both adults were available to the child. The results were consistent across these studies: although infants did develop attachments to their day-care providers, they spent more time near the mother, sought her assistance in a problem-solving situation, chose her as a social interaction partner, and preferred her as a source of comfort, compared with the day-care provider. Developing an emotional bond to the day-care provider did not usurp the mother's position as a primary attachment figure.

Children in day care can use their care provider as a "secure base" from whom they derive comfort, and information, and interaction. They apparently develop an "attachment hierarchy" within the day-care setting, such that they seek out a certain care provider more often than others in the same setting. The most significant ways in which these relationships with care providers differ from relationships with mother is in their stability and the depth of the child's feeling: children in day care do not usually mourn the loss of a day-care provider in the way that Bowlby described the despair and detachment behavior of children who lost their mothers. It is a different thing to lose a secondary attachment object and to lose the primary or sole attachment figure.

Although little empirical research on the benefits of these secondary relationships has been conducted, the studies that have been carried out provide confirmation that secure relationships with care providers are beneficial to children in some of the same ways that secure child–mother attachments are beneficial. Compared with children rated as insecure or less involved with their day-care providers, children with secure attachments engage in more exploratory behavior, are more engaged and competent with their peers, play in more sophisticated ways with their peers, and are better able to handle separations from their parents, easily engaging in play and exploration upon their parents' departure from the day-care setting.

As an outgrowth of the line of research examining the quality of children's relationships with nonparental care providers, researchers have considered whether secure attachments with day-care providers can play a compensatory role when attachments with parents are insecure. Theoretically, a child is better off having a secure attachment relationship with at least one person—even if it is not the mother—than having no secure attachment relationships at all. This has been confirmed by empirical study: children rated as secure in their interactions with day-care providers but insecure with their mothers are more socially competent than children whose relationships with both mother and caregiver are insecure. Children whose relationships with both adults are secure are even more socially competent. This suggests that a secure relationship with the care provider can provide benefits in the area of social development even for children who are not at risk for social problems as a consequence of having an insecure attachment to their mother.

But not all children in day care form secure relationships with their day-care providers. What factors mediate the quality of the relationship with the caregiver? Not surprisingly, the single most important predictor of attachment quality is the sensitivity and responsiveness of the caregiver herself: when day-care providers are warm, involved, positive (smiling, hugging, holding, speaking in a warm tone), responsive, and in tune with children's needs and signals, children are more likely to develop secure relationships with them. In fact, when caregivers are emotionally remote and detached, the children in their care tend to prefer interacting with an adult female stranger than with the familiar day-care provider. Settings that feature fewer competing demands for the caregiver's attention (a smaller total group size, a more favorable adult–child ratio) allow the care provider to be more respon-

sive to individual children, who in turn are more likely to form secure attachments with them. Caregiver stability is also related to the quality of the attachment relationship: when caregivers have been in the care setting longer, children are more likely to direct both distress and nondistress attachment behaviors toward them and are better able to tolerate separations from their parents at drop-off time in the day-care setting. The amount of time per week children spend with their day-care providers and the age at which they enter care have a similar effect: the more hours per week the two interaction partners spend together, the more likely the child is to form a secure attachment relationship, and the younger the child is when he or she enters care, the more positively engaged is he or she with the caregiver. In high-quality day-care settings, these three factors (caregiver stability, amount of care, and age of entry) combine to give the care provider a chance to get to know the child and read his or her most subtle cues and for the child to learn the care provider's interaction style and experience her behavior as predictable.

Children are also more likely to develop secure relationships with care providers whom they observe to be well-regarded by their mothers. Several studies have shown that children whose mothers have more contact with the caregiver are more likely to be securely attached to the caregiver.

B. Cognitive and Language Development

Day care has long been recognized as a potential intervention setting for children from less advantaged home environments, and a number of studies have confirmed that in a high-quality day-care setting, these children show accelerations in cognitive and language development that in some cases are sustained into middle childhood and beyond. Somewhat less clear are the short- and longer-term effects of day care as it is regularly experienced by most children in the United States—in care arrangements other than specialized, high-quality day care intervention programs focusing on cognitive enrichment. [See COGNITIVE DEVELOPMENT.]

1. Day-Care versus Non-Day-Care Group Comparisons

Although most research on the effects of day care on children's cognitive development has focused on day-care *enrichment* programs, some studies have investigated the effects of experience in more typical day-care settings. These studies show that when children enter care as infants, no differences are found in their cognitive ability through age 12 months. This has been shown even in studies where the day-care providers were less stimulating than mothers. Thus, even though the day-care children spent the day in the care of a less stimulating adult (the day-care provider) than non-day-care children (who spent the day with their mothers), no differences were observed in the cognitive ability of these two groups. This suggests that day-care children's mothers provide adequate (or even compensatory) stimulation for their children during the times when they are together.

2. Contributions of Day-Care Quality

Variations in day-care quality have a major influence on children's cognitive and language development. When day-care quality is high, children have higher scores on standardized intelligence tests, advanced language skills, and, later, higher school achievement. These positive effects have been shown to extend from infancy into early adolescence. Characteristics of the day-care environment found to be associated with these gains include an educationally oriented curriculum as well as caregiver stimulation, verbal interaction, provision of educational experiences, responsiveness to child questions, and authoritative management. Caregivers with more extensive formal training and with fewer children in the day-care group are more likely to provide these types of stimulating and developmentally supportive experiences for the children in their care.

With respect to day-care intervention programs, this same pattern of cognitive advances is seen. Children's language development appears to be particularly malleable to intervention efforts: programs focusing on early literacy training, for example, have yielded advances in children's language skills that persist through late adolescence. However, these longer term positive effects of day-care intervention programs are not always found. Because children targeted for intervention programs typically come from less advantaged home environments, the challenge becomes to sustain the gains of the cognitively enriching day-care environment after the child leaves the program. Programs that include a family intervention component are generally more successful in producing these longer term benefits.

3. Child and Family Variables

The fact that difficulties are encountered in sustaining cognitive gains from intervention day-care programs for children from less advantaged home environments implies that family factors moderate the effects of day care on children's cognitive development. In fact, some researchers have found that children's verbal ability is better predicted by the quality of the home environment than by the quality or type of day-care environment. Other studies, however, have shown that stimulating verbal interactions with caregivers predict both verbal and cognitive skills even after family background variables are controlled. Still other studies suggest that although day care has a positive effect on the cognitive development of children from impoverished homes, it may have a *negative* effect on children from more advantaged homes, particularly when care is initiated before the first birthday.

C. Social Competence with Peers

Over the preschool years, children grow in social skills and develop social relationships. They progress in interacting with their peers from simply staring to approaching and exploring, to smiling and offering toys, to interactions that are intense and reciprocal. They learn to play complex games, to act out roles, and to participate in cooperative activities in groups. They make friends with special playmates. A large number of researchers have focused on day-care children's relations with their peers, expecting that because these children have so much more experience with other children, this must make a difference in their social relations with agemates. They have observed children in their day-care settings as they interact with other children after greater or lesser amounts of time in day care. They have brought unacquainted pairs of children who are in either day-care or parental care into a set-up play situation in the laboratory and watched their interactions with one another. They have tested children from different care arrangements on their willingness to cooperate and help each other. The results of their studies suggest that day care also makes a difference in peer relations.

Day-care children are more at ease socially when they meet a new child. In unfamiliar situations, children attending day-care centers or nursery schools are more outgoing, less timid and fearful, and more helpful and cooperative than children who spend their time at home. They are more likely to share materials and behave empathically toward other children. Their interactions with peers are also more complex and mature. They can sustain their play longer and respond more appropriately and immediately to the other children's behavior. They are more knowledgeable about the social world. They know more about social and moral rules—for example, they know that it is worse to hit another child than it is to talk when the teacher is talking. When they start school, children who have attended day care or nursery school are better adjusted, more persistent at their tasks, and more likely to be leaders.

These differences in social competence do not appear in all studies of all day-care programs for all children, but when differences do appear, children in day care are, on average, more advanced.

Many researchers have attempted to deconstruct the "day care vs. non-day care" grouping variable to look at variations in child social competence outcomes based on more refined aspects of day-care experience including age of entry, amount, stability, type, and quality of care. With respect to age of entry, most studies seem to support the generalization that early exposure to the peer group via early entry to day care has positive effects on children's social competence. Compared with children who began nonmaternal care later in life or not at all, children who began care as infants have been observed to have fewer behavior problems as toddlers, to be more positive in their social interactions as preschoolers, to exhibit greater facility in entering the peer group, to have more friends and be more involved in social activities in the primary grades, and to be more assertive through the sixth grade. However, not all studies paint such a rosy picture. There has been research finding that early entry into day care is associated with less compliance and poorer peer relations in grade school. Perhaps other aspects of the day-care experience can help explain this apparent discrepancy in the research findings.

A second moderator of the effects of early day care on children's social competence is the amount of care children have experienced. In general, research indicates that children spending greater amounts of time in day care are more likely to show advanced social competence. With respect to type of care, there is some evidence that center care (compared with sitter or family day care) is associated with advanced social competence in the preschool years. Stability of care ar-

rangements has also been shown to affect children's social development: children who are more competent with peers experience stable arrangements.

The quality of the day-care program and environment has been found to be consistently related to children's social competence. When caregivers provide a moderate amount of structure and a day-care "curriculum" that encourage children's cooperation, independence, self-expression, and social interaction, the children are more likely to be cooperative, self-confident, and assertive. Quality of care is a better predictor of concurrent and later social functioning than is age of entry into care.

Once again, however, day-care characteristics alone do not predict the course of children's social development: family factors also play an important role. For example, in one study, mothers' anxiety about placing their children in day care predicted children's later social adjustment in the day-care setting: children whose mothers had initially been reluctant to place their children in day care were more compliant, cooperative, persistent, and prosocial than children whose mothers had not expressed such concern.

IV. CONCLUSIONS AND FUTURE DIRECTIONS

Significant progress has been made over the past 25 years in understanding the effects of day care on children's development. Nevertheless, more research, using complex models of potential contributors to child outcomes, is needed in order to untangle and understand the effects of day care completely. What does seem clear from the research that has been conducted is that high-quality day care is not harmful to the cognitive or social development of preschool-aged children, and it can be beneficial to children, especially those from disadvantaged home environments. Evidence is mounting to suggest that the same is true for infant care: day care in and of itself, especially if it is of high quality, is not detrimental for children's development.

More and more, however, we are beginning to see that the determinants of the effects of day care on children's development go beyond factors directly related to children's day-care attendance (e.g., quality of the day-care environment, age of entry into day care, stability of care, number of hours in care, etc.). Characteristics of the family environment (e.g., parental sensitivity and responsiveness, opportunities for stimulation in the home environment, parental role satisfaction, etc.) contribute at least as much as the day-care environment in directing the course of child social and cognitive development. Moreover, it may be the case that families who place their children in day care compared to those who do not, or families who choose one type of day care versus another, vary systematically on family characteristics that might themselves explain observed differences among groups. Parents may simply choose day-care experiences for their children that provide more of the same types of experiences the child receives at home; thus day care merely reinforces (or perhaps magnifies) certain developmental outcomes for which the child was destined as a result of experiences in the home environment.

Comprehensive, longitudinal studies such as the NICHD Study of Early Child Care show researchers, policymakers, and parents that the question "Is day care good or bad for children?" is indeed hopelessly simplistic and naive. The results of such studies help illuminate our understanding of the complex ways in which child, family, and day-care characteristics interact to shape the course of development. Sometime in the not-too-distant future these studies may yield results that have practical and policy implications, such as how many hours per week of care is too many, how many children in a group is detrimental for development, what is the ideal day-care setting for a child with a difficult temperament. Until these questions have answers, day-care research will continue.

BIBLIOGRAPHY

Booth, A. (Ed.). (1992). *Child care in the 1990s: Trends and consequences.* Hillsdale, NJ: Erlbaum.

Chehrazi, S. (Ed.). (1990). *Psychosocial issues in day care.* Washington, DC: American Psychiatric Press.

Clarke-Stewart, K. A. (1989). Infant day care: Maligned or malignant? *American psychologist, 44,* 266–273.

Clarke-Stewart, K. A., Gruber, C. P., & Fitzgerald, L. M. (1994). *Children at home and in day care.* Hillsdale, NJ: Erlbaum.

Gamble, T. J., & Zigler, E. (1986). Effects of infant day care: Another look at the evidence. *American Journal of Orthopsychiatry, 56,* 26–42.

Hayes, C. D., Palmer, J. L., & Zaslow, M. J. (Eds.). (1990). *Who cares for America's children? Child care policy for the 1990s.* Washington, DC: National Academy Press.

Lamb, M. E., & Sternberg, K. J. (1990). Do we really know how day care affects children? *Journal of Applied Developmental Psychology, 11,* 351–379.

Phillips, D. A. (Ed.). (1987). *Quality in child care: What does research tell us? Research Monographs of the National Association for the Education of Young Children* (Vol. 1). Washington, DC: National Association for the Education of Young Children.

Scarr, S., & Eisenberg, M. (1993). Child care research: Issues, perspectives, and results. *Annual Review of Psychology, 44,* 613–644.

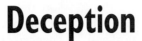

Deception

Bella M. DePaulo and Jenny S. Törnqvist

University of Virginia

Deception   Deliberately leading another person or persons to form a belief or impression that the deceiver believes to be false.

Lying   Deliberately leading another person or persons to form a belief or impression that the deceiver believes to be false. Sometimes defined as limited to verbal or written statements.

Machiavellianism   A personality trait characterized by manipulativeness, cynicism, and a low level of concern with conventional morality.

Motivational Impairment Effect   People who are highly motivated to get away with their lies are ironically more likely actually to get caught whenever others can observe their nonverbal cues.

Other-Oriented Lies   Lies told to benefit others.

Self-Centered Lies   Lies told to benefit oneself.

Self-Presentation   The attempt to shape, through our actions and personal styles, the way we are seen by others.

DECEPTION is a common occurrence in everyday life, despite the common belief that honesty is a virtue above all other virtues. In this article, deception will be examined in terms of the mental health implications of (a) telling lies; (b) being told lies; (c) being skilled at getting away with one's lies; and (d) being skilled at detecting lies.

I. INTRODUCTION

From a purely scientific point of view, questions about the mental health implications of deception can be answered most compellingly through experimental research. For example, to understand the effects of telling many lies (compared to very few lies, or even none at all) on mental health and well-being, it would be useful, methodologically, to randomly assign people to tell either many lies or hardly any lies in their everyday lives, and then measure the consequences. But of course this study would be both unethical and impossible to conduct, as would the parallel study in which some people are randomly assigned to be told many lies by other people in their everyday lives, whereas others would be assigned to a condition in which they are told hardly any lies. Similarly, we cannot conduct studies in which people are randomly assigned to be skilled liars, or skilled lie detectors. Therefore, to begin to learn about the mental health implications of deception, we need to take a more indirect route. We can look at the kinds of data that can and have been collected, and draw from those results some hints about the answers to our questions. For example, we will review research that compares people who tell many lies to those who tell very few lies, and see whether they differ in their satisfaction with their interpersonal relationships. If they do differ, we still cannot know for sure that they differ because of their different rates of lying, but such a finding would add to the plausibility of that conclusion.

The prevalent view of lying in Western society is a rather harsh one. Lying is viewed as unethical and liars are seen as cold, calculating, and exploitative. From this vantage point, lying would be expected to occur very infrequently, and people who tell lies should be chastised and shunned. The most serious lies that people tell, which are often deep betrayals of trust, may fit this dark view of deceit. But research on the little lies of everyday life suggests an entirely different perspective on liars and their lies. Little lies are not extraordinary or unusual events; instead, they are part of the fabric of everyday social discourse. In daily life, lies are told to accomplish the most basic goals of social life, such as influencing other people, making a good impression, and reassuring and protecting others.

II. LYING IN EVERYDAY LIFE

A. Pervasiveness of Lying

Lying is a fact of everyday life. From studies in which people have kept daily records of all of the lies that they tell, the most conservative estimate is that people tell a lie nearly every day. Typically, they lie in at least one out of every five of their interactions with other people that last 10 minutes or more. Over the course of a week, people lie to at least 30% of the people they see.

B. Kinds of Lies

There are many ways to categorize the different kinds of lies that people tell, but the distinction that has been most enduring over many decades, and across diverse disciplines such as philosophy, ethics, and psychology, is based on the liars' reasons or motivations for telling their lies. Most fundamentally, lies can be categorized as either self-centered or other-oriented. Self-centered lies are lies told to benefit the liars, whereas other-oriented or altruistic lies benefit someone other than the liar. There are many possible subtypes of both self-centered and other-oriented lies, but the two most

basic ones are lies told for reasons of personal advantage and lies told for more psychological reasons. Self-centered lies told for reasons of personal advantage are those lies told by liars for their own personal gain. These are the lies told in pursuit of the liars' own financial or material advantage, and to protect the liars' property or assets. They are the lies that people tell to get what they want and to spare themselves from being bothered or annoyed or from doing something that they do not want to do. Self-centered lies told for psychological reasons include the lies told to protect the liars from embarrassment, disapproval, worry, conflict, or from having their feelings hurt. They can also protect the liars' privacy, and make the liars appear better than they think they really are. Similarly, other-oriented lies can be told for reasons of other people's personal advantage or to benefit or protect them psychologically.

What is noteworthy about the goals that motivate deceptive presentations is that they are among the same goals that motivate nondeceptive ones. Both when people are lying and when they are telling the truth, they are often trying to get what they want, to make a positive impression on other people, to protect themselves from being embarrassed or hurt, and to be supportive and kind to others. Honest self-presentations are not necessarily ones in which people tell all nor even ones in which people evenhandedly present some of their good qualities and some of their bad ones. People can edit their self-presentations in ways that underscore the aspects of themselves that are most relevant to the topic at hand without trying to mislead anyone. For example, a person from Kansas who has traveled only to Paris can contribute personal anecdotes to a conversation about European travel without ever mentioning that the trip to Paris was the only time she was not in Kansas and still be basically honest. In contrast, if she also tries to convey the impression that Paris was just one of her many worldwide adventures, then she has crossed the line into deliberate deceit. If two people have the same goal of impressing others with their sophistication and worldliness during a conversation about travel, the person who actually has traveled widely will find it easier to achieve that goal without straying from the truth than will someone who has hardly ever traveled.

The conventional and harsh view of lying would predict that lies are more often told to benefit the liars themselves than to benefit other people, and that lies told for reasons of personal advantage would be even more prevalent than lies told for psychological reasons. But studies have shown that this expectation is only partly correct. People do tell many more self-centered lies than other-oriented ones. But of the self-centered lies, many more of them are told for psychological reasons than for materialistic reasons or for reasons of personal convenience. In everyday life, people lie far more often to make themselves look better and to protect themselves from being embarrassed or hurt than to procure illicitly a better grade or a raise or promotion.

C. Cognitive and Emotional Significance of Everyday Lies

If the little lies of everyday life are routine occurrences rather than extraordinary events, then we might expect to find that they are of only minor consequence to the people who tell them. That is, in fact, what people say about their everyday lies. They do not plan those lies very carefully and they do not regard them as serious. Before they tell their everyday lies, people do not worry much about getting caught, and a week or so after telling them, they usually report that they in fact were not caught. Everyday lies also tend to be lies of little or no regret. When asked whether, if given a second chance, they would tell their lies again, the participants said that they would do so more than 70% of the time.

D. The Discomfort of Deceit

Although the little lies of everyday life typically fit smoothly into the fabric of social life, there are still some bumps. There are cultural proscriptions against lying, and these are likely to leave their mark. One suggestive indication that people may feel uncomfortable about their lies is that people's rate of telling lies in face-to-face interaction is lower than it is in the more distant modality of telephone conversations. More directly relevant are people's reports of how they felt before, during, and after the telling of their everyday lies. Although people report only low to moderate degrees of discomfort, they do feel worse while telling their lies, and immediately afterwards, than they had just before.

III. WHO LIES?

A. Personality Differences

Although it is probably true that everyone lies, some people lie much more frequently than others. Similarly, although the fundamental goals of social life are probably important to everyone, there are striking differences in the degree to which different people care about different goals. The more people care about a social interaction goal that can be attained by lying, the more likely they should be to lie frequently in everyday life.

I. Manipulativeness

One important social interaction goal that can be attained by lying is that of pursuing one's own self-interests. A personality dimension that is especially relevant to that goal is manipulativeness, as indexed, for example, by measures of "Machiavellianism" and "social adroitness." Manipulative people show little concern for conventional morality and are willing to use other people to get what they want. These people add credence to the stereotypical view of liars as selfish and exploitative. They lie significantly more than people who are less manipulative, and they are especially likely to tell the kinds of lies that benefit themselves.

2. Impression Management

A very different social interaction goal is that of self-presentation. People who are "publicly self-conscious" or "other-directed" are not out to exploit other people; they are out to impress them. They care deeply about what other people think of them, and so they may be willing to lie to appear to be the kind of person they only wish they were. Research supports this prediction. People who care more about the impressions they convey to other people tell more lies than people who are less concerned about their self-presentations.

3. Relationship Quality

When impression management is the goal, people care about others, but in a self-centered way; that is, they care about what others think of *them*. A more genuinely altruistic concern about other people might be characteristic of people who have warm, satisfying, and enduring interpersonal relationships. Perhaps people who are more selflessly concerned with other people will tell fewer lies. And, in fact, research has shown that people who have high quality relationships with people of the same sex as themselves (but not the opposite sex) tell fewer lies in their everyday lives. Moreover, when these people do tell lies, they are relatively more likely to tell altruistic lies than self-centered ones.

4. Socialization

We have argued that the view of lying as an everyday social interaction process is at odds with the public view of lying as reprehensible. It is the public view, rather than our own, that should govern people's actual lie telling. The more people ascribe to the conventional morality that condemns lying, the less likely they should be to tell lies in their everyday lives. And in fact, this is exactly what the data have shown. People who score high on a personality scale measuring responsibility describe themselves as dependable, conscientious, and straightforward. These people tend to lie less frequently than less responsible individuals, and they are especially unlikely to tell self-serving lies.

5. Psychopathology

Although mentally healthy people tell lies almost every day, the lies that they tell are not so frequent, so blatant, or so pointless as to be self-defeating. In contrast, people with psychiatric disorders such as narcissistic, antisocial, compulsive, borderline, or histrionic personalities, lie in ways that undermine their normal development and compromise their quality of life.

B. Sex Differences

In Western society, women are in many ways the socioemotional specialists. They spend more time socializing with other people than men do, and they do so in more intimate ways. They also think about other people more than men do, and they may even reminisce about other people more. Women are also nonverbally warmer than men, more supportive, and more self-disclosing. Although it might seem to follow from women's more open and more intimate interpersonal style that women might lie less often than men in their everyday lives, there is no support for this position. In their overall rates of telling lies, men and women are equals. The sexes do differ, however, in the kinds of lies they tell and in the persons to whom they tell their lies. The key distinction again involves self-centered versus other-oriented lies. When women are lying to men, or when men are lying to women or to men, they tell many more self-centered lies than other-oriented ones. But when women are interacting with other women, their rate of telling altruistic lies is about the same as their rate of telling self-centered lies. "You did the right thing"; "You look great"; "What a wonderful dinner"; "What a thoughtful present—I love it"; "I understand"; and "I agree" are all the kinds of lies that are especially likely to be told by one woman to another woman.

C. Age Differences

I. Childhood

When adults are asked how often particular children tell lies, they are likely to think of the kinds of lies told to conceal transgressions such as stealing, cheating, and fighting. If these adult reports are then used to predict children's subsequent life experiences, it is sometimes discovered that boys who frequently lied during childhood were more likely to get into trouble (for example, with drugs or with the law) as adolescents and adults. (These kinds of studies are conducted less often with girls.) Perhaps it should not be surprising that lying to cover transgressions early in life predicts more transgressions later in life. This research is important, but it tells only part of the story about lying in childhood.

The broader view of the development of lying begins with the recognition that there are different kinds of lies that children tell other than ones that are used to dodge punishment and blame. For example, children learn to tell lies to protect and reassure others. Even when they are only preschoolers, girls will sometimes pretend to like a disappointing present given to them by an adult, apparently to spare the adult's feelings. In research with older children, it has been reported that between the ages of 8 and 12, the number of boys who will lie to protect another boy from punishment increases.

From a cognitive perspective, the attainment of the ability to tell lies is a developmental milestone. Lie telling involves a sophisticated form of perspective taking in which the liars realize that they can influence others to come to a particular understanding that the liars themselves believe to be false. Successful lie telling also represents a psychological victory in the domain of autonomy and relatedness. Children who attempt to lie and who lie successfully recognize that they have thoughts and feelings that are separate from those of other people, and that can be hidden. In telling lies, they may be developing a sense of privacy and a sense of self.

2. Adulthood

There are no life-span longitudinal studies of lying in everyday life. However, there are suggestive data from a pair of diary studies conducted by the same researchers and involving the same methodology. The participants in one of the studies were college students and in the other, they were an older (and also more demographically diverse) group of people from the community. The participants in the older group lied less frequently than the college students on every measure: They told only one lie per day (compared to two for the college students), they lied in one in every five of their social interactions (compared to one in three for the college students) and they lied to 30% of the people with whom they interacted (compared to 38% for the college students). Further, within the community group, which ranged in age from 18 to 71, the older people told significantly fewer lies than the younger ones.

D. Cultural Differences

We do not yet know whether there are differences across cultures in the frequency with which people tell everyday lies. However, there is evidence to suggest that the kinds of lies that people tell are different in different cultures. One of the most important distinctions may be whether a culture is collectivist or individualist. In collectivist cultures, the needs and values of the group are primary. In individualist cultures, individual freedom and autonomy are more central. People from collectivist cultures, compared to those from individualist ones, report that they are more willing to lie when their family or other important social group would benefit from the lie.

Subcultural variations may also be important to our understanding of the kinds of lies that people tell. The special patterns of lying that occur when women interact with other women may be an example of a subcultural pattern. Beginning in childhood, when girls interact primarily with other girls and boys with other boys, separate subcultures seem to develop. The

"culture of girls" is characterized by close interpersonal bonds and norms of equality and supportiveness. Perhaps the effects of this early socialization are evident in the patterns of lie-telling that occur in adulthood when women are especially likely to tell kind and supportive lies to other women.

IV. TO WHOM ARE LIES TOLD?

A. Casual and Close Relationship Partners

In studies in which people are asked to describe a time when they were dishonest with a close relationship partner, almost no one ever says that they cannot recall such a time. People do tell everyday lies to friends, relatives, and lovers. But because people typically interact with close relationship partners more often than with acquaintances and strangers, they also have more opportunities to lie to them. Taking opportunities into account, people's rate of lying (number of lies told to a person relative to the number of social interactions with that person) to their close relationship partners is lower than to casual partners such as acquaintances and strangers. People may lie less often to the people to whom they feel closer because they care more about those people. Consistent with this explanation is the fact that when people do lie to their close relationship partners, relatively more of the lies they tell are altruistic lies than self-centered ones. However, it is also possible that people tell fewer everyday lies to their closer relationship partners because they are less likely to get away with their lies when the other person knows about their past and will continue to interact with them in the future. There is evidence for this possibility as well: People report that the everyday lies they told to their close relationship partners were more likely to have been discovered than the lies they told to their more casual acquaintances.

Kindhearted lies may have an important place not only in close relationships that are well established, but also in those that are just beginning to develop. For example, when people are discussing paintings with art students whom they are meeting for the first time, those people who already feel fondness for the art students, compared to those who do not, are less likely to be truthful about the paintings of theirs that they do not like. It is apparently more difficult for people to convey a hurtful truth to people they like than to people they do not like, even when the target is someone they hardly even know. By conveying more enthusiasm for the liked artists' work than they really do feel, and by withholding their criticisms, they may feel that they are giving a potentially desirable relationship a better chance to develop and flourish.

Lies that are dangerous rather than benign are also told in casual relationships, such as during the first few dates with romantic partners. In dating contexts, lies about sexual histories and about health are not rare. In a survey of college students, a third of the men and 10% of the women said that they had told a lie in order to have sex, and an even greater proportion of them reported that they had been lied to for purposes of sex. A fifth of the men and 4% of the women said that they would be willing to lie about their HIV status.

B. People with High Expectations

Close relationship partners often have high expectations for each other. These expectations are an expression of their high regard for each other, and so they can be a source of comfort and pride. However, there is also a potential hazard. When people feel that they have violated the expectations of a person who is dear to them, they may be reluctant to make that known. Therefore, to shield their partner from disappointment and to maintain the regard that their partner has for them, they may lie. Because close relationship partners probably have more expectations, and more diverse expectations, for each other than do more casual acquaintances, it should follow that the rate of lying to them is higher. But for everyday lies, it is not. It is in the domain of serious lies that positive expectations have their power to act as deterrents of the truth.

Other people who may have high expectations are those in positions of authority, such as bosses, teachers, and supervisors. If a superior has high expectations of a subordinate, the subordinate might work hard to live up to those expectations. However, the subordinate might also be tempted to lie to cover mistakes or poor performances that might jeopardize the superior's high regard.

C. People Who Care

There are contexts in which honest communications can be of great instrumental value. For example, when supervisors are evaluating employees, or when teach-

ers are appraising students, their feedback can help in the development and refinement of skills. But people in evaluative roles are reluctant to provide such feedback, especially when it is negative, and they often put off doing so. There are communication barriers in less formal contexts as well. For example, even though honesty and openness are highly valued characteristics of friendships, friends are not totally forthcoming in conveying their evaluations of each other, and they are especially hesitant when their evaluations are critical.

The temptation to tell lies in evaluative situations has been systematically investigated in a series of studies in which participants discussed paintings with an art student. The participants first picked out their most and least favorite paintings from those that were on display, and only then did they learn that they were to discuss those paintings with the art student. Just before discussing one of the paintings that the participant most detested, the art student mentioned that the painting was special to her in some way—either it was one of her favorites, or she had painted it herself. She also said that one of the paintings that participant liked the most was of her favorites or one of her own. In these studies, the more invested the art student was in the paintings, the more difficult it was for the participants to tell the truth about what they really did think of them—especially when what they thought was very critical. It was more difficult for the participants to tell the truth when the paintings were the art student's favorites than when the art student had no special investment in the paintings at all, and it was the most difficult when the paintings were the art student's own work. Sometimes the participants dealt with these difficult situations by telling outright lies; for example, they sometimes said that they really liked the paintings that they had already admitted in writing that they hated. But they used other deceptive strategies as well. They sometimes stonewalled—that is, they tried to avoid making any evaluative statements at all. They also amassed misleading evidence, as when they mentioned many aspects of the paintings that they really did like, while neglecting to mention many of the aspects they really disliked. In addition, they used a very creative strategy of communicating positive evaluations by implication. They did this by being very forthcoming about how much they disliked paintings created by other art students, while saying little about the present art student's paintings that they disliked just as much.

In the stereotypical view of deception, liars tell their lies to hurt and exploit other people, but in the art studies, a very different motivation seemed to be evident. The liars seemed to be telling their lies in order to protect the art students from having their feelings hurt.

D. Men and Women

We noted previously that although men and women do not differ in the frequency with which they tell lies, there are more subtle differences. Specifically, when women are interacting with other women (compared to when men are involved as liars or targets), the kinds of lies that are likely to be told are more likely to be kindhearted ones. Although the telling of altruistic lies to women is especially characteristic of women, men also tell more altruistic lies to women than to men. Both men and women note that the women to whom they lie, more so than the men, would feel even worse if they heard the truth instead of the lie. In that sense, too, they feel that their lies are protective of women. Conversely, when women and men are interacting with men, they are more likely to tell self-promoting lies than when they are interacting with women. Generally, then, people tell their lies to protect and reassure women and to impress men.

V. LYING IN SPECIAL CONTEXTS

A. Accepted and Expected Lies

There are certain contexts in which lie telling is expected, sanctioned, and condoned. For example, in many card games, board games, and sports, deception is essential. If basketball players were not allowed to look one way while tossing the ball the other way, or if poker players were not allowed to bluff, the players would no longer feel that they were playing basketball or poker. Athletes and cardplayers who are skilled deceivers and detectors of deceit are admired and rewarded.

In the grimmer context of the military, lies are also expected and accepted. To the extent that miliary action is condoned, then lying to the enemy, and sometimes even to one's countrymen and women, is condoned as well.

Lying can also be part of one's job description. Undercover agents, for example, live a lie; it is their job

to do so. Deception can also be part of one's job in a way that is less obvious, but still quite important. For example, part of the work that flight attendants and employees of Disney's Magic Kingdom do is "emotion work": They are to appear pleasant and cordial, regardless of how they really do feel.

B. Dangerous and Disgraceful Lies

At the other extreme are lies that are condoned by virtually no one. Because it is the mission of scientists to seek the truth, scientific fraud is considered especially noteworthy and disgraceful. Some lies can even be deadly, as when criminals dress as delivery people in order to be allowed into the homes of their victims, or when dating partners lie about their HIV status.

C. Lies in Medical Contexts

Currently in the United States, the vast majority of physicians report that they truthfully disclose diagnoses even of very serious diseases such as cancer to their patients. Such disclosure is faithful to the doctrine of informed consent, and respectful of patients' autonomy. Yet this norm of disclosure is very new. As recently as the early 1960s, the vast majority of the doctors in the United States said that they would *not* reveal a diagnosis of cancer to a patient. Moreover, that norm of nondisclosure was one which had persisted for about 2500 years, since the time of Hippocrates. Even today, nondisclosure is often practiced in other countries such as Japan and Italy. In the United States, although disclosure may be the norm for discussions of diagnoses and treatment, there is still much withholding and softening of information about grim prognoses.

In times and places where nondisclosure is common practice, it has been justified in terms of benefits to the patients. From the physicians' point of view, what they are doing is not telling lies but offering hope. Some offer this hope with the belief that it might actually heal. Others feel that the telling of painful truths is improper and cruel, and in violation of their obligation to protect and care for their patients. Those who believe in disclosure argue instead that it is primarily the physicians who are protected by the withholding of dire diagnoses, for disclosure is more emotionally challenging and perhaps more time-consuming.

The ethical question of whether patients should be told the whole truth cannot be answered with data.

However, there is a scientific question at the crux of this controversy, and that is whether hope can indeed heal, or at least slow the rate of progressive diseases. Although such questions may sound more spiritual than scientific, the mechanisms may be quite straightforward. For example, hopeful people may work harder at maintaining a healthier lifestyle, or hopefulness may have physiological correlates that are consistent with more positive health outcomes. More research is needed to address these important questions.

VI. SKILL AT DECEIVING

In laboratory studies of the communication of deception, communicators (sometimes called "senders") lie and tell the truth and other people ("judges") try to determine whether the communicators are lying or telling the truth. In these studies the senders have lied and told the truth about many different topics, such as their opinions, their emotions, and their life experiences. Typically, the judges perform better than chance at distinguishing the truths from the lies, but not much better. For example, when the senders are lying and telling the truth equally often, and judges would be right by chance 50% of the time, accuracy is typically better than 50% but is rarely better than 60%. According to these studies, then, it would appear that human lie-detectors have the edge over human liars, in that the liars are caught more often than they get away with their lies. However, in these studies the judges are asked explicitly to consider the possibility that the senders might be lying. In more naturalistic situations outside of the lab, there may be many situations in which people never even think of the possibility that the other person might be lying. And in fact, in studies in which people kept track of all of their lies every day for a week, and then reported another week later whether their lies had been detected, the participants said that to their knowledge, the vast majority of their lies had never been uncovered. It may be, then, that in everyday life, it is the liars and not the detectors who have the edge.

One possible explanation for why the senders in the laboratory studies are not more successful at getting away with their lies is that they are not sufficiently invested in them. Often there are no rewards for success or punishments for failure. To test this explanation, Bella DePaulo and her colleagues conducted a series of studies in which some of the senders were more highly motivated to get away with their lies, and others were less highly motivated. For example, the motivated senders might be lying about a personally important issue, or they might be communicating to people who are especially attractive or important to them, or they may have heard that the ability to lie successfully is linked to professional success. These more highly motivated senders, rather than becoming more successful at getting away with their lies, instead became less successful, particularly when the judges could see their facial expressions and body movements or listen to the tone of their voices. When the senders were especially motivated to tell successful lies, they seemed to try too hard to control their nonverbal behaviors. Their performances seemed overcontrolled, as if they were trying to hide something, which of course they were.

Not everyone is susceptible to the motivational impairment effect that typically occurs when people are especially motivated to get away with their lies. Some people, when the pressure is on to tell a successful lie, will rise to the occasion and lie even more convincingly than they do ordinarily. People who are confident in their skill at lying fit this description, as do people who are physically attractive. It is also likely that people who are very practiced at telling certain kinds of lies, and who believe that their lies are justified, are impervious to the motivational impairment effect. For example, in a study in which judges watched experienced salespersons pitching products they liked and products they disliked, the judges were completely unsuccessful at determining when the salespersons were lying and when they were telling the truth.

People who make a living at marketing or selling may find that it literally pays to be a good liar. Whether there might be costs as well, such as guilt at taking advantage of a trusting customer, remains to be determined. Similarly, there is evidence that boys, girls, and men (but not women) who are especially dominant and influential in their interactions with their peers are also especially skilled at appearing convincing when they are actually telling lies. But even getting one's way can have its costs, at least for some people. For example, in a study in which children were rewarded if they could convince their peers that bitter crackers were actually quite tasty, the children who felt most uncomfortable afterwards were the successful girls and the unsuccessful boys.

VII. SKILL AT DETECTING LIES

When liars get away with their lies, judges have failed to detect those lies, and when liars get caught, judges have been successful. Thus, research on skill at detecting lies is the flip side of the research on skill at deceiving. In laboratory studies in which judges are asked explicitly to determine whether another person is lying, the judges succeed more often than would be expected by chance. However, in everyday life situations, in which people have to figure out for themselves when to suspect another person, liars may have the advantage. There is a presumption of honesty in everyday communications, and that presumption is helpful to those who violate it. So strong is the presumption that even in laboratory studies in which judges are told explicitly that some of the people they will see might be lying, and in fact half of them are lying, the judges almost always guess that more than half of the communications they observed were truths. Further, there may be a presumption of honesty built into the human information-processing system. Daniel Gilbert has argued that the first step in understanding information is to believe it. This happens almost effortlessly. It takes another step, which is an effortful one, to disbelieve. If this model is correct, then liars are also advantaged by the ease of believing, compared to the extra time and effort required for disbelief.

Even if people were to put forth the effort required to disbelieve a communication, they still might not report that what they had just heard was a lie. Attributing deceit is not a bloodless act of information processing; it is calling someone a liar. Even when people really do think that another person is lying, they may refrain from saying so unless they are very sure. It is possible that even certainty is not enough. People may refrain from labeling other people's communications as lies if, for example, they think that social interactions will proceed more smoothly when people do not challenge each other's credibility. Or they may feel that if they behave as if they really did believe the other person, then the other person might feel liked or that person might like the believer more. If, over time, people who notice lies habitually act as if they believed the liar, then they might eventually fail even to notice the lies.

The many possible reasons for lie-detection failures may be especially pertinent to our understanding of a curious set of findings in the realm of sex differences.

In many domains of interpersonal perception, women are more skilled and more successful than are men. For example, women are better than men at recognizing faces, and they are also better at reading nonverbal cues in honest communications. However, they are not better than men at detecting deception. By some measures, they are even worse. For example, when watching videotapes from the art studies in which participants were sometimes claiming to like the paintings more than they really did, women report believing that more of the expressed liking is genuine than do men. Similarly, when women and men listen to others pretending to like people they really dislike, women again are more inclined than the men to believe that the speakers really do like the people they are describing.

Across the different kinds of interpersonal perception tasks that have been studied, it appears that women are especially more accurate than men at understanding the kinds of messages that other people want them to see and not more accurate than men, and sometimes even less accurate, at understanding the kinds of messages that others might not want them to discern. The findings suggest, but do not show definitively, that women may be trying to be accommodating to other people. This pattern of sex differences has been reported in the United States, and in numerous other countries as well. For some countries, however, the effect is more compelling than for others, and the differences are systematic. In the countries in which the women are especially likely to read overt cues and to miss covert ones, the women seem to be more oppressed. For example, those countries have proportionately fewer women in higher education and fewer women's groups.

Even within the United States, not all women show the pattern of nonverbal accommodation, and of those who do, not all show it equally strongly. Again, the differences are telling. Those women who are especially likely to be better at reading overt cues than covert ones tend *not* to be assertive, manipulative, intrusive, or hostile. Their personal styles appear to be consistent with traditional sex roles. In many segments of society, it can still be rewarding for women to behave in accord with conventional standards (that others might consider outmoded). Perhaps it is for this reason that women who seem more accommodating in the way they read nonverbal cues also report somewhat better interpersonal outcomes. For example, in high school, those women are seen as more popular by their teachers, and in college, the more nonverbally accommodating women report feeling more satisfied with the quality of their relationships with other people.

The sex differences findings suggest the counterintuitive conclusion that it may not always be advantageous to be a skilled detector of lies. Because so many of the lies of everyday life are little lies of little consequence, they may be better left undetected. People who notice the insincerity of polite replies, or who recognize the dubiousness of others' overstated achievements, may find it more difficult to enjoy the interaction and to maintain easy, cordial relationships with others than do people who are more oblivious. There may also be other personal costs to being too skilled at detecting deceit. For example, if a friend pretends to like a painting you love and have hung on the wall of your study, do you really want to see through the deception and realize that she actually hates the painting? The cost is that in the privacy of your own study where only your own tastes should matter, you may come to enjoy the painting less once you have so perceptively recognized your friend's loathing. The benefits of such perceptiveness seem negligible.

VIII. CONCLUSIONS

The arguments against lying are well known and in no need of repetition. For some kinds of lies, such as serious lies that are deep betrayals of trust, we agree with the conventional wisdom that abhors them. Yet for many the little lies that told in everyday life, we think that the verdict should be more complex.

Although honesty is often desirable and healthy, it is not always the best policy. The common coupling of the words "brutal" and "honesty" underscores the hazards of telling the whole truth. The risks are both intrapersonal and interpersonal. Should we feel obligated, in the name of honesty, to reveal painful information that we have not yet come to terms with ourselves? Should we, in the name of truthfulness, feel compelled to respond honestly even to inappropriate inquiries that violate our privacy and our dignity?

Should we feel honor-bound to tell nothing but the truth to the ailing cancer patient who in the midst of chemotherapy treatments asks how she looks? Should we be honest about our feelings about a loathed gift to the person who offered it in friendship and love? The answers to these questions are no longer merely speculative. We now know that people tell relatively more of these altruistic lies than self-centered lies to the people in their lives to whom they feel emotionally closer. We also know that people who tell relatively more altruistic lies than selfish lies have more satisfying relationships with people of the same sex. We do *not* know that kind lies are *responsible* for better relationships, and we probably never will. But we do know that there is a connection.

It is also important to recognize that the telling of lies, including even very serious and reprehensible lies, is governed by ordinary principles of human behavior. As Leonard Saxe has noted, if the consequences of owning up to damning truths are dire, we cannot expect honesty to prevail.

What about the perspective of the person who could potentially be the target of a lie? Is it always desirable to be told the truth instead? If other people lie to you, does that mean that they are trying to manipulate or exploit you? Sometimes it does, and in those instances, the truth is, of course, preferable. But in other instances, the appeal of the truth is not so obvious. David Nyberg gives this example: "Your two closest friends offer to tell you, with unchecked candor and without regard for your feelings, everything they think about you. Would you want them to do it?" If you go to a doctor for what you think is a sore shoulder, would you really want to hear all at once and in unvarnished terms that what you really have is a malignant melanoma that will probably prove fatal?

At least in some countries, such as the United States, people have strong beliefs about deception and its links to mental health. They believe that lying is a bad thing, and that it is better to know, than not to know, when others are speaking dishonestly. Research indicates that in some important ways, these intuitions are wrong.

BIBLIOGRAPHY

Barnes, J. A. (1994). *A pack of lies: Towards a sociology of lying.* Cambridge, UK: Cambridge University Press.
DePaulo, B. M., Kashy, D. A., Kirkendol, S. E., Wyer, M. M., &

Epstein, J. A. (1996). Lying in everyday life. *Journal of Personality and Social Psychology, 70,* 979–995.

DePaulo, B. M., Stone, J. I., & Lassiter, G. D. (1985). Deceiving and detecting deceit. In B. R. Schlenker (Ed.), *The self and social life* (pp. 323–370). New York: McGraw-Hill Book Company.

Ekman, P. (1985). *Telling lies.* New York: Norton.

Ford, C. V., King, B. H., & Hollender, M. H. (1988). Lies and liars: Psychiatric aspects of prevarication. *American Journal of Psychiatry, 145,* 554–562.

Kashy, D. A., & DePaulo, B. M. (1996). Who lies? *Journal of Personality and Social Psychology, 70,* 1037–1051.

Lewis, M., & Saarni, C. (1993). *Lying and deception in everyday life.* New York: Guilford Press.

Nyberg, D. (1993). *The varnished truth: Truth-telling and deceiving in ordinary life.* Chicago: The University of Chicago Press.

Saxe, L. (1991). Lying: Thoughts of an applied social psychologist. *American Psychologist, 46,* 409–415.

Taylor, S. E. (1989). *Positive illusions.* New York: Basic Books.

Defense Mechanisms

Phebe Cramer

Williams College

Anxiety An unpleasant emotional state, often including a feeling of threat, in which the nature of the threat is unknown.

Ego A descriptive term encompassing those aspects of the psyche that are most in touch with external reality, including cognition, perception, reality testing, reasoning, and judgment. Defense mechanisms are also considered to be ego functions.

Fear An intense emotion in response to present or anticipated danger or pain. In contrast to anxiety, the stimulus producing the reaction is known.

Guilt An unpleasant feeling resulting from having violated the principles of one's own conscience, often accompanied by a lessened sense of self-worth.

Id A descriptive term encompassing those aspects of the psyche that are in contact with the inner body but not directly with the external world, including the instinctual drives.

Superego A descriptive term encompassing those aspects of the psyche derived from the moral standards of the parents or of society, including conscience and the ego ideal.

DEFENSE MECHANISMS are mental operations which disguise or otherwise modify the content of the mind and/or the perception of reality. The purpose of these ego functions is to protect the individual from being disturbed by excessively painful feelings, drives, or ideas. The operation of defense mechanisms is generally unconscious—that is, unknown to the individual—for the function of disguise is effective only if the individual is unaware of the deception. Because of the distortions involved, the operation of defense mechanisms may interfere with the veracity of the individual's view of internal or external reality.

I. HISTORY OF THE CONCEPT

In Sigmund Freud's early explorations of psychopathology, he noted that the human mind has the capacity to keep certain painful feelings hidden from consciousness. Prior to 1900, this capacity was thought of as a general mental function, in which one type of mental material was used to screen or conceal other more painful material.

During the period from 1900 to 1923, Freud's interest shifted away from the role of affect and of external reality as factors in determining the use of defenses. Instead, his work focused on the importance of inner, instinctual drives in understanding human behavior. With this new direction, the idea of defense mechanisms was also modified. At this time, defense was conceptualized as a kind of counterforce which prevented the open and unchecked discharge of the drives. This idea of a single counterforce, termed repression, was used to replace the several different varieties of defense mechanisms which had been previously identified. However, after 1926, Freud found it useful to reintroduce the idea of multiple defense mechanisms, of which repression was one variety. At this time, Freud had developed his tripartite model of the personality as consisting of id, ego, and superego. The concept of defense mechanism was considered to be one of the ego functions.

Thus, in the development of the concept of defense mechanism, there were changing ideas about two problematic issues. The first was concerned with whether defenses were directed against painful affect emanating from experiences with the environment (objective anxiety), or whether the defense was against the pressure of instinctual drives (instinctual anxiety). The second issue involved the question of whether there was one single defense function, or whether there were multiple, qualitatively distinct defense mechanisms. To some degree, these issues remain unsettled today.

II. MOTIVES FOR DEFENSE

The issue of the source of the anxiety—objective or instinctual—was reconciled in the work of Anna Freud, who proposed that defenses against painful feelings and defenses against instinctual drives are based on the same motives—namely, to "ward off" feelings of anxiety and guilt. [See ANXIETY.]

Early in life, the individual has little capacity to protect against excessive stimulation or excitement resulting from the discharge of instinctual drives; when excessive, this discharge produces a state of anxiety, or, when more extreme, of panic. Later in development, the individual becomes able to anticipate the possible occurrence of this painful stimulation. This anticipation is expressed in the form of an anxiety signal, which instigates the use of a defense mechanism. The motive in this case for the use of defenses is the warding off of instinctual anxiety.

A second motive for defense—the warding off of feelings of guilt—has a different origin. In the course of development, the individual experiences satisfaction and pleasure as a result of the nurturance and benevolent caretaking of an important other. In time, the individual's sense of well-being and security becomes tied to the reception of these narcissistic supplies, either from the external caretaker or, later, from the internal representation of that caretaker—i.e., from the development of conscience which provides a sense of nurturance or disapproval, much as the original caretaker

once did. Initially, the infant's continuing existence depends on receiving these narcissistic supplies; in their absence, there is a threat of annihilation. At this stage, the threat of loss of these supplies is experienced as objective anxiety—i.e., as emanating from the environment. Later, with the development of conscience, the loss of self-approval is experienced as superego anxiety, or guilt. In order to protect the self from the ensuing loss of self-esteem which occurs when the dictates of conscience are violated, defense mechanisms may be called into play. [See SELF-ESTEEM.]

Defense mechanisms thus function to "ward off" dangers to the ego from two directions. The ego is defended against inner dangers—the discharge of instinctual drives and the related instinctual anxiety. It is also defended against dangers based on external prohibitions and the related objective anxiety, and against dangers emanating from the mental representations of those prohibitions (conscience) that produce feelings of guilt and loss of self-esteem (superego anxiety). These three motives—instinctual anxiety, objective anxiety, and superego anxiety, or guilt—prompt the use of defense mechanisms to protect the ego from being disrupted by instinctual impulses and to protect the self from the loss of self-esteem.

III. VARIETIES OF DEFENSE MECHANISMS

Although Freud originally thought of only a single defense function, in the development of psychoanalytic theory he came to recognize some 17 qualitatively different mental operations that provided a defensive function. Subsequently, there have been several attempts to provide an exhaustive cataloguing of the many varieties of defense, with incomplete agreement across the various listings. As many as 44 different defense mechanisms have been described, although most listings focus on a smaller number of operations. Attempts to provide definitive listings of defenses are complicated by issues such as whether normal developmental processes (such as introjection, or identification) should be included, or whether successful coping mechanisms, such as suppression and humor, should be considered defense mechanisms. Some attempts have been made to classify defenses in terms of cognitive complexity, level of abstraction, developmental maturity/immaturity, and degree of psychopathology, but no single classificatory system has been agreed upon.

Among the most frequently cited defense mechanisms are repression, denial, displacement, projection, reaction formation, undoing, isolation, rationalization, intellectualization, and sublimation. While it is not possible in the present brief essay to provide a comprehensive description of each of these mechanisms, a few examples of certain distinctions and relationships between mechanisms may be given. For example, *repression* is generally thought of as being directed against painful internal thoughts or impulses, while *denial* is directed against disturbing external stimuli, the perception of which would arouse painful feelings. However, this distinction is relative, for repression may be directed against the memory of a painful external event, while denial may play a role in the adherence to inner, wish-fulfilling fantasies. In its prototypical form, the mechanism of denial is cognitively rather simple, involving only the attachment of a negative sign to a perception: for example, "the night is frightening" is changed into "the night is *not* frightening."

In contrast, the mechanisms of *displacement* and *projection* are cognitively more complex. In displacement, thoughts or feelings about one person are transferred or displaced onto another (who is often less powerful, or less important to the individual). Thus the feeling "I am angry at my boss" is displaced and becomes "I am angry at my son." Cognitively, this defense involves a change in the object to whom the emotion is attached, but the subject, or owner of the feeling remains the same. In contrast, in projection, the owner of an unacceptable thought or feeling projects the thought outward and attributes it to some other individual: the unacceptable thought "I hate Tom" becomes "Tom hates me." For both displacement and projection, the object of the unacceptable feeling is changed (anger at boss changed to anger at son; anger at Tom changed to anger at me) but projection involves additionally a change in the subject of the emotion ("I hate" becomes "Tom hates"). Projection is thus cognitively more complex than displacement.

IV. DEFENSE MECHANISMS AND PSYCHOPATHOLOGY

The concept of defense mechanism was originally developed in the exploration of psychopathology. Neurotic symptoms were explained as the manifestation of particular defense mechanisms, and the diagnosis of a

particular neurosis was based on the presence of these defenses. For example, use of the defense of repression is associated with a diagnosis of hysteria, while the presence of undoing and rationalization contributes to a diagnosis of obsessive-compulsive neurosis. Within the range of psychosis, excessive use of projection is a diagnostic indicator of paranoia.

From this origin, it was easy to infer that the use of defense mechanisms was necessarily associated with psychopathology. This conception of defenses, however, involves both an overgeneralization and an oversimplification. While the use of defenses may sometimes be pathological, in other instances defenses are adaptive and promote psychological adjustment. Defenses are pathological when they are used in an overly rigid fashion, occur in connection with too many people or situations, significantly distort reality perception, and interfere with other ego functions. Pathological defenses are also inappropriate, in the sense of being out of phase with the developmental level of the individual or maladaptive for the current situation.

However, insofar as defense mechanisms function to reduce anxiety and thus contribute to psychological adjustment, they also have a positive, nonpathological function. Just what the relationship is between defense mechanisms and other mechanisms used for coping or adaptation is not clear. It has been suggested that the same mechanisms may be used either for defense or for coping purposes, depending on the demands of the situation. Alternatively, it may be that one type of mechanism evolves out of the other, or the two may be entirely separate in origin. [See PSYCHOPATHOLOGY.]

V. DEFENSES AND DEVELOPMENT

While defenses may be associated with psychopathology, they are also a necessary part of normal development. Because the child's developing ego is weak, it is the presence of defense mechanisms that prevents painful affects from disrupting its functioning and interfering with its development. This view was early presented by S. Freud and was amplified by A. Freud. Subsequently, attempts have been made to describe the relationship between defenses and development. At the core of this work is the assumption that the choice of defenses changes over time. In this case, it should be possible to specify a developmental continuum showing a chronological ordering of the emergence of the different defenses over the lifespan. In this conception, different defenses are conceived of as age- or stage-related and can be characterized as age appropriate or inappropriate.

A second conception of defense development refers to the idea that individual defenses have a developmental history of their own, with early beginnings in reflex behaviors which are gradually transformed into voluntary motor behavior and then internalized into mental operations. The relative strength of any one defense waxes and wanes over the lifespan, with individual defenses reaching their zenith at different stages of development.

Two different models have been used to characterize the developmental relationships among defense mechanisms. The "horizontal" approach uses a time line as a point of reference; the appearance of different defenses is ordered chronologically along this time line. This approach encompasses both the idea that different defenses emerge at different points in time, or at different developmental stages, and the conception that each defense has its own developmental history. The "vertical" approach orders defenses in terms of a hierarchy, based on some principle of classification, such as degree of complexity or reality distortion. While the vertical approach may use a dimension such as maturity/immaturity to classify defenses, and may arrange a hierarchy based on this dimension, such models are not truly developmental because the levels within the hierarchy are not related to age or developmental stage. Rather, the model describes different levels of defense used by individuals of the same age.

Research evidence from empirical studies supports the horizontal model of defense mechanisms development. Denial, a cognitively simple defense, is used frequently in early childhood; its use decreases across middle and later childhood and adolescence. Projection, somewhat more complex, cognitively, increases in use from early childhood to later childhood and adolescence. The use of identification as a defense is relatively infrequent in childhood but increases during adolescence. These trends may be seen in Figure 1, which is based on the projective test findings of 320 children, ages 3 to 18 years.

Similar results have been found for children's *understanding* of the functioning of defense mechanisms. These findings are relevant to the issue of defense mechanisms development since, in order for the disguise function of a defense to be effective, the operation of the mechanism cannot be understood. Once it is understood, the defense is no longer effective. Thus, the use

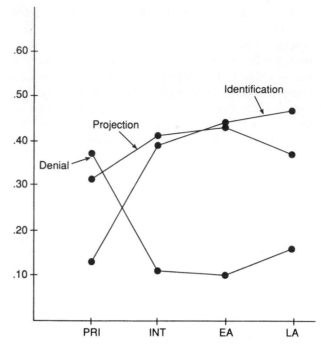

Figure 1   The use of defense mechanisms by children and adolescents of four age groups: primary (PRI)—mean age = 5 years, 8 months; intermediate (INT)—mean age = 9 years, 10 months; early adolescent (EA)—mean age = 14 years, 6 months; and late adolescent (LA)—mean age = 16 years.

of a defense must precede its understanding, and a developmental progression of defense use, followed by defense understanding, is an expected repetitive pattern. Cognitively simple forms of defense, such as denial, are used by young children until they are figured out or understood. When the defense is understood, it becomes ineffective. At this point, an increase in cognitive capacities allows the child to use a more complex defense, such as displacement, the functioning of which is not yet understood. When this defense becomes understood by the child, it, too, becomes ineffective and is replaced with another more complex defense, such as projection, which is not yet understood.

Other research studies have related the use of different defense mechanisms to different levels of ego development, with results consistent with the age-related findings reported above.

VI. MEASURES OF DEFENSE

One of the most difficult issues in the study of defense mechanisms is the problem of observation and measurement. Since a defense is effective only if the individual is unaware of its occurrence (i.e., it is unconscious) this raises the problem of how the defense may be known or studied. While some attempts to measure defense are based on direct questioning of the individual, this approach clearly runs into a logical dilemma: if the defense is effective, the individual using the defense is unaware of its existence and so cannot report on its use. A solution to this dilemma is to note that, while the person using the defense may not be conscious of the defensive behavior, another observer of the behavior could be aware of its defensive function. These two approaches—direct report and indirect observation—have formed the basis of the some 58 different measures that have been used to study defense mechanisms. Direct report measures include questionnaire items which may bear no obvious relationship to the defense being studied but have been shown empirically to correlate with defense use. Other direct measures ask subjects to self-report on the use of various manifestations of different defenses. While this method may seem to involve the logical contradiction discussed above, supporters of this approach indicate that a person may be capable of reporting on the use of defensive behaviors without realizing that the behavior serves a defensive purpose. While there are clear advantages to using such structured-inquiry, structured-response approaches—they are straightforward, objective, and easily scored without rater bias—there are equally obvious limitations. The information collected is limited to the questions asked and the range of responses allowed by the test format. Further, the request for the individual to comment on his own behavior creates a substantial possibility for reporter bias: the wish to appear in a positive light, and the use of one's customary defenses in reaction to the somewhat stressful situation of reporting on oneself may confound the results obtained.

More indirect measures of defense mechanisms have included story-completion tasks and clinical interviews. Both of these methods involve a structured inquiry, but there is generally more latitude provided for the individual to give responses, which may be relatively open-ended and unstructured. This allows a free-flowing sample of the individual's thought processes to be obtained, in which the actual use of defenses may be manifest. However, the relatively unstructured nature of the response material raises issues of observer bias or subjectivity. Problems stemming from the wish to appear in a socially desirable light are not eliminated, but

may be recognized in this format as a manifestation of a defense mechanism.

Other indirect measures of defense mechanisms largely circumvent problems relating to social desirability by using techniques for which there are no clearly desirable responses. These approaches, consisting of projective tests, such as the Thematic Apperception Test, and perceptual defense paradigms, in which stimulus material is presented below the visual threshold level, utilize an unstructured or ambiguous inquiry, and call for an open-ended response. It is the way in which the individual goes about formulating a response that provides the material for judging defensive functioning. Problems of possible observer or rater bias are also present in this approach.

VII. SELECTED CONTEMPORARY RESEARCH

As mentioned above, research with children has shown that cognitively simpler defenses, such as denial, are used more frequently by younger children, while more complex defenses, such as identification, occur more frequently among adolescents and young adults. Long-term studies of adult males have found that the use of defenses continues to change with age. Between late adolescence and adulthood, the use of immature defenses, such as turning against the self, denial, and reaction formation, decreased, while mature defenses, such as sublimation and suppression, increased with age. Further, the use of mature defenses, such as altruism, suppression, and sublimation, was found to be associated with positive psychological adjustment, marital success, happiness, and objective physical health, while the use of immature defenses, such as denial and projection, was associated with psychiatric illness. In addition, within a sample of working-class men, the use of mature, as compared to immature, defenses appeared to causally contribute to the men's upward social mobility.

Self-report measures of defense mechanisms have found systematic differences between men and women in the choice of defense, with men scoring higher on the outwardly directed defenses of projection and turning against the object, and women scoring higher on the inwardly directed defenses of turning against the self and reversal. Defense use has also been found to be related to sexual orientation, regardless of biological gender. Persons with a feminine orientation use defenses more often associated with females, and vice versa.

While the use of immature defenses has been found

to be associated with psychopathology, clinical improvement in psychiatric status following on a course of psychotherapy has been shown to be accompanied by a decrease in the use of these defenses. A similar change in defense use has been found during the recovery period of heroin addicts. Other types of intervention, such as experimentally induced failure experiences and naturally occurring trauma, have been shown to increase the use of defense mechanisms, presumably to protect the individual from the negative emotions associated with the experience.

This article has been reprinted from the *Encyclopedia of Human Behavior, Volume 2.*

BIBLIOGRAPHY

Blum, H. P. (Ed.) (1985). "Defense and Resistance." International Universities Press, New York.

Cramer, P. (1988). The Defense Mechanism Inventory: A review of research and discussion of the scales. *J. Pers. Assess.* **52,** 142–164.

Cramer, P. (1991). "The Development of Defense Mechanisms: Theory, Research, and Assessment." Springer-Verlag, New York.

Dorprat, T. L. (1985). "Denial and Defense in the Therapeutic Situation." Jason Aronson, New York.

Giovacchini, P. L. (1987). "A Narrative Textbook of Psychoanalysis." Aronson, Northvale, N.J.

Ihilevich, D., & Gleser, G. C. (1986). "Defense Mechanisms. Their Classification, Correlates, and Measurement with the Defense Mechanisms Inventory." DMI Associates, Owosso, MI.

Lerner, P. M., & Lerner, H. D. (1980). Rorschach assessment of primitive defenses in borderline personality structure. In "Borderline Phenomena and the Rorschach Test" (J. S. Kwawer, H. Lerner, P. Lerner, & A. Sugarman, Eds.), pp. 257–274. International Universities Press, New York.

Perry, J. C., & Cooper, S. H. (1989). An empirical study of defense mechanisms. *Arch. Gen. Psych.* **46,** 444–452.

Sandler, J. (1985). "The Analysis of Defense. The Ego and the Mechanisms of Defense Revisited" (with A. Freud). International Universities Press, New York.

Smith, G. J. W., & Danielsson, A. (1982). "Anxiety and Defense Strategies in Childhood and Adolescence." International Universities Press, New York.

Swanson, G. E. (1988). "Ego Defenses and the Legitimization of Behavior." Cambridge University Press, New York.

Vaillant, G. E. (1986). "Empirical Studies of Ego Mechanisms of Defense." American Psychiatric Press, Inc., Washington, DC.

Vaillant, G. E. (1992). The historical origins and future potential of Sigmund Freud's concept of the mechanisms of defence. *Int. Rev. Psycho-anal.* **19,** 35–50.

Dementia

John L. Woodard

Emory University School of Medicine*

Agnosia   Inability to recognize the symbolic meaning of stimulus material.

Aphasia   Impairment of expressive and/or receptive language skills producing communication difficulty.

Apraxia   An acquired inability to perform learned, purposeful motor acts.

Ataxia   Impairment of smooth coordinated muscle movement.

Athetosis   Involuntary movements characterized by a continuous slow, writhing, dancelike quality, often seen in Huntington's disease.

Basal Ganglia   A collection of nuclei in the forebrain, typically considered to include the caudate nucleus, putamen, parts of the thalamus, and the lentiform nucleus.

Bradykinesia   A condition often seen in Parkinson's disease produced by muscular rigidity that results in slowed movement, particularly on tasks involving fine motor coordination (e.g., writing).

Chorea   Involuntary rapid, jerky, complex movements, often seen in Huntington's disease, together with athetosis.

Delirium   A state of clouded consciousness, typically associated with fluctuating alertness and confusion.

Dementia   A persistent decline in intellectual functioning in multiple cognitive domains relative to a previous level of performance.

Dysarthria   Difficulty with articulation due to impairment of the oral musculature.

Encephalitis   Infection and inflammation of brain tissue.

Encephalopathy   Dysfunction of the brain due to any cause.

General Paresis   Chronic syphilitic meningoencephalitis, associated with a progressive dementia and generalized paralysis.

Korsakoff's Syndrome   Disturbance of orientation, confusion, delusions, and hallucinations associated with chronic alcoholism.

Meningitis   Inflammation of the meninges of the brain.

Ophthalmoplegia   Paralysis or weakness of the eye muscles.

Prions   Subviral, infectious, unencapsulated protein particles that are thought to be associated with diseases such as kuru, Creutzfeld-Jacob disease, Gerstmann-Straussler-Scheinker syndrome, and Fatal Familial Insomnia.

Wernicke's Encephalopathy   A clinical syndrome associated with thiamine deficiency (frequently related to alcoholism) resulting in ophthalmoplegia, ataxia, and dementia.

---

*Present address: Memory Assessment Clinic and Alzheimer's Disease Program, Georgia State University.

DEMENTIA, as it is used in this article, refers to a persistent decline in intellectual functioning in multiple cognitive domains relative to a previous level of performance. A separate article discusses Alzheimer's

Copyright © 1998 by Academic Press.
All rights of reproduction in any form reserved.

Disease. Although Alzheimer's disease (AD) accounts for 45 to 80% of all dementias, the absence of a definite biological marker of AD in living patients continues to necessitate the exclusion of less common but sometimes treatable dementing conditions and differentiation among degenerative dementias. Given that some non-Alzheimer's dementias are potentially treatable (i.e., further cognitive deterioration can be avoided or minimized) and/or reversible (i.e., cognitive functioning can be improved), a thorough consideration of all potential etiologies is imperative. This article will describe the non-Alzheimer's dementias along a continuum of relatively untreatable, progressive disorders to treatable and potentially reversible causes. Many of these conditions represent diagnostic challenges given their rarity, and clinical diagnostic criteria for these disorders are either nonexistent or highly variable. The degenerative, non-Alzheimer's dementias will be considered first, the majority of which have limited treatment options available. Next, dementias due to cerebrovascular disease will be surveyed, some of which may be treated to avoid further progression of cognitive impairment. Dementias due to infectious processes will be reviewed subsequently, many of which may also be treatable if discovered in their early stages. Dementia due to toxic or metabolic conditions may be among the most treatable etiologies and are potentially reversible if detected and corrected relatively early. Finally, dementia due to other causes, many of which are treatable and reversible, will be examined.

I. DEGENERATIVE DEMENTIAS

A. Frontal Lobe Degeneration and Pick's Disease

1. Clinical Features

Patients with degenerative changes confined principally to bilateral frontal or fronto-temporal brain regions often demonstrate a characteristic clinical pattern with early onset of personality changes associated with inappropriate social or personal behavior, followed by cognitive deficits that are evident later in the course of the disorder. With the exception of elicitation of primitive reflexes (e.g., grasp, suck, snout), neurological signs are typically absent. Computed tomog-

raphy (CT) and magnetic resonance imaging (MRI) scans commonly reveal prominent atrophy of the frontal or fronto-temporal cerebral cortex. Positron emission tomography (PET) and SPECT (single photon emission computed tomography) typically reveal diminished glucose metabolism and cerebral blood flow in the frontal and fronto-temporal cortex. [*See* Brain Scanning/Neuroimaging.]

Frontal lobe dementia tends to first become manifest in younger individuals in their 50s or early 60s, although cases have been reported in patients as young as 20. Women are affected nearly twice as often as men. Approximately half of patients diagnosed with frontal lobe degeneration have a first-degree relative who has shown similar behavioral and cognitive changes. Because of the striking and frequently problematic personality changes, frontal lobe degeneration is often misdiagnosed as a psychiatric disorder. Impaired judgment and lack of insight commonly lead to inability to manage instrumental activities of daily living, together with occupational impairment. Personality changes may reflect prominent apathy and lack of motivation at one extreme, or disinhibited, reckless, and hyperactive behavior at the other extreme. Language changes sometimes reflect terse, stereotyped, repetitive phrases, gradually progressing to echolalia (repetition of phrases said by others) and palilalia (repetition of single syllables uttered by themselves or others). Memory and orientation, visuospatial skills, and basic language abilities are surprisingly well-preserved during the early stages of this disorder, although neuropsychological measures of executive functioning may reveal perseveration, diminished word list generation, cognitive rigidity, and difficulty formulating and sequencing complex behaviors. [*See* Personality.]

Pick's disease is a specific type of frontal lobe degeneration that is characterized by the presence of distinctive neuropathological markers known as "Pick bodies" that disrupt neuronal cytoskeletal organization and displace the neuronal nucleus toward the periphery of the cell body. Approximately half of the patients diagnosed with frontal lobe degeneration show evidence of Pick bodies at biopsy or autopsy.

2. Treatment

Frontal lobe degeneration may be treated only symptomatically. Behavioral agitation and aggression are typically treated pharmacologically with neuroleptics. Activities of daily living must be routinized, and frequent supportive guidance and reality orientation may be used in an attempt to minimize disruptive behavior.

B. Parkinson's Disease

1. Clinical Features

Parkinson's Disease (PD), a degenerative disorder mainly involving the pigmented cells in the substantia nigra and other pigmented brain stem nuclei, affects approximately 1% of all individuals over the age of 65. Dopamine depletion in the frontal cortex and striatum (particularly in the anterodorsal portion of the head of the caudate nucleus), is the major neurochemical deficit associated with PD, although reduced levels of norepinephrine, acetylcholine, and somatostatin, and diminished serotonin receptors have also been reported. The cause of PD is not known, although toxic agents such as manganese poisoning in industrial workers and injection of 1-methyl-4-phenyl 1,2,3,6 tetrahydropyridine (MPTP) in drug abusers, are known to produce PD symptoms and pathology, suggesting the possibility that an environmental factor could play a role in the etiology. Although CT and MRI exhibit little predictive value for diagnosis of PD in an individual case, PET studies using fluorodeoxyglucose may show hypometabolism in the basal ganglia and frontal cerebral cortex. Regional cerebral blood flow studies have shown reductions in frontal cortical blood flow.

PD is most prominently associated with motor abnormalities involving a resting tremor, loss of postural reflexes, stooped posture, bradykinesia (slowed movement), cogwheel rigidity, and slow shuffling gait. Small handwriting, dysarthria, reduced vocal volume, and a tendency to speak in a monotone fashion may also be seen. Between 25 and 40% of PD patients may develop dementia. When present, PD dementia typically occurs during the later stages of the disorder.

Bradyphrenia (cognitive slowing) is typically one of the earliest features of PD dementia. Language deficits tend to involve motor components of speech (e.g., dysarthria, diminished phrase length, dysprosody, micrographia) more severely than linguistic aspects of speech, such as naming and comprehension. Memory and learning deficits are also seen in the early stages of PD dementia. For example, procedural learning (ability to acquire a new perceptual-motor skill) tends to be impaired. Effortful memory and spontaneous free recall are also generally impaired in PD dementia, although recognition memory is often preserved. Deficits in visuospatial abilities involving both visuoperceptual and visuoconstructional aspects have been well documented. Executive functioning deficits involving establishing, maintaining, and shifting cognitive set also are common in PD dementia and are similar to deficits in patients with discrete lesions of the frontal lobes. Depression may occur in 25 to 40% of PD patients.

2. Treatment

PD is most commonly treated with medication designed to ameliorate the central dopamine deficiency. Levodopa, a dopamine precursor that readily crosses the blood–brain barrier and is metabolized to dopamine, is the most common pharmacologic agent used to treat PD. Following levodopa administration, symptomatic improvement in movement abnormalities is seen in approximately 60% of patients, and cognitive impairment has also been shown to improve following pharmacotherapy. However, this form of treatment becomes ineffective after 1 to 4 years, presumably due to progressive neuronal loss and inability of remaining neurons to convert levodopa to dopamine. Depression in PD is not affected by levodopa therapy and sometimes may be a side effect of the medication. Tricyclic antidepressants and electroconvulsive therapy have been used successfully to improve mood and motor disability.

Surgical treatment of PD has a long history and a promising future. Before dopaminergic medications were available, the accepted method of treatment involved surgical placement of a lesion in the ventrolateral thalamus. Although this procedure improved tremor and reduced rigidity, this procedure had little effect on the akinesia associated with PD. Surgical intervention using placement of a lesion in the globus pallidus (pallidotomy) had also been attempted, although wide variability in the accuracy of lesion placement produced inconsistent and often devastating results. Using new microelectrode-guided lesion placement techniques, pallidotomy has reemerged as a potential treatment for PD with much fewer complications. Pallidotomy produces relatively rapid and substantial improvement in the motor symptoms, although there tends to be little effect on neuropsychological and psychiatric status postsurgically.

C. Diffuse Lewy Body Disease

1. Clinical Features

This disorder has received considerable attention within recent years as an important cause of dementia with parkinsonian features, although it has also been considered by some to be a variant of Alzheimer's disease. The occurrence of diffuse Lewy body disease appears to be linked to a genetic mutation in the beta-amyloid precursor protein gene on chromosome 21. Approximately 20% of patients with a clinical diagnosis of Alzheimer's disease are thought to have concomitant diffuse Lewy body disease. This disease thus appears to reflect an overlap between Parkinson's disease and Alzheimer's disease.

A progressive dementia, consisting of impaired attention, memory, language (e.g., verbal fluency, praxis, and naming), and visuospatial/visuoperceptual skills, typically appears first, followed by parkinsonian features, including akinesia, tremor, and rigidity. A cognitive hallmark of early diffuse Lewy body disease is a fluctuating cognitive state in which patients can be cognitively impaired on one day and cognitively intact on the next day. Sensitivity to the effects of neuroleptic medications, sometimes resulting in obtundation or stupor, has also been reported in this dementia. Neuropsychiatric disturbances, including paranoid delusions and auditory and visual hallucinations, are present in approximately half of all patients with diffuse Lewy body disease and tend to occur early in the disease course.

Histologically, Lewy bodies are inclusion bodies (similar to Pick bodies) that disrupt neuronal cytoskeletal organization. In diffuse Lewy body disease, Lewy bodies are diffusely present in surviving cortical neurons, although they tend to favor layers V and VI of cingulate and entorhinal cortex, and they are also found in the brain stem and substantia nigra. Spongioform changes restricted to the temporal lobe help to differentiate diffuse Lewy body disease from prion diseases (described later in this article) in which the spongioform changes are diffusely located. However, there is no current evidence that diffuse Lewy body disease is transmissible. Efforts are currently underway to understand the nature of different Lewy body disease and its relationship with Alzheimer's disease and with Parkinson's disease.

2. Treatment

Symptomatic pharmacological treatment of the Parkinsonian features of this disorder is the only therapeutic option at this time. The dementia associated with diffuse Lewy body disease currently is not amenable to treatment.

D. Huntington's Disease

1. Clinical Features

Huntington's disease is a genetically inherited autosomal dominant condition that affects approximately 5 out of 100,000 patients. Persons with an affected parent have a 50% chance of developing the disease. The genetic locus for the disease appears on the short arm of chromosome 4. Males and females are equally likely to inherit the disorder. The disorder typically becomes manifest in persons between the ages of 25 and 45, although juvenile forms of the disease also occur. The disorder is characterized by choreiform (dancelike) movements involving the limbs and trunk, bradykinesia, and psychiatric disturbances (particularly affective disorders). Neuropathologically, a characteristic loss of the medium-sized spiny neurons in the caudate and putamen, which project to the globus pallidus and pars reticulata of the substantia nigra, occurs in Huntington's disease. Neuronal loss also occurs in the globus pallidus, ventrolateral thalamus, and subthalamic nucleus. This neuronal loss is associated with marked neurotransmitter reductions in the GABA-synthetic enzyme glutamate decarboxylase, neuropeptides (enkephalin, substance P, cholecystokinin), acetylcholine, and choline acetyltransferase. CT and MRI scans generally show a bilateral "wasting" of the caudate nucleus (although the entire striatum is typically involved), with concomitant dilatation of the anterior horns of the lateral ventricles. Cortical atrophy is also commonly present. SPECT scans show decreased blood flow in the basal ganglia and frontal cortex, and PET studies also demonstrate diminished glucose utilization in these regions. For a number of years, Huntington's disease was considered to be a prototypical "subcortical" dementia, with the greatest pathological changes occurring in subcortical structures such as the basal ganglia. However, it is now clear that pathological changes occur in cortical regions as well, thereby blurring the distinction between the terms "cortical" and "subcortical" dementia.

Early signs of Huntington's disease include alterations in memory, affect, or movement. As the disease progresses, impaired attention and concentration and executive dysfunction become prominent. Memory is also impaired and is characterized by deficient retrieval of new information during the early stages. Cues are generally effective in facilitating patients' recognition performance, although deficient encoding of new information becomes evident as the diseases progresses. Procedural learning tends to be impaired. Language abilities (e.g., comprehension, naming) are usually unaffected until the later stages of the disorder, although impairment in the motor aspects of speech may be associated with dysarthria and impaired writing. Diminished word list generation is also commonly seen. Approximately 50% of patients with Huntington's disease may develop affective disturbances, and there is a high risk of depression and suicide in this population. Impulsive aggressive or sexual behavior, irritability, angry outbursts, and anxiety are also common psychiatric manifestations.

A presymptomatic genetic test was recently developed to determine whether an individual carries the abnormal gene and hence will eventually manifest the disease. However, prior to undergoing such testing, genetic counseling is extremely important, as there is a high risk of suicide in persons who test positive.

2. Treatment

Huntington's disease has a progressive course that cannot be altered, although some control can be gained over the choreiform movements. Neuroleptic medications and tetrabenazine (a dopamine antagonist) may be helpful in this regard. The findings of reduced GABA in the basal ganglia in Huntington's disease patients have prompted the use of GABA-ergic agents, such as isoniazid, which have also had limited success in treating choreiform movements. Intravenous injection of physostigmine has been demonstrated to reduce the movement abnormalities in Huntington's disease, although oral administration of cholinergic compounds has not shown significant efficacy. The dementia associated with Huntington's disease is not improved with medication. However, it is important to note that the affective disturbances, including depression, irritability, angry outbursts, and psychosis, are amenable to pharmacologic treatment. Electroconvulsive therapy has also been effective in treating the depression associated with Huntington's disease. Psychosocial interventions, including genetic counseling, personal counseling, patient and caregiver support groups, and management of psychiatric disturbances, play a significant role in the treatment of these patients.

E. Progressive Supranuclear Palsy

1. Clinical Features

Progressive supranuclear palsy (PSP) is a relatively rare disorder that shares many of the same motoric abnormalities seen in Parkinson's disease. However, PSP also affects brainstem nuclei, producing progressive loss of volitional eye movements, swallowing difficulties, and dysarthria associated with pseudobulbar palsy, together with rigidity in the neck and trunk, and hypererect posture with neck extension. Voluntary downward gaze is generally lost first, followed by loss of upward gaze, and finally loss of horizontal eye movements. Approximately 60 to 80% of PSP patients exhibit dementia. PET studies have shown prominent hypometabolism and hypoperfusion in the superior frontal lobes, and hypometabolism has also been observed in the caudate, putamen, thalamus, and pons.

Cognitive changes associated with PSP dementia include bradyphrenia, impaired learning, memory consolidation, and retrieval, personality changes including apathy and depression, impaired motor aspects of speech (e.g., hypophonia, dysarthria, diminished verbal output), and impaired executive functioning on tasks such as word list generation. Aphasia, apraxia, and agnosia are typically not seen in PSP.

2. Treatment

PSP has a relatively rapid, progressive course that is minimally amenable to treatment. Motor abnormalities, such as dyskinesia and rigidity, and extraocular movements are occasionally responsive to treatment with dopamine precursors and dopamine receptor agonists, although the dementia associated with PSP is generally unaffected. As with Parkinson's disease, pharmacotherapy becomes less effective as the disease progresses.

F. Cortical-Basal Ganglionic Degeneration

1. Clinical Features

This degenerative disorder is typically associated with asymmetric neurological findings together with an overlay of cortical and subcortical neuropsychological deficits. Asymmetric rigidity and akinesia of the arms is typically seen, together with myoclonic jerking, tremor, and dystonic movements. From a neuropsychological perspective, a profound apraxia is associated with the affected limb, which gradually progresses to a loss of all executive functions associated with limb movement. Cognitive slowing, perseveration, and difficulty with cognitive flexibility is also seen. Generalized cerebral atrophy is typically present on CT and MRI scans. Asymmetric metabolic and blood flow abnormalities are often observed in the basal ganglia and associated fronto-parietal cortex on PET and SPECT.

2. Treatment

There are no effective treatments for this progressive disorder.

G. Hallervorden-Spatz Syndrome

1. Clinical Features

Hallervorden-Spatz syndrome is a rare autosomal recessive condition that first becomes manifest in late childhood or early adolescence. It is characterized by motoric spasticity and rigidity, dystonia, or chorea, together with a progressive dementia. Moodiness, depression, and angry outbursts may presage the cognitive decline. Increased deposition of iron in blood vessels and cells of the basal ganglia is associated with this disorder. The globus pallidus and pars reticulata of the substantia nigra are typically discolored, appearing rusty brown, and partially destroyed. Magnetic resonance imaging (MRI) may show hypodensity in the globus pallidus, putamen, or substantia nigra, or a gradual wasting of the basal ganglia similar to that found in Huntington's disease may also be seen.

2. Treatment

There are no effective treatments for this condition.

H. Wilson's Disease

1. Clinical Features

Wilson's disease is another autosomal recessive condition that occurs in approximately 1/30,000 patients.

It typically becomes manifest in the late teens or early 20s and affects males and females equally. This disorder is associated with abnormal copper metabolism, and increased deposition of copper is found in the liver, brain, and eyes. Motor symptoms include tremor, rigidity, dystonia, chorea, and dysarthria. Progressive dementia, characterized by impaired memory, poor concentration, impaired abstract reasoning and concept formation, and bradyphrenia, and psychiatric disturbances, such as psychosis, emotional lability, and childishness, occur in Wilson's disease. Language functions are commonly spared. The cognitive and motor symptoms of Wilson's disease are likely to be the result of the toxic effects of copper on cerebral tissue. Characteristic features of Wilson's disease include the brownish-green *Kayser-Fleischer ring* found in the limbus of the cornea, low serum ceruloplasmin (a copper-carrying protein) concentration, and elevated copper excretion. CT and MRI scans frequently reveal hypodensity in the lenticular nuclei. PET scans may also demonstrate diffuse hypometabolism, together with marked hypometabolism in the lenticular nuclei.

2. Treatment

Early diagnosis is essential, as this disorder is one degenerative condition that can be effectively treated with reduction of dietary copper, administration of the copper chelating agent D-penicillamine, and administration of pyridoxine to prevent anemia, thereby inhibiting further progression and reversing both hepatic and neurological signs.

I. Cerebellar and Olivopontocerebellar Degeneration

1. Clinical Features

A heterogeneous spectrum of disorders involving progressive ataxia, some of which are genetically inherited, are also associated with dementia. Symptoms associated with cerebellar dysfunction, such as ataxic gait, hypotonia, limb unsteadiness, intention tremor, and dysarthria, are common. Extracerebellar signs, such as ophthalmoplegia, deafness, hyperreflexia, and extensor plantar responses, may also occur and tend to be more indicative of olivopontocerebellar atrophy. Cerebellar degeneration may be evident on CT or MRI scans, while PET scans may show hypometabolism in the cerebellar hemispheres, cerebellar vermis, and brain stem. The inferior olivary and pontine nuclei often appear atrophied. Choline acetyltransferase and acetylcholinesterase tend to be diminished in olivopontocerebellar degeneration. The dementia syndrome is characterized by impaired attention and memory, apathy, and psychomotor retardation.

2. Treatment
There are no effective treatments for this disorder.

II. DEMENTIA DUE TO CEREBROVASCULAR DISEASE

In contrast to the degenerative dementias in which the specific etiology is generally uncertain, dementia due to ischemic, anoxic, or hemorrhagic events can often be traced to known risk factors, such as cigarette smoking, hyperlipidemia, cardiac arrhythmia, or platelet aggregation. Given knowledge of these risk factors, early diagnosis of vascular dementia may potentially minimize further cognitive deterioration. Vascular dementia can be attributed to the cumulative effect of cerebrovascular events largely confined to the cerebral cortex (multi-infarct dementia), vascular lesions in specific subcortical structures (thalamic vascular dementia and lacunar state), or to accumulated, small vessel vascular lesions confined mainly to the periventricular white matter regions (Binswanger's disease or subcortical arteriosclerotic encephalopathy).

A. Multi-Infarct Dementia

I. Clinical Features
Multi-infarct dementia is associated with accumulated vascular damage that preferentially affects cortical gray matter areas. Men are typically affected more often than women. A rapid disease onset and stepwise clinical course characterized by plateaus and sharp declines in functioning are both associated with multi-infarct dementia, although more gradual and progressive diminution in mentation may also be seen as well. Nocturnal confusion, previous hypertension, and a history of transient ischemic attacks are also associated with multi-infarct dementia. Neurological examination typically reveals focal or bilateral pyramidal or extrapyramidal signs, including plantar extensor response, limb rigidity or spasticity, hyperreflexia, gait disturbance, or urinary incontinence. There is wide variation in the types and severity of cognitive

deficits associated with multi-infarct dementia, depending on the location and number of infarcts. The prototypic neuropsychological profile is a "patchy" presentation, with relative preservation of some abilities and loss of other skills. Frequent deficits are seen in the areas of orientation and attention, recent memory, abstract reasoning and problem solving, and language deficits, such as impaired writing, frequent literal paraphasias (e.g., saying "tome" for comb), apraxia, and difficulty with complex comprehension. Coronary insufficiency with systemic hypotension tend to produce more diffuse deficits. Psychiatric features, most notably depression and emotional lability, are also common in cerebrovascular dementia.

2. Treatment
Early diagnosis is important in order to prevent or retard further progression of the dementia. Recognition of the presence of multiple risk factors for vascular disease can also facilitate diagnosis and identify targets for treatment. Controllable risk factors include cigarette smoking, hyperlipidemia, diabetes, and hypertension. Agents that inhibit platelet aggregation, such as aspirin or warfarin, may also reduce the risk of thrombotic infarction. Speech therapy may be helpful for patients who have developed aphasia, and occupational and physical therapy are beneficial to maximize the potential for continued independent living.

B. Thalamic Vascular Dementia

I. Clinical Features
Vascular lesions to the thalamus may produce a range of neurological and neuropsychological deficits depending on the specific thalamic nuclei involved. From a neurological perspective, thalamic hemorrhage may be associated with greater sensory than motor loss, memory impairment, impaired vertical gaze, and aphasic symptoms, if the lesion occurred in the dominant hemisphere. Variable arousal, including hypersomnia and loss of consciousness, have been reported with lesions (usually bilateral) to the paramedian thalamus. Disturbed attention on less-structured tasks may also be seen in thalamic lesions. Deficits that are typically characteristic of frontal lobe lesions are frequently associated with thalamic lesions as well, possibly in the region of the dorsomedial nucleus. These deficits include perseveration, increased susceptibility to interference, difficulty in sequencing information,

and personality changes such as apathy, abulia, lack of concern, and euphoria. Language following ventrolateral and ventroanterior thalamic lesions is generally characterized by intact repetition, comprehension, reading, and writing, contrasted with impaired speech initiation, diminished content of speech, reduced word list generation, dysprosody, dysarthria, perseveration, and hypophonia. Lesions in the pulvinar and posterolateral thalamus have been associated with anomia, normal or increased speech output, and impaired comprehension. Visuospatial deficits may follow bilateral or unilateral right thalamic damage. Memory impairment has been attributed to lesions affecting the dorsomedial nucleus, mammillary bodies, and/or mammilothalamic tract.

2. Treatment

Thalamic vascular lesions are not reversible. Treatment involves reducing or eliminating modifiable vascular risk factors plus supportive measures including speech, occupational, or physical therapy, and managing neuropsychiatric conditions should they occur.

C. Lacunar State

1. Clinical Features

Small infarctions ranging from 0.5 to 1.5 mm in diameter that are located primarily in the basal ganglia, thalamus, internal capsule, and brain stem are referred to as *lacunes*. Lacunes are thought to result primarily from hypertension-related fibrinoid necrosis of arterioles resulting in occlusion, although some lacunes may be associated with hemorrhage. The lenticulostriate branches of the middle cerebral artery or the thalamogeniculate, choroidal, and thalamoperforator branches of the posterior communicating and posterior cerebral arteries are commonly involved. The term *lacunar state* describes the condition in which multiple lacunes are present. Hypertension, diabetes, and atherosclerotic emboli have been noted to contribute to the formation of lacunes. Lacunar state is generally associated with combined motoric and cognitive impairment. The motor symptoms include rigidity and bradykinesia (which are seen in Parkinson's disease), spasticity, hyperreflexia, limb weakness, pseudobulbar palsy, and extensor plantar responses. Given the many motor abnormalities that are similar to Parkinson's disease, the term "arteriosclerotic parkinsonism" was used until recently to describe deficits

associated with lacunar state. Cognitive deficits typically involve impaired memory, apathy, psychomotor retardation, impaired mental control and orientation, and frontal-lobe type deficits. Mood changes and fluctuations in mental state are also observed. Lacunes may be evident on CT or MRI, although many lacunes are too small to be visualized using either imaging technique. PET scans may reveal areas of hypometabolism at the site of the lacune as well as in cortical locations receiving projections from the affected region.

2. Treatment

Once present, the cognitive and motor impairment associated with lacunar state cannot be reversed, although preventative measures such as correction of modifiable risk factors will help to reduce or retard progression.

D. Binswanger's Disease (Subcortical Arteriosclerotic Encephalopathy)

1. Clinical Features

When ischemic damage is confined to the periventricular white matter regions, the term Binswanger's disease or subcortical arteriosclerotic encephalopathy is applied. Occlusion of small blood vessels is commonly associated with this condition. Binswanger's disease may resemble a degenerative dementia such as Alzheimer's disease by virtue of its insidious onset and gradual progression. It may lack the abrupt onset and stepwise decline associated with other vascular dementias. Hypertension and smoking are the most common risk factors for Binswanger's disease. Clinical deficits vary depending on the extent of the lesions, although incontinence, pseudobulbar palsy, asymmetric weakness, gait disturbance, parkinsonism, and dysarthria have been described. Mood disturbances include irritability, apathy, mania with hyperactivity, depression with suicidal ideation, and psychosis with paranoid delusions. From a cognitive perspective, memory deficits are usually only mild in Binswanger's disease, although poor judgment, perseveration, abulia, and increased response latency are seen more frequently. Loss of white matter is most severe in the frontal lobes. The short arcuate "U" fibers are generally spared. Lacunar state may coexist with Binswanger's disease. Enlarged ventricles and evidence of periventricular lucency associated with white matter ischemia are typically noted on CT and MRI.

Varying degrees of periventricular lesions have been reported in "normal" asymptomatic elderly individuals without neurological complaints, suggesting that the amount of white matter ischemia has little correlation with the extent of cognitive impairment. This finding has stimulated controversy regarding the radiologic diagnosis of Binswanger's disease. However, there are also data to suggest that persons with radiologic evidence of white matter lesions have significantly lower intellectual performance and more motor abnormalities than persons without diffuse white matter lesions, suggesting that periventricular lucencies may be a harbinger of deficits associated with Binswanger's disease even in asymptomatic individuals.

2. Treatment

As with the other vascular dementias, prevention of further deterioration through careful monitoring of vascular risk factors (particularly smoking and hypertension) and antiplatelet treatment with agents such as aspirin, warfarin, and ticlopidine are the only treatment strategies for this condition at this juncture.

E. Vasculitis

Dementia may also be associated with inflammation of the cranial arteries due to systemic illnesses, such as giant cell (temporal) arteritis, sarcoidosis, systemic lupus erythematosus, granulomatous arteritis, and polyarteritis nodosa, or to chemical arteritis associated with use of amphetamines, "crack" cocaine, or oral contraceptives. Amyloid angiopathy is often associated with hemorrhages but may also be associated with dementia. Dementia due to vasculitis generally presents acutely in a manner consistent with a confusional state, although gradually progressive dementia is not uncommon. Cerebral arteriography and brain biopsy are often necessary for diagnosis. Treatment with anti-inflammatory agents is frequently prescribed.

III. DEMENTIA DUE TO INFECTIOUS AGENTS

The central nervous system can be vulnerable to infection from a variety of agents. Infectious agents producing dementia include viruses, bacteria, fungi, parasites, and atypical *proteinaceous infectious agents* called prions. Given an intact immune system, infection of the central nervous system is relatively rare, although infection by herpes simplex or cryptococcus can occur in immunocompetent hosts. However, in cases of immune system compromise, the brain may become vulnerable to a variety of infectious agents, some of which may be treatable if discovered early in the course of the disorder. The term encephalitis refers to inflammation and infection of brain tissue associated with any of the infectious agents described above. The term encephalopathy is broader, encompassing dysfunction of the brain due to any cause.

A. Viral Infections

A *virus* is a small particle of protein-encapsulated DNA or RNA that infects a host cell and replicates itself therein. Two groups of viruses that may produce dementia have been described. The first group is termed the neurotropic viruses, such as those causing rabies and poliomyelitis, which have a special affinity for central nervous system cells. The second group is known as the pantropic viruses, such as mumps, measles, and herpes simplex, which invade cells throughout the body, in addition to central nervous system cells.

1. HIV Encephalopathy

a. Clinical Features   The dementia associated with infection by the Human Immunodeficiency Virus (HIV) which produces Acquired Immunodeficiency Syndrome (AIDS) has been well-characterized, and central nervous system involvement is present in virtually all AIDS patients at autopsy. Central nervous system compromise is produced in two ways. First, by weakening the immune system, the brain becomes susceptible to rare infectious agents, such as parasites and fungi. On a second level, the virus invades and destroys neurons, glia, subcortical nuclear structures, and white matter of the brain. Numbness, tingling, muscular weakness, and coordination difficulty may frequently be indications of direct central nervous system involvement by HIV. Other early neurological manifestations may include ataxia, action tremor, dysarthria, and exaggerated lower extremity reflexes. Headache, seizures, incontinence, and rigidity may appear with later disease progression. Early cognitive features may include forgetfulness, fluctuations in attention and concentration, and difficulty maintaining a coherent stream of thought. Apathy and depression may also become prominent during the early stages of infection. Frank memory deficits emerge later, in addition to visuospatial impairment, diminished fine motor coordination, decreased cognitive flexibility, and intact simple reaction time contrasted with impaired choice reaction time. Naming and vocabulary are typically preserved throughout the disease. Confusion and disorientation, psychomotor slowing, mutism, and apathy are frequently seen in the preterminal stages. Some patients may exhibit psychotic features and/or prominent affective symptoms. Cortical atrophy with ventricular enlargement and sulcal widening is generally evident on CT or MRI scans, although MRI scans will typically also reveal deep white matter lesions. In the early stages of HIV infection, reduced cerebral glucose metabolism and cerebral blood flow is generally evident in subcortical structures, including the basal ganglia and thalamus on PET or SPECT. More prominent and focal cortical hypometabolism and hypoperfusion are noted in the later stages and is quite distinct from the pattern observed in primary degenerative dementias, such as Alzheimer's disease. [*See* HIV/AIDS.]

b. Treatment Medical management of opportunistic infections with antimicrobials, control of affective disorders with psychotherapy and medication, and careful monitoring of potential toxic and/or metabolic disruptions is important for limiting progression due to these secondary causes of dementia. Although it has significant side effects, the drug azidothymidine (AZT) has been beneficial in limiting viral replication within the individual and improving cognitive function. Individuals with mild to moderate dementia associated with HIV infection have shown improvement in cognition and in cerebral glucose metabolism following AZT treatment. The benefits from AZT are time-limited, however, typically lasting several months before the virus continues to progress. Reduction of the risk factors associated with contraction of HIV through community education, particularly related to intravenous drug abuse and unprotected and promiscuous sexual relations, should also be helpful in reducing the spread of this disease.

2. Subacute Sclerosing Panencephalitis (SSPE)

a. Clinical Features The measles virus may sometimes cause an acute encephalitis, although it may also produce a slowly developing degenerative process

known as subacute sclerosing panencephalitis (SSPE). Progressive Rubella Panencephalitis is another viral encephalitis that is clinically similar to SSPE. SSPE typically presents during childhood or adolescence several years following measles infection and produces a rapid deterioration leading to death in from 3 to 10 months. Boys are affected more frequently than girls. Behavioral changes, including oppositional behavior and angry outbursts, together with slow cognitive decline and a deterioration in school performance typically are the earliest features of SSPE. Onset of seizures and movement abnormalities, such as myoclonic jerking (short, rapid involuntary muscular contractions), gait disturbance, and rigidity, are also seen in SSPE. End stages of the disease are characterized by hypothalamic dysfunction and autonomic failure and decerebrate posturing. Cognitive features include visuospatial deficits, distractibility, inability to self-dress, apraxia, alexia, aphasia, and agnosia. General intellectual functioning declines steadily throughout the course of SSPE. The electroencephalogram (EEG) demonstrates a characteristic burst-suppression pattern exemplified by periodic high amplitude waveform complexes, making it particularly helpful in diagnosis. MRI scans may reveal hyperintensities on T2-weighted images in the basal ganglia. PET may show hypermetabolism in the basal ganglia contrasted with cortical hypometabolism in the early stages of the disorder.

b. Treatment SSPE typically progresses to death within several months, although periods of remissions and exacerbations are common. Amantadine, isoprinosine, and intraventricular administration of interferon have been reported to be effective in prolonging life and in bringing about periods of remission. Fortunately, the number of SSPE cases has been significantly reduced by the introduction of the measles vaccine. Thus, this devastating childhood dementia is potentially preventable.

3. Herpes Simplex Encephalitis

a. Clinical Features The Herpes Simplex Virus (HSV I) can produce an acute, severe encephalitis that results in destruction of the medial temporal and orbitofrontal cortical regions, with relative sparing of white matter. Following initial infection, HSV resides in cell bodies of the trigeminal nerves innervating cutaneous regions of the face. Reactivation of the virus can lead to viral migration along the trigeminal nerve with subsequent encephalitis. Headache and fever may be associated with early stages of the HSV encephalitis, followed by acute mental status changes, seizures, and coma. The disease is often fatal. However, in survivors, there is usually prominent memory impairment, reflecting damage to the medial temporal regions. A human condition resembling the so-called Kluver-Bucy syndrome seen in monkeys, represented by diminished responsiveness to social and emotional stimuli, increased oral exploratory behavior, reduced aggression and fearfulness, and difficulty recognizing the meaning or significance of common objects ("psychic blindness"), is sometimes associated with bilateral temporal lobe destruction. Aphasia may also be a cognitive sequel of HSV encephalitis. CT or MRI scans may show areas of lucency in the temporal lobe, and EEG may reveal diffuse or focal slowing or periodic sharp and slow-wave complexes.

b. Treatment Early treatment with acyclovir and adenine arabinoside may substantially diminish the morbidity and mortality associated with HSV encephalitis.

4. Viral Infections Associated with Underlying Systemic Illness

a. Clinical Features Progressive Multifocal Leukoencephalopathy (PML) is associated with infection by the papova viruses in immunocompromised persons (e.g., AIDS) or individuals with chronic lymphoproliferative, myeloproliferative, or granulomatous diseases. This disease affects many different areas of cerebral and cerebellar white matter and may be associated with motor weakness, gait disturbance, dysarthria, blindness and other visual disorders, and seizures. The dementia associated with PML includes behavioral changes, memory deficits, poor concentration, and language deficits. MRI may show multifocal hyperintensities in the white matter associated with subcortical demyelination. Microscopic changes include abnormal oligodendrocytes that are large and contain intranuclear inclusion bodies. Abnormally shaped, multinuclear astrocytes are also found in the areas of the lesions. PET studies reveal cortical hypometabolism in regions associated with white matter changes. Simian virus 40 (SV 40) is one of the most common papova viruses associated with PML.

b. Treatment Treatment of PML remains uncertain. There are some reports of improvement following cy-

tarabine therapy, although clinical trials with other antiviral agents have produced mixed results.

5. Limbic Encephalitis

a. Clinical Features Limbic Encephalitis involves a progressive cognitive decline over 1 to 2 years in individuals with an underlying malignancy. Oat cell carcinoma of the lung is one neoplasm that is frequently associated with limbic encephalitis, although the syndrome has been described in a variety of other cancers. Characteristic features include marked disturbance of affect, commonly involving anxiety and depression, in addition to prominent memory impairment. Hallucinations and variable alertness may also be seen. Pathological changes include neuronal loss and inflammatory changes concentrated in hippocampus and medial temporal lobe, although lateral temporal cortex, and other widespread brain regions may also be involved. Limbic encephalitis may result from an autoimmune response producing an attack on temporal lobe neurons, given the relatively acute presentation, inflammatory changes, and occasional presence of intranuclear inclusion bodies.

b. Treatment There are no effective treatments for this paraneoplastic dementia.

B. Bacterial Infections

1. Bacterial Meningitis

a. Clinical Features Most forms of bacterial meningitis (infectious inflammation of the meninges surrounding the brain) typically have a rapid onset and are associated with fever, headache, and stiff neck. Although not common, certain bacteria produce a chronic meningitis that is associated with a gradual or subacute cognitive decline. For example, tuberculosis can be associated with central nervous system involvement manifested by pyramidal, extrapyramidal, and cerebellar signs, involuntary movements, poor insight, impaired memory, and personality changes. Lyme disease is caused by a tick-transmitted spirochete (*Borrelia burgdorferi*). A red rash around the bite area is typically followed by mild flu-like symptoms. Arthritis, cardiac symptoms, and neurological symptoms, including meningoencephalitis may appear months later.

b. Treatment Although it was previously a fatal condition, tuberculosis meningitis is now generally treatable and curable. Common treatments include combination therapy with isoniazid, streptomycin, and para-aminosalicylic acid or isoniazid and rifampin. However, some treatment-resistant strains of tuberculosis have been reported recently, posing a significant challenge for future treatment of this disease. Oral penicillin or tetracycline is typically used to treat Lyme disease in the early stages, although intravenous administration of antibiotics may be required in the later stages.

2. Syphilis

a. Clinical Features The spirochete, *Treponema pallidum,* is responsible for syphilitic infection. If not treated, symptomatic neurosyphilis may develop in approximately 10% of cases. Symptomatic neurosyphilis tends to be more common in men. Meningovascular syphilis, a condition associated with multiple strokes, may appear approximately 2 to 10 years after the initial syphilitic infection. The condition known as general paresis may appear 7 to 15 years after the initial infection and is characterized by prominent dementia, either with or without psychiatric manifestations, such as mania, depression, or psychosis. In addition to impaired memory, some individuals with general paresis may become severely disoriented and may confabulate. Other cognitive deficits include anomia, apraxia, verbal paraphasias, and dysarthria. Coarse tremors of the jaw and tongue are common. Diagnosis of syphilitic infection is facilitated by serum detection of specific treponemal antibodies (fluorescent treponemal antibody absorption; FTA-abs), together with pleocytosis (white blood cells) present in the cerebrospinal fluid (CSF). On autopsy, significant frontotemporal cortical atrophy is evident.

b. Treatment Standard treatment involves intravenous administration of penicillin G, although dosage recommendations and treatment duration vary. Close monitoring of CSF every three months for the first year and every six months during the second year following treatment is recommended.

3. Brain Abscesses

a. Clinical Features A variety of bacteria may produce small pockets of pus known as abscesses in or around brain tissue. They are commonly the result of secondary infections and generally originate from middle ear infections, sinusitis, or pulmonary conditions. With increasing size, the abscess behaves as an expanding mass and may produce elevated intracranial pressure. The abscess may also produce necrosis or cell death, destroying neural tissue in the vicinity of the abscess.

b. Treatment Abscesses may be treated with antibiotics, and they often require surgical drainage.

C. Mycotic (Fungal) Infections

1. Clinical Features

Fungal CNS infections are relatively rare. They occur most commonly in immunocompromised individuals (e.g., HIV infection, immunosuppressant therapy, systemic malignancies). Examples of such infections include cryptococcal meningitis, histoplasmosis, aspergillus, blastomycosis, and candida. These fungi may produce a chronic meningitis that has an insidiously progressive course associated with compromised intellectual functioning, variable arousal, impaired attention and orientation, and poor memory. Cranial nerve palsies are often seen.

2. Treatment

Once established, fungal infections are difficult to treat and often result in a high mortality.

D. Parasitic Infections

1. Clinical Features

The parasite *Entamoeba histolytica* (responsible for producing amoebiasis or amoebic dysentery) and several other protozoan and helminthic parasites may produce encephalitis, chronic meningitis, and brain abscesses. The parasite *Plasmodium falciparum,* responsible for producing cerebral malaria, is associated with infection of capillaries within the brain producing local hemorrhages, demyelination, and neuronal degeneration.

2. Treatment

Antimalarial agents and steroid therapy are effective in completely reversing the effects of cerebral malaria if they are administered early in the course of the infection.

E. Prion Disease

Prions are subviral, infectious, unencapsulated protein particles that resist most known forms of inactivation. They are resistant to boiling, ultraviolet light, and formalin, but they are susceptible to proteolytic treatments, such as autoclaving or immersion in a strong alkali solution. Human prion diseases include Creutzfeldt-Jacob disease (CJD), Gerstmann-Straussler-Scheinker (GSS) syndrome, kuru and fatal familial insomnia (FFI). Animal prion diseases include bovine spongioform encephalopathy (BSE; "mad cow disease"), and scrapie (seen in sheep). These neurodegenerative diseases were previously thought to be due to "slow viruses." Prion disease can be infectious (kuru, infectious CJD), sporadic (CJD with or without apparent somatic DNA mutation), or familial due to prion protein gene mutation (familial CJD, GSS syndrome, and FFI).

The common denominator among all of the prion diseases is an aberrant metabolism of the prion protein (PrP) usually leading to an accumulation of an abnormal isoform of intracellular PrP. All infectious prions are composed of this abnormal PrP isoform. The prion diseases are referred to as the "spongioform encephalopathies" by virtue of the characteristic "spongy" appearance of the postmortem cerebral tissue on microscopic examination. This appearance results from the formation of ubiquitous vacuoles induced by rupture of neuronal and glial membranes.

The transmissibility of prion disease via intracerebral inoculation with fresh-frozen brain tissue from humans with spongioform encephalopathy to primates is well established. Human-to-human transmission of CJD has also been documented through corneal transplants, human pituitary growth hormone therapy, human pituitary gonadotropin therapy, dura mater grafts, contaminated electroencephalographic electrode implants, and other neurosurgical procedures. Kuru was once common and was the leading cause of death among the Fore tribe in New Guinea. This disease also is associated with human-to-human transmission, as it is thought to be related to the cannibalistic consumption of dead family members. In addition to dementia, kuru is associated with gait ataxia, followed by limb ataxia, a shiverlike tremor, and dysarthria.

The recently reported epidemic of Bovine Spongioform Encephalopathy (BSE or prion disease affecting cattle) in the United Kingdom has caused increased attention to be focused on the intraspecies transmission of prion disease. There has been some speculation that byproducts of sheep infected with scrapie may have been incorporated into cattle feed and may be associated with the apparent increase of BSE in British cattle. Transmission of prion disease from cattle to humans is not well documented, although two cases of CJD in individuals who were occupationally exposed to BSE have been reported in England and Wales. Thus far, the concurrence of CJD and BSE is less than that which could have occurred by chance, and the incidence of CJD in Europe has remained static over recent years.

CJD is perhaps the most prototypical of the prion diseases with an incidence of approximately 1 case per million. In a series of 230 neuropathologically verified cases of CJD, up to 8% of the cases appear to be familial. CJD typically presents with subacute, rapidly progressive dementia and myoclonus, and in most cases, eventually demonstrates a characteristic EEG pattern of periodic sharp wave complexes that are predominantly triphasic. Cognitive deficits include concentration difficulty, fatigue, forgetfulness and depression during the early stages of illness, followed by marked aphasia and other cortical signs of dementia such as amnesia, agnosia, apraxia, and rapid intellectual decline. CT and MRI may be normal, or generalized atrophy or focal hyperintensities may be observed. PET and SPECT studies show multifocal areas of hypometabolism and hypoperfusion.

GSS is a familial disorder that typically occurs between the ages of 40 and 70, with a duration ranging from 4 to 10 years. It presents as a cerebellar syndrome and dementia. Early motor features are consistent with cerebellar dysfunction, including impaired smooth pursuit eye movements, coordination difficulty, ataxia, and ophthalmoplegia. Parkinsonian symptoms are also sometimes reported. Bradykinesia, rigidity, and extensor plantar responses are also observed during the later stages. Cognitive difficulties are more prominent toward the latter stages of the disease and typically include impaired memory, dysnomia, poor judgment, psychomotor slowing, and affective disorders.

FFI is also a familial disorder that is associated with selective degeneration of specific regions of the thalamus. Individuals with FFI exhibit an untreatable insomnia and impaired regulation of the autonomic nervous system. FFI is sometimes referred to as "thalamic CJD."

Familial CJD, GSS syndrome, and FFI have been associated with specific mutations on the short arm of chromosome 20 in the prion protein (PrP) gene. The mutations are tightly linked to the expression of the disease. The PrP is a normal cellular protein that is synthesized by neurons and glial cells throughout life. PrP has been referred to as a "housekeeping" gene that is necessary for basic cellular functioning. PrP is located in the cellular membrane and is present in evolutionarily diverse organisms. It is thought that prion diseases are associated with a conformational change in PrP, resulting in an abnormal, protease-resistant isoform that is referred to as PrP^P. PrP^P may result from either a genetic mutation causing synthesis of this new isoform or from post-translational modification in the gene product. The abnormal PrP^P is thought to lead to cellular death by producing vacuoles and amyloid deposition.

IV. DEMENTIA DUE TO TOXIC OR METABOLIC CONDITIONS

Metabolic derangements and toxic exposure are frequently overlooked causes of dementia, possibly due to the fact that these conditions often present acutely as confusional states, characterized by a fluctuating level of arousal, distractibility, increased motor and verbal response latencies, disorientation, and hallucinations (predominantly visual). Tremor, myoclonus, and asterixis are the most common motor findings associated with these acute conditions. However, metabolic changes or toxic exposure may also occur very slowly, producing a symptom resembling dementia. There are many causes of toxic/metabolic disorders, and a thorough description of each cause is beyond the scope of this article. However, some of the more common systemic illnesses associated with dementia syndromes include endocrine (e.g., thyroid disease, parathyroid disease, disorders of the adrenal medulla and pituitary gland), cardiovascular (e.g., congestive heart failure, hyperviscosity states including polycythemia and hyperlipidemia, anemia), pulmonary (e.g., pulmonary insufficiency, sleep apnea, postanoxic states), renal (e.g., uremia, dialysis encephalopathy), and hepatic (e.g., cirrhosis) dysfunction. Metabolic deficiencies and excesses (e.g., alterations in serum sodium, calcium, magnesium), and vitamin deficiency states (e.g., thiamine (B$_1$), niacin (B$_2$), cyanocobalamin (B$_{12}$), folate) are also important considerations in the dementia evaluation. Finally, exposure to a variety of toxic agents may produce encephalopathies. These substances include medications (e.g., psycho-

tropic medications, anticholinergic medications, antihypertensive agents), drugs of abuse (alcohol, barbiturates, solvent vapor, amphetamines), heavy metals, and industrial cleaners and solvents. If discovered early and treated aggressively, the progression of a large number of these conditions may be arrested or slowed, and the cognitive disorders may be reversed in some cases. These conditions represent perhaps the most treatable etiologies associated with cognitive impairment, although they are much less common than the degenerative or vascular dementias.

A. Systemic Illnesses

I. Thyroid Dysfunction

a. Clinical Features   Thyroid dysfunction accounts for a sizable number of metabolic disturbances, and most of these disorders are highly treatable. Hyperthyroidism tends to be most frequently seen in the late teens or early 20's, although it may also mimic a progressive dementia in the elderly. Idiopathic thyroid overactivity accounts for most cases of hyperthyroidism, although other causes may include thyroid cancer, goiter, or pituitary adenoma that results in overproduction of thyroid stimulating hormone. In younger persons, hyperthyroidism may first present with personality changes including depression, restlessness, anxiety, emotional lability, and irritability, together with concentration and memory deficits, tremor, and tachycardia. Weight loss, skin changes, shortness of breath, and heat intolerance may also occur. These symptoms may progress to cognitive deterioration, apathy, somnolence, and coma in advanced stages. In contrast, the initial personality changes (e.g., anxiety and restlessness), tremor, and tachycardia may be completely absent in elderly persons with hyperthyroidism, and they may instead present with apathy, lethargy, and psychomotor slowing. Hypothyroidism also has prominent neurobehavioral effects including variable attention and orientation, memory deficits, psychomotor slowing, paranoia, and hallucinations. Cold intolerance and weight gain are common. Psychosis may occur in as many as 5 to 15% of individuals with hypothyroidism, while dementia may occur in 5% of hypothyroid individuals.

b. Treatment   Restoration of normal levels of thyroid hormones, most frequently through oral administration of synthetic thyroid supplementation (hypothyroidism) or through surgical or radioactive ablation of the thyroid gland (hyperthyroidism), commonly leads to improved cognitive and physical functioning.

2. Parathyroid Dysfunction

a. Clinical Features Hyperparathyroidism is frequently associated with elevated serum levels of calcium. Apathy, depression, weakness, and a tendency to tire easily are seen in the early stages. As progression ensues, disorientation, poor memory, fluctuations in attention, paranoia and hallucinations may occur. Hypoparathyroidism and associated low serum levels of calcium commonly result in basal ganglia calcification that may produce parkinsonian motor features (e.g., bradykinesia and limb rigidity) or choreic movement abnormalities. Dementia associated with hypoparathyroidism includes variable orientation and concentration, apathy, and hallucinations.

b. Treatment Restoration of normal serum calcium levels in these two metabolic disorders can reverse the cognitive and motor abnormalities in some patients, particularly if discovered early.

3. Cushing's Disease and Addison's Disease

a. Clinical Features Overproduction (Cushing's disease) or underproduction (Addison's disease) of glucocorticoids from the adrenal gland may also produce symptoms of dementia. Cushing's disease most commonly results from pituitary tumors (adenomas), although adrenal tumors may also be associated with this disorder. Depression, psychomotor slowing, disturbed sleep patterns, irritability, and diminished attention, concentration, and memory are seen in this disease and are correlated with the degree of serum cortisol elevation. Addison's disease may produce apathy, impaired memory, depression, paranoia, and irritability, together with weight loss, easy fatigue, and electrolyte imbalances.

b. Treatment Restoration of normal serum cortisol levels improves cognitive functioning in most cases.

4. Cardiovascular Disease

a. Clinical Features Cardiac insufficiency resulting from congestive heart failure, chronic arrhythmias, or occlusion of the major cerebral arteries from atherosclerosis is associated with diminished cerebral perfusion. As a result, decreased oxygen can be supplied to the brain, and an accumulation of cellular metabolic by-products (e.g., carbon dioxide) and a corresponding decrease in pH in surrounding neural tissue take place. Somnolence, irritability, disorientation and confusion, and memory deficits are common. Repeated, prolonged vascular events may result in a stepwise deterioration. Hyperviscosity and hypercoagulable conditions such as hyperlipidemia and polycythemia (a proliferation of red blood cells) may produce sluggish blood flow and occlusive microvascular infarctions. Anemia may also produce cerebral anoxia due to the low concentration of oxygen-carrying hemoglobin in the blood. Myoclonus, restlessness, generalized cognitive deficits, and inattention are associated with chronic anemia.

b. Treatment Improvement in cardiac output and correction of hyperviscosity and hypercoagulable states often lead to improved cognitive functioning. Treatment of anemia, often through dietary iron supplementation, commonly leads to reversal of the associated neurological and cognitive symptoms.

5. Pulmonary Disease and Anoxic States

a. Clinical Features Chronic pulmonary encephalopathy may result from a variety of diseases that produce pulmonary insufficiency such as emphysema and chronic obstructive pulmonary disease. Tremor and asterixis, headache, and papilledema may reflect physical manifestations of pulmonary encephalopathy. Disorientation, drowsiness, forgetfulness, and variable attention are common mental status changes associated with this condition. As in cardiovascular disease, decreased cerebral oxygen and increased carbon dioxide buildup in neuronal tissue is thought to be associated with the clinical manifestations of the disorder. A similar cognitive presentation has been described in hypoxia associated with living at high altitudes for extended periods. Sleep apnea has been cited as a common cause of cognitive impairment, particularly in the elderly, by producing chronic hypoxia and sleep deprivation. Finally, postanoxic states caused by cardiopulmonary arrest, carbon monoxide poisoning, hanging, and strangulation may produce a gradient of cerebral damage ranging from complete brain death, persistent vegetative state characterized by return of autonomic functioning without apparent higher cognitive activity, or variable deficits of higher cognitive functions, depending on the extent of cerebral damage.

Amnesia, aphasia, agnosia, visuospatial and visuoconstructional deficits, together with spasticity, dystonia, and ataxia have been described in variable combinations in postanoxic cases. Milder cases may present with impaired judgment, memory deficits, and disinhibition.

b. Treatment If discovered early, improvement in pulmonary function may reverse neurological and cognitive deficits. Sleep apnea is highly responsive to treatment using a continuous positive airway pressure (CPAP) device during sleep. In survivors of postanoxic states, rehabilitation, including occupational, speech, and physical therapies, may often be necessary.

6. Renal Disease and Dialysis
a. Clinical Features Any disease affecting renal function may produce a wide range of metabolic abnormalities. In addition to a spectrum of medical conditions, a variety of drugs may also impair renal functioning. Tremor, myoclonus, and asterixis are commonly associated with this condition. Disorientation, memory disturbance, variable arousal, irritability, hallucinations, and paranoia or affective lability occur as a result of the metabolic changes produced by chronic renal failure. Uremic encephalopathy is associated with increased serum creatinine and elevated blood urea nitrogen (BUN). The EEG can be a good index of uremic encephalopathy and is commonly characterized by background slowing and disorganization, although paroxysmal bilaterally synchronous bursts of slow wave activity may also be seen. Dialysis encephalopathy produces a progressive cognitive decline, myoclonus, depression, markedly abnormal EEG, and a distinctive progressive difficulty with expressive and motor aspects of speech (including difficulty with initiation, dysarthria, and anarthria) contrasted with relatively preserved naming and comprehension. Cognitive deficits may be seen on visuospatial and timed psychomotor tasks. Paroxysmal slow wave bursts and generalized background slowing are seen in the earlier stages of the disease, although bifrontal bursts of slow and sharp waves, and spike activity may be seen in later stages. The cause of dialysis dementia remains uncertain, although a variety of metabolic etiologies and aluminum intoxication have been proposed as possibilities.

b. Treatment There have been no successful treatments for dialysis encephalopathy, and the condition typically progresses to death within one to two years. Benzodiazepine administration has been temporarily effective in ameliorating the EEG, cognitive, and speech abnormalities, although these benefits subsequently abate and deterioration resumes. Desfuroximes may sometimes be used as an aluminum chelating agent.

7. Hepatic Disease
a. Clinical Features Elevated levels of ammonia and short-chain fatty acids are commonly associated with hepatic encephalopathy and may underlie the associated cognitive impairment. There are a variety of diseases associated with hepatic encephalopathy, although alcoholic cirrhosis is the most common of these disorders. Approximately 5% of patients with cirrhosis may develop hepatic encephalopathy. Neuropsychiatric manifestations are frequent in hepatic encephalopathy and may be associated with euphoria, depression, and bizarre behavior. Variable arousal, visuoconstructional deficits, impaired attention and concentration, and memory deficits, together with irregular action tremor, asterixis, gait ataxia, exaggerated reflexes, and motor impersistence are characteristic cognitive and neurological features.

b. Treatment Treatment typically involves strict dietary reduction of protein intake and absorption because proteins are commonly metabolized to ammonia.

B. Vitamin Deficiencies

Vitamin deficiencies can be seen in persons with poor or variable diets due to severe depression, anorexia nervosa, bulimia, social isolation in elderly persons, starvation, appetite loss associated with systemic illness (e.g., cancer), Crohn's disease, and chronic alcoholism. Gastrointestinal malabsorption syndromes (e.g., sprue or celiac disease) is another major cause of vitamin deficiency. [*See* FOOD, NUTRITION, AND MENTAL HEALTH.]

1. Thiamine (Vitamin B_1)
a. Clinical Features Thiamine deficiency is most common in chronic alcoholism, but it may be seen in other nutritionally deficient states, including gastrointestinal malabsorption syndromes. The deficiency is due to consumption of a poor diet rather than to the effects of alcohol itself. Chronic thiamine deficiency

produces a condition known as Korsakoff's Psychosis. This syndrome presents with ocular movement abnormalities, ataxia (particularly of gait), and a confusional state. Impaired recent memory generally appears following resolution of the confusional state. Complete amnesia for new information is common, and existing memory exhibits a characteristic temporal gradient, with remote memory being relatively intact compared to recent memory. Confabulation (i.e., providing irrelevant, unnecessary information that was not part of the original to-be-recalled material) may be seen in the early stages of this disorder, but it tends to be less common in later stages. Personality changes are often present, and docility with relative lack of concern with their deficits (anosognosia) are common. Pathological changes are seen in the mammillary bodies and the dorsomedial nucleus of the thalamus, in addition to the periventricular gray matter surrounding the third and fourth ventricles. The mammillary bodies are often shrunken and discolored, and this structural change is sometimes evident on CT or MRI scan.

b. Treatment   Thiamine administration may reverse the eye movement abnormalities and ataxia, although it does little to reverse the memory deficit. However, thiamine supplementation is important to prevent further memory decline. Vasopressin, clonidine, and methylphenidate have been reported to improve memory performance in some patients, although there has been no treatment that has been consistently effective.

2. Vitamin B$_{12}$

a. Clinical Features   Vitamin B$_{12}$ (cyanocobalamin) deficiency is associated with pernicious anemia. A lack of intrinsic factor in the gastrointestinal tract results in deficient absorption of dietary B$_{12}$ and is the most common cause of B$_{12}$ deficiency. Prolonged B$_{12}$ deficiency can produce peripheral neuropathy, optic atrophy, and a dementia syndrome characterized by slowed mental processing, memory impairment, depression, and confusion. Neuropsychiatric manifestations, including delusions, hallucinations, paranoia, and agitation may also be seen.

b. Treatment   Monthly intramuscular vitamin B$_{12}$ injections are used to treat this deficiency, and most of the neurological symptoms improve or resolve during the first month of treatment, if it is initiated relatively early.

3. Folate Deficiency

a. Clinical Features   This deficiency state is common in Western countries but only rarely produces dementia. Diminished dietary intake or gastrointestinal malabsorption of folate are the most common causes, although the deficiency may be seen following chronic phenytoin or primidone administration. The condition may mimic B$_{12}$ deficiency in many ways. Poor concentration, disorientation, memory deficits, difficulty with cognitive flexibility, perseveration, and apathy have been reported to occur in folate deficiency.

b. Treatment   Maintenance oral folate administration generally reverses the cognitive deficits.

4. Niacin (B$_2$) Deficiency (Pellagra)

a. Clinical Features   Symptoms of this deficiency state have been referred to as the three D's: dermatitis, diarrhea, and dementia, indicating the prominent effects on the skin, gastrointestinal tract, and central nervous system. This deficiency can result from low dietary intake, malabsorption syndromes, or chronic systemic illnesses. The dementia associated with pellagra is manifested by apathy, confabulation, psychomotor slowing, irritability, and memory impairment. Cogwheel rigidity and frontal release signs (sucking and grasping signs) are seen in acute niacin deficiency.

b. Treatment   Consumption of a diet with adequate niacin is a standard treatment, although niacin supplements may be necessary for several days in severe cases. Most symptoms resolve gradually over several weeks after initiating treatment.

C. Toxic Conditions

There are numerous substances known to be toxic to the central nervous system, and exposure to such substances continues to increase as technology advances. Many industrial pollutants in the air and water, pesticides, herbicides, food additives, and household supplies such as cleaners, paints, and organic solvents have been reported to produce potentially toxic effects on the central nervous system. Although many of these substances require a prolonged, continuous exposure to be harmful, the long-term effects of a number of chemicals are not known. In addition, medications can produce toxicity if they are overused or if alterations in the individual's metabolism prevent toxic by-products from being adequately cleared from the body. The elderly are particularly susceptible to toxic effects of drugs, due to greater variability in metabolic rates, decreased body mass, and lower drug-binding protein levels. Thus, close monitoring for toxicity and modification of drug dosages are often necessary in older persons. Finally, drugs of abuse have frequently been associated with dementia, and the neurotoxic effects of alcohol reflect perhaps the most common dementia associated with substance abuse.

1. Occupational and Environmental Toxic Exposure

a. Clinical Features A number of metals may interfere with cellular metabolism, producing dementia after prolonged or accumulated exposure. Lead, inorganic and organic mercury, manganese, arsenic, thallium, tin, bismuth, nickel, and cadmium have all been associated with dementia syndromes. Organic solvents can enter the body through inhalation or skin contact. They are often used in various cleaning supplies and include carbon tetrachloride, trichloroethane, trichloroethylene, methyl chloride, and ethylene glycol. These substances may produce irritability, depression, impaired concentration, memory deficits, and peripheral neuropathy. Organochlorine insecticides may produce anxiety and irritability, but dementia syndromes are somewhat rarer. In contrast, prolonged or continuous exposure to organophosphate insecticides may produce memory impairment, sleep disturbance, distractibility and anxiety.

b. Treatment/Prevention The use of protective clothing and devices may be effective in eliminating or minimizing exposure to these hazardous toxic substances, thereby preventing intoxication.

2. Toxic Effects of Medications

a. Clinical Features Medications frequently have side effects that may produce dementia following prolonged use. Tricyclic antidepressants have anticholinergic properties that may exacerbate memory impairment in vulnerable persons, and their use in the elderly must be carefully monitored. Lithium has also been associated with a dementia syndrome manifested by disorientation, impaired attention and concentration,

and comprehension deficits. A high-frequency tremor is often associated with lithium use as well. Benzodiazepines (e.g., diazepam, lorazepam, and alprazolam) are associated with impairment in memory functioning that is characterized by an inability to learn new information. Neuroleptic medications (e.g., haloperidol and the phenothiazines) may also produce chronic confusional states and dementia syndromes following long term use. Use of benzodiazepines and neuroleptics are also associated with increased risk of falling and hip fracture in the elderly. Some dementia syndromes have occasionally been associated with antihypertensive medications such as alpha-methyldopa and propanolol presumably through disruption of catecholaminergic synaptic functioning. Recent studies of anticonvulsants suggest that the barbiturates have the greatest impact on cognitive functioning, while anticonvulsants such as phenytoin, carbamazepine, and valproic acid do not commonly produce major cognitive effects at therapeutic serum levels. Dementia syndromes have also been associated with several drugs used in chemotherapy for cancer.

3. Toxic Effects of Drugs of Abuse

a. Clinical Features Chronic polydrug abuse has been associated with dementia syndromes, particularly when barbiturates and analgesics are combined. Intravenous drug use using unsterile needles may produce multi-infarct dementia through bacterial endocarditis, although spread of HIV through sharing needles constitutes a much greater risk. An irreversible parkinsonian syndrome was produced in a small group of intravenous drug users who injected themselves with the compound MPTP (described in Degenerative Dementias—Parkinson's Disease). Intentional solvent inhalation (e.g., "glue sniffing") is also associated with significant central nervous system effects resulting in motor and cranial nerve abnormalities and dementia. [See Substance Abuse.]

Alcohol is the most common substance associated with abuse and consequently has been widely studied. At least three mechanisms are thought to underlie cognitive deficits in alcohol abuse: thiamine deficiency through dietary neglect (described in the section on vitamin deficiencies), hepatic dysfunction through cirrhosis (described in the section on systemic illnesses—hepatic disease), and direct neurotoxic effects of alcohol on the central nervous system. Alcoholic dementia accounts for approximately 7% of dementias among patients evaluated for cognitive decline, and it tends to be seen in older patients after a number of years of abuse. According to Cummings and Benson, daily alcohol intake of 150 ml of absolute alcohol constitutes the definition of excessive alcohol use, which corresponds to two bottles of wine, seven pints of beer, or one-half bottle of distilled spirits. Neuropsychological deficits are seen in the following cognitive domains: memory, visuospatial functioning, abstract reasoning, and verbal fluency. Disorientation, circumstantiality, perseveration, psychomotor slowing and impaired attentional deployment are also typical. CT and MRI scans show cerebral atrophy manifested by enlarged lateral ventricles and widening of the cortical sulci. Atrophy of the cerebellar vermis is also commonly seen. Abnormal EEG slowing is also common in this patient group. Atrophy of the white matter and of the cerebral cortex have been reported at autopsy, together with atrophy of the mammillary bodies, dorsomedial nucleus of the thalamus, the mammilothalamic tract, and the cerebellar vermis. [*See* ALCOHOL PROBLEMS.]

b. Treatment Abstinence from alcohol, together with improved dietary nutrition, results in at least partial reversal of many cognitive deficits, with recovery being dependent both on the chronicity of abuse and on the length of abstinence. However, it is rare for an alcoholic to return to their baseline level of cognitive functioning.

V. DEMENTIA DUE TO OTHER CAUSES

A. Hydrocephalus

I. Clinical Features

Although this condition is not a common cause of dementia, it can be effectively treated if discovered early. An accumulation of cerebrospinal fluid (CSF) in the brain leads to enlargement of the ventricles. The nature of this CSF accumulation is unclear, but possible causes include excessive CSF secretion from the choroid plexus (e.g., choroid plexus papilloma), obstruction of CSF outflow from the ventricles to the cerebral subarachnoid space (e.g., obstructive noncommunicating hydrocephalus), or obstruction of the CSF flow from the subarachnoid space to the saggital sinus region (e.g., obstructive communicating hydrocepha-

lus). Intracranial pressure can be normal or high in any of these conditions. The clinical triad of gait disturbance, cognitive impairment, and urinary incontinence are commonly associated with communicating hydrocephalus. The cognitive impairment is manifested by disorientation, memory impairment, psychomotor slowing, poor abstract reasoning, and bradyphrenia.

2. Treatment

Communicating hydrocephalus may be treated by placement of a shunt tube to divert CSF from intracranial spaces to an extracranial site. Maintaining patency of the shunt tube can be problematic and may require shunt replacement. Nonobstructive hydrocephalus (e.g., hydrocephalus ex vacuo) refers to ventricular enlargement due to cerebral atrophy typically due to degenerative conditions, and is not amenable to surgical intervention.

B. Head Trauma

I. Closed Head Injury

a. Clinical Features Severe closed head injury may produce a posttraumatic dementia. The cognitive deficits may be due to a variety of mechanisms, including diffuse axonal injury, subdural or intracerebral hematoma, and cerebral contusions. The range of deficits following head injury is dependent on the location of cerebral damage and on the severity and mechanism of the trauma. Degree and duration of coma have been shown to correlate with functional outcome. Following loss of consciousness, a period of posttraumatic confusion and disorientation typically ensues, which may last days to weeks. Delirium, agitation, irritability, apathy, or withdrawal may be seen during this period. The duration of posttraumatic and retrograde amnesia duration are sometimes useful prognostic indicators, with longer amnestic periods associated with poorer outcomes. The duration of posttraumatic amnesia refers to the period between the injury and the resumption of continuous memory. The duration of retrograde amnesia refers to the period between the accident and the first clear memory prior to the accident. Longer durations of posttraumatic amnesia have been found to correlate with poorer cognitive outcomes in some studies. Other indices of severity, such as oculocephalic disturbances, are also prognostic of return to work and cognitive recovery. Minor head injury with no or minimal (less than 20 minutes) loss of consciousness, no focal neurologic deficits, and no positive neuroradiologic findings typically does not result in significant cognitive sequelae longer than three months postinjury in persons with no pre-injury history of head trauma, neuropsychiatric disturbance, or drug or alcohol abuse.

b. Treatment Rehabilitation programs are frequently helpful in developing strategies to compensate for cognitive and motor deficits.

2. Dementia Pugilistica

a. Clinical Features Repeated minor head blows, such as those that occur in boxing, result in the condition known as dementia pugilistica. Degeneration of the substantia nigra, neuronal loss in the cortex and cerebellum, neurofibrillary tangle formation and diffuse deposition of beta-amyloid plaques are seen at autopsy. Initial clinical features include mild coordination difficulty and affective dyscontrol, followed by apraxia, aphasia, agnosia, apathy, blunted affect and focal neurologic signs. End stages of the disease are characterized by global cognitive deterioration and the development of parkinsonism.

b. Treatment Anti-parkinsonian medications may be helpful in treating the movement abnormalities, although this condition is considered to be progressive.

C. Tumors

1. Clinical Features

Depending on their location and extent, tumors can cause only discrete cognitive deficits, or they may produce global cognitive impairment characteristic of a dementia syndrome. Tumors in the thalamus, hypothalamus, or frontal or temporal cortex are more often associated with dementia. As noted above, chemotherapy can sometimes be associated with development of dementia independent of the tumor.

2. Treatment

The clinical course of patients with tumors is highly variable, depending on the pathology of the tumor and its location. However, with improved imaging methods, treatment can frequently be initiated early, thereby improving prognosis.

D. Psychiatric Conditions

1. Depression

a. Clinical Features Severely depressed individuals may manifest impaired attention and concentration, disorientation, and memory deficits, which may frequently be difficult to differentiate from a dementia. In addition, a "dementia syndrome of depression" has been recognized. Some reports have suggested that individuals with this syndrome may exhibit greater cortical volume loss, greater anxiety, and more frequent delusions relative to depressed patients without cognitive impairment. Difficulty abstracting and grasping the meaning of situations, increased response latency, and impaired attention, concentration, and recall but relatively preserved recognition memory are common neuropsychological features. The memory deficit associated with depression is thought to be related to fluctuations in attention and concentration and is less severe than that seen in Alzheimer's disease. Aphasia, apraxia, and inability to name objects are generally not present. The etiology of depression and the dementia syndrome of depression remains elusive, but it is relatively clear that multiple neurotransmitter systems are involved. Disturbed functioning of nigrostriatal and frontal-limbic connections may also be involved in producing variable alertness and attention. [*See* Depression.]

b. Treatment Cognitive deficits associated with depression are highly treatable with conventional antidepressant pharmacotherapy, or with electroconvulsive therapy in the case of pharmacologic nonresponse. Cognitively oriented psychotherapy has also been a highly effective treatment for depression. Antidepressants with potent anticholinergic properties should be avoided, as these medications may potentially exacerbate the severity of memory impairment. [*See* Cognitive Therapy; Psychopharmacology.]

2. Schizophrenia

a. Clinical Features Schizophrenia (dementia praecox) affects approximately 1% of the general population. Initial presentation is that of psychosis, which generally begins in adolescence or young adulthood. Clinical features include "positive" symptoms such as delusions, hallucinations, and formal thought disorder, and "negative" symptoms such as apathy, blunted affect, and anhedonia. Negative symptoms tend to emerge later in the disorder and are associated with dementia ("deficit syndrome"). Exacerbations and remissions of psychotic features characterize the course of the illness. Cognitive deficits are more common during exacerbations of the disease and include difficulty with abstract reasoning, memory impairment, disorientation, perseveration, impaired judgment, and tangentiality. The mechanism of cognitive decline in schizophrenia has not been determined. Ventricular enlargement and sulcal widening on CT and MRI scans correlate with the severity of cognitive impairment, raising the possibility that neuronal loss may account for the dementia. However, disordered monoamine function has also been proposed to underlie the cognitive deficits in schizophrenia. [*See* SCHIZOPHRENIA.]

b. Treatment Treatment with the phenothiazines, butyrophenones, and thioxanthenes has been used to reduce the positive symptoms. Negative symptoms tend to be unaffected by these three classes of medications, although clozapine has shown some promise.

ACKNOWLEDGMENTS

The author thanks Dr. Felicia C. Goldstein, Dr. Robert C. Green, and Dr. Alexander P. Auchus of Emory University School of Medicine for reviewing this manuscript. Support for this research was provided by the Emory Alzheimer's Disease Center (NIA Grant #P30AG10130).

BIBLIOGRAPHY

Cummings, J. L., & Benson, D. F. (1992). *Dementia: A clinical approach* (2nd ed.). Boston: Butterworth-Heinemann.

Heilman, K. M., & Valenstein, E. (1993). *Clinical neuropsychology* (3rd ed.). New York: Oxford.

Kolb, B., & Whishaw, I. Q. (1990). *Fundamentals of human neuropsychology* (3rd ed.). New York: W. H. Freeman.

Mann, D. M. A., Neary, D., & Testa, H. (1994). *Color atlas and text of adult dementias*. London: Mosby-Wolfe.

Roberts, G. W., Leigh, P. N., & Weinberger, D. R. (1993). *Neuropsychiatric disorders*. London: Mosby-Wolfe.

Dependent Personality

Robert F. Bornstein

Gettysburg College

Authoritarian Parenting A parenting style wherein the primary caretakers impose rigid and inflexible rules and expectations on the child, and the child is expected to conform completely and without question to these rules and expectations.

Dependent Personality Disorder A psychiatric disorder characterized by long-standing, extreme dependency which causes significant interpersonal and/or occupational impairment for the afflicted individual.

Diathesis Predisposition or risk factor; the term is typically used in psychiatric or medical settings to refer to any form of vulnerability which places an individual at increased risk for physical or psychological illness.

Disease-Prone Personality A hypothetical construct referring to a set of personality traits, attitudes, and behaviors which place an individual at risk for disease.

Interactionism A framework for conceptualizing personality dynamics wherein behavior is understood as reflecting the interaction of stable personality traits and immediate situational influences.

Oral Dependency A psychoanalytic term referring to a set of traits which simultaneously reflect a passive, helpless outlook and a predisposition to cope with stress and anxiety via food- and mouth-related activities (e.g., cigarette smoking).

Self-Concept One's mental representation of the self, which is relatively stable and not strongly affected by changes in mood state; the self-concept may have both conscious and unconscious components, and is often associated with a strong affective (i.e., emotional) response.

Suggestibility The degree to which a person's attitudes or opinions are easily swayed by the expressed opinions of others.

The term **DEPENDENCY,** as it is used in personality theory and research refers to a personality orientation (or "style") wherein an individual: (1) perceives him- or herself as helpless, powerless, and ineffectual, and therefore (2) turns to others for support, advice, and reassurance rather than attempting to cope with tasks and challenges in an autonomous, self-directed manner. Individuals who consistently display a passive, help-seeking orientation in a variety of situations and circumstances are described as having a *dependent personality*. During the past several decades there have been hundreds of published studies examining the antecedents, correlates, and consequences of dependent personality traits. These investigations may be grouped into three broad areas: developmental, social, and clinical. Research in each of these areas is discussed in this article.

Encyclopedia of Mental Health
Volume 1

I. HISTORICAL OVERVIEW OF DEPENDENCY THEORY AND RESEARCH

Although Freud made little mention of the psychodynamics of dependent personality traits, several prominent psychoanalytic theorists (e.g., Karl Abraham, Otto Fenichel, Edward Glover) published papers on the dependent personality during the first few decades of the 20th century. These seminal papers stimulated clinicians' and researchers' interest in the topic of dependency, and not surprisingly, much of the early research on dependency came from a psychoanalytic perspective. Early psychoanalytic studies tested the hypothesis that a dependent personality orientation in adolescence or adulthood could be traced to events that occurred during the infantile "oral" period (i.e., during the first 1 to 2 years of life).

Specifically, the psychoanalytic model hypothesized that high levels of dependency resulted from overgratification or frustration during breastfeeding and weaning. Infantile experiences of frustration or overgratification were presumed to result in "oral fixation" and an inability to accomplish the developmental tasks associated with the infantile, oral stage (i.e., the development of a stable self-concept, along with feelings of autonomy, self-efficacy, and self-sufficiency). Although later studies indicated that dependency in adulthood was not directly related to infantile feeding or weaning experiences, the psychoanalytic model played a central role in bringing dependency research into mainstream psychology.

During the 1950s and 1960s, social learning models began to influence dependency theory and research, supplanting (to some degree) the classical psychoanalytic model. These social learning models differed in certain respects, although they shared the fundamental hypothesis that high levels of dependency result from the reinforcement of passive, dependent behavior in the context of the infant–caretaker relationship. Social learning models of dependency further hypothesized that—insofar as passive, help-seeking behavior was reinforced by the parents (and other authority figures) during early and middle childhood—the individual would continue to show high levels of dependency later in life.

By the early 1970s, the social learning view of dependency began to give way to ethological (i.e., attachment) theory, which was becoming increasingly influential in a number of domains within psychology. In contrast to the classical psychoanalytic and social learning models of dependency, attachment theory emphasized the innate, biological underpinnings of the infant–mother relationship as a primary factor in the development of dependent personality traits. Attachment models of dependency have not yet achieved the same status and influence as have the psychoanalytic and social learning models. Nonetheless, attachment theory stimulated a great deal of research examining the etiology and development of dependent personality traits, including some noteworthy studies examining infant–mother bonding in infrahuman subjects. Recent research in this area has focused on exploring the similarities between dependency and various forms of attachment behavior (e.g., insecure attachment) in children and adults. [See ATTACHMENT.]

During the 1980s researchers took a more eclectic view of dependent personality traits, combining aspects of the psychoanalytic, social learning, and attachment models in order to arrive at a more integrated, comprehensive perspective on dependency. Thus, relatively few studies during the past decade have focused exclusively on one theoretical framework. Rather, researchers have built upon the strengths of different theoretical models, integrating and synthesizing these models to formulate hypotheses that account for aspects of dependency which are best explained via attention to multiple theoretical perspectives. Recent research on dependency has emphasized the importance of unconscious, unexpressed dependency needs (a concept typically associated with the psychoanalytic model), along with an exploration of the impact of early learning and socialization experiences in the development dependent personality traits (an area of inquiry which originated in social learning theory). During the past decade there have also been increasing efforts to integrate the results of developmental, social, and clinical studies of dependency in order to understand the ways in which findings from these three areas of dependency research complement (and contradict) each other.

II. THE DEVELOPMENT OF DEPENDENCY

Developmental studies of dependency can be divided into three areas: (1) studies of the acquisition of dependent personality traits in infancy and early childhood; (2) investigations of the development of dependency during adolescence and adulthood; and (3) studies of dependency in older adults.

A. Childhood Antecedents of Dependency

The results of numerous studies indicate that overprotective, authoritarian parenting is a primary cause of exaggerated dependency needs during adolescence and adulthood. Prospective and retrospective studies of the parenting style–dependency link have produced highly similar results, allowing strong conclusions to be drawn regarding the etiology of dependent personality traits. Findings in this area confirm that when parents show one of these qualities (i.e., overprotectiveness or authoritarianism), the likelihood that their children will show high levels of dependency increases significantly. When parents show both of these qualities, high levels of dependency in their offspring are particularly likely to result.

It appears that overprotective, authoritarian parenting produces high levels of dependency in children largely because overprotective, authoritarian parents prevent the child from engaging in the kinds of trial-and-error learning that help to provide a sense of mastery, autonomy, and self-sufficiency in children. Consequently, the child of overprotective, authoritarian parents comes to perceive him- or herself as powerless and ineffectual, and continues to rely on others—especially figures of authority—for advice, guidance, and protection. As numerous researchers have noted, the child's inability (or unwillingness) to behave in an assertive, autonomous manner exacerbates the situation, in that behaving in a passive, helpless way encourages figures of authority (e.g., parents, teachers) to continue to perform tasks for the child which the child is actually capable of doing on his or her own. Thus, the child's expressions of dependency come to serve as cues which continue to elicit helping and caretaking behavior on the part of others, further reinforcing the child's passive, dependent behavior and ultimately resulting in even greater levels of helplessness and dependency. Recent research confirms that the overt expression of dependency strivings does in fact serve as a help-eliciting cue in both children and adults. [See PARENTING.]

B. Dependency in Adolescence and Adulthood

During adolescence, substantial sex differences in dependency emerge, with girls showing significantly higher levels of dependency than boys. This pattern of results is consistent across different cultures (e.g., American, British, Japanese, Indian, German, Israeli), and across different cultural groups within American society. Moreover, the finding that females show higher levels of dependency than do males has been replicated numerous times. Recent studies further suggest that traditional sex-role socialization practices may be largely responsible for the higher levels of dependency typically found in women relative to men. Insofar as traditional sex-role socialization practices tend to encourage passive, help-seeking behavior in girls to a greater extent than boys, these socialization practices would be expected to produce higher levels of dependency in women than in men. Not surprisingly, empirical studies confirm that—to the extent that a girl grows up in a household which emphasizes traditional sex-role socialization practices—she is likely to show high levels of dependency during adolescence and adulthood. Conversely, to the extent that a boy is exposed to traditional sex-role socialization practices (which emphasize assertive, autonomous behavior in boys), he is likely to show low levels of dependency later in life.

Not only do sex-role socialization practices play an important role in determining the expression of dependency needs in adolescents, but studies confirm that the object of an individual's dependency strivings (i.e., the person toward whom dependency needs are expressed most readily) changes from childhood to adolescence. Although dependency needs in childhood are typically directed toward the parents and other authority figures (e.g., teachers), during adolescence the dependent individual directs his or her dependency strivings toward members of the peer group rather than toward figures of authority. This shift continues to occur throughout early adulthood, at which point romantic partners become primary outlets for the expression of an individual's dependency needs. In addition, adults often express dependency strivings toward various "pseudo-parental" authority figures (e.g., supervisors, physicians, therapists), and (to a lesser extent) toward peers, parents, and siblings.

C. Dependency in Older Adults

There have been no published studies examining individual differences in level of dependency in older adults. However, research suggests that, in general, older adults tend to exhibit more pronounced dependency needs than do younger adults. To some extent, the higher levels of dependency shown by older adults relative to younger adults reflects the fact that older adults as a group are more dependent on others to carry out tasks associated with daily living (e.g., cooking, shopping, driving). In this context, it is not surprising to learn that those older adults who live in environments which encourage autonomy and independence tend to show lower levels of dependency than do those older adults who live in environments where passivity and dependency are permitted or encouraged. Several investigations have demonstrated that changes in older adults' frequency of dependent behaviors can be traced directly to the contingencies which characterize the environments in which they live: Environments that directly or indirectly encourage the overt expression of dependency needs (e.g., certain nursing home environments and residential treatment facilities) actually appear to cause significant, long-term increases in the dependency levels of older adults.

III. INTERPERSONAL CORRELATES OF DEPENDENCY

In general, studies of the interpersonal correlates of dependency indicate that dependent persons adopt a passive, helpless stance in interpersonal interactions. Specifically, laboratory and field investigations indicate that individuals with a dependent personality orientation show high levels of suggestibility, cooperativeness, compliance, and interpersonal yielding. These results are not surprising when one considers the underlying goals and motivations of the dependent person. Clearly, being helped, nurtured, and protected is very important to the dependent person. In this context, one would expect that the dependent individual would exhibit behaviors that serve to strengthen and reinforce ties to potential nurturers and caretakers. Thus, dependent persons (1) tend to yield to the opinions of others in laboratory conformity experiments; (2) show high levels of suggestibility in both laboratory

and field studies; and (3) are cooperative and compliant in social, academic, psychiatric, and medical settings.

Although the dependent person is generally suggestible, cooperative, compliant, and yielding, it is noteworthy that these dependency-related behaviors are even more pronounced when the dependent person is interacting with a figure of authority than when he or she is interacting with a peer. Apparently, figures of authority are perceived by the dependent individual as being particularly good protectors and caretakers. Consequently, the kinds of ingratiation strategies used by the dependent person with peers (e.g., compliance and interpersonal yieldings) are exhibited even more readily around figures of authority.

Dependent persons in social settings also show high levels of help-seeking behavior. The dependency–help-seeking relationship is found in both men and women, and is consistent across different age groups (i.e., children, adolescents, adults), and across different measures of help-seeking. The dependency–help-seeking relationship found in adults clearly reflects the early developmental experiences of the dependent person. To the extent that help-seeking behavior during childhood was reinforced by the parents and other authority figures, the dependent adolescent or adult will continue to show exaggerated help-seeking behaviors in a variety of situations and settings.

Performance anxiety and fear of negative evaluation might also play a role in encouraging the dependent individual to behave in a help-seeking manner in social situations. Although there have been relatively few studies examining directly the dependency-performance anxiety relationship, studies in this area indicate that (1) dependent persons show higher levels of performance anxiety (and fear of negative evaluation) than do nondependent persons; and (2) there is a positive relationship between the degree to which a dependent person reports high levels of performance anxiety and the degree to which that person shows high levels of help-seeking behavior in various situations and settings.

One final set of findings regarding the interpersonal correlates of dependency warrants mention in the present context. In a series of investigations conducted during the 1970s and 1980s, researchers demonstrated that dependent persons exhibit higher levels of interpersonal sensitivity (i.e., sensitivity to subtle verbal and nonverbal cues) than do nondependent persons. In fact, dependent persons are able to infer with surprising accuracy the attitudes and personal beliefs of strangers, roommates, teachers, and therapists. Although at first glance these results seem inconsistent with the oft-reported finding that dependency is associated with passivity and helplessness, findings regarding the dependency–interpersonal sensitivity relationship are actually quite consistent with these other findings. Clearly, to the extent that a dependent person is able to infer accurately the attitudes and personal beliefs of teachers, roommates, and therapists, the dependent person will be better able to develop strong ties to these potential nurturers, protectors, and caretakers.

IV. DEPENDENCY AND PSYCHOPATHOLOGY

Because dependency has typically been conceptualized as a flaw or deficit in functioning, numerous studies have examined the relationship between level of dependency and risk for psychopathology. Studies of the dependency–psychopathology relationship can be divided into four areas: (1) studies of dependency and depression; (2) investigations of the dependency–substance use disorders relationship; (3) studies of dependency, obesity, and eating disorders; and (4) research on dependent personality disorder.

A. Dependency and Depression

Although laboratory and field studies confirm that there is a positive relationship between level of dependency and level of depression in children, adolescents, and adults, the dependency–depression relationship is more complex than early researchers had thought. On the one hand, exaggerated dependency needs do in fact place an individual at increased risk for the subsequent onset of depression. However, it is also the case that the onset of depressive symptoms results in increases in dependent thoughts, feelings, and behaviors in a variety of subject groups. Presumably, the feelings of helplessness, hopelessness, anhedonia, and anergia that are frequently associated with depression can manifest themselves in increases in overt dependent behaviors in depressed subjects [See DEPRESSION.]

The mechanism by which dependent personality traits place an individual at risk for depression is not completely understood, but initial findings suggest that dependency increases risk for depression by causing the dependent person to be particularly upset and threatened by experiences of interpersonal loss. To be sure, interpersonal stressors affect everyone to some degree. However, the dependent person's lifelong tendency to look to others for nurturance, guidance, and protection may cause him or her to become extremely sensitive to the possibility that a potential caretaker will no longer be available to fulfill their protective and nurturing role. In this respect, dependency represents a vulnerability (or diathesis) that—when combined with interpersonal stressors—places the dependent person at increased risk for depression.

B. Dependency and Substance Use Disorders

Dozens of studies have examined the possibility that dependent persons might be at elevated risk for substance use disorders. The results of these investigations have been decidedly mixed. For example, although studies confirm that dependent persons are at increased risk for tobacco addiction, numerous investigations have failed to obtain the hypothesized relationship between dependency and risk for alcoholism. In fact, longitudinal studies of the dependency–alcoholism link indicate that the onset of alcoholism is followed by increases in dependent thoughts, feelings, and behaviors. However, there is no evidence that dependency actually places individuals at risk for alcohol abuse or dependence. [See SUBSTANCE ABUSE.]

Similar findings have emerged in studies of dependency and other types of substance use disorders. Researchers have examined possible links between dependency and risk of opiate, cocaine, barbiturate, marijuana, and poly-drug abuse. The results of these studies have been relatively clear-cut: Dependent individuals do not show elevated risk for these substance use disorders, although—consistent with earlier findings regarding the dependency–alcoholism link—research confirms that the onset of an addictive disorder is often associated with elevations in dependent feelings, thoughts, and behaviors.

C. Dependency, Obesity, and Eating Disorders

The hypothesis that dependent personality traits would be associated with obesity and other eating disorders (i.e., anorexia and bulimia) can be traced to the classical psychoanalytic hypothesis (described earlier) that the etiology of dependency lies in "oral fixation." There have been numerous studies examining the dependency–obesity relationship, and in general these investigations have found only weak relationships between dependency and obesity. Moreover, the dependency–obesity link (when it occurs at all) is somewhat stronger in women than in men. The disappointing results obtained in this area have caused researchers to shift their attention from examining the dependency-obesity relationship to examining the relationship between dependency and eating disorders such as anorexia and bulimia.

Studies of the relationship between dependency and anorexia and bulimia have produced much stronger and more consistent findings than did studies of the dependency–obesity link. Anorexic and bulimic subjects almost invariably show higher levels of dependency than do matched control subjects who do not have these disorders. The dependency–bulimia link appears to be somewhat stronger than the dependency–anorexia link, although additional studies will be needed to confirm and clarify these preliminary results. Studies in this area also suggest that interpersonal stressors (e.g., the breakup of a romantic relationship) might increase the dependent person's risk for anorexia and bulimia in much the same way as they increase the dependent person's risk for depression. Thus, a diathesis–stress conceptualization of the dependency–eating disorders relationship holds considerable promise for future research in this area. [*See* ANOREXIA NERVOSA AND BULIMIA NERVOSA.]

D. Dependent Personality Disorder

Although the vast majority of studies of the dependency–psychopathology relationship have explored possible links between dependency and other forms of psychopathology (e.g., depression), in recent years there has been an increasing emphasis on conceptualizing exaggerated dependency needs as a separate and distinct form of psychological illness. The most prominent framework used to examine the pathological aspects of the dependency is the concept of "dependent personality disorder" as this disorder is described in the *Diagnostic and Statistical Manual of Mental Disorders* (*DSM*). The *DSM* framework argues that individuals who show exaggerated, inflexible dependency needs which cause social or occupational impairment

may be diagnosed as having a dependent personality disorder. Unfortunately, because the diagnostic category of dependent personality disorder was first discussed in 1980, with the publication of the third edition of the *DSM* series, there has been relatively little research on this disorder. Initial findings regarding the correlates and consequences of dependent personality disorder can be grouped into three areas and summarized simply. [*See* PERSONALITY DISORDERS.]

First, studies confirm that individuals with dependent personality disorder are at increased risk for a wide range of psychopathologies, including depression, anxiety disorders, eating disorders, and somatization disorders. Individuals diagnosed with dependent personality disorder also show elevated risk for certain other personality disorders (e.g., border-line, avoidant, passive–aggressive). To some extent, findings regarding the links between dependent personality disorder and other forms of psychopathology dovetail with findings regarding the dependency–psychopathology relationship in general: As discussed earlier, studies to date suggest that dependent individuals show increased risk for a wide range of psychopathologies.

Second, epidemiological research suggests that the prevalence of dependent personality disorder in community samples is relatively low, with about 5% of community subjects showing clinically significant dependent personality disorder symptoms. As expected, the frequency of dependent personality disorder symptoms and diagnoses in clinical (i.e., psychiatric inpatient or outpatient) samples is somewhat higher, with many studies reporting base rates of this disorder in clinical subjects of about 10–15%. Although dependent personality disorder appears to be somewhat more prevalent in women than in men, the magnitude of the sex difference in dependent personality disorder diagnosis rates is not great.

Third, studies confirm that dependent personality disorder symptoms predict some important aspects of psychological treatment. For example, clinicians report elevated rates of help-seeking behaviors (e.g., requests for emergency sessions, requests for feedback and advice) among dependent personality disorder patients relative to nondependent patients. Along slightly different lines, recent research in this area suggests that dependent personality disorder is associated with cooperativeness and compliance with therapeutic regimens. Finally, several studies indicate that patients diagnosed with dependent personality disorder remain in psychological and medical treatment significantly longer than do nondependent patients, presumably because treatment termination involves giving up a relationship with an important caretaking figure, which the dependent person is reluctant to do.

V. DEPENDENCY AND PHYSICAL DISORDERS

One of the most interesting and noteworthy findings to emerge from recent studies of the dependent personality has to do with risk for physical disorders. Research indicates that dependent persons are at increased risk for a wide variety of physical illnesses, including infectious diseases, ulcers, heart disease, and cancer. Longitudinal (i.e., prospective) studies and archival (retrospective) studies have produced highly consistent findings in this area. The dependency–disease link has been found in men and women, and in both children and adults. Furthermore, the magnitude of the dependency–disease relationship is quite substantial. In fact, a recent direct comparison of the magnitude of the disease risk associated with dependency and the magnitude of the disease risk associated with other "illness-related" personality variables (e.g., hostility, compulsiveness, introversion) revealed that the magnitude of the relationship between dependency and risk for physical illness is actually larger than the personality–illness risk relationship found for all other illness-related personality variables. Clearly, dependency must be regarded as an important component of the "disease-prone personality."

The mechanism by which dependency increases an individual's risk for physical illness parallels closely the mechanism by which dependency increases an individual's risk for depression. Specifically, it appears that dependency acts as a diathesis which—when coupled with experiences of interpersonal stress or loss—increases an individual's risk for various forms of illness. Preliminary findings in this area further suggest that the dependency–interpersonal stress–illness relationship may be mediated by the immune system: Dependent persons who experience significant interpersonal stressors show measurable deficits in immune function. The diminished immunocompetence associated with dependency and interpersonal stress may represent the common pathway through which the de-

pendent individual is placed at increased risk for various forms of illness. However, additional studies will be needed to confirm and extend these initial results. [*See* PSYCHONEUROIMMUNOLOGY.]

Ironically, although the dependent person is at increased risk for physical illness, the personality traits associated with dependency (e.g., cooperativeness, compliance, help-seeking) may actually help the dependent person to respond well to various treatment regimens. Physicians and other healthcare professionals consistently report that dependent individuals are compliant, cooperative patients who adhere particularly well to difficult treatment regimens. In addition, the dependent person is inclined to seek the advice and help of a physician relatively quickly when physical symptoms appear. This "medical help-seeking" tendency is certainly consistent with findings regarding the help-seeking behaviors of dependent persons in social settings. In addition, the help-seeking tendencies of the dependent person clearly represent a positive, adaptive quality of dependency. To the extent that the dependent person seeks help relatively quickly when physical symptoms appear, the likelihood of successful treatment should increase.

VI. THE DEPENDENT PERSONALITY: PAST, PRESENT, AND FUTURE

Early research on the dependent personality was concerned primarily with two issues: (1) the exploration of personality traits and behaviors that were hypothesized to be associated with dependency (e.g., passivity, low self-esteem); and (2) the examination of psychoanalytic hypotheses regarding the etiology and dynamics of dependency (i.e., studies of oral fixation and oral dependency). Needless to say, the focus of dependency research has changed considerably during the past several decades. It is worthwhile to review some of these changes in order to get a sense of the directions in which dependency research is likely to head during the coming years.

One important shift in this area has occurred with respect to the focus of dependency research. Whereas early studies in this area tended to focus on understanding the antecedents of dependent personality traits, recent studies have instead focused on understanding the consequences of dependency. Many of these recent investigations have examined the interpersonal (i.e., social) consequences of dependency, although other studies have assessed the effects of dependent personality traits on risk for physical or psychological illness.

A second shift characterizing the study of dependency has involved the research methodologies used in this area. Many early investigations of the dependent personality employed correlational designs. Moreover, many of these early studies took place in field settings (e.g., schools) rather than in the laboratory. In contrast, recent research in this area has tended to use experimental (rather than correlational) designs, and most recent investigations of dependency have taken place in laboratory rather than field settings.

A third shift characterizing research in this area has to do with clinicians' and researchers' conceptualization of dependency. For most of this century, dependency has been regarded primarily as a flaw or deficit in functioning. However, in recent years researchers have begun to examine the positive, adaptive qualities of dependency (e.g., compliance with medical regimens, willingness to seek help when symptoms appear). Thus, psychologists have moved from conceptualizing dependency solely in terms of deficit and dysfunction to conceptualizing dependency in a way which recognizes that dependency is associated with both positive and negative qualities.

Fourth, the emphasis in dependency research has shifted from a more-or-less exclusive focus on dependency-related behaviors (e.g., help-seeking), to the study of dependency-related emotions and cognitions. Recent studies in this area have suggested that the disparate behaviors of dependent individuals can be understood more completely (and predicted more accurately) if the dependent individual's cognitive style is assessed directly. As researchers have increasingly emphasized the ways in which the dependent person's self-concept and perceptions of other people mediate his or her behavior, many apparent inconsistencies in previous studies of dependency-related behaviors have been resolved.

Finally, researchers are beginning to examine more closely the interaction of dependent personality traits and aspects of the situation or setting in which behavior is exhibited. Although dependency is often associated with passivity and helplessness, recent studies suggest that situational variables (e.g., the status of the person with whom the dependent individual is interacting, the type of environment in which an interaction occurs) also play a significant role in directing the behavior of the dependent person. In this respect, traditional trait models are beginning to give way to interactionist models of dependency. This shift has already generated some noteworthy findings, and the interactionist perspective on dependency is likely to produce many more important advances in dependency theory and research during the coming years.

This article has been reprinted from the *Encyclopedia of Human Behavior, Volume 2.*

BIBLIOGRAPHY

Birtchnell, J. (1988). Defining dependence. *Br. J. Med. Psychol.* **61**, 111–123.

Birtchnell, J. (1991). The measurement of dependence by questionnaire. *J. Pers. Disorders* **5**, 281–295.

Blatt, S. J., & Homann, E. (1992). Parent–child interaction in the etiology of dependent and self-critical depression. *Clin. Psychol. Rev.* **12**, 47–91.

Bornstein, R. F. (1992). The dependent personality: Developmental, social and clinical perspectives. *Psychol. Bull.* **112**, 3–23.

Bornstein, R. F. (1993). "The Dependent Personality." Guilford, New York.

Hirschfeld, R. M. A., Shea, M. T., & Weise, R. (1991). Dependent personality disorder: Perspectives for DSM-IV. *J. Pers. Disorders* **5**, 135–149.

Overholser, J. C. (1992). Interpersonal dependency and social loss. *Pers. Individual Diff.* **13**, 17–23.

Zuroff, D. C., Igrega, I., & Mongrain, M. (1990). Dysfunctional attitudes, dependency and self-criticism as predictors of depressive mood states. *Cog. Ther. Res.* **14**, 315–326.

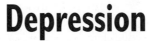

Depression

Rick E. Ingram

San Diego State University

Christine Scher

San Diego State University
and
University of California, San Diego

Bipolar Disorder An affective disorder that is characterized by at least one episode of mania. Used to be referred to as manic-depression.

Comorbidity The occurrence of more than one disorder at the same time. For example, depression and anxiety are often comorbid, meaning that an individual will experience both of these states simultaneously.

Double Depression Refers to dysthymia and major depressive disorder occurring at the same time.

Epidemiology Information about the prevalence of disorders in a population. In the case of disorders such as depression, a prevalence rate refers to the number of people who have the disorder during a particular time period (e.g., the percentage of people in given location diagnosed with Major Depressive Disorder within a 1-year period of time).

Etiology References to the cause of the disorder. An etiological theory would be a theory about what causes a disorder.

Hypomania Episodes characterized by the same symptoms as manic episodes, but that are shorter and are associated with less impairment.

Melancholia A very severe form of depression that can be associated with psychotic features such as delusions (i.e., false beliefs) and hallucinations (i.e., sensory experiences which have no basis in reality).

Negative Affectivity The tendency to be chronically distressed and to chronically view oneself negatively. Negative affectivity may be a precursor to both depression and anxiety.

Negative Cognition Subtype of Depression A proposal that there is a specific kind of depression that is caused by negative and dysfunctional thinking patterns.

Nosology The diagnosis of disorders into discrete entities with the assumption that each disorder that is nosologically classified will have a different cause, course, prognosis, and treatment response.

Unipolar Disorder An affective disorder that is characterized by depression without any evidence for the occurrence of manic episodes.

DEPRESSION means different things to different people. For some, depression means feelings of unhappiness that are uncomfortable but do not seem to hinder daily activities. For others, the depression connotes a sickness characterized by severely depressed mood, loss of appetite, lack of concentration, and an inability to function on one's own.

Even for professionals the use of the term depression can vary. In 1987, Kendall and colleagues noted that "The professional use of the term *depression* has several levels of reference: symptom, syndrome, nosologic disorder. . . . Depression itself can be a symptom—for example, being sad. As a syndrome, depression is a constellation of signs and symptoms that cluster together. . . . The syndrome of depression is itself a psychological dysfunction but can also be present, in secondary ways, in other diagnosed disorders. Finally, for depression to be a nosologic category careful diagnostic procedures are required during which other potential diagnostic categories are excluded. The presumption, of course, is that a discrete nosologic entity will ultimately prove to be etiologically distinct from other discrete entities, with associated differences likely in course, prognosis, and treatment response." It is this likely nosologic disorder of depression that we will discuss.

I. DEFINITION OF DEPRESSION

A. Symptoms of Depression

Any definition of depression must begin with the fourth edition of the *Diagnostic and Statistical Manual of Mental Disorders (DSM-IV)*. The *DSM-IV* represents the official diagnostic classification system of the American Psychiatric Association and provides the criteria that are used to diagnosis depression. These criteria consist of the symptoms of depression. In order to make a diagnosis of depression, at least five out of nine possible symptoms must be present. These include (1) depressed mood; (2) diminished pleasure or interest in activities; (3) significant weight loss or weight gain; (4) insomnia or hypersomnia; (5) agitation; (6) fatigue or loss of energy; (7) thoughts of worthlessness or inappropriate guilt; (8) diminished concentration ability; and (9) thoughts of death or suicide.

Symptoms of depression may vary according to an individual's age and culture. Children who are depressed, for instance, may express symptoms of irritability rather than sadness. They may also fail to make expected weight gains rather than lose weight. On the other end of the age continuum, older adults are more likely than younger adults to experience symptoms such as loss of appetite, loss of interest, and thoughts of death. Cultural differences also exist in report of depressive symptoms. One study, for example, found that depressed Jewish patients reported more somatic symptoms, and less guilt, than did non-Jewish patients. Another study that examined depressive symptomatology in American, Korean, Philippine, and Taiwanese college students found that Taiwanese students reported the lowest numbers of

somatic symptoms and the highest numbers of affective symptoms. The other ethnic groups reporting similar levels of these symptoms. One's age and culture thus seems to affect how depression is expressed.

B. Comorbidity: The Relationship between Depression and Anxiety

Comorbidity refers to the occurrence of more than one disorder at the same time. Although researchers and clinicians generally acknowledge depression as a distinct disorder, it does overlap with a variety of other difficulties. Much current research on this overlap has focused on the relationship between anxiety and depression. This is not surprising, given the high rates of comorbidity found in studies of the two disorder types. For example, one study found that 63% of a group of patients with panic disorder also experienced major depression. One possible explanation provided for such overlap lies in the concept of "negative affectivity." In 1984, Watson and Clark described individuals with high levels of negative affectivity as having a tendency "to be distressed and upset and have a negative view of self, whereas those low on the dimension are relatively content and secure and satisfied with themselves." Other characteristics of high negative affectivity include nervousness, tension, worry, anger, scorn, revulsion, guilt, self-dissatisfaction, rejectedness, and sadness.

Both anxiety and depression seem to consist of high negative affectivity. There are however, important differences between depression and anxiety. While both depression and anxiety are characterized by high levels of negative affect, only depression is related to lowered levels of positive affect. Thus, depressed individuals tend to display both high negative affect and low positive affect, whereas anxious individuals display high negative affect and may or may not have lowered positive affect—the level of positive affect is unrelated to one's anxiety state. Research on negative affect as a link between anxiety and depression is continuing at a rapid pace. [*See* ANXIETY.]

II. DIAGNOSTIC CLASSIFICATION

Earlier we noted the *DSM-IV*. The *DSM-IV* is the most widely used classification scheme for psychiatric disorders in North America. According to this manual, there are five types of mood disorders that include depression as a significant component. These are (1) Major Depressive Disorder; (2) Dysthymic Disorder; (3) Bipolar I Disorder; (4) Bipolar II Disorder; and (5) Cyclothymic Disorder. Each of these classifications differs in terms of etiology, course, and symptomatology. [*See* MOOD DISORDERS.]

A. Major Depressive Disorder

For a diagnosis of Major Depressive Disorder (MDD), *DSM-IV* specifies that at least five symptoms must occur for a period of at least 2 weeks. Chief among these symptoms is depressed mood that occurs most of the day, nearly every day for at least 2 weeks, or significantly diminished interest or pleasure in virtually all activities most of the day, nearly every day for the 2-week period.

MDD can be further classified according to *severity* (i.e., mild, moderate, severe without psychotic features, severe with psychotic features), *course* (e.g., single episode versus recurrent episodes), and *presentation* (e.g., with catatonic features, with melancholic features). Psychotic features of depression include such experiences as delusions (i.e., false beliefs) and hallucinations (i.e., sensory experiences that have no basis in reality). A delusion, for example, would be a person who believes that she is dead. Catatonic features of depression involve psychomotor disturbances such as excessive movement or stupor. Melancholic features include the inability to experience pleasure even when good things happen and a lack of interest in previously pleasurable activities. No matter what the specific characteristics of a given individual's disturbance, MDD is, by definition, extremely distressing to the sufferer and is associated with significant impairment in important areas of the person's life (e.g., at work, home or school).

B. Dysthymic Disorder

Dysthymic Disorder is characterized by a chronic depressed mood that lasts at least 2 years in adults and at least 1 year in children and adolescents. This depressed mood is accompanied by at least two of the following six depressive symptoms: (1) poor appetite or overeating; (2) insomnia or hypersomnia; (3) low energy or fatigue; (4) low self-esteem; (5) poor concentration or difficulty making decisions; and (6) feel-

ings of hopelessness. As fewer depressive symptoms are required to make a diagnosis, Dysthymic Disorder is often considered a milder form of depression than MDD. However, it can be just as upsetting to the sufferer and can cause just as much impairment. In addition, Dysthymic Disorder may occur in combination with episodes of major depression. When Dysthymic Disorder occurs along with major depression, the individual is considered to be suffering from a "double depression." The cooccurrence of MDD and dysthymia is not uncommon.

C. Bipolar I Disorder

The hallmark characteristic of Bipolar I Disorder is mania. According to *DSM-IV*, a manic episode is characterized by elevated, expansive, or irritable mood that is persistent and distinctly different from normal elevated or irritable moods. This period is accompanied by at least three of seven possible symptoms. These symptoms include (1) inflated self-esteem; (2) a decreased need for sleep; (3) unusual talkativeness; (4) the feeling that one's thoughts are racing; (5) increased distractibility; (6) increased activity; (7) involvement in pleasurable but potentially harmful activities (e.g., sexual indiscretions).

Bipolar I Disorder is typically recurrent; according to *DSM-IV*, additional episodes occur in more than 90% of individuals who have had a single manic episode. The manic episodes of those with Bipolar I Disorder are often intermixed with periods of depression. Like those with MDD, people with Bipolar I Disorder may exhibit psychotic, catatonic, and melancholic features as part of either their mania or their depression.

D. Bipolar II Disorder

Bipolar II Disorder is characterized by periods of hypomania intermixed with periods of depression. Hypomanic episodes are characterized by the same symptoms as manic episodes. However, hypomanic episodes are shorter (e.g., 4 days in duration) and are associated with less impairment. While manic episodes may include psychotic features, interrupt daily functioning, and require hospitalization, hypomanic episodes typically do not. The depression experienced as part of Bipolar II Disorder, however, can be just as severe as that experienced in MDD and Bipolar I Disorder.

E. Cyclothymic Disorder

Cyclothymic disorder is characterized by hypomanic periods intermixed with depressive periods that are not as severe as those experienced in MDD, Bipolar I Disorder, and Bipolar II Disorder. In Cyclothymia, the periods of mood disturbance may alternate rapidly, with little respite from affective difficulties. For a diagnosis of Cyclothymia these periods of shifting moods must be problematic for at least 2 years in adults and at least 1 year in children and adolescents.

In addition to the five official diagnoses, *DSM-IV* has denoted four classifications for further study that include depression as a significant component. Such classifications are not yet considered to be disorders and more information is needed on factors such as symptom presentation, etiology, and degree of impairment to sufferers before these might be considered disorders in their own right. Nevertheless, these may represent serious problems and even though they are currently exploratory, we describe them here. They are: (1) Premenstrual Dysphoric Disorder; (2) Minor Depressive Disorder; (3) Recurrent Brief Depressive Disorder; and (4) Mixed Anxiety-Depressive Disorder.

III. EXPLORATORY CATEGORIES OF DEPRESSIVE DISORDERS

A. Premenstrual Dysphoric Disorder

Premenstrual Dysphoric Disorder is characterized by several hallmark symptoms of depression (e.g., decreased interest in usual activities, depressed mood, difficulty sleeping or sleeping too much) in addition to symptoms such as affective lability, feelings of being overwhelmed or out of control, and food cravings. In order to meet the criteria that have been proposed for this diagnosis, such symptoms must have occurred during the late luteal phase of most of a woman's menstrual cycles in the past year. As a number of authors have pointed out, such a classification has potentially serious social, political, and legal ramifications for women. For example, some have argued that if this classification is adopted as an official diagnosis then women might be stigmatized as more unstable than or inferior to men. Arguments such as this keep the classification of Premenstrual Dysphoric Disorder a topic of considerable debate. [*See* PREMENSTRUAL SYNDROME (PMS).]

B. Minor Depressive Disorder

Minor Depressive Disorder is characterized by fewer depressive symptoms than are seen in MDD. The level of impairment is also less than that associated with MDD. To meet the proposed criteria for Minor Depressive Disorder, a person must demonstrate either a depressed mood or loss of interest and two additional symptoms of a Major Depressive Episode. If this classification were included in future DSM editions as a disorder, it would constitute a residual category to be used only after the other mood disorders have been ruled out.

C. Recurrent Brief Depressive Disorder

The principle difference between Recurrent Brief Depressive Disorder and MDD is one of duration. Recurrent Brief Depressive Disorder is characterized by periods of depression that meet all of the criteria for a Major Depressive Episode except for the duration requirement. While in major depressive episodes, symptoms must last at least 2 weeks, in recurrent brief depressive episodes, symptoms must last at least 2 but less than 14 days. In addition, these brief episodes must occur at least once a month for 12 months to meet criteria for the classification of Recurrent Brief Depressive Disorder. Recurrent Brief Depressive Disorder is quite similar to MDD in its age of onset and family incidence rates, thus raising questions as to whether this should be considered a distinct disorder.

D. Mixed Anxiety-Depressive Disorder

The impetus behind a mixed anxious-depressed category lies in the finding that there are many people suffering from symptoms of anxiety and depression who do not meet criteria for any DSM anxiety or mood disorder, but who are nonetheless significantly impaired by their difficulties. The classification of Mixed Anxiety-Depressive Disorder is characterized by a dysphoric mood for at least 1 month in addition to at least four additional symptoms that primarily reflect anxiety (e.g., mind going blank, worry, hypervigilance). The primary argument in favor of adopting this proposed disorder is that it would cover the large number of people who have significant impairment linked to depression and anxiety but who do not fall into any currently existing diagnostic category. The primary argument against this classification is that people suffering from both depression and anxiety could in fact be categorized into already existing disorders with the use of more precise assessment methods.

IV. EPIDEMIOLOGY

Epidemiology refers to information about the incidence and prevalence of disorders in a population. A prevalence rate refers to the number of people who have a given disorder during a particular time period (e.g., the percentage of people in given location diagnosed with MDD within a 1-year period of time). An incidence rate refers to the number of new cases of a disorder which occur during a given time period (e.g., the number of people diagnosed with Dysthymic Disorder during April 1996). Because the distribution of a disorder can be examined to determine whether it correlates with other factors, epidemiological information can be important for understanding some of the possible causes and correlates of depression. [*See* Epidemiology: Psychiatric.]

A. Prevalence

1. National Prevalence

Two recent large-scale surveys of psychopathology in the United States have provided differing prevalence data on depression. Using diagnostic criteria from the revised 3rd Edition of the *DSM* (*DSM-III-R*), the Epidemiologic Catchment Area (ECA) study examined the rates of depression in five sites: New Haven, Baltimore, St. Louis, Los Angeles, and Durham. The ECA study found the lifetime prevalence of major depression (i.e., the number of people experiencing major depression during any point in life) to be 4.9% and the lifetime prevalence of dysthymia to be 3.2%. Alternatively, the National Comorbidity Survey (NCS) reported much higher prevalence rates: 14.9% for lifetime major depression and 6.4% for dysthymia. The discrepancies between these two studies may be accounted for by the different assessment instruments used, slightly different diagnostic criteria employed, and different age ranges studied (i.e., the ECA sample was 18 years of age or older, whereas the NCS sample ranged in age from 15 to 54 years). According to the ECA study, prevalence rates for bipolar disorders were much lower; lifetime prevalence of these disorders was

.8% for Bipolar I and .5% for Bipolar II. The NCS lifetime prevalence for manic episode was somewhat higher: 1.6%. Even though these epidemiological studies reported somewhat discrepant rates, they are in agreement that mood disorders are relatively common in the United States.

2. International Prevalence

A number of studies have examined the community prevalence of major depression in countries besides the United States. International lifetime prevalence rates vary widely, from a low of 3.3% in Seoul to a high of 15.1% among New Zealand residents aged 25 to 46. While such differences may indeed reflect true international differences in the occurrence of depression, other factors such as cultural differences in the sensitivity of the instruments used to assess disorder and different sample ages may also account for this range. In prevalence studies focusing on bipolar illness, ranges from .07% in Sweden to 7% in Ireland have been reported. Most studies, however, place prevalence at about 1% for bipolar illnesses, consistent with data from the ECA and NCS studies.

B. Age Differences

The ECA study also reported incidence rates of depression for various age groups. For men, major depression was highest among those aged 18 to 29. A large decline in incidence was noted for men aged 45 and older. For women, the incidence of major depression was highest in the group aged 30 to 44 and did not decline until age 65. [*See* Aging and Mental Health.]

C. Sex and Ethnic Differences

According to the ECA study, lifetime prevalence rates of major depression, dysthymia, and all mood disorders are approximately twice as high for women as for men. Women's lifetime rates were 7.0%, 4.1%, and 10.2%, respectively, while rates for men were 2.6%, 2.2%, and 5.2%, respectively. These differences occur across a variety of ethnic groups (e.g., African American, Hispanic, Caucasian) even when differences in education, income, and occupations are controlled. Sex differences are also found in countries besides the United States. While sex differences in depression are among the most stable of findings across studies, no sex differences in the rates of bipolar disorder are reliably found. [*See* GENDER DIFFERENCES IN MENTAL HEALTH.]

Although sex difference in the incidence of depression occur across different ethnic groups, there are some differences among these groups overall. For instance, the ECA study found higher rates of Major Depression and Dysthymia among Caucasians and Hispanics than among African Americans. However, few difference in the rates of bipolar disorders among the three groups were found. [*See* ETHNICITY AND MENTAL HEALTH.]

D. Environmental Correlates

The ECA study also examined a number of environmental correlates of depression and bipolar disorders. This study found that people who were separated or divorced had higher 1-year prevalence rates of major depression (6.3%) than those who were never married (2.8%), currently married (2.1%), or widowed (2.1%). This was also true of those with bipolar disorders, although the rates for those separated or divorced versus never married were nearly identical (1.7% versus 1.6%). The 1-year prevalence rate of major depression was also higher among the unemployed than the employed (3.4% versus 2.2%), but the rate was nearly identical for those with bipolar disorders (1.1% versus 1.0%). In addition, the ECA study found higher rates of major depression among white-collar workers and those with at least 12 years of education, but lower rates of depression among those with annual incomes of $15,000 or more. Consistent with the major depression findings, bipolar disorders were also less prevalent among those with annual incomes of $15,000 or more. Bipolar disorders were also found to be the most prevalent among none-white-collar workers with less than 12 years of education. Overall, these socioeconomic status differences were quite small.

V. ETIOLOGICAL THEORIES OF DEPRESSION

A variety of different psychological theories of the causes of depression have been proposed. These can be grouped in psychoanalytic, interpersonal, and cognitive.

A. Psychological Theories

I. Psychoanalytic Approaches

The first psychoanalytic writers to theorize about the etiology of depression were Sigmund Freud and his student, Karl Abraham. As would be expected, there are a number of similarities in the theories proposed by Freud and Abraham. First, both Freud and Abraham believed that some people are predisposed to experience depression. For Abraham, this predisposition consisted of anatomical anomalies that allowed a person to experience a great deal of oral eroticism. For Freud, this predisposition consisted of narcissistic object choices (e.g., object choices which are so similar to the self that love of the object is truly love of self). Second, both believed that a predisposition to experience depression was not, in and of itself, enough to cause depression. In order to experience a depression, a predisposed individual must also experience the loss of a loved object (e.g., through death or rejection).

Despite these basic similarities, the two theorists diverge somewhat on how depression occurs once a loss has been experienced. For Abraham, the loss of a loved object in a person predisposed to depression triggers a regression to the oral stage of psychosexual development. Such a regression is meant to achieve three purposes: (1) to increase pleasure; (2) to hold on to the object through oral incorporation; and (3) to discharge one's aggressive impulses on to the object. Such a regression manifests itself most saliently in the depressive symptoms of eating too much or too little. For Freud, the loss of a loved object possesses different implications. Since the lost object was a narcissistic choice and thus represented the self, loss of the object means loss of the self. This loss of self triggers feelings of anger and depression. The energy associated with these negative feelings is withdrawn from the lost object and brought inward, in a process called introjection. Thus, depression as conceptualized by Freud is often summarized as "anger turned inward." For Freud, the difference between sadness and "true" depression was the difference between "this is awful" and "I am awful." Freud further extended his theory to account for the mania characteristic of bipolar depressive disorders. He hypothesized that, once the feelings of anger and depression over loss of the object are resolved, the energy associated with these negative feelings is freed for other purposes. In a person with bipolar disorder, this freed energy is used to zealousy search for new objects, thus accounting for the symptoms of mania.

More recent psychoanalytic theorists have focused on the superego's role in depression. Some theorists, for example, have suggested that depression is distinguished from other states such as shame, apathy, or resentment by the presence of guilt. As guilt results only from an intrapsychic conflict of the superego, the superego is necessarily implicated in depression. One result of these differences in etiological focus has been the proposition of two forms of depression: anaclitic and introjective. Anaclitic depression is characterized by feelings of helplessness, inferiority, and being unloved. Anaclitic depression is proposed to be associated with the earlier stages of development and is most closely associated with the theorizing of Abraham and Freud. Alternatively, introjective depression focuses on feelings of unworthiness and failure to measure up to expectations and standards. It is associated with later stages of development, and more closely aligned with the works of later psychoanalytic theorists. Although much of psychoanalytic theory has been criticized on grounds that it has not been empirically tested, the distinction between anaclitic and introjective depressions has been empirically examined and found to be valid. Psychoanalytic theorists have accounted for the development of bipolar disorders as well. Most notable amongst these theorists is Melanie Klein, who expanded upon the work of Freud. [*See* Psychoanalysis.]

2. Interpersonal Approaches

Interpersonal approaches to the etiology and maintenance of depression focus on the interplay between a depressed person and his or her relations with others. Empirical research in this area has taken several directions. For example, some researchers focus on the role of social skills in depression, asking such questions as whether depressed people have poor social skills and whether the lack of such skills results in decreased reinforcement from others and consequent depression. Other research has evaluated the types of communications depressed people emit (e.g., sadness, hopelessness) and the effects these communications have on others. If others find the communications of depressed persons aversive, they will likely avoid such persons, which may then exacerbate depressive symptoms such as isolation and loneliness. Still others address the interplay between stress, social support, and depression.

All of these lines of research have found some support; interpersonal research highlights the fact that depression is caused by a multitude of factors in interplay with one another.

Much of the research converges on the theoretical idea that depression is maintained by a vicious cycle that is caused by disruptions in interpersonal interactions. For instance, many depressed individuals quite understandably seek out social support from others. If this support does not alleviate the negative feelings, further support is sought. This intensified support seeking, however, has the paradoxical effect of pushing away those who have been supportive. That is, as individuals begin to feel that their support capacity has been exhausted they pull back from the depressed person, leading to an even further intensification of social support seeking, and the further distancing of potentially supportive people.

Interpersonal factors in the etiology of bipolar depressive disorders have not received as much research attention as such factors in unipolar depressive disorders. Nonetheless, persons with both types of depressive disorders seem to have difficulties in retaining social support. Indeed, in one recent study, people with bipolar disorder perceived their social supports as less available to them and as less adequate in the amount of support received than people in a community sample. Furthermore, perceptions of social support availability seemed to decrease as the duration of illness increased. Thus, it seems likely that social support plays a role in bipolar as well as unipolar depressive disorders.

3. Cognitive Approaches

Currently, cognitive approaches are among the most widely studied theories in the etiology of depression. One of the most influential of these theories was proposed by Aaron Beck in 1967. Beck argued that all individuals possess cognitive structures called schemas that guide the ways information in the environment is attended to and interpreted. Such schemas are determined from childhood by our interactions with the external world. For example, a child who is constantly criticized may begin to believe she is worthless. She might then begin to interpret every failure experience as further evidence of her worthlessness. If this negative processing of information is not changed, it will become an enduring part of her cognitive organization, that is, a schema. When this schema is activated (e.g., by a poor grade on a test or any other failure experience), it will predispose her to depressive feelings (e.g., I'm no good). Beck stated that, as a result of this faulty information processing, depressed persons demonstrate a cognitive triad of negative thoughts about themselves, the world, and the future. He further extended his argument to include the manic phases of bipolar depressive disorders. Beck stated that such phases are characterized by a manic triad of irrationally positive thoughts about oneself, the world, and the future. Like the depressive triad in unipolar depressive disorders, the manic triad in bipolar depressive disorders was hypothesized to lead to the symptoms of mania, such as inflated self-esteem and extremely elevated mood. [*See* COGNITIVE THERAPY.]

There is widespread agreement that depression can be caused by different factors. Some theorists have argued that dysfunctional cognitions cause only a subset of depressions. Termed the "negative cognition" subtype, this type of depression is brought about by either the kinds of schemas discussed by Aaron Beck or by dysfunctional attributional patterns that lead depressed people to take responsibility for the occurrence of negative events, and to avoid taking responsibility for positive events. This dysfunctional attributional pattern can lead to a sense of hopelessness that results in a "hopelessness depression," a component of negative cognition depression.

B. Biological Theories

Although there are a variety of biologically based theories of depression, they can be broken down into two general approaches: genetic and neurotransmitter.

1. Genetic Approaches

Genetic approaches suggest that depression is the result of inheriting genes that predispose to occurrence of depression. Three types of studies that are used to investigate genetic inheritance of depression illustrate this approach. These studies consist of family studies, twin studies, and adoption studies. In a typical family study, families with a depressed member are interviewed to determine how many other family members have or had an affective disorder. In twin studies, the concordance rate of affective disorder between monozygotic and dizygotic twin pairs is compared. Because monozygotic twins have identical genes, if genetic theories are correct then concordance rates of depression should be higher than for dizygotic twins (who

have similar but not identical genes). In adoption studies, two strategies are most often used. In the first, the rate of depressive disorder in the biological parents of adopted persons with and without affective disorders is compared. In the second, the rate of depressive disorders is compared between adopted children with and without affectively disordered biological parents. Adoption studies have an advantage over family and twin studies, as the effects of environment on affective disorder are reduced in this design. However, adoption studies constitute the least-used approach to investigating genetic factors in depression; the difficulty of obtaining complete records on adoptees and their biological parents makes this design quite prohibitive.

Despite design differences, all three genetic approaches to the etiology of depression have yielded similar results: depression is heritable to at least some degree. A recent review of the research literature, for example, found rates of affective disorders among first-degree relatives of unipolar-disordered individuals ranging from 11.8% to 32.2%. Rates of affective disorders among first-degree relatives of bipolar-disordered individuals ranged from 10.6% to 33.1%. Rates of affective disorder among first-degree relatives of normal individuals ranged from 4.8% to 6.3. In twin studies of unipolar and bipolar depression, concordance rates ranged from .04 to 1.0 for monozygotic twins, and from 0.0 to .43 to dizygotic twins, with the majority of studies reviewed reporting no concordance for dizygotic twins. The results of genetic investigations clearly suggest that there is a genetic component to depression, although the exact nature and functioning of this component is thus far still unknown. [*See* GENETIC CONTRIBUTORS TO MENTAL HEALTH.]

2. Neurotransmitter Approaches

Research on brain chemistry as an etiological factor in unipolar depression has focused on two monoamine neurotransmitters: norepinephrine (NE) and serotonin (5-HT). Initially, researchers believed that depression was due to a lack of NE in the brain, and later, to a lack of both NE and 5-HT. However, several difficulties with these hypotheses arose: (1) While the effects of antidepressants on monoamine levels start within hours of taking the medication, decreased depression levels do not become apparent until weeks later. (2) Some drugs that do not affect monoamine levels alleviate depression. (3) Some drugs that increase monoamine levels do not alleviate depression.

Thus, researchers have directed their efforts to investigating more complicated relations between these neurotransmitters and depression. Recent efforts have included the study of receptor site hyposensitivity, relationships between NE and 5-HT, and relationships between 5-HT and the neurotransmitter dopamine (DA).

Research on brain chemistry as in etiological factor in bipolar depression has followed much the same course as such research on unipolar depression. Initially, researchers believed that the mania characteristic of bipolar disorders was due to excesses of the neurotransmitters NE and 5-HT, exactly opposite the belief for depression. However, difficulties arose with this hypothesis, including findings that (1) lithium, the medical treatment of choice for bipolar disorder which seems to affect both NE and 5-HT, was effective at controlling both depression and mania, and (2) both depression and mania may be characterized by lower levels of 5-HT. Thus, as with unipolar depression, researchers of bipolar depression have begun investigating more complicated relationships between bipolar depression and neurotransmitters. Similar to the recent efforts concerning unipolar depression, researchers have investigated interactions between 5-HT and DA, interactions between NE and DA, and receptor site hypersensitivity. These types of investigations represent promising areas of research in elucidating the multifaceted etiology of depression. Certainly, biology and psychology are implicated in the causes of depression, both unipolar and bipolar forms.

VI. PROTECTIVE FACTORS

Given the potentially devastating effects of depression, many researchers have devoted their efforts to studying factors that decrease the likelihood of becoming depressed or decrease the amount of time spent in depressive episodes. Among the most widely studied of such protective factors are social support and coping styles. [*See* PROTECTIVE FACTORS IN DEVELOPMENT OF PSYCHOPATHOLOGY.]

A. Social Support

There are numerous facets to the concept of social support. For example, social support can be conceived as the number of persons one can rely on for support. Social support can also be conceived as the amount of support received, regardless of the number of persons

one receives support from. In addition, socially supportive relationships can be conceptualized on a continuum of quality from very poor to very good. Examination of all these facets has proven important in understanding relationships between depression and social support.

Overall, people in contact with numerous socially supportive persons are less likely to have mental health difficulties, including depression. In addition, those who perceive a great deal of support from others are less likely to be negatively affected by stressors that might lead to depression. For people who have become depressed, having a confidant such as a spouse or best friend and a supportive family is related to greater success in treatment. The quality of such relationships is also important to treatment. In one study, for example, depressed persons with good-quality confidant relationships needed shorter periods of treatment than those with poor-quality confidant relationships.

The effects of social support for people with bipolar depressive disorders have not been as well studied as the effects for people with unipolar depressive disorders. Nonetheless, research suggests that social support is indeed beneficial for people with bipolar disorders. In one study, for example, a great deal of available social support was related to fewer psychological symptoms, better social adjustment, and better overall functioning. [*See* SOCIAL SUPPORT.]

B. Coping Styles

Ways of coping with stressors can be roughly divided into two categories: approach strategies and avoidance strategies. Approach strategies are characterized by identifying the problematic situation, devising reasonable solutions to it, an implementing those solutions. Avoidance strategies include trying not to think about the problem, wishing the problem did not exist, and fantasizing about life without the problem. Overall, approach strategies seem to help people cope with stressors that might otherwise lead to depression. In addition, use of approach strategies is associated with better treatment outcome for those who become depressed. Conversely, people who use avoidance strategies to cope with stress seem more likely to become depressed and to have poorer treatment outcomes.

As with the effects of social support, research on coping styles among people with bipolar depressive disorders is scarce. Nonetheless, one recent study that examined differences in coping between high- and low-functioning people with bipolar disorders suggested that avoidant coping styles are associated with poorer functioning. Thus, relationships between coping styles and bipolar depressive disorders and coping and unipolar depressive disorders may be similar. [*See* COPING WITH STRESS.]

BIBLIOGRAPHY

Beck, A. T. (1967). *Depression: Causes and treatment*. Philadelphia: University of Pennsylvania Press.

Beckham, E. E., & Leber W. R. (1995). (Eds.). *Handbook of depression* (2nd ed.). New York: Guilford Press.

Cicchetti, D., & Toth, S. L. (1992). (Eds.). *Developmental perspectives on depression*. Rochester, NY: University of Rochester Press.

Craig, K. D., & Dobson, K. S. (1995). (Eds.). *Anxiety and depression in children and adults*. Thousand Oaks, CA: Sage.

Kendall, P. C., Hollon, S. D., Beck, A. T., Hammen, C. L., & Ingram, R. E. (1987). Issues and recommendations regarding use of the Beck Depression Inventory. Cognitive Therapy and Research, 11, 289–299.

Ingram, R. E., Miranda, J., & Segal, Z. V. (in press). *Cognitive vulnerability to depression*. New York: Guilford Press.

Robins, L. N., & Regier, D. A. (1991). (Eds.). *Psychiatric disorders in America*. New York: The Free Press.

Depression—Applied Aspects

Ricardo F. Muñoz

University of California, San Francisco

I. Types of Depression
II. Depression as a Disorder
III. Prevention of Depression
IV. Treatment of Major Depression
V. Maintenance
VI. Healthy Mood Management:
   A Developmental Perspective
VII. Conclusion

Depressed Mood A feeling state consisting of dejection, sadness, and demoralization, usually accompanied by diminished reaction to pleasurable events.
Depressive Disorder A condition in which an individual exhibits a specified number of depressive symptoms of enough severity and duration to meet well-delineated and widely accepted diagnostic criteria.
Emotion A noticeable subjective feeling, usually lasting on the order of minutes, in reaction to internal or external stimuli.
Mood A relatively persistent feeling state, lasting for hours or days.

The term DEPRESSION can be used in a number of ways. As commonly used, it refers to a normative, usually transient and generally dejected, dispirited, or sad mood state. It can also be a symptom related to several emotional or physical disorders. It can refer to a syndrome (a collection of symptoms that usually occur together) and is also used as the official name for a specific mental disorder in the current psychiatric nomenclature. As the latter, depression is considered to be a psychopathological entity hypothesized to have distinctive etiological mechanisms, prognosis,

and treatment implications. This entry describes these types of depression, discusses the prevalence of the more common types studied, and presents prevention, treatment, and maintenance interventions currently suggested for persons with depression. The final section examines the concept of healthy mood management from a developmental perspective.

I. TYPES OF DEPRESSION

A. Depressed Mood

Depressed mood states appear to be a normal part of human subjective experience. Most individuals have a personal understanding of depressed mood, in contrast with, say, psychotic experiences or addictions. Depressed mood states usually involve the emotion of sadness, a subjective lack of energy, reduced motivation to engage in formerly pleasant activities, reduced desire to have positive interactions with other people, and a belief that one's lot in life is difficult. Such states color one's reactions to external events, but they can themselves be modified by such events. Normal states of depressed mood last hours or days. Once they become more chronic and start affecting one's ability to function, they are often conceptualized as part of a pathological process, which can ultimately meet criteria for a diagnosis of a clinical depressive disorder.

It is useful to examine the relationship between emotions, such as sadness, and mood states. Emotion researchers generally conceptualize emotions as relatively short-lived reactions to external or internal stimuli. These reactions appear to be relatively autonomous, that is, not ordinarily subject to conscious planning. They have physiological, expressive, and subjective elements. They usually occur within seconds of the triggering stimulus and last on the order of minutes. As the subjective feeling which is part of an emotional response lasts longer, it can become a mood state. Alternatively, the emotion can fade away or change into a different emotion; for example, in response to being surprised, one can exhibit a startle response, then fear, anger, and finally amusement and relief. The trigger for these kinds of changes can be external (the availability of new information) as well as internal (the subjective interpretation of the new information).

Although, under normal circumstances, the initial emotional response to specific triggers appears to be too quick to be under conscious control, once the emotion begins to develop, the modulation of the emotional response does seem to be amenable to planned influences. Part of the developmental process in humans involves the regulation of emotion. Maturity is judged in part on the individual's ability to control his or her emotional responses. [*See* EMOTIONAL REGULATION.]

The role of mood states in the development of psychopathology has yet to be adequately elucidated. It is well known that prior to having a major depressive episode, there is usually a period of gradually increasing depressed mood and symptoms. If these symptoms develop into a major depressive episode, they are retrospectively considered a prodrome of the clinical episode. However, most individuals with high depressive symptoms do not go on to a clinical episode of depression. It may be that naturally occurring events in daily life may increase or decrease the probability of pathological depression. Or perhaps different coping mechanisms, when put into practice, afford differential degrees of protectiveness. Alternatively, it may be that those who are predisposed, because of genetic or other biological factors, are the ones who are most likely to fall prey to the pathological process. As of now, the answers to these questions are not yet in. [*See* COPING WITH STRESS; PROTECTIVE FACTORS IN DEVELOPMENT OF PSYCHOPATHOLOGY.]

B. Depression as a Symptom

Depression can be viewed as a dichotomous concept: it is present or it is not. It can also be conceptualized as a continuum: one can be more or less depressed.

The former conceptualization is compatible with the disorder view of depression, and is covered later. The latter concept has been much used in epidemiologic studies and in clinical studies, particularly in those focused on treatment outcome. The general strategy for measuring the level of depression that an individual is experiencing has been to construct a questionnaire or a structured interview that inquires about several aspects of the depressive state, usually focusing on duration and/or intensity of several symptoms of depression. The questionnaire or interview is then scored, yielding a single continuous variable. Higher scores reflect a greater level of depression. Depression symptom scales have been useful in providing normative data on the experience of depression in community samples and in helping to evaluate the effect of treatment on level of depression. Depression symptom scales are usually not intended to diagnose depression.

Epidemiological studies provide evidence that depressive symptoms are prevalent in the general population. High levels of depressive symptomatology, as measured by self-report symptom scales, have sometimes been referred to as demoralization. Demoralization appears to be more prevalent in low-income minority populations than in white middle-class samples. It is unclear whether the difference is due primarily to ethnicity or to social class, but the preponderance of the evidence indicates that when controls are implemented for socioeconomic factors, the differences in depression levels diminish or disappear. [*See* ETHNICITY AND MENTAL HEALTH; SOCIOECONOMIC STATUS.]

The interpretation of similar differences in depression scores showing higher levels for women has also been controversial. Disentangling the role of socioeconomic issues between men and women is much harder, because married women, especially those who do not have a paying job outside the home, are generally assigned their husband's social class, even though they may not have the same type of independence or control over resources that their husbands do. [*See* GENDER DIFFERENCES IN MENTAL HEALTH.]

The relationship between age and depressive symptoms is not clear. Most studies have found no difference, others have found higher rates in younger persons, and still others found higher rates in older persons. [*See* AGING AND MENTAL HEALTH.]

There is a relatively clear connection between depressed symptoms and substance abuse. Studies of national samples have found that individuals with negative mood states, including depression, are more likely to use cigarettes and alcohol. They are also less likely to quit smoking, and if they quit, are more likely to relapse. The direction of causality is not easy to disentangle, however. Use of drugs, including alcohol, can increase the likelihood of depressed states. The physiological effects of drugs on the nervous system is probably implicated in this process, but it is also true that the disruption to the individual's life caused by drug abuse probably produces significant psychological stress. [See ALCOHOL PROBLEMS, SUBSTANCE ABUSE; SMOKING.]

C. Depression as a Syndrome

Major depressive episode is the most common depressive syndrome. A syndrome is a configuration of symptoms that often occur together and constitute a recognizable condition. Although the presence of a major depressive syndrome is a necessary characteristic of major depressive disorder, it is not sufficient. The syndrome can occur for other reasons. For example, medications or drugs of abuse, as well as general medical conditions, can have direct physiological effects which can trigger the symptoms of a major depressive episode. Similarly, the loss of a loved one can result in this configuration of symptoms. In the latter case, unless the symptoms persist for longer than 2 months, or produce marked functional impairment, suicidality, or psychosis, they are considered to be part of the normal course of bereavement. [See BEREAVEMENT.]

The implication is that major depressive syndrome is much more prevalent than major depressive disorder. Currently, major depressive disorder is conceptualized as a clinical entity that may have genetic, other biological, and psychosocial sources, much like a specific illness. Major depressive syndrome is a condition that may be triggered by specific life events or by physical influences on the body, but it does not necessarily imply an underlying psychopathological process. These assumptions reflect a basic dilemma in the mental health field, namely, whether there is a qualitative difference between "normal" conditions (such as depressed mood or major depressive syndrome) and the officially recognized mental disorders (such as major depressive disorder), or whether the latter are merely quantitatively more intense and longer lasting manifestations of normal mood fluctuations.

D. Depressive Disorders

The most commonly used diagnostic system in the United States is the Diagnostic and Statistical Manual of Mental Disorders, fourth edition (*DSM-IV*). Depression is implicated primarily in what are termed the mood disorders. The mood disorders are themselves divided into two major categories: the depressive disorders and the bipolar disorders. The depressive disorders are sometimes referred to as unipolar depressions, that is, mood disorders in which changes from normal mood occur in only one direction, toward depressed mood. Bipolar disorders exhibit bidirectional fluctuations, either to depressed mood or to abnormally euphoric (manic) mood states. It is recognized that mood disorders can be the result of general medical conditions as well as the result of the use or abuse of drugs and other substances. Mood disorders caused by drug use or abuse are not considered primary mood disorders. In the following section, the *DSM-IV* diagnostic criteria for the more common mood disorders are presented. [See MOOD DISORDERS.]

II. DEPRESSION AS A DISORDER

A. Major Depression

Major depression is the most common of the mood disorders. The key diagnostic criterion for major depressive *disorder* is the presence of a major depressive *episode*.

There are nine symptoms that define a major depressive episode. Of the nine, at least five must have been present during a 2-week period. They must represent a change from previous functioning and they must cause significant impairment in daily functioning. At least one of the five symptoms must be either the first or the second symptom in the following list:

1. Depressed mood most of the day, nearly every day
2. Reduced interest or pleasure in all or almost all activities
3. Significant weight loss or weight gain, or a significant decrease or increase in appetite
4. Trouble sleeping or sleeping too much
5. Psychomotor agitation or retardation
6. Fatigue or loss of energy
7. Feeling worthless or guilty in an excessive or inappropriate manner

8. Problems in thinking, concentrating, or making decisions
9. Recurrent thoughts of death, suicidal ideation, specific suicidal plan, or a suicide attempt

B. Dysthymia

Dysthymia differs from major depression in that it is generally more chronic and is defined by fewer symptoms. The *DSM-IV* criteria for dysthymic disorder include a depressed mood for most days for at least 2 years in adults or at least 1 year in children and adolescents. In addition, two or more of the following six symptoms must be present: poor appetite or overeating, trouble sleeping or sleeping too much, low energy or fatigue, low self-esteem, poor concentration or difficulty making decisions, and feelings of hopelessness. The initial 2-year period must not have included a major depressive episode and the 2-year period of depression must not have been broken by a period of normal mood lasting more than 2 months.

C. Bipolar Disorder

Depressed mood and a major depressive episode may be part of bipolar disorders. However, what characterizes bipolar disorders is the occurrence of one or more manic episodes. The *DSM-IV* criteria for manic episode include a period of abnormally elevated, expansive, or irritable mood lasting at least 1 week, plus three or more of the following seven symptoms:

1. Inflated self-esteem or grandiosity
2. Decreased need for sleep
3. More talkative than usual or pressured to keep talking
4. Flight of ideas or racing thoughts
5. Distractibility
6. Marked increased in goal-directed activity or psychomotor agitation
7. Excessive involvement in pleasurable activities with a high potential for painful consequences

There are two subtypes of bipolar disorders: Bipolar I involves full-blown manic episodes, and Bipolar II involves less intense, manic-like episodes, known as hypomanic episodes. There is also a bipolar disorder that parallels dysthymia, called cyclothymia. It is a chronic disorder that is characterized by the presence of both hypomanic periods and depressive periods

most of the time for at least 2 years. Both depressive and bipolar disorders include residual categories called, respectively, "depressive disorder not otherwise specified" and "bipolar disorder not otherwise specified." In both cases, the disorders do not meet the full criteria for either depressive or bipolar diagnoses.

III. PREVENTION OF DEPRESSION

In its major 1994 report, *Reducing Risks for Mental Disorders,* the Institute of Medicine put forward a framework for mental health interventions that has three major levels: prevention, treatment, and maintenance. The most commonly known level of intervention is the treatment of acute cases of mental disorders. The Institute of Medicine also wanted to highlight the need for interventions that occur before the onset of the disorder, namely, preventive interventions, and interventions that occur after an acute episode has ended, that is, "maintenance" interventions intended to reduce relapse or recurrence or to help the individual regain the highest possible level of functioning. Each of these three levels is divided into the following subcategories.

A. Levels of Preventive Intervention

1. Universal Preventive Interventions
Universal preventive interventions for mental disorders are targeted to the general public or to a whole population group that has not been identified on the basis of individual risk. These interventions are believed to have a preventive effect on the population as a whole, and are believed to be protective of several types of psychological disorders. In general, such interventions should be of relatively low cost and easily disseminated.

2. Selective Preventive Interventions
Selective preventive interventions for mental disorders are targeted to subgroups of the population whose risk of developing mental disorders is significantly higher than average. Risks factors used to identify these groups may be biological, psychological, or social. The important factor is that they are associated with the onset of a mental disorder. Selective interventions could include interventions targeted to widows, people who are getting married for the first time, chil-

dren going into the school system or graduating from the school system, individuals who have been laid off from work, women about to have their first child, or victims of trauma.

3. Indicated Preventive Interventions

Indicated preventive interventions are targeted to high-risk individuals who are identified as having minimum but detectable signs or symptoms foreshadowing a mental disorder or who have biological markers indicating predisposition for mental disorders. As in all of the preventive interventions, the individuals or groups targeted do not meet the full diagnostic criteria for the particular disorder being prevented at the time of being recruited into a preventive intervention program.

B. Attributable Risk

To engage in preventive interventions, one must identify the risk and/or protective factors that increase or decrease the probability of developing a particular disorder. An important concept from epidemiology is that of attributable risk. *Attributable risk* refers to the proportion of cases of a specific condition or disorder that are attributable to a specific factor. For instance, it is commonly known that tobacco smoking is related to lung cancer. However, lung cancer can also be caused by other factors. If we were to eradicate tobacco, a large proportion of lung cancer would be prevented, but not all cases. The proportion prevented would be the proportion of cases attributable to smoking, or the attributable risk.

Many factors have been linked to depression. Some of them are demographic factors that cannot be changed for the individual, such as sex, death of a parent during early childhood, or a family history of the disorder. Therefore it is important to focus on *modifiable* risk factors, especially those with a high level of attributable risk. From a preventive standpoint, one possible risk factor that is related to later episodes of major depression is the evidence of deficits in mood regulation. A potential strategy, therefore, is to identify individuals who have high symptom levels of depression, but who do not meet the criteria for a depressive disorder, and to teach such individuals methods to manage their moods. Such methods can come, for example, from cognitive–behavioral techniques that have been found to be useful in the treatment of depression. Some studies have already shown that de-

pressive symptoms can be reduced in nonclinical populations that nevertheless show high depressive symptom levels when recruited. As of this writing, there have not been enough randomized controlled prevention trials to be able to say conclusively that new cases of major depression can be prevented. The development and evaluation of preventive interventions for depression and other mental disorders may be the next important stage in the development of mental health interventions.

IV. TREATMENT OF MAJOR DEPRESSION

Treatment interventions are divided into two sublevels: (1) case identification, to provide early treatment for cases of major depression that have not been identified previously; and (2) standard treatment, which accounts for the bulk of mental health intervention efforts.

The need for case identification efforts arises from the underdiagnosis of major depression and other depressive disorders in primary care clinics. Only 20% of individuals who meet criteria for major depression seek mental health services. However, more than 70% of those who meet criteria for major depression do seek health care, generally from a primary care physician. Yet, only about a third of individuals with major depression are so identified by their primary care providers. It is imperative, therefore, that primary care physicians and other health care providers learn to identify cases of depression so that individuals suffering from them may receive appropriate interventions.

Major depression is eminently treatable. Between 60% and 80% of individuals with major depression respond to either psychological or pharmacological treatments. Other less common types of treatment, such as light therapy and electroconvulsive therapy, have also been found effective for certain cases of major depression.

Treatments for depression vary in their theoretical assumptions and in the specific interventions used with patients. Certain common elements include an explicit helping relationship between the therapist and the patient, the identification of depression as a clinical disorder that requires treatment (as opposed to some type of "personal weakness"), an explanatory framework for the mechanisms that trigger and maintain the depression, and implicit or explicit recommendations for patient behaviors that are expected to bring about improvement.

Many types of psychological approaches are currently used in the treatment of depression. Those that have been most often subjected to randomized controlled outcome trials are the cognitive–behavioral therapies. Cognitive–behavioral therapies for depression are based on the hypothesis that mood is influenced by a person's cognitive and behavioral patterns. These patterns have been learned, usually in a social context, and can be modified. The purpose of therapy is to work with the patient to identify the cognitions (thoughts, assumptions, other mental processes) and behaviors (activity levels, interpersonal skills, and other physical or observable actions) that are most related to specific mood states. The goal of therapy is to reduce cognitions and behaviors that increase the probability of depressed states and augment those that decrease the probability of depression. [See BEHAVIOR THERAPY; COGNITIVE THERAPY.]

Another psychological approach to depression that has been repeatedly evaluated in randomized trials is interpersonal psychotherapy. This approach focuses on the influence that the interpersonal context has on triggering and maintaining depressive mood. The therapist reviews with the patient current and past interpersonal relationships as they relate to depressive symptoms. The focus of therapy usually centers on one or more of four major areas: grief, interpersonal disputes, role transitions, and interpersonal deficits.

Other psychological treatments have not been studied as extensively. However, brief approaches to therapy that specifically target depression have generally shown encouraging results.

Pharmacotherapy for depression has also been subjected to many randomized controlled trials. There are several types of antidepressants, all of which have approximately the same efficacy. Those developed most recently tend to have fewer side effects and lower lethality if used to attempt suicide. Pharmacotherapy is probably the most commonly used form of evidence-based treatment for depression in the United States, in part, because it is much more available than the psychotherapies. Antidepressants are prescribed at least as often by nonpsychiatric physicians as by psychiatrists. This has led to a strong (and controversial) emphasis on educating primary care providers to detect and treat depression in their setting before re-ferring to mental health care providers. [See PSYCHO-PHARMACOLOGY.]

Results of randomized trials do not always agree. Nevertheless, the preponderance of the evidence indicates that pharmacotherapy, cognitive–behavioral therapy, and interpersonal psychotherapy are all significantly effective in the treatment of major depression. The rate of improvement is generally faster for pharmacotherapy, but total improvement over a 20-week treatment is generally comparable across treatments, especially for mild and moderate cases of major depression. There appears to be some advantage to pharmacotherapy for more severe cases of depression, and clearly so for cases of depression with psychotic features in which antidepressants and antipsychotics may be prescribed simultaneously. A combination of psychotherapy and pharmacotherapy is often used in the treatment of depression. Most controlled studies have shown either additional improvement or no detectable difference in efficacy when both treatments are used. There appears to be no general disadvantage to the use of combined treatment. A major problem with treatment for depression is the high rate of relapse. This leads to a focus on maintenance strategies.

V. MAINTENANCE

The third large segment of mental health interventions identified by the Institute of Medicine is the area of *maintenance*. Even though the treatment of acute episodes of depression and other disorders may be quite effective, relapse or recurrence of such an episode can be not only as disruptive as the first experience of clinical depression, but, at times, even more demoralizing. The fear that this painful condition will recur can have a major impact on a person's outlook. Approximately 50% of persons who have had one major depressive episode have a second; 70% of those with two have a third; and 90% of those with three have a fourth. These figures suggest two important goals for the mental health field: preventing the first episode (as described earlier) and, if the first episode occurs, providing interventions that will maintain a healthy mood state, thus forestalling relapse and recurrence.

Current convention uses the terms relapse and recurrence in relatively well-defined ways. When treatment with antidepressants is effective, depressive symptoms diminish within a few weeks. In the 1980s, it was found that if antidepressant therapy was ended, a large proportion of patients began to exhibit symptoms again. The conclusion was that the processes underlying the mood dysregulation were still active, but that the medication was able to control the symptoms. Once medication ended, the symptoms reappeared. This reappearance was thought to be part of the same episode of depression. Now, the reappearance of symptoms within a year of the start of the episode is called relapse. Once the person has been free of clinical symptoms of depression for a year or more, the depressive episode is considered to be over. If symptoms reappear in the future, such an event is a recurrence.

Studies in which individuals who responded well to pharmacotherapy were followed for 1 or 2 years after treatment ended have found rates of relapse or recurrence as high as 70%. This has led to the recommendation that pharmacotherapy be continued for several months, and perhaps years, after the acute depressive episode has subsided. Some clinicians now state that for certain patients, lifetime maintenance pharmacotherapy is indicated.

Similar studies in which individuals who responded well to cognitive therapy have been followed have found much lower relapse rates of approximately 35% after 1 or 2 years. This has led to speculation that cognitive therapy may have an advantage in terms of reducing relapse or recurrence rates. More studies designed specifically to answer this question are needed.

What is clear at this time is that individuals who have had a depressive episode are at high risk for repeated episodes of clinical depression. These individuals should be taught to monitor their mood state and to obtain treatment as soon as possible after the onset of significant depressive symptoms in the future.

VI. HEALTHY MOOD MANAGEMENT: A DEVELOPMENTAL PERSPECTIVE

The development of effective mood management is an essential aspect of individual human growth. It is also a major factor in the health of a community. Among the major causes of death are several causes that appear to be influenced by mood problems. The top nine preventable causes of death, which account for about

one half of all deaths in the United States, are tobacco, diet and exercise patterns, alcohol, microbial agents, toxic agents, firearms, sexual behavior, motor vehicles, and illicit use of drugs. Consider for a moment how many of these might be exacerbated by depressed mood.

The relationship between negative mood states and smoking and drinking has already been described. It is highly likely that illicit use of drugs follows a similar pattern. Diet and exercise certainly are affected by depressed mood. Deaths from firearms present an interesting illustration of how strong, and yet invisible to most of us, the impact of depression is on our society: few people are aware that for several decades over half the deaths from firearms in the United States have been suicides. Unprotected sexual behavior not only exposes individuals to sexually transmitted diseases, but also to unplanned pregnancies. And some proportion of motor vehicle accidents are related to alcohol and other substance abuse, or to reckless driving, which may be the result of desperate states of mind. The proportion of these factors that is attributable to depression is yet unknown, but is likely to be significant.

Many factors have been implicated in the development of deficits in emotion regulation. None appear to be necessary or sufficient to cause depression, nor are there known factors that offer complete protection from depression.

There appears to be a substantial genetic component in the more severe forms of depression, such as bipolar disorders and major depression. How this genetic influence is manifested physiologically is not yet known. Several biological abnormalities have been identified in subgroups of individuals exhibiting depression. However, most of them appear to occur during a depressed episode and to subside once a normal mood state is attained. None appear to be universally shared by clinically depressed individuals. Developmental influences also appear to be risk factors for depression, such as being born to a mother who is currently depressed, the loss of parents in childhood, and a high number of stressful life events. Social and environmental factors also have well-documented effects on depression. For example, poverty has been shown to account for approximately 10% of new cases of major depression. [*See* GENETIC CONTRIBUTORS TO MENTAL HEALTH.]

The emotion regulation literature suggests that certain mechanisms can be used to affect whether a given emotion occurs or to modulate the intensity, duration, and tone of the emotion once it has been triggered. Factors that can come into play prior to the triggering of the emotion include changes in either the external or the internal environment, that is, either in the environment in which the individual is located (including the people in such an environment) or in the mind of the individual. Attention, memory, mental rehearsal, and the interpretation of the material brought into consciousness via these avenues, all can set the probabilities of certain emotions being triggered. Once an emotion is triggered, the responses of the individual to the emotion can maintain or diminish the intensity and duration of the emotion.

Developmental aspects of emotion regulation include the basic survival aspects of emotion expression in infants, including the instrumental functions of crying or smiling, cooing, and vocalizing; the development of language and its role in modulating emotional response when used by others and by the child; the differential reinforcement and punishment of specific emotions; acquiring expectations regarding which kinds of emotion regulation are possible by observing role models; and, as the individual moves into adolescence and adulthood, gaining greater ability to shape one's environment, choosing one's friends, activities, and school and work settings. Certain professional training includes fairly specific instructions regarding the types of emotional expression that are preferred, discouraged, or prohibited.

The development of healthy mood management or emotion regulation is a key prerequisite of mental health. As individuals develop, a large proportion attempt to modulate their mood by maladaptive methods, including the use of psychoactive substances. If these methods become part of the person's usual repertoire, they can have serious long-term consequences. The delineation of mood management strategies and their consequences deserves further study and dissemination.

Mood management skills are important in at least three broad contexts: work, relationships, and aloneness. The ability to maintain a healthy mood state in each of these situations appears to be necessary to good mental health. The theoretical factors that have been important in the development of treatment modalities can be integrated into a concept of mood management. Each addresses a different level of analysis: biological approaches focus on the neurochemical bases of emotion regulation, cognitive–behavioral approaches focus on psychological mediators of emotion regulation, and interpersonal approaches emphasize the influences of interpersonal relations on emotion regulation and dysregulation.

VII. CONCLUSION

Depression is an experience that has been shared by most human beings at one time or another. Thus, it can be thought of as a feeling state that is within the realm of normal functioning. If the frequency, intensity, and duration of this feeling increase, it can become a pathological process. After it crosses a certain threshold, criteria for which are now well-defined, it is diagnosed as a specific mental disorder. Mental health interventions that focus on this disorder include preventive, treatment, and maintenance interventions, of which treatment is the most developed and the most available. The public health impact of depression is considerable. Advances in the identification and dissemination of effective mood management strategies could have a major impact in the health of our societies.

BIBLIOGRAPHY

Akiskal, H. S., & McKinney, W. T. J. (1973). Depressive disorders: Toward a unified hypothesis. *Science, 182,* 20–29.

American Psychiatric Association. (1994). *Diagnostic and statistical manual of mental disorders* (4th ed.). Washington, DC: American Psychiatric Association.

Beck, A. T., Rush, A. J., Shaw, B. F., & Emery, G. (1979). *Cognitive therapy of depression.* New York: Guilford Press.

Beckham, E. D., & Leber, W. R. (Eds.). (1995). *Handbook of depression: Treatment, assessment, and research* (2nd ed.). New York: Guilford Press.

Bruce, M. L., Takeuchi, D. T., & Leaf, P. J. (1991). Poverty and psychiatric status: Longitudinal evidence from the New Haven Epidemiologic Catchment Area Study. *Archives of General Psychiatry, 48,* 470–474.

Depression Guideline Panel. (1993). *Depression in primary care: Vol. 1. Detection and diagnosis* (Clinical Practice Guideline No. 5 AHCPR Publication No. 93-0550). Rockville, MD: Department of Health and Human Services, Public Health Service, Agency for Health Care Policy and Research.

Depression Guideline Panel. (1993). *Depression in primary care: Vol. 2. Treatment of major depression* (Clinical Practice Guideline No. 5, AHCPR Publication No. 93-0551). Rockville, MD: Department of Health and Human Services, Public Health Service, Agency for Health Care Policy and Research.

Frank, E., Prien, R. F., Jarret, J. B., Keller, M. B., Kupfer, D. J., Lavori, P., Rush, A. J., & Weissman, M. M. (1991). Conceptualization and rationale for consensus definitions of terms in major depressive disorder: response, remission, recovery, relapse, and recurrence. *Archives of General Psychiatry, 48,* 851–855.

Gross, J. J., & Muñoz, R. F. (1995). Emotion regulation and mental health. *Clinical Psychology: Science and Practice, 2,* 151–164.

Lewinsohn, P. M., Hoberman, H., Teri, L., & Hautzinger, M. (1985). An integrative theory of depression. In S. Reiss & R. Bootzin (Eds.), *Theoretical issues in behavior therapy* (pp. 331–359). New York: Academic Press.

McGrath, E., Keita, G. P., Strickland, B. R., & Russo, N. F. (Eds.). (1990). *Women and depression: Risk factors and treatment issues.* Washington, DC: American Psychological Association.

Mrazek, P. J., & Haggerty, R. J. (Eds.). (1994). *Reducing risks for mental disorders: Frontiers for preventive intervention research.* Washington, DC: National Academy Press.

Muñoz, R. F., Hollon, S. D., McGrath, E., Rehm, L. P., & VandenBos, G. R. (1994). On the AHCPR Depression in Primary Care Guidelines: Further considerations for practitioners. *American Psychologist, 49,* 42–61.

Muñoz, R. F., & Ying, Y. (1993). *The prevention of depression: Research and practice.* Baltimore, MD: Johns Hopkins University Press.

Whybrow, P. C., Akiskal, H. S., & McKinney, W. T. (1984). *Mood disorders: Toward a new psychobiology.* New York: Plenum Press.

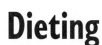

Dieting

Traci McFarlane, Janet Polivy, and C. Peter Herman

University of Toronto

Dieting　An attempt, either successful or unsuccessful, to restrict caloric intake with the intention of losing or maintaining weight or altering body shape.

Physiological Deprivation　The experience of a lack of some substance needed by the body.

Psychological Deprivation　The experience of frustration caused by the inaccessibility of a desired goal object (e.g., food).

Restrained Eaters　Individuals who are concerned with their weight and/or shape and who have a history of attempting to restrict their caloric intake to control this aspect of their appearance (chronic dieters).

Restraint Scale　A ten-item self-report instrument that inquires about weight fluctuations and concern for dieting. This scale is used to classify subjects as either unrestrained or restrained eaters.

Serotonin　A neurotransmitter that functions in many of the mechanisms of sleep and emotional arousal.

State Measures (e.g., anxiety, self-esteem)　Self-report instruments that ask subjects to complete the questionnaire based on how they are feeling or thinking at the present moment.

Trait Measures (e.g., anxiety, self-esteem)　Self-report instruments that ask subjects to complete the questionnaire based on how they feel or think in general, represents an enduring characteristic in an individual.

Tryptophan　An amino acid that is the precursor for serotonin.

Unrestrained Eaters　Individuals who are not unduly concerned with their weight and/or shape and who do not attempt to control their weight/shape through dietary restriction.

This article reviews the largely negative mental health consequences of **DIETING** in four specific areas: emotional responsiveness, self-esteem, cognition, and disordered eating. Dieting over the life span is discussed along with the effects of certain foods (or lack of certain foods) on mental health. Finally, we examine a healthy eating pattern that is nonhazardous and health-promoting rather than detrimental to physical and mental health.

I. INTRODUCTION

Dieting may be defined as the attempt to restrict one's food intake with the intention of reducing or maintaining one's weight or body size. Thus, any effort to restrict food intake for this purpose, no matter how temporary or how unsuccessful, is considered dieting. One would expect that dieters will lose weight and experience some physiological deprivation as a result of caloric restriction. Indeed, there are people who do successfully lose weight and maintain their thinner physiques. However, successful dieters make up only a small proportion of those who attempt to lose

Encyclopedia of Mental Health
Volume 1

weight. What is more typical is that the dieter loses some weight initially, but finds that the lost weight rapidly returns; often, there is a net weight gain. The body reacts to caloric restriction by adjusting to use less energy (i.e., calories) to run its vital functions. As a result of this drop in metabolism the body retains more calories and promotes weight gain. Up to 95% of dieters regain their weight within 2 years, and as many as 99% of dieters have reached or surpassed their prediet weight within a 5 year period. The dieter will typically attempt another diet in responses to this weight gain. Repeated attempts at weight loss following weight gain (yo-yo dieting) is counterproductive to successful weight loss, and can lead to a variety of health problems.

One study showed that chronic dieters (or restrained eaters) did not lose any weight over a 6-week period, nor had they lost any weight at the 6-month follow-up. In the same study, restrained subjects showed greater short-term weight fluctuations than did nondieters (or unrestrained eaters). These results suggest that attempts to restrain caloric intake are often followed by compensatory eating that cancels out the initial restriction. The typical dieter does not experience a significant overall nutritional depletion. Thus, it is unlikely that physiological deprivation plays a significant role in dieters' daily functioning. Chronic dieting is more likely to be characterized by psychological deprivation (or frustration) than by caloric depletion. Interestingly, new evidence shows that restrained eaters have lower bone density than unrestrained eaters, indicating that chronic dieting negatively affects nutritional status and physical well-being. This area is not widely explored and requires more research.

For the most part, dieting has proven to be an ineffective method of weight loss. Nonetheless, dieting remains widespread in our society. American surveys between 1950 and 1966 reported that 7% of men and 15% of women were trying to lose weight. By 1978, 16% of all adults were dieting, and in 1985, 25% of men and 45% of women were dieting to lose weight. Recently, two large national surveys indicated that approximately 24% of men and 40% of women are dieting at any one time.

Although dieting occurs across the entire life span, it appears that young women are most likely to engage in dieting. As early as 1977, one survey revealed that three quarters of American college women had dieted in an attempt to control their weight. Dieting has been reported by 40% of 18-year-old girls in Sweden, and has been shown to be a well-established behavior in British girls as young as 12 years old. Many researchers have found that for adolescent girls and young women, dieting is more common than not dieting. These statistics indicate that "normal" eating for young Western women is characterized by dieting attempts.

It has been suggested that those who choose to diet may possess certain preexisting psychological characteristics that differ from those who do not become involved in dieting. Future dieters are generally less satisfied with their appearance and are more likely to strive to achieve external ideas. As a result, they are more susceptible to external pressures to achieve the thin ideal and are more likely to diet.

Regardless of any predisposing vulnerabilities, dieting in and of itself can lead to negative mental health consequences. Repeated attempts at restriction in the face of numerous temptations leads to strong feelings of deprivation or frustration. The frustration created from even a temporary caloric restriction can lead to impaired psychological functioning. Specifically, dieting can increase negative emotionality, lead to further deficits in self-esteem, and impair cognitive abilities and the normal regulation of eating.

II. EFFECTS OF DIETING ON MENTAL HEALTH

A. Emotionality

People on diets have been characterized as irritable, dysphoric, and emotionally unstable. Investigations of restrained eating have found positive correlations between restraint (as measures by the Restraint Scale) and measures of depression, social anxiety, stress, neuroticism, maladjustment, and emotional lability. Moreover, laboratory studies have shown repeatedly that chronic dieters report feeling more depressed and anxious than do nondieters. This is sometimes true under normal baseline conditions (i.e., when subjects are asked to complete self-report measures in the absence of any experimental manipulation or provocation) and is intensified after ego-threatening manipulations or events. In a representative series of studies, subjects were assigned to either a control or an anxiety-provoking condition. To create anxiety, the experimenter told subjects that they would be required to present an impromptu speech that would be evaluated by others. As predicted, all subjects reported feeling more anxious in anticipation of having to make a speech. In other words, participants' state anxiety had increased in response to the speech threat. However, the speech threat was particularly effective at creating distress among restrained eaters. Restrained eaters exposed to the speech threat reported higher state anxiety scores than all other groups. An interesting pattern emerged in a study that also assessed trait anxiety. For unrestrained eaters, trait anxiety was unaffected by the speech threat, but speech-threatened restrained eaters reported significantly higher trait anxiety than did unthreatened restrained eaters. Apparently, the speech threat affected the restrained eaters' perception about how they feel in general and rendered them unable to perceive any difference between their present dysphoric state and how they usually feel. [See ANXIETY.]

False feedback about weight has recently been used in the laboratory to manipulate mood in restrained and unrestrained eaters. One study weighed subjects as either 5 pounds heavier or 5 pounds lighter than their actual weight. As predicted, the emotional state of unrestrained eaters was not at all affected by this feedback. For restrained eaters who were weighed to be lighter, there was no significant change. However, when they were weighed to be 5 pounds heavier, the impact was rather dramatic. The restrained eaters who were informed that they had gained 5 pounds reported feeling more upset, disappointed, anxious, nervous, sad, depressed, and guilty than did either the unrestrained eaters or the restrained eaters in the weighed-light condition. Weight gain, whether real or imagined, is thus a source of distress for dieters.

Some researchers have demonstrated that restrained eaters (and overweight people as well) are also more likely to experience extremes in positive emotions. The experience of emotional extremes in dieters may be a consequence of certain predisposing characteristics shared by dieters as a group. Specifically, it has been suggested that dieters are more reliant on their environment and look to external cues to provide them with information about how they should look, act, and feel. This external orientation may account for

the extremes in positive emotions experienced by dieters (e.g., a dieter may think, "This party is a joyous occasion, therefore I feel extremely happy," or, in the case of laboratory studies, "These slides are extremely attractive and positive, therefore I feel happy").

Conversely, dieting itself appears to contribute to negative emotional extremes. Reliance on external cues may have some effect on how the dieter feels, but the frustration associated with dieting also contributes to the negative emotions experienced by dieters. Thus, we would predict that if a psychologically healthy non-dieter were asked to diet, he or she would experience increased negative emotions without corresponding increases in positive emotions. Partial support for this prediction comes from Keys' classic study conducted at the University of Minnesota in the 1940s. In this study, male volunteers were exposed to a 6-month starvation diet in which they ate approximately one half of their usual dietary intake. On a variety of screening tests, these volunteers were found to be physically and psychologically healthy. Over the course of the study, the men experienced depression, outbursts of anger, irritability, anxiety, and apathy. They became progressively more withdrawn, isolated, and less interested in spending time with others. There were no reports of any increase in the frequency or intensity of positive emotions. This study demonstrates that dieting can lead to negativity in psychologically healthy people. One problem with applying these results to dieters in general is that unlike most dieters, Keys' subjects experienced true physiological deprivation and were successful in losing weight. Thus, it becomes impossible to determine how much of the negative affect was produced by psychological deprivation and how much was produced by physiological deprivation. Interestingly, once the study was over, some of the subjects began overeating and initially regained more weight than they had lost.

Another study supports the notion that psychological deprivation leads to increases in negative affect. This 4-month prospective study involved teenaged girls who were not physiologically deprived. The authors attempted to uncover the causal connection between stress, poor psychological adjustment, and dieting behavior. As predicted, dieting was significantly correlated with psychological symptoms and level of stress. More importantly, the authors found that dieting status could predict the degree of stress

4 months later. However, the level of stress or symptomatology was not an accurate predictor of dieting behavior. Taken together, the evidence from these two studies indicates that the negative hyperemotionality experienced by dieters is at least partly a response to the frustration associated with dieting, rather than any predisposition characterological flaw of the dieter.

More significant mental health problems have been reported in the clinical dieting literature. Some studies of dieters undergoing diet treatments have reported serious episodes of depression or anxiety requiring psychiatric intervention and even psychotic episodes necessitating hospitalization. Such severe reactions to weight loss treatments tend to be rare in behavioral treatments but more common in psychiatric, surgical, or jaw-wiring patients. This could reflect either sampling differences or effects of more severe treatments, but there does seem to be a greater risk of psychiatric dysfunction in patients who diet in more drastic manners.

B. Self-Image

Another characteristic associated with dieting is low self-esteem. When people succeed at important tasks they tend to feel better about themselves. On the other hand, when people fail, they generally feel worse about themselves, especially if they fail at a task that they believe is important. We know that dieters usually fail at dieting, and we can safely assume that dieters regard dieting and weight loss as an important part of their lives. There is a pervasive myth in society that people can change their weight and shape if enough willpower is exerted. In reality, this task is not easily accomplished and may be impossible for most dieters. The likely failure of the dieter leads to feelings of inadequacy and worthlessness.

Several studies have examined the emphasis that dieters place on weight and shape. In two recent experiments, subjects were asked to rate the importance of their weight and shape when evaluating themselves as a person. Ratings were made on a seven-point scale, with 1 representing "not at all important" and 7 representing "the most important aspect." Not surprisingly, restrained eaters scored significantly higher than unrestrained eaters on this measure. On average, dieters considered their weight and shape to be as im-

portant to their self-image as most other things in their life. Many dieters saw their weight and shape as being critical, and rated it as the most important aspect when evaluating themselves as a person. Given the importance of weight loss to the dieter, failed weight change attempts can be devastating to the dieter's overall self-image.

A number of studies have shown that dieters report lower self-esteem than do nondieters. This is true for both state and trait self-esteem. (Like anxiety, lowered state self-esteem in restrained eaters has been shown to generalize in the laboratory to lowered trait self-esteem following certain manipulations, i.e., speech threat.) One commonly used state self-esteem scale subdivides total self-esteem into performance, social, and appearance subscales. In most cases, the lower-than-average self-esteem in dieters can be accounted for by the appearance subscale. However, in some circumstances (i.e., speech threat, weighed 5 pounds heavier), restrained eaters' social self-esteem and to a lesser extent their performance self-esteem are also lower than that of unrestrained eaters'. Other studies have found that restrained eaters are also more likely to complete sentence fragments with negative self-referent completions than are unrestrained eaters. Also, restrained eaters have been shown to rate themselves as more ashamed, out of control, bad, passive, unhealthy, lazy, weak, and unattractive than unrestrained eaters. [See SELF-ESTEEM.]

It is possible that having a low opinion of oneself predisposes individuals to be less satisfied with their appearance and makes them more likely to diet. Alternatively, it may be that those who decide to diet and then find themselves failing at each dieting effort may feel progressively worse about themselves, lowering their self-esteem with each dieting failure. Thus, lowered self-esteem could be a precursor or cause of dieting, or it could be an outcome of unsuccessful dieting.

There is no direct evidence to demonstrate that dieters experience lowered self-esteem after dietary failures. However, there is evidence that therapeutic interventions designed to stop dieting behaviors can lead to increased self-esteem. If it is true that each dietary failure produces lower self-esteem, then individuals who undertake chronic dieting may experience a spiral, where each failure at dieting produces greater negative affect and prevents either successful acceptance of one's body or successful weight loss. Clearly, more research is needed to examine the interaction between dieting and self-image.

C. Cognitive Effects

1. General Cognitive Impairment

Some evidence has indicated that dieters experience some impairment in cognitive performance, as evidenced by general distractibility and an inability to concentrate. For example, one study included a demanding vigilance task and an immediate memory task. Compared with nondieters, dieters reported significantly fewer correct responses and displayed slower reaction times on the vigilance task. Dieters also recalled significantly fewer items than nondieters on an immediate free-recall test. Moreover, restrained eaters have also been reported to show impaired performance on less demanding tasks under conditions of high arousal or stress. It has been suggested that the stressful effects of maintaining dietary restraint result in dieters being more easily distracted when performing mental tasks. The effects of chronic stress or anxiety are particularly evident on highly demanding tasks, whereas performance on simple tasks or in situations of low arousal might actually be improved.

2. Preoccupation with Food and Weight/Shape

It would seem reasonable for a dieter to use the following strategy: Avoid thinking about food and focus on your new and improved future body. Thinking about certain qualities of food seems likely to be a trigger for eating. It is commonly believed that dieters stand a better chance of dietary success if they can manage to avoid thinking about food. Weight reduction clinics and the ever helpful "tips to lose weight" section of women's magazines suggest that people distract themselves by reading the newspaper or taking a bath if they start to think about food and eating. However, the difficulty of inhibiting thoughts has been demonstrated in a series of studies. These authors asked some of their subjects not to think about a particular topic (i.e., a white bear) while other subjects were instructed to think about it as much as possible. The subjects asked to suppress the thought wound up thinking about white bears almost half as often as those who were thinking about it as much as

they could. Moreover, suppression of the thought was followed by a rebound effect such that thoughts of white bears increased. The authors concluded that attempted thought suppression has the paradoxical effect of producing a preoccupation with the inhibited thought, which is expressed both immediately by intrusions of the forbidden thought and in a delayed manner by an increase in the thought when the prohibition is lifted. Even when subjects were asked to apply a distraction strategy, they were unable to suppress successfully a simple thought regarding a white bear.

Dieters do not normally think about or encounter white bears in their environment, but they are exposed to food on a daily basis. For dieters, food thoughts are undoubtedly even more difficult to ignore than any thoughts about white bears. When the dieter attempts to suppress a food thought in an attempt to preserve dietary restraint, the thought is likely to emerge eventually into consciousness with even more force and frequency. Restrained eaters often report experiencing intrusive thoughts about food and attempt to suppress these diet-sabotaging thoughts. Once the dieter finally surrenders to food thoughts and decides that restriction is no longer an option, the preoccupation with food becomes overwhelming.

Other evidence of the link between dieting and food preoccupation can be found in reports of disordered eating and in the Keys study. In the Keys study, the dieting male subjects found concentration on their usual activities increasingly difficult. They were absorbed by persistent thoughts of food and eating. Food became a principal topic of conversation, reading, and fantasy. After the study, some participants even changed their occupation to be involved in the food industry. Similarly, anorexia and bulimia nervosa patients have been characterized as preoccupied or even obsessed with food. They exhibit an almost exclusive mental focus on food and food-related matters. This includes what some authors have described as a morbid interest in cooking and providing food for others. [See ANOREXIA NERVOSA AND BULIMIA NERVOSA.]

It has been suggested that attempted weight loss elicits cognitive processes that motivate individuals to seek out food to restore or maintain their weight at the appropriate biological level. Presumably, dwelling on images of food (and of oneself consuming it) stimulants deprived individuals to redouble their efforts to obtain food. Thus, a preoccupation with food is a natural response to deprivation. Attempts to suppress this preoccupation are likely to exaggerate it.

Another common dieting strategy is to focus on the desired goal state—one's thin, beautiful body. Women (and to a lesser extent men) are confronted with an on-slaught of messages from the media indicating that beauty, success, happiness, and self-worth are all predicated on achieving a slender body shape. Media images of unrealistically thin people offer the sugges-tion that it is possible to reshape one's body. This myth produces feelings of failure and frustration in people confronted with these images as they discover that they cannot attain them. However, many dieters con-tinue to expose themselves to fashion magazines and television programs featuring unrealistic, unattainable body shapes. The research on the effects of media im-ages is inconsistent, showing that dieters only some-times report negative affect following exposure to the thin-ideal. Moreover, it is possible that dieters persist in their exposure to media because these images assist their attempts to focus on the desired goal; they still believe they will be able to reach the ideal. Also, diet-ers may temporarily immerse themselves in fantasies about all the wonderful things that will happen once they achieve a smaller or lighter body. For example, dieters may picture themselves wearing the same sexy outfit as the model in the picture, or attracting a ro-mantic partner, or simply achieving overall success and happiness through slimness. It could be argued that this process is adaptive in that preoccupation with a goal can motivate individuals to gather their resources to obtain the desired goal. Unfortunately, a thin physique is not as easy to achieve as the me-dia leads people to believe. Certain body shapes are physiologically and genetically impossible to obtain for most individuals. With this obstacle in place, it is inevitable that the fantasy will eventually give way to frustration.

This progression from fantasy to frustration may explain the conflicting results in the literature regard-ing the effects of exposure to the thin-ideal. Perhaps some type of enjoyment is felt during the fantasy epi-sodes, which may be followed by periods of frustra-tion and strong negative emotions. Some experienced dieters and eating-disordered patients learn that me-dia images cause psychological pain and eventually they forgo voluntary exposure to the thin-ideal. It is

at this point that chronic dieters and eating-disordered patients may switch their strategy from intensely fo-cusing and fantasizing on weight and shape to des-perately trying to suppress their weight and shape thoughts. As a result, they will experience the effects of attempted thought suppression and be invaded by intrusive rebound cognitions related to weight and shape. Thus, depending on dieters' beliefs in their ability to obtain the thin-ideal, their weight and shape cognitions may be either voluntary or intrusive.

3. Selective Attention and Memory

Because restrained eaters spend more time thinking about food and body shape, they process stimuli re-lated to these topics differently than do unrestrained eaters. Specifically, they pay more attention to infor-mation connected to food, eating, weight, and shape. For example, when asked to reproduce an essay about a fictitious person, restrained eaters are more likely to recall eating- and food-related information than neu-tral information, whereas unrestrained eaters do not show this memory bias.

Many investigators have used the Stroop paradigm to study attentional biases in dieters. Subjects are shown words of varying emotional or cognitive sig-nificance and are asked to name the colors the words are printed in; optimal color-naming performance re-quires ignoring the actual meaning of the words. De-lays in color naming occur when the word meaning attracts the subjects' attention despite efforts to attend only to the color of the word. People with full-blown eating disorders show dramatic color-naming delays when words related to food or body shape are used (e.g., chocolate, obese). Studies conducted explicitly on dieters find color-naming delays, only when sub-jects have had their weight concerns primed before-hand by being weighed or by being induced to con-sume high-calorie food. Thus, it appears that chronic dieters demonstrate a memory bias and an attentional bias toward food- and weight/shape-related material.

D. Eating Behavior

Another consequence of dieting is that eating behavior can become disturbed, making the dieter vulnerable to disinhibition and overeating. Dietary inhibition re-quires that one's eating behaviors come under delib-erate control. Thus, according to the requirements of the diet, the dieter decides when to eat, what to eat, and how much to eat. After neglecting physiology in favor of conscious caloric restriction, normal regulation of eating eventually deteriorates. In effect, the dieter has difficulty recognizing and responding to internal hunger and satiety cues. Laboratory research has focused on the disinhibition of restrained eating in a variety of conditions, including forced preloading, distress, intoxication, and weighing subjects heavier than their actual weight.

After being induced to consume a high caloric or forbidden food, dieters become disinhibited and go on to overindulge. This is a pattern that has been reliably demonstrated in "taste perception experiments," in which subjects believe that they are sampling and rating a test food (e.g., ice cream). Subjects are told that the experimenter is interested only in how the ice cream tastes after a preload (e.g., milkshake). The purpose of this deception is to convince subjects that the experimenter is not interested in how much ice cream they eat. For this reason, the ice cream is secretly weighed before and after the "taste perception task." Typically, nondieters behave in a straightforward manner, eating less ice cream after a preload than when not given a preload. This predictable pattern indicates that nondieting individuals compensate for the prior consumption by reducing further intake. By contrast, dieters who have consumed a preload actually eat more ice cream than dieters who have eaten nothing. In fact, preloaded dieters eat more ice cream than all other groups studied. This phenomenon has been labeled *counterregulation,* because the pattern of consumption displayed by dieters runs counter to normal regulation.

Once dieters have eaten something fattening or forbidden, they seem to believe that they have ruined their caloric regimen for the day. This state of violation allows the dieter to overeat and/or eat forbidden foods, and has been termed the "what-the-hell effect." This temporary permission to indulge often leads to excessive, fast-paced eating episodes. Dieters engage in this unrestricted eating with the understanding that they will reinstate their diet at a later time. [See CONTROL.]

A similar pattern emerges after experimental exposure to anxiety. As expected, unrestrained eaters eat less when they are anxious than when they are calm, presumably because of the appetite-suppressing effects of stress on the sympathetic nervous system. However, when restrained eaters become distressed,

they abandon their restraint and indulge in the food that has been provided. Interestingly, the overeating of distressed dieters is provoked more by threats to the ego or self-image, such as failure and performance anxiety, than by actual fear of physical harm. Although ego threats slightly suppress eating in unrestrained eaters, they significantly increase consumption of food by restrained eaters. Related studies have found that clinical depression was associated with decreased appetite and weight loss in unrestrained eaters, but with increased appetite and weight gain in restrained eaters. [See DEPRESSION.]

Although it is not clear exactly why anxiety and other negative affective states led to overeating in dieters, two types of theories—functional and externality—have been proposed to explain this interesting response. On the one hand, *functional theories* claim that distressed dieters actively and purposefully seek out food in an attempt to counteract anxiety. One of the earliest functional theories suggests that eating provides comfort to distressed dieters. A related alternative suggests that eating may serve as a distraction from one's worries. Both the comfort and distraction explanations apply more obviously to dieters than to nondieters, who apparently do not derive enough benefits from eating to use it as a defense against distress. Another proposal suggests that overeating serves a "masking" function for dieters. Rather than dwell on a direct threat to their self-image, dieters put themselves in a position to misattribute their distress to the overeating instead of to the actual threat. This redirection of anxiety is functional because the distress of overeating is usually easier to deal with than the distress arising from more serious threats to one's self-image. Each of these functional explanations maintains that the purpose of distress-induced overeating is to counteract, even if only temporarily, the original distress.

In contrast, *externality theories* suggest that the overeating observed in distressed dieters is an automatic, almost reflexive response to the external orientation created by the distress. It has been suggested that distress makes dieters more externally responsive to environmental cues. For the distressed dieter, prominent food cues gain control over eating, which may easily become excessive. A related theory suggests that the painful self-awareness induced by ego-threat is particularly distressing for dieters, whose self-esteem is low to begin with. Dieters seek to escape aversive self-awareness by focusing their attention on salient external stimuli and immersing themselves in the activities suggested by such stimuli. Should food be salient at the moment, the probability of eating will increase appreciably. Both types of theories account for anxiety-induced overeating in dieters, and attribute the suppressed eating displayed by nondieters to the physiological correlates of anxiety that inhibit hunger.

Laboratory studies of restrained eaters have also identified alcohol as a disinhibitor of eating. However, the disinhibition occurs only when dieters realize that they have consumed alcohol. As with other disinhibitors, alcohol suppresses eating in unrestrained eaters, probably because of the high caloric density of alcohol. Restrained eaters, however, eat diet-maintaining amounts when given a placebo but eat large amounts following actual alcohol consumption. It has been suggest that alcohol may alter the dieter's balance of motivation such that immediate attractions override the delayed gratification involved in diet maintenance.

Another disinhibitor that has recently been studied in the laboratory is the altered-scale manipulation. When unrestrained eaters are weighed as 5 pounds heavier than their actual weight, their eating is unaffected. In contrast, when restrained eaters are weighed as 5 pounds heavier, they eat significantly more than both restrained eaters who have not been weighed and unrestrained eaters in either condition. In this situation, it seems as if dieters are reacting as they do to the forced preload—"I gained 5 pounds, so I might as well indulge" (i.e., the what-the-hell effect). Alternatively, the distress created from this false weight gain could lead restrained eaters to overeat for the same reasons that other sources of distress induce overeating in dieters.

Chronic dieting has often been cited as a contributing factor in the development of binge eating and eating disorders. Dieting and subsequent frustration may alter the dieter's perceptual reactivity to attractive food cues, making them more irresistible. Furthermore, the cognitively regulated eating behavior entailed by the dieter renders the dieter more susceptible to temporary disinhibitions of restraint and consequent binge eating. In addition, both attempted deprivation and distress over their dietary failures may render dieters more aroused and emotionally labile. In vulnerable individuals, dieting can lead to the onset of eating disorders. Although restrained eating does not necessarily lead to an eating disorder, most cases of eating disorders are preceded by dieting. Many authors have related the increased incidence of anorexia nervosa to cultural pressures toward slimness and to the dieting that is believed to be required to achieve this goal. Similarly, bulimia nervosa has been strongly linked to dieting.

III. DIETING ACROSS THE LIFE SPAN

Dieting occurs across the entire life span. For girls, the preoccupation with thinness and dieting often begins before puberty and increases linearly with age, reaching a maximum at around age 18. The number of adolescents who are dieting has increased dramatically over the last three decades. Given the cultural bias toward thinness in women, it is not difficult to see how young girls might believe that losing weight will increase their popularity. Adolescence is a period of social, cognitive, and physical changes that strongly influence the development of body image and weight concerns. Succumbing to external pressures to diet at an early age may predispose the teenager to a lifetime of body dissatisfaction and harmful dietary patterns. In fact, early onset of dieting is a reliable predictor of eating disorder pathology.

The major psychological and physical changes of adolescence require proper nutrition for optimum development. Because most adolescent girls are of normal weight, and are still developing physically and should be gaining weight, trying to lose weight is likely to be an extremely frustrating—not to mention dangerous—endeavor. In comparison with nondieting adolescents, dieters reported more feelings of failure, higher levels of depression and social anxiety, and lower levels of self-esteem. Furthermore, daily life stressors are likely to be increased in dieters who are required to change their lifestyles to maintain their diet (e.g., making up excuses to avoid eating). Indeed, in the prospective study mentioned earlier, it was demonstrated that dieting successfully predicted higher stress levels in teenage girls. In addition to these psychological consequences, there is evidence of physical health hazards as a result of adolescent dieting, especially in those who are not overweight. These hazards include arrested physical growth, amenorrhea, weakness, constipation, and lack of concentration.

There is a marked decrease with age in both weight dissatisfaction and dieting behavior among women. One study on Canadian adults found that the number of normal-weight women who said they would like to weigh less decline sharply with age, dropping from 37% in the 18 to 24 age group to 6% in the 65 to 74 age group. However, the fact that the proportion of women who said they had never tried to lose weight increased with age, suggests that this age-related decline of dieting reflects historical changes in norms for body weight among women in our society rather than a declining concern about slimness with age.

The reasons for dieting may differ with age. One study found that women under 35 years were more likely to state that they dieted for appearance-related reasons rather than for health-related reasons. Those 35 to 44 years old cited each of these reasons in equal proportions. Only at age 45 and above was improving health more likely to be mentioned than attractiveness.

Although the preoccupation with slimness and dieting has traditionally been associated with young women, it has been recently suggested that this preoccupation can also extend to postmenopausal women. These cases include women who have been preoccupied with their weight throughout their lives and women who have acquired the preoccupation late in life, usually after an environmental stressor (e.g., bereavement). Older women (and women and men of all ages) are also at risk of suffering negative psychological (e.g., depression, anxiety) and physical effects (e.g., osteoporosis) as a consequence of dieting.

IV. EFFECTS OF CERTAIN FOODS ON MENTAL HEALTH

In examining the effects of dieting, it is important to consider the effect that starving and eating—and in particular, eating specific types of food—has on emotion and mental health. It has been demonstrated that brain serotonin synthesis can be affected by changes in the macronutrient content of a diet, such that low levels of carbohydrate might produce disturbances in serotonergic function, which might contribute to depression. This suggests that the depression noted in dieters might be at least partly the result of suppressing their carbohydrate intake. To test this hypothesis, a study compared low calorie diets either with or without carbohydrate. No differences in mood or appetite were found based on the nutrient content of the 827 kcal diet provided to these subjects. The authors concluded that carbohydrate-free diets do not depress or elevate mood.

Several other investigators have studied the effect of carbohydrates on mood. An investigation of the effect of the macronutrient content of food on mood attempted to resolve conflicting reports of mood changes during dieting. Half the subjects were assigned to eat a vegetarian diet for 6 weeks, and half were asked to eat a mixed diet (meat and other foods), with both groups instructed to restrict their caloric intake to approximately 1000 kcal per day. The mixed-diet group was asked to eat equal amounts of all foods and to include 500 g of meat or fish each week, whereas the vegetarian group was asked to avoid meat, fish, and poultry, to restrict their intake of milk, dairy products, and eggs to a minimum, and to eat primarily vegetables, fruits, and whole-meal products. Subjects rated their moods daily and kept nutritional diaries. They lost an average of approximately 6.5 kg of body weight. Macronutrient intake changed such that the vegetarian group ate proportionally more carbohydrates during the diet phase, whereas the mixed group ate proportionally more protein during this time. Mood declined significantly for the mixed-diet group, supporting the hypothesis that carbohydrate reduction during caloric restriction contributes to depressed mood.

There is evidence that some subjects, often overweight individuals, crave and consume large amounts of foods containing primarily carbohydrate, whereas others do not. The effect of carbohydrates on mood is different for these two types of individuals. For carbohydrate cravers, eating a high carbohydrate food results in a reduction in feelings of depression; noncravers, on the other hand, report feeling more depressed, as well as more tired. Cravers were also much more numerous than noncravers in the sample tested, suggesting that many individuals are likely to display this responsivity to carbohydrates. It is not clear from this research who is likely to become a craver and who is not, or why.

Another researcher attempted to be more explanatory and argued that protein foods compete for the same receptor sits as serotonin, so that protein consumption reduces levels of serotonin in the brain. Carbohydrates do not compete for these receptor sites, which allows more serotonin to be released, thus alleviating depression and helping to reduce hunger. Carbohydrate craving may thus be the body's method of trying to control both depression and hunger. This combination may create (in our slimness-oriented society) a vicious cycle of overeating carbohydrates, restricting carbohydrate intake to compensate, feeling depressed, craving more carbohydrates, overeating, and dieting again.

An examination of high versus low food-cravers (not just carbohydrate cravers) revealed some differences in both chronic moods and responses to eating. Subjects were likely to feel hungry before they began to crave food. Negative mood and the sensory qualities of food (conditions that make eating likely or imminent) also seem to make cravings more likely. Most of the subjects craved sweet foods (carbohydrates). The authors speculated that cravings, particularly cravings for sweets, may serve a function. Those who reported that they generally indulge their cravings and eat the foods they desire also reported feeling more positive moods in response. The authors recognize the possibility, however, that the positive mood shift reported by these cravers may simply reflect relief from their hunger.

Another group of researchers posited that undereating contributes to the depression seen in dieting and eating-disordered patients. They found that fasting produces depression; even in the absence of low body weight, patients with elevated biological indices of starvation had more depressive symptoms. The authors also compared a vegetarian diet with a mixed-food diet and found that mood correlated with the carbohydrate content of diet and tryptophan levels in the food. Again, it appears that reduced carbohydrate intake leads to dysphoric mood. Others have reviewed the evidence on the link between eating disorders and depression and agreed that starvation and weight fluctuations can cause depression.

A study of the general effect of food showed that for Mexican American males aged 10 to 14, food was most likely to be associated with excitement, energy, and stimulation, especially for subjects with a higher percentage of body fat; for female subjects, food was associated with cravings and pleasure from handling it, particularly for the larger subjects. These non-nutritive uses or effects of food are assumed to influence motivations to eat or even overeat. This accords with the

earlier description of obese patients' responses to food prior to beginning a hospital starvation regimen. Before starvation, all subjects reported that food was the focus of their lives, and many binged. Moreover, eating (even binge eating) produced intense pleasurable affect, and most also said that it relieved anxiety and frustration.

Overall then it appears that the existing literature does not demonstrate a consistent relation between mood and carbohydrate intake. Where a relation is found, it is in the direction of carbohydrate intake leading to more positive mood (or, conversely, lack of carbohydrates being associated with more negative mood).

V. HEALTHY EATING: THE UNDIETING APPROACH

Evidence is mounting that some frustrated dieters may be interested in learning to stop dieting and start eating in response to their bodies' "natural" signals again. Books that attempt to educate readers about the downside of dieting have been selling slowly but steadily and the authors have received numerous requests for more information on ways to stop dieting. A recent dissertation study exploring an educational group approach to helping people to stop dieting drew hundreds of responses. Programs to educate women about the negative effects of dieting and to help them substitute internally driven "natural" eating for cognitively mediated (and easily disrupted) dieting have been developed and tested in the last 5 years. Giving up dieting results in improved feelings about the self (self-esteem, self-efficacy), improved mood, and less disordered eating patterns.

Natural eating entails reeducating the dieter to pay attention to internal signals of hunger and satiety, signals which had to be ignored if the dieter were to diet successfully and eat less than the body demanded. Without these internal cues, dieters have less feedback telling them to stop eating once they have begun and to know when it is physiologically appropriate for them to eat or to refrain from eating. Natural eating involves eating when one is hungry, eating the foods for which one feels hungry, and stopping eating as soon as one is satisfied (not stuffed!).

One way to learn to respond to hunger and satiety

cues is to consume meals and snacks on a regular basis. A rule of thumb is to eat breakfast no longer than one hour after awakening, lunch two to three hours later, and dinner sometime in the early evening. One or two snacks could be incorporated. Meals and snacks should consist of around 2000 calories per day for an average women, or 2700 calories per day for an average man. Eventually the body will start to experience hunger and satiety signals.

Once the dieter is able to recognize hunger and satiety cues, it is important to teach her to ask what it is that she wants to eat when she feels hungry. Dieters who crave a particular food report being less satisfied by other foods, so it seems likely that they will be satisfied sooner if they eat the foods that they want. Psychological deprivation (not being allowed to eat one's favorite foods) may well contribute to the well-documented tendency of dieters to overeat or even binge eat when presented with attractive foods. It is thus important to eliminate this sort of deprivation by including one's favorite foods in one's daily diet.

Learning to stop eating when one is satisfied is probably the most difficult aspect of natural eating. It is often helpful to stop frequently during a meal and reassess one's current level of hunger. It also takes time for satiety cues to build, so this strategy helps to slow down consumption and give satiety signals a chance to become noticeable.

What else can we do to help restrained eaters to eat in a more healthy and natural manner? One alternative is to recognize which dieters should be advised to give up their caloric restrictions and learn to eat a balanced, healthy diet. Those whose weights are within the normal to moderately above normal range, and who are already eating a varied diet are unlikely to suffer medical problems related to weight, and should be so advised. These individuals can be helped to establish a healthy lifestyle incorporating moderate exercise, balanced diet, and no restrictions on any particular food.

Those whose weights are lower than normal, on the other hand, should be educated more vigorously about the hazards of dieting and encouraged to eat and exercise in a healthy manner. For those individuals whose weights fall into the obese range, and show some signs of developing health problems associated with weight, some restrictions of intake may be necessary. Even with obese patients, however, the dangers of psychological deprivation leading to overindulgence must be remembered. These people should be encouraged to increase their caloric expenditure through gradual increments in physical activity, while learning to eat naturally. The goal for all should be a healthy lifestyle that can be maintained indefinitely.

VI. CONCLUSIONS

Individuals who choose to diet soon encounter psychological deprivation that arises directly from attempted food restriction. This frustration leads to aversive consequences such as negative emotionality, lowered self-esteem, impaired cognitive functioning, and disturbed eating patterns. Attempts to restrict one's caloric intake are disrupted by a variety of events, including threats to self-esteem, negative affect, preoccupation with food thoughts, and weight fluctuations. Because dieting actually increases the probability of these events, dieters are destined to engage in disinhibited eating and subsequently fail at dieting. The regular bouts of overeating demand more dieting to offset the effects of the extra calories consumed, and more dieting leads to further disinhibition and overeating. The cycle becomes self-perpetuating, with each failure increasing the negative mental health consequences of dieting. Although dieting occurs throughout the life span, it appears that young girls are particularly at risk for the negative mental health consequences of dieting. Early education regarding the elusiveness of the thin-ideal and the negative consequences of dieting may be crucial in reducing the incidence of dieting. We recommend that most dieters give up dieting and permanently adopt a way of eating that promotes both physical and psychological health.

BIBLIOGRAPHY

Ciliska, D. (1990). *Beyond dieting.* New York: Brunner/Mazel.

Crowther, J. H., Hobfall, S. E., Stephens, M. A. P., & Tennenbaum, D. L. (Eds.). (1992). *The etiology of bulimia: The individual and familial context.* Washington, DC: Hemisphere Publishers.

Fairburn, C. G. (Ed.). (1993). *Binge eating.* London: Guilford Press.

Fairburn, C. G., & Wilson, G. T. (Eds.). (1993). *Binge eating:*

Nature, assessment and treatment. New York: Guilford Press.

Herman, C. P., & Polivy, J. (1991, November). Fat is a psychological issue. *New Scientist, 16,* 41–45.

Polivy, J., & Herman, C. P. (1983). *Breaking the diet habit.* New York: Basic Books.

Polivy, J., & Herman, C. P. (1985). Dieting and binging: A causal analysis. *American Psychologist, 40,* 193–201.

Polivy, J., & Herman C. P. (1987). Diagnosis and treatment of normal eating. *Journal of Consulting and Clinical Psychology, 55,* 635–644.

Rosen, J. C., Tacy, B., & Howell, D. (1990). Life stress, psychological symptoms, and weight reducing behavior in adolescent girls: A prospective analysis. *International Journal of Eating Disorder, 9,* 17–26.

Wegner, D. M., & Pennebaker, J. W. (Eds.). (1993). *Handbook of mental control.* Engelwood Cliffs, NJ: Prentice Hall.

Dissociative Disorders

Richard P. Kluft

Temple University School of Medicine and Harvard Medical School

Amnesia An inability to recall important personal information that is too extensive to be explained by ordinary forgetfulness.

Depersonalization A feeling of detachment or estrangement from one's self, such as a feeling of detachment from one's self, the sensation one is an outside observer of one's body, or a feeling that one is like an automaton or is living in a dream.

Derealization An alteration in the perception of one's surroundings so that a sense of the reality of the external world is lost.

Dissociation A disruption in the usually integrative functions of consciousness, memory, identity, or perception of the environment.

Fugue Sudden unexpected travel away from home or one's customary place of work, with inability to recall one's past.

Identity, Personality State, Alter (synonyms) An entity with a relatively persistent and well-founded sense of self and a relatively characteristic and consistent pattern of behavior and feelings to given stimuli.

Switching Changing from one personality state to another.

Trance The capacity to sustain an attentive, receptive, and intensely focused concentration with diminished peripheral awareness. The more peripheral awareness fades in relation to focused attention, the deeper the trance.

Dissociation and the **DISSOCIATIVE DISORDERS** constitute one of the most compelling and controversial fields of study in the mental health sciences. Dissociation is a failure or a disruption in the usually integrative functions of consciousness, memory, identity, or perception of the environment. Such symptoms and experiences challenge, indeed threaten, one's customary sense of one's self and one's experience. Dissociation includes both phenomena within the normal range, and phenomena that are distinctly psychopathological. Some dissociative manifestations have a relatively universal distribution, while others are more or less culture bound. Recent findings indicate that abnormal dissociative phenomena are most often associated with trauma, overwhelming stress, and/or intolerable intrapsychic conflict. Several distinct dissociative disorders have been identified as discrete conditions, while others are grouped in an overflow category called dissociative disorder not otherwise specified, or are under consideration for adoption, such as dissociative trance disorder. The distinct conditions are dissociative amnesia, dissociative fugue, depersonalization disorder, and dissociative identity disorder (formerly known as multiple personality disorder). Each will be explored in view of contemporary advances. Controversial areas will be dealt with as they arise, with one exception. The complex relationship between dissociation and memory will receive separate discussion.

I. DISSOCIATION

The concept of dissociation appears in the mental health literature as early as the work of Benjamin Rush, but did not rise to prominence until the work of Pierre Janet, who first used the term *désagregation.* Broadly defined, dissociation indicates that two or more mental processes or contents are not associated or integrated in the normally expected manner. Disruptions of the integrative functions of consciousness, memory, identity, or perception of the environment fall under the rubric of dissociation in the *Diagnostic and Statistical Manual of Mental Disorders,* Fourth Edition. Disruptions of motor behavior are included among the dissociative disorders in some other classification systems.

Dissociation has proven an elusive concept to define, and has had different referents in different contexts. Dissociation has been understood as constituting a spectrum of phenomena. Within a normal spectrum are experiences of absorption, focused concentration, meditation, hypnosis, and some mild depersonalization. Within the pathological spectrum are disruptions of memory, identity, consciousness, and perception of the environment and self. Scholars disagree as to whether the normal and abnormal dissociative phenomena are on a single continuum, or whether there are two disjunctive continua.

Dissociation has been used as an explanatory or descriptive concept for a wide array of phenomena, including hypnosis, automatic behaviors, a mechanism of defense, distinguishing certain forms of memory, describing some forms of psychopathology, a number of cognitive phenomena, and to account for many findings in psychology laboratories. In an attempt to move toward clarification, Cardena described several domains of dissociation. In the first, dissociation as nonconscious or nonintegrated mental modules or systems, he includes dissociation as (1) the absence of conscious awareness of impinging stimuli or ongoing behaviors; (2) the coexistence of separate mental systems or identities that should be integrated in the person's consciousness, memory, or identity; and (3) ongoing behaviors or perceptions that are inconsistent with a person's introspective verbal report. It is important to appreciate that dissociation has as well both cognitive and often psychophysiologic aspects. Dissociation allows the segregation of some sets of data from other sets of data in a relatively rule-bound way. Numerous studies of dissociative identity disorder patients demonstrate that both the different identities and the switch process by which one is replaced by another have neuropsychophysiologic correlates.

Dissociation appears to have a series of functions. It automatizes behavior so that some actions and thought processes can occur without direct conscious attention, and hence with increased efficiency. It may permit a form of resolution for irreconcilable conflicts by keeping dissonant issues in different areas or levels of consciousness. Dissociation may allow an escape from reality, giving the illusion of mastery or escape from intolerable circumstances. Dissociation can isolate catastrophic experiences until an individual is better able to integrate them into mainstream consciousness. Dissociation can facilitate cathartic discharge, by putting aside the prohibition against the expression of certain feelings under most circumstances in some cultures.

II. DISSOCIATION AS A RESPONSE TO TRAUMA

Although dissociation may occur spontaneously or in response to deliberate efforts, such as meditation, pursuit of mystical experiences, mediumistic trance, culture-bound rituals and practices, and autohypnosis, and may result from profound intrapsychic conflict, in the modern literature there has been a deep interest in the connection of dissociation and trauma. Reviews of the literature demonstrate that dissociative phenomena have long been associated with the experience of trauma. For example, rape victims and persons experiencing beatings not infrequently see themselves from above, and may even feel sorry for the unfortunate victim of the assault. Combat soldiers not infrequently have considerable amnesia for their actual experience of combat. Survivors of childhood abuse may block out their recollection in whole or in part. Victims of natural disasters commonly experience a variety of dissociative as well as posttraumatic symptoms. [*See* POSTTRAUMATIC STRESS.]

Modern studies have confirmed and expanded upon clinical and anecdotal informations. In a series of studies, David Spiegel and several colleagues studied normal populations exposed to natural disasters such as an earthquake and a firestorm, and the reactions of witnesses to executions. They discovered that dissociative as well as anxiety symptoms are part of the trauma response for many individuals, and that the proximity of exposure to and degree of involvement with the trauma are determinants of the intensity of symptomatology. Dissociative responses to trauma are predictors for the development of posttraumatic stress disorder, and high hypnotizability, a construct different from but in some ways related to dissociation, is associated with chronicity of severe posttraumatic symptomatology. Spiegel observed that dissociative defenses, which allow the compartmentalization of perceptions and memories, both help victims separate themselves from the full impact of trauma while it is occurring, and may delay the necessary working through and putting into perspective of these experiences once they have occurred. They may help trauma victims maintain a sense of control while they are feeling helpless, but then they become a mechanism by which the individual feels psychologically helpless once physical control is reestablished. The short-term assistance afforded by dissociation may, if its mechanism persists in other circumstances, become a major disadvantage.

III. THE SPECTRUM OF DISSOCIATIVE SYMPTOMATOLOGY

Many efforts have been made to describe the wide range of dissociative manifestations. Many are flawed by a failure to distinguish between the phenomenology of dissociation and those of hypnosis. Here only manifestations associated with dissociative psychopathology will be included.

Detachment and/or withdrawal from one's present circumstances can occur when an individual either blocks out awareness of his or her environment, or narrows his or her focus very dramatically to focus on a particular stimulus to the exclusion of the rest of the environment. This is a common symptom in overwhelmed individuals, and constitutes the essential feature of some forms of dissociative trance disorder.

Steinberg has offered a model of dissociation that includes five symptom areas: amnesia, depersonalization, derealization, identity confusion, and identity alteration. Amnesia is the forgetting of personal information that is more extensive than can be explained by ordinary forgetfulness. Typically it takes the form of either (1) the subjective awareness that one has lost or is missing time; (2) appreciation that there are periods of one's life for which one cannot account (e.g., "my memory begins when I was in high school"); or (3) a realization upon reflection or in response to questioning that one cannot recall particular aspects or time periods of one's life. Amnesia is a core phenomenon of all forms of dissociative disorder except some forms of dissociative disorder not otherwise specified and depersonalization disorder. Many consider it the quintessential dissociative symptom.

Depersonalization occurs when one's experience and perception of one's self is disrupted and/or distorted. Those who suffer depersonalization may feel detached from their selves, experience their selves as strange or unreal, feel detached from parts of their bodies and/or their emotions, or may feel like automatons or robots. They may see themselves as if they were watching themselves at a distance, or in a movie. As Steinberg notes, common mild depersonalization occurs as a symptom, is an isolated event or one of a few episodes, and is brief, often seconds to minutes. It often is precipitated by fatigue, stress, sensory deprivation, intoxication, illness, or hypnogogic or hypnopompic states. Transient depersonalization is an isolated symptom occurring in a single episode in response to life-threatening danger or severe psychological trauma. It may last from minutes to weeks. Abnormal depersonalization occurs in a constellation of other psychological symptoms, is persistent or recurrent, and may be chronic and persistent, lasting for weeks to years. It may be precipitated by stress or a traumatic memory, but it persists and recurs in the absence of stressors. While depersonalization occurs in many dissociative disorders, abnormal depersonalization is the essence of depersonalization disorder.

Derealization involves a sense of estrangement or detachment from the environment rather than the self. The environment may be experienced as unreal; familiar locations and others may seem strange and/or unfamiliar. It usually occurs in connection with other dissociative phenomenology. When it occurs in isolation, it is a form of dissociative disorder not otherwise specified.

Identity confusion is a subjective feeling of uncertainty, puzzlement, or conflict about one's own identity. It often is associated with considerable inner turmoil about struggles or even battles over one's identity. It usually occurs with other dissociative symptoms, and is not the core of any particular dissociative disorder.

Identity alteration involves a person's shift in role or identity that is observable by others through changes in a person's observable behavior. Some manifestations involve the use of different names, possession of knowledge or skills for which one cannot account, and the discovery of strange or unfamiliar personal items in one's possession. Identity alteration is often accompanied by episodes of amnesia such that one has no recollection of the out-of-character behavior. It is quite developed in dissociative identity disorder. Identity alteration is an essential aspect of those forms of dissociative trance disorder in which another identity is enacted, and is the cardinal feature of dissociative identity disorder. It is found in many cases of dissociative fugue, and in many forms of dissociative disorder not otherwise specified that closely resemble dissociative identity disorder.

IV. DEPERSONALIZATION DISORDER

Although depersonalization is an extremely common experience and psychiatric symptom, it usually is encountered in connection with other disorders, such as anxiety disorders in phobic patients with panic attacks and agoraphobia, depression, schizophrenia, borderline personality disorder, substance abuse (and withdrawal), seizure disorders (especially partial complex seizures), organic illness, and medication side effects. Depersonalization is experienced transiently by many persons in connection with severe stress or danger. Depersonalization Disorder itself is rarely diagnosed, and has been little studied. Its diagnostic criteria are given in Table I.

Depersonalization disorder is characterized by persistent or recurrent episodes of feeling of detachment

Table I Diagnostic Criteria for Depersonalization Disorder

A. Persistent or recurrent experiences of feeling detached from, and as if one is an outside observer of, one's mental processes or body (e.g., feeling like one is in a dream).

B. During the depersonalization experience, reality testing remains intact.

C. The depersonalization causes clinically significant distress or impairment in social, occupational, or other important areas of functioning.

D. The depersonalization experience does not occur exclusively during the course of another mental disorder, such as Schizophrenia, Panic Disorder, Acute Stress Disorder, or another Dissociative Disorder, and is not due to the direct physiological effects of a substance (e.g., a drug of abuse, a medication) or a general medical condition (e.g., temporal lobe epilepsy).

or estrangement from one's self. The afflicted person may feel detached from his/her body or mental processes, and may feel as if he/she were an external observer of his/her own life and actions, as if he or she were an automaton, or watching a movie of him/herself. Often his/her emotions are numb, with the exception of anxiety and depression, often related to the depersonalization experiences. He/she may feel as if in a fog or trance, have difficulty recognizing him/herself in the mirror, may feel that behavior and emotions are not under his/her control, and may experience body parts as detached or distorted in size or unreal. Others may seem unfamiliar or unreal. Derealization, the sense that the external world is strange or unreal, may be present. Because these experiences often are difficult to describe and understand, the sufferer may be unable or unwilling to communicate them, fearing that they mean that he/she is crazy.

The course of depersonalization disorder is often chronic, marked by remissions and exacerbations. Exacerbations are often associated with stress, subjective, or in response to external events.

A. Epidemiology

Although up to 50 to 80% of the population has experienced depersonalization, and this symptom is found in from 40 to 80% of psychiatric inpatients, depersonalization disorder remains uncommonly diagnosed, and of unknown incidence and prevalence. Many series indicate a 2–4:1 female to male ratio, but these studies antedate modern diagnostic criteria.

Childhood cases have been reported, but most series indicate a mean age at diagnosis of 24 to 27 years. Most cases are diagnosed between ages 15 and 30. The late onset of depersonalization disorder is rare. Neither familial nor cultural factors have been identified. [*See* EPIDEMIOLOGY: PSYCHIATRIC.]

B. Etiology

The cause of depersonalization disorder, like that of depersonalization, remains obscure, with most authorities acknowledging several theories, and some speculating that all models must ultimately affect the temporal lobe and its cerebral connections. Steinberg noted five models: (1) physiologic or anatomical disturbances, as in temporal lobe disturbances, metabolic and toxic states; (2) a "preformed functional response of the brain" adaptive to overwhelming trauma, as in psychiatric disorders and stress responses; (3) defense against painful and conflictual affects; (4) splits between the observing and experiencing ego, so that the patient becomes a detached observer of the self; and (5) when a child is reared in an environment that fails to acknowledge some aspect of the child, who experiences that aspect as not quite real.

C. Diagnosis

The differential diagnosis of depersonalization is complex, and includes a range of medical and psychological disorders. A complete review of records is indicated, as well as a physical examination, a mental status, and perhaps neurological consultation. Screening blood chemistries should include a complete blood count, electrolytes, thyroid studies, chemistries (including liver studies, blood sugar, etc.), and possibly toxicology studies. Electroencephalograms (with nasopharyngeal leads if temporal lobe epilepsy is suspected) and possibly brain imaging studies are indicated.

The baseline mental status examination should be performed, but it is not a good screen for dissociative phenomena. An expanded dissociative mental status may be used. Depersonalization phenomena are inquired after in the Dissociative Experiences Scale (DES), but examination of individual items may be more revealing than the overall score, because depersonalization is only one of the dissociative phenomena it explores. Steinberg's Revised Structured Clinical Interview for the Diagnosis of *DSM-IV* Dissociative Disorders (SCID-D) is an excellent structured interview for dissociative disorders, and has 95% interrater reliability (weighted kappa of .88) for depersonalization items.

In making the diagnosis it should be clear that the depersonalization is in fact severe and symptomatic rather than transient, and is not better explained by some more common mental disorder.

D. Treatment

The treatment of depersonalization per se is the treatment of the underlying disorder. Depersonalization Disorder often proves difficult to treat. Although many therapies have been employed to treat one or more patients with this condition, the literature remains anecdotal, with no approach having achieved wide success. This probably speaks to the diversity of this group of patients, and the diversity of the etiology of their symptoms.

The psychodynamic approach assumes the depersonalization is a defense from low self-esteem, with feelings of worthlessness and helplessness, and with traumatic memories. The origins of these feelings and issues, and of the depersonalization that has resulted, are explored and worked through. The patient becomes able to see that unrealistic expectations are related to these feelings, and more realistic standards, when accepted, can allow the patient's sense of and experience of self to become acceptable.

Cognitive education about the symptoms may be helpful. Behavioral approaches, including flooding, performing aversive tasks when depersonalization occurs, and contingent rewards for symptom absence, have been successful or somewhat successful in studies of one or two patients. Hypnosis may be used to demonstrate to patients how to initiate and control depersonalization experiences. [*See* BEHAVIOR THERAPY; HYPNOSIS AND THE PSYCHOLOGICAL UNCONSCIOUS.]

Some depersonalization has responded to single intravenous administration of amphetamines. Half responded, and half of the responders rapidly relapsed. Tricyclic antidepressants have occasionally been useful, as has fluoxetine in six female patients. Some patients respond to either clozapine or phenazepam.

Patients have also responded to clonazepam. [*See* Psychopharmacology.]

I. Example

A 32-year-old woman sought treatment because she felt no connection with her body and her feelings. She often saw her body as if she were outside of herself, observing her actions as if she were watching a movie of her life. She had no reaction to situations that usually evoked strong emotional reactions. She was terrified that she never would feel again, and planned to kill herself if her situation could not be corrected. She withdrew from all social contacts because she did not know what she really felt about them. In fact, at times she felt that the people in her life had become strangers to her, and doubted if they were real. She experienced her home as having changed and become unfamiliar. Her parents were very controlling, and she was stifled and dependent. Initially doubtful that therapy could help her, she reluctantly accepted fluoxetine, which, at 60 mg/day, offered her much relief, although she still remained uncomfortably symptomatic. She allowed her therapist to recreate her dissociative symptoms with hypnosis, and learned to control many of her symptoms autohypnotically. Then she was able to allow a psychodynamic exploration of the circumstances that led to her becoming symptomatic. As she addressed these inner conflicts and family difficulties, her symptoms became progressively less frequent and less severe. She moved from her parents' home and developed a social life of her own. After having been without depersonalization symptoms for a year, she was tapered off of her medication and she was seen infrequently in follow-up sessions. She retained her gains and made many improvements in her life. After a mild recurrence, she was placed on fluoxetine again, and she was seen for a series of sessions. She has been asymptomatic for a year, maintained on fluoxetine and monthly visits.

V. DISSOCIATIVE AMNESIA

Amnesia is both a symptom of mental disorders and a free-standing mental disorder, dissociative amnesia, in its own right. It is among the diagnostic criteria for dissociative fugue, dissociative identity disorder, somatization disorder, acute stress disorder, and posttraumatic stress disorder.

An inability to recall important personal information is the core feature of dissociative amnesia. What is forgotten is usually traumatic or stressful, and is too extensive to be explained by normal forgetfulness. (Unfortunately, there is no consensus regarding the domain of normal forgetfulness.) The memory impairment is reversible. Autobiographic material cannot be retrieved in a verbal form; if temporarily accessed, it cannot be completely retained in awareness. The most common presentation of amnesia is a retrospectively reported gap or series of gaps of the individual's life history. In some cases, what has been forgotten may manifest itself in nightmares, reenactments, intrusive imagery, and somatoform symptoms. Although acute, florid and dramatic episodes of amnesia, often associated with wartime trauma or natural disasters, may be recognized at once, most patients ultimately given the dissociative amnesia diagnosis did not have their symptoms recognized as such, and may be in treatment an average of four years before the diagnosis is rendered. Diagnostic criteria are given in Table II.

Several subtypes of amnesia are recognized in *DSM-IV*. In *localized amnesia,* there is an inability to recall events related to a circumscribed period of time, usually surrounding a disturbing event. In *selective amnesia,* an individual can recall some, but not all, of the events during a circumscribed period of time. Less common are some other forms. *Generalized amnesia* is a failure to recall one's whole life. *Continuous am-*

Table II Diagnostic Criteria for Dissociative Amnesia

A. The predominant disturbance is one or more episodes of inability to recall important personal information, usually of a traumatic or stressful nature, that is too extensive to be explained by ordinary forgetfulness.

B. The disturbance does not occur exclusively during the course of Dissociative Identity Disorder, Dissociative Fugue, Posttraumatic Stress Disorder, Acute Stress Disorder, or Somatization Disorder and is not due to the direct physiological effects of a substance (e.g., a drug of abuse, a medication) or a neurological or other general medical condition (e.g., Amnestic Disorder Due to Head Trauma).

C. The symptoms cause clinically significant distress or impairment in social, occupational, or other important areas of functioning.

---

nesia involves an ongoing inability to recall events after a particular time, including the present, such that the patient continues to fail to recall events even as they continue to occur. In *systematized amnesia*, there is a loss of memory for certain categories of information, such as memories relating to one's family or to a particular person.

Until Coons' systematic 1992 study, it had been thought that the onset of amnesia was acute, of sudden onset, and that the condition resolved rapidly and rarely recurred. It now is clear that some amnesia is chronic—it involves the loss of large blocks of time and does not resolve rapidly. Furthermore, 24 to 40% have multiple episodes of amnesia. While older studies emphasized dramatic acute amnesias, Coons found 46% had amnesia for recent events, 60% had amnesia for remote events, and 24% had both recent and remote memory loss. Recent amnesias range from minutes to four hours (mean, 1.2 hours). Remote amnesias range from one month to many years (mean, 7.7 years). Remote amnesia is usually selective, but may be generalized.

Dissociative amnesia patients may suffer from a number of other symptoms: depression (84%), headaches (64%), sexual dysfunction (60%), somatization (44%), depersonalization (40%), and many others.

The subjective experience of amnesia may include: blackouts or "time loss"; reports by others of disremembered behaviors; the appearance of unexplained possessions; perplexing changes in relationships; fragmentary recall of one's life history; evidence of unusual fluctuations in skills, habits, tastes, and knowledge; fuguelike episodes; recurrent, unexplained mistaken identity experiences; and brief, trancelike amnesia episodes ("microamnesias"). Not uncommonly, in acute amnesias, there may be a period of confusion before the individual realizes that he/she has suffered a memory loss, and is able to organize his/her understanding of his/her circumstances around that construct.

A. Epidemiology

Many older studies report on amnesia as a symptom rather than dissociative amnesia as it is currently defined. Nonetheless, studies done in civilian academic hospital and clinic settings indicate a prevalence of amnesia as a serious symptom or primary diagnosis in

from 0.26% to 1.8% of cases, while studies of combat veterans have shown a prevalence of 5 to 14.4%, and suggest that the percentage increases with exposure to more severe and sustained combat. These suggest that dissociative amnesia will be more common in populations exposed to massive trauma. Recently Ross and his colleagues examined 1005 randomly selected citizens of Winnipeg, Canada, and followed up half with a structured interview. Seven percent of the interviewees fulfilled criteria for dissociative amnesia. Although it is conceivable that some organic amnesias may have been inadvertently included, this demonstrates that this condition is quite common, and usually goes undiagnosed.

B. Etiology

Although some authorities continue to conceptualize amnesia as malingering, as an artifact of therapy, as a social role designed to escape responsibility, and so on, most experienced scholars and clinicians understand dissociative amnesia to be a basic aspect of the psychobiology of the human trauma response: a protective activation of altered states of consciousness in reaction to overwhelming psychological trauma. Memories, affects, sensations, and cognitions associated with trauma are encoded in an altered state; upon return to baseline conditions, access to this material is blocked in whole or in part. Nonetheless, as noted above, it may covertly influence behavior and mentation.

Profound intrapsychic distress and conflict with or without exogenous trauma may play an etiologic role. Coons described possible precipitants in his series (some cases had multiple precipitants): child abuse (60%); marital trouble (24%); disavowed sexual behavior (16%); suicide attempts (16%); criminal behavior (12%); death of relative (4%); psychotherapy (4%); runaway behavior (4%); unknown (16%). He further noted that his dissociative amnesia patients had a strong history of childhood trauma. Seventy-two percent had childhood trauma: sexual abuse (52%); physical abuse (40%); neglect (16%); abandonment (12%).

Despite contemporary controversy about amnesia for trauma, virtually every systematic study and comprehensive review has demonstrated not only that trauma is extremely prevalent in the history of those with dissociative amnesia, and that studies of traumatized populations consistently document the presence of amnesia among their clinical phenomenology. This is further buttressed by numerous cross-cultural studies demonstrating that dissociative amnesia is a instead, widely-recognized response across cultures to psychological trauma.

As of this writing there is considerable interest in studies demonstrating that there is a distinct psychophysiology to traumatic amnesia, and that there is a decrease in the size of the hippocampus in the brains of combat veterans with posttraumatic stress disorder and survivors of childhood abuse. It remains to be seen whether this line of research will cast further light on the origins and mechanisms of dissociative amnesia. There is also some interest in whether dissociative amnesia is related to the hypnotizability and dissociativity of traumatized individuals.

C. Diagnosis

No particular test or examination can unequivocally demonstrate whether an impairment of memory is organic, malingered, associated with a mental disorder, or some combination of the above. The differential diagnosis of dissociative amnesia includes: dementia, delirium, and amnestic syndromes; discrete memory loss in organic disorders (posttraumatic amnesia, amnesia associated with seizure disorders, anmesia due to psychoactive substances, transient global amnesia); other dissociative disorders; other mental disorders of which dissociative amnesia is a symptom (posttraumatic stress disorder, somatoform disorder, borderline personality disorder, acute stress disorder); malingered amnesia.

Therefore, a comprehensive examination is crucial. It must include a complete history, involving attention to developmental concerns and inquiry about trauma in childhood and adult life. When possible, it is useful to obtain prior medical records and collateral interviews. Assessment must include a complete physical and neurological examination with cognitive testing, and baseline laboratory studies with an electrocardiogram, toxicology, and blood alcohol level. Additional studies may be warranted: dementia workup, electroencephalogram, computed axial tomography, magnetic resonance imaging studies, and neuropsychological studies. On occasion prolonged electroencephalographic monitoring in a specialized teleme-

try unit may be needed to rule out occult seizure disorders. Most situations are relatively straightforward unless there are superimposed organic and psychogenic components. The relatively new Structured Clinical Interview for *DSM-IV* Dissociative Disorders–Revised is a useful diagnostic approach.

D. Treatment

Treatment is facilitated by using a triphasic trauma therapy model. Herman speaks of a phase of safety followed by a phase of remembrance and mourning, and finally a phase of reintegration. The first stage attempts to make the individual safe, offers stabilizing interventions, and builds his or her strength as a therapeutic alliance with the clinician is formed. In the second, if it has been possible to achieve the goals of the first, the disowned material is accessed and processed. Then the patient is helped to reintegrate him or herself, and to reconnect with life, moving the patient beyond the focus on trauma into a renewed life.

The therapy never is simply a matter of "getting out the trauma." The stressors that are powerful enough to sever the continuity of autobiographic memory are not simply the events or conflicts themselves. Overwhelming affects and the personal meaning of the trauma reinforce the persistence of the amnesia. Despair, grief, guilt, shame, self-hatred, helplessness, and terror often play powerful roles. Furthermore, the events shrouded by amnesia may have caused profound shifts in the patient's view of him/herself and others, and his/her view of the world. The meaning of the trauma and the amnesia for it must be explored and addressed in order to prevent the patient from remaining symptomatic.

Uncovering efforts always must be undertaken cautiously, and paced carefully, with a profound respect for the patient's vulnerability. While usually recent amnesias can be resolved in short order, more chronic amnesias with childhood onsets must be approached with extreme circumspection. Some such patients can be retraumatized and destabilized if efforts to overcome amnesia are too hasty.

If a supportive environment can be established in the treatment of recent acute amnesia, often spontaneous remission of the amnesia will occur, the material will return in the course of history taking or treatment, or permissive suggestions that memory recovery will occur when the patient is ready, and at a pace that the patient can tolerate, will be successful. With more chronic situations, it often is more important to establish a more long-term therapy that addresses the sequelae of whatever led to the amnesia. Such patients are often at considerable risk for self-harm, self-destructive relationships, alcohol or substance abuse, and so on, as the treatment continues. Some hospital stays may prove necessary for restabilization or to address difficult issues in a safe environment. Uncovering dissociated memories may be contraindicated for patients with instabilities in their ego strength, personal circumstances, or therapeutic alliance.

The use of hypnosis and drug-facilitated interviews have a venerable history in the resolution of dissociative amnesia. However, it is appreciated that many procedures designed to enhance the recovery of memory may also lead to the recovery of confabulated memories that the patient will subjectively experience as genuine and compelling. Therefore, in any circumstance in which a patient may be involved in legal proceedings, it is essential to withhold their use prior to assessing the implications of such interventions, lest the patient be considered to have had his/her memory distorted by these processes, and be compromised as a witness to his/her own circumstances.

If there is no contraindication, hypnosis may be used to contain and titrate the experience of distressing symptoms, facilitate the recovery of memories in an orderly and titrated manner, offer ego-strengthening to the patient, and assist in the processing and integration of dissociated material. Permissive amnesia can be suggested for material that emerges prematurely or precipitously. Drug-facilitated interviews often can lower the inhibitions and defenses of the dissociative amnesia patient. Often the amnesia created by the barbiturate chemicals usually used allows revelations to be made without the patient's recalling the revelation. Such sessions are best taped or videotaped.

I. Example

A woman in her late twenties was admitted to a general hospital unit, acutely depressed. She had amnesia for a period of approximately 2 hours of the previous evening. She had gone over to her fiance's home planning to finalize some details of their upcoming wedding and returned home much earlier than she was expected. She went to bed with a severe headache, and awakened the next morning suicidally depressed. Antidepressants and suicide precautions were begun. Medical and neurological workups and lab studies were normal, and an electroencephalogram was unremarkable. Her depression had come "out of a clear blue sky," with no antecedent psychobiological changes or known stressors. Her psychiatrist worked to establish a warm supportive relationship with her, and was successful in making her feel safe and cared about. On the third hospital day he happened to inquire about her visitors. When she sadly observed that her fiance had not come to see her, the psychiatrist began to inquire about their relationship. She became acutely upset, and began to strike her head with her fists, shouting "No!" repeatedly. The psychiatrist took her hands to prevent self-injury. After about 15 minutes of screaming "No!" and trying to attack herself, she collapsed, sobbing. Several minutes later she was able to whisper that she had just remembered that when she had gone to visit her fiance, she had found him in the company of a mutual female friend. Her lipstick was smudged and her blouse had been hastily and incorrectly buttoned. Confronted with clear evidence that her fiance had been with this other woman, she left, not having said a word. In therapy sessions it was discovered that her sense of shame and rejection (the wedding date was near, wedding invitations had already been printed) had generated an incredible rage in which she experienced strong homicidal urges, which were completely alien to her character. These had been turned against herself, a character style of the patient's, and the overwhelming experience and its profound implications for her life had been dissociated. Only the depression remained accessible to the conscious mind. After ventilating her grief and outrage, and making a safety contract not to harm herself or others, she was transferred to outpatient treatment.

VI. DISSOCIATIVE FUGUE

The essential feature of dissociative fugue is sudden unexpected travel away from one's home or one's customary place of work, with an inability to recall one's past (Criterion A). There is either confusion about one's personal identity or the assumption of a new identity, either partial or complete (Criterion B). The diagnostic criteria are given in Table III. The travel and identity alteration may be brief, running its course in hours or days, with a minimal amount of travel.

Table III   Dissociative Fugue

A. The predominant disturbance is sudden, unexpected travel away from home or one's customary place of work, with inability to recall one's past.

B. Confusion about personal identity or assumption of a new identity (partial or complete).

C. The disturbance does not occur exclusively during the course of Dissociative Identity Disorder and is not due to the direct physiological effects of a substance (e.g., a drug of abuse, a medication) or a general medical condition (e.g., temporal lobe epilepsy).

D. The symptoms cause clinically significant distress or impairment in social, occupational, or other important areas of functioning.

However, it may continue for weeks, months, or even years, and involve a complicated pattern of travel extending over thousands of miles and many national boundaries. Usually both the onset and recovery are rapid and sudden, and often the recovery occurs upon arising from sleep. Recurrences once were thought rare, but it is clear that some patients who suffer dissociative fugues may have recurrences, and many have other dissociative symptoms at other points in time. Most fugues do not involve the formation of elaborate alternate identities. When a new identity is formed, it often but not inevitably is more gregarious and uninhibited than was the baseline identity. This expectation may be based on the sociocultural aspects of the societies in which famous classic cases were discovered. The person may assume a new name, establish a new domicile, and develop a complex set of activities that appear well integrated. There may be no hint of mental illness. However, considerable agitation and distress may accompany the recovery of the baseline identity, coming to grips with the lost time and the behaviors attributed to the person in his/her alternate identity and/or the period for which he/she was amnestic, and the reactions of those effectively abandoned by the patient during the fugue.

Often fugues occur in stressful situations in which remaining in one's baseline identity and occupation involves real risk and danger, such as in military settings.

A. Epidemiology

It is virtually impossible to use older studies as a guide, because the boundaries between the dissocia-

tive and posttraumatic states with amnestic symptoms are not clearly drawn. In a modern study using *DSM-III-R* criteria, Ross and colleagues found that approximately 1% of a nonpatient population acknowledged the symptoms of dissociative fugue on a structured interview. However, many times reports of fugue behavior ultimately is attributed to an underlying dissociative identity disorder; this may be an overestimation. There is general consensus that dissociative fugue is relatively uncommon compared to dissociative amnesia and dissociative identity disorder, and that it appears to be more common in war, natural disasters and in other settings in which violence and extreme social disruption are common.

B. Etiology

The same factors that are associated with dissociative amnesia are relevant. In addition, the literature is divided as to the relevance of individual psychopathology and difficult family backgrounds. Dissociative fugue often occurs under circumstances that raise a suspicion of malingering, because the fugue may appear to reduce accountability, responsibility, or exposure to danger (such as evading combat). Psychodynamic factors often appear more relevant than trauma per se. Many patients with fugues have intense separation anxiety, suicidal or homicidal impulses, and primitive denial. Furthermore, many fugues have the quality of wish fulfillments. Many fugues begin in association with fatigue, sleep, or sleep deprivation; some observe that heavy alcohol use may be a predisposing factor.

C. Diagnosis

The approach to diagnosis is similar to that for dissociative amnesia. It is useful to recall, however, that in the middle of a dissociative fugue, if the patient has developed another identity, he or she may not have either an awareness of the past or an awareness of amnesia for the past. Consequently, they may be without symptoms or distress, and are unlikely to come to the attention of the mental health professions. When they revert to their former identities they can become very distressed over their amnestic gaps and their circumstances. Malingering is often in the differential diagnosis, because many individuals in fugues leave situations that it would be desirable to leave for one's own safety or benefit.

D. Treatment

The approach to treatment is similar to that for dissociative amnesia; when alternated identities are encountered, approaches similar to that for dissociative identity disorder may be useful. However, there may be considerable real world consequences associated with the life the person has led while in an alternate identity or a confused state, and these must be addressed. Often there are considerable issues with guilt and shame.

In the unusual circumstance that the patient is still in a fugue when treated, one must recover information about the baseline identity, learn what led to its being abandoned, and facilitate its restoration. When the patient is encountered after having returned to the baseline identity, both the amnesia and the alternative identity (if it persists covertly) must be addressed.

I. Example

The friendly and outgoing 32-year-old assistant manager of a fast food restaurant retired to his office saying he was beginning to feel "weird," and planned to take a nap. When a coworker went to check on him a few minutes later, he found the manager in an agitated state, wondering what he was doing there. When addressed by the name by which he was known, he corrected the coworker, claiming a different first name and a slightly different last name as his own. He claimed to be a fireman in a large city several states away. He thought the date was 3 months earlier than the calendar date. Having returned home, he entered psychotherapy. His psychiatrist learned that this man was known as a worried, fretful, and anxious but contained man, socially inhibited, but as a fireman, willing to take risks and highly regarded for his bravery in difficult situations. Under hypnosis, it emerged that his counterphobic behavior covered over a deeper pervasive insecurity. On the last shift before he vanished, he and a new firefighter had been briefly trapped in a dangerous situation that he had decided to enter. A roof had fallen in, injuring the rookie firefighter and narrowly missing the patient. He had been terribly frightened, and guilty that he had exposed the rookie to injury. He began to have profound uncertainty and insecurity. He suffered several panic attacks. However, he determined to continue his work and to disregard his concern. When he next drove to the station, he instead wound up several hundred miles away, and

began an alternative life. Hypnosis never succeeded in obtaining more than a patchy recollection of the missing time period, and never could access any trace of the alternative identity under which he had lived. Psychotherapy helped him discover the sources of his insecurity and need to prove himself strong and brave over and over again. He found a different career and had no recurrent difficulties.

VII. DISSOCIATIVE IDENTITY DISORDER

Dissociative identity disorder is a chronic complex dissociative psychopathology characterized by disturbances of memory and identity. Its manifestations are often polysymptomatic, pleiomorphic, and fluctuating. Often in the course of its natural history there are periods in which the condition is apparently latent and can only be diagnosed by history, and often the overt manifestations fall short of dissociative identity disorder criteria, and the condition's phenomenology is more appropriately described as dissociative disorder not otherwise specified.

The essential features of dissociative identity disorder are the presence of two or more distinct identities or personality states that recurrently take control of the patient's behavior, accompanied by amnesia. The diagnostic criteria are presented in Table IV. This condition demonstrates a failure to integrate identity, memory, and consciousness. The personality states may vary considerably in their degrees of awareness of the existence, activities, and thoughts of one another. They may also differ considerably in their de-

Table IV Diagnostic Criteria for Dissociative Identity Disorder

A. The presence of two or more distinct identities or personality states (each with its own relatively enduring pattern of perceiving, relating to, and thinking about the environment and self).

B. At least two of these identities or personality states recurrently take control of the person's behavior.

C. Inability to recall important personal information that is too extensive to be explained by ordinary forgetfulness.

D. The disturbance is not due to the direct physiological effects of a substance (e.g., blackouts or chaotic behavior during alcohol intoxication) or a general medical condition (e.g., complex partial seizures). Note: In children, the symptoms are not attributable to imaginary playmates or other fantasy play.

gree of elaboration and distinctness. Each personality state has its own identity, self-representation, autobiographical memory, and sense of ownership of its own activities. Separate names are commonly, but not inevitably present, and often are more a title than a name (e.g., "The Evil One," "Rage," "Mother," etc.). Modern studies indicate that female patients have, on the average, from 16 to 18 alters, while males average approximately 8. Patients with very large numbers of personalities have been described. Approximately half of contemporary cases have 10 or fewer identities.

The personalities are not separate people. In many ways it is more accurate to understand the dissociative identity disorder patient as deprived of a single identity than as in possession of many identities. All of the personality states and their interaction constitute the patient's personality in the conventional use of the term; i.e., the dissociative identity disorder patient's identity is to have multiple identities. Although the dramatic differences across the personality states often are the focus of curiosity about this condition, it is actually their common feature of being alternative ways of adapting to difficult circumstances that is more central.

Usually the primary identity that carries the legal name is depressed, constricted, guilty, and somewhat masochistically passive. The alternate identities often have different names and contrasting characteristics. They commonly are represented as emerging in response to particular circumstances and/or stressors, and may differ in reported age, gender, knowledge, coping style, dominant affects and concerns, and so on. They not infrequently contain an inner world of alters that replicates significant aspects of the intrafamilial and/or interpersonal aspects of the patient's childhood circumstances. Typically, but not inevitably, the system of personality states will include parts designed to cope in general and with specific circumstances, parts based on abusers, parts based on real or wished-for protectors, and parts that hold the memory and experience of traumatic experiences. In complex cases personality states may be created to hold specific traumata and very specialized skills.

Not infrequently the inner world of the personalities, in which they are imagined to interact, has a subjective reality equally or more compelling than the external world. In this world, the personality states are experienced as having complex relationships, involving both enmities and alliances of various sorts. On occasion, the patient can mistake what has occurred in his or her inner world for what has occurred in the outer world, and vice versa.

The personality states may take control to take advantage of one another, may make critical comments on one another (heard as internal voices), and may be in open conflict, sometimes so intense that one tries to kill the other, often inflicting harm on the body with the misapprehension that thereby they will kill the other, but not themselves. Their degree of conviction of their being genuinely separate may be intense enough to be considered delusional.

Gaps in memory for both recent and remote events is characteristic. Often the amnesia is asymmetrical; that is, part A has a far greater degree of memory for the actions of part B than part B has for the actions of part A. Typically protective alters and alters that are identified with aggressors have more extensive memories. Some patients have personality states that have the role of maintaining a reasonably continuous memory, for the whole life or for some period of life.

Although personality states' influences are most obvious when they actually take overt control, it is more common for them to influence from behind the scenes by producing hallucinations such as a voice giving instructions, or by imposing a feeling, thought, or action that is felt as an unwilled intrusion by the personality ostensibly in charge of the body at the time.

The personality states take control from one another in response to psychosocial stressors, particular circumstances, or inner arrangements or conflicts among the personality states. The transfer of control need not be complete—situations in which more than one personality state is out and/or influencing behavior ("copresence") are commonplace. The process of transition, or "switch" phenomenon, may occur within seconds or less, but, it may occur gradually. When there is conflict between the personality state in apparent control with the effort of another personality state to emerge, the switch may be accompanied with much agitation and discomfort, and, not infrequently, headaches and physical gestures indicating conflict or distress (psychomotor agitation, facial features and expressions showing the two states in fluctuating degrees of presence, hands raised to the face, and expostulations, etc.).

Dissociative identity disorder patients commonly have many depressive, somatoform, and posttraumatic symptoms (such as nightmares, startle responses, and flashbacks). Self-mutilation, suicide attempts, and, less frequently, aggressive behavior, may occur. Numerous anxiety symptoms are common. Substance abuse, sexual dysfunction, conversion symptoms, eating disorders, and sleep disorders may cooccur. Many times the abusive relationships of their childhood are repeated in chronic experiences of revictimization. These patients are highly hypnotizable as a group, and have many capacities associated with this talent, such as the capacity to block out pain, and to hallucinate and to negatively hallucinate (e.g., to not see what is before them). Their many difficulties often lead to the picture of borderline personality disorder, but sophisticated psychological testing indicates that for most patients, the superficial picture of borderline features is not matched by a borderline structure.

A. Epidemiology

Long considered rare, apocryphal, or iatrogenic, it now is clear that dissociative identity disorder is a relatively common condition, and that often its features are clearly apparent long before the diagnosis is made and treatment begun. Two types of studies have been done to assess its contemporary prevalence—studies of clinical populations and studies of nonpatient populations. Studies in the United States, Canada, the Netherlands, and Norway have used screening tests such as the Dissociative Experiences Scale to screen inpatient psychiatric populations from which known dissociative disorder patients have been excluded. They studied patients with screening test scores that suggested the possibility of a dissociative disorder with structured interviews such as the SCID-D or DDIS. These studies indicate that between 3 and 5% of psychiatric inpatients have previously undiagnosed dissociative identity disorder. Similar studies of partial hospitalization and drug treatment settings have identified an even higher prevalence. Ross and his colleagues have studied a stratified sample (1055 persons) of the population of Winnipeg, Canada, with the Dissociative Experiences Scale, and followed up as many as possible (43%) with DDIS interviews. They concluded that 3.1% fulfilled criteria for dissociative identity disorder. However, they determined that only approximately 1% were actually clinical dissociative identity disorder patients. It is unclear whether this reflects problems with the instrument or the diagnostic criteria, whether there

are nonpathological endogenous forms of dissociative identity disorder, or whether patients remaining completely amnestic for childhood abuse were less symptomatic.

In modern clinical studies dissociative identity disorder is most commonly discovered in women among adult populations, at a ratio of 8 to 9:1 in most studies. However, among children the gender distribution is close to 1:1. It remains unclear whether females are harder to diagnose among youngsters and males among adults, or whether gender differences in adults seeking and remaining in treatment plays a role in this discrepancy. Many speculate that many males with this disorder enter the legal rather than the mental health treatment system, but there is no hard data to demonstrate this. [*See* GENDER DIFFERENCES IN MENTAL HEALTH.]

Although the average age at diagnosis is in the early-to-mid 30s, this condition has been identified in patients ranging from 3 years to over 80 years of age. Much remains to be learned about its recognition in various age groups.

B. Etiology

Many models for the development of dissociative identity disorder have been offered. Kluft noted 11 basic models: (1) supernatural/transpersonal; (2) psychological; (3) sociological; (4) role-playing/malingering/iatrogenesis; (5) trance state/autohypnotic; (6) split brain/hemispheric laterality; (7) neurologic (temporal lobe/complex partial seizures/kindling); (8) behavioral states of consciousness; (9) neural network or memory/information processing; (10) neodissociation/ego states; and a (11) basic affects model. None essentially precludes the operation of another, and none explains dissociative identity disorder rather than illustrates a potential possible mechanism.

Generally it is agreed by those who perceive dissociative identity disorder as a naturalistically occurring disorder that dissociative identity disorder occurs in connection with a child's being overwhelmed, usually repeatedly, and often by abuse. Those who dispute its legitimacy and/or dispute its origin in the context of childhood trauma emphasize the importance of an iatrogenesis model. As of this writing, the iatrogenesis hypothesis is a matter of opinion rather than a proven fact. However, a number of studies have documented that most patients who develop dissociative identity disorder were indeed abused. Surveys that accept the patients' accounts as data report childhood abuse in the histories of up to 97 or 98%. Studies that document abuse or investigate abuse allegations have documented abuse in 95% of children and adolescents and in up to 85 to 89% of adults. [See CHILD SEXUAL ABUSE.]

Kluft's four-factor theory holds that dissociative identity disorder occurs in (factor 1) a dissociation-prone child (a biological capacity) who experiences (factor 2) overwhelming stressors that cannot be managed with nondissociative defenses. While child abuse is the most frequent stressor in North American studies, this may not be universally the case. Exposure to death, vicarious traumatization (by witnessing the intentional or accidental death or mistreatment of others), the loss of significant persons, cultural dislocation, dysfunctional family pressures (often in the context of divorce), childhood illness and injury, and repeated childhood surgeries have been cited as instrumental overwhelming stressors as well.

The child makes use of (factor 3) various shaping influences and substrates to form the kernel of the various alters. These may include life experiences and crucial persons in the child's life space (via introjection, internalization, and identification), imaginary companionship, developmental lines, extrinsic interpersonal influences from childhood (encouragement of role-playing and acting, contradictory caretaker demands or reinforcement systems, or identification with a dissociative parent) and from contemporary sources (previous therapy, the media and literature, errors in technique, autohypnotic coping). Finally, the situation is reinforced by (factor 4) the inadequate provision of stimulus barriers and restorative experiences by significant others. This approach to etiology is consistent with clinical experience.

C. Diagnosis

Numerous studies demonstrate that on the average dissociative identity disorder patients have been in treatment for just under 7 years before their condition is diagnosed, and have received over three inaccurate or comorbid diagnoses before it is recognized. Most standard mental status and interview schedules are not constructed to make adequate inquiry about the dissociative phenomena that play a role in the phenomenology of dissociative identity disorder. This is especially problematic because many of its manifestations are subtle and covert much of the time.

Until the last few years it had been customary to make inquiries about signs suggestive of dissociative identity disorder. These include: (1) prior treatment failure; (2) three or more prior diagnoses; (3) concurrent psychiatric and somatic symptoms; (4) fluctuating symptoms and levels of function; (5) severe headaches and/or other pain syndromes; (6) time distortion, time lapses, or frank amnesia; (7) being told of disremembered behaviors; (8) others noting observable changes; (9) the discovery of objects, productions, or handwriting in one's possession that one cannot account for or recognize; (10) the hearing of voices (80% experienced as within the head) that are experienced as separate, urging the patient toward some activity; (11) the patient's use of "we" in a collective sense and/or making self-referential statements in the third person; (12) the eliciting of other entities through hypnosis or a drug-facilitated interview; (13) a history of child abuse; and (14) an inability to recall childhood events from the years 6 to 11.

Recently Loewenstein published a special mental status that makes inquiry about six areas of symptomatology commonly demonstrated in dissociative identity disorder patients: (1) indications of the dissociative processes at work (e.g., differences in behavior, linguistic indications, switching; (2) signs of the patient's high hypnotic potential (e.g., enthrallment, trance logic, out-of-body experiences); (3) amnesia; (4) somatoform symptoms; (5) posttraumatic stress disorder symptoms; and (6) affective symptoms.

Many clinicians ask directly to meet an alter if they have reason to believe that dissociative identity disorder is present. Other strategies involve: (1) asking the patient to journal for 20 to 30 minutes a day, because other personalities may make entries; (2) extending the interview to 2.5 to 3 hours, because often spontaneous dissociation will be observed. At times the use of hypnosis or drug-facilitated interviews is warranted and useful.

The most modern strategy involves the use of structured diagnostic interviews if either there are clinical indications that dissociation may be present of if a screening test of dissociation, such as the Dissociative Experiences Scale indicates the need for further assessment. Clinicians generally use a score of 20 or more as suggestive, while researchers recently have advocated a score of 30. Two structured interviews are available, the Dissociative Disorders Interview Schedule (DDIS) of Colin Ross, and the Structured Clinical Interview for *DSM-IV* Dissociative Disorders–Revised (SCID-D-R) of Marlene Steinberg. The DDIS involves an array of forced choice questions that permit the interviewee to endorse the symptoms of many psychiatric disorders (including the dissociative disorders), the experience of abuse, and many symptoms associated with dissociative identity disorder. It takes from 45 to 75 minutes to administer. The SCID-D-R is a semistructured interview allowing the clinician considerable discretion and at times several options. It may take from 45 minutes to over 2 hours to administer. It includes items of observation made during the interview. Amnesia, depersonalization, derealization, identity confusion, and identity alteration are rated. Dissociative identity disorder patients generally score 3 or above in each category (although derealization may be weak), for a score of from 15 to 20. Both instruments are highly sensitive (over 90%) and have few false positives. The DDIS makes wider inquiries and asks for some history; the SCID-D-R gives a much richer and more comprehensive portrait of the patient's experience of his or her disorder.

D. Treatment

A curious dichotomy pervades writing on the treatment of dissociative identity disorder. On the one hand, experienced clinicians have developed a form of therapy that has resulted in many successful outcomes. On the other, those skeptical of the condition's legitimacy fulminate against that treatment, and maintain it has the potential to create and/or worsen it. They opine that it should be treated by nonreinforcement of the dissociative psychopathology and by focusing on contemporary problems of living. The compelling weight of evidence is that dissociative identity disorder is a naturalistically occurring disorder that responds better to specific therapy for dissociative identity disorder than nonspecific therapy or a regimen of nonreinforcement and redirection. However, it is also clear that many patients have not prospered in specific treatments that were inattentive to their particular vulnerabilities and needs. The treatment of this group of patients must be individualized thoughtfully.

Ideally, the treatment should address alleviating the problems of identity and memory; that is, they should attempt to bring the patient to a subjective sense of a unified identity by integrating the personality states, and amnesia should be relieved by achieving a confluent identity in the here and now, and by uncovering amnesia for past events. It is understood that what is uncovered in the treatment of the traumatized may not consist exclusively of material that is historically accurate and can be verified. Considerable controversy surrounds the nature and accuracy of traumatic memory. Some authorities hold that it is reconstructive and unreliable, while others hold that it involves both retrieved and reconstructive elements. Some demonstrations of the recovery of verifiable memories have been published, which appear to have only minor reconstructive elements. However, regardless of this controversy, which remains unresolved, it is understood that processing the mind's representation of its past appears essential to the achievement of an integrated identity and memory.

While the unification of the dissociative identity disorder patient is the optimal goal, it is only one aspect of the treatment of a suffering individual, and may have a lower priority than other goals in many treatments, and even at many times in a treatment that is attempting to pursue integration. Integrationalist therapies set as their goal the integration of the individual in the course of resolving problematic symptoms and difficulties in living. Personality-focused therapies attempt a problem-solving approach among the personality states, which are encouraged to collaborate more harmoniously without necessarily ceding their separateness. Adaptationalism focuses primarily on managing here-and-now difficulties and maximizing function. Although a vocal minority of therapists and many patients oppose working toward integration, as of this writing, it appears that the long-term stability of integrated patients is superior to that of patients who do not integrate.

The triphasic approach to the traumatized patient, described above, applies to the treatment of dissociative identity disorder. The stages of the treatment of dissociative identity disorder (Table V) are consistent with this model. Stages 1 to 3 are consistent with the phase of safety, stage 4 is consistent with the phase of remembrance and mourning, and stages 5 to 9 are consistent with the phase of reconnection. In practice, the stages discussed below as if they were discrete blend into and overlap with one another. For ex-

Table V   The Stages of the Psychotherapy of Dissociative Identity Disorder

---

1. Establishing the therapy
2. Preliminary interventions
3. History gathering and mapping
4. Metabolism of the trauma
5. Moving toward integration/resolution
6. Integration/resolution
7. Learning new coping skills
8. Solidification of gains and working through
9. Follow-up

---

ample, some identities may have integrated before others have even been discovered.

Establishing the psychotherapy involves the creation of an atmosphere of safety in which the diagnosis can be made and confirmed, the security of the treatment frame can be established, the therapeutic alliance is begun, the patient is informed of the nature of the treatment, and sufficient hope and confidence is established.

Preliminary interventions involve gaining access to the more readily reached personality states; establishing contracts against terminating treatment prematurely, self-harm, suicide, and so on; fostering communication and cooperation among the alters; expanding the therapeutic alliance; and maximizing symptomatic relief safely. New coping skills are taught, many of which may involve hypnotic or auto-hypnotic methods, in order to help the patient deal with intrusive traumatic material, calm unsettled personality states, and recover his/her equilibrium.

In *history-gathering and mapping* one learns more about the personality states, their origins, and their relationships to one another. The inner world of the personalities is clarified. Working with this enhanced knowledge, further efforts are made to deal with the personality states' issues and interactions, and to gain more cooperation and collaboration.

Without achieving the goals of these first three stages, it is not advisable to proceed to *metabolism of the trauma*, which involves accessing and dealing with the overwhelming events alleged to be at the sources of the dissociative identity disorder. A precipitous and/or premature entry into this work is often associated with the decompensation of the patient. Patients who cannot achieve the goals of the stages prior to metabolism of the trauma should remain in a supportive and preliminary therapy that builds ego strength and focuses on adaptational and personality-oriented issues. Integration should not be pursued.

When a patient is able to move into the trauma work, this work should be done in a very circumspect, cautious, and gradual fashion. Even in this stage, trauma work should not be the focus of every session, and care is given to restabilize the patient as much as possible at the end of each session. Some personality states will integrate spontaneously in this process.

Moving toward integration/resolution involves working through the traumatic material across the personality states and facilitating still further cooperation, communication, mutual identification, and empathy among them. At this stage often the personality states may show signs that their identities are fading or blurring.

Integration/resolution consists of the patient's coming to a new and more solid stance toward both self and the world. Integration is the blending of the personality states into a unity. Resolution is a smooth collaboration among personality states that retain their separateness.

Learning new coping skills involves appreciating and mastering how to deal with life without dissociative defenses. *Solidification of gains and working through* is a long and difficult stage in which the patient must learn to live in the world. Often working through in the transference what has been learned about the past is quite helpful. Characterologic issues may become accessible for the first time. Relationship issues and stress management are crucial, as is dealing with intercurrent traumata. [*See* COPING WITH STRESS.]

Follow-up rather than termination is advised in order to sequentially reassess the stability of the outcome, especially for those patients who achieved resolution rather than integration. It is not uncommon to find minor or partial relapses, or the discovery of personality states that were not accessible previously, in the first 27 months after integration.

Several aspects of treatment require special consideration. Medication is useful for target symptoms or comorbid conditions, but is ineffective for the treatment of the core symptoms of dissociative identity disorder. Hospitalization may be required when a patient becomes self-destructive/suicidal or aggressive to others, overwhelmed by traumatic material to the point of dysfunction, or unable to contain alters' inappropriate activities. The creative arts therapies (movement therapy, art therapy, music therapy, etc.) are very helpful for this group of patients. Although they often are disruptive to general therapy groups, carefully conducted groups specifically for this patient group have been very beneficial.

Hypnosis plays a major role in the treatment of dissociative identity disorder, whether the therapist introduces it or not. Spontaneous trance and autohypnotic phenomena abound, even in the absence of trance induction. Many hypnotic techniques are useful for symptom relief, attenuating the impact of powerful events and affects, ego strengthening, giving comfort to overwhelmed or anxious alters, modulating abreactions, and accessing personality states to make them available to the therapy. This is in addition to the venerable use of hypnosis to retrieve dissociated materials, which is currently the source of some controversy. A recent study validated many memories that were retrieved with the use of hypnosis, but there is ample reason to be circumspect about material recovered in this manner, because it may be confabulated in whole or in part. Clinicians utilizing hypnosis for this purpose should have explained this concern prior to undertaking the procedure, and should have their patient's informed consent. Hypnosis should be avoided in instances in which the state of the patient's memory may be crucial for forensic matters. Often individuals who have been hypnotized may be held by the courts to have had their memories contaminated by the process; this may seriously damage the legal standing of the patient in court proceedings.

Although no controlled studies of the treatment of dissociative identity disorder are available, there is an ample body of literature to indicate that most of those patients who can involve themselves in a definitive therapy with a therapist experienced in the treatment of this condition have a reasonably good prognosis. Recent studies demonstrate that there are three subgroups of dissociative identity disorder patients. One has relatively little comorbid pathology and relatively good ego strength, and usually gets well within a few years. A second has more ego weakness and comorbidity and runs a longer and often more crisis-filled treatment, but makes slow and gradual progress. Many in this group will integrate, and many others will ultimately have a good resolution. A third group has more ego weakness and comorbidity, and/or may remain enmeshed with alleged abusers. This group rarely can move toward definitive treatment and their treatment must remain adaptationalist

and personality-oriented for long periods. Many may never integrate or reach stable resolutions, but a minority makes dramatic gains, even after long periods of instability.

I. Example

Nancy, a 36-year-old nurse, had been in treatment for depression and posttraumatic stress for several years before her increasing complaints of headaches, hearing voices in her head, and amnesia led to an evaluation for dissociative identity disorder. She had given a history of father–daughter incest. Nancy's sisters and coworkers described out-of-character angry outbursts for which she had no memory. At times men she did not know called her or even arrived at her door maintaining they had a date for that night. Her closet contained several garments she did not recall buying, and their style was more revealing than her customary garb. Her diary contained entries in a handwriting she was sure was not hers. Her score on a dissociative experiences scale was 42. On an early version of the SCID-D interview she scored 18 (amnesia 4, depersonalization 4, derealization 3, identity confusion 3, identity alteration 4). During the SCID-D, an inquiry about internal dialogs (the voices heard within her head) prompted a spontaneous switch into another personality, Jill, which identified itself as the owner of the more revealing garments, and described an active social life unbeknownst to Nancy, whom she disparaged. This personality attributed the angry outbursts to still another personality, Liz, and mentioned the existence of several others as well. Liz emerged upon request and vociferously attacked Nancy as a "wimp" who had allowed herself to be abused as a child and dominated in contemporary work, family, and social situations. Liz stated that she punished Nancy for her failures by inflicting injuries to the body, and tried to prevent Jill from being sexual, because she considered all sex abusive.

Nancy was transferred to the consultant for treatment. For several months her therapy focused on enhanced coping, safety, increased mutual tolerance and cooperation across the many personalities. Although the main thrust of her therapy was psychodynamic, she was taught many autohypnotic, cognitive, and behavioral approaches to stress and the management of painful material. Safety contracts with all known alters were obtained, and her personality system was explored without probing traumatic material in detail or in depth. Then, slowly, each personality was allowed to tell, abreact, and process its experiences. Some alters integrated spontaneously after doing their work, while others responded to suggestions to integrate employing hypnosis and imagery. Nancy had a few serious crises in which she became suicidal while she dealt with the traumatic material; she twice inflicted cuts on her forearms, and several times overused medication to "take away the pain." On one occasion she lost 2 weeks of work because she was so disorganized by work on her traumata. However, with some emergency sessions and telephone support, these crises were weathered. Her sisters and mother were able to confirm many of the memories of abuse recovered from her alters. In her fourth year of therapy she achieved complete integration. Treatment continued to work through her traumata in a unified self, and to enhance her coping. Two years after her integration, she visited her then terminally ill father, and told him she forgave him, even if he could not admit his transgressions. He admitted his misuse of her and begged her to pray for him lest he go to hell.

VIII. DISSOCIATIVE DISORDER NOT OTHERWISE SPECIFIED

This category is utilized for those patients suffering from dissociative symptoms whose symptoms do not fulfill the diagnostic criteria for the specific designated dissociative disorders. Currently it includes the research category, Dissociative Trance Disorder, which is discussed separately here. Typical examples are listed in Table VI. The natural history of many patients with Dissociative Identity Disorder involves many periods of time in which their overt symptoms are vague, and their phenomenology is more accurately described under this heading. In Coons' study of 50 patients with Dissociative Disorder Not Otherwise Specified, 17 were found to have disorders with separate ego-states or identities, 16 had a spectrum of dissociative symptoms he termed "not further specified" (in which a wide variety of dissociative symptoms were present without any reaching a diagnosable threshold for a dissociative disorder), 10 suffered dissociative psychoses (many dissociative features with psychotic dimensions in association with another psychosis), 3 had gender identity disorders with dissociative features (personas with different genders, but without an amnestic barrier between them), one had the Ganser syndrome, and one a nocturnal dissociative disorder (in which separate identities are noted, but only nocturnally, arising from apparent sleep, but with wake electroencephalograms). As a group, 96% of these patients reported histories of childhood abuse or neglect. 82% suffered depression. In clinical practice, many patients who achieve

Table VI Description of Dissociative Disorder Not Otherwise Specified

This category is included for disorders in which the predominant feature is a dissociative symptom (i.e., a disruption in the usually integrated functions of consciousness, memory, identity, or perception of the environment) that does not meet criteria for any specific Dissociative Disorder. Examples include:

1. Clinical presentations similar to Dissociative Identity Disorder that fail to meet full criteria for this disorder. Examples include presentations in which a) there are not two or more distinct personality states, or b) amnesia for important personal information does not occur.

2. Derealization unaccompanied by depersonalization in adults.

3. States of dissociation that occur in individuals who have been subjected to periods of prolonged and intense coercive persuasion (e.g., brainwashing, thought reform, or indoctrination while captive).

4. Dissociative trance disorder: single or episodic disturbances in the state of consciousness, identity, or memory that are indigenous to particular locations and cultures. Dissociative trance involves narrowing of awareness of immediate surroundings or stereotyped behaviors or movements that are experienced as being beyond one's control. Possession trance involves replacement of the customary sense of personal identity by a new identity, attributable to the influence of a spirit, power, deity, or other person, and associated with stereotyped "involuntary" movements or amnesia. Examples include *Amok* (Indonesia), *bebainan* (Indonesia), *latah* (Malaysia), *pibloktoq* (Arctic), *ataque de nervios* (Latin America), and possession (India). The dissociative or trance disorder is not a normal part of a broadly accepted collective cultural or religious practice.

5. Loss of consciousness, stupor, or coma not attributable to a general medical condition.

6. Ganser syndrome: The giving of approximate answers to questions (e.g., "2 plus 2 equals 5") when not associated with Dissociative Amnesia of Dissociative Fugue.

this diagnosis appear to have autohypnotically based symptoms resembling trance phenomena gone out of control.

1. Example 1. (Ego-State Disorder)

A woman presented with depersonalization, derealization, inner voices, and depression. Behind these voices were over a dozen apparent identities, most of which were not very elaborate. Usually she experienced their voices and feelings as intrusive symptoms. There was no contemporary amnesia, nor did the other identities directly assume executive control. In her predominant personality she had amnesia for documented childhood abuse.

2. Example 2. (Dissociative Disorder Not Further Specified)

A woman with recurrent major depression had amnesia for some aspects of her childhood abuse, rare episodes of time loss, depersonalization, and one or two brief fugues. Several evaluations for Dissociative Identity Disorder were negative.

As dissociative disorders continue making their way into the clinical mainstream, it is likely that some of these symptom complexes will be accorded recognition as separate mental disorders.

The treatment of the various forms of Dissociative Disorder Not Otherwise Specified usually follows the approaches helpful for the types of dissociative disorder they most resemble. Ego-state disorders respond nicely to the therapy used for Dissociative Identity Disorders, for example. Patients whose symptoms resemble trance phenomena often respond well to approaches that teach them autohypnotic self-regulation, allowing the restructuring of their dysfunctional dissociative experiences.

IX. DISSOCIATIVE TRANCE DISORDER

This diagnostic entity is included in *DSM-IV* among those conditions that have not been accepted, but are considered worthy of further study. Its essential feature is an involuntary state of trance that is not a normal aspect of cultural or religious practice that causes clinically significant distress or impairment. Those afflicted either manifest an altered response to their environment, or feel or appear to be possessed or taken over by some other identity, usually a spirit, power,

Table VII Research Criteria for Dissociative Trance Disorder

A. Either (1) or (2):
1. Trance, i.e., temporary marked alteration in the state of consciousness or loss of customary sense of personal identity without replacement by an alternate identity, associated with at least one of the following:
   a. narrowing of awareness of immediate surroundings, or unusually narrow and selective focusing on environmental stimuli;
   b. Stereotyped behaviors or movements that are experienced as being beyond one's control.
2. Possession trance, a single or episodic alternation in the state of consciousness, characterized by the replacement of customary sense of personal identity by a new identity. This is attributed to the influences of a spirit, power, deity, or other person, as evidenced by one (or more) of the following:
   a. stereotypic and culturally determined behaviors or movements that are experienced as being controlled by the possessing agent;
   b. Full or partial amnesia for the event
B. The trance or possession trance state is not accepted as a normal part of a collective cultural or religious practice.
C. The trance or possession trance state causes clinically significant distress or impairment in social, occupational, or other important areas of functioning.
D. The trance or possession trance state does not occur exclusively during the course of a Psychotic Disorder (including Mood Disorder With Psychotic Features and Brief Psychotic Disorder) or Dissociative Identity Disorder and is not due to the direct physiological effects of a substance or a general medical condition.

deity, or person. In the latter case, there usually is amnesia for the possession experience. Diagnostic criteria are in Table VII. These conditions tend to be episodic with a duration from minutes to hours.

Although pathological trance phenomena appear to be ubiquitous and most aspects of them appear reasonably uniform across cultures, possession trance states often are profoundly influenced by culture both with regard to the identity of the entities encountered, the nature of the behaviors performed in the altered state, associated sensory alterations (such as anesthesia to pain, blindness, etc.), and the nature and degree of amnesia. Many have sufficient distinctness to be regarded as culture-bound syndromes.

Trance phenomena often appear to have an autohypnotic or dissociative mechanism. They appear related to dissociated memories and/or intense intrapsychic conflicts out of conscious awareness. Trance possession states appear to share these substrates, but achieve their unique forms of expression from the patient's cultural and social surround.

A. Trance

The patients are clearly out of contact with the environment and are preoccupied with inner experiences. In general they do not communicate with those who attempt to speak to them, do so in a rudimentary manner, or reveal that they are disoriented to the contemporary environment, and are reacting to events of the past or inner preoccupations. They often are still, and may be mistaken as catatonic. However, some rock, engage in stereotyped behaviors or movements, or appear to be reenacting a past scenario. Some verbalize, often with distress and/or agitation, and may be hard to understand. These episodes are self-limited, but may recur. The patient usually is amnestic for the trance; for some there is a dreamlike or depersonalized recollection.

1. Example

A woman whose young son died tragically some years ago periodically lapses into altered states during which she appears to be rocking a baby in her arms and crooning a silent lullaby. At these times she is unresponsive to others' conversation and physical efforts to attract her attention.

B. Possession Trance State

Here the manifestations dramatize the patient's experience of being taken over by another entity. Commonly, the patient is amnestic while another entity controls behavior, but cases exist in which the patient is aware of the entity's intrusion and contends with it for the control of behavior. Some such circumstances are ego-syntonic and sought out, such as when the patient speaks in the voice of a benign advisor or mentor, as in mediumistic trance, and do not come under the aegis of this condition if they do not cause dysfunction. However, in circumstances when the entities are not benign, the experience of the patient may be terrifying. The actions of the entity may lead to self-injury or suicide. Nemiah holds that those who feel they are possessed by evil spirits have guilt-laden conflicts over personal transgressions, but many cases demon-

strate other dynamics, such as identification with an aggressor.

1. Example

A professional man from Haiti was noted to periodically lapse into states in which his voice and behavior changed, and he spoke in a French dialect. At such times he assembled a series of objects, impervious to others' attempts to intervene, and chanted over them. He was amnestic for these episodes, which endangered his career. A physician who spoke French examined him under hypnosis and found that in these altered states he experienced himself as an evil spirit trying to call up still other evil spirits.

C. Treatment

Dissociative trance disorder usually responds to the same sort of treatment strategies used for the more familiar dissociative disorders. A supportive therapeutic environment must be established, and the pace of the therapy must respect the vulnerability of the patient to being overwhelmed in the process of reacquiring access to the dissociated material. The dissociated mental contents must be explored with techniques that can reaccess them and manage the abreaction of whatever painful emotions are associated with them. Hypnosis and drug-facilitated interviews may prove useful. Patients are helped to gradually work through the traumata and/or conflicts, to retain what had been dissociated in conscious awareness, and to master new strategies of managing their residual impacts. Often autohypnotic strategies can restructure pathological dissociative trances, and teach patients to master them.

When dealing with many possession trance states, the strategies useful in managing dissociative identity disorder, informed by a sensitivity to the cultural elements of the condition, are often effective.

D. Comment

Often as traditional societies with indigenous possession trance states become industrialized, and as their citizens are educated to accept worldviews that are more universal and secular, the incidence of these conditions decreases except in remote areas and ethnic enclaves that preserve old beliefs and practices. When this occurs, often dissociative identity disorder, a laicized expression of the older trance possession states, and related forms of dissociative disorder not otherwise specified, begin to occupy the psychopathological niche once held by them.

X. DISSOCIATION AND MEMORY

One of the most complex and controversial aspects of the study of the dissociative disorders is the relationship between dissociation and memory. While many traumatized individuals remember what has befallen them, many individuals with dissociative disorders, posttraumatic stress, and related conditions have either blocked out memory of their traumatization or only have partial, fragmentary, and/or intermittent recollection. Williams demonstrated that as many as 38% of girls with documented childhood abuse did not report a documented episode of abuse when reinterviewed at 17-year follow-up. Kluft found many instances in which long-forgotten abuses recovered in psychotherapy, often with hypnosis, could be documented. Additionally, genuinely traumatized individuals may have and/or recover distorted and/or inaccurate recollections of abuse. Both relatively accurate and relatively inaccurate memories may be found in the same patient.

As a consequence, although there is consensus that many dissociative disorder patients have suffered severe traumatization, the only test of the accuracy of an apparent recollection of abuse is external corroboration by some form of documentation or by some witness whose corroboration or failure to corroborate the allegation would not be patently self-serving. A denial by an alleged perpetrator has no more face validity than the accusation made against him/her.

The study of this area has been compromised by a failure to distinguish between the constructs of "truth" that are useful in psychotherapy, science, and the court of law. Neither of these constructs are necessarily consistent with historical truth, but all are useful in particular contexts.

BIBLIOGRAPHY

Cardena, E. (1994). The domain of dissociation. In S. J. Lynn & J. W. Rhue (Eds.), *Dissociation: Clinical and theoretical perspectives* (pp. 15–31). New York: Guilford.

Coons, P. M. (1992). Psychogenic amnesia: A clinical investigation of 25 cases. *Dissociation,* **5,** 73–79.

Coons, P. M. (1992). Dissociative disorder not otherwise specified: A clinical investigation of 50 cases with suggestions for typology and treatment. *Dissociation,* **5,** 187–195.

Hermon, J. L. (1992). *Trauma and recovery.* New York: Basic Books.

Kluft, R. P. (1995). The confirmation and disconformation of memories of abuse in DIO patients: A naturalistic study. *Dissociation,* **8,** 253–258.

Kluft, R. P., & Fine, C. G. (1993). *Clinical perspectives on multiple personality disorder.* Washington, DC: American Psychiatric Press.

Michelson, L. K., & Ray, W. J. (Eds.).(1996). *Handbook of dissociation.* New York: Plenum.

Putnam, F. W. (1989). *Diagnosis and treatment of multiple personality disorder.* New York: Guilford.

Ross, C. A. (1997). *Dissociative identity disorder: Diagnosis, clinical features, and treatment of multiple personality disorder* (2nd ed.). New York: Wiley.

Spiegel, D. (Section Editor). (1991). Dissociative disorders. In A. Tasman & S. M. Goldfinger (Eds.), *American Psychiatric Press review of psychiatry* (Vol. 10) (pp. 141–275). Washington, DC: American Psychiatric Press.

Steinberg, M. (1994). Interview guide to the *Structured Clinical Interview for the Diagnosis or DSM-IV Dissociative Disorders—revised.* Washington, DC: American Psychiatric Press.

Divorce

Matthew D. Johnson and Thomas N. Bradbury

University of California, Los Angeles

Annulment A ruling that a marriage was never properly formed.

Binuclear family Divorced families with coparenting arrangements.

Coparenting Cooperation between divorced parents in the raising of their children.

Divorce A judicial declaration dissolving a marriage.

Divorce Mediation The process of spouses meeting together with an impartial third party to identify, discuss, and ultimately resolve divorce disputes.

Marital Quality Spouses' perceptions of the quality of their marriage (syn. marital satisfaction).

Marital Stability The status of the marriage (i.e., whether spouses are married, separated, or divorced).

Morbidity (1) The proportion of afflicted individuals in a certain population or geographical area. (2) The percentage of deaths associated with a specific condition.

Primary Parent Designates the custodial parent when ex-spouses are unable to "coparent."

Separation Cessation of conjugal cohabitation. With married couples this is a temporary state ending in either divorce or reconciliation.

Single Parent Designates the custodial parent when there is no foreseeable contact with the other spouse (i.e., widowed, severe abuse, or abandonment).

The prevalence of **DIVORCE** makes its impact on society unavoidable, and one of the most stressful life events a person may experience. Spouses experiencing divorce are likely to face emotional distress, legal questions, monetary concerns, parenting and custodial changes, community and friendship disruption, and an alteration of their perceived autonomy. Divorce has had a severe economic impact on our society, increasing the number of families needing government assistance. These economic deficits are being shouldered by children, who more than any other demographic group in the United States live below the poverty line. However, divorce has been considered either a virulent influence on society, resulting in a generation of angry, apathetic, and angst-filled adult children of divorce; or a relatively innocuous phenomenon, which adds to a dynamic cultural landscape by changing our conception of family. Understanding and exploring divorce is the goal of this article.

I. DEMOGRAPHICS OF DIVORCE

Marital dissolution over the last two centuries has increasingly been the result of divorce and decreasingly the result of death. Analyses of divorce rates in the twentieth century have noted an overall increase in the divorce rate; however, the rate of increase has not remained constant. The most striking changes were in the 1950s and 1960s when the rate went down, and in the late 1960s and early 1970s when the divorce rate rose sharply. There are several explanations for these two shifts, many of which tend to focus on the economic and social factors of the time. For example, there were sharp contrasts between these two periods, particularly with regard to women in the workplace. In the 1950s and 1960s wages were relatively high, one income per household was often enough to support a family, and the career options of women were more limited. These factors changed in the late sixties, and for many couples who entered the 1960s in less than satisfying marriages the cultural revolution of the sixties seemed inviting. The loosening of social rules and increased economic opportunities allowed partners and parents to extricate themselves from unhappy situations and start over.

The proportion of first marriages in the United States likely to end in divorce has stayed between 50 and 55% since the middle of the 1970s. This represents a significant long-term increase from the 1860s when approximately 5% of all marriages ended in divorce. Another statistic used to describe the amount of divorce in the United States is the annual divorce rate, which is the number of divorces per 1000 existing marriages. In the 1860s the rate was between one and two, and in the 1980s the rate was between 21 and 23. Although the divorce rate appears to be leveling off now, it remains relatively high. According to the 1990 U.S. Bureau of the Census, these figures represent the highest divorce rate of any major industrialized country; this fact has drawn attention to the consequences and causes of divorce.

II. CONSEQUENCES OF DIVORCE

The consequences of marital separation have long been viewed as damaging and disruptive to individuals and to society. As a result, religious and civic institutions have a history of discouraging marital dissolution. The fears of the societal chaos that would result if marriages dissolved prompted early Christians to forbid annulment. In England, even when the state came to oversee the contract of marriage, prompted by King Henry VIII seeking an annulment, the state did not immediately recognize the right to divorce until sometime between 1660 and 1857 (through the Matrimonial Causes Act passed by the English Parliament). Divorce was so rare in colonial America that individual divorce settlements were discussed in Congress. However, the process of marital separation has become less restrictive in time, with most states allowing for "no fault" divorces, and now most divorce agreements may be settled without a formal judicial hearing. Nevertheless, there is still significant evidence that divorce involves increased stress and disruption, which often are associated with negative repercussions for spouses and children. Below we review the findings of research on the consequences of divorce on spouses and children, and consider the theoretical implications of these data. However, care should be taken in interpreting these data, as correlational findings are potentially misleading. Correlational research indicates only an association between variables that, while informative, does not necessarily indicate the direction of causality between those variables.

A. For Spouses

As a result of the prevalence of divorce in the United States, and the obvious distress of spouses in the process of divorce, there have been many attempts to explore the impact of divorce on spouses. Much of the research has been correlational, but the findings suggest that divorce is a profoundly stressful event that has a powerful influence on the physical and mental well-being of spouses. Compared to married spouses, divorced spouses tend to experience a lower standard of living, higher rates of stress, higher rates of depression and other mental health problems.

There is strong evidence associating divorce and psychopathology. For example, divorced or separated individuals are overrepresented in psychiatric populations, a finding that is consistent across age, sex, and race. In one study, first admissions to psychiatric hospitals in Pueblo, Colorado, were nine times higher for males with disrupted marriages than with intact marriages, and females were three times as likely to be divorced or separated. Stated otherwise, although divorced or separated males constituted only 6.5% of ever-married males age 14 and over in the Pueblo, Colorado, population, they constituted 46% of ever-married psychiatric patients; for women the percentages were 8% and 32%, respectively. It is notable that the findings are stronger for men than women, which is contrary to the commonly held belief that marital disruption is usually far more difficult for women than men. One implication of this finding is that many of the difficulties faced by divorced women are more apparent than the psychological challenges that men experience. However, it should be noted that women who have experienced three or more marriages are more likely to report symptoms of psychopathology than women with one or fewer divorces; this finding did not hold for men. The impact of divorce on mental health has been substantiated by studies demonstrating an increase in symptoms of depression during and following marital dissolution.

In addition to being associated with psychopathology, divorce is associated with poor health outcomes. After adjusting for age, persons who experienced marital dissolution have higher rates of illness and disability than married or never-married individuals. Separated and divorced persons, especially women, are particularly vulnerable to severe short-term medical conditions. In addition, the stressful nature of divorce leads to health problems specifically associated with stress (e.g., heart disease). Given the association of divorce and disease, it is not surprising that divorced individuals have a higher rate of morbidity than individuals with differing marital status (e.g., single, married, widowed). The higher mortality rate may also be related to factors such as greater prevalence of alcoholism and a greater vulnerability to motor vehicle accidents among divorced individuals. Indeed, divorce is associated with higher age-adjusted death rates for all causes combined compared to married people of the same age, sex, and ethnicity.

In a related vein, the percentage of people who have committed suicide who are divorced or separated is more than double the percentage of the general population. However, there is no difference between married and divorced in the number of attempts, indicating that divorced persons are underrepresented among those who survive a suicide attempt. The suicide rate is highest for divorced persons among all marital categories. This finding holds regardless of ethnicity, except among non-White females, for whom it is the second highest (behind widowed; still more than double that of married persons). The discrepancy is even larger for homicide; for both genders and across ethnicity death from homicide happens far more to divorced persons than any other marital classification. [*See* SUICIDE.]

Four hypotheses have been offered to explain the relationship between divorce and poor mental and physical health outcomes. First, the premarital disability hypothesis suggests that persons with physical or emotional deficits are less likely to maintain a successful marriage. Second, the postmarital disability hypothesis contends that the likelihood of marital disruption will increase as a consequence of disabilities arising during the marriage. Third, the protectiveness of marriage hypothesis asserts that the status of being married reduces vulnerability to a very wide variety of illnesses and may decrease the likelihood of hospitalization. Fourth, the stress generation hypothesis that states that marital disruption constitutes a significantly stressful event that negatively affects health. Several longitudinal and retrospective studies have suggested the presence of two distinct yet interdependent components of a comprehensive model: First, mental or physical health problems can precede and may precipitate marital distress. Second, marital disruption may precipitate health difficulties that may have been otherwise avoided. These studies suggest that a diathesis-stress model may best explain the relationship of divorce and health. According to this model, individuals bring varying levels of physical and emotional vulnerabilities to marriage (diathesis), and marital difficulties (stress) induce the development of these vulnerabilities into significant health and behavioral problems.

B. For Children

> Sharing kids with a person you have come to despise must be a bit like getting caught in a messy car wreck and then being forced to spend the rest of your life paying visits to the paraplegic in the other vehicle: You are never allowed to forget your mistake. (Elizabeth Wurtzel, 1994, *Prozac Nation: Young and Depressed in America*)

Given the association of divorce and negative outcomes for spouses, it is logical that parental activities and the family environment may be influenced by divorce, thus affecting the health of children. This section summarizes the findings of a large body of research on the immediate and long-term effects of divorce on children, including academic achievement, behavioral problems, psychopathology, and social skills. These effects are examined with three etiological models: (a) children experience a loss of opportunities (e.g., less disposable income); (b) children have difficulty adjusting to a new family structure (e.g., father moving out); (c) children experience an increase in familial stress (e.g., parental conflict) leading to poor adjustment. In 1991, Amato and Keith conducted a quantitative review of relevant research that revealed some support for the first two models, but the most consistent support was found for the familial stress model.

I. Loss of Opportunities

One developmental perspective of the impact of divorce on children suggests that divorced families have fewer economic resources, so that the children of divorce have fewer opportunities for activities and experiences that encourage growth. These lost opportunities are believed to adversely affect intellectual and social development, lowering the well-being of children.

A simple way of testing whether this is an important factor in child outcomes would be to compare outcomes of children of divorce to those in intact families before and after controlling for family income. Only one study has done this (see Amato & Keith, 1991): without controlling for family income children of divorce did worse on 27 of 34 outcomes measured than intact families, but when researchers controlled for income the number decreased to 13. Other studies have found some support for this perspective, with some indicating that intact families with limited financial resources had better child outcomes than divorced families in the same financial situation. There are also indications that a perceived decline in socioeconomic status is associated with poorer parent–child relationships.

Although these findings demonstrate modest support for this perspective, there are also contradictory findings. The addition of a stepparent, which usually raises the economic situation of families, does not consistently improve child outcomes. Overall these findings suggest inconsistent and only modest support for the view that the diminished resources and opportunities associated with divorce lead to maladjustment in children.

2. Disruption of Family Structure

A second perspective on the effect of divorce on children is based on the premise that the family is the primary social institution charged with raising children, and that it is generally better to have a two-parent family than a one-parent family. Living with only one parent has been associated with certain disadvantages, especially in terms of socialization deficits. Although this model has been criticized for emphasizing family composition and implicitly devaluing family process, the concept is straightforward: Parents are developmentally important resources; thus, assuming parity among other variables, two parents are better than one. Findings regarding this model have been somewhat weak and appear related to the gender of the child.

A review of relevant research found that children who lost a father by death had poorer academic achievement, conduct, psychological adjustment, and self-esteem than children in intact two-parent families. However, children who no longer lived with their father due to divorce did worse than children who lost a father to death on academic achievement and conduct. This evidence does not unequivocally support the perspective that the loss of a father due to divorce is the factor leading to poorer outcomes for children.

Another way of approaching this perspective would be to compare single-parent homes resulting from divorce to homes with a stepparent. A review of studies with these data revealed that children in families with a stepparent had poorer outcomes than intact two-parent families. However, the comparison of single-parent families and families with stepparents yielded a gender interaction. The six studies that examined this question only included families with stepfathers, not families with stepmothers living in the primary family. Having a stepfather improved the outcome for boys but worsened the outcome for girls, relative to single-parent families.

Another hypothesis derived from this perspective is that increased frequency of contact with the noncustodial parent will increase a child's well-being. The results of studies examining this question have varied markedly, with some studies indicating that increased contact is associated with better outcomes on some measures, others finding no effects, and still others finding that increased contact may be associated with increased problems. Therefore, this specific hypothesis is not well supported in the research literature, except that having a male parental figure appears to have some benefit for boys and having a stepfather appears to be somewhat detrimental for girls.

3. Familial Stress

A third perspective assumes that the events leading up to and associated with divorce involve stresses that are not only felt by parents but are experienced by the entire family. Examples of events that are considered stressful surrounding divorce are moving, changes in contact with extended family, and parental conflict.

Of these, parental conflict is the most well-supported etiological agent. The role of family conflict can be assessed by testing four hypotheses derived from this perspective.

First, children in divorced and low-conflict intact families should have better outcomes than children in high-conflict intact families. Eight studies have compared child outcomes of low-conflict intact families, high-conflict intact families, and divorced families. Comparing low conflict to high conflict: high conflict had more problems with conduct, psychological adjustment, and self-concept. Comparing divorced to high-conflict intact families: high conflict had more problems with psychological adjustment and self-esteem. When all outcomes are combined children in high-conflict intact families fare worse than low-conflict intact families and divorced families.

A second hypothesis would be that, assuming the level of parental conflict subsides following the divorce, children's well-being should improve after the divorce. There is some evidence to support this hypothesis indicating differences in children of intact and divorced families become less pronounced over time. In addition, a comparison of studies examining the well-being of children within 2 years of the divorce had greater effect sizes than studies using families that divorced more than 2 years previously. (There is some evidence that the well-being of spouses improves in a similar manner over time.) Examinations of cross-sectional studies provided less supporting evidence, but should be interpreted more cautiously than the longitudinal studies. [See WELLNESS IN CHILDREN.]

A third hypothesis would be that the amount of parental conflict preceding a divorce will correspond to children's negative outcomes following a divorce. The longitudinal effects of divorce on children were studied using two very large surveys conducted in Great Britain and the United States. Results indicated that the effects of divorce were mitigated when the outcome variables were controlled for at predivorce. In other words, these data suggest that the effects of divorce on children can be largely related to conditions existing well before marital separation. It is notable that this finding, and those describing more specifically the impact of marital conflict on children, is more profound for boys than girls. One compelling explanation for this gender difference is the greater predisposition of boys to externalize symptoms by acting out, thus making their symptoms more apparent.

A fourth hypothesis stemming from this perspective is that children's difficulty adjusting to divorce is associated with the level of postdivorce parental conflict. There was support for this hypothesis in several studies, with some evidence that the effect is more reliable for boys than girls.

Several theories have been offered to clarify the mechanism by which parental conflict influences childhood well-being; two of these have been supported through empirical research. First, a modeling mechanism suggests that parental conflict interferes with a child's imitation of the same-sex parent, or that viewing parental conflict may lead to a child's rejection of both parents. Several other modeling hypotheses have been suggested and tested. The research has also found that boys tend to model aggressive behavior more than girls, possibly explaining the aforementioned gender difference.

A second mechanism that has been supported in the empirical literature is that parental conflict leads to alterations and inconsistencies in disciplinary practices. Several specific theories involving discipline practices have been suggested, but a common theme is the idea that arguing about discipline in front of the child is perceived as confusing and will lead to an increase in behavior problems. The fact that boys tend to be disciplined about equally by mothers and fathers, and girls are disciplined mostly by mothers, would also partly explain the fact that boys tend to be affected by parental conflict more than girls because parental coordination of discipline is likely to be hampered by conflict.

C. Summary

Research documents the difficulties and problems associated with divorce. For spouses, evidence appears to support a diathesis-stress model of the negative consequences associated with divorce. Research to date indicates that individuals with attributes generally associated with increased risk for psychological and physiological health difficulties are more likely to experience interpersonal difficulties and marital conflict, thus forming a diathesis for poor psychological and physical health outcomes. Moreover, it has been noted that the process of divorce is one of the most stressful events people may experience and that the stress of marital discord often leads to increased psychopathology, disease morbidity, and mortality. Of course, the stress of divorce affects children as well as spouses, and much has been written about the impact of divorce on children. It appears the most damaging aspect of divorce on children stems from the high level of family conflict associated with marital separation.

The long-term consequences of divorce on children were examined in 1991 by Amato and Keith, who quantitatively examined the research literature on the effects of parental divorce on adults. Their findings did not support the contention that the effects of divorce on children are relatively short-term. The data indicate that adults who experienced parental divorce as children have more psychological problems (e.g., depression), lower marital quality, more divorce, lower educational attainment, lower income, lower occupational prestige, and lower physical health. Ultimately, divorce appears to have pervasive, permanent, and generally negative effects on the family.

III. CAUSES OF DIVORCE

Far less is known about the causes of divorce than the consequences of divorce. This section will summarize the findings of research on marital instability. Methodologically, this research can be categorized into three groups: cross-sectional studies, retrospective studies, and prospective (i.e., longitudinal) studies. Cross-sectional studies will not be considered because of their limited ability to address etiological questions; retrospective studies sample couples who are divorced (or divorcing) and ask participants what factors caused their marriage to end. The reliance on memory in the retrospective method is a major shortcoming of this research. Several studies have demonstrated the fallibility of retrospective reports, specifically noting that people tend to forget some past events, remember events as occurring earlier than they actually did, and reconstruct the past to make sense of their current situation. Specifically, patterns of marital satisfaction over time measured with cross-sectional and retrospective methods have not been substantiated by research using more rigorous prospective methodologies. The best way to understand the development of marital discord and the processes leading to divorce is to examine the links of events, characteristics, and behaviors to changes in marital satisfaction and stability. The optimal method for studying these changes is through the use of longitudinal research. There-

fore, the findings discussed in this section will focus on results from the longitudinal studies of marital development.

In 1995, Karney and Bradbury conducted a quantitative review of 115 longitudinal studies of marital quality and instability. They noted that factors influencing marital quality are highly correlated with factors affecting marital dissolution, thus marital satisfaction predicts couples staying married more than any other variable. However, it is likely that other factors influence whether or not couples choose to end their marriage, by first influencing marital satisfaction or other variables. Therefore, marital quality and marital dissolution will be examined independently followed by a discussion of possible models of marital instability.

The effects of several factors on marriage have been explored in the research literature, including spousal similarity, personality, age, premarital cohabitation, parenting satisfaction, income, stress, and behavior. Only one study to date has examined the effects of *spousal similarities* on marriage while controlling for possibly confounding variables, and it found that homogamy did not affect the marriage. However, similarity was limited to job status. Fifty-six *personality* traits have been examined in the marital literature. Personality traits are commonly categorized into five factors: neuroticism, extraversion, impulsivity, agreeableness, and conscientiousness. Of these, neuroticism has demonstrated the most influence on marital satisfaction and stability. However, there are no studies examining the effects of other personality variables when accounting for neuroticism. *Age* has been found to be positively associated with marital stability; however, this is a variable that is not well understood because age at the time of the study is confounded with age when wed and with the aforementioned variable of marital duration. No study to date has employed controls allowing a better understanding of the effects of age on marriage. *Premarital cohabitation* is correlated with later marital dissolution; however, this finding should be interpreted with caution due to evidence suggesting the relationship may not be causal. In a 1995 review by Erel and Burman the emotions and behaviors associated with *parenting satisfaction* were found to be related to marital satisfaction and behavior; however, a later study by Kurdek did not support this finding. The relationship between *income* and marital dissolution appears to be moderated by the gender of the employed spouse. Husbands' employment and income are correlated with less marital dissolution, while wives' employment and income are positively associated with divorce. However, it is unclear if this finding is related to financial independence lowering the barriers to divorce or if wives' financial independence precipitates lower marital satisfaction. Other research has suggested that the level of income is not as important as the stability of the income that is associated with marital stability. Finally, there is some evidence that the effects of economic hardship on marital quality and stability are mediated by the expression of affect in marital interactions. The last two factors to be addressed, stress and behavior, encompass a broad range of variables, thus will be considered in more detail. [*See* PARENTING; PERSONALITY.]

The effects of *stress* on marital stability and quality have not been studied to the extent that would be expected, given the diversity of stresses that exist. Nevertheless, the prospective studies that have been completed suggest that the presence of stressful experiences leads to less stable and satisfying marriages. However, one stressful life event that has unique effects on marriage, and has been studied extensively in terms of the effects on marriage, is the transition to parenthood. The process of becoming a parent appears to be associated with lower marital satisfaction, yet it also appears to lessen the likelihood of divorce. The increased sense of responsibility and the normative nature of having children may explain the stabilizing affect of this stressful life event, and distinguish it from other events (e.g., car accidents). It should also be noted that the effects of the transition to parenthood appear to be moderated by the degree to which the couple's expectations about parenting are realistic. More research designed to understand moderating factors affecting the impact of stressful events on marriage appears to be an important next step with important implications for intervention strategies. [*See* STRESS.]

The *behavior* of spouses during marital interactions has been theorized to be an important causal factor in the development of marital instability, leading to the study of over 50 behavioral variables. The Karney and Bradbury review aggregated these into five broad factors: positive behavior, negative behavior, avoidance, positive reciprocity, and negative reciprocity. The results of the studies of behavior have varied somewhat, making interpretations of these data

difficult. One of the most variable and counterintuitive findings is the effect of negative behavior on marital quality and stability. There is some evidence that negative behavior by both spouses is negatively correlated with marital satisfaction concurrently, but positively correlated longitudinally. Although these findings have replicated, the meta-analytic results do not fully support this finding; the weight of evidence supports the view that negativity in interaction foreshadows decline in marital quality and, in turn, marital stability. In addition to negativity, other behavioral variables had relatively modest effects on marital stability and satisfaction. These findings may indicate either that the effects of behavior are not as longitudinally important as once thought, or that the effects of behavior on marriage are moderated by other factors. Finally, it bears noting that most of the longitudinal research on marriage involves established couples. As a result it is not clear if predictive variables provide information about the onset of marital difficulties or the continuing course of already distressed relationships.

In summary, the longitudinal data on marriage do not account for much of the marital outcome variance. In addition, the cumulative findings do not identify one theoretical perspective while refuting others. Part of the reason for this is the atheoretical nature of much of this work. It has been suggested that more theory testing be part of the longitudinal studies of marital dissolution. For example, one model being tested was posited by Karney and Bradbury as part of their 1995 review. They proposed a "vulnerability-stress-adaptation model of marriage" in which the combination of enduring vulnerabilities, stressful life events, and adaptive processes have reciprocal influence on marital quality, which in turn affects the likelihood of divorce.

IV. DIVORCE-RELATED INTERVENTIONS

Despite the lack of a comprehensive understanding of the development of marital discord and the processes leading to divorce, various interventions have been designed to prevent the development of marital distress, address and modify marital discord, aid the adjustment of children, and facilitate the process of divorce. Psychological interventions may be considered either primary, secondary, or tertiary. Primary interventions are those focusing on prevention, serving to inoculate people from potential mental health problems. Secondary approaches identify individuals with preliminary signs of mental health problems or who are deemed "at-risk," and interventions are devised to decrease the likelihood of further problems. Tertiary interventions are treatments for existing problems. These three levels of intervention—corresponding to "before it happens," "before it gets worse," and "before it's too late"—encompass the following opportunities for intervention in marriage, divided into four developmental phases: premarital counseling (a primary or secondary intervention), marital therapy (a tertiary intervention), interventions for children of divorce or conflictive marriages (a secondary or tertiary intervention), and divorce mediation (a tertiary intervention).

A. Premarital Counseling

The rationale for interventions designed to prevent marital dysfunction is derived from the fact that all couples will experience problems and stressful events. Intervening before the onset of difficulties may help alleviate tension in the time between the onset of the problems and the point at which a tertiary intervention is sought. Primary prevention interventions may promote couples' ability to effectively address marital problems while they are still relatively minor. In addition, one of the advantages of primary prevention programs could be their ability to address a larger segment of the population, especially if the programs were administered by professionals and paraprofessionals in community settings. This is particularly important given that most couples seeking relationship related interventions do not visit a clinical psychologist or psychiatrist, but instead turn to clergy or primary care physicians for assistance.

Several programs aimed at the primary prevention of marital dysfunction have been developed and are currently offered to the public. Only the Prevention and Relationship Enhancement Program (PREP) is based on empirical findings of marital researchers and long-term follow-up data. PREP focuses on the acquisition of marital communication and problem-solving skills. This program is offered in an extended (6 week, 2.5 hours per week) version and a weekend version. The program consists of didactic training, consultation, and practice. Studies of the efficacy of PREP are encouraging, although it remains unclear how helpful

this program will be for couples at elevated risk for marital instability.

Numerous other prevention programs are currently available; three major programs are briefly described here. The Relationship Enhancement (RE) program is described as integrating elements of communication skills training, empathy training, client-centered therapy, and behavioral techniques. The efficacy of this program has only been demonstrated using measures designed by the developers of the intervention, over relatively short spans of time, leaving the program's effectiveness unclear. The Practical Application of Intimate Relationship Skills (PAIRS) is a 12- to 16-week program involving one therapist per couple. The program includes both components of individual and group therapy in addition to skills training. There have been no long-term outcome studies, precluding an assessment of program effectiveness. Marriage Encounter is a weekend retreat run by other couples, and organized by the Association for Couples in Marriage Enrichment (ACME). The intervention focuses on raising and addressing marital issues such as problem solving, communication, spirituality, intimacy, and sexuality. Outcome research has indicated couples experience increased marital satisfaction and trust; however, other findings indicate that some couples experience an increase in marital conflict as a result of unresolved issues raised during the retreat.

Having reviewed a sample of primary intervention programs that are available, it is important to note research that suggests couples who are most at risk for divorce may not be particularly likely to participate in prevention programs. Given this finding, and the expense involved in administering these programs, it has been suggested that targeting at-risk couples for prevention programs may be a more efficient use of resources. By disseminating some of these programs through existing organizations, such as religious organizations and the military, some steps have been taken to broaden the reach of programs and to make them available to couples without as many economic resources. Studies are currently underway to assess how this method of dissemination affects the efficacy of these programs.

B. Marital Therapy

The growing acceptance of tertiary conjoint therapy as an aid to resolving marital difficulties, thus preventing divorce, over the last 25 years has fueled an increase in the number of theoretical orientations to marital therapy. These treatments have emphasized different aspects of marital processes, including the exchange of behaviors, the role of cognitions, the family system, spouses' unconscious desires and fantasies, the ability to problem-solve, the attachment style of each spouse, and the role of emotional expression. In addition, recently developed treatments have sought to integrate aspects of more than one established treatment. However, the proliferation of approaches to marital therapy has not been followed by research indicating which of the approaches is most effective. Controlled studies tend to suggest that about half of all couples improve with therapy, although many of these couples subsequently relapse. However, the efficacy of Behavioral Marital Therapy appears to be significantly higher. Little is known about the effectiveness of marital therapy as it is provided typically in community settings. Furthermore, it appears that, for reasons that are not fully understood, the effects of marital therapy vary widely. [See COUPLES THERAPY.]

C. Interventions for Children

In 1992 Grych and Fincham reviewed interventions designed to prevent or reduce the negative effects of divorce on children. The review compared the findings regarding factors that protect children from stressors to the factors targeted by various treatments. The "triad of protective factors" for children include positive personality factors, an emotionally supportive family, and extended support systems outside the family. As noted previously, research suggests that an important step in minimizing the deleterious effects of divorce on children is for the parents to maintain low levels of conflict and to remain consistent and warm in their relationships with their children. However, the majority of interventions designed to moderate the effects of divorce on children are focused on the child, as opposed to the family or the broader support system. Thus, as expected, the child-focused interventions demonstrated only modest success at modifying the effects of parental divorce, especially in high-conflict families. Furthermore, because there are so few family oriented approaches (i.e., involving participation of the whole family system) specifically designed to moderate the effects of divorce, there is relatively little research on their effectiveness.

D. Mediation

Divorce mediation is a form of conflict resolution in which both spouses meet with an impartial third party to identify, discuss, and resolve their disputes pertaining to marital separation. Often the third party has a background as a mental health worker. Couples are either self-referred or have been referred by a judge. Arriving at a mutually acceptable child custody arrangement is one of the most difficult processes in divorce, and this is the area in which mediation may be most beneficial. Given the negative consequences of parental conflict on children, mediation may be less detrimental than determining custody through traditional legal channels. It has been noted that mediation is likely to involve less overt conflict between the spouses. This is partly due to the cooperative atmosphere encouraged in mediation, as opposed to the adversarial environment of a courtroom. In traditional courtroom hearings nearly any derogatory evidence about a spouse may be introduced to the court to help a judge determine the "best interests" of the child, often increasing the acrimony between spouses.

Research on the effectiveness of mediation is generally positive, with evidence indicating that people participating in mediation are more satisfied than those participating in courtroom settlements. In addition, there is evidence that mediation decreases the likelihood of postdivorce litigation. However, the psychological benefits of mediation are less clear, with some indications that it may increase the depression of mothers. This is possibly a result of increased opportunity for power in the relationship to be exploited in the process of mediation. A better understanding of the benefits and costs of mediation is needed before stronger conclusions are drawn about its effect on family members.

V. CONCLUSION

In summary, a large body of research addressing the consequences of divorce has indicated that there appear to be significant and profound negative implications of divorce on the psychological and physical well-being of spouses and children. The precise mechanisms that lead to these negative consequences are still unclear. However, empirical evidence does indicate that the effects of divorce are very similar to the effects of other severe stressful life events, with the implication that lessening the stress associated with the process of divorce may lessen the consequences. Furthermore, it appears evident that the most detrimental factor of the process of divorce on children is family conflict. This finding has several important implications. First, it means that if a divorce will lessen severe conflict in a family it may not be contraindicated. Second, lessening the impact of divorce-related conflict on children through tertiary interventions, such as mediation, is most likely beneficial. Third, more emphasis should be placed on understanding the development of severe marital conflict. Fourth, with greater understanding of the causes of conflict, more effective interventions can be designed, evaluated, disseminated, and implemented to prevent marital discord.

BIBLIOGRAPHY

Amato, P. R. (1996). Explaining the intergenerational transmission of divorce. *Journal of Marriage and the Family, 58,* 628–640.

Amato, P. R., & Keith, B. (1991). Parental divorce and adult well-being: A meta-analysis. *Journal of Marriage and the Family, 53,* 43–58.

Amato, P. R., & Keith, B. (1991). Parental divorce and the well-being of children: A meta-analysis. *Psychological Bulletin, 110,* 26–46.

Bloom, B. L., Asher, S. J., & White, S. W. (1978). Marital disruption as a stressor: A review and analysis. *Psychological Bulletin, 85,* 867–894.

Cherlin, A. J. (1992). *Marriage, divorce, remarriage.* Cambridge, MA: Harvard University Press.

Cherlin, A. J., Furstenberg, F. F., Chase-Lansdale, P. L., Kiernan, K. E., Robins, P. K., Morrison, D. R., Teitler, J. O. (1991). Longitudinal studies of effects of divorce on children in Great Britain and the United States. *Science, 252,* 1386–1389.

Emery, R. E., & Wyer, M. M. (1987). Divorce mediation. *American Psychologist, 42,* 472–480.

Emery, R. E. (1982). Interparental conflict and the children of discord and divorce. *Psychological Bulletin, 92,* 310–330.

Grych, J. H., & Fincham, F. D. (1992). Interventions for children of divorce: Toward greater integration of research and action. *Psychological Bulletin, 111,* 434–454.

Karney, B. R., & Bradbury, T. N. (1995). The longitudinal course of marital quality and stability: A review of theory, method, and research. *Psychological Bulletin, 118,* 3–34.

Wurtzel, E. (1994). *Prozac nation: Young and depressed in America.* Boston: Houghton Mifflin.

ISBN 0-12-226676-5